# KINESIOLOGY
## *of the*
# MUSCULOSKELETAL
# SYSTEM

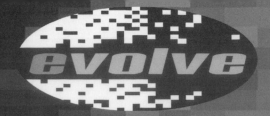

# The Latest *Evolution* in Learning.

Evolve provides online access to free learning resources and activities designed specifically for the textbook you are using in your class. The resources will provide you with information that enhances the material covered in the book and much more.

Visit the Web address listed below to start your learning evolution today!

▶▶ *LOGIN:* **http://evolve.elsevier.com/Neumann/**

Evolve Student Learning Resources for Neumann: *Kinesiology of the Musculoskeletal System* offers the following features:

- **WebLinks**
  Links to places of interest on the web specific to your classroom needs.

- **Suggestion Box**
  An opportunity to submit your suggested improvements to the text to the author for possible inclusion in the next edition.

# Think outside the book...*evolve*.

# KINESIOLOGY
## *of the*
# MUSCULOSKELETAL SYSTEM

## *Foundations for Physical Rehabilitation*

### DONALD A. NEUMANN, PT, PhD

*Associate Professor*
*Department of Physical Therapy*
*Marquette University*
*Milwaukee, Wisconsin*

*Artwork by*
### ELISABETH E. ROWAN, BSc, BMC

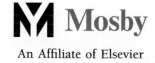

An Affiliate of Elsevier

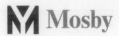

*Publishing Director:*   Andrew M. Allen
*Senior Acquisitions Editor:*   Maureen Pfeifer
*Senior Developmental Editor:*   Scott Weaver
*Manuscript Editor:*   Mary Anne Folcher
*Production Manager:*   Betty Taylor
*Illustration Specialist:*   Peg Shaw
*Illustrator:*   Karen Giacomucci

**Library of Congress Cataloging-in-Publication Data**

Neumann, Donald A. Kinesiology of the musculoskeletal system: foundations for physical rehabilitation/
   Donald A. Neumann; artwork by Elisabeth E. Rowan.—1st ed.
      p.; cm.
   Includes bibliographical references and index.
   ISBN 0–8151–6349–5
   1. Kinesiology. 2. Human mechanics. 3. Musculoskeletal system—Diseases—Patients—Rehabilitation.
I. Title.
   [DNLM: 1. Kinesiology, Applied. 2. Biomechanics. 3. Movement. 4. Musculoskeletal Physiology. WB 890
N492k 2002]
   QP303. N465 2002                                                                                612.7′6—dc21
                                                                                                        2001032610

Mosby, Inc.
*An Affiliate of Elsevier*
11830 Westline Industrial Drive
St. Louis, Missouri 63146

Printed in the United States of America

**Last digit is the print number:   9   8   7   6   5   4   3**

*To those whose lives have been changed*
*by the struggle and joy of learning*

# Donald A. Neumann

Donald Neumann began his career in 1972 as a licensed, physical therapy assistant in Miami, Florida. In 1976, he received a Bachelor of Science degree in physical therapy from the University of Florida. By 1986, he received both Master of Science and PhD degrees from the University of Iowa. His areas of graduate study included science education, exercise science, and kinesiology. While a graduate student at the University of Iowa, Donald received the Mary McMillan Scholarship Award from the American Physical Therapy Association (APTA).

Donald accepted his first job as a staff physical therapist in 1976, at Woodrow Wilson Rehabilitation Center in Virginia, where he specialized in the treatment of persons with spinal cord injuries. Because of his interest in teaching, he became the Coordinator of Clinical Education within the Physical Therapy Department at this facility. To this day, Dr. Neumann remains involved in the rehabilitation of persons with spinal cord injuries. In 2002, he produced a series of educational videos funded by the Paralyzed Veterans Association. The videos describe many of the kinesiologic principles used to enhance the movement potential in persons with quadriplegia.

Since finishing graduate school in 1986, Donald has been on faculty at the Department of Physical Therapy at Marquette University in Milwaukee. His primary areas of teaching are kinesiology, anatomy, and spinal cord injury rehabilitation. In 1994, Dr. Neumann received Marquette University's Teacher of the Year Award. In 1997, the APTA awarded Dr. Neumann the Dorothy E. Baethke—Eleanor J. Carlin Award for Excellence in Academic Teaching. He has also presented numerous seminars on the clinical relevance of kinesiology to a wide range of health care professionals. In 2002, Dr. Neumann was awarded a Fulbright Scholarship to teach Kinesiology in Lithuania.

Dr. Neumann has received funding by the National Arthritis Foundation to conduct research that focused on the biomechanics of the hip joint. He studied methods of protecting an unstable or a painful hip from potentially large and damaging forces. In 1989, he was the first recipient of the Steven J. Rose Endowment Award for Excellence in Orthopedic Physical Therapy Research. In 1991, he received the Eugene Michels New Investigator Award from the APTA. In 2000, Dr. Neumann received the APTA's Jack Walker Award for the best article on clinical research published in *Physical Therapy* in 1999. Dr. Neumann is currently an Associate Editor of the *Journal of Orthopaedic & Sports Physical Therapy*.

## *About the Illustrator: Elisabeth E. Rowan*

When she was 8 years old, Elisabeth knew she wanted to be an illustrator. As a child, she spent many hours illustrating the books that she had read. Her interest in medical illustration grew as she studied the biologic sciences. She was especially interested in the form and function of the human body.

Elisabeth's formal education in art consists of a Bachelor of Fine Arts in Drawing and Painting from the University of Wisconsin, Milwaukee, and a Bachelor of Science in Biomedical Communications (Medical Illustration) from the University of Toronto. Elisabeth now works at Kalmbach Publishing Company, Waukesha, Wisconsin, as a magazine illustrator. Her work is featured regularly in *Astronomy* and *Birder's World*. She currently lives in Milwaukee.

# *About the Illustrations*

Most of the more than 650 illustrations that appear within this volume are original, produced by the combined efforts of Donald Neumann and Elisabeth Rowan. The illustrations were first conceptualized by Dr. Neumann and then rendered by Ms. Rowan with meticulous attention to detail. As a team, Don and Elisabeth met weekly

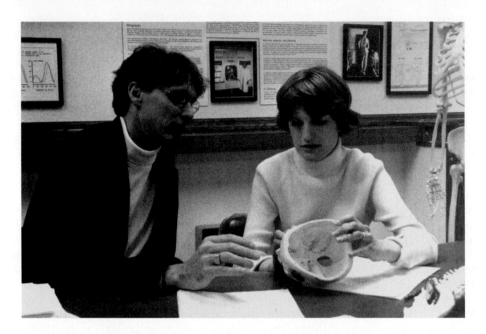

for 6½ years to complete this project. Dr. Neumann states that "The artwork really drove the direction of much of my writing. I really needed to understand a particular kinesiologic concept at its most essential level in order to effectively explain to Elisabeth what needed to be illustrated. In this way, the artwork kept me honest; I wrote only what I truly understood."

Neumann and Rowan produced two primary forms of artwork for this text (see the following samples). Elisabeth depicted the anatomy of bones, joints, and muscles by hand, creating very detailed pen-and-ink drawings (Fig. 1). These drawings started

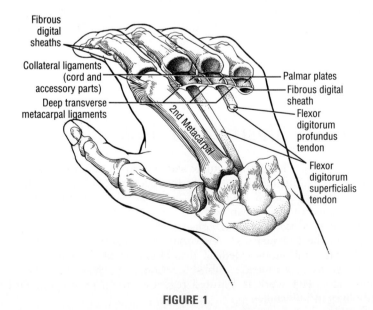

**FIGURE 1**

with a series of pencil sketches, often based on anatomic specimens dissected by Dr. Neumann. The pen-and-ink medium was chosen to give the material an organic, classic feeling.

The second form (Fig. 2) used a layering of artistic media, integrated with the use of computer software. Many of the pieces started with a digital photograph transformed into a simplified outline of a person performing a particular movement. Images of bones, joints, and muscles were then electronically embedded within the human outline. Overlaying various biomechanical images further embellished the resultant illustration. The final design displayed specific and often complex biomechanical concepts in a relatively simple manner, while preserving human form and expression.

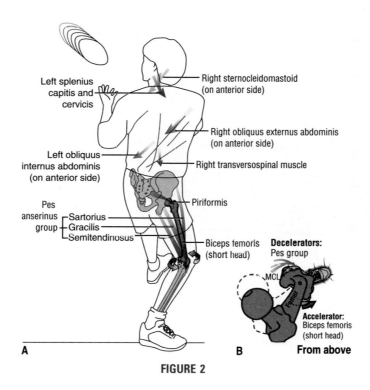

**FIGURE 2**

# ABOUT THE CONTRIBUTORS

**A. JOSEPH THRELKELD, PT, PhD**

Associate Professor, Chair, Department of Physical Therapy; Director, Biodynamics Laboratory, Department of Physical Therapy, Creighton University, Omaha, Nebraska

A 1976 physical therapy graduate of the University of Kentucky, Lexington, Dr. Threlkeld has been involved in the clinical management of musculoskeletal dysfunctions, particularly arthritis and related disorders. In 1984, he completed his doctoral work in anatomy with a focus on the remodeling of articular cartilage. Since then, he has conducted research on the abnormal kinematics associated with musculoskeletal and neuromuscular impairments as well as the neuromusculoskeletal responses to therapeutic intervention. His teaching areas have been kinesiology, anatomy, and histology.

*Basic Structure and Function of the Joints* (Chapter 2)

**DAVID A. BROWN, PT, PhD**

Assistant Professor, Department of Physical Therapy and Human Movement Sciences and Department of Physical Medicine and Rehabilitation, Northwestern University Medical School, Chicago, Illinois

Dr. David Brown is the son of a physical therapist (Elliott). David graduated with a master's degree in physical therapy from Duke University, Durham, in 1983 and then received a PhD in exercise science from the University of Iowa, Iowa City, in 1989. His primary area of clinical expertise is neurorehabilitation with a special emphasis on locomotor impairment following stroke. He has published research in journals such as *Journal of Neurophysiology, Brain, Stroke,* and *Physical Therapy.* Dr. Brown has presented his research at both national and international conferences. His highest ambition is to contribute to the discovery of innovative intervention strategies for the amelioration of neuromuscular impairments and for the restoration of locomotor function.

*Muscle: The Ultimate Force Generator in the Body* (Chapter 3)

**DEBORAH A. NAWOCZENSKI, PT, PhD**

Associate Professor, Department of Physical Therapy, Ithaca College's Rochester Campus, Rochester, New York

Dr. Nawoczenski received both a Bachelor of Science degree in physical therapy and a Master of Education degree from Temple University, Philadelphia. She also received a PhD in Exercise Science (Biomechanics) from the University of Iowa, Iowa City. Dr. Nawoczenski is co-director of the Movement Analysis Laboratory at Ithaca College's Rochester Campus. She is engaged in research on the biomechanics of the foot and ankle. Dr. Nawoczenski also holds a position as an Adjunct Assistant Professor of Orthopaedics in the School of Medicine and Dentistry at the University of Rochester, Rochester, New York. She has served as an Editorial Board Member for the *Journal of Orthopaedic & Sports Physical Therapy* and was co-editor of the two-part special issue on the foot and ankle. Dr. Nawoczenski has co-authored and co-edited two textbooks: Buchanan LE, Nawoczenski DA (eds): *Spinal Cord Injury: Concepts and Management Approaches,* and Nawoczenski DA, Epler ME (eds): *Orthotics in Functional Rehabilitation of the Lower Limb.*

*Biomechanical Principles* (Chapter 4)

## GUY G. SIMONEAU, PT, PhD, ATC

Associate Professor, Marquette University, Department of Physical Therapy, Milwaukee, Wisconsin

Dr. Simoneau received a Bachelor of Science in physiothérapie from the Université de Montréal, Canada, a Master of Science degree in sports medicine from the University of Illinois at Urbana-Champaign, Illinois, and a PhD in exercise science (locomotion studies) from The Pennsylvania State University, State College. He teaches orthopaedic physical therapy and pursues research on gait and the ergonomic design of computer keyboards. Dr. Simoneau has been the recipient of several teaching and research awards from the American Physical Therapy Association, including the 2000 Education Award of the Orthopaedic Section, the 1998 Education Award of the Sports Section, the 1997 Eugene Michels New Investigator Award, and the 1996 Margaret L. Moore New Academic Faculty Award. He has been funded by the National Institutes of Health and the Foundation for Physical Therapy, among others, to study walker-assisted ambulation and by the National Institute of Occupational Safety and Health (NIOSH) and the Arthritis Foundation to study the design of computer keyboards. Dr. Simoneau is currently Editor-in-Chief of the *Journal of Orthopaedic & Sports Physical Therapy*.

*Kinesiology of Walking* (Chapter 15)

# REVIEWERS

Paul Andrew, PT, PhD
Department of Physical Therapy
Ibaraki Prefectural University of Health
  Sciences
Ibaraki-ken, Japan

Susana Arciga, PT
St. Mary's Hospital
Outpatient Orthopedic and Sports
  Medicine Center
Milwaukee, WI

Cindi Auth, PT
Physical Therapy Department
Zablocki VA Medical Center
Milwaukee, WI

Marilyn Beck, RDH, MEd
Department of Dental Hygiene
Marquette University
Milwaukee, WI

Teri Bielefeld, PT, CHT
Physical Therapy Department
Zablocki VA Medical Center
Milwaukee, WI

Peter Blanpied, PT, PhD
Physical Therapy Program
University of Rhode Island
Kingston, RI

Ann M. Brophy, PT
NovaCare Outpatient Rehabilitation
Milwaukee, WI

Frank L. Buczek, Jr., PhD
Motion Analysis Laboratory
Shriners Hospital for Children
Erie, PA

Daniel J. Capriani, PT, MEd
Department of Physical Therapy
Medical College of Ohio
Toledo, OH

Anya Carlisle, MPT
Physical Therapy Department
Zablocki VA Medical Center
Milwaukee, WI

Leah Cartwright, PT
Physical Therapy Department
Zablocki VA Medical Center
Milwaukee, WI

Gary Chleboun, PT, PhD
School of Physical Therapy
Ohio University
Athens, OH

Mary A. Cimrmancic, DDS
Marquette University School of
  Dentistry
Milwaukee, WI

Adam M. Davis, PT
Quad Med, LLC
Sussex, WI

Brian L. Davis, PhD
Department of Biomedical Engineering
The Lerner Research Institute
The Cleveland Clinic Foundation
Cleveland, OH

Sara M. Deprey, PT, MS
Department of Allied Health
Carroll College
Waukesha, WI

Sara Jean Donegan, DDS, MS
Marquette University School of
  Dentistry
Milwaukee, WI

William F. Dostal, PT, PhD
Department of Rehabilitation Therapies
University of Iowa Hospitals and
  Clinics
Iowa City, IA

Joan E. Edelstein, PT, MA
Physical Therapy
Columbia University
New York, NY

Timothy Fagerson, PT, MS
Orthopaedic Physical Therapy Services,
  Inc.
Wellesley Hills, MA

Kevin P. Farrell, PT, OCS, PhD
Physical Therapy
Saint Ambrose University
Davenport, IA

Esther Haskvitz, PT, PhD
Notre Dame College
Physical Therapy Program
Manchester, NH

Jeremy Karman, PT
Physical Therapy Department
Sports Medicine Institute
Aurora Sinai Medical Center
Milwaukee, WI

Michelle Lanouette, PT, MS
Physical Therapy Department
Zablocki VA Medical Center
Milwaukee, WI

Paula M. Ludewig, PT, PhD
Program in Physical Therapy
University of Minnesota
Minneapolis, MN

Jon D. Marion, OTR, CHT
Marshfield Clinic
Marshfield, WI

Brenda L. Neumann, OTR, BCIAC
Clinic for Neurophysiologic Learning
Milwaukee, WI

Janet Palmatier, PT, MHS, CHT
Work Injury Care Center
Glendale, WI

Randolph E. Perkins, PhD
Physical Therapy and Cell and
  Molecular Biology
Northwestern University Medical
  School
Chicago, IL

Christopher M. Powers, PT, PhD
Department of Biokinesiology and
  Physical Therapy
University of Southern California
Los Angeles, CA

Kathryn E. Roach, PT, PhD
Division of Physical Therapy
University of Miami School of
  Medicine
Coral Gables, FL

Michelle G. Schuh, PT, MS
Department of Physical Therapy and
  Program in Exercise Science
Marquette University
Milwaukee, WI

**Christopher J. Simenz, MS, CSCS**
Department of Physical Therapy and
    Program in Exercise Science
Marquette University
Milwaukee, WI

**Guy G. Simoneau, PT, PhD, ATC**
Department of Physical Therapy
Marquette University
Milwaukee, WI

**Carolyn Wadsworth, PT, MS, OCS,
    CHT**
Department of Rehabilitation Therapies
University of Iowa Hospitals and
    Clinics
Iowa City, IA

**David Williams, MPT, ATC, CSCS**
Physical Therapy Program
Iowa City, IA

**Chris L. Zimmermann, PT, PhD**
Physical Therapy Program
Concordia University, Wisconsin
Mequon, WI

# FOREWORD

To be the author of a text is a major undertaking and, possibly, appreciated only by those who have completed such a venture. The author has a responsibility not only for providing accurate information but also for delivering the material in a format conducive to comprehension. A significant confounding factor is the perpetual explosion of knowledge for which the author is responsible for inclusion in the work.

Perhaps in his earlier days, Don Neumann never anticipated the creation of this volume on the *Kinesiology of the Musculoskeletal System,* but the work has been intrinsic to him since his days as a physical therapy assistant in the early 1970s. He received both the Outstanding Clinical Award and the Outstanding Academic Award as an undergraduate student at the University of Florida under the tutelage of faculty including Martha Wroe, Fred Rutan, and Claudette Finley. He then pursued his master's and doctoral degrees. He has never strayed far from the clinic, however, where he still treats patients with spinal cord injuries.

Dr. Neumann excels as a true teacher. In this capacity, he has demonstrated his love for teaching others and sharing his excitement for the subject matter. Don has gone beyond teaching, however. He has also made a contribution as a scholar by focusing his attention on the hip joint and the influence of the arthritic process. His efforts in this domain have been recognized in terms of awards such as the American Physical Therapy Association's Eugene Michels New Investigator Award (1991) and the Jack Walker Award (2000), which recognizes published clinical research in *Physical Therapy*.

All of these aspects reveal only part of the picture, however, because you must know the man to appreciate him.

Quiet in manner and complimentary by nature, he gives his energies to excellence in the projects that he undertakes. All his personal qualities would take too long to describe and would only embarrass this humble author. I have had the distinct privilege of having him as a graduate student and teaching assistant and as a critic of my work. Although unsuccessful in attempts to hire him, I recognize that others have gained from his presence.

Don should be congratulated on the completion of *Kinesiology of the Musculoskeletal System: Foundations for Physical Rehabilitation.* The osteology, arthrology, and neurology, and the muscle—as a functional unit—provide a meaningful blend for a text on kinesiology, a science fundamental to the student and practicing clinician. Of special merit are the illustrations, which uniquely convey a blending of kinesiologic and anatomic material. *Kinesiology of the Musculoskeletal System* is also invaluable for its inclusion of Special Focus issues and other features that provide clinical relevance to the presentation.

Don has been successful in developing a useful textbook not only for physical therapists but also for many in other disciplines. His work is comprehensive and readable and contributes greatly to the pool of literature available to students and professionals alike.

Gary L. Soderberg, PT, PhD, FAPTA
Professor and Director of Research
Department of Physical Therapy
Southwest Missouri State University
Springfield, Missouri

# PREFACE

Kinesiology is the study of human movement, typically pursued within the context of sport, art, or medicine. To varying degrees, *Kinesiology of the Musculoskeletal System: Foundations for Physical Rehabilitation,* relates to all three areas. It is intended, however, primarily as a foundation for the practice of physical rehabilitation. The phrase "physical rehabilitation" is used in a broad sense, referring to therapeutic efforts that restore optimal physical function. Although kinesiology can be presented from many different angles, I and my contributing authors have focused primarily on the mechanical interactions between the muscles and joints of the body. These interactions are described for normal movement and, in the case of disease, trauma, or otherwise altered tissue, for abnormal movement. I hope that this textbook provides a valuable educational resource for a wide range of health- and medical-related professions, both for students and clinicians.

This textbook places a large emphasis on the anatomic detail of the musculoskeletal system. By applying surprisingly few principles of physics and physiology, the reader should be able to mentally transform a static anatomic image into a dynamic, three-dimensional, and relatively predictable movement. The illustrations created for *Kinesiology of the Musculoskeletal System* are designed to encourage this mental transformation. This approach to kinesiology reduces the need for rote memorization and favors reasoning based on mechanical analysis. This type of reasoning can assist the clinician in developing proper evaluation, diagnosis, and treatment related to dysfunction of the musculoskeletal system.

The completion of this textbook represents the synthesis of more than 25 years of experience as a physical therapist. This experience includes a rich blend of clinical, research, and teaching activities that are related, in one form or another, to kinesiology. Although I was unaware of it at the time, my work on this textbook began the day I prepared my first kinesiology lecture as a college professor at Marquette University in 1986. Since then, I have had the good fortune of being exposed to intelligent and motivated students. Their desire to learn has continually fueled my ambition to teach. As a way to encourage my students to listen actively rather than to transcribe my lectures passively, I developed an extensive set of kinesiology lecture notes. Year after year, my notes evolved, forming the blueprints of this text. Now complete, this text embodies my knowledge of kinesiology as well as my experiences while teaching the subject. The book contains many clear and exciting illustrations, as well as a compelling list of references that support my teaching.

The organization of this textbook reflects the overall plan of study used in my two-semester kinesiology course sequence. The textbook contains 15 chapters, divided into four major sections. *Section I* provides the essential topics of kinesiology, including an introduction to terminology and basic concepts, a review of basic structure and function of the musculoskeletal system, and an introduction to biomechanical and quantitative aspects of kinesiology. *Sections II* through *IV* present the specific anatomic details and kinesiology of the three major regions of the body. *Section II* focuses entirely on the upper extremity, from the shoulder to the hand. *Section III* covers the kinesiology of the axial skeleton, which includes the head, trunk, and spine. A special chapter is included within this section on the kinesiology of mastication and ventilation. *Section IV* presents the kinesiology of the lower extremity, from the hip to the ankle and foot. The final chapter in this section, the *Kinesiology of Walking,* functionally integrates and reinforces much of the kinesiology of the lower extremity.

This textbook is specifically designed for the purpose of *teaching.* To that end, concepts are presented in layers, starting with Section I, which lays much of the scientific foundation for chapters contained in Sections II through IV. The material covered in these chapters is also presented layer by layer, building both clarity and depth of knowledge. Most chapters begin with *osteology*—the study of the morphology and subsequent function of bones. This is followed by *arthrology*—the study of the anatomy and the function of the joint, including the associated periarticular connective tissues. Included in this study is a thorough description of the regional kinematics, both from an arthrokinematic and osteokinematic perspective.

The most extensive component of most chapters within Sections II through IV highlights the *muscle and joint interactions.* This topic begins by describing the skeletal attachments of muscles within a region, including a summary of the innervation to both the muscles and the joint structures. Once the shape and physical orientation of the muscles are established, the mechanical interplay between the muscles and the joints is presented. Topics presented include strength and movement potential of muscles, muscular-produced forces imposed on joints, intermuscular and interjoint synergies, important functional roles of muscles, and functional relationships that exist between the muscles and underlying joints.

Clinical examples and corollaries are used extensively throughout to help narrow the gap between what is often taught in the classroom and what is experienced in clinical practice. Clinical examples pertain to a wide range of issues, typically relating to how pathology, trauma, and other conditions contribute to functional impairments or limitations. Discussions are frequently related to issues involving prolonged immobilization of limbs; instability or malalignment of joints; abnormal posture or limited range of motion; paralysis and muscular force imbalances; and trauma and inflammation of the muscles, joints, and periarticular connective tissues.

Several special educational features are included. Foremost are the high quality anatomic and kinesiologic *illustrations.* This artwork is intended to excite and simplify, without compromising the depth of the material. The textbook is accompanied by an Evolve website that features an electronic image collection, which includes the majority of the figures in the book. The images, which can be be printed out or transformed into PowerPoint slides, are available as a teaching tool for instructors who adopt the book for use in their classes. (Instructors should check with their sales representative for further information.) *Special Focus* features are used to highlight areas of special interest. Topics in a Special Focus include notable clinical corollaries, distinctive structural and functional relationships, and "reach-out" concepts designed to stimulate further interest or provide additional background. *Appendices* at the end of each of the four sections provide useful reference materials. Appendices II through IV, for example, provide a readily accessible reference to the detailed bony attachments of muscles. This information is useful in laboratory exercises designed to study a muscle's action based on its specific attachments. One very

instructive activity involves having students use a skeleton model and a piece of string to mimic a muscle's line-of-force. Groups of students can discuss a muscle's potential action by observing the line-of-force of the "string" relative to an imaginary axis of rotation through a particular joint. This exercise helps students to understand the three-dimensional nature of muscle actions and how the actions and strength of a muscle can change with different positions of a limb. Multiple *tables* and *summary boxes* are provided to help organize the material to facilitate learning.

My original intention in writing this text was to present kinesiology in a comprehensive, relevant, logical, and clear manner. This textbook will hopefully inspire others to further pursue a fascinating and important subject matter. I intend this first edition to be the beginning of a lifelong endeavor.

*DAN*

# ACKNOWLEDGMENTS

I welcome this opportunity to acknowledge a great number of people who have provided me with kind and thoughtful assistance throughout this long project. I am sure that I have inadvertently overlooked some people and, for that, I apologize.

The best place to start with my offering of thanks is with my immediate family, especially my wife Brenda who, in her charming and unselfish style, paved the way for the completion of this project. I thank my son, Donnie, and stepdaughter, Megann, for their patience and understanding. I also thank my caring parents, Betty and Charlie Neumann, for the many opportunities that they have provided me throughout my life.

Four persons significantly influenced the realization of *Kinesiology of the Musculoskeletal System: Foundations for Physical Rehabilitation.* Foremost, I wish to thank Elisabeth E. Rowan, the primary medical illustrator of the text, for her years of dedication and her uncompromisingly high standard of excellence. I also extend my gratitude to Drs. Lawrence Pan and Richard Jensen, present and past directors, respectively, of the Department of Physical Therapy at Marquette University. These gentlemen unselfishly provided me with the opportunity to fulfill a dream. And, finally, I wish to thank Scott Weaver, Managing Editor at Harcourt Health Sciences, for his patience and guidance through the final, and most challenging, phases of the project.

I am also indebted to the following persons who contributed special chapters to this textbook: David A. Brown, Deborah A. Nawoczenski, Guy G. Simoneau, and A. Joseph Threlkeld. I am also grateful to the many persons who reviewed chapters, most of whom did so without financial remuneration. These reviewers are all listed elsewhere in previous sections.

Several people at Marquette University provided me with invaluable technical and research assistance. I thank Dan Johnson for much of the digital photography contained within this book. I appreciate Nick Schroeder, graphic artist, for always fitting me into his busy schedule. I also wish to thank Ljudmila ("Milly") Mursec and Rebecca Eagleeye for their important help with library research.

Many persons affiliated directly or indirectly with Marquette University provided assistance with a wide range of activities, including proofreading, verifying references or concepts, posing for or supplying photographs, taking x-rays, and providing clerical assistance. I am grateful to Santana Deacon, Monica Diamond, Gregg Fuhrman, Barbara Haines, Douglas Heckenkamp, Lisa Hribar, Erika Jacobson, Davin Kimura, Stephanie Lamon, John Levene, Lorna Loughran, Christopher Melkovitz, Melissa Merriman, Alexander Ng, Michael O'Brien, Ellen Perkins, Gregory Rajala, Elizabeth Shanahan, Pamela Swiderski, Donald Taylor, Michelle Treml, Stacy Weineke, Sidney White, and David Williams.

I am very fortunate to have this forum to acknowledge those who have made a significant, positive impact on my professional life. In a sense, the spirit of these persons is interwoven within this text. I acknowledge Shep Barish for first inspiring me to teach kinesiology; Martha Wroe for serving as an enduring role model for my practice of physical therapy; Claudette Finley for providing me with a rich foundation in human anatomy; Patty Altland for emphasizing to Darrell Bennett and myself the importance of not limiting the functional potential of our patients; Gary Soderberg for his overall mentorship and firm dedication to principle; Thomas Cook for showing me that all this can be fun; and Mary Pat Murray for setting such high standards for kinesiology education at Marquette University.

I wish to acknowledge several special people who have influenced this project in ways that are difficult to describe. These people include family, old and new friends, professional colleagues, and, in many cases, a combination thereof. I thank the following people for their sense of humor or adventure, their loyalty, and their intense dedication to their own goals and beliefs, and for their tolerance and understanding of mine. For this I thank my four siblings, Chip, Suzan, Nancy, and Barbara; Brenda Neumann, Tad Hardee, David Eastwold, Darrell Bennett, Tony Hornung, Joseph Berman, Robert Morecraft, Bob Myers, Debbie Neumann, Guy Simoneau, and the Mehlos family, especially Harvey, for always asking "How's the book coming?"

Finally, I want to thank all of my students, both past and present, for making my job so rewarding.

*DAN*

# CONTENTS

# SECTION IV

## Lower Extremity                                           385

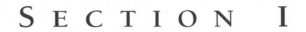

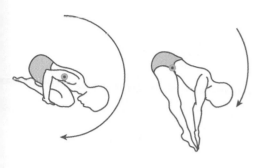

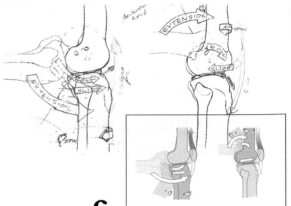

# Essential Topics of Kinesiology

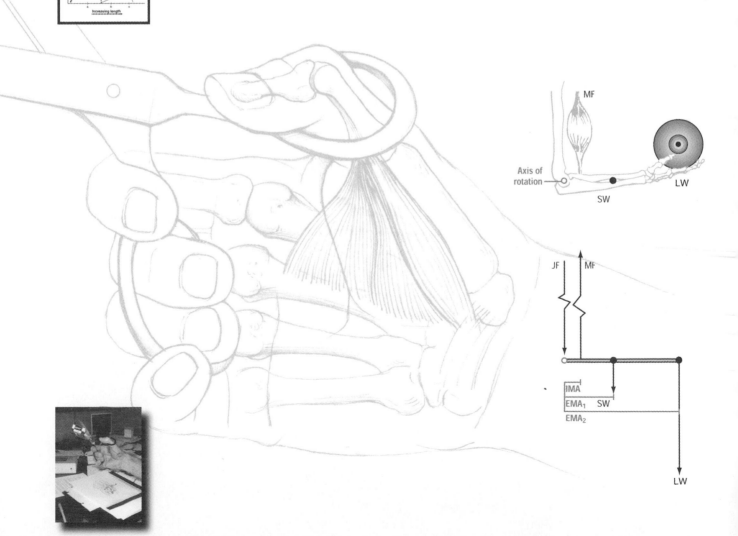

MF

Axis of
rotation

LW

SW    JF    MF

IMA
EMA₁   SW
EMA₂

LW

# SECTION I

# Essential Topics of Kinesiology

**Section I** is divided into four chapters, each describing a different topic related to kinesiology. This section provides the background for the more specific kinesiologic discussions of the various regions of the body (Sections II to IV). Chapter 1 provides introductory terminology and biomechanical concepts related to kinesiology. Chapter 2 presents the basic anatomic and functional aspects of joints—the pivot points for movement of the body. Chapter 3 reviews the basic anatomic and functional aspects of skeletal muscle—the source that produces active movement and stabilization of the joints. More detailed discussion and quantitative analysis of many of the biomechanical principles introduced in Chapter 1 are provided in Chapter 4.

# CHAPTER 1

# Getting Started

## DONALD A. NEUMANN, PT, PhD

### TOPICS AT A GLANCE

## INTRODUCTION

### What Is Kinesiology?

The origins of the word *kinesiology* are from the Greek *kinesis*, to move, and *ology*, to study. *Kinesiology of the Musculoskeletal System: Foundations for Physical Rehabilitation* serves as a guide to kinesiology by focusing on the anatomic and biomechanical interactions within the musculoskeletal system. The beauty and complexity of these interactions have inspired the work of two great artists: Michelangelo Buonarroti (1475–1564) and Leonardo da Vinci (1452–1519). Their work likely inspired the creation of the classic text *Tabulae Sceleti et Musculorum Corporis Humani* published in 1747 by the anatomist Bernhard Siegfried Albinus (1697–1770). A sample of this work is presented in Figure 1–1.

The primary intent of this book is to provide students and clinicians with a *foundation for the practice of physical rehabilitation*. A detailed review of the anatomy of the musculoskeletal system, including its innervation, is presented as a background to the structural and functional aspects of movement and their clinical applications. Discussions are presented on both normal conditions and abnormal conditions that result from disease and trauma. A sound understanding of kinesiology allows for the development of a rational evaluation, a precise diagnosis, and an effective treatment of musculoskeletal disorders. These abilities represent the hallmark of high quality for any health professional engaged in the practice of physical rehabilitation.

This text of kinesiology borrows heavily from three bodies of knowledge: anatomy, biomechanics, and physiology. *Anatomy* is the science of the shape and structure of the human body and its parts. *Biomechanics* is a discipline that uses principles of physics to quantitatively study how forces interact within a living body. *Physiology* is the biologic study of living organisms. This textbook interweaves an extensive review of musculoskeletal anatomy with selected principles of biomechanics and physiology. This approach allows the kinesiologic functions of the musculoskeletal system to be reasoned rather than purely memorized.

The remainder of this chapter provides fundamental biomechanical concepts and terminology related to kinesiology. The glossary at the end of the chapter summarizes much of the essential terminology. A more in-depth and quantitative approach to the biomechanics applied to kinesiology is presented in Chapter 4.

## KINEMATICS

*Kinematics* is a branch of mechanics that describes the *motion* of a body, without regard to the forces or torques that may produce the motion. In biomechanics, the term *body* is used rather loosely to describe the entire body, or any of its parts or segments, such as individual bones or regions. In general, there are two types of motions: translation and rotation.

3

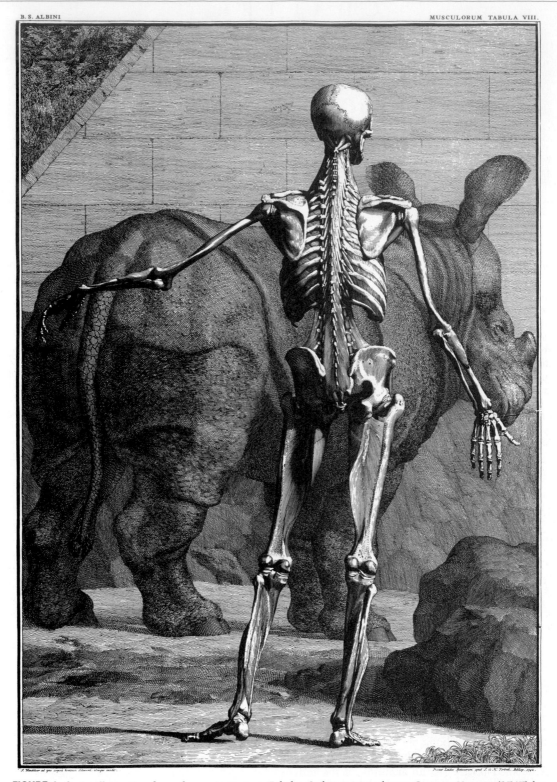

**FIGURE 1–1.** An illustration from the anatomy text *Tabulae Sceleti et Musculorum Corporis Humani* (1747) by Bernhard Siegfried Albinus.

## Translation Compared with Rotation

*Translation* describes a linear motion in which all parts of a rigid body move parallel to and in the same direction as every other part of the body. Translation can occur in either a *straight line (rectilinear)* or a *curved line (curvilinear)*. While walking, for example, a point on the head moves in a general curvilinear manner (Fig. 1–2).

*Rotation*, in contrast, describes a motion in which an assumed rigid body moves in a circular path about some pivot

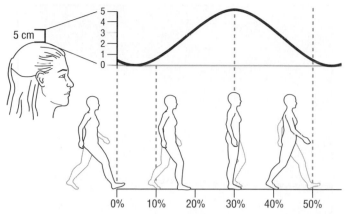

**FIGURE 1–2.** A point on the top of the head is shown translating upward and downward in a curvilinear fashion while walking. The X axis shows the percentage of completion of one entire gait (walking) cycle.

| TABLE 1–1. Common Conversions Between Units of Kinematic Measurements | |
|---|---|
| 1 meter (m) = 3.28 feet (ft) | 1 ft = .305 m |
| 1 m = 39.37 inches (in) | 1 in = .0254 m |
| 1 centimeter (cm) = .39 in | 1 in = 2.54 cm |
| 1 m = 1.09 yards (yd) | 1 yd = .91 m |
| 1 kilometer (km) = .62 miles (mi) | 1 mi = 1.61 km |
| 1 degree = .0174 radians (rad) | 1 rad = 57.3 degrees |

rotating body is zero. For most movements of the body, the axis of rotation is located within or very near the structure of the joint.

Movement of the body, regardless of translation or rotation, can be described as active or passive. *Active movements* are caused by stimulated muscle. *Passive movements,* in contrast, are caused by sources other than muscle, such as a push from another person, the pull of gravity, and so forth.

The primary variables related to kinematics are position, velocity, and acceleration. Specific units of measurement are needed to indicate the quantity of these variables. Units of meters or feet are used for translation, and degrees or radians are used for rotation. In most situations, *Kinesiology of the Musculoskeletal System* uses the *International System of Units,* adopted in 1960. This system is abbreviated SI, for Système International, the French name. This system of units is widely accepted in many journals related to kinesiology and rehabilitation. The kinematic conversions between the more common SI units and other measurement units are listed in Table 1–1.

point. As a result, all points in the body simultaneously rotate in the same angular direction (e.g., clockwise and counterclockwise) across the same number of degrees.

Movement of the human body, as a whole, is often described as a translation of the body's *center of mass,* located generally just anterior to the sacrum. Although a person's center of mass translates through space, it is powered by muscles that *rotate the limbs.* The fact that limbs rotate can be appreciated by watching the path created by a fist while flexing the elbow (Fig. 1–3). (It is customary in kinesiology to use the phrases "rotation of a joint" and "rotation of a bone" interchangeably.)

The pivot point for the angular motion is called the *axis of rotation.* The axis is at the point where motion of the

## Osteokinematics

### PLANES OF MOTION

*Osteokinematics* describes the *motion of bones* relative to the three cardinal (principal) planes of the body: sagittal, frontal, and horizontal. These planes of motion are depicted in the context of a person standing in the *anatomic position* as in Figure 1–4. The *sagittal plane* runs parallel to the sagittal suture of the skull, dividing the body into right and left sections; the *frontal plane* runs parallel to the coronal suture of the skull, dividing the body into front and back sections. The *horizontal (or transverse) plane* courses parallel to the horizon and divides the body into upper and lower sections. A sample of the terms used to describe the different osteokinematics is shown in Table 1–2. More specific terms are defined in the chapters that describe the various regions of the body.

### AXIS OF ROTATION

Bones rotate about a joint in a plane that is perpendicular to an *axis of rotation.* The axis is typically located through the convex member of the joint. The shoulder, for example, allows movement in all three planes and, therefore, has three axes of rotation (Fig. 1–5). Although the three orthogonal axes are depicted as stationary, in reality, as in all joints, each axis shifts throughout the range of motion. The axis of rotation remains stationary only if the convex member of a

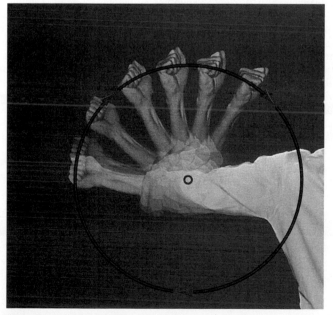

**FIGURE 1–3.** Using a stroboscopic flash, a camera is able to capture the rotation of the forearm. If not for the anatomic constraints of the elbow, the forearm could, in theory, rotate 360 degrees about an axis of rotation located at the elbow (red circle).

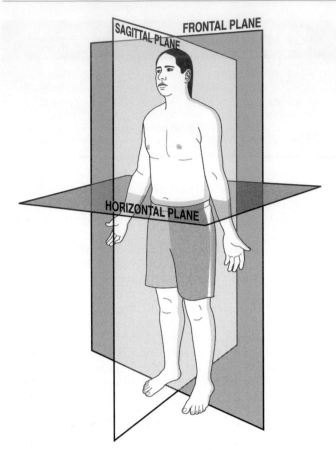

**FIGURE 1–4.** The three cardinal planes of the body are shown as a person is standing in the anatomic position.

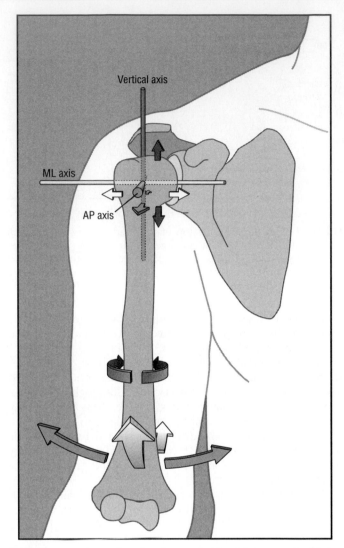

**FIGURE 1–5.** The right glenohumeral (shoulder) joint highlights three orthogonal axes of rotation and associated planes of angular motion: flexion and extension (white curved arrows) occur about a medial-lateral (ML) axis of rotation; abduction and adduction (red curved arrows) occur about an anterior-posterior (AP) axis of rotation; and internal and external rotation (gray curved arrows) occur about a vertical axis of rotation. Each axis of rotation is color-coded with its associated plane of movement. The straight arrows shown parallel to each axis represent the slight translation potential of the humerus relative to the scapula. This illustration shows both angular and translational degrees of freedom. (See text for further description.)

joint were a perfect sphere, articulating with a perfectly reciprocally shaped concave member. The convex members of most joints, like the humeral head at the shoulder, are imperfect spheres with changing surface curvatures. The issue of a migrating axis of rotation is discussed further in Chapter 2.

## DEGREES OF FREEDOM

*Degrees of freedom* are the number of independent movements allowed at a joint. A joint can have up to three degrees of angular freedom, corresponding to the three dimensions of space. As depicted in Figure 1–5, for example,

---

| TABLE 1–2. A Sample of Common Osteokinematic Terms | | |
| --- | --- | --- |
| **Sagittal Plane** | **Frontal Plane** | **Horizontal Plane** |
| Flexion and extension | Abduction and adduction | Internal (medial) and external (lateral) rotation |
| Dorsiflexion and plantar flexion | Lateral flexion | Axial rotation |
| Forward and backward bending | Ulnar and radial deviation | |
| | Eversion and inversion | |

Many of the terms are specific to a particular region of the body. The thumb, for example, uses different terminology.

the shoulder has three degrees of angular freedom, one for each plane. The wrist allows two degrees of freedom, and the elbow only one.

Unless specified differently throughout this text, the term degrees of freedom indicates the number of permitted *planes of angular motion* at a joint. From a strict engineering perspective, however, degrees of freedom applies to angular as well as translational movements. All synovial joints in the body possess at least some translation, driven actively by muscle, or passively owing to the natural laxity within the structure of the joint. The slight passive translations that occur in most joints are referred to as *accessory motions* and are defined in three linear directions. From the anatomic position, the directions correspond to those of the three axes of rotation. In the relaxed glenohumeral joint, for example, the humerus can be passively translated anterior-posteriorly, medial-laterally, and superior-inferiorly (see Fig. 1–5). At many joints, especially the knee and ankle, the amount of translation is used clinically to test the integrity of ligaments.

## OSTEOKINEMATICS: A MATTER OF PERSPECTIVE

In general, the articulations of two body segments constitute a joint. Movement at a joint can therefore be considered from two perspectives. (1) the proximal segment can rotate against the relatively fixed distal segment, and (2) the distal segment can rotate against the relatively fixed proximal segment. These two perspectives are shown for knee flexion in Figure 1–6. A term such as knee flexion, for example, describes only the *relative motion* between the thigh and leg. It does not describe which of the two segments is actually rotating. Often, to be clear, it is necessary to state the bone that is considered the primary rotating segment. As in Figure 1–6, for example, the terms tibial-on-femoral movement or femoral-on-tibial movement adequately describe the osteokinematics.

Most routine movements performed by the upper extremities involve distal-on-proximal segment kinematics. This reflects the need to bring objects held by the hand either toward or away from the body. The proximal segment of a joint in the upper extremity is usually stabilized by muscles or gravity, whereas the distal, relatively unconstrained, segment rotates.

Feeding oneself or throwing a ball are two common examples of distal-on-proximal segment kinematics employed by the upper extremities. The upper extremities are certainly capable of performing proximal-on-distal segment kinematics, such as flexing and extending the elbows while performing a pull-up.

The lower extremities routinely perform both distal-on-proximal and proximal-on-distal segment kinematics. These kinematics reflect, in part, the two primary phases of walking: the *stance phase,* when the limb is planted on the ground under the load of body weight, and the *swing phase,* when the limb is advancing forward. Many other activities, in addition to walking, use both kinematic strategies. Bending the knee in preparation to kick a ball, for example, is a type of distal-on-proximal segment kinematics (Fig. 1–6A). Descending into a squat position, in contrast, is an example of proximal-on-distal segment kinematics (Fig. 1–6B). In this last example, a relatively large demand is placed on the quadriceps muscle of the knee to control the gradual descent of the body.

The terms open and closed kinematic chain are frequently used in the physical rehabilitation literature and clinics to describe the concept of relative segment kinematics.[4,10] A kinematic chain refers to a series of articulated segmented links, such as the connected pelvis, thigh, leg, and foot of the lower extremity. The terms "open" and "closed" are typically used to indicate whether the distal end of an extremity is fixed to the earth or some other immovable object. An *open kinematic chain* describes a situation in which the distal segment of a kinematic chain, such as the foot in the lower limb, is *not fixed* to the earth or other immovable object. The distal segment, therefore, is free to move (see Fig. 1–6A). A *closed kinematic chain* describes a situation in which the distal segment of the kinematic chain is *fixed* to the earth or another immovable object. In this case, the proximal seg-

**Knee flexion**

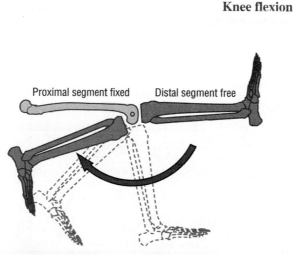
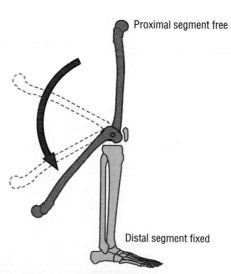

**FIGURE 1–6.** Sagittal plane osteokinematics at the knee show an example of (A) distal-on-proximal segment kinematics and (B) proximal-on-distal segment kinematics. The axis of rotation is shown as a circle at the knee.

Proximal segment fixed    Distal segment free

Proximal segment free

Distal segment fixed

**A  Tibial-on-femoral perspective**

**B  Femoral-on-tibial perspective**

ment is free to move (see Fig. 1–6B). These terms are employed extensively to describe methods of applying resistance to muscles and ligaments, especially in the knee.[2,3]

Although very convenient terminology, the terms open and closed kinematic chains are often ambiguous. From a strict engineering perspective, the terms open and closed kinematic chains apply more to the *kinematic interdependence* of a series of connected rigid links, which is not exactly the same as the previous definitions given here. From this engineering perspective, the chain is "closed" if *both ends* are fixed to a common object, much like a closed circuit. In this case, movement of any one link requires a kinematic adjustment of one of more of the other links within the chain. "Opening" the chain by disconnecting one end from its fixed attachment interrupts this kinematic interdependence. This more precise terminology does not apply universally across all health-related and engineering disciplines. Performing a one-legged partial squat, for example, is often referred to clinically as the movement of a closed kinematic chain. It could be argued, however, that this is a movement of an open kinematic chain because the contralateral leg is not fixed to ground (i.e., the circuit formed by the total body is open). To avoid confusion, this text uses the terms open and closed kinematic chains sparingly, and the preference is to explicitly state which segment (proximal or distal) is considered fixed and which is considered free.

## Arthrokinematics

### TYPICAL JOINT MORPHOLOGY

*Arthrokinematics* describes the *motion* that occurs between the *articular surfaces* of joints. As described further in Chapter 2, the shapes of the articular surfaces of joints range from flat to curved. Most joint surfaces, however, are curved, with one surface being relatively convex and one relatively concave (Fig. 1–7). The convex-concave relationship of most articulations improves their congruency, increases the surface area for dissipating contact forces, and helps guide the motion between the bones.

### FUNDAMENTAL MOVEMENTS BETWEEN JOINT SURFACES

Three fundamental movements exist between joint surfaces: roll, slide, and, spin.[11] These movements occur as a convex surface moves on a concave surface, and vice versa (Fig.

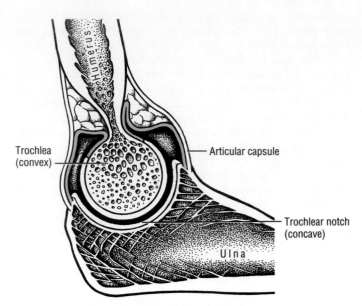

**FIGURE 1–7.** The humeroulnar joint at the elbow is an example of a convex-concave relationship between two articular surfaces. The trochlea of the humerus is convex, and the trochlear notch of the ulna is concave.

1–8). Although other terms are used, these are useful for visualizing the relative movements that occur within a joint. The terms are formally defined in Table 1–3.

#### *Roll-and-Slide Movements*

One primary way that a bone rotates through space is by a *rolling* of its articular surface against another bone's articular surface. The motion is shown for a convex-on-concave surface movement at the glenohumeral joint in Figure 1–9A. The contracting supraspinatus muscle rolls the convex humeral head against the slight concavity of the glenoid fossa. In essence, the roll directs the osteokinematic path of the abducting shaft of humerus.

A rolling convex surface typically involves a concurrent, oppositely directed slide. As shown in Figure 1–9A, the inferior-directed *slide* of the humeral head offsets most of the potential superior migration of the rolling humeral head. The offsetting roll-and-slide kinematics is analogous to a tire on a car that is spinning on a sheet of ice. The potential for the

| TABLE 1–3. Three Fundamental Arthrokinematics: Roll, Slide, and Spin | | |
|---|---|---|
| **Movement** | **Definition** | **Analogy** |
| Roll* | *Multiple points* along one rotating articular surface contact *multiple points* on another articular surface. | A tire rotating across a stretch of pavement. |
| Slide† | A *single point* on one articular surface contacts *multiple points* on another articular surface. | A stationary tire skidding across a stretch of icy pavement. |
| Spin | A *single point* on one articular surface rotates on a *single point* on another articular surface. | A rotating toy top on one spot on the floor. |

*Also termed rock.
†Also termed glide.

**Convex-on-concave arthrokinematics**

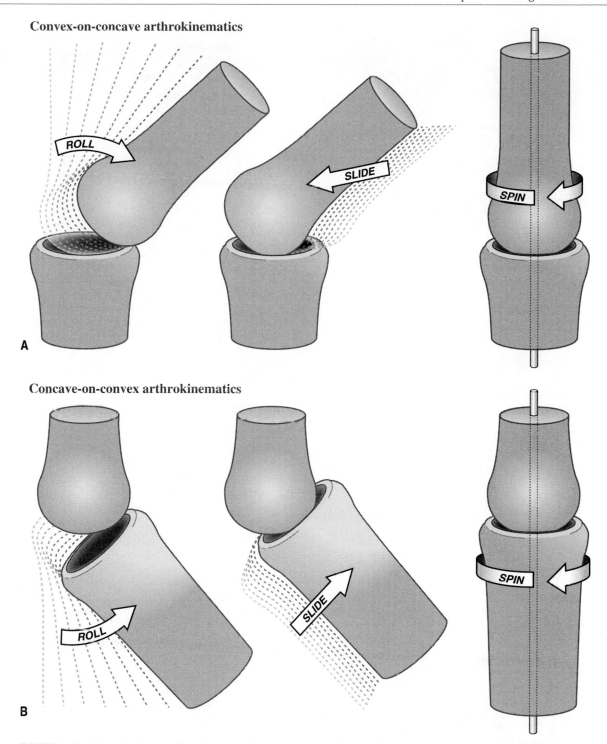

**Concave-on-convex arthrokinematics**

**FIGURE 1–8.** Three fundamental movements between joint surfaces: roll, slide, and spin. *A,* Convex-on-concave arthrokinematics; *B,* concave-on-convex arthrokinematics.

tire to rotate forward on the icy pavement is offset by a continuous sliding of the tire in the opposite direction to the intended rotation. A classic pathologic example of a convex surface rolling *without* an off-setting slide is shown in Figure 1–9*B*. The humeral head translates upward and impinges the delicate tissues in the subacromial space. The migration alters the relative location of the axis of rotation, thereby

changing the leverage of the muscles that cross the glenohumeral joint. As shown in Figure 1–9*A*, the concurrent roll and slide maximizes the angular displacement of the abducting humerus, and minimizes the net translation between joint surfaces. This mechanism is particularly important in joints in which the articular surface area on the convex member exceeds that of the concave member.

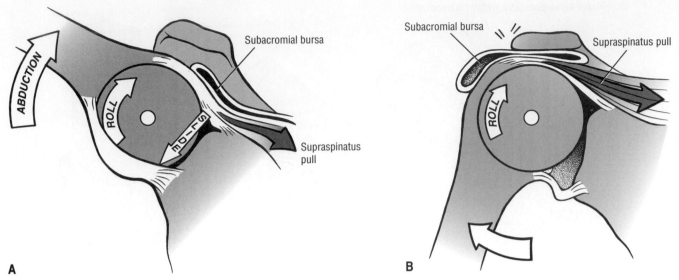

**FIGURE 1–9.** Arthrokinematics at the glenohumeral joint during abduction. The glenoid fossa is concave, and the humeral head is convex. *A*, Roll-and-slide arthrokinematics typical of a convex articular surface moving on a relatively stationary concave articular surface. *B*, Consequences of a roll occurring without a sufficient off-setting slide.

### Spin

Another primary way that a bone rotates is by a *spinning* of its articular surface against the articular surface of another bone. This occurs as the radius of the forearm spins against the capitulum of the humerus during pronation of the forearm (Fig. 1–10). Other examples include internal and external rotation of the 90-degree abducted glenohumeral joint and flexion and extension of the hip. Spinning is the primary mechanism for joint rotation when the longitudinal

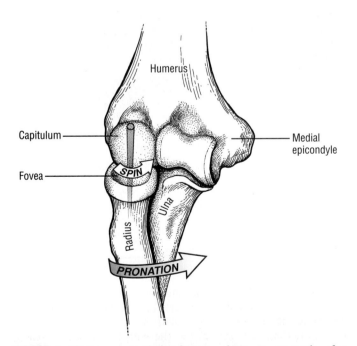

**FIGURE 1–10.** Pronation of the forearm shows an example of a spinning motion between the head of the radius and the capitulum of the humerus.

axis of the long bone intersects the surface of its articular mate at right angles.

### Motions That Combine Roll-and-Slide and Spin Arthrokinematics

Several joints throughout the body combine roll-and-slide with spin arthrokinematics. A classic example of this combination occurs during flexion and extension of the knee. As shown during femoral-on-tibial knee extension (Fig. 1–11*A*), the femur spins internally slightly, as the femoral condyle rolls and slides relative to the fixed tibia. These arthrokinematics are also shown as the tibia extends relative to the fixed femur in Figure 1–11*B*. In the knee, the spinning motion that occurs with flexion and extension occurs automatically and is mechanically linked to the primary motion of extension. As described in Chapter 13, the obligatory spinning rotation is based on the shape of the articular surfaces at the knee. The conjunct rotation helps to securely lock the knee joint when fully extended.

### PREDICTING AN ARTHROKINEMATIC PATTERN BASED ON JOINT MORPHOLOGY

As previously stated, most articular surfaces of bones are either convex or concave. Depending on which bone is moving, a convex surface may rotate on a concave surface or vice versa (compare Fig. 1–11*A* with 1–11*B*). Each scenario presents a different roll-and-slide arthrokinematic pattern. As depicted in Figure 1–11*A* and 1–9*A* for the shoulder, during a *convex-on-concave* movement, the convex surface rolls and slides in *opposite directions*. As previously described, the contradirectional slide offsets the translation tendency inherent to the rolling convex surface. During a *concave-on-convex movement,* as depicted in Figure 1–11*B*, the concave surface rolls and slides in *similar directions*. These two principles are very useful for visualizing the arthrokinematics during a movement. In addition, the principles serve as a basis for

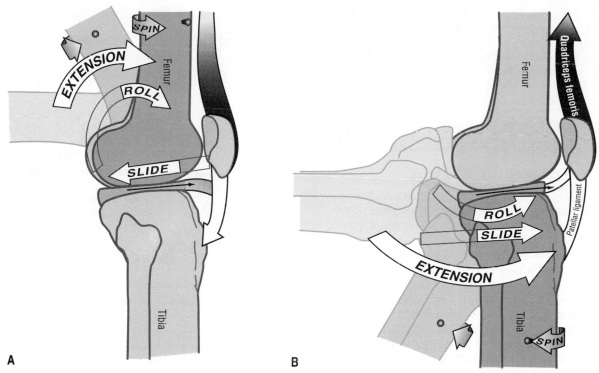

**FIGURE 1–11.** Extension of the knee demonstrates a combination of roll-and-slide with spin arthrokinematics. The femoral condyle is convex, and the tibial plateau is slightly concave. *A,* Femoral-on-tibial (knee) extension. *B,* Tibial-on-femoral (knee) extension.

some manual therapy techniques. External forces may be applied by the clinician that assist or guide the natural arthrokinematics at the joint. For example, in certain circumstances, glenohumeral abduction can be facilitated by applying an inferior-directed force at the proximal humerus, simultaneously with an active-abduction effort. The arthrokinematic principles do, however, require a knowledge of the joint surface morphology.

---

**Arthrokinematic Principles of Movement**

1. For a *convex-on-concave surface movement,* the convex member rolls and slides in *opposite directions.*
2. For a *concave-on-convex surface movement,* the concave member rolls and slides in *similar directions.*

---

## CLOSE-PACKED AND LOOSE-PACKED POSITIONS AT A JOINT

The pair of articular surfaces within most synovial joints "fit" best in only one position, usually in or near the very end range of a motion. This position of maximal congruency is referred to as the joint's *close-packed position.* In this position, most ligaments and parts of the capsule are pulled taut, providing an element of natural stability to the joint. Accessory motions are minimal in a joint's close-packed position.

For many joints in the lower extremity, the close-packed position is associated with a habitual function. At the knee, for example, the close-packed position is full extension—a position that is typically approached while standing. The

combined effect of the maximum joint congruity and stretched ligaments helps to provide transarticular stability to the knee.

All positions other than a joint's close-packed position are referred to as the joint's *loose-packed positions.* In these positions, the ligaments and capsule are relatively slackened, allowing an increase in *accessory movements.* The joint is generally least congruent near its mid range. In the lower extremity, the loose-packed positions of the major joints are biased toward flexion. These positions are generally not used during standing, but frequently are preferred by the patient during long periods of immobilization, such as extended bed rest.

## KINETICS

*Kinetics* is a branch of mechanics that describes the effect of forces on the body. The topic of kinetics is introduced here as it applies to the musculoskeletal system. A broader and more detailed explanation of this subject matter is provided in Chapter 4.

From a kinesiologic perspective, a *force* can be considered as a "push or pull" that can produce, arrest, or modify movement. Forces therefore provide the ultimate impetus for movement and stabilization of the body. As described by Newton's second law, the quantity of a force (F) can be measured by the product of the mass (m) that received the push or pull, multiplied by the acceleration (a) of the mass. The formula $F = ma$ shows that, given a constant mass, a force is directly proportional to the acceleration of the mass—measuring the force yields the acceleration and vice versa. A force is zero when the acceleration of the mass is zero and vice versa.

Based on the SI, the unit of force is a *newton (N)*: 1 N = 1 kg × 1 m/sec². The English equivalent to the newton is the pound (lb): 1 lb = 1 slug × 1 ft/sec² (4.448 N = 1 lb).

## SPECIAL FOCUS 1–1

### Body Weight Compared with Body Mass

A kilogram (kg) is a unit of *mass* that indicates the number of particles within an object. A kilogram is *not* a unit of force or weight. Under the influence of gravity, however, a 1-kg mass weighs 9.8 N. This is the result of gravity acting to accelerate the 1-kg mass toward the center of earth at a rate of about 9.8 m/s². If a person weighs 150 lb, gravity is pulling the center of mass of the person toward the center of earth with a force equal to 150 lb (667 N).

Often, however, the weight of the body is expressed in kilograms. The assumption is that the acceleration due to gravity acting on the body is constant and, for practical purposes, is ignored. Technically, however, the weight of a person varies inversely with the square of the distance between the mass of the person and the center of the earth. A person on the summit of Mt. Everest at 29,035 ft (≈8,852 m) weighs slightly less than a person with identical mass at sea level.[5] The acceleration due to gravity on Mt. Everest is 9.782 m/s² compared with 9.806m/s² at sea level.[4]

## Musculoskeletal Forces

### IMPACT OF FORCES ON THE MUSCULOSKELETAL TISSUES: INTRODUCTORY CONCEPTS AND TERMINOLOGY

The same forces that move and stabilize the body also have the potential to deform and injure the body. The manner by which forces or loads are most frequently applied to the musculoskeletal system is illustrated in Figure 1–12. (See the glossary at the end of this chapter for definitions.) Healthy tissues are able to resist changes in their shape. The tension force that stretches a healthy ligament, for example, is met by an intrinsic tension generated within the elongated tissue. Any tissue weakened by disease or trauma may not be able to adequately resist the application of the loads depicted in Figure 1–12. The proximal femur weakened by osteoporosis, for example, may fracture from the impact of a fall owing to *compression or torsion (twisting), shearing* or *bending* of the neck of the femur.

The inherent ability of connective tissues to tolerate loads can be observed experimentally by plotting the amount of force required to deform an excised tissue.[6] Figure 1–13 shows the tension generated by an excised ligament that has been stretched to a point of mechanical failure. The vertical axis of the graph is labeled *stress,* a term that denotes the internal resistance generated as a tissue resists its deforma-

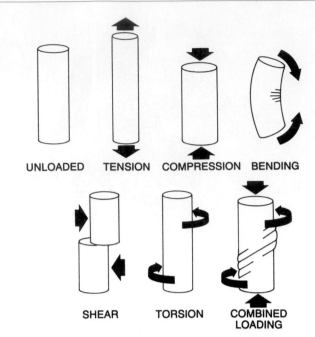

**FIGURE 1–12.** The manner by which forces or loads are most frequently applied to the musculoskeletal system is shown. The combined loading of torsion and compression is also illustrated. (With permission from Nordin M, Frankel VH: Biomechanics of bones. Basic Biomechanics of the Musculoskeletal System, 2nd ed. Philadelphia, Lea & Febiger, 1989.)

tion, divided by its cross-sectional area. The horizontal axis is labeled *strain,* which is the ratio of the tissue's deformed length to its original length.[8] A similar procedure may be performed by *compressing,* rather than by stretching, an excised slice of cartilage or bone, for example, and then plotting the amount of stress within the tissue.

Figure 1–13 shows five zones (A to E). In *zone A,* the slightly stretched or elongated ligament produces only a small amount of tension. This nonlinear region of low tension reflects the fact that the collagen fibers within the ligament must first be drawn taut before significant tension is measured. *Zone B* shows the linear relationship between stress and strain in a normal ligament. The ratio of stress to strain in an elastic material is a measure of its *stiffness*. All normal tissues within the musculoskeletal system exhibit some degree of stiffness. The clinical term "tightness" usually implies a pathologic condition of abnormally high stiffness.

Zone B in Figure 1–13 is often referred to as the *elastic zone* of the stress-strain plot. The amount of stretch (strain) applied to the ligament in this zone is significant and likely experienced during many natural movements of the body. Within this zone, the tissue returns to its original length or shape once the deforming force is removed. The area under the curve (red) represents *elastic deformation energy*. Most of the energy utilized to deform the tissue is released when the force is removed. Even in a static sense, elastic energy can do useful work for the body. When stretched even a moderate amount within the elastic zone, ligaments and other connective tissues surrounding muscles perform important joint stabilization functions.

*Zone C* in Figure 1–13 shows a mechanical property of stretched connective tissue called *plasticity*. At this extreme

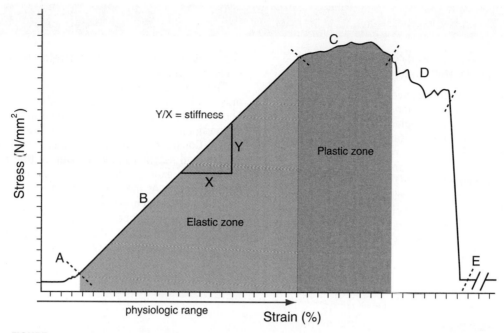

**FIGURE 1–13.** The stress-strain curve of an excised ligament is shown that has been stretched to a point of mechanical failure (disruption). The ligament is considered an elastic tissue. *Zone A* shows the nonlinear region. *Zone B* (elastic zone) shows the linear relationship between stress and strain, demonstrating the *stiffness* of the tissue. *Zone C* indicates the mechanical property of *plasticity*. *Zones D* and *E* demonstrate the points of progressive mechanical failure of the tissue. (Modified with permission from Neumann DA: Arthrokinesiologic considerations for the aged adult. In Guccione AA (ed): Geriatric Physical Therapy, 2nd ed. Chicago, Mosby-Year Book, 2000.)

and abnormally large stretch, the tissue generates only marginal increases in tension as it continues to elongate. At this point, the ligament is experiencing microscopic failure and remains permanently deformed. The area under the curve (gray) represents *plastic deformation energy*. Unlike the elastic deformation energy (region B), the plastic energy is not recoverable in its entirety when the deforming force is released. As elongation continues, the ligament reaches its initial point of failure in *zone D* and complete failure in *zone E*.

The graph in Figure 1–13 does *not* indicate the variable of time. Tissues in which the stress-strain curve changes as a function of time are considered *viscoelastic*. Most tissues within the musculoskeletal system demonstrate at least some degree of viscoelasticity (Fig. 1–15). One phenomenon of a viscoelastic material is creep. As demonstrated by the tree branch in Figure 1–15, *creep* describes a progressive strain of a material when exposed to a constant load over time. The phenomenon of creep explains why a person is taller in the morning than at night. The constant compression caused by body weight on the spine throughout the day literally squeezes fluid out of the intervertebral discs. The fluid is reabsorbed at night while the sleeping person is in a non-weight-bearing position.

The stress-strain curve of a viscoelastic material is also sensitive to the *rate* of loading of the tissue. In general, the slope of a stress-strain relationship when placed under tension or compression increases throughout its elastic range as the rate of the loading increases.[8] The rate-sensitivity nature of viscoelastic connective tissues may protect surrounding structures within the musculoskeletal system. Articular carti-

lage in the knee, for example, becomes stiffer as the rate of compression increases,[7] such as during running. The increased stiffness affords greater protection to the underlying bone at a time when joint forces are greatest.

## INTERNAL AND EXTERNAL FORCES

The principal forces acting to move and stabilize the musculoskeletal system can be conveniently divided into two sets: internal and external. *Internal forces* are produced from structures located *within* the body. These forces may be "active" or "passive." Active forces are generated by stimulated muscle, generally under volitional control. Passive forces, in contrast, are typically generated by tension in stretched periarticular connective tissues, including the intramuscular connective tissues, ligaments, and joint capsules. Active forces produced by muscles are typically the largest of all internal forces.

*External forces* are typically produced by forces acting from *outside* the body. These forces usually originate from either *gravity* pulling on the mass of a body segment or an external load, such as that of luggage or "free" weights, or *physical contact*, such as that applied by a therapist against the limb of a patient. Figure 1–16A shows an opposing pair of internal and external forces: an internal force (muscle), pulling the forearm, and an external (gravitational) force, pulling on the center of mass of the forearm. Each force is depicted by an arrow that represents a vector. By definition, a *vector* is a quantity that is completely specified by its magnitude and its direction. (Quantities such as mass or

## SPECIAL FOCUS 1-2

### Productive Antagonism: The Body's Ability to Convert Passive Tension into Useful Work

As previously described, connective tissue produces tension when stretched. Since tension is a force, it has the ability to do work. Several examples are presented throughout this text in which the tension produced by stretched connective tissues performs useful functions. This phenomenon is called *productive antagonism* and is demonstrated for a pair of muscles in the simplified model in Figure 1–14. As shown in the middle, part of the energy produced by active contraction of muscle A is transferred and stored as an elastic energy in the stretched connective tissues within muscle B. The elastic energy is released as muscle B actively contracts to drive the nail into the board (lower). Part of the contractile energy produced by muscle B is used to stretch muscle A, and the cycle is repeated.

This transfer and storage of energy between opposing muscles is useful in terms of overall metabolic efficiency. This phenomenon is often expressed in different ways by multiarticular muscles (i.e., muscles that cross several joints). Consider the rectus femoris, a muscle that flexes the hip and extends the knee. During the upward phase of jumping, for example, the rectus femoris contracts to extend the knee. At the same time, the extending hip stretches the active rectus femoris across the front of the hip. As a consequence, the overall shortening of the rectus femoris is minimized, thereby maintaining a low level of useful passive tension within the muscle.

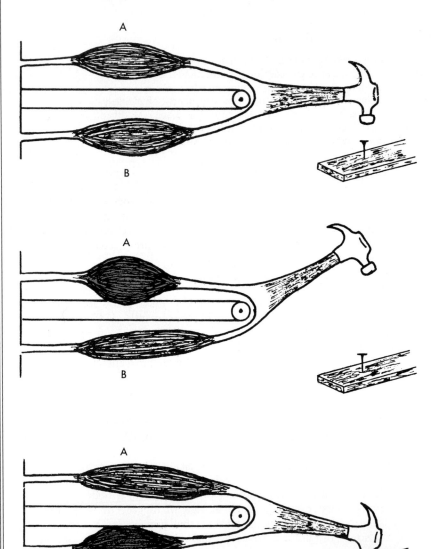

**FIGURE 1–14.** A simplified model showing a pair of opposed muscles surrounding a joint. Muscles A and B in the *top* are shown in their relaxed state. In the *middle,* muscle A (red) is contracting to provide the force needed to lift the hammer in preparation to strike the nail. In the *lower* view, muscle B (red) is contracting, driving the hammer against the nail, while simultaneously stretching muscle A. (Modified with permission from Brand PW: Clinical Biomechanics of the Hand. St Louis, CV Mosby, 1985.)

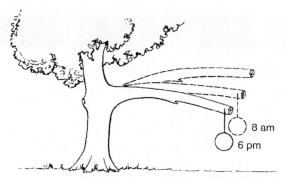

**FIGURE 1–15.** The branch of the tree is demonstrating a time-dependent property of creep associated with a *viscoelastic material.* Hanging a load on the branch at 8 AM creates an immediate deformation. By 6 PM, the load has caused additional deformation in the branch. (With permission from Panjabi MM, White AA: Biomechanics in the Musculoskeletal System. New York, Churchill Livingstone, 2001.)

serts to the bone. The *angle-of-insertion* describes the angle formed between a tendon of a muscle and the long axis of the bone to which it inserts. In Figure 1–16A, the angle-of-insertion is 90 degrees. The angle-of-insertion changes as the elbow rotates into flexion or extension. The point of application of the external force depends on whether the force is the result of gravity or the result of a resistance applied by physical contact. Gravity acts on the *center of mass* of the body segment (see Fig. 1–16A, dot at the forearm). The point of application of a resistance generated from physical contact can occur anywhere on the body.

> **Factors Required to Completely Describe a Vector in Most Biomechanical Analyses**
> - Magnitude
> - Direction (line-of-force or line-of-gravity)
> - Sense
> - Point of application

speed are scalars not vectors. A scalar is a quantity that is completely specified by its magnitude and has no direction.)

In order to completely describe a vector in a biomechanical analysis, its magnitude, direction, sense, and point of application must be known. The forces depicted in Figure 1–16A indicate these four factors.

1. The *magnitude* of each force vector is indicated by the length of the shaft of the arrow.

2. The *direction* of both force vectors is indicated by the spatial orientation of the shaft of the arrows. Both forces are oriented vertically, commonly referred to as the **Y** direction. The direction of a force can also be described by the angle formed between the shaft of the arrow and a reference line. Throughout this text, the direction of a muscle force and the direction of gravity are commonly referred to as their *line-of-force* and *line-of-gravity,* respectively.

3. The *sense* of each force vector is indicated by the orientation of the arrowhead. In the example depicted in Figure 1–16A, the internal force acts upward in a *positive* **Y** *sense;* the external force acts downward in a *negative* **Y** *sense.*

4. The *point of application* of the vectors is where the base of the vector arrow contacts the part of the body. The point of application of the muscle force is where the muscle in-

As a push or a pull, all forces acting on the body cause a potential translation of the segment. The direction of the translation depends on the net effect of all the applied forces. Since in Figure 1–16A the muscle force is three times greater than the weight of the forearm, the net effect of both forces would accelerate the forearm vertically upward. In reality, however, the forearm is typically prevented from accelerating upward by a *joint reaction force* produced between the surfaces of the joint. As depicted in Figure 1–16B, the distal end of the humerus is pushing *down* with a reaction force against the proximal end of the forearm. The magnitude of the joint reaction force is equal to the difference between the muscle force and external force. As a result, the sum of all vertical forces acting on the forearm is balanced, and net acceleration of the forearm in the vertical direction is zero. The system is therefore in *static linear equilibrium.*

## Musculoskeletal Torques

Forces exerted on the body can have two outcomes. First, as depicted in Figure 1–16A, forces can potentially translate a body segment. Second, the forces, if acting at a *distance* from

**FIGURE 1–16.** A sagittal plane view of the elbow joint and associated bones. *A,* Internal (muscle) and external (gravitational) forces are shown both acting vertically, but each in a different sense. The two vectors each have a different magnitude and different points of attachment to the forearm. *B,* Joint reaction force is added to prevent the forearm from accelerating upward. (Vectors are drawn to relative scale.)

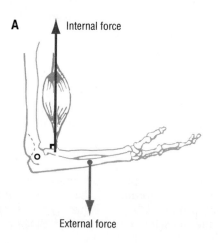

**A**   Internal force

External force

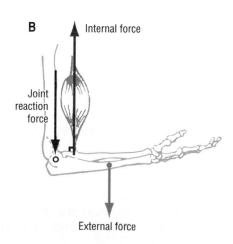

**B**   Internal force

Joint reaction force

External force

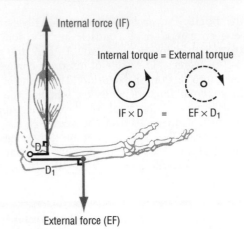

**FIGURE 1–17.** The balance of internal and external torques acting in the sagittal plane about the axis of rotation at the elbow (small circle) is shown. The *internal torque* is the product of the internal force multiplied by the internal moment arm (D). The internal torque has the potential to rotate the forearm in a counterclockwise direction. The *external torque* is the product of the external force (gravity) and the external moment arm (D₁). The external torque has the potential to rotate the forearm in a clockwise direction. The internal and external torques are equal, demonstrating a condition of static rotary equilibrium. (Vectors are drawn to relative scale.)

the axis of rotation at the joint, produce a potential rotation of the joint. The shortest distance between the axis of rotation and the force is called a *moment arm*. The product of a force and its moment arm is a *torque* or a *moment*. Torque can be considered as a rotatory equivalent to a force. A force pushes and pulls an object in a linear fashion, whereas a torque rotates an object about an axis of rotation.

Torques occur in planes about an axis of rotation. Figure 1–17 shows the torques produced within the sagittal plane by the internal and external forces introduced in Figure 1–16. The *internal torque* is defined as the product of the internal force (muscle) and the internal moment arm. The *internal moment arm* (see Fig 1–17,D) is the distance between the axis of rotation and the perpendicular intersection with the internal force. As depicted in Figure 1–17, the internal torque has the potential to rotate the forearm in a counterclockwise, or flexion, direction.

The *external torque* is defined as the product of the external force (gravity) and the external moment arm. The *external moment arm* (see Fig 1–17,D₁) is the distance between the axis of rotation and the perpendicular intersection with the external force. The external torque has the potential to rotate the forearm in a clockwise, or extension, direction. The internal and external torques happen to be equal in Figure 1–17, and therefore no rotation occurs at the joint. This condition is referred to as *static rotary equilibrium*.

## Muscle and Joint Interaction

The term *muscle and joint interaction* refers to the overall effect that a muscle force may have on a joint. This topic is revisited repeatedly throughout this textbook. A force produced by a muscle that has a moment arm causes a torque, and a potential to rotate the joint. A force produced by a muscle that lacks a moment arm (i.e., the muscle force

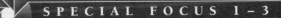

**Torque Makes the World Go 'Round**

Torques are experienced by everyone, in one way or another. Muscles and gravity are constantly competing for dominance of torque about the axis of rotation at joints. The direction of rotation of a bone about a joint can indicate the more dominant torque. Furthermore, manual contact forces applied against objects in the environment are frequently converted to torques. Torques are used to unscrew a cap from a jar, turn a wrench, swing a baseball bat, and open a door. In the last example, the door is opened by the product of the push on the door knob multiplied by the perpendicular distance between the door knob and the hinge. Trying to open a door by pushing only a couple of centimeters from the hinge of the door is very difficult, even when applying a large pushing force. In contrast, a door can be opened with a slight push, provided the push is applied at the door knob, which is purposely located at a distance far from the hinge. *A torque is the product of a force and its moment arm.* Both variables are equally influential.

Torques are involved in most therapeutic situations with patients, especially when physical exercise or strength assessment is involved. A person's "strength" is the product of their muscle's force, and, equally important, the distance between the muscle's line-of-force and the axis of rotation. As explained further in Chapter 4, the length of a muscle's moment arm changes constantly throughout a range of motion. This partially explains why a person is naturally stronger in certain parts of a joint's range of motion.

Clinicians frequently apply manual resistance against their patients as a means to assess, facilitate, and challenge a particular muscle activity. The *force* applied against a patient's extremity is usually perceived as an external *torque* by the patient's musculoskeletal system. A clinician can challenge a particular muscle group by applying an external torque by way of a small manual force exerted a great distance from the joint or a large manual force exerted close to the joint. Either means can produce the same external torque against the patient. Modifying the force and external moment arm variables allows different strategies to be employed based on the strength and skill of the clinician.

passes *through* the axis of rotation) will not cause a torque or a rotation. The muscle force is still important, however, because it usually provides a source of stability to the joint.

## TYPES OF MUSCLE ACTIVATION

A muscle is considered activated when it is stimulated by the nervous system. A muscle produces a force through three types of activation: isometric, concentric, and eccentric. The physiology of the three types of activation is described in greater detail in Chapter 3 and briefly summarized subsequently.

*Isometric activation* occurs when a muscle is producing a force while maintaining a constant length. This type of activation is apparent by the origin of the word isometric (from the Greek *isos,* equal; and *metron,* measure or length). During an isometric activation, the internal torque produced at a joint is equal to the external torque; hence, there is no muscle shortening or rotating at the joint (Fig. 1–18A).

*Concentric activation* occurs as a muscle produces a force as it contracts (shortens) (Fig. 1–18B). Literally, concentric means "coming to the center." During a concentric activation, the internal torque at the joint exceeds the opposing external torque. This is reflected by the fact that the muscle contracted and accelerated a rotation of the joint in the direction of the activated muscle.

*Eccentric activation,* in contrast, occurs as a muscle produces an active force while being elongated. The word eccentric literally means "away from the center." During an eccentric activation, the external torque about the joint exceeds the internal torque. In this case, the joint rotates in the direction dictated by the relatively larger external torque, such as that produced by the cable in Figure 1–18C. Many common activities employ eccentric activations of muscle. Slowly lowering a cup of water to a table, for example, is caused by the pull of gravity on the forearm and water. The activated biceps slowly elongates in order to control their descent. The triceps muscle, although considered as an elbow "extensor," is most likely inactive during this particular process.

The term "contraction" is often used synonymously with "activation," regardless of whether the muscle is actually shortening, lengthening, or remaining at a constant length. The term "contract" literally means to be *drawn together* and, therefore, its use can be confusing when describing either an isometric or eccentric activation. Technically, a contracting muscle occurs during a concentric activation only.

## A MUSCLE'S ACTION AT A JOINT

A *muscle's action at a joint* is defined as its potential to cause a torque in a particular rotation direction and plane. The actual naming of a muscle's action is based on an established nomenclature, such as flexion or extension in the sagittal plane, abduction or adduction in the frontal plane, and so forth. The terms "muscle action" and "joint action" are used interchangeably throughout this text, depending on the context of the discussion. If the action is associated with a nonisometric muscle activation, the resulting osteokinematics may involve distal-on-proximal segment kinematics, or vice versa, depending on the relative stability of the two segments that comprise the joint.

Kinesiology allows one to determine the action of a muscle, without relying purely on memory. Suppose the student desires to determine the action of the *posterior deltoid* at the glenohumeral (shoulder) joint. In this particular analysis, two assumptions are made. First, it is assumed that the humerus is the freest segment of the joint, and that the scapula is fixed, although the reverse assumption could have been made. Second, it is assumed that the body is in the anatomic position at the time of the muscle activation.

The first step in the analysis is to determine the planes of rotary motion (degrees of freedom) allowed at the joint. In this case, the glenohumeral joint allows rotation in all three planes (see Fig. 1–5). Figure 1–19A shows the potential for the posterior deltoid to rotate the humerus in the frontal plane. The axis of rotation at the joint passes in an anterior-posterior direction through the humeral head. In the anatomic position, the line-of-force of the posterior deltoid passes inferior to the axis of rotation. By assuming that the scapula is stable, the posterior deltoid would rotate the humerus toward adduction, with a strength equal to the product of the muscle force multiplied by its internal moment arm. This same logic is next applied to determine the muscle's action in the horizontal and sagittal planes. As depicted in Figure 1–19B and C, it is apparent that the muscle is also

### Three types of muscle activation

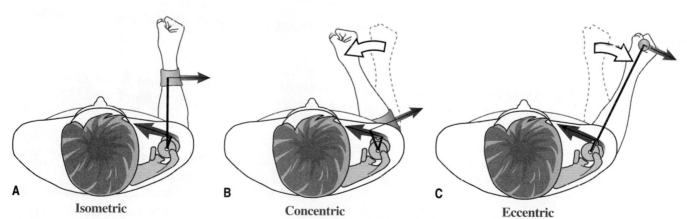

**FIGURE 1–18.** Three types of muscle activation are shown as the pectoralis major actively attempts to internally rotate the shoulder (glenohumeral) joint. In each of the three illustrations, the internal torque is the product of the muscle force (red) and its moment arm; the external torque is the product of the force in the cable (gray) and its moment arm. Note that the external moment arm and, therefore, the external torque is different in each illustration. A, Isometric activation is shown as the internal torque matches the external torque. B, Concentric activation is shown as the internal torque exceeds the external torque. C, Eccentric activation is shown as the external torque exceeds the internal torque. (Vectors are *not* drawn to scale.)

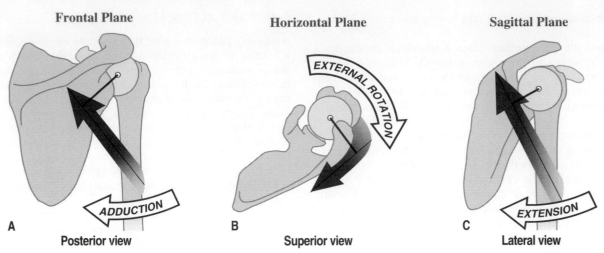

**Frontal Plane**     **Horizontal Plane**     **Sagittal Plane**

EXTERNAL ROTATION

ADDUCTION

EXTENSION

**A**     **B**     **C**
**Posterior view**     **Superior view**     **Lateral view**

**FIGURE 1–19.** The multiple actions of the posterior deltoid are shown at the glenohumeral joint. *A,* Adduction in the frontal plane. *B,* External rotation in the horizontal plane. *C,* Extension in the sagittal plane. The internal moment arm is shown extending from the axis of rotation (small circle through humeral head) to a perpendicular intersection with the muscle's line-of-force.

an external (lateral) rotator and an extensor of the glenohumeral joint.

The logic so presented can be used to determine the action of *any muscle* in the body, at any joint. If available, an articulated skeleton model and a piece of string that mimics the line-of-force of a muscle is helpful in applying this logic. This exercise is particularly helpful when analyzing a muscle whose action switches, depending on the position of the joint. One such muscle is the posterior deltoid. From the anatomic position, the posterior deltoid is an *adductor* of the glenohumeral joint. If the arm is lifted (abducted) fully overhead, however, the line-of-force of the muscle shifts just to the *superior side* of the axis of rotation. As a consequence, the posterior deltoid actively abducts the shoulder. This shift can be visualized with the aid of Figure 1–19A. The example shows how one muscle can have opposite actions, depending on the position of the joint at the time of muscle activation. It is important, therefore, to establish a reference position for the joint when analyzing the actions of a muscle. One common reference position is the anatomic position (see Fig. 1–4). Unless otherwise specified, the actions of muscles described throughout Sections II to IV are based on the assumption that the joint is in the anatomic position.

### Terminology Related to the Actions of Muscles

The following terms are often used when describing the actions of muscles:

1. The *agonist* is the muscle or muscle group that is most directly related to the initiation and execution of a particular movement. For example, the tibialis anterior is the agonist for the motion of dorsiflexion of the ankle.

2. The *antagonist* is the muscle or muscle group that is considered to have the opposite action of a particular agonist. For example, the gastrocnemius and soleus muscles are considered the antagonists to the tibialis anterior.

3. A pair of muscles are considered *synergists* when they cooperate during the execution of a particular movement.

Actually, most meaningful movements of the body involve multiple muscles acting as synergists. Consider, for example, the flexor carpi ulnaris and flexor carpi radialis muscles during flexion of the wrist. The muscles act synergistically because they cooperate to flex the wrist. Each muscle, however, must neutralize the other's tendency to move the wrist in a side-to-side (radial and ulnar deviation) fashion. Paralysis of one of the muscles significantly affects the overall action of the other.

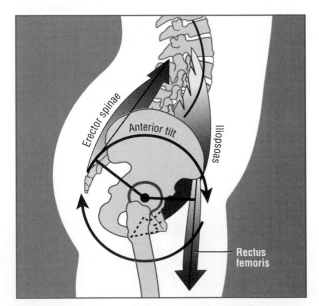

**FIGURE 1–20.** Side view of the force-couple formed between two representative hip flexor (rectus femoris and iliopsoas) muscles and back extensor (erector spinae) muscles, as they contract to tilt the pelvis in an anterior direction. The internal moment arms used by the muscles are indicated by the dark black lines. The axis of rotation runs through both hip joints.

Another example of muscle synergy is described as a muscular force-couple. A muscular *force-couple* is formed when two or more muscles simultaneously produce forces in different linear directions, although the torques act in the same rotary direction. A familiar analogy of a force couple occurs between the two hands while turning a steering wheel of a car. Rotating the steering wheel to the right, for example, occurs by the action of the right hand pulling down and the left hand pulling up on the wheel. Although the hands are producing forces in different linear directions, they cause a torque on the steering wheel in a common rotary direction. The hip flexor and low back extensor muscles, for example, form a force-couple to rotate the pelvis in the sagittal plane about both hip joints (Fig. 1–20).

## Musculoskeletal Levers

### THREE CLASSES OF LEVERS

A lever is a simple machine consisting of a rod suspended across a pivot point. The seesaw is a classic example of a lever. One function of a lever is to convert a force into a torque. As shown in the seesaw in Figure 1–21, a 672-N (about 150-lb) man sitting 0.91 m (about 3 ft) from the pivot point produces a torque that balances a boy weighing half his weight, who is sitting twice the distance from the pivot point. In Figure 1–21, the opposing torques are equal:

$$BW_m \times D = BW_b \times D_1.$$

As indicated, the boy has the greatest leverage ($D_1$). *Leverage* describes the relative moment arm length possessed by a particular force.

Internal and external forces produce torques throughout the body through a system of bony levers. The most important forces involved with musculoskeletal levers are those produced by muscle, gravity, and physical contacts within the environment. Levers are classified as either *first, second,* or *third class.*

**First-Class Lever.** As depicted in Figure 1–21, the first-class lever has its axis of rotation positioned *between* the opposing forces. An example of a first-class lever in the body is the head-and-neck extensor muscles that control the posture of the head in sagittal plane (Fig. 1–22A). As in the seesaw example, the head is held in equilibrium when the product of the muscle force (MF) multiplied by the internal moment arm (IMA) equals the product of head weight (HW) multiplied by its external moment arm (EMA). In first-class levers, the internal and external forces typically act in similar

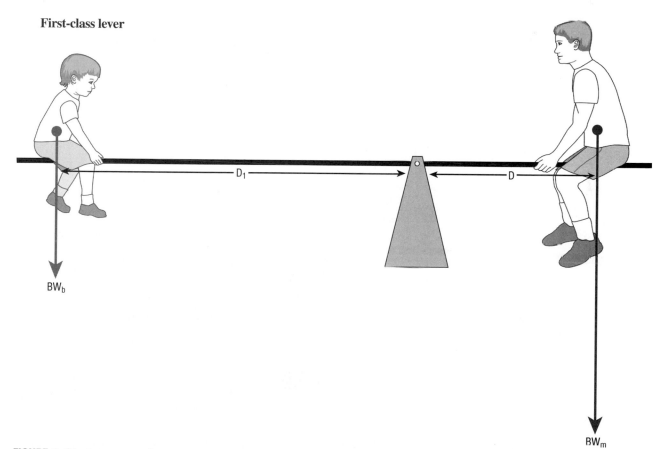

**First-class lever**

**FIGURE 1–21.** A seesaw is shown as a typical first-class lever. The body weight of the man ($BW_m$) is 672 N (about 150 lb). He is sitting .91 m (about 3 ft) from the pivot point (D). The body weight of the boy ($BW_b$) is only 336 N (about 75 lb). He is sitting 1.82 m (about 6 ft) from the pivot point ($D_1$). The seesaw is balanced since the clockwise torque produced by the man is equal in magnitude to the counterclockwise torque produced by the boy: 672 N × .91 m = 336 N × 1.82 m.

## First-class lever

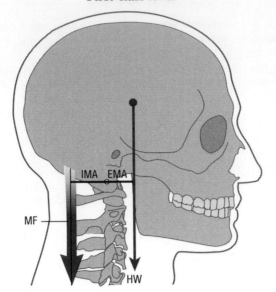

**Data for first-class lever:**
Muscle force (MF) = unknown
Head weight (HW) = 46.7 N (10.5 lbs)
Internal moment arm (IMA) = 4.0 cm
External moment arm (EMA) = 3.2 cm
*Mechanical advantage = 1.25*

$MF \times IMA = HW \times EMA$
$MF = \dfrac{HW \times EMA}{IMA}$
$MF = \dfrac{46.7 \text{ N} \times 3.2 \text{ cm}}{4.0 \text{ cm}}$
$MF = 37.4 \text{ N (8.4 lbs)}$

**A**

## Second-class lever

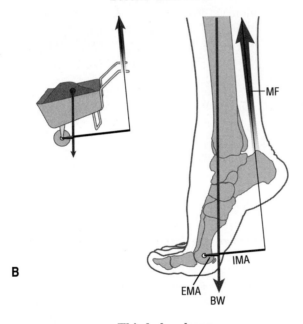

**Data for second-class lever:**
Muscle force (MF) = unknown
Body weight (BW) = 667 N (150 lbs)
Internal moment arm (IMA) = 12.0 cm
External moment arm (EMA) = 3.0 cm
*Mechanical advantage = 4.0*

$MF \times IMA = BW \times EMA$
$MF = \dfrac{BW \times EMA}{IMA}$
$MF = \dfrac{667 \text{ N} \times 3.0 \text{ cm}}{12.0 \text{ cm}}$
$MF = 166.8 \text{ N (37.5 lbs)}$

**B**

## Third-class lever

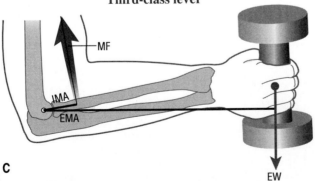
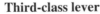

**Data for third-class lever:**
Muscle force (MF) = unknown
External weight (EW) = 66.7 N (15 lbs)
Internal moment arm (IMA) = 5.0 cm
External moment arm (EMA) = 35.0 cm
*Mechanical advantage = .143*

$MF \times IMA = EW \times EMA$
$MF = \dfrac{EW \times EMA}{IMA}$
$MF = \dfrac{66.7 \text{ N} \times 35.0 \text{ cm}}{5.0 \text{ cm}}$
$MF = 467.0 \text{ N (105.0 lbs)}$

**C**

**FIGURE 1–22.** Anatomic examples are shown of first- (*A*), second- (*B*), and third- (*C*) class levers. (The vectors are *not* drawn to scale.) The data contained in the boxes to the right show how to calculate the muscle force required to maintain static rotary equilibrium. Note that the mechanical advantage is indicated in each box. The muscle activation is isometric in each case, with no movement occurring at the joint.

linear directions, although they produce torques in opposing rotary directions.

**Second-Class Lever.** A second-class lever has two unique features. First, its axis of rotation is located at one end of a bone. Second, the muscle, or internal force, possesses greater leverage than the external force. As illustrated in Figure 1–22B, a calf muscle group uses a second-class lever to produce the torque needed to stand on tiptoes. The axis of rotation for this action is through the metatarsophalangeal joints. The internal moment arm used by calf muscles greatly exceeds the external moment arm used by body weight. Second-class levers are rare in the musculoskeletal system.

**Third-Class Lever.** As in the second-class lever, the third-class lever has its axis of rotation located at one end of a bone. The elbow flexor muscles use a third-class lever to produce the flexion torque required to support a barbell (Fig. 1–22C). Unlike the second-class lever, the external weight supported by a third-class lever always has greater leverage than the muscle force. The third-class lever is the most common lever used by the musculoskeletal system.

## MECHANICAL ADVANTAGE

The *mechanical advantage* (MA) of a musculoskeletal lever is defined as the ratio of the internal moment arm to the external moment arm. Depending on the location of the axis of rotation, the first-class lever can have an MA equal to, less than, or greater than one. Second-class levers always have an MA greater than one. As depicted in the boxes associated with Figure 1–22A and B, lever systems with an MA greater than one are able to balance the torque equilibrium equation by an internal (muscle) force that is *less than* the external force. Third-class levers always have an MA less than one. As depicted in Figure 1–22C, in order to balance the torque equilibrium equation, the muscle must produce a force much *greater than* the opposing external force.

---

**Mechanical Advantage (MA) is equal to the Internal Moment Arm/External Moment Arm**

- First-class levers may have an MA less than 1, equal to 1, or more than 1.
- Second-class levers always have an MA more than 1.
- Third-class levers always have an MA less than 1.

---

The majority of muscles throughout the musculoskeletal system function with a mechanical advantage of much *less than one,* and, actually, it may be more appropriate to call this a mechanical disadvantage! Consider, for example, the biceps at the elbow, the quadriceps at the knee, and the supraspinatus and deltoid at the shoulder. Each of these muscles attaches to bone relatively close to the joint's axis of rotation. The external forces that oppose the action of the muscles typically exert their influence considerably *distally* to the joint, such as at the hand or the foot. Consider the force demands placed on the supraspinatus and deltoid muscles to maintain the shoulder abducted to 90 degrees while

holding an external weight of 35.6N (8 lb) in the hand. For the sake of this example, assume that the muscles have an internal moment arm of 2.5 cm (about 1 in) and that the center of mass of the external weight has an external moment arm of 50 cm (about 20 in). (For simplicity, the weight of the limb is ignored.) The 1/20 MA requires that the muscle would have to produce 711.7N (160 lb) of force, or *twenty times* the weight of the external load! As a general principle, skeletal muscles produce forces several times larger than the external loads that oppose them. Depending on the shape of the muscle and configuration of the joint, a certain percentage of the muscle force produces large compression or shear forces at the joint surfaces. Periarticular tissues, such as articular cartilage, fat pads, and bursa, must partially absorb or dissipate these large *myogenic (muscular-produced) forces.* In the absence of such protection, joints may partially degenerate and become painful and chronically inflamed. This presentation is the hallmark of severe osteoarthritis.

### *Dictating the "Trade-off" between Force and Distance*

As previously described, most muscles are obligated to produce a force much greater than the resistance applied by the external load. At first thought, this design may appear flawed. The design is absolutely necessary, however, when the large distances and velocities experienced by the more distal points of the extremities are considered.

*Work* is the product of force times distance (see Chapter 4). In addition to converting a force to a torque, a musculoskeletal lever converts the work of a contracting muscle to the work of a rotating bone. The mechanical advantage of a musculoskeletal lever dictates how the work is converted — through either a relatively large force exerted over a short distance or a small force exerted over a large distance. Consider the small mechanical advantage of 1/20 described earlier for the supraspinatus and deltoid muscles. This mechanical advantage implies that the muscle must produce a force 20 times greater than the weight of the external load. What must also be considered, however, is that the muscles need to contract only 5% (1/20) the distance that the center of mass of the load would be raised by the abduction action. A very short contraction distance of the muscles produces a very large angular displacement of the arm.

Although all points throughout the abducting arm share the same *angular* displacement and velocity, the more distal points on the arm move at an even greater *linear* displacement and velocity. The ability of a short contraction range to generate large velocities of the limb may have an important physiologic advantage for the muscle. As explained in Chapter 3, a muscle produces its maximal force within only a relatively narrow range of its overall length.

In summary, most muscle and joint systems in the body function with a mechanical advantage of less than one. The muscles and underlying joints must, therefore, "pay the price" by generating and dispersing relative large forces, respectively, even for seemingly low-load activities. Obtaining a high linear velocity of the distal end of the extremities is a necessity for generating large contact forces against the environment. These high forces can be used to rapidly accelerate objects held in the hand, such as a tennis racket, or to accelerate the limbs purely as an expression of art and athleticism, such as dance.

## SPECIAL FOCUS 1 – 4

### Surgically Altering a Muscle's Mechanical Advantage: Dealing with the Trade-off

A surgeon may perform a muscle-tendon transfer operation as a means to partially restore the loss of internal torque at a joint. Consider, for example, complete paralysis of the elbow flexor muscles following poliomyelitis. Such a paralysis can have profound functional consequences, especially if it occurs bilaterally. One approach to restoring elbow flexion is to surgically reroute the fully innervated triceps tendon to the anterior side of the elbow (Fig. 1–23). The triceps, now passing anteriorly to the medial-lateral axis of rotation at the elbow, becomes a flexor instead of an extensor. The length of the internal moment arm for the flexion action can be exaggerated, if desired, by increasing the perpendicular distance between the transferred tendon and the axis of rotation. By increasing the muscle's mechanical advantage, the activated muscle produces a *greater torque per level of muscle force.* This may be a beneficial outcome, depending on the specific circumstances of the patient.

An important mechanical trade-off exists whenever a muscle's mechanical advantage is increased. Although a greater torque is produced per level muscle force, a given amount of muscle shortening results in a *reduced angular displacement of the joint.* As a result, a full muscle contraction may produce an ample torque, however, the joint may not complete its full range of motion. In essence, the active range of motion "lags" behind the muscle contraction. The reduced angular displacement and velocity of the joint may have negative functional consequences. This mechanical trade-off needs to be considered before the muscle's internal moment arm is surgically exaggerated. Often, the greater torque potential gained by increasing

the moment arm functionally "outweighs" the loss of the speed and distance of the movement.

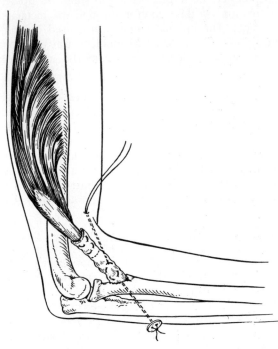

**FIGURE 1–23.** An anterior transfer of the triceps following paralysis of the elbow flexor muscles. The triceps tendon is elongated by a graft of fascia. (From Bunnell S: Restoring flexion to the paralytic elbow. J Bone Joint Surg 33A:566, 1951.)

## GLOSSARY

**Acceleration:** change in velocity of a body over time, expressed in linear (m/s²) and angular (°/s²) terms.

**Accessory movements:** slight, passive, nonvolitional movements allowed in most joints (also called "joint play").

**Active force:** push or pull generated by stimulated muscle.

**Active movement:** motion caused by stimulated muscle.

**Agonist muscle:** muscle or muscle group that is most directly related to the initiation and execution of a particular movement.

**Angle-of-insertion:** angle formed between a tendon of a muscle and the long axis of the bone to which it inserts.

**Antagonist muscle:** muscle or muscle group that has the action opposite to a particular agonist muscle.

**Arthrokinematics:** motions of roll, slide, and spin that occur between the articular surfaces of joints.

**Axis of rotation:** an imaginary line extending through a joint about which rotation occurs (also called the pivot point or the center of rotation).

**Axial rotation:** angular motion of an object in a direction perpendicular to its longitudinal axis, often used to describe a motion in the horizontal plane.

**Bending:** effect of a force that deforms a material at right angles to its long axis. A bent tissue is compressed on its concave side and placed under tension on its convex side. A bending moment is a quantitative measure of a bend. Similar to a torque, a bending moment is the product of the bending force and the perpendicular distance between the force and the axis of rotation of the bend.

**Center of mass:** point at the exact center of an object's mass (also referred to as center of gravity when considering the weight of the mass).

**Close-packed position:** unique position of most joints of the body where the articular surfaces are most congruent, and the ligaments are maximally taut.

**Compression:** application of one or more forces that press an object or objects together. Compression tends to shorten and widen a material.

**Concentric activation:** activated muscle that shortens as it produces a force.

**Creep:** a progressive strain of a material when exposed to a constant load over time.

**Degrees of freedom:** number of independent movements allowed at a joint. A joint can have up to three degrees of translation and three degrees of rotation.

**Displacement:** change in the linear or angular position of an object.

**Distal-on-proximal segment kinematics:** type of movement in which the distal segment of a joint rotates relative to a fixed proximal segment (also called an open kinematic chain).

**Distraction:** movement of two objects away from one another.

**Eccentric activation:** activated muscle that is elongating as it produces a force.

**Elasticity:** property of a material demonstrated by its ability to return to its original length after the removal of a deforming force.

**External force:** push or pull produced by sources located outside the body. These typically include gravity and physical contact applied against the body.

**External moment arm:** distance between the axis of rotation and the perpendicular intersection with an external force.

**External torque:** product of an external force and its external moment arm (also called external moment).

**Force:** a push or a pull that produces, arrests, or modifies a motion.

**Force-couple:** interaction of two or more muscles acting in different linear directions, but producing a torque in the same rotary direction.

**Force of gravity:** potential acceleration of a body to the center of the earth due to gravity.

**Friction:** resistance to movement between two contacting surfaces.

**Internal force:** push or pull produced by a structure located within the body. Most often internal force refers to that produced by an active muscle.

**Internal moment arm:** distance between the axis of rotation and the perpendicular intersection with a muscle (internal) force.

**Internal torque:** product of an internal force and its internal moment arm.

**Isometric activation:** activated muscle that maintains a constant length as it produces a force.

**Joint reaction force:** push or pull produced by one joint surface against another.

**Kinematics:** branch of mechanics that describes the motion of a body, without regard to the forces or torques that may produce the motion.

**Kinematic chain:** series of articulated segmented links, such as the connected pelvis, thigh, leg, and foot of the lower extremity.

**Kinetics:** branch of mechanics that describes the effect of forces on the body.

**Leverage:** relative moment arm length possessed by a particular force.

**Line-of-force:** direction of a muscle's force.

**Line-of-gravity:** direction of the gravitational pull on a body.

**Load:** general term that describes the application of a force to a body.

**Longitudinal axis:** axis that extends within and parallel to a long bone or body segment.

**Loose-packed positions:** positions of most joints of the body where the articular surfaces are least congruent, and the ligaments are slackened.

**Mass:** quantity of matter in an object.

**Mechanical advantage:** ratio of the internal moment arm to the external moment arm.

**Muscle action:** potential of a muscle to produce an internal torque within a particular plane of motion and rotary direction (also called *joint action* when referring specifically to a muscle's potential to rotate a joint). Terms that describe a muscle action are flexion, extension, pronation, supination, and so forth.

**Osteokinematics:** motion of bones relative to the three cardinal, or principal, planes.

**Passive force:** push or pull generated by sources other than stimulated muscle, such as tension in stretched periarticular connective tissues, physical contact, and so forth.

**Passive movement:** motion produced by a source other than activated muscle.

**Plasticity:** property of a material demonstrated by remaining permanently deformed after the removal of a force.

**Pressure:** force divided by a surface area (also called stress).

**Productive antagonism:** phenomenon in which relatively low-level tension within stretched connective tissues performs a useful function.

**Proximal-on-distal segment kinematics:** type of movement in which the proximal segment of a joint rotates relative to a fixed distal segment (also referred to as a closed kinematic chain).

**Roll:** multiple points along one rotating articular surface contact multiple points on another articular surface. (Also called rock.)

**Rotation:** angular motion in which a rigid body moves in a circular path about a pivot point or an axis of rotation.

**Scalar:** quantity, such as speed and temperature, that is completely specified by its magnitude and has no direction.

**Segment:** any part of a body or limb.

**Shear:** forces on a material that act in opposite but parallel directions (like the action of a pair of scissors).

**Shock absorption:** ability to dissipate forces.

**Slide:** single point on one articular surface contacts multiple points on another articular surface. (Also called glide.)

**Spin:** single point on one articular surface rotates on a single point on another articular surface (like a toy top).

**Static linear equilibrium:** state of a body at rest in which the sum of all forces is equal to zero.

**Static rotary equilibrium:** state of a body at rest in which the sum of all torques is equal to zero.

**Stiffness:** ratio of stress (force) to strain (elongation) within an elastic material.

**Strain:** ratio of a tissue's deformed length to its original length.

**Stress:** force generated as a tissue resists deformation, divided by its cross-sectional area (also called pressure).

**Synergists:** two muscles that cooperate to execute a particular movement.

**Tension:** application of one or more forces that pulls apart or separates a material. (Also called a distraction force.) Used to denote the internal stress within a tissue as it resists being stretched.

**Torque:** a force multiplied by its moment arm; tends to rotate a body or segment about an axis of rotation.

**Torsion:** application of a force that twists a material about its longitudinal axis.

**Translation:** linear motion in which all parts of a rigid body move parallel to and in the same direction as every other point in the body.

**Vector:** quantity, such as velocity or force, that is completely specified by its magnitude and direction.

**Velocity:** change in position of a body over time, expressed in linear (m/s) and angular (degrees/s) terms.

**Viscoelasticity:** property of a material expressed by a changing stress-strain relationship over time.

**Weight:** gravitational force acting on a mass.

## SUMMARY

Many of the basic biomechanical principles and essential terms and concepts used to communicate the subject matter of kinesiology are provided. Chapters 2 to 4 give additional background on the essential topics of kinesiology. This material then sets the foundation for the more anatomic-based chapters, starting with the shoulder complex in Chapter 5.

## REFERENCES

1. Brand PW: Clinical Biomechanics of the Hand. St Louis, CV Mosby, 1985.
2. Bynum EB, Barrack RL, Alexander AH: Open versus closed chain kinetic exercises after anterior cruciate ligament reconstruction. Am J Sports Med 23:401–406, 1995.
3. Fitzgerald GK: Open versus closed kinetic chan exercises: After anterior cruciate ligament reconstructive surgery. Phys Ther 77:1747–1754, 1997.
4. Gowitzke BA, Milner M: Scientific Bases of Human Movement, 3rd ed. Baltimore, Williams & Wilkins, 1988.
5. Hardee EB III: Personal communication. Afton, VA, 2002.
6. Neumann DA: Arthrokinesiologic considerations for the aged adult. In Guccione AA: Geriatric Physical Therapy, 2nd ed. Chicago, Mosby-Year Book, 2000.
7. Nordin M, Frankel VH: Basic Biomechanics of the Musculoskeletal System, 2nd ed. Philadelphia, Lea & Febiger, 1989.
8. Panjabi MM, White AA: Biomechanics in the Musculoskeletal System. New York, Churchill Livingstone, 2001.
9. Rodgers MM, Cavanagh PR: Glossary of biomechanical terms, concepts, and units. Phys Ther 64:1886–1902, 1984.
10. Steindler A: Kinesiology of the Human Body: Under Normal and Pathological Conditions. Springfield, Charles C Thomas, 1955.
11. Williams PL, Bannister LH, Berry M, et al: Gray's Anatomy, 38th ed. New York, Churchill Livingstone, 1995.

# CHAPTER 2

# Basic Structure and Function of the Joints

A. JOSEPH THRELKELD, PT, PhD

## TOPICS AT A GLANCE

## INTRODUCTION

A *joint* is the junction or pivot point between two or more bones. Movement of the body as a whole occurs primarily through rotation of bones about individual joints. Joints also transfer and dissipate forces owing to gravity and muscle activation throughout the body.

*Arthrology*—the study of the classification, structure, and function of joints—is an important foundation for the overall study of kinesiology. Aging, long-term immobilization, trauma, and disease all affect the structure and ultimate function of joints. These factors also significantly influence the quality and quantity of human movement.

This chapter focuses on the general anatomic structure and function of joints. The chapters contained in Sections II to IV review the specific anatomy and detailed function of the individual joints throughout the body. This detailed information is a prerequisite for the effective rehabilitation of persons with joint dysfunction.

## CLASSIFICATION AND DESCRIPTION OF JOINTS

### Classification Based on Anatomic Structure and Movement Potential

One common method to classify joints focuses primarily on anatomic structure and their subsequent movement potential

(Table 2–1).[27] Based on this scheme, three types of joints exist in the body and are defined as *synarthrosis, amphiarthrosis,* and *diarthrosis.*

### SYNARTHROSIS

A *synarthrosis* is a junction between bones that is held together by dense irregular connective tissue. This relatively rigid junction allows little or no movement. Examples of synarthrodial joints include the sutures of the skull, the teeth embedded in the mandible and maxillae, the distal tibiofibular joint, and the interosseous membranes of the forearm and leg. The epiphysial plate of a growing bone is also classified as a synarthrodial "joint" by some.[27] Because the function of an epiphysis is skeletal growth rather than motion, this classification is not used here.

The function of a synarthrosis is to bind bones together and to transmit force from one bone to the next with minimal joint motion. A synarthrodial joint allows forces to be dispersed across a relatively large area of contact, thereby reducing the possibility of injury.

### AMPHIARTHROSIS

An *amphiarthrosis* is a junction between bones that is formed primarily by fibrocartilage and/or hyaline cartilage. Perhaps the most familiar example of an amphiarthrosis is the interbody joint of the spine. This joint uses an intervertebral disc

**TABLE 2–1. Classification of Joints Based on Anatomic Structure and Movement Potential**

| | Joint Material | Available Motion | Primary Function | Examples |
|---|---|---|---|---|
| Synarthrosis | Dense, irregular connective tissue | Negligible | Binds bones within a functional unit; disperses forces across the joined bones | Sutures of the skull<br>Teeth embedded in sockets of the maxillae and mandible<br>Interosseous membrane of the forearm and leg<br>Distal tibiofibular joint |
| Amphiarthrosis | Hyaline cartilage or fibro-cartilage | Minimal to moderate | Provides a combination of relatively restrained movement and shock absorption | Intervertebral disc (within the interbody joints of the spine)<br>Xiphisternal joint<br>Pubic symphysis<br>Manubriosternal joint |
| Diarthrosis (synovial joint) | True joint space filled with synovial fluid and surrounded by a capsule | Extensive | Provides the primary pivot points for movement of the musculoskeletal system | Glenohumeral joint<br>Tibiofemoral (knee) joint<br>Interphalangeal joint<br>Apophyseal (facet) joint of the spine |

and embedded nucleus pulposus to provide a rugged, resilient cushion that absorbs and disperses forces between adjacent vertebrae. Other examples of amphiarthrodial joints are the pubic symphysis and the manubriosternal joint. These joints allow relatively restrained movements. They also transmit and disperse forces between bones.

## DIARTHROSIS: THE SYNOVIAL JOINT

A *diarthrosis* is an articulation that contains a fluid-filled joint cavity between bony partners. Because of the presence of a synovial membrane, diarthrodial joints are more frequently referred to as *synovial joints*. Synovial joints are the majority of the joints of the upper and lower extremities.

Diarthrodial, or synovial, joints are specialized for movement and always exhibit seven elements (Fig. 2–1). The joint cavity is filled with (1) *synovial fluid*. This provides nutrition and lubrication for the (2) *articular cartilage* that covers the ends of the bones. The joint is enclosed by a peripheral curtain of connective tissue that forms the (3)

*articular capsule.* The articular capsule is composed of two histologically distinct layers. The internal layer consists of a thin (4) *synovial membrane,* which averages three to ten cell layers thick. The membrane acts as a barrier to adjacent capillaries, permitting only the fluid and solutes of blood plasma into the synovial fluid of a normal joint. Blood cells and large proteins, such as antibodies, are normally excluded from the synovial space. The cells of the synovial membrane also manufacture and add hyaluronate and lubricating glycoproteins (i.e., lubricin) to the joint fluid.[26]

The external, or fibrous, layer of the articular capsule of the synovial joint is composed of dense irregular connective tissue. The articular capsule provides support between the bones and containment of the joint contents. Certain regions of the fibrous capsule are thicker in order to resist or control specific motions. The thickened regions of connective tissue represent (5) *capsular ligaments.* Examples of prominent capsular ligaments are the anterior glenohumeral ligaments and the medial collateral ligament of the knee. The joint capsule is supplied with small (6) *blood vessels* with capillary beds

Elements ALWAYS associated with diarthrodial (synovial) joints.
• Synovial fluid
• Articular cartilage
• Articular capsule
• Synovial membrane
• Capsular ligaments
• Blood vessels
• Sensory nerves
Elements SOMETIMES associated with diarthrodial (synovial) joints.
• Intraarticular discs or menisci
• Peripheral labrum
• Fat pads
• Synovial plicae

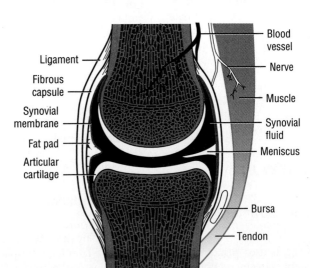

**FIGURE    2–1.** Elements associated with a typical diarthrodial (synovial) joint. The synovial plicae are not depicted.

that penetrate as far as the junction of the fibrous capsule and synovial membrane. The (7) *sensory nerves* also supply the fibrous capsule with appropriate receptors for pain and proprioception.

To accommodate the wide spectrum of joint shapes and functional demands, other elements may sometimes appear in synovial joints (see Fig. 2–1). *Intraarticular discs,* or *menisci,* are pads of fibrocartilage imposed between the articular surfaces of synovial joints. These structures increase articular congruency and improve force dispersion. Intraarticular discs and menisci are found in several joints of the body (see Box). Menisci are occasionally found in the apophyseal joints of the spine, but their function, constancy, and frequency remain controversial.[1,8,29,30]

---

**Intraarticular Discs (Menisci) Are Found in Several Synovial Joints of the Body**
- Tibiofemoral (knee)
- Distal radioulnar
- Sternoclavicular
- Acromioclavicular
- Temporomandibular

---

Two large synovial joints of the body possess a *peripheral labrum* of fibrocartilage. The labrum extends from the bony rims of both the glenoid cavity of the shoulder and the acetabulum of the hip. These specialized structures deepen the concave member of these joints and support and thicken the attachment of the joint capsule. *Fat pads* are variable in size and positioned within the substance of the joint capsule, interposed between the fibrous capsule and the synovial membrane. Fat pads are most prominent in the elbow and the knee joints. They thicken the joint capsule, causing the inner surface of the capsule to fill nonarticulating synovial spaces (i.e., recesses) formed by incongruent bony contours. In this sense, fat pads reduce the volume of synovial fluid necessary for proper joint function. If these pads become enlarged or inflamed, they may alter the mechanics of the joint.

*Synovial plicae* (i.e., synovial folds, synovial redundancies, or synovial fringes) are slack, overlapped pleats of tissue composed of the innermost layers of the joint capsule. They occur normally in joints with large capsular surface areas such as the knee and elbow. Plicae increase synovial surface area and allow full joint motion without undue tension on the synovial lining. If these folds are too extensive or become thickened or adherent due to inflammation, they can produce pain and altered joint mechanics.[3,4,15]

## Classification of Synovial Joints Based on Mechanical Analogy

Thus far, joints have been classified into three broad categories according to the anatomic structure and subsequent movement potential: synarthrosis, amphiarthrosis, and diarthrosis. Because an in-depth understanding of synovial joints is so crucial to an understanding of the mechanics of movement, they are here further classified using an analogy to familiar mechanical objects or shapes (Table 2–2).

---

**TABLE 2–2. Classification of Synovial Joints by Analogy**

| | Primary Angular Motions | Mechanical Analog | Anatomic Examples |
|---|---|---|---|
| Hinge joint | Flexion and extension only | Door hinge | Humeroulnar joint Interphalangeal joint |
| Pivot joint | Spinning of one member around a single axis of rotation | Door knob | Proximal radioulnar joint Atlantoaxial joint |
| Ellipsoid joint | Biplanar motion (flexion-and-extension and abduction-and-adduction) | Flattened convex ellipsoid paired with a concave trough. | Radiocarpal joint |
| Ball-and-socket joint | Triplanar motion (flexion-and-extension, abduction-and-adduction, and internal-and-external rotation) | Spherical convex surface paired with a concave cup. | Glenohumeral joint Coxofemoral (hip) joint |
| Plane joint | Typical motions include a slide (translation) or a combined slide and rotation. | Relatively flat surfaces apposing one another, like a book on a table. | Intercarpal joints Intertarsal joints |
| Saddle joint | Biplanar motion; a spin between the bones is possible but may be limited by the interlocking nature of the joint. | Each member has a reciprocally curved concave and convex surface oriented at right angles to one another, like a horse rider and a saddle. | Carpometacarpal joint of the thumb Sternoclavicular joint |
| Condyloid joint | Biplanar motion; either flexion-and-extension and abduction-and-adduction, or flexion-and-extension and axial rotation (internal-and-external rotation) | Mostly spherical convex surface that is enlarged in one dimension like a knuckle; paired with a shallow concave cup. | Metacarpophalangeal joint Tibiofemoral (knee) joint |

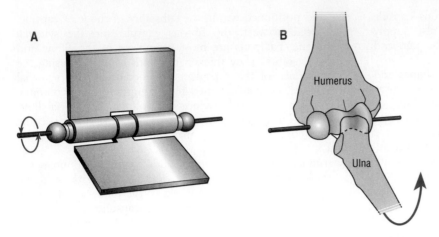

**FIGURE 2-2.** A hinge joint (A) is illustrated as analogous to the humeroulnar joint (B). The axis of rotation (i.e., pivot point) is represented by the pin.

A *hinge joint* is analogous to the hinge of a door, formed by a central pin surrounded by a larger hollow cylinder (Fig. 2-2A). Angular motion at hinge joints occurs primarily in a plane located at right angles to the hinge, or axis of rotation. The humeroulnar joint is a clear example of a hinge joint (Fig. 2-2B). As in all synovial joints, slight translation (i.e., sliding) is allowed in addition to the rotation. Although the mechanical similarity is less complete, the interphalangeal joints of the digits are also classified as hinge joints.

A *pivot joint* is formed by a central pin surrounded by a larger cylinder. Unlike a hinge, the mobile member of a pivot joint is oriented parallel to the axis of rotation. This mechanical orientation produces the primary angular motion of spin, similar to a doorknob's spin around a central axis (Fig. 2-3A). Two excellent examples of pivot joints are the proximal radioulnar joint, shown in Figure 2-3B, and the atlantoaxial joint between the dens of the second cervical vertebra and the anterior arch of the first cervical vertebra.

An *ellipsoid joint* has one partner with a convex elongated surface in one dimension that is mated with a similarly elongated concave surface on the second partner (Fig. 2-4A). The elliptic mating surfaces severely restrict the spin between the two surfaces but allow biplanar motions, usually defined as flexion-extension and abduction-adduction. The

radiocarpal joint is an example of an ellipsoid joint (Fig. 2-4B). The flattened "ball" of the convex member of the joint (i.e., carpal bones) cannot spin within the elongated trough (i.e., distal radius) without dislocating.

A *ball-and-socket joint* has a spherical convex surface that is paired with a cuplike socket (Fig. 2-5A). This joint provides motion in three planes. Unlike the ellipsoid joint, the symmetry of the curves of the two mating surfaces of the ball-and-socket joint allows spin without dislocation. Ball-and-socket joints within the body include the glenohumeral joint and the hip joint.

A *plane joint* is the pairing of two flat or relatively flat surfaces. Movements combine sliding and some rotation of one partner with respect to the other—much like a book can be slid over a tabletop (Fig. 2-6A). As depicted in Figure 2-6B, most of the intercarpal joints are considered to be plane joints. The internal forces that cause or restrict movement between carpal bones are supplied by tension in muscles or ligaments.

Each partner of a *saddle joint* has two surfaces: one surface is concave, and the other is convex. These surfaces are oriented at approximate right angles to one another and are reciprocally curved. The shape of a saddle joint is best visualized using the analogy of a horse's saddle and rider (Fig. 2-7A). From front to back, the saddle presents a concave surface reaching from the saddle horn to the back of the saddle. From side to side, the saddle is convex stretching from one stirrup across the back of the horse to the other stirrup. The rider is also doubly curved, presenting convex and concave curves to complement the shape of the saddle. The carpometacarpal joint of the thumb is the clearest example of a saddle joint (Fig. 2-7B). The reciprocal, interlocking nature of this joint allows ample biplanar motion, but limited spin between the trapezium and the first metacarpal.

A *condyloid joint* is much like a ball-and-socket joint except that the concave member of the joint is very shallow (Fig. 2-8A). Condyloid joints usually allow 2 degrees of freedom. Ligaments or bony incongruity restrains the third degree. Condyloid joints often occur in pairs, such as the knee (Fig. 2-8B), the temporomandibular joints, and the atlantooccipital joints (i.e., occipital condyles with the first cervical vertebra). The metacarpophalangeal joint of the finger is also an example of a condyloid joint. The root word of the term "condyle" actually means "knuckle."

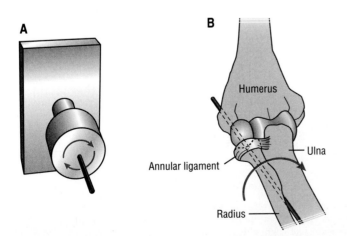

**FIGURE 2-3.** A pivot joint (A) is shown as analogous to the proximal radioulnar joint (B). The axis of rotation is represented by the pin.

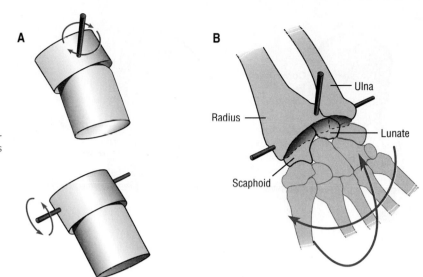

**FIGURE 2–4.** An ellipsoid joint (*A*) is shown as analogous to the radiocarpal joint (wrist) (*B*). The two axes of rotation are shown by the intersecting pins.

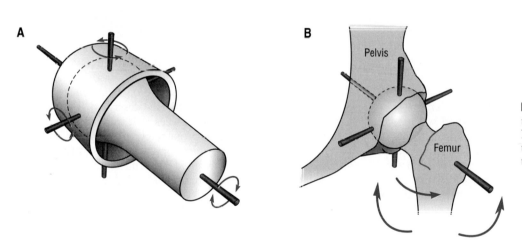

**FIGURE 2–5.** A ball-in-socket articulation (*A*) is drawn as analogous to the hip joint (*B*). The three axes of rotation are represented by the three intersecting pins.

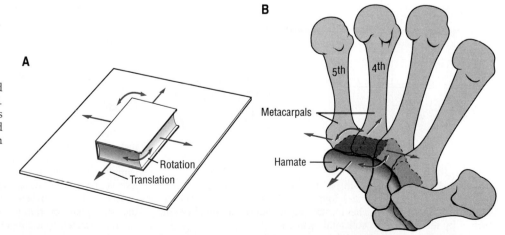

**FIGURE 2–6.** A plane "joint" is formed by opposition of two flat surfaces (*A*). The book moving on the table top is depicted as analogous to the combined slide and spin at the fourth and fifth carpometacarpal joints (*B*).

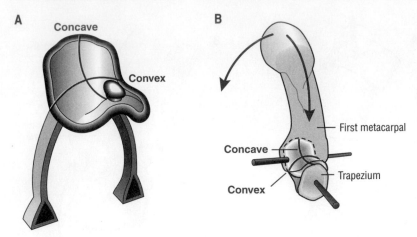

**FIGURE 2–7.** A saddle joint (*A*) is illustrated as analogous to the carpometacarpal joint of the thumb (*B*). The saddle in *A* represents the trapezium bone. The "rider," if present, would represent the base of the thumb's metacarpal. The two axes of rotation are shown in *B*.

The kinematics at condyloid joints vary based on joint structure. At the knee, for example, the femoral condyles fit within the slight concavity provided by the tibial plateau. This articulation allows flexion-extension and axial rotation (i.e., spin). Abduction and adduction, however, are restricted primarily by ligaments.

## Simplifying the Classification of Synovial Joints: Ovoid and Saddle Joints

It is often difficult to classify synovial joints based on an analogy to mechanics alone. The metacarpophalangeal joint (condyloid) and the glenohumeral joint (ball-and-socket), for example, have similar shapes but differ considerably in the relative magnitude of movement and overall function. Joints always display subtle variations that make simple mechanical descriptions less applicable. A good example of the difference between mechanical classification and true function is seen in the gentle undulations that characterize the intercarpal and intertarsal joints. These joints produce complex multiplanar movements that are inconsistent with their simple "planar" mechanical classification. To circumvent this difficulty, a simplified classification scheme recognizes only two articular forms: the ovoid joint and the saddle joint (Fig. 2–9). Essentially all synovial joints with the notable exception of planar joints can be categorized under this scheme.

An *ovoid joint* has paired mating surfaces that are imperfectly spherical, or egg-shaped, with adjacent parts possessing a changing surface curvature. In each case, the articular surface of one bone is convex and the other is concave.

A *saddle joint* has been previously described. Each member presents paired curved surfaces that are opposite in direction and oriented at approximately 90 degrees to each other. This simplified classification system allows the generalization to the arthrokinematic patterns of movement as a roll, slide, or spin (see Chapter 1). This generalization is used throughout this text.

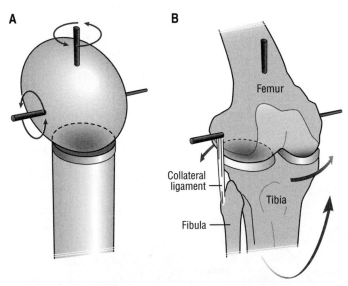

**FIGURE 2–8.** A condyloid joint is shown (*A*) representing an analogy to the tibiofemoral (knee) joint (*B*). The two axes of rotation are shown by the pins. The frontal plane motion at the knee is blocked by tension in the collateral ligament.

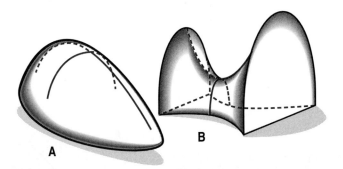

**FIGURE 2–9.** Two basic shapes of joint surfaces. *A*, The egg-shaped *ovoid surface* represents a characteristic of most synovial joints of the body (for example, hip joint, radiocarpal joint, knee joint, metacarpophalangeal joint). The diagram shows only the convex member of the joint. A reciprocally shaped concave member would complete the pair of ovoid articulating surfaces. *B*, The *saddle surface* is the second basic type of joint surface, having one convex surface and one concave surface. The paired articulating surface of the other half of the joint would be turned so that a concave surface is mated to a convex surface of the partner.

## AXIS OF ROTATION

In the analogy using a door hinge (see Fig. 2–2A), the axis of rotation (i.e., the pin through the hinge) is *fixed*, because it remains stationary throughout the rotation of the door. With the axis of rotation fixed, all points on the door experience equal arcs of rotation. In anatomic joints, however, the axis of rotation is rarely, if ever, fixed during bony rotation. Finding the exact position of the axis of rotation in anatomic joints is therefore not as obvious. A simplified method of estimating the position of the axis of rotation in anatomic joints is shown in Figure 2–10A. The intersection of the two perpendicular lines drawn from a-a′ and b-b′ defines the *instantaneous axis of rotation* for the 90-degree arc of knee flexion. The term instantaneous indicates that the location of the axis holds true only for the particular arc of motion. The smaller the angular range used to calculate the instantaneous axis, the more accurate the estimate. If a series of line drawings are made for a sequence of small angular arcs of motion, the location of the instantaneous axes can be plotted for each portion within the arc of motion (Fig. 2–10B). The path of the serial locations of the instantaneous axes of rotation is called the *evolute*. The path of the evolute is longer and more complex when the mating joint surfaces are less congruent or have greater changes in their radii of curvature, such as the knee. The smaller the individual arcs used for calculation, the more accurate is the resulting evolute.

In many practical clinical situations it is necessary to make simple estimates of the location of the axis of rotation of a joint. These estimates are necessary when performing *goniometry*, measuring torque about a joint, or when constructing a prosthesis or an orthosis. A series of x-ray measurements are required to precisely identify the instantaneous axis of rotation at a joint. This method is not practical in ordinary clinical situations. Instead, an *average axis* of rotation is assumed to occur throughout the entire arc of motion. This axis is located by an anatomic landmark that coincides with the *convex member* of the joint.

## BIOLOGIC MATERIALS THAT FORM CONNECTIVE TISSUES WITHIN JOINTS

The composition, proportion, and arrangement of biologic materials that compose the connective tissue within joints strongly influence their mechanical performance. The fundamental materials that make up the connective tissues of a joint are *fibers, ground substance,* and *cells*. These biologic materials are blended in various proportions based on the mechanical demands of the joint.

| **Biologic Materials That Form the Connective Tissues within Joints** |
|---|
| 1. Fibers |
|     Collagen (types I and II) |
|     Elastin |
| 2. Ground substance |
|     Glycosaminoglycans |
|     Water |
|     Solutes |
| 3. Cells |

## Fibers

Various types of collagen fibers and elastic fibers occur in joints. *Collagen fibers* are made of short subunits (fibrils), which are wound in a helical structure much like short threads. These threads are placed together in a strand, several of which are spirally wound into a rope. Twelve collagen types have been described,[27] but two types make up the

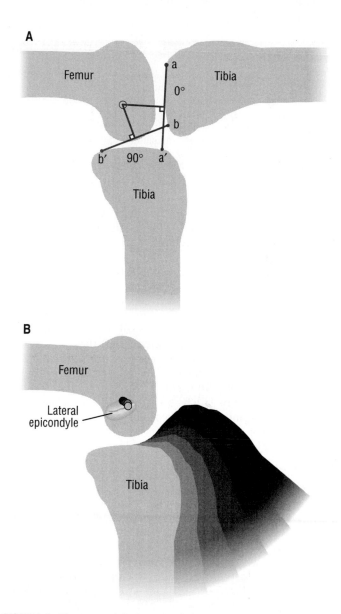

**FIGURE 2–10.** A simplified method for determining the instantaneous axis of rotation for 90 degrees of knee flexion (*A*). With the use of x-ray, two points (a and b) are identified on the tibial plateau. With the position of the femur held stationary, the same two points are identified following 90 degrees of flexion (a′ and b′). Next, two perpendicular lines are drawn from a-a′ and b-b′. The point of intersection of these two perpendicular lines identifies the instantaneous axis of rotation for the 90-degree arc of motion. This same method can be repeated for many smaller arcs of motion, producing several slightly different axes of rotation (*B*). The path of the "migrating" axes is called the evolute. At the knee, the average axis of rotation is oriented in the medial-lateral direction, piercing the lateral epicondyle of the femur.

majority of collagen in normal joints—type I and type II. *Type I collagen fibers* are thick, rugged fibers that are gathered into bundles and elongate very little when placed under tension. Being relatively stiff, type I collagen fibers are ideal for binding and supporting the articulations between bones. Type I collagen is therefore the primary protein found in ligaments, fascia and fibrous joint capsules. This type of collagen also makes up the parallel fibrous bundles that compose tendons—the structures that transmit the force of muscle to bone.

---

**Two Predominant Types of Collagen Fibers in Normal Joints**
- *Type I:* thick, rugged fibers that elongate very little when stretched; compose ligaments, tendons, fascia, and fibrous capsules.
- *Type II:* thinner and less stiff than type I fibers; provide a flexible woven framework for maintaining the general shape and consistency of structures such as hyaline cartilage.

---

*Type II collagen fibers* are thinner than type I and possess slightly less tensile strength. These fibers provide a flexible woven framework for maintaining the general shape and consistency of more complex structures, such as hyaline cartilage. Type II collagen still provides internal strength to the tissue in which it resides.

In addition to collagen, the connective tissues within joints have varying amounts of *elastin fibers*. These fibers are composed of a netlike interweaving of small elastin fibrils that resist tensile (stretching) forces, but they have more "give" when elongated. Tissues with a high proportion of elastin readily return to their original shape after being deformed. This property is useful in structures that undergo significant deformation, such as the cartilage of the ear, or in certain spinal ligaments that help return a bone to its original position after movement.

## Ground Substance

Collagen and elastin fibers are embedded within a water-saturated matrix known as *ground substance*. The ground substance of joint tissues is made of *glycosaminoglycans (GAGs), water,* and *solutes*. The GAGs are highly branched and negatively charged amino sugars that are strongly bonded with water. Structurally, the GAGs resemble long bottle brushes that are strongly hydrophilic due to their negative charge (Fig. 2–11). Water provides a fluid medium for diffusion of nutrients within a tissue. In addition, water assists with the mechanical properties of tissue. The tendency of GAGs to imbibe and hold water causes the tissue to swell. Swelling is limited by embedded collagen or elastin fibers anchored into an adjacent supporting structure, such as bone or dense bands of fibers. The interaction between the restraining fibers and the swelling GAGs provides a turgid structure that resists compression, much like a balloon or a water-filled mattress. An example of such a structurally dynamic material is articular cartilage. This important tissue provides an ideal surface covering for joints and is capable of dispersing the millions of repetitive forces that have an impact on joints throughout a lifetime.

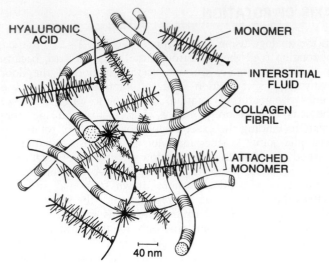

**AGGREGATE IN COLLAGEN MESHWORK**

**FIGURE 2–11.** Schematic drawing of the molecular organization of cartilage. A glycosaminoglycan (GAG) molecule is formed by a hyaluronic acid center thread to which proteoglycan monomers are attached, forming a bottle brush configuration. The GAG molecule is shown interlacing between collagen fibrils. Water fills much of the space within the matrix. (From Nordin M, Frankel VH: Basic Biomechanics of the Musculoskeletal System, 2nd ed. Philadelphia, Williams & Wilkins, 1989.)

## Cells

The *cells* within connective tissues of the joints are responsible for maintenance and repair. In contrast to skeletal muscle cells, these cells do not confer significant mechanical properties on the tissue. Damaged or aged components are removed, and new components are manufactured and remodeled. Cells of connective tissues of the joints are generally sparse and interspersed between the strands of fibers or embedded deeply in regions of high GAG content. This sparseness of cells in conjunction with limited blood supply often results in poor or incomplete healing of damaged or injured joint tissues.

## TYPES OF CONNECTIVE TISSUES THAT FORM THE STRUCTURE OF JOINTS

Four types of connective tissues predominate in joints: *dense irregular connective tissue, articular cartilage, fibrocartilage,* and *bone*. Anatomic and functional details of the four connective tissues are listed in Table 2–3. The table also includes clinical correlates associated with each tissue.

### Dense Irregular Connective Tissue

*Dense irregular connective tissue* is found in the fibrous external layer of the articular capsule, ligaments, fascia, and tendons. Structurally, this connective tissue has a high proportion of type I collagen fibers that are arranged in bundles and aligned to resist the natural stresses placed on the tissue. The connective tissue bundles function most effectively when they are stretched parallel to their long axis. After the initial

## TABLE 2-3. Types of Connective Tissues that Form the Structure of Joints

| | Anatomic Location | Fibers | Ground Substance (GAGs + Water + Solutes) | Cells | Mechanical Specialization | Clinical Correlate |
|---|---|---|---|---|---|---|
| **Dense irregular connective tissue** | Composes the external fibrous layer of the joint capsule<br>Forms ligaments, fascia, and tendons | High type I collagen fiber content<br>Most tissues have low elastin fiber content<br>Parallel fibers are arranged in bundles oriented in several directions | Low ground substance content | Sparsely located cells tightly packed between fibers | Ligament: Binds bones together and restrains unwanted movement at the joints; resists tension in several directions<br>Tendon: attaches muscle to bone | Rupture of the lateral collateral ligament complex of the ankle can lead to medial-lateral instability of the talocrural joint. |
| **Articular cartilage** | Covers the ends of articulating bones in synovial joints | High type II collagen fiber content; fibers help anchor cartilage to subchondral bone and restrain the ground substance. | High ground substance content | Moderate number of cells; flattened near the articular surface and rounded in deeper layers of the cartilage | Resists and distributes compressive forces (joint loading) and shear forces (surface sliding); very low coefficient of friction | During early stage of osteoarthritis, GAGs are released from deep in the tissue, reducing the force distribution capability; adjacent bone thickens to absorb the increased force, often causing the formation of osteophytes (bone spurs). |
| **Fibrocartilage** | Composes the intervertebral discs and the disc within the pubic symphysis<br>Forms the intra-articular discs (menisci) of the tibiofemoral, sternoclavicular, acromioclavicular, and distal radioulnar joints<br>Forms the labrum of the glenoid fossa and the acetabulum | Multidirectional bundles of type I collagen | Moderate ground substance content | Moderate number of cells that are rounded and dwell in cellular lacunae | Provides some support and stabilization to joints; primary function is to provide "shock absorption" by resisting and distributing compressive and shear forces | Tearing of the intervertebral disc can allow the central nucleus pulposus to escape (herniate) and press on a spinal nerve or nerve root. |
| **Bone** | Forms the internal levers of the musculoskeletal system | Specialized arrangement of type I collagen to form lamellae and osteons and to provide a framework for hard mineral salts (e.g., calcium crystals) | Low GAG content | Moderate number of flattened cells embedded between the layers of collagen; many progenitor cells found on the fibrous external (periosteal) and internal (endosteal) layers. | Resists deformation; strongest resistance is applied against compressive forces due to body weight and muscle force.<br>Provides a rigid lever to transmit muscle force to move and stabilize the body | Osteoporosis of the spine produces a loss of bony trabeculae and mineral content in the vertebral body of the spine; may result in fractures of the vertebral body during walking or even coughing. |

slack is pulled tight, the ligaments and joint capsule provide immediate tension that restrains undesirable motion between bony partners.

The fibrous joint capsule and ligaments resist forces from several directions. To accomplish this, the fiber bundles within the connective tissues are arranged in several dominant directions, unlike the parallel alignment of collagen bundles found in a tendon (Fig. 2–12).[6,20] The GAGs and elastin fiber content are usually low in dense irregular connective tissue.

When trauma or disease produces laxity in the ligament or capsules, muscles take on a more dominant role in restraining joint movement. Even if muscles surrounding a ligamentously lax joint are strong, there is loss of joint stability. Compared with ligaments, muscles are slower to supply force due to the electromechanical delay necessary to build active force. Muscle forces often have a less than ideal alignment for restraining undesirable joint movements, and they often cannot provide the most optimal deterrent force.

## Articular Cartilage

*Articular cartilage* is a specialized type of hyaline cartilage that forms the load-bearing surface of joints. Articular cartilage covering the ends of the articulating bones has a thickness that ranges from 1 to 4 mm in the areas of low compression force and 5 to 7 mm in areas of high compression.[16,25] The tissue is avascular and aneural. Unlike regular hyaline cartilage, articular cartilage lacks a perichondrium. This allows the opposing surfaces of the cartilage to form ideal load-bearing surfaces. Similar to periosteum on bone, perichondrium is a layer of connective tissue that covers most cartilage. It contains blood vessels and a ready supply of primitive cells that maintain and repair underlying tissue. This is an advantage not available to articular cartilage.

Chondrocytes of various shapes are located within the ground substance of different layers or zones of articular cartilage (Fig. 2–13A). These cells are bathed and nourished by nutrients within the synovial fluid. Nourishment is facilitated by the "milking" action of articular surface deformation during intermittent joint loading. The chondrocytes are surrounded by predominantly type II collagen fibers. As depicted in Figure 2–13B, the fibers are arranged to form a restraining network or "scaffolding" that adds structural stability to the tissue. The deepest fibers in the calcified zone are firmly anchored to the subchondral bone. These fibers are linked to the vertically oriented fibers in the adjacent deep zone which, in turn, are linked to the obliquely oriented fibers of the middle zone, and finally to the transversely oriented fibers of the superficial tangential zone. The series of chemically interlinked fibers form a netlike fibrous structure that entraps the large GAG molecules beneath the articular surface. The GAGs in turn attract water that provides a unique element of rigidity to articular cartilage. The rigidity increases the ability of cartilage to adequately withstand loads.

Articular cartilage distributes and disperses compressive forces to the subchondral bone. It also reduces friction between joint surfaces. The coefficient of friction between two surfaces covered by articular cartilage and wet with synovial fluid is extremely low, ranging from 0.005 to 0.02 in the human knee for example. This is 5 to 20 times lower and more slippery than ice on ice, which has a coefficient of 0.1.[17] The impact of normal weight-bearing activities, therefore, is reduced to a stress that typically can be absorbed without damaging the skeletal system.

The absence of a perichondrium on articular cartilage has the negative consequence of eliminating a ready source of primitive perichondrial fibroblastic cells used for repair. Even

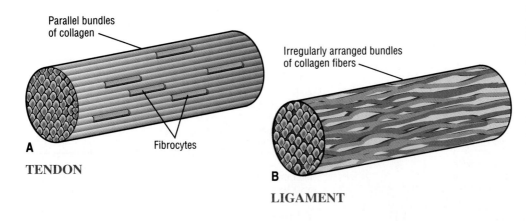

Parallel bundles
of collagen

Fibrocytes

**A**

**TENDON**

Irregularly arranged bundles
of collagen fibers

**B**

**LIGAMENT**

**FIGURE 2–12.** Diagrammatic representation of the fibrous organization of tendons and ligaments. *A,* The bundles of collagen in a *tendon* are tightly packed and arranged parallel to one another. The arrangement allows the tendon to transmit unidirectional tensile forces from a muscle without having to take up slack in the bundles. The cells that maintain this connective tissue (fibrocytes) are few in number and flattened between the collagen bundles. *B,* A *ligament* has collagen bundles that are less parallel to one another. This allows the ligament to accept tensile forces from several different directions while holding two bones together. Bundles may be organized parallel to the most common lines of tension. The fibrocytes of the ligament are not shown in this drawing but are few in number and flattened.

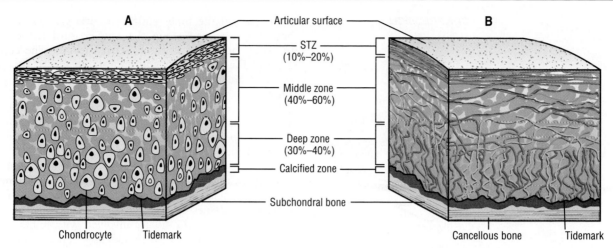

**FIGURE 2–13.** Two schematic diagrams of hyaline articular cartilage. A, The organization of the *cells* (chondrocytes) is shown located through the ground substance of the articular cartilage. The flattened chondrocytes near the articular surface are within the *superficial tangential zone* (STZ) and are oriented parallel to the joint surface. The STZ comprises about 10% to 20% of the articular cartilage thickness. The cells in the *middle zone* are more rounded and become increasingly arranged in columns in the *deep zone*. A region of calcified cartilage (*calcified zone*) joins the deep zone with the underlying subchondral bone. The edge of the calcified zone that abuts the deep zone is known as the *tidemark* and forms a diffusion barrier between the articular cartilage and the underlying bone. Nutrients and gasses must pass from the synovial fluid through all the layers of articular cartilage to nourish the chondrocytes including the cells at the base of the deep zone. The diffusion process is assisted by intermittent compression ("milking" action) of the articular cartilage. B, The organization of the *collagen fibers* in articular cartilage is shown in this diagram. In the superficial tangential zone, the collagen is oriented parallel to the articular surface, forming a fibrous grain that helps resist abrasion of the joint surface. The fibers become less tangential and more obliquely oriented in the middle zone, finally becoming almost perpendicular to the articular surface in the deep zone. The deepest fibers are anchored into the calcified zone to help tie the cartilage to the underlying subchondral bone.

though articular cartilage is capable of normal maintenance and replenishment of its matrix, significant damage to adult articular cartilage is often repaired very poorly or not at all.

## Fibrocartilage

As its name implies, fibrocartilage has a much higher fiber content than other types of cartilage. The tissue functionally shares properties of both dense irregular connective tissue and articular cartilage. Dense bundles of type I collagen travel in many directions with a moderate number of GAGs. As depicted in Figure 2–14, round chondrocytes reside within lacunae that are embedded within a dense collagen network.

Fibrocartilage forms much of the substance of the intervertebral discs, the labrum, and the discs located within the pubic symphysis and other joints of the extremities (for example, the menisci of the knee). These structures help support and stabilize the joints, as well as dissipate compression forces. As depicted in Figure 2–14A, the menisci of the knee dissipate compression forces by spreading out radially. The dense interwoven collagen fibers also allow the tissue to resist tensile and shearing forces in multiple planes. Fibrocartilage is therefore an ideal shock absorber in regions of the body that are subject to high multidirectional forces. This function is best realized in the menisci of the knee and the intervertebral discs of the spinal column.

The perichondrium surrounding fibrocartilage is poorly organized and contains small blood vessels located only near the peripheral rim of the tissue. Fibrocartilage is largely aneural and thus does not produce pain or participate in proprioception, although a few neural receptors may be found at the periphery where fibrocartilage abuts a ligament or joint capsule.

The nourishment of adult fibrocartilage is largely dependent on diffusion of nutrients through the synovial fluid in synovial joints. In amphiarthrodial joints, such as the adult intervertebral disc, nutrients are diffused across the fluid contained in the adjacent trabecular bone. The diffusion of nutrients and removal of metabolic wastes in the fibrocartilage of amphiarthrodial joints is assisted by the "milking" action of intermittent weight bearing.[13] This principle is readily apparent in adult intervertebral discs that are insufficiently nourished when the spine is held in fixed postures for extended periods. Without proper nutrition, the discs may partially degenerate and lose part of their protective function.

A direct blood supply penetrates the outer rim of fibrocartilaginous structures where they attach to ligaments (e.g., the spine) or to joint capsules (e.g., the knee). In adult joints, some repair of damaged fibrocartilage can occur near the vascularized periphery, such as the outer one third of menisci of the knee and the outermost lamellae of intervertebral discs. The innermost regions of fibrocartilage structures, much like articular cartilage, demonstrate poor or negligible healing owing to the lack of a ready source of undifferentiated fibroblastic cells.[13,21,23]

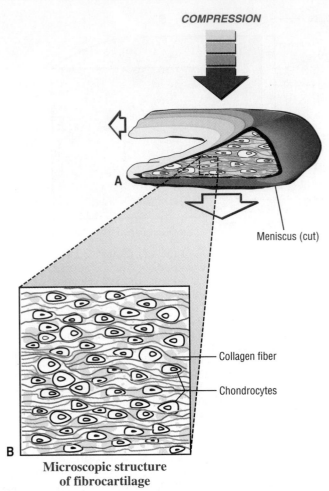

**COMPRESSION**

Meniscus (cut)

Collagen fiber

Chondrocytes

B

**Microscopic structure
of fibrocartilage**

**FIGURE 2–14.** Histologic organization of fibrocartilage. *A,* This is a cut section of a compressed, wedge-shaped piece of fibrocartilage (i.e., meniscus) taken from the knee. The meniscus partially dissipates the compression force by spreading out in a radial direction indicated by *arrows. B,* Schematic illustration of a microscopic section from the middle of the sample of fibrocartilaginous meniscus.

## Bone

*Bone* provides rigid support to the body and equips the muscles of the body with a system of levers. The outer cortex of the long bones of the adult skeleton has a shaft composed of thick, compact cortical bone (Fig. 2–15). The ends of long bones, however, are lined with a thin layer of compact bone that covers an interconnecting network of cancellous bone. Bones of the adult axial skeleton, such as the vertebral body, possess an outer shell of cortical bone that is filled with a supporting core of cancellous bone.

The structural subunit of cortical bone is the *osteon* or *haversian system,* which organizes the collagen fibers, predominantly type I, into a unique series of concentric spirals that form lamellae (Fig. 2–16). The matrix of bone contains calcium phosphate crystals, which allow bone to accept tremendous compressive loads. The cells of bone are confined within narrow lacunae (i.e., spaces) positioned between the lamellae of the osteon. Because bone deforms very little, blood vessels can pass into its substance from the outer

periosteal and the inner endosteal surfaces. The vessels can then turn to travel along the long axis of the bone in a tunnel at the center of the haversian canals. The connective tissue of the periosteum and endosteum are richly vascularized and are innervated with sensory receptors for pressure and pain.

Bone is a very dynamic tissue. Remodeling constantly occurs in response to forces applied through physical activity and in response to hormonal influences that regulate systemic calcium balance. The large scale removal of bone is carried out by osteoclasts—specialized cells that originate from the bone marrow. Primitive fibroblasts for bone repair originate from the periosteum and endosteum and from the perivascular tissues that are woven throughout the vascular canals of bone. Of the tissues involved with joints, bone has by far the best capacity for remodeling, repair, and regeneration.

Bone demonstrates its greatest strength when compressed along the long axis of its shaft, which is comparable to loading a straw along its long axis. The ends of long bones receive multidirectional compressive forces through the weight-bearing surfaces of articular cartilage. Stresses are spread to the subjacent subchondral bone and then into the

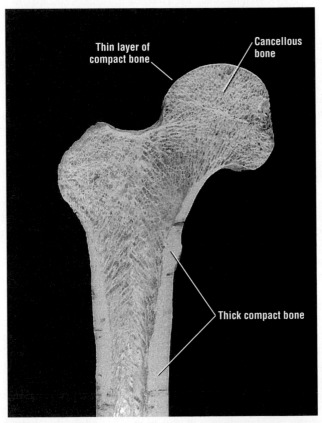

Thin layer of compact bone

Cancellous bone

Thick compact bone

**FIGURE 2–15.** A cross-section showing the internal architecture of the proximal femur. Note the thicker areas of compact bone around the shaft and the lattice-like cancellous bone occupying most of the medullary region. (From Neumann DA: An Arthritis Home Study Course: The Synovial Joint: Anatomy, Function, and Dysfunction. The Orthopedic Section of the American Physical Therapy Association, La Crosse, WI, 1998.)

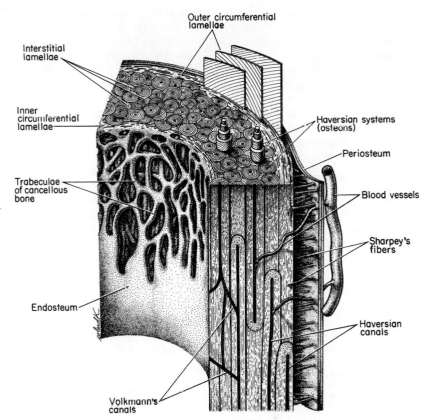

**FIGURE 2–16.** Histologic organization of cortical bone. (From Fawcett DW: A Textbook of Histology, 12th ed. New York, Chapman & Hall. Redrawn after Benninghoff A: Lehrbuch der Anatomie des Menschen. Berlin, Urban and Schwarzenberg, 1994.)

network of cancellous bone, which in turn acts as a series of struts to redirect the forces into the long axis of the cortical bone of the shaft. This structural arrangement redirects forces for absorption and transmission by taking advantage of bone's unique architectural design.

## EFFECTS OF AGING

Aging is associated with histologic changes in connective tissue that, in turn, may produce mechanical changes in joint function. The rate and process by which tissue ages is highly individual and can be modified, positively or negatively, by the types and frequency of activities and by a host of medical and nutritional factors.[2] In the broadest sense, aging is accompanied by a slowing of the rate of fiber and GAG replacement and repair.[2,11] The effects of microtrauma can accumulate over time to produce subclinical damage that may progress to a structural failure or a measurable change in mechanical properties. A clinical example of this phenomenon is the age-related deterioration of the ligaments and capsule associated with the glenohumeral joint. Reduced structural support provided by these tissues may eventually culminate in tendonitis or tears in the rotator cuff muscles.[22]

Aging also influences the mechanical resilience of GAGs within connective tissue. The GAG molecules produced by aging cells are fewer in number and smaller in size than those produced by young cells.[2,11] This change in the GAGs results in decreased water-binding capacity that reduces the hydration of connective tissues. The less hydrated tissue has

lower compressive strength. The dryer connective tissues do not slide across one another as easily. As a result, the bundles of fibers in ligaments do not align themselves with the imposed forces as readily, hampering the ability of the tissue to maximally resist a rapidly applied force. The likelihood of adhesions forming between previously mobile tissue planes is increased; thus, aging joints may lose range of motion more quickly than younger joints. Aged articular cartilage contains less water and is less able to attenuate and distribute imposed forces to the adjacent bone.

The age-related alteration of connective tissue metabolism in bone contributes to the slower healing of fractures. The altered metabolism also contributes to osteoporosis, particularly type II or senile osteoporosis—a type that thins both trabecular and cortical bone in both genders.[9]

## EFFECTS OF IMMOBILIZATION ON THE STRENGTH OF THE CONNECTIVE TISSUES OF A JOINT

The amount and arrangement of fibers and GAGs in connective tissues are influenced by physical activity. At a normal level of physical activity, the connective tissues are able to adequately resist the natural range of forces imposed on the musculoskeletal system. A joint immobilized for an extended period demonstrates marked changes in the structure and function of its associated connective tissues. The mechanical strength of the tissue is reduced in accord with the decreased forces of the immobilized condition. This is a normal response to an abnormal condition. Placing a body part in a cast and confining a person to a bed are examples in which immobilization dramatically reduces the level of force imposed on the musculoskeletal system. Although for different reasons, muscular paralysis or weakness also reduces the force on the musculoskeletal system.

The rate of decline in the strength of connective tissue is somewhat dependent on the normal metabolic activity of the specific tissue. Immobilization produces a marked decrease in tensile strength of the ligaments of the knee, for example, in a period of weeks.[19,28] The earliest biochemical markers of this remodeling can be detected within days after immobilization.[12,18] Even after the cessation of the immobilization and after the completion of an extended post-immobilization exercise program, the ligaments continue to have lower tensile strength than ligaments that were never subjected to immobilization.[12,28] Other tissues such as bone and cartilage also show a loss of mass, volume, and strength following immobilization.[14,24] The results from experimental studies imply that tissues rapidly lose strength in response to reduced loading. Full recovery of strength following restoration of loading is much slower and often incomplete.

Immobilizing a joint for an extended period is often necessary to promote healing following an injury such as a fractured bone. Clinical judgment is required to balance the potential negative effects of the immobilization with the need to promote healing. The maintenance of maximal tissue strength around joints requires judicious use of immobilization, a quick return to loading, and early rehabilitative intervention.

## JOINT PATHOLOGY

Trauma to connective tissues of a joint can occur from a single overwhelming event (acute trauma), or in response to an accumulation of lesser injuries over an extended period (chronic trauma). *Acute trauma* often produces detectable pathology. A torn or severely stretched ligament or joint capsule causes an acute inflammatory reaction. The joint may also become structurally unstable when damaged connective tissues are not able to restrain the natural extremes of motion.

Joints frequently affected by acute traumatic instability are typically associated with the longest lever arms of the skeleton and, therefore, are exposed to high external torques. For this reason, the tibiofemoral, talocrural, and glenohumeral joints are frequently subjected to acute ligament damage with resultant instability.

Acute trauma can also result in intraarticular fractures involving articular cartilage and subchondral bone. Careful reduction or realignment of the fractured fragments helps to restore the smooth, low-friction sliding functions of articular surfaces. This is critical to maximal recovery of function. Although the bone adjacent to a joint has excellent ability to repair, the repair of fractured articular cartilage is often incomplete and produces mechanically inferior areas of the joint surface that are prone to degeneration. Focal increases in stress due to poor surface alignment in conjunction with impaired articular cartilage strength can lead to post-traumatic osteoarthritis.

The repair of damaged fibrocartilaginous joint structures depends on the proximity and adequacy of a blood supply. A tear of the outermost region of the meniscus of the knee adjacent to blood vessels embedded with the capsule may completely heal.[21,23] In contrast, tears of the innermost circumference of a meniscus do not typically heal completely. This is also the case in the inner lamellae of the adult intervertebral disc that does not have the capacity to heal following significant damage.[13]

*Chronic trauma* is often classified as a type of "overuse syndrome" and reflects an accumulation of unrepaired, relatively minor damage. Chronically damaged joint capsules and ligaments gradually lose their restraining functions, although the instability of the joint may be masked by a muscular restraint substitute. In this case, joint forces may be increased owing to an exaggerated muscular "guarding" of the joint. Only when the joint is challenged suddenly or forced by an extreme movement does the instability become readily apparent.

Recurring instability may cause abnormal loading conditions on the joint tissues, which can lead to their mechanical failure. The surfaces of articular cartilage and fibrocartilage may become fragmented with a concurrent loss of GAGs and subsequent lowered resistance to compressive and shear forces. Early stages of degeneration often demonstrate a roughened or "fibrillated" surface of the articular cartilage (Fig. 2–17). A fibrillated region of articular cartilage may later develop cracks, or clefts, that extend from the surface into the middle or deepest layers of the tissue. These changes may reduce the shock absorption quality of the tissue.

Two disease states that commonly cause joint dysfunction are osteoarthritis (OA) and rheumatoid arthritis (RA). *Osteoarthritis* is characterized by a gradual erosion of articular cartilage with a low inflammatory component.[7] Some refer to OA as "osteoarthrosis" to emphasize the lack of a distinctive inflammatory component. As erosion of articular cartilage progresses, the underlying subchondral bone becomes more mineralized and, in severe cases, becomes the weight-bearing surface when the articular cartilage pad is completely worn. The fibrous joint capsule and synovium become distended and thickened. The severely involved joint may be completely unstable and dislocate or may fuse allowing no motion.

The frequency of OA increases with age and has several manifestations. *Idiopathic OA* occurs in the absence of a specific cause; it affects only one or a few joints, particularly those that are subjected to the highest weight-bearing loads: hip, knee, and lumbar spine. *Familial OA* or *generalized OA* affects joints of the hand and is more frequent in women. *Post-traumatic OA* may affect any synovial joint that has been exposed to a trauma of sufficient severity.

*Rheumatoid arthritis* differs markedly from OA, as it is a systemic, autoimmune connective tissue disorder with a strong inflammatory component.[10] The destruction of multiple joints is a prominent manifestation of RA. The joint dysfunction is manifested by significant inflammation of the capsule, synovium, and synovial fluid. The articular cartilage is exposed to an enzymatic process that can rapidly erode the articular surface. The joint capsule is distended by the recurrent swelling and inflammation, often causing marked joint instability and pain.

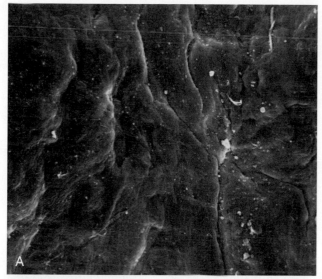

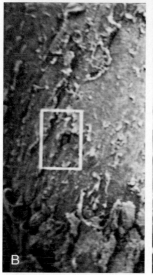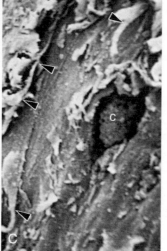

**FIGURE 2–17.** A scanning electron micrograph of the articular surface of a femoral condyle of a knee in a 71-year-old embalmed male cadaver, contrasting levels of degeneration. *A,* Articular cartilage from an apparently "normal"-looking region of the lateral femoral condyle. The wavy but smooth surface texture represents the normal aging process in hyaline cartilage (200×). *B,* Fibrillated articular cartilage from a region of the medial femoral condyle from the same knee as *A* (225×). *C,* Higher magnification of *B* (600×) shows the roughened or frayed region of the cartilage *(arrowheads).* The lower case "c" indicates an exposed chondrocyte, which is usually concealed within the matrix. (Micrographs courtesy of Dr. Robert Morecraft, University of South Dakota School of Medicine, Sioux Falls, South Dakota.)

## SUMMARY

Joints provide the foundation of musculoskeletal motion and permit the stability and dispersion of internal and external forces. Several classification schemes exist to categorize joints and to allow discussion of their mechanical and kinematic characteristics. Motions of anatomic joints are often complex owing to their asymmetrical shapes and incongruent sur-

faces. The axis of rotation is often estimated for purposes of clinical measurement.

The function and resilience of joints are determined by the architecture and the types of tissues that make up the joints. The ability to repair damaged joint tissues is strongly related to the presence of a direct blood supply and the availability of progenitor cells. The health and longevity of joints are affected by age, loading, trauma, and certain disease states.

## REFERENCES

1. Bogduk N, Engel R: The menisci of the lumbar zygapophyseal joints. A review of their anatomy and clinical significance. Spine 9:454–460, 1984.
2. Buckwalter JA, Woo SL, Goldberg VM, et al: Soft-tissue aging and musculoskeletal function. J Bone Joint Surg Am 75:1533–1548, 1993.
3. Clarke RP: Symptomatic, lateral synovial fringe (plica) of the elbow joint. Arthroscopy 4:112–116, 1988.
4. Dandy DJ: Anatomy of the medial suprapatellar plica and medial synovial shelf. Arthroscopy 6:79–85, 1990.
5. Dupont JY: Synovial plicae of the knee. Controversies and review. Clin Sports Med 16:87–122, 1997.
6. Fawcett DW: Connective tissue. In Bloom W, Fawcett DW (eds): A Textbook of Histology, 12th ed. New York: Chapman & Hall, 1994.
7. Fife RS, Hochberg MC: Osteoarthritis. In Klippel JH (ed): Primer on the Rheumatic Diseases, 11th ed. Atlanta, Arthritis Foundation, 1997.
8. Giles LG: Human lumbar zygapophyseal joint inferior recess synovial folds: A light microscope examination. Anat Rec 220:117–124, 1988.
9. Glaser DL, Kaplan FS: Osteoporosis. Definition and clinical presentation. Spine 22 (Suppl):12S–16S, 1997.
10. Goronzy JJ, Weyand CM, Anderson RJ: Rheumatoid arthritis. In Klippel JH (ed): Primer on the Rheumatic Diseases, 11th ed. Atlanta, Arthritis Foundation, 1997.
11. Hamerman D: Aging and the musculoskeletal system. Ann Rheum Dis 56:578–585, 1997.
12. Hayashi K: Biomechanical studies of the remodeling of knee joint tendons and ligaments. J Biomech 29:707–716, 1996.
13. Humzah MD, Soames RW: Human intervertebral disc: Structure and function. Anat Rec 220:337–356, 1988.
14. Jortikka MO, Inkinen RI, Tammi MI, et al: Immobilisation causes long-lasting matrix changes both in the immobilised and contralateral joint cartilage. Ann Rheum Dis 56:255–261, 1997.
15. Kim SJ, Choe WS: Arthroscopic findings of the synovial plicae of the knee. Arthroscopy 13:33–41, 1997.
16. Kurrat HJ, Oberlander W: The thickness of the cartilage in the hip joint. J Anat 126:145–155, 1978.
17. Mow VC, Flatow EL, Foster RJ, et al: Biomechanics. In Simon SR (ed). Orthopaedic Basic Science. Rosemont, IL, American Academy of Orthopaedic Surgeons, 1994.
18. Muller FJ, Setton LA, Manicourt DH, et al: Centrifugal and biochemical comparison of proteoglycan aggregates from articular cartilage in experimental joint disuse and joint instability. J Orthop Res 12:498–508, 1994.
19. Noyes FR: Functional properties of knee ligaments and alterations induced by immobilization. Clin Orthop Rel Res 123:210–242, 1977.
20. O'Brien SJ, Neves MC, Arnoczky SP, et al: The anatomy and histology of the inferior glenohumeral ligament complex of the shoulder. Am J Sports Med 18:449–456, 1990.
21. O'Meara PM: The basic science of meniscus repair. Orthop Rev 22:681–686, 1993.
22. Panni AS, Milano G, Lucania L, et al: Histological analysis of the coracoacromial arch: Correlation between age-related changes and rotator cuff tears. Arthroscopy 12:531–540, 1996.
23. Rubman MH, Noyes FR, Barber-Westin SD: Arthroscopic repair of meniscal tears that extend into the avascular zone. A review of 198 single and complex tears. Am J Sports Med 26:87–95, 1998.
24. Sato Y, Fujimatsu Y, Kikuyama M, et al: Influence of immobilization on bone mass and bone metabolism in hemiplegic elderly patients with a long-standing stroke. J Neurol Sci 156:205–210, 1998.
25. Stockwell RA: The interrelationship of cell density and cartilage thickness in mammalian articular cartilage. J Anat 109:411–421, 1971.

26. Swann DA, Silver FH, Slayter HS, et al: The molecular structure and lubricating activity of lubricin isolated from bovine and human synovial fluids. Biochem J 225:195–201, 1985.

27. Williams PL, Bannister LH, Berry MM, et al (eds): The skeletal system. In Gray's Anatomy, 38th ed. New York, Churchill Livingstone, 1995.

28. Woo SL-Y, Gomez MA, Sites TJ, et al: The biomechanical and morphological changes in the medial collateral ligament of the rabbit after immobilization and remobilization. J Bone Joint Surg 69A:1200–1211, 1987.

29. Xu GL, Haughton VM, Carrera GF: Lumbar facet joint capsule: Appearance at MR imaging and CT. Radiology 177:415–420, 1990.

30. Yu SW, Sether L, Haughton VM: Facet joint menisci of the cervical spine: Correlative MR imaging and cryomicrotomy study. Radiology 164:79–82, 1987.

# CHAPTER 3

# Muscle: The Ultimate Force Generator in the Body

DAVID A. BROWN, PT, PHD

## TOPICS AT A GLANCE

## INTRODUCTION

Stable posture results from a balance of competing forces. Movement, in contrast, occurs when competing forces are unbalanced. Force generated by muscles is the primary means for controlling the intricate balance between posture and movement. Muscle controls posture and movement in two ways: (1) stabilization of bones, and (2) movement of bones.

This chapter considers the role of muscle and tendon in generating, modulating, and transmitting force. These functions are necessary to fix and/or move skeletal structures. How muscle stabilizes bones by generating an appropriate amount of force at a given length is investigated. Force generation occurs both passively (i.e., by a muscle's resistance to stretch) and, to a much greater extent, actively (i.e., by active contraction).

Ways in which muscle modulates or controls force so that bones move smoothly and forcefully are investigated next. Normal movement is highly regulated and refined, regardless of the infinite environmental constraints imposed on a given task.

The approach herein enables the student of kinesiology to understand the multiple roles of muscles in controlling the postures and movements that are used in daily tasks. In addition, the clinician also has the information needed to form clinical hypotheses about muscular impairments that interfere with functional activities. This understanding can lead to the judicious application of interventions to improve a person's abilities.

## MUSCLE AS A SKELETAL STABILIZER: GENERATING AN APPROPRIATE AMOUNT OF FORCE AT A GIVEN LENGTH

Bones support the human body as it interacts with its environment. Although many tissues that attach to the skeleton support the body, only muscle can adapt to both immediate and long-term external forces that can destabilize the body. Muscle tissue is ideally suited for this function because it is coupled both to the external environment and to the internal control mechanisms offered by the nervous system. Under the fine control of the nervous system, muscle generates the force needed to stabilize skeletal structures under an amazingly wide array of conditions. For example, muscle exerts fine control to stabilize fingers wielding a tiny scalpel during eye surgery. It can also generate large forces during the final seconds of a "dead-lift" weightlifting task.

Understanding the special role of muscle in generating stabilizing forces begins with an appreciation of how muscle morphology and muscle-tendon architecture affect the range of force available to a given muscle. The components of muscle are explored that produce passive tension when a muscle is elongated (or stretched), or active force when a

**TABLE 3–1. Major Concepts: Muscle as a Skeletal Stabilizer**

1. Muscle morphology
2. Structural organization of skeletal muscle
3. Connective tissues within muscle
4. Physiologic cross-sectional area
5. Pennation angle
6. Passive length-tension curve
7. Parallel and series elastic components of muscle and tendon
8. Elastic and viscous properties of muscle
9. Active length-tension curve
10. Histology of the muscle fiber
11. Total length-tension curve
12. Isometric force and internal torque-joint angle curve development
13. Mechanical and physiologic properties affecting internal torque-joint angle curve

muscle is stimulated by the nervous system. The relationship between muscle force and length and how it influences the isometric torque generated about a joint are then examined. Table 3–1 is a summary of the major concepts addressed in this section.

## Muscle Morphology: Shape and Structure

Muscle morphology describes the basic shape of a whole muscle. Muscles have many shapes, reflecting their ultimate function. Figure 3–1 shows two common shapes of muscle: fusiform and pennate (from the Latin penna, meaning feather). *Fusiform muscles,* such as the biceps brachii, have fibers running parallel to each other and to the central tendon. In *pennate muscles,* the fibers approach the central tendon obliquely. Pennate muscles may be further classified as unipennate, bipennate, or multipennate, depending on the number of similarly angled sets of fibers that attach into the central tendon.

The *muscle fiber* is the structural unit of muscle, ranging in thickness from about 10 to 100 micrometers, and length from about 1 to 50 cm.[17] Each muscle fiber is actually an individual cell with multiple nuclei. The connective tissue that surrounds and supports muscle serves many roles. Similar to connective tissue throughout other bodily structures, the connective tissue within muscle consists of fibers embedded in an amorphous ground substance. Most fibers are collagen, and the remaining fibers are elastin. The combination of these two proteins provides strength, structural support, and elasticity to muscle.

Three different, although structurally related, sets of connective tissue occur in muscle: epimysium, perimysium, and endomysium (Fig. 3–2). The *epimysium* is a tough structure that surrounds the entire surface of the muscle belly and separates it from other muscles. In essence, the epimysium gives form to the muscle belly. The epimysium contains tightly woven bundles of collagen fibers that are highly resistive to stretch. The *perimysium* lies beneath the epimysium, and divides muscle into fascicles that provide a conduit for blood vessels and nerves. This connective tissue, like epi-

mysium, is tough and thick and resistive to stretch. The *endomysium* surrounds individual muscle fibers. It is composed of a relatively dense meshwork of collagen fibrils that are partly connected to the perimysium. Through lateral connections to the muscle fiber, the endomysium conveys part of the contractile force to the tendon.

Although the three types of connective tissues are described as separate entities, they are interwoven in such a way that they may be considered as a continuous sheet of connective tissue. All connective tissue that encases a muscle, directly or indirectly, contributes to the tendons of the muscle.

## Muscle Architecture

Each muscle and its tendons have different architecture and, as a consequence, are able to generate different ranges of force. Understanding muscle architecture allows the prediction of the functional role of a given muscle. Physiologic cross-sectional area and pennation angle are major determinants of the range and the force produced by the muscle.

The *physiologic cross-sectional area* of a muscle reflects the amount of contractile protein available to generate force. Generally speaking, the cross-sectional area (cm²) of a fusiform muscle is determined by dividing the muscle's volume (cm³) by its length (cm). A fusiform muscle with many thick fibers has a greater cross-sectional area than a muscle of similar length and morphology with fewer thinner fibers. *Maximal force potential of a muscle is, therefore, proportional to the sum of the cross-sectional area of all the fibers.* Under normal conditions, the thicker the muscle, the greater the force potential. Measuring the cross-sectional area of a fusiform muscle is relatively simple because all fibers run paral-

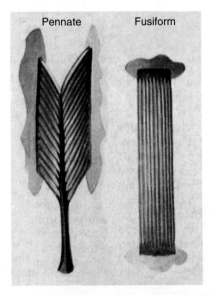

**FIGURE 3–1.** Two common shapes of muscle, fusiform and pennate, are shown. Different shapes are formed by different fiber orientation relative to the connecting tendon. (Modified from Williams PL: Gray's Anatomy: The Anatomical Basis of Medicine and Surgery, 38th ed. New York, Churchill Livingstone, 1995.)

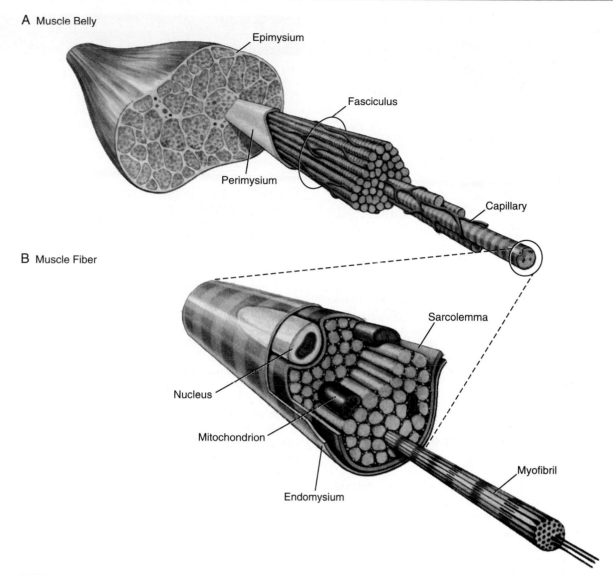

**FIGURE 3–2.** Three sets of connective tissue are identified in muscle. *A,* The muscle belly is enclosed within the *epimysium* and then further subdivided into individual fasciculi by the *perimysium. B,* Each muscle fiber contains myofibrils that are enclosed within the *endomysium.* (Modified from Williams PL: Gray's Anatomy: The Anatomical Basis of Medicine and Surgery, 38th ed. New York, Churchill Livingstone, 1995.)

lel. Caution needs to be used, however, when measuring the cross-section of pennate muscles, because fibers run at different angles to each other.

*Pennation angle* refers to the angle of orientation between the muscle fibers and tendon (Fig. 3–3). If muscle fibers attach parallel to the tendon, the pennation angle is defined as 0 degrees. In this case, essentially all of the force generated by muscle fibers is transmitted to the tendon and across a joint. If, however, the pennation angle is greater than 0 degrees (i.e., oblique to the tendon), then less of the force produced by the muscle fiber is transmitted to the tendon. Theoretically, a muscle with a pennation angle close to 0 degrees transmits full force to the tendon, whereas the same muscle with a pennation angle close to 30 degrees transmits

86% of its force to the tendon. (The cosine of 30 degrees is 0.86.)

In general, pennate muscles produce greater maximal force than fusiform muscles of similar size. By orienting fibers obliquely to the central tendon, a pennate muscle can fit more fibers into a given length of muscle. This space-saving strategy provides pennate muscles with a relatively large physiologic cross-sectional area and, hence, a relatively large capability for generating high force. Consider the multipennate gastrocnemius muscle that must generate very large forces during jumping, for example. Interestingly, the reduced transfer of force from the pennate fiber to the tendon, due to the greater pennation angle, is small compared with the large force potential furnished by the gain in

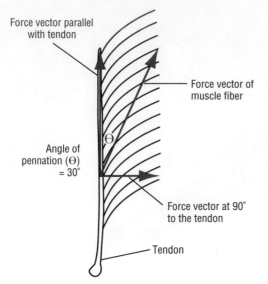

**FIGURE 3–3.** Unipennate muscle is shown with the muscle fibers oriented at a 30-degree angle of pennation (*θ*).

physiologic cross-sectional area. As shown in Figure 3–3, a pennation angle of 30 degrees still enables the fibers to transfer 86% of their force through the long axis of the tendon.

## Muscle and Tendon: Generation of Force

### PASSIVE LENGTH-TENSION CURVE

Muscle contains contractile proteins that are embedded within a network of connective tissues, namely, the epimysium, perimysium, and endomysium. Table 3–2 lists the functions of these tissues. Connective tissues are slightly elastic and, like a rubber band, generate resistive force (i.e., tension) when elongated.

For functional rather than anatomic purposes, the connective tissues within the muscle and tendon have been described as the *parallel elastic component* and the *series elastic component*. Elongation or stretch of the whole muscle lengthens the connective tissue elements (Fig. 3–4). The parallel elastic component refers to the connective tissues

**TABLE 3–2. Functions of Connective Tissue within Muscle**

1. Provides gross structure to muscle
2. Serves as a conduit for blood vessels and nerves
3. Generates passive tension by resisting stretch
4. Assists muscle to regain shape after stretch
5. Conveys contractile force to the tendon and across the joint

that surround or lie parallel to the proteins that cause the muscle to contract. The series elastic component, in contrast, refers to the connective tissues within the tendon. Because the tendon lies in series with the contractile proteins, active forces produced by these proteins are transferred directly to the bone and across the joint. Stretching a muscle by extending a joint elongates both the parallel elastic component and the series elastic component, generating a springlike resistance, or stiffness, in the muscle. The resistance is referred to as a *passive tension* because it is does not depend on active or volitional contraction. The concept of parallel and serial elastic components is a simplified description of the anatomy; however, it is useful to explain the levels of resistance generated by a stretched muscle.

The tendon has several unique mechanical properties. Because of the longitudinal orientation and thickness of its collagen fibers, the tendon can resist large forces that might otherwise damage the muscle tissue. Muscle fibers decrease in diameter by as much as 90% as they blend with the tendon tissue.[12] As a result, the force through a muscle fiber per cross-sectional area (i.e., stress) increases significantly. At each end of a muscle fiber is an extensive folding of the plasmalemma (i.e., the membrane surrounding the muscle fiber), which interdigitates with the connective tissue of the tendon. This folding ensures that high forces can be distributed over a large area, thus reducing the stress on the muscle.

When the parallel and series elastic components are stretched within a muscle, a generalized *passive length-tension curve* is generated (Fig. 3–5). The curve is similar to that obtained by stretching a rubber band. Approximating the shape of an exponential mathematical function, the passive

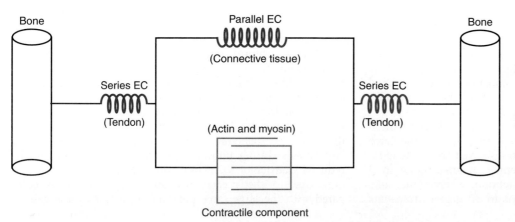

**FIGURE 3–4.** Contractile components and elastic components (EC) that generate force in muscle tissue are shown. The contractile component represents the actin and myosin crossbridge structures. The parallel elastic component (parallel to the contractile component) represents muscle connective tissue. The series elastic component (in series with the whole muscle) represents the connective tissues within the tendon. The parallel and series connective tissues act in a manner similar to a spring.

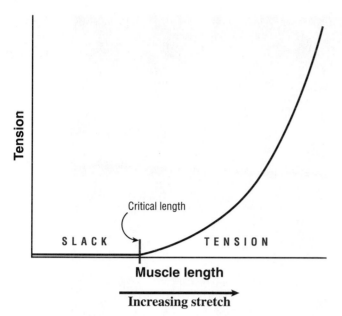

**FIGURE 3–5.** A generalized passive length-tension curve is shown. As a muscle is progressively stretched, the tissue is slack during its initial shortened lengths until it reaches a critical length where it begins to generate tension. Beyond this critical length, the tension builds as an exponential function.

elements within the muscle begin generating passive tension after the critical length where all of the relaxed (i.e., slack) tissue has been brought to an initial level of tension. After this critical length has been reached, tension progressively increases until it reaches levels of extremely high stiffness. At higher tension, the tissue fails. The simple passive length-tension curve represents an important component of force-generating capability in muscle and tendon tissue. This capability is especially important at very long lengths where muscle fibers begin to lose their active force-generating capability. Passive tension stabilizes skeletal structures against gravity and responds to perturbations and other imposed loads. Passive elongation of the Achilles tendon of the ankle during the downstroke of bicycle pedaling, for example, allows for transmittal of hip and muscular forces to the bicycle crank.[6] This capability, however, is limited because of the slow adaptability of the tissue to rapidly changing external forces and because of the significant amount of initial lengthening that must occur before tissue can generate sufficient passive tension.

Stretched muscle tissue exhibits the properties of elasticity and viscosity. Both properties influence the amount and rate of passive tension developed within a stretched muscle. A stretched muscle exhibits *elasticity* because it can temporarily store part of the energy that created the stretch. Stored energy, although relatively slight when compared with the full force potential of the muscle, helps prevent a muscle from being damaged during maximal elongation. *Viscosity,* in this context, describes the rate-dependent resistance encountered between the surfaces of adjacent fluid-like tissues. Viscosity is rate dependent; thus, a muscle's internal resistance to elongation increases with the rate of stretch. Viscosity

helps protect a muscle from being damaged by a quick and forceful stretch. The viscous properties of muscle prolong the application of force to allow a more gradual elongation, reducing the risk of tissue rupture. In summary, both elasticity and viscosity serve as damping mechanisms that protect the structural components of the muscle and tendon.

## ACTIVE LENGTH-TENSION CURVE

Muscle tissue is uniquely designed to generate force actively in response to a stimulus from the nervous system. This section describes the means for generating active force. Active force is produced by the muscle fiber. Ultimately, active force and passive tension must be transmitted to the skeletal structures. The interaction between active and passive forces is explored in the next section.

As explained earlier, muscle fibers constitute the basic functional element of muscle. Furthermore, each muscle fiber, or cell, is composed of many tiny strands called myofibrils. *Myofibrils* are the contractile elements of the muscle fiber and have a distinctive structure. Each myofibril is 1 to 2 micrometers in diameter and consists of many *myofilaments*. The primary structures within myofilaments are two types of proteins: *actin* and *myosin*. The regular organization of myofilaments produces the characteristic banded appearance of the myofibril as seen under the microscope (Fig. 3–6). The actin and myosin physically interact through cross-bridges (i.e., projections from the myosin filament) and other connective structures. By way of the endomysium, myofibrils ultimately connect with the tendon. This elegant connective web, formed between myofilaments and connective tissues, allows force to be evenly distributed throughout muscle and efficiently transmitted to skeletal structures.

Upon inspection of the muscle fiber, a distinctive light and dark banding is apparent (Fig. 3–7). The dark bands, the *A-bands,* correspond to the presence of *myosin*—the thick filaments. Myosin also contains projections, called *cross-bridges,* which are arranged in pairs (Fig. 3–8). The light bands, the *I-bands,* contain *actin*—the thin filaments (see Fig. 3–7). In a resting muscle fiber, actin filaments partially overlap myosin filaments. Under an electron microscope, the bands reveal a more complex pattern that consists of H bands, M lines, and Z discs (Table 3–3).

The banding pattern repeats along the length of the mus-

| TABLE 3–3. Regions Within a Sarcomere | |
|---|---|
| A bands | Dark bands caused by presence of thick myosin filament |
| I bands | Light bands caused by presence of thin actin filament |
| H band | Region within A band where actin and myosin do not overlap. |
| M lines | Mid region thickening of thick myosin filament in the center of H band |
| Z discs | Region where successive actin filaments mesh together. Z disc helps anchor the thin filaments. |

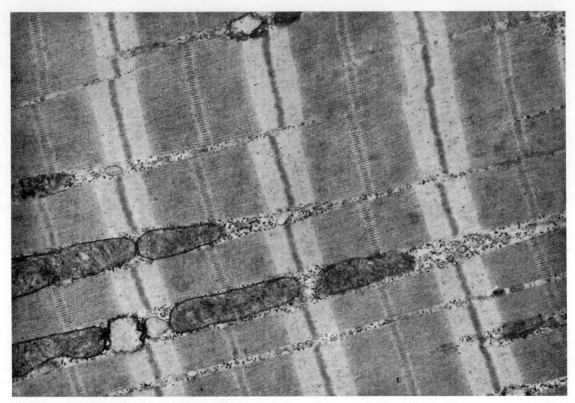

**FIGURE 3–6.** Electron micrograph of muscle myofibrils demonstrates the regularly banded organization of myofilaments—actin and myosin. (From Fawcett DW: The Cell. Philadelphia, W.B. Saunders, 1981.)

cle. Each individual banding unit is called a *sarcomere*, extending from one Z disc to the next. The sarcomere is considered the active force generator of the muscle fiber. By understanding the active contractile events that take place in

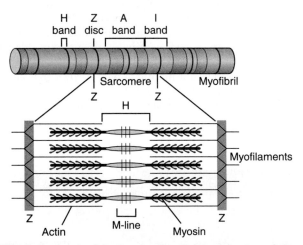

**FIGURE 3–7.** Detail of the regular, banded organization of the myofibril showing the position of the A band, I band, H band, and Z disc. The expanded view of a single sarcomere demonstrates how the actin and myosin filaments contribute to the banded organization. (Modified from Guyton AC, Hall JE: Textbook of Medical Physiology, 10th ed. Philadelphia, W.B. Saunders, 2000. Modified in Guyton from Fawcett DW: Bloom and Fawcett: A Textbook of Histology. Philadelphia, W.B. Saunders, 1986. *Original art by Sylvia Colard Keene.* Reproduced by permission of Edward Arnold Limited.)

the sarcomere, it is possible to understand the mechanics of muscle contraction since this process is repeated from one sarcomere to the next.

The currently accepted model for describing active force generation is called the *sliding filament hypothesis* and was developed independently by Hugh Huxley[8] and Andrew Huxley (no relation).[9] In this model, active force is generated as actin filaments slide past myosin filaments, causing approximation of the Z discs and narrowing of the H band. This action results in progressive overlap of actin and myosin filaments so that sarcomere length is effectively shortened even though the filaments themselves do not shorten (Fig. 3–9). Each cross-bridge attaches to its adjacent actin filament so that the force generated depends on the number of simultaneous cross-bridge/actin attachments. The greater the number of cross-bridge attachments, the greater the amount of active force generated within the sarcomere.

As a consequence of the arrangement between the actin and myosin within a sarcomere, the amount of active force depends, in part, on the instantaneous length of the muscle fiber. A change in fiber length—either by active contraction or by passive elongation—alters the amount of overlap between cross-bridges and actin filaments. The active length-tension curve for a sarcomere is presented in Figure 3–10. The ideal *resting length* of a muscle fiber or sarcomere is the length that allows the greatest number of cross-bridge attachments and, therefore, the greatest potential active force. As the sarcomere is lengthened or shortened from its resting length, the number of potential cross-bridge attachments decreases so that lesser amounts of active force are generated, even under conditions of full activation. The resulting active

**FIGURE 3–8.** Further detail of a sarcomere showing the cross-bridge structure created by the myosin heads and their attachment to the actin filaments. Note that the actin filament also contains the proteins troponin and tropomyosin. Troponin is responsible for exposing the actin filament to the myosin head, thereby allowing crossbridge formation. (Modified from Berne RM, Levy MN: Principles of Physiology, 2nd ed. St. Louis, Mosby, 1996.)

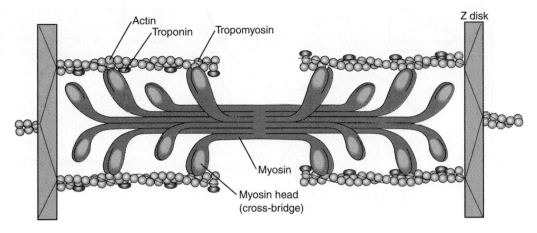

length-tension curve is described by an inverted U-shape with its peak at the ideal resting length.

The term length-force relationship is more appropriate for considering the terminology established in this text (see definition of force and tension in Chapter 1). The phrase *length-tension* is, however, used because of its wide acceptance in the physiology literature.

## SUMMATION OF ACTIVE FORCE AND PASSIVE TENSION: THE TOTAL LENGTH-TENSION CURVE

The active length-tension curve, when combined with the passive length-tension curve, yields the total length-tension curve of muscle. The combination of active force and passive tension allows for a large range of muscle force over a wide range of muscle length. Consider the total length-tension curve for the muscle shown in Figure 3–11. At shortened lengths (a), below active resting length, and below the length that generates passive tension, active force dominates the force generating capability of the muscle. Thus, force rises rapidly as the muscle is lengthened (stretched) toward its resting length. As the muscle fiber is stretched beyond its resting length (b), passive tension begins to contribute so that the decrement in active force is offset by increased passive tension, effectively flattening this part of the total length-tension curve. This characteristic portion of the passive length-tension curve allows muscle to maintain high

levels of force even as the muscle is stretched to a point where active force generation is compromised. As the muscle fiber is further stretched (c), passive tension dominates the curve so that connective tissues are under near maximal stress. High levels of passive tension are most apparent in two-joint muscles placed in overelongated positions. For example, as the wrist is extended, typically the fingers passively flex slightly owing to the stretch placed on the finger flexor muscles as they cross the front of the wrist. The amount of passive tension depends in part on the natural stiffness of the muscle.

## Isometric Force: Development of the Internal Torque-Joint Angle Curve

As defined in Chapter 1, isometric activation of muscle is a process by which the muscle produces force without a signif-

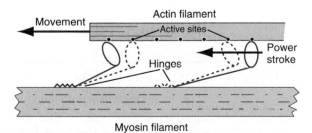

**FIGURE 3–9.** The sliding filament action that occurs as myosin heads attach and then release from the actin filament is illustrated. Contractile force is generated during the power stroke of the cycle. (From Guyton AC, Hall JE: Textbook of Medical Physiology, 10th ed. Philadelphia, W.B. Saunders, 2000.)

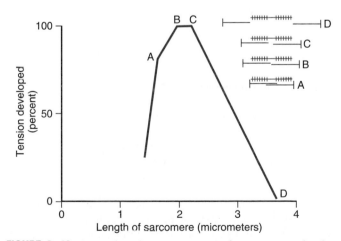

**FIGURE 3–10.** Active length-tension curve of a sarcomere for four specified sarcomere lengths (upper right, A through D). Actin filaments (A) overlap so that the number of crossbridge attachments is reduced. In B and C, actin and myosin filaments are positioned to allow an optimal number of crossbridge attachments. In D, actin filaments are positioned out of the range from the myosin heads so that no crossbridge attachments are possible. (From Guyton AC, Hall JE: Textbook of Medical Physiology, 10th ed. Philadelphia, W.B. Saunders, 2000.)

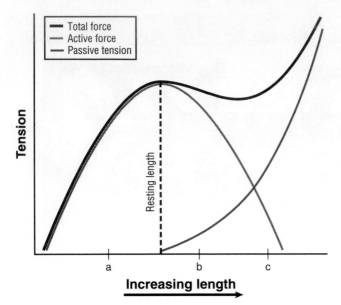

**FIGURE 3–11.** Total length-tension curve for a typical muscle. At shortened lengths (a), all force is generated actively. As the muscle fiber is stretched beyond its resting length (b), passive tension begins to contribute to the total force. In c, the muscle is further stretched and passive tension accounts for most of the total force.

icant change in length. This occurs naturally when the joint over which a stimulated muscle crosses is constrained from movement. Constraint often occurs from a force produced by an antagonistic muscle. Isometrically produced forces provide the necessary stability to the joints and body as a whole. The amplitude of an isometrically produced force from a given muscle reflects the summation of both length-dependent active and passive forces.

Maximal isometric force of a muscle is often used as a general indicator of a muscle's peak strength and can indicate motor recovery.[3,10,16] In clinical settings, it is not possible to directly measure length or force of maximally activated muscle. However, a muscle's internal *torque* generation can be measured isometrically about several different joint angles. Figure 3–12 shows the internal torque versus the joint angle curve ("torque-angle curve") of two muscle groups under isometric, maximal effort conditions. The torque-angle curve is the rotational equivalent to the total length-tension curve of a muscle group. The internal torque produced isometrically by a muscle group can be determined by asking an individual to produce a maximal effort contraction against a known external torque. As described in Chapter 4, an external torque can be determined by using an external force-sensing device (dynamometer) at a known distance from the joint's axis of rotation. Because the measurement is done in the muscle's isometric state, the internal torque is assumed to be equal to the external torque.

The shape of a maximal effort torque angle curve is very specific to each muscle group (see Fig. 3–12A and B). Its shape yields important information about the physiologic and mechanical factors that determine the torque produced by the muscle group. Consider the following two factors shown in Figure 3–13. First, *muscle length* changes as joint angle changes. As previously described, a muscle's force out-

put—in both active and passive terms—is highly dependent on muscle length. Second, the changing joint angle alters the length of the moment arm, or *leverage,* that is available to the muscle. Because both length and leverage are altered simultaneously by joint rotation, it is not always possible to know which is more influential in determining the final shape of the torque-angle curve. A change in either variable—mechanical or physiologic—alters the clinical expression of a muscular-produced internal torque (Table 3–4).

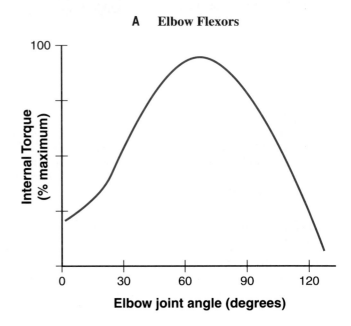

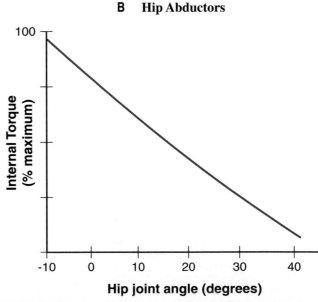

**FIGURE 3–12.** Internal torque versus joint angle curve of two muscle groups under isometric, maximal effort conditions is shown. The shape of the curves are very different for each muscle group. *A,* Internal torque of the elbow flexors is greatest at an angle of about 75 degrees of flexion. *B,* Internal torque of the hip abductors is greatest at a frontal plane angle of −10 degrees (i.e., 10 degrees toward adduction).

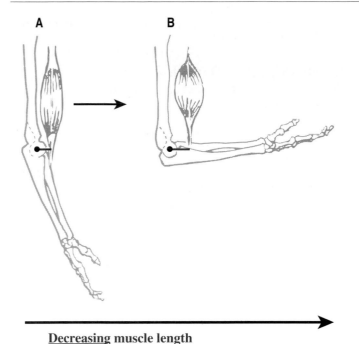

**A**          **B**

<u>Decreasing</u> muscle length

<u>Increasing</u> muscle moment arm

**FIGURE 3–13.** Muscle length and moment arm have an impact on the maximal effort torque for a given muscle. *A*, Muscle is at its near greatest length, and muscle moment arm (red line) is at its near shortest length. *B*, Muscle length is shortened, and muscle moment arm length is greatest. (Modified from LeVeau BF: Williams & Lissner's Biomechanics of Human Motion, 3rd ed. Philadelphia, W.B. Saunders, 1992.)

The torque-angle curve of the hip abductors demonstrated in Figure 3–12*B* depends primarily on muscle length, as shown by the linear reduction of maximal torque produced at progressively greater abduction angles of the

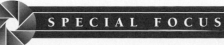

**SPECIAL FOCUS 3 – 1**

**Exploring the Reasons for the Unique "Signature" of a Muscle Group's Isometric Torque-Angle Curve**

Consider the functional implications associated with the shape of a muscle group's torque-angle curve. Undoubtedly, the shape is related to the nature of *external force* demands on the joint. For the elbow flexors, for example, the maximal internal torque potential is greatest in the mid ranges of elbow motion, and least near full extension and full flexion (see Fig. 3–12*A*). Not coincidentally, the external torque-effect due to gravity on hand-held objects is also typically greatest in the mid ranges of elbow motion, and least in the extremes of this motion.

For the hip abductor muscles, the internal torque potential is greatest near neutral (0 degrees of abduction) (see Fig. 3–12*B*). This joint angle coincides with the approximate angle where the hip abductor muscles are most needed for frontal plane stability while walking. Large amounts of hip abduction torque are rarely required in a position of maximal hip abduction.

hip. Regardless of the muscle group, however, the combination of high total muscle force (based on muscle length) and great leverage (based on moment arm length) results in the greatest relative internal torque.

In summary, isometric torque measures differ depending upon the joint angle, regardless of maximal effort. It is therefore important that clinical measurements of isometric torque include the joint angle so that future comparisons are valid. The testing of isometric strength at different joint angles enables the characterizing of the functional range of a mus-

**TABLE 3 – 4. Clinical Examples and Consequences of Changes in Mechanical or Physiologic Variables that Influence the Production of Internal Torque**

| Changed Variable | Clinical Example | Effect of Internal Torque | Possible Clinical Consequence |
|---|---|---|---|
| *Mechanical:* Increased internal moment arm | Surgical displacement of greater trochanter to increase the internal moment arm of hip abductor muscles | Decrease in the amount of muscle force required to produce a given level of hip abduction torque | Decreased hip abductor force can reduce the force generated across an unstable or a painful hip joint; considered a means of "protecting" a joint from damaging forces |
| *Mechanical:* Decreased internal moment arm | Patellectomy following severe fracture of the patella | Increase in the amount of knee extensor muscle force required to produce a given level of knee extension torque | Increased force needed to extend the knee may increase the wear on the articular surfaces of the knee joint |
| *Physiological:* Decreased muscle activation | Damage to the deep portion of the peroneal nerve | Decreased strength in the dorsiflexor muscles | Reduced ability to walk safely |
| *Physiological:* Significantly decreased muscle length at the time of neural activation | Damage to the radial nerve with paralysis of wrist extensor muscles | Decreased strength in wrist extensor muscles causes the finger flexor muscles to flex the *wrist* while making a grasp | Ineffective grasp due to overcontracted (shortened) finger flexor muscles |

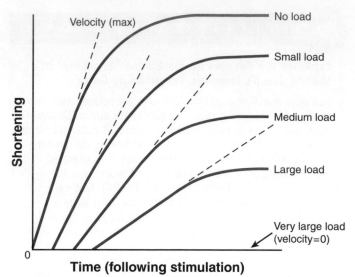

**FIGURE 3–14.** Relationship between muscle load (external resistance) and maximal shortening velocity. (Velocity is equal to the slope of the dotted line.) At a no load condition, a muscle is capable of shortening at a high velocity. As a muscle becomes progressively loaded, the maximal shortening velocity decreases. Eventually, at some very large load, the muscle is incapable of shortening and the velocity is 0. (Redrawn from McComas AJ: Skeletal Muscle: Form & Function. Champaign, IL, Human Kinetics, 1996.)

cle's strength. This information may be required to determine the suitability of a person for a certain task at the workplace, especially if the task requires a critical internal torque to be produced at certain joint angles.

## MUSCLE AS A SKELETAL MOVER: FORCE MODULATION

The previous section considers how an isometrically activated muscle can stabilize the skeletal system; this next section considers how muscles actively grade forces while changing lengths, which is necessary to move the skeletal system. Active grading of muscle force requires a mechanism to control excitation of muscle tissue. The nervous system acts as a "controller" that can vary the activation of muscle according to the particular demands of the task. For example, if the task is to point accurately at a small target, the controller must be able to make split-second adjustments in activation levels to a relatively small number of muscle fibers. With this control strategy, the pointing finger does not veer off course when external perturbations or resistance are imposed. If the task is to produce a forceful motion, the controller must then rapidly and efficiently activate large numbers of muscle fibers.

Understanding the role of muscle activation in generating movement begins with an appreciation of how muscle force is modulated while the muscle is either shortening or lengthening. The ways in which force is graded by neural activation are explored. The reduction in force that occurs with muscular fatigue is examined. Finally, the use of electromy-

ography as a tool for understanding muscle activation during movement is introduced.

## Modulating Force Through Concentric or Eccentric Activation: Force-Velocity Relationship

The nervous system stimulates a muscle to generate or resist a force by concentric, eccentric, or isometric activation. During concentric activation, the muscle shortens (contracts); during eccentric activation, the muscle elongates; and during isometric activation, the length of the muscle remains constant. During concentric and eccentric activation, the *rate of change* of length is significantly related to the muscle's maximal force potential. During concentric activation, for example, the muscle contracts at a maximum velocity when the load is negligible (Fig. 3–14). As the load increases, the maximal contraction velocity of the muscle decreases. At some point, a very large load results in a contraction velocity of zero (i.e., the isometric state).

Eccentric activation needs to be considered separately from concentric activation. With eccentric activation, a load that barely exceeds the isometric force level causes the muscle to lengthen slowly. Speed of lengthening increases as a greater load is applied. There is a maximal load that the muscle cannot resist, and beyond this load level the muscle uncontrollably lengthens.

The theoretical force-velocity curve for muscle across concentric, isometric, and eccentric activations is often shown with the force on the Y (vertical) axis and shortening and lengthening velocity on the X (horizontal) axis (Fig. 3–15). In general, during a maximal effort concentric activation, the amount of muscle force is *inversely proportional* to the velocity of muscle shortening. During a maximal effort eccentric activation, the muscle force is, to a point, *directly proportional* to the velocity of muscle lengthening. The clinical expression of a force-velocity relationship of muscle is a torque-joint

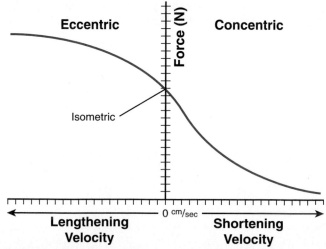

**FIGURE 3–15.** Theoretic force-velocity curve of an activated muscle is shown. Concentric activation is shown on the right and eccentric activation on the left. Isometric activation occurs at the zero velocity point on the graph.

angular velocity relationship. This type of data can be derived through *isokinetic dynamometry* (see Chapter 4).

The inverse relationship between a muscle's maximal force potential and its shortening velocity is related to the concept of power. *Power,* or the rate of work, can be expressed as a product of force times contraction velocity, (i.e., the area under the curve on the right hand side of Figure 3–15). A constant power output of a muscle can be sustained by increasing the load (resistance) while proportionately decreasing the contraction velocity, or vice versa. This is very similar in concept to switching gears while riding a bicycle.

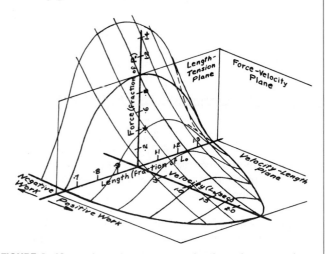
A muscle undergoing a concentric contraction against a load is doing *positive work* on the load. In contrast, a muscle undergoing eccentric activation against an overbearing load is doing *negative work.* In the latter case, the muscle is storing energy that is supplied by the load. A muscle, therefore, can act as either an active accelerator of movement against a load while contracting (i.e., through concentric activation), or it can act as a "brake" or decelerator when a load is applied and the activated muscle is lengthening (i.e., through eccentric activation).

## Activating Muscle via the Nervous System

Several important mechanical mechanisms underlying muscle force generation have been examined. Of utmost importance, however, is the fact that muscle is excited by impulses that are generated within the nervous system, specifically by alpha motoneurons that are located in the ventral horn of the spinal cord. Each alpha motoneuron has an axon that extends out of the spinal cord and connects with multiple muscle fibers located throughout a whole muscle. The alpha motoneuron and all muscle fibers that are innervated by it are called a *motor unit.* Because of this arrangement, the nervous system can produce a muscle force from small contractions involving only a few muscle fibers, and large contractions that involve most of the fibers. Excitation of alpha motoneurons may come from many sources, for example, afferents, spinal interneurons, and cortical descending neurons. Each source can activate an alpha motoneuron by first *recruiting* the motoneuron and then by driving it to higher rates of sequential activation. The sequence of driving motoneurons to higher rates, known as *rate coding,* allows recruited muscle to generate greater amounts of force. Both of these issues of driving motoneurons are discussed further.

### RECRUITMENT

Recruitment refers to the initial activation of a specific set of motoneurons resulting in the generation of action potentials that excite target muscle fibers. The nervous system recruits a motor unit by altering the voltage potential across the alpha motoneuron membrane surface. The facilitation process is the summation of competing inhibitory and facilitatory input that ultimately results in a threshold action potential that drives the motoneuron to propagate excitation to the muscle fibers. Once the muscle fiber is activated, a muscle twitch occurs and a small amount of force is generated. Table 3–5 lists the major sequence of events underlying muscle fiber activation. By recruiting more motoneurons, more muscle fibers are activated, and, therefore, more force is generated within the whole muscle.

Motoneurons come in different sizes and are connected with muscle fibers of different contractile characteristics (Fig. 3–17). The size of the motoneuron influences the order with which it is recruited by the nervous system (i.e., smaller motoneurons will be recruited before larger motoneurons). This principle is called the *Henneman Size Principle.* It was first experimentally demonstrated and developed by Elwood Henneman in the late 1950s.[7] The principle accounts for the orderly recruitment of motor units, specified by size, which allows for smooth and controlled force development.

---

**TABLE 3–5. Major Sequence of Events Underlying Muscle Fiber Activation**

1. Action potential initiated and propagated down a motor axon.
2. Acetylcholine released from axon terminals at neuromuscular junction.
3. Acetylcholine bound to receptor sites on motor endplate.
4. Sodium and potassium ions enter and depolarize muscle membrane.
5. Muscle action potential propagated over membrane surface.
6. Transverse tubules depolarized leading to release of calcium ions surrounding the myofibrils.
7. Calcium ions bind to troponin, which leads to the release of inhibition over actin and myosin binding.
8. Actin combines with myosin adenosine triphosphate (ATP), an energy-providing molecule.
9. Energy released to produce movement of myosin cross-bridges.
10. Thick and thin filaments slide relative to each other.
11. Actin and myosin bond is broken and re-established if calcium concentration remains sufficiently high.

---

Muscle fibers that are connected with small motoneurons have twitch responses, that are relatively long in duration and small in amplitude (see Fig. 3–17, right). Motor units associated with these fibers are classified as *S* (slow) because the fibers are slow to respond to a stimuli, or *SO* (slow, oxidative). The *O* reflects the histochemical profile. SO fibers show relatively little fatigue (i.e., loss of force during sustained activation).

Muscle fibers that are connected with large motoneurons have twitch responses that are relatively brief in duration and high in amplitude (Fig. 3–17, left). Motor units associated with these fibers are classified as *FF* (fast and easily fatigued), or *FG* (fast and glycolytic), reflecting the histochemical profile. FG fibers fatigue relative easily.

An entire spectrum of intermediate motor units exists that shows physiologic and histochemical profiles somewhere between slow and fast type motor units (Fig. 3–17, middle). Motor units associated with these fibers are termed *FR* (fatigue resistant). The fibers are termed *FOG* to represent the combined utilization of oxidative and glycolytic energy sources.

The motor unit types depicted in Figure 3–17 allow for a wide range of physiologic responses from fibers within skeletal muscles. The earlier (smaller) recruited motoneurons produce longer duration, small force contractions. Later recruited (larger) motoneurons add successively greater forces of shorter duration. Through this spectrum, the nervous system is able to activate muscle fibers that sustain stable postures over a long period of time, and, when needed, produce high, short duration bursts of force for more impulsive movements.

## RATE CODING

After a specific motoneuron is recruited, muscle force is modulated by an increase in the rate of its excitation, a concept called *rate coding*. Although a single action potential in a skeletal muscle fiber lasts 1 to 2 milliseconds (ms), a muscle fiber contraction (commonly called a twitch) may last for as long as 130 ms in an S fiber. Because of the long twitch duration, it is possible for a number of subsequent action potentials to begin during the initial twitch.[4] If a fiber is allowed to relax completely before the subsequent action potential, the second fiber twitch generates equivalent force to the first twitch (Fig. 3–18). If the next action potential arrives before the preceding twitch has relaxed, however, the muscle twitches summate and generate an even greater level of peak force. Alternatively, if the next action potential arrives closer to the peak force level of the initial twitch, the force is even greater.

A set of repeating action potentials, separated by a suitable time interval, generates a series of summated mechanical twitches, termed *unfused tetanus*. As the time interval shortens, the unfused tetanus generates greater force until the successive peaks and valleys of mechanical twitches fuse into a single, stable level of muscle force, termed *fused tetanus* (or *tetanization*) (see Fig. 3–18). Fused tetanus represents the greatest force level that is possible for a muscle fiber. Motor units, therefore, activated at high rates are capable of generating greater overall force than the same number of motor units activated at lower rates. Because motor units are distributed across an entire muscle, fiber contractile forces summate across the entire muscle and ultimately are transmitted to the tendon and across the joint.

## Muscle Fatigue

As muscle fibers are repeatedly stimulated, the force generated by a fiber eventually decreases, even though the rate of activation remains the same (Fig. 3–19). The decline in muscle force under conditions of stable activation is termed *muscle fatigue*. In theory, muscle fatigue can occur from metabolic processes, or from failure in physiologic mechanisms involved with the neuromuscular system. Normally, the nervous system compensates for muscle fatigue by either increasing the rate of activation (i.e., rate coding) or recruiting assistive motor units (i.e., recruitment), thereby maintaining a stable force level. When an exercising muscle begins to fatigue and performance begins to degrade, a rest period allows that muscle to resume its normal performance level. The rest period that is required depends on the type and intensity of the fatiguing contraction.[1] For example, a muscle that is rapidly fatigued by high intensity and short duration exercise recovers after a rest of seconds to minutes. In contrast, a muscle that is slowly fatigued by low intensity, long duration exercise requires up to 24 hours for recovery.

Fatigue involves a variety of elements located throughout the neuromuscular system. It is convenient to think of fatigue as occurring primarily within central or peripheral neuromuscular elements. *Central fatigue* may be affected by psychological factors, such as sense of effort, and/or neurophysiological factors, such as descending control over interneurons and motoneurons located in the spinal cord. With central fatigue, voluntary efforts at activating the motoneuron pool become suboptimal when an individual is asked to generate a maximum muscle contraction.[13] During a maximal effort, the nervous system may initiate inhibitory pathways to prevent the efficient activation of motoneuron pools.

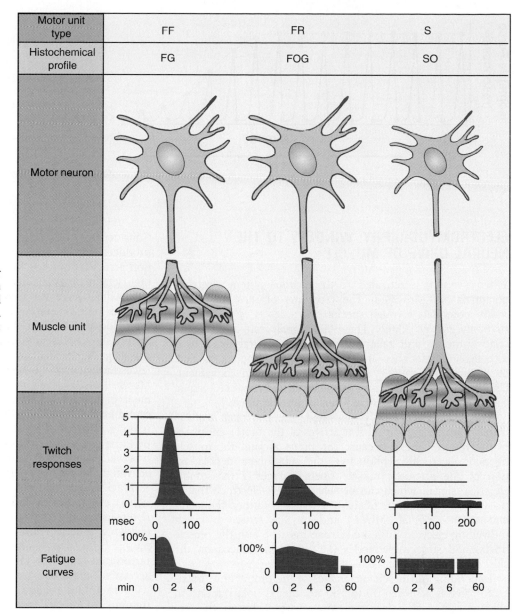

**FIGURE 3–17.** Classification of motor unit types from a muscle based on histochemical profile, size, and twitch (contractile) characteristics. (Modified from Berne RM, Levy MN: Principles of Physiology, 3rd ed. St. Louis, Mosby, 1996.)

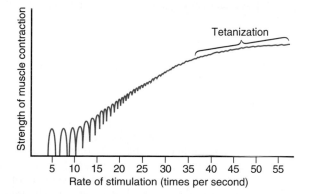

**FIGURE 3–18.** Summation of individual muscle twitches (contractions) are recorded over a wide range of stimulation frequencies. Note that at low frequencies of stimulation (5–10 per second), the initial twitch is relaxed before the next twitch can summate. At progressively higher frequencies, the twitches summate to generate higher force levels until a fused twitch (tetanization) occurs. (From Guyton AC, Hall JE: Textbook of Medical Physiology, 10th ed. Philadelphia, W.B. Saunders, 2000.)

Neural pathway conduction delays or blocks, such as in multiple sclerosis, may impair the ability to activate motoneuron pools.[15] When central fatigue is a suspected mechanism contributing to low muscle force output, verbal encouragement or loud commands can momentarily enhance output.

*Peripheral fatigue* may result from neurophysiologic factors related to action potential propagation in motor nerves and transmission of activation to muscle fibers. The motor nerve terminal, where the motor nerve innervates the muscle fibers, may exhibit transmission failure so that the action potential is not propagated across to the plasmalemma.[11] Repetitive activation of motor units can result in a gradual reduction of acetylcholine release.[2] Since acetylcholine is the essential transmitter responsible for activating plasmalemma, a gradual reduction in its release lessens the size of the resultant twitch for a given muscle. Biochemical factors may be involved in peripheral fatigue. The chemical composition of muscle fiber cytoplasm may undergo a variety of changes that reduce force output over time.[5]

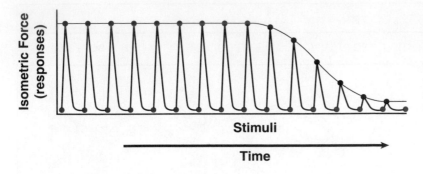

**FIGURE 3–19.** Muscle fatigue is demonstrated by a reduction in force over a sustained isometric activation. As the stimuli continue over time, the force responses of the muscle lessen.

## ELECTROMYOGRAPHY: WINDOW TO THE NEURAL DRIVE OF MUSCLE

When a muscle is activated via the nervous system, electrical potentials are generated. The recording of these amplified action potentials through special electrodes is referred to as *electromyography (EMG)*. The EMG signals can indicate the relative timing and relative level of the neural drive to a muscle, and thus they are useful in understanding the role of a particular muscle in controlling a given movement. Under certain conditions, the magnitude of the EMG signal can also indicate the relative levels of muscle force.

When a motor unit is activated, the electrical impulse travels along the axon until it arrives at the motor endplates of the muscle fibers. Because the tissue around the muscle fibers is electrically conductive, the subsequent depolarization of the activated muscle fibers induces a measurable electrical signal, which can be sensed by an electrode that is placed near the muscle fibers. The signal is termed the *motor unit action potential (MUAP)* and can be sensed by both indwelling electrodes (i.e., electrode inserted into the muscle fibers) and surface electrodes (i.e., electrode placed on the skin overlying the muscle).

Depending on the characteristics of the motor unit, maximum force is achieved 20 to 150 ms after depolarization. An electromechanical delay, therefore, exists between the appearance of muscle electrical activity and the mechanical force generation.[14,18] As described, two mechanisms exist to modulate muscle force: recruitment and rate coding. As the number of active motor units in the muscle is increased via recruitment, greater numbers of MUAPs occur. The sum of these signals generates an overall greater amplitude EMG signal. As the firing rate of active motor units is increased, greater numbers of MUAPs occur within a given time period. A greater amplitude EMG signal also results, typically indicating a greater force level in the active contractile component of muscle.

Caution is advised when interpreting changes in EMG amplitude under conditions other than isometric activation. When an activated muscle is lengthening or shortening, the source for the electrical signal changes its orientation in relation to the electrode that picks up the signal. The signal, therefore, may represent a compilation of MUAPs from different regions of a muscle or even from different muscles.

Because of the length-tension and force-velocity relationships of muscle, the EMG amplitude may vary considerably as a muscle produces a force via nonisometric activations.

Consider the following two extreme examples. Muscle A produces a given submaximal force via an eccentric activation across its optimal force-generating length, at a relatively high lengthening velocity. Muscle B produces an equivalent submaximal force via a concentric activation across its nonoptimal force-generating length, at a relatively high shortening velocity. Based on the length-tension and force-velocity relationships, Muscle A is operating at a relative *physiologic advantage* for producing force. Muscle A, therefore, requires fewer motoneurons to be recruited, and at slower rates, than Muscle B. EMG levels would therefore be less for the movement performed by Muscle A, although both muscles produced equivalent submaximal forces. Using EMG magnitude is not a valid tool for comparing the internal force produced by these two muscles. EMG is a useful tool for this purpose, however, if the two muscles are operating under similar activation, length, and velocity conditions.

EMG can be performed with surface or fine wire (insertional) electrodes. Surface electrodes are easy to apply and noninvasive, and they can detect signals from a large area overlying muscle. Fine wire electrodes, inserted into the muscle belly, allow greater specificity in terms of the muscle region and allow the choice of deeper muscles that are not accessible when using surface electrodes. Nevertheless, fine wire electrodes require a high level of technical skill and training before safe implementation; therefore, surface electrodes are more commonly used in clinical practice.

Because EMG signals originate as very small signals, there is a high risk for extraneous electrical noise. Noise signal can be controlled in several ways. Differential electrode configurations (two pick-up electrodes that are electrically coupled) are used to subtract the noise signal that is commonly recorded by both electrodes. Adequate skin preparation ensures that the tiny EMG signals are recorded efficiently rather than being overly impeded by unprepared skin. The recording environment can be electrically isolated so that extraneous noise is kept far from the equipment. Electrical signals can be preamplified at the electrode source, rather than amplified after the signal is conducted to a distant amplifier, so that intervening noise from movement of the electrode cable is minimized. Signal filtering (i.e., eliminating specific frequencies of electrical signals) can be used to reduce known sources of interfering electrical signals. Low frequency noise, for example, may be present from power sources coupled to the wall outlet. A filter that is designed to eliminate most of the electrical signal at and under 60 Hz significantly reduces the noise from these sources.

The EMG signal requires processing to be useful for kinesiologic interpretation. Raw or raw-filtered signals refer to the original biphasic waveform that is picked up by the electrode. Often, the raw signal is smoothed and/or integrated. *Smoothing* refers to the flattening of the peaks and valleys that occurs in a biphasic electrical signal. Smoothing is performed to allow moment-to-moment quantification of the signal because it eliminates the transient changes in peak values of the signal. *Integration* is a mathematical term that refers to measuring the area under the curve. This process allows for cumulative EMG quantification or averaging EMG over a fixed period of time. Signals that are smoothed and/or integrated can be used in biofeedback devices, such as visual meters or audio signals, and to drive other devices, such as electrical stimulators, to assist in muscle activation at a preset threshold of voluntary activation.

When comparing the intensity of a processed EMG signal between different muscles, it is often necessary that the signal be *normalized* to some common reference signal. This is especially necessary when the magnitude of the EMG is being compared between persons or between sessions, requiring that the electrodes be reapplied. One common method of normalization involves referencing the raw EMG signal from a muscle to the signal produced as a person performs a *maximal voluntary isometric contraction*. Meaningful comparisons can then be made on the relative intensity, expressed as a percent, of the muscle's neural drive during some activity.

The collection of EMG signals during movement, when supplemented by kinematic and kinetic measures, can provide a comprehensive method for analyzing how muscles contribute to a movement. EMG can also provide insight into the neural control of purposeful movements. A clinician can use EMG to aid in the understanding of physical impairments underlying dysfunctional movement. This understanding can then lead to identification of diagnoses associated with movement dysfunction and to appropriate intervention strategies.

## REFERENCES

1. Andrews BJ: Reducing FES muscle fatigue. In Pedotti A, Ferrarin M (eds): Restoration of Walking for Paraplegics. Amsterdam, Ios Press, 1992, pp 197–202.
2. Asmussen E: Muscle fatigue. Med Sci Sports Exerc 25:412–420, 1993.
3. Brouwer B, Wheeldon RK, Stradiotto-Parker N, Allum J: Reflex excitability and isometric force production in cerebral palsy: The effect of serial casting. Dev Med Child Neurol 40:168–175, 1998.
4. Burke R, Levine D, Tsairis P, Zajac F: Physiological types and histochemical profiles in motor units of the cat gastrocnemius. J Physiol 234:723–748, 1973.
5. Fitts RH, Metzger JM: Mechanisms of muscular fatigue. In Poortmans JR (ed): Principles of Exercise Biochemistry, 2nd revised ed. 1993, pp 248–268.
6. Fregly B, Zajac F: A state-space analysis of mechanical energy generation, absorption, and transfer during pedaling. J Biomech 29:81–90, 1996.
7. Henneman E, Mendell LM: Functional organization of motoneuron pool and its inputs. In Brookhart, JM, Mountcastle, VB, Brooks, VB (eds): Handbook of Physiology, vol. 2. Bethesda, American Physiological Society, 1981, pp 423–507.
8. Huxley H, Hanson J: Changes in the cross-striations of muscle during contraction and stretch and their structural interpretation. Nature 173:973–976, 1954.
9. Huxley A, Niedergerke R: Structural changes in muscle during contraction. Interference microscopy of living muscle fibres. Nature 173:971–973, 1954.
10. Jaramillo J, Worrell TW, Ingersoll CD: Hip isometric strength following knee surgery. J Orthop Sports Phys Ther 20:160–165, 1994.
11. Krnjevic K, Miledi R: Failure of neuromuscular propogation in rats. J Physiol 140, 1958.
12. Loeb G, Pratt C, Chanaud C, Richmond F: Distribution and innervation of short, interdigitated muscle fibers in parallel-fibered muscles of the cat hindlimb. J Morph 191:1–15, 1987.
13. McKenzie DK, Biglandritchie B, Gorman RB, Gandevia SC: Central and peripheral fatigue of human diaphragm and limb muscles assessed by twitch interpolation. J Physiol 454:643–656, 1992.
14. Merletti R, Knaflitz M, Deluca CJ: Electrically evoked myoelectric signals. Crit Rev Biomed Eng 19:293–340, 1992.
15. Sandroni P, Walker C, Starr A: Fatigue in patients with multiple sclerosis—motor pathway conduction and event-related potentials. Arch Neurol 49:517–524, 1992.
16. Wessel J, Kaup C, Fan J, et al: Isometric strength measurements in children with arthritis: Reliability and relation to function. Arthr Care Res 12:238–246, 1999.
17. Yamaguchi G, Sawa A, Moran D, et al: A survey of human musculotendon actuator parameters. In Winters J, Woo S-Y (eds): Multiple Muscle Systems: Biomechanics and Movement Organization. New York, Springer-Verlag, 1990, pp 717–773.
18. Zhou S, Lawson DL, Morrison WE, Fairweather I: Electromechanical delay in isometric muscle contractions evoked by voluntary, reflex and electrical stimulation. Eur J Appl Physiol 70:138–145, 1995.

## ADDITIONAL READINGS

Biewener A, Roberts T: Muscle and tendon contributions to force, work, and elastic energy savings: A comparative perspective. Exerc Sport Sci Rev 28:99–107, 2000.
Brown DA, Kautz SA: Increased workload enhances force output during pedaling exercise in persons with poststroke hemiplegia. Stroke 29:598–606, 1998.
Brown DA, Kautz SA: Speed-dependent reductions of force output in people with poststroke hemiparesis. Phys Ther 79:919–930, 1999.
Enoka R, Fuglevand A: Motor unit physiology: Some unresolved issues. Muscle Nerve 24:4–17, 2001.
Gordon A, Homsher E, Regnier M: Regulation of muscle contraction in striated muscle. Physiol Rev 80:853–924, 2000.
Herzog W: Muscle properties and coordination during voluntary movement. J Sports Sci 18:141–152, 2000.
Hill A: The heat of shortening and the dynamic constants of muscle. Proc R Soc Lond (Biol) 126:136–195, 1938.
Hof A, Van den Berg J: EMG to force processing I: An electrical analogue of the Hill muscle model. J Biomech 14:747–758, 1981.
Hof AL, Pronk CNA, Best JA: Comparison between EMG to force processing and kinetic analysis for the calf muscle moment in walking and stepping. J Biomech 20:167–178, 1987.
Huijing PA: Muscle, the motor of movement: Properties in function, experiment and modelling. J Electromyogr Kinesiol 8:61–77, 1998.
Kautz S, Brown D: Relationships between timing of muscle excitation and impaired motor performance during cyclical lower extremity movement in post-stroke hemiplegia. Brain 121:515–526, 1998.
Komi PV: Stretch-shortening cycle: A powerful model to study normal and fatigued muscle. J Biomech 33:1197–1206, 2000.
Lieber R, Friden J: Clinical significance of skeletal muscle architecture. Clin Orthop 383:140–151, 2001.
Lippold O: The relationship between integrated action potentials in a human muscle and its isometric tension. J Physiol 117:492–499, 1952.
Siegler S, Hillstrom HJ, Freedman W, Moskowitz G: Effect of myoelectric signal processing on the relationship between muscle force and processed EMG. Am J Phys Med 64:130–149, 1985.
Woods JJ, Bigland-Ritchie B: Linear and nonlinear surface EMG/force relationships in human muscles. Am J Phys Med 62:287–299, 1983.

# CHAPTER 4

# Biomechanical Principles

DEBORAH A. NAWOCZENSKI, PT, PhD
DONALD A. NEUMANN, PT, PhD

## TOPICS AT A GLANCE

## INTRODUCTION

It can be overwhelming to consider all the factors that may have an impact on human movement. And, many treatment approaches used in physical rehabilitation depend on an accurate description of movement and a reliable assessment of a person's response to intervention. The justification for and the successful outcome of surgical and nonsurgical interventions are also frequently measured by changes in the quality and quantity of movement. In response to these factors, a variety of analysis techniques may be utilized to assess movement, ranging from visual observation to sophisticated motion analyses and imaging techniques. Most often, the complexity of movement analysis is simplified by starting with a basic evaluation of the forces on a single rigid body segment. Newton's laws of motion help to explain the relationship between forces and their impact on individual joints, as well as on total body motion. Even at the basic level of analysis, this information can be used to understand mechanisms of injury, as well as to guide treatment approaches. Technologic advances continue to enhance the ability to understand and influence human performance.

## NEWTON'S LAWS: APPLICATION TO MOVEMENT ANALYSIS

The outcome of all movement analysis is ultimately determined by the forces applied to the body being moved. In the 17th century, Sir Isaac Newton observed that forces were related to mass and motion in a predictable fashion. His *Philosophiae Naturalis Principia Mathematica* (1687) provided the basic laws and principles of mechanics that form the cornerstone of human movement analysis. These laws, referred to as the law of inertia, the law of acceleration, and the law of action and reaction, are collectively known as the *laws of motion* and form the framework from which advanced motion analysis techniques are derived.

# Newton's Laws of Motion

This chapter uses Newton's laws of motion to introduce techniques of analysis for describing the relationship between the forces applied to the body and the consequences of those forces on human motion. (Throughout the chapter, the term "body" is used when elaborating on the concepts related to the laws of motion and the methods of quantitative analysis. The reader should be aware that this term could also be used interchangeably with the entire human body; a segment or part of the body, such as the forearm segment; an object, such as a weight that is being lifted; or the system under consideration, such as the foot-floor interface. In most cases, the simpler term, body, is used when describing the main concepts.) Newton's laws are described for both linear and rotational (angular) motion (Table 4–1).

## NEWTON'S FIRST LAW: LAW OF INERTIA

Newton's first law states that a body remains at rest or in constant linear velocity except when compelled by an external force to change its state. A force is required to start, stop, or alter *linear motion*. The application of Newton's first law to *rotational motion* states that a body remains at rest or in constant angular velocity about an axis of rotation unless compelled by an external torque to change its state. Whether the motion be linear or rotational, Newton's first law describes the case in which a body is in equilibrium. A body is in *static equilibrium* when its velocity is zero, or in *dynamic equilibrium* when its velocity is not zero, but constant. In either case, the acceleration of the body is zero.

---

**Key Terms Associated with Newton's First Law**
- Static equilibrium
- Dynamic equilibrium
- Inertia
- Center of mass
- Mass moment of inertia
- Radius of gyration

---

Newton's first law is also called the law of inertia. *Inertia* is related to the amount of energy required to alter the velocity of a body. The inertia within a body is directly proportional to its *mass* (i.e., the amount of matter constituting the body). For example, if two bodies have different masses but are moving at similar linear velocities, a greater force is required to alter the motion of the more massive body.

Each body has a point about which its mass is evenly distributed. The point, called the *center of mass,* can be considered where the acceleration of gravity acts on the body. When subjected to gravity, the center of mass of a body is often described as its *center of gravity*. For the entire upright human body, the center of mass lies just anterior to the second sacral vertebra (Fig. 4–1A). The center of mass for an individual's thigh and leg segments is shown in Figure 4–1B and C, respectively. During movement, the center of mass is continually changing—its location being a function of the location and size of the individual body segments. Additional information regarding the center of mass of body segments is discussed later in this chapter under the topic of "Anthropometry."

The *mass moment of inertia* of a body is a quantity that indicates its resistance to a change in *angular velocity*. Unlike mass, its linear counterpart, the mass moment of inertia depends not only on the mass of the body, but also on the distribution of its mass with respect to an axis of rotation.[6] Because most human motion is angular, rather than linear, it is important to understand the concept of mass moment of inertia. The mass moment of inertia (I) is defined in the box, where n indicates the number of particles in a body, $m_i$ indicates the mass of each particle in the body, and $r_i$ is the distribution or distance of each particle from the axis of rotation.

---

**Mass Moment of Inertia**

$$I = \sum_{i=1}^{n} m_i r_i^2 \qquad \text{(Equation 4.1)}$$

---

The average distance between the axis of rotation and the center of mass of a body is called the *radius of gyration*. The Greek letter rho ($\rho$) is used to indicate the radius of gyration. Substituting $\rho$, the radius of gyration, for r in the moment of inertia equation (Equation 4.1), yields the sim-

---

**TABLE 4–1. Newton's Laws: Linear and Rotational Components**

| Law | Linear Component | Rotational Component |
|---|---|---|
| First: Law of Inertia | A body remains at rest or in constant linear velocity except when compelled by an external force to change its state. | A body remains at rest or in constant angular velocity about an axis of rotation unless when compelled by an external torque to change its state. |
| Second: Law of Acceleration | The linear acceleration of a body is directly proportional to the force causing it, takes place in the same direction in which the force acts, and is inversely proportional to the mass of the body. | The angular acceleration of a body is directly proportional to the torque causing it, takes place in the same rotary direction in which the torque acts, and is inversely proportional to the mass moment of inertia of the body. |
| Third: Law of Action-Reaction | For every force there is an equal and opposite directed force. | For every torque there is an equal and opposite directed torque. |

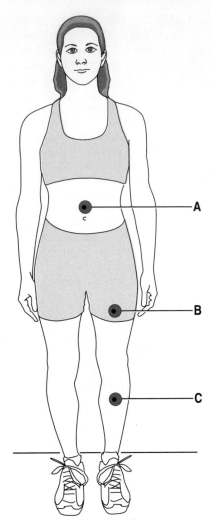

**FIGURE 4–1.** The center of mass of the whole body (*A*) is shown with respect to the frontal plane. The center of mass is also shown for the thigh segment (*B*) and the leg segment (*C*).

pler Equation 4.2 shown in the box. The units of I are kilograms-meters squared (kgm²). The equation describes that a body's resistance to a change in angular velocity is proportional to the mass of the object (m) and the squared distance between the center of mass of the object and the axis of rotation ($\rho^2$).

---

| **Mass Moment of Inertia** | |
| :--- | ---: |
| $I = m \times \rho^2$ | (Equation 4.2) |

---

The fact that $\rho$ is squared in Equation 4.2 has important biomechanical implications. Consider, for example, that during the swing phase of walking the entire lower limb shortens owing to the combined movements of hip and knee flexion and ankle dorsiflexion. A functionally shortened limb reduces the average distance of the mass particles within the limb relative to the hip joint's medial-lateral axis of rotation. The reduced mass moment of inertia reduces the force required by the hip flexor muscles to accelerate the limb

forward. Alternatively, a given muscle force can advance the lower limb more quickly while walking when the lower extremity is flexed as compared with straightened. The change in joint position (i.e., increased hip and knee flexion and ankle dorsiflexion) used to decrease the resistance to angular motion becomes even more apparent as a person changes from walking to running.

Athletes often attempt to control the mass moment of inertia of their entire body by altering the position of their individual body segments. This concept is well illustrated by divers who reduce their moment of inertia in order to successfully complete multiple somersaults while in the air (Fig. 4–3*A*). The athlete can assume an extreme "tuck" position by placing the head near the knees, holding the arms and legs tightly together, thereby bringing more body mass closer to the axis of rotation. Based on the principle of "conservation of angular momentum," reducing the resistance to the angular motion increases the angular velocity. Conversely, the athlete could slow or stop the rotation by assuming a "pike" position, or by straightening the extremities (Fig. 4–3*B*). The mass of the extremities is positioned farther from the medial-lateral axis of rotation, thereby increasing the resistance to angular motion and decreasing the rate of spin.

## NEWTON'S SECOND LAW: LAW OF ACCELERATION

### Force (Torque)-Acceleration Relationship

Newton's second law states that the acceleration of a body is directly proportional to the force causing it, takes place in the same direction in which the force acts, and is inversely proportional to the mass of the body. Newton's second law generates an equation that relates the force (F), mass (m), and acceleration (a) (see Equation 4.3). Conceptually, Equation 4.3 defines a *force-acceleration relationship*. Considered a cause-and-effect relationship, the left side of the equation, force (F), can be regarded as a cause because it represents the interaction between a body and its environment. The right side, m × a, represents the effect of the interaction on the system. In this equation, ΣF designates the sum of or "net" forces acting on a body. If the sum of the forces acting on a body is zero, acceleration also is zero and the body is in linear equilibrium. As previously discussed, this case is described by Newton's first law. If, however, the net force produces an acceleration, the body travels in the direction of the resultant force.

---

| **Newton's Second Law of Linear Motion Quantifying a Force** | |
| :--- | ---: |
| $\Sigma F = m \times a$ | (Equation 4.3) |
| 1 Newton (N) = 1 kgm/s² | |

---

The angular counterpart to Newton's second law states that a *torque (T)* produces an angular acceleration ($\alpha$) of the body that is proportional to, and in the rotary direction of the torque, and is inversely proportional to the mass moment of inertia of the body (I) (see Equation 4.4 in the box). (This chapter uses the term "torque." The reader should be aware

**SPECIAL FOCUS 4–1**

### A Closer Look at Mass Moment of Inertia

Figure 4–2 illustrates the concept of mass moment of inertia. A rectangular object is considered to consist of five point masses ($M_1$–$M_5$), each with a mass of 0.5 kg. The object is free to rotate in the horizontal plane. In this example, the rectangular object is able to rotate separately about two vertical axes of rotation ($Y_1$ and $Y_2$). Distances ($r_1$–$r_5$) are each 0.1 m long, representing the distance between each mass particle ($M_1$–$M_5$) and between the indicated mass particles and the two axes of rotation. The axis of rotation $Y_2$ runs through the center of mass of the entire object ($M_3$). The following calculations demonstrate how the distribution of the mass particles, relative to a given axis of rotation, dramatically affects the mass moment of inertia of the rotating object. Consider $Y_1$ as the axis of rotation. The mass moment of inertia is

determined using Equation 4.1 and substituting known values (see the box). Next, consider $Y_2$ as the axis of rotation. The mass particles are distributed differently if each axis is considered separately. As seen in the calculations, the mass moment of inertia, if considering $Y_2$ as the axis, is 5.5 times less than that if considering $Y_1$ as the axis. One reason for the reduced moment of inertia is that the $M_3$ mass particle, which is coincident with the axis $Y_2$, offers zero resistance to the rotation of the rectangular object. As a general principle, therefore, the mass moment of inertia about an axis of rotation that passes through the center of mass of a body is always smaller than the moment of inertia about any parallel axis.

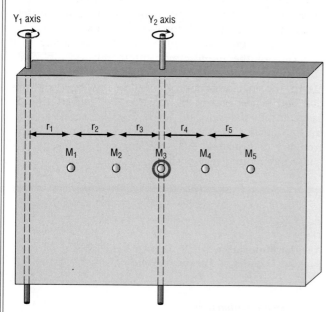

$Y_1$ axis        $Y_2$ axis

$r_1$    $r_2$    $r_3$    $r_4$    $r_5$

$M_1$    $M_2$    $M_3$    $M_4$    $M_5$

**$Y_1$ Axis**

$$I = \sum_{i=1}^{n} m_i r_i^2$$

$$= m_1 r_1^2 + m_2 (r_{1+2})^2 + m_3 (r_{1+2+3})^2 + m_4 (r_{1+2+3+4})^2$$

$$+ m_5 (r_{1+2+3+4+5})^2$$

$$= 0.5 \text{ kg } (0.1 \text{ m})^2 + 0.5 \text{ kg } (0.2 \text{ m})^2 + 0.5 \text{ kg } (0.3 \text{ m})^2$$

$$+ 0.5 \text{ kg } (0.1 \text{ m})^2 + 0.5 \text{ kg } (0.5 \text{ m})^2$$

$$= 0.275 \text{ kgm}^2$$

**$Y_2$ Axis**

$$I = \sum_{i=1}^{n} m_i r_i^2$$

$$= m_1 (r_{2+3})^2 + m_2 (r_3)^2 + m_3 r^2 + m_4 (r_4)^2 + m_5 (r_{4+5})^2$$

$$= 0.5 \text{ kg } (0.2 \text{ m})^2 + 0.5 \text{ kg } (0.1 \text{ m})^2 + 0.5 \text{ kg } (0 \text{ m})^2$$

$$+ 0.5 \text{ kg } (0.1 \text{ m})^2 + 0.5 \text{ kg } (0.2 \text{ m})^2$$

$$= 0.05 \text{ kgm}^2$$

**FIGURE 4–2.** A rectangular object is shown with a potential to rotate about two separate axes of rotation ($Y_1$, $Y_2$). The two sets of calculations associated with each axis of rotation show how the distribution of mass within a body affects the mass momentum of inertia. The object is assumed to consist of five equal mass points ($M_1$–$M_5$), located at set distances ($r_1$–$r_5$) from each other and from the axes of rotation. The center of mass of the entire object is located at $M_3$ (red circle).

Each segment in the human body is made up of different tissues, such as bone, muscle, fat, and skin, and is not of uniform density. This makes calculation of the mass moment of inertia more challenging than the calculation of the mass. Values for the mass moment of inertia for each body segment have been generated from cadaver studies, mathematical modeling, and various imaging techniques.[2,4,7,8,15]

that this term is interchangeable with moment and moment of force.) In this equation, $\Sigma T$ designates the sum of or "net" torques acting to rotate a body. Conceptually, Equation 4.4 defines a *torque-angular acceleration relationship*. Within the musculoskeletal system, the primary torque producer is muscle. The contracting biceps muscle, for example, produces a net flexion torque at the elbow as the hand is accelerated to the mouth. The flexion torque is directly proportional to the angular acceleration of the rotating elbow, as well as directly

proportional to the mass moment of inertia of the rotating forearm and hand segments.

---

**Newton's Second Law of Rotary Motion Quantifying a Torque**

$$\Sigma T = I \times \alpha \qquad \text{(Equation 4.4)}$$

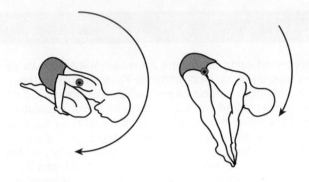

**A  Increased angular
velocity**

**B  Decreased angular
velocity**

**FIGURE 4–3.** A diver illustrates an example of how the mass moment of inertia about a medial-lateral axis (black dot) can be altered through changes in the position of the trunk and extremities. In position A, the diver decreases the mass moment of inertia, which increases the angular velocity of the spin. In position B, a change in the position of the extremities causes a greater mass moment of inertia and decreases the angular velocity of the spin.

### Impulse-Momentum Relationship

Additional relationships can be derived from Newton's second law through the broadening and rearranging of Equations 4.3 and 4.4. One such relationship is specified as the *impulse-momentum relationship.*

Acceleration is the rate of change of velocity ($\Delta$v/t). Substituting this expression for linear acceleration in Equation 4.3 results in Equation 4.5 (see the box). Equation 4.5 can be further rearranged to Equation 4.6. The product of mass and velocity on the right side of Equation 4.6 defines the momentum of a moving body. *Momentum* describes the quantity of motion possessed by a body. Momentum is generally represented by the letter p and is in units kgm/s. The product of force and time on the left side of Equation 4.6 is called an *impulse,* and it measures what is required to change the momentum of a body. The momentum of an object can be changed by a large force delivered for a brief instant or a

small force delivered over a longer time. Equation 4.6 defines the linear *impulse-momentum relationship.*

| | |
|---|---|
| $F = m\,\Delta v/t$ | (Equation 4.5) |
| $Ft = m \times v$ | (Equation 4.6) |

**Linear Momentum (p) = Mass × Linear Velocity**

**Linear Impulse = Force × Time**

The impulse-momentum relationship provides another perspective from which to study human performance, as well as to gain insight into injury mechanisms. The concept of an impulse-momentum relationship is often utilized in the design features of sports and recreation equipment for the purpose of protecting users from injury. Running footwear with shock-absorbing outsoles and bike helmets with protective padding are examples of designs intended to reduce injuries by increasing the time, or duration, of impact in order to minimize the peak force of the impact.

Newton's second law involving torque can apply to the rotary case of the impulse-momentum relationship. Similar to the substitutions and rearrangements for the linear relationship, the angular relationship can be expressed by substitution and rearrangement of Equation 4.4. Substituting $\Delta\omega$/t (change in angular velocity) for $\alpha$ (angular acceleration) results in Equation 4.7 (see the box). Equation 4.7 can be rearranged to Equation 4.8—the angular equivalent of the impulse-momentum relationship.

| | |
|---|---|
| $T = I\,\Delta\omega/t$ | (Equation 4.7) |
| $Tt = I \times \omega$ | (Equation 4.8) |

**Angular Momentum = I × Angular Velocity**
**Angular Impulse = Torque × Time**

### Work-Energy Relationship

To this point, Newton's second law has been described using (1) the force (torque)-acceleration relationships (Equations 4.3 and 4.4), and (2) the impulse-momentum relationships (Equations 4.5 through 4.8). Newton's second law can be restated to provide a *work-energy relationship.* This third approach can be used to study human movement by analyzing the extent to which a force or torque can move or rotate an object over some distance. *Work* (W) in a linear sense is equal to the product of the magnitude of the *force* (F) applied against an object and the *distance* that the object moves in the direction of force while the force is being applied (Equation 4.9 in box). If no movement occurs, no mechanical work is done. The most commonly used units to describe work are equivalent units: the Newton-meter (Nm) and the joule (J). Similar to the linear case, angular work can be defined as the product of the magnitude of the torque (T) applied against the object, and the angular distance in degrees or radians that the object rotates in the direction of torque, while the torque is being applied (Equation 4.10).

---

**SPECIAL  FOCUS  4 – 2**

**Mass Moment of Inertia and Prosthetic Design**

The mass moment of inertia is taken under consideration in prosthetic design for the person with an amputation. The use of lighter components in foot prosthesis, for example, not only reduces the overall mass of the prosthesis, but also results in a change in the distribution of the mass to a more proximal location in the leg. As a result, less resistance is imposed upon the remaining limb during the swing phase of gait. The benefit of these lighter components is realized in terms of lessened energy requirements for the person with an amputation.

## SPECIAL FOCUS 4–3

### A Closer Look at the Impulse-Momentum Relationship

Numerically, an impulse can be calculated as the product of the average force (N) and its time of application. Impulse can also be represented graphically as the area under a force-time curve. Figure 4–4 displays a force-time curve of the horizontal component of the anterior-posterior shear force applied by the ground against the foot *(ground reaction force)* as an individual ran across a force plate embedded in the floor. The curve is biphasic:

the posterior-directed impulse during initial floor contact is negative, and the anterior-directed impulse during propulsion is positive. If the two impulses (i.e., areas under the curves) are equal, the net impulse is zero, and there is no change in the momentum of the system. In this example, however, the posterior-directed impulse is greater than the anterior, indicating that the runner's forward momentum is decreased.

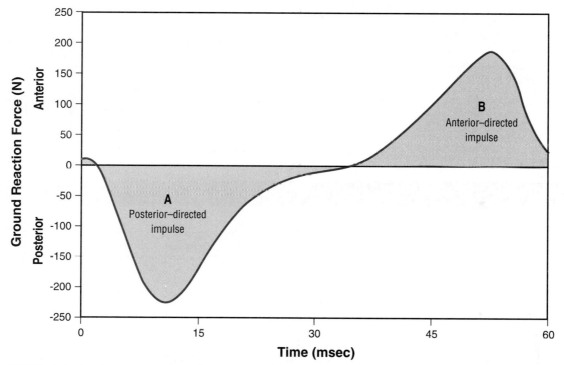

**FIGURE 4–4.** Graphic representation of the areas under a force-time curve showing the (A) posterior-directed and (B) anterior-directed impulses of the horizontal component of the ground reaction force while running.

---

| Work (W) | | |
| --- | --- | --- |
| W (linear) = F × distance | (Equation 4.9) | |
| W (angular) = T × degrees | (Equation 4.10) | |

The work-energy relationship describes mechanical work in terms of the expenditure of energy. Energy can be considered as the measure of the "fuel" available to the system to perform work. The work-energy relationship has been particularly helpful to the study of walking in humans. The mechanical work of walking is often the global indicator of the metabolic demands on the body, without the detailed account of the intricacies of the movement.

The work-energy relationships previously described in Equations 4.9 and 4.10 do not take into account the time

over which the forces or torques are applied. Yet, in most daily activities, it is often the rate at which a force does work that is important. The rate of work is defined as power. The ability for muscles to generate adequate power may be critical to the success of movement or to the understanding of the impact of a treatment intervention. On the basketball court, for example, it is often the speed at which a player can jump for a rebound that determines success. Another example of the importance of the rate of work can be appreciated in an elderly person with Parkinson's disease who must cross a busy street in the time determined by a pedestrian traffic signal.

*Power* (P) is work (W) divided by time (see Equation 4.11 in box on the following page). Because work is the product of force (F) and distance (d), the rate of work can be restated in Equation 4.12 as the product of force and velocity (d/t). Angular power may also be defined as in the linear

**Using Angular Power as a Measure of Muscle Performance**

The concept of angular power is often used as a clinical measure of muscle performance. The mechanical power produced by the quadriceps, for example, is equal to the net internal torque produced by the muscle times the average angular velocity of knee extension. The power is often used to designate the net transfer of energy between active muscles and external loads. *Positive power* reflects the rate of work done by *concentrically active muscles* against an external load. *Negative power,* in contrast, reflects the rate of work done by the external load against *eccentrically active muscles.* This information can be utilized as research and diagnostic tools for comparisons of normal and pathologic function.

case, using the angular analogs of force and velocity, torque (T) and angular velocity ($\omega$), respectively (Equation 4.13).

**Power (P)**

$$P = W/t \qquad \text{(Equation 4.11)}$$

$$P \text{ (linear)} = F \times d/t \text{ or } F \times v \qquad \text{(Equation 4.12)}$$

$$P \text{ (angular)} = T \times \omega \qquad \text{(Equation 4.13)}$$

Table 4–2 summarizes the definitions and units needed to describe many of the physical measurements related to Newton's second law.

## NEWTON'S THIRD LAW: LAW OF ACTION-REACTION

Newton's third law of motion states that for every action there is an equal and opposite reaction. This law implies that every effect one body exerts on another is counteracted by an effect that the second body exerts on the first. The two

**TABLE 4 – 2. Physical Measurements Associated with Newton's Second Law**

| Physical Measurement | Linear Application | | Rotational Application | |
|---|---|---|---|---|
| | *Definition* | *Units* | *Definition* | *Units* |
| Distance | Linear displacement | Meter (m) | Angular displacement | Degrees (°)* |
| Velocity | Rate of linear displacement | Meters per second (m/s) | Rate of angular displacement | °/s |
| Acceleration | Rate of change in linear velocity | m/s² | Rate of change in angular velocity | °/s² |
| Mass | Quantity of matter in an object; influences the object's resistance to a change in linear velocity | kilogram (kg) | Not applicable | |
| Mass moment of inertia | Not applicable | | Quantity *and* distribution of matter in an object; influences an object's resistance to a change in angular velocity | kgm² |
| Force | A push or pull; mass times linear acceleration | kgm/s² (N) | Not applicable | |
| Torque | Not applicable | | A force times a moment arm; mass moment of inertia times angular acceleration | kgm²°/s² (or Nm) |
| Impulse | Force times time | Ns | Torque times time | Nms |
| Momentum | Mass times linear velocity | kgm/s | Mass moment of inertia times angular velocity | kgm²°/s |
| Work | Force times linear displacement | Nm (joules) | Torque times angular displacement | Nm (joules) |
| Power | Rate of linear work | Nm/s or J/s (watts) | Rate of angular work | Nm/s or J/s (watts) |

* Radians, which are unitless, may be used instead of degrees.

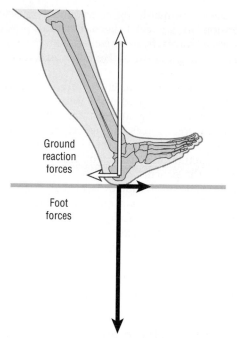

Ground
reaction
forces

Foot
forces

**FIGURE 4–5.** The forces between the ground and foot are depicted during the early part of the walking cycle. The ground reaction forces (red arrows) act superiorly and posteriorly, whereas the foot forces (black arrows) act inferiorly and anteriorly.

bodies interact simultaneously, and the consequence is specified by the law of acceleration: $\Sigma F = ma$. That is, each body experiences a different effect and that effect depends on its mass. For example, a person who falls off the roof of a second-story building exerts a force on the ground, and the ground exerts an equal and opposite force on the person. Because of the discrepancies in mass between the ground and the person, the effect, or acceleration experienced by the person, is much greater than the effect "experienced" by the ground. As a result, the person may sustain significant injury.

Perhaps the most direct application of Newton's law of action-reaction is the reaction force provided by the surface upon which one is walking. The foot produces a force against the ground owing to the accelerations of all superincumbent body segments. In accord with Newton's third law, the ground generates a *ground reaction force* in the opposite direction but of equal magnitude (Fig. 4–5). The ground reaction force changes in magnitude, direction, and point of application on the foot/shoe throughout the period of gait. Ground reaction forces can be measured via force platforms (see section on Kinematic and Kinetic Measurement Systems later in this chapter), and the forces are commonly used as input data for the quantitative analysis of human motion.

## INTRODUCTION TO MOVEMENT ANALYSIS: SETTING THE BACKGROUND

The previous section describes the nature of the cause and effect relationship between force and motion as outlined by Newton's laws. Although it may be relatively simple to con-

ceptualize the role of muscles in human movement, it is also important to understand the added impact of gravity and other external forces. The observation and analysis of movement must take into consideration the net effect of muscle activity, the resulting internal forces, as well as all the external forces on the quantity and quality of motion. The following section illustrates methods for basic analysis of movement, beginning with an introduction to anthropometry— the measurement of the design characteristics of the human body. This section also demonstrates how changes in external forces and torques can have an impact on muscle response, joint motion, and joint reaction force.

## Anthropometry

Anthropometry is derived from the Greek root *anthropos* (man) and *metron* (measure). In the context of human movement analysis, anthropometry may be broadly defined as the measurement of certain physical design features of the human body, such as length, mass, volume, density, center of mass, radius of gyration, and mass moment of inertia. These body segment parameters are essential to conduction of kinematic and kinetic analyses for both normal and pathologic motion. Analysis of movement frequently requires information regarding the mass of individual segments or the distribution of mass within a given segment. These factors determine the inertial properties that muscles must overcome to generate movement. Anthropometric information is also valuable in the design of the work environment, furniture, tools, and sports equipment.

Much of the information regarding the body segments' center of mass and mass moment of inertia has been derived from cadaver studies.[4] Refer to Table 1 in Appendix IA for anthropometric data on weights of different body segments and locations of the centers of mass. Other methods for deriving this information have included mathematical modeling and imaging techniques, such as computed tomography and magnetic resonance imaging.

## Free Body Diagram

The analysis of movement requires that all forces that act on the body be taken into account. Prior to any analysis, a *free body diagram* is constructed to facilitate the process of solving biomechanical problems. The free body diagram is a "snapshot" or simplified sketch that represents the interaction between a system and its environment. The system under consideration may be a single rigid segment, such as the foot, or it may be several segments, such as the head, arms, and trunk. These can be regarded together as a single rigid system.

A free body diagram requires that all relevant forces acting upon the system are carefully drawn. These forces may be produced by muscle; gravity, as reflected in the weight of the segment; fluid; air resistance; friction; and ground reaction forces. Arrows are used to indicate force vectors.

How a free body diagram is defined depends on the intended purpose of the analysis. Consider the example presented in Figure 4–6. In this example, the free body diagram represents the *external forces* acting on the body of an individual during the push off, or the propulsive, phase of

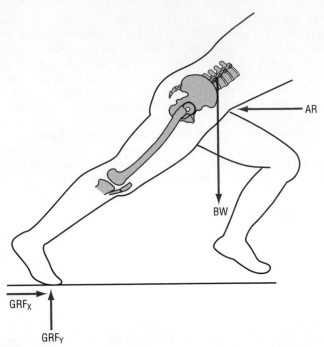

**FIGURE 4–6.** A free body diagram of a sprinter. The external forces on the system include the force due to the body weight (BW) of the runner and contact forces: the ground reaction force (GRF) in vertical (Y) and horizontal directions (X), and the force created by air resistance (AR). (The force vectors are not drawn to scale.)

running. In this example, the "system" under consideration is defined as the lower trunk and lower extremities. The external force vectors include the weight of the combined body segments, which have been reduced to a single vector referred to as body weight (BW), and the contact forces. The contact forces include the ground reaction forces (GRF), in both vertical (Y) and horizontal (X) directions, and the air resistance (AR).

The system so described can be specified differently, depending on the analysis. Assume that it is of interest to examine the major vertical forces acting on the foot and ankle region while standing on tiptoes (Fig. 4–7). The system of interest is redefined as the foot, and it is represented as a simplified single rigid link that is isolated from the remainder of the body. The free body diagram involves figuratively "cutting through" the desired joint. The effects of muscle force are usually distinguished from the effects of other soft tissues, such as the joint capsule and ligaments. Although the contribution of the individual muscles acting across a joint may be determined, a single resultant muscle force (MF) vector is often used to represent the sum total of all muscle forces. In order to complete the free body diagram, the ground reaction force (GRF) and weight of the foot (FW) are indicated in a manner similar to that described for the analysis in Figure 4–6.

As shown in the free body diagram of Figure 4–7, an additional contact force is identified: the *joint reaction force (JRF)*. The term reaction implies that one joint surface pushes back against the other joint surface. The joint reaction force represents the net or cumulative effect of forces transmitted from one segment to another.[5] Joint reaction

forces are caused primarily by activation of muscle and by passive tension in stretched ligaments and gravity (body weight). Passive forces from stretched soft tissues are relatively small in magnitude and are often excluded from the analysis.

Clinically, reducing joint reaction force is a major focus in treatment programs designed to lessen pain and prevent joint degeneration. Frequently, treatments are directed toward reducing joint forces through changes in the magnitude of muscle activity and their activation patterns or through a reduction in the weight transmitted through a joint. Consider the patient with osteoarthritis of the hip joint as an example. The magnitude of joint reaction force may be decreased by having the person reduce walking velocity, thereby lessening the magnitude of muscle activation. Alternatively, a cane may be used to reduce forces through the hip joint.[11] If obesity is a factor, a weight-reduction program could be recommended.

## INITIAL STEPS FOR SETTING UP THE FREE BODY DIAGRAM

The key elements needed to begin problem solving in human movement are to determine the purpose of the analysis, identify the body, and indicate all the forces that act on that body. The following example presents steps to assist with construction of a free body diagram.

Consider the situation in which an individual is holding a weight out to the side, as shown in Figure 4–8. This system is assumed to be in static equilibrium, and the sum of all opposing forces and torques are equal. One goal of the analysis might be to determine how much muscle force is required by the glenohumeral joint abductor muscles to keep the arm abducted to 90 degrees; another goal might be to determine the magnitude of the glenohumeral joint reaction force during this same activity.

*Step I,* in setting up the free body diagram, is to identify and isolate the system under consideration. In this example, the system is the entire arm and weight combination.

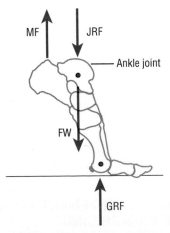

**FIGURE 4–7.** A free body diagram of the system defined as the foot. The following vertical forces are shown: resultant plantar flexor muscle force (MF); joint reaction force (JRF); weight of foot (FW); and ground reaction force (GRF). Vectors are not drawn to scale.

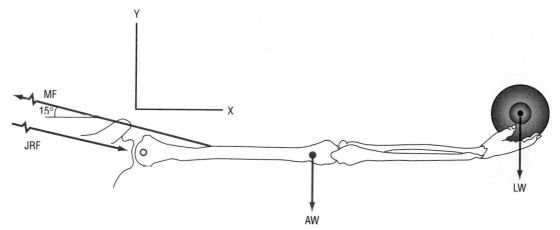

**FIGURE 4–8.** Free body diagram isolating the system as a right arm and weight combination: resultant shoulder abductor muscle force (MF); glenohumeral joint reaction force (JRF); arm weight (AW); and load weight (LW). The axis of rotation is shown as an open red circle at the glenohumeral joint. (Modified from LeVeau BF: Williams & Lissner's Biomechanics of Human Motion, 3rd ed. Philadelphia, WB Saunders, 1992.)

*Step II* involves setting up a reference frame that allows the position and movement of a body to be defined with respect to a known point, location, or axis (see Fig. 4–8, X-Y reference). More detail on establishing a reference frame is discussed in the next section.

*Step III* illustrates the internal and external forces that act on the system. Internal forces are those produced by muscle (MF). External forces include the gravitational pull of both the weight of the load (LW), as well as the weight of the arm (AW). The external forces are drawn on the figure at the approximate point of application of these forces. The location of the vector (AW) acts at the center of mass of the upper extremity and is determined using anthropometric data, such as those presented in Appendix IA.

The direction of the internal MF is drawn in a direction that opposes the potential motion produced by the external forces. In this example, the rotation produced by the external forces, AW and LW together with their moment arms, tends to move the arm in a clockwise or adduction direction. Thus, the line-of-force of MF, in combination with its moment arm, tends to rotate the arm in a counterclockwise or abduction direction.

*Step IV* of the procedure is to show the contact forces that act on the system. Because this system is assumed to be in static equilibrium, contact forces such as air resistance are ignored. Another contact force to consider is a push or pull applied to the external aspect of the body, such as the manual resistance delivered by a therapist or by an opposing player in a sporting event. In this example, the only relevant contact force is the joint reaction force (JRF) created across the glenohumeral articulation. Initially, the direction of the joint force may not be known but, as explained later, is typically drawn in a direction opposite to the pull of the dominant muscle force. The precise direction of the JRF can be determined after static analysis is carried out and unknown variables are calculated. This method of analysis is discussed in detail in the following section of this chapter. The box summarizes the key steps in setting up the free body diagram.

> **Initial Steps in Setting Up the Free Body Diagram**
>
> *Step I:* Identify and isolate the system under consideration.
>
> *Step II:* Establish a reference frame.
>
> *Step III:* Illustrate the internal (muscular) and external (gravitational) forces that act on the system.
>
> *Step IV:* Illustrate the contact forces that act on the system, typically including the joint reaction force.

## REFERENCE FRAMES

In order to accurately describe motion or solve for unknown forces, a reference frame and an associated coordinate system need to be established. This information allows the position and movement direction of a body, a segment, or an object to be defined with respect to some known point, location, or segment's axis of rotation. If a reference frame and coordinate system are not identified, it becomes very difficult to interpret and compare measurements in clinical and research settings.

A reference frame is arbitrarily established and may be placed inside or outside the body. Reference frames used to describe position or motion may be considered either relative or global. A *relative reference frame* describes the position of one limb segment with respect to an adjacent segment, such as the foot relative to the leg, the forearm relative to the upper arm, or the trunk relative to the thigh, as shown in Figure 4–9A. A measurement is made by comparing motion between an anatomic landmark or coordinates of one segment with an anatomic landmark or coordinates of a second segment. Goniometry provides one example of a relative coordinate system used in clinical practice. Elbow joint range of motion, for example, describes a measurement using a relative reference frame defined by the long axes of the upper arm and forearm segments, with an axis of rotation through the elbow.

Relative reference frames, however, lack the information needed to define motion with respect to a fixed point or

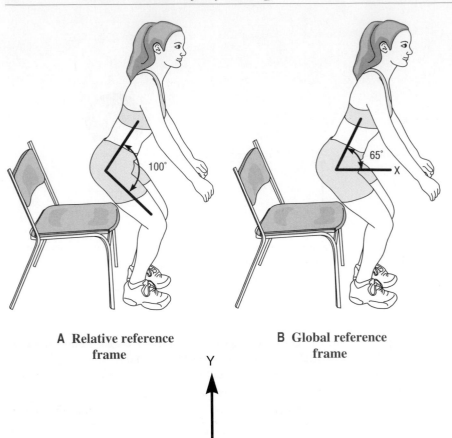

**A  Relative reference
frame**

**B  Global reference
frame**

**FIGURE 4–9.** Two types of reference frames. *A* depicts a relative reference frame showing the trunk rotated 100 degrees relative to the thigh; *B* depicts a global reference frame showing the trunk rotated 65 degrees with respect to the horizontal plane (X).

location in space. To analyze motion with respect to the ground, direction of gravity, or another type of externally defined reference frame in space, a *global or laboratory reference frame* must be defined. The position of the trunk with respect to a horizontal reference is an example of a measurement made with respect to a global reference frame (Fig. 4–9*B*).

Use of one type of reference frame over another may result in different outcome measures. Figure 4–9 illustrates how a relative and global reference frame can be used to describe the position of the trunk during the sit-to-stand activity, but the outcome measures are different. The use of two distinct reference frames for describing the same "snapshot" of an activity, but having different results, emphasizes the importance of identifying the reference frame when describing human movement.

Whether motion is measured via a relative or global reference frame, the location of a point or segment in space can be specified using a coordinate system. In human movement analysis, the *Cartesian coordinate system* is most frequently employed. The Cartesian system utilizes coordinates for locating a point on a plane by identifying the distance of the point from each of two intersecting lines or, in space, by the distance from each of three planes intersecting at a point. This system, therefore, is either two-dimensional (2D) or three-dimensional (3D). A 2D system is defined by two imaginary axes arranged perpendicular to each other. The two axes (X, Y) are usually positioned such that one is

horizontal (X) and the other vertical (Y), although they may be oriented in any manner that facilitates quantitative solutions. A 2D system is frequently utilized when the motion being described is predominantly planar (i.e., in one plane), such as knee flexion and extension during gait.

In most cases, human motion occurs in more than one plane. Even the knee, whose motion is considered to occur predominantly in the sagittal plane while walking, also undergoes small rotations in both horizontal and frontal planes. In order to adequately describe the motions that occur in more than one plane, a 3D reference system is necessary. A 3D system has three axes, each perpendicular or *orthogonal* to each other. In contrast to the planar description of the 2D system, the coordinates in a 3D system can designate any point or vector in space relative to the X, Y, and Z axes.

A coordinate system needs to indicate direction of motion as well as position—in both a linear and a rotational sense. By convention, most coordinate systems are constructed such that linear movements to the right, up, and forward are defined as positive, whereas movements to the left, down, and backward are negative. The direction of a force producing a motion can be defined by the direction that the object is being accelerated. Rotary or angular movements are described in the plane (sagittal, frontal, horizontal) that a segment is moving, which is perpendicular to the axis of rotation. A segment's rotation direction may be described as clockwise or counterclockwise or as flexion or extension (see Chapter 1), depending on the situation. In this text, the

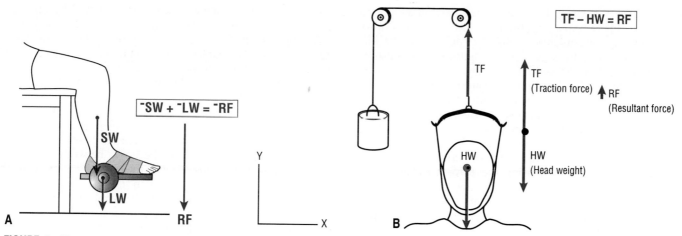

**FIGURE 4–10.** Vector composition of parallel, coplanar forces. *A,* Two force vectors are acting on the knee: the segment (leg) weight (SW) and the load weight (LW) applied at the ankle. These forces are added to determine the resultant force (RF). The negative sign indicates a downward pull. *B,* The weight of the head (HW) and traction force (TF) act along the same line but in opposite directions. The resultant force (RF) is the algebraic sum of these vectors.

direction of the torque that is producing a rotation is designated by the direction (e.g., counterclockwise, flexion) of the segment being accelerated. A more mathematically based convention for designating the direction of a torque uses the *right-hand rule.*[5] This convention is described in Appendix IB.

In closing, 3D analysis is more complicated than 2D analysis, but it does provide a more comprehensive profile of human movement. There are excellent resources available that describe techniques for conducting 3D analysis, and some of these references are provided at the end of the chapter.[1,3,17,18] The quantitative analysis discussed in this chapter focuses on 2D analysis techniques.

## Representing Forces

Force vectors can be represented in different manners, depending on the context of the analysis. Several vectors can be combined to represent a single vector. This method of representation is called *vector composition.* Alternatively, a single vector may be resolved or "decomposed" into several components. This technique is termed *vector resolution.*

The representation of vectors using composition and resolution provides the means of understanding how forces rotate or translate body segments and subsequently cause rotation, compression, shear, or distraction at the joint surfaces.

Composition and resolution of forces can be accomplished using graphic methods of analysis or right-angle trigonometry. These techniques are needed to represent and subsequently calculate muscle and joint forces.

### GRAPHIC METHODS OF FORCE ANALYSIS

#### *Composition of Forces*

Vector composition allows several parallel, coplanar forces to be simply combined graphically as a single *resultant force* (Fig. 4–10). In Figure 4–10A, the weight of the leg segment (SW) and the weight of the load (LW) are added graphically

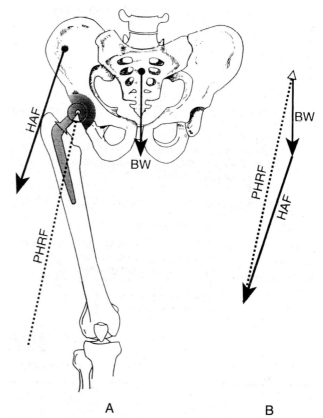

**FIGURE 4–11.** *A,* Three forces are shown acting on a pelvis that is involved in single-limb standing over a right prosthetic hip joint. The forces are hip abductor force (HAF), body weight (BW), and prosthetic hip reaction force (PHRF). *B,* The polygon (or "tip-to-tail") method is used to determine the magnitude and direction of the PHRF, based on the magnitude and direction of HAF and BW. (From Neumann DA: Hip abductor muscle activity in persons who walk with a hip prosthesis while using a cane and carrying a load. Phys Ther 79:1163–1176, 1999, with permission of the Physical Therapy Association.)

by means of a ruler and a scale factor determined for the vectors. In this example, the resultant force (RF) acts downward and has the tendency to distract (pull apart) the knee joint, if unopposed by other forces. Figure 4–10B illustrates a cervical traction device that employs a weighted pulley system, acting in the direction opposite to the force created by the weight of the head. Simple addition yields the value of the resultant force. The positive sign of RF indicates a slight net upward distraction force on the head and neck.

Force vectors acting on a body may be coplanar, but they may not always act parallel. In this case, the individual vectors may be composed using the *polygon method.* Figure 4–11 illustrates how the polygon method can be applied to a frontal plane model to estimate the reaction force on a prosthetic hip while standing on one limb. With the arrows drawn in proportion to their magnitude and in the correct orientation, the vectors of body weight (BW) and hip abductor force (HAF) are added in a "tip-to-tail" fashion (Fig. 4–11B). The combined effect of the BW and HAF vectors is determined by placing the tail of the HAF vector to the tip of the BW vector. Completing the polygon yields the resultant prosthetic hip reaction force (PHRF), showing its magnitude and direction (see Fig. 4–11B, dotted line). In this case, the resultant vector represents a reaction force and, therefore, is directed in a sense that opposes the sum of the other two vectors.

A *parallelogram* can also be constructed to determine the resultant of two coplanar but nonparallel forces. Instead of placing the force vectors tip-to-tail, as discussed in the previous example, the resultant vector can be found by drawing a parallelogram based on the magnitude and direction of the two component force vectors. Figure 4–12A provides an illustration of the parallelogram method to combine several component vectors into one resultant vector. The component force vectors, $F_1$ and $F_2$ (black solid arrows), are generated by the pull of the flexor digitorum superficialis and profundus, as they pass palmar (anterior) to the metacarpophalangeal joint. The diagonal, originating at the intersection of $F_1$ and $F_2$, represents the resultant force (RF) (see Fig. 4–12A, thick red arrow). Because of the angle between $F_1$ and $F_2$, the resultant force tends to raise the tendons away from the joint. Clinically, this phenomenon is described as a *bowstringing force* due to the tendons' resemblance to a pulled cord connected to the two ends of a bow. In rheumatoid arthritis, the bowstringing force may rupture the ligaments and dislocate the metacarpophalangeal joints (Fig. 4–12B).

In many cases, especially when analyzing muscle forces, the parallelogram method can be described as a rectangle, such that the components of the resultant force are oriented at right angles to each other. As shown in Figure 4–13, the two right-angle forces are referred to as *normal* and *tangential components* ($MF_N$ and $MF_T$). The hypotenuse of the right triangle is the resultant muscle force (MF).

In summary, when two or more forces applied to a segment are combined into a single resultant force, the magnitude of the resultant force is considered equal to the sum of the component vectors. The resultant force can be determined graphically as summarized in the box.

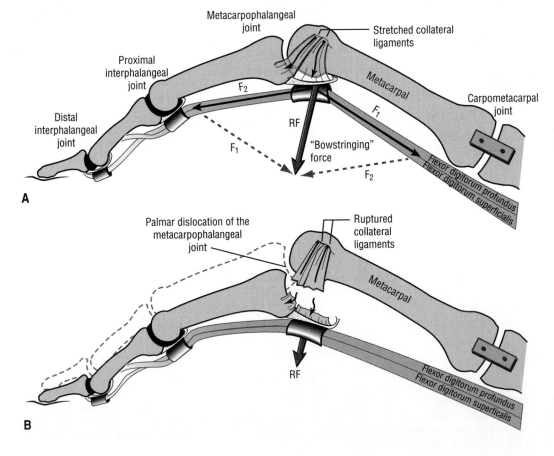

**FIGURE 4–12.** *A,* Parallelogram method is used to illustrate the effect of two force vectors ($F_1$ and $F_2$) produced by contraction of the flexor digitorum superficialis and profundus muscles across the metacarpophalangeal (MCP) joint. The resultant force (RF) vector creates a bowstringing force on the connective tissues at the MCP joint. *B,* In a digit with rheumatoid arthritis, the resultant force can, over time, rupture ligaments and cause palmar dislocation of the metacarpophalangeal joint.

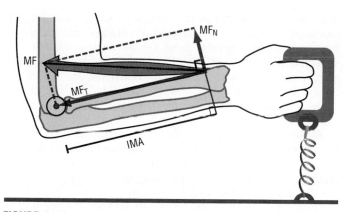

**FIGURE 4–13.** The muscle force (MF) produced by the brachioradialis is represented as the hypotenuse (diagonal) of the rectangle. The normal force (MF$_N$) and tangential force (MF$_T$) are also indicated. The internal moment arm (IMA) is the perpendicular distance between the axis of rotation (red circle) and (MF$_N$).

> **Summary of How to Graphically Compose Force Vectors**
> * Parallel forces vectors can be combined by using simple vector addition (Fig. 4–10).
> * Nonparallel, coplanar force vectors can be composed by using the polygon ("tip-to-tail") method (Fig. 4–11), or the parallelogram method (Figs. 4–12 and 4–13).

## Resolution of Forces

The previous section illustrates the composition method of representing forces, whereby multiple coplanar forces acting on a body are replaced by a single resultant force. In many clinical situations, a knowledge of the effect of the *individual components* that produce the resultant force may be more relevant to an understanding of the impact of these forces on joint motion and joint loading, as well as developing specific treatment strategies. *Vector resolution* is the process of replacing a single resultant force by two or more forces that, when combined, are equivalent to the original resultant force.

One of the most useful applications of the resolution of forces involves the description and calculation of the rectangular components of a muscle force. As depicted in Figure 4–13, the rectangular components of the muscle force are shown at right angles to each other and are referred to as the normal and tangential components (MF$_N$ and MF$_T$). The normal component represents the component of the muscle's resultant force that acts perpendicularly to the long axis of the body segment. Because of the internal moment arm (see Chapter 1) associated with this force component, one effect of the normal force of a muscle is to cause a rotation (i.e., produce a torque). The normal force may also cause a translation of the bony segment.

The tangential component represents the component of the muscle's resultant force that is directed parallel to the long axis of the body segment. The effect of this force is to compress and stabilize the joint or, in some cases, distract or separate the segments forming the joint. The tangential component of a muscle force does not produce a torque when it

passes through the axis of rotation because it has no moment arm (see Fig. 4–13, MF$_T$). Table 4–3 summarizes the characteristics of the tangential and normal force components of a muscle, as in Figure 4–13.

### Contrasting Internal versus External Forces and Torques

The examples presented to this point on methods of resolving forces into normal and tangential components have focused on the forces and torques produced by muscle. As described in Chapter 1, muscles, by definition, produce internal forces or torques. The resolution of forces into normal and tangential components can also be applied to *external forces* acting on the human body, such as those from gravity, external load or weight, and manual resistance, as applied by a clinician. In the presence of an external moment arm, external forces produce an *external torque*. Generally, in the condition of equilibrium, the external torque acts about the joint's axis of rotation in the opposite direction to a given internal torque.

Figure 4–14 illustrates the resolution of both internal and external forces for an individual who is performing an isometric knee extension exercise. Three resultant forces are depicted in Figure 4–14A: knee extensor muscle force (MF), leg segment weight (SW), and external load weight (LW) applied at the ankle. The weight of the leg segment and external load acts at the center of the respective masses. Figure 4–14B shows the resultant internal forces and external forces broken into their normal and tangential components.

### Influence of Changing the Angle of the Joint

The relative magnitude of the normal and tangential components of force applied to a bone depends on the position of the limb segment. Consider first how the change in angular position of a joint alters the *angle-of-insertion of the muscle* (see Chapter 1). Figure 4–15 shows the biceps muscle force (MF) at four different elbow joint positions, each with a different angle-of-insertion ($\alpha$) to the forearm. Each angle-of-

**TABLE 4–3. Normal versus Tangential Force Components of a Muscle Force**

| Normal Force Component | Tangential Force Component |
|---|---|
| Acts perpendicular to a bony segment | Acts parallel to a bony segment |
| Often indicated as F$_N$ but may be indicated as F$_Y$, depending on the choice of the reference frame | Often indicated as F$_T$ but may be indicated as F$_X$, depending on the choice of the reference frame |
| Can cause rotation and/or translation: A rotation may occur if the moment arm > 0. A translation may occur as a compression, distraction, or shearing between articulating surfaces. | A translation may occur as a compression or distraction between articulating surfaces. |

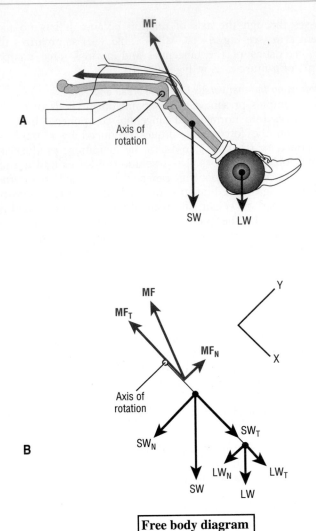

**FIGURE 4–14.** Resolution of internal forces (red) and external forces (black) for an individual performing an isometric knee extension exercise. *A,* The following resultant force vectors are depicted: muscle force (MF) of the knee extensors; leg segment weight (SW); and load weight (LW) applied at the ankle. *B,* A free body diagram shows the resultant vectors resolved into their rectangular components: normal component of the muscle force ($MF_N$); tangential component of the muscle force ($MF_T$); normal component of the segment weight ($SW_N$); tangential component of the segment weight ($SW_T$); normal component of the load weight ($LW_N$); and tangential component of the load weight ($LW_T$). In both *A* and *B,* the open red circles mark the medial-lateral axis of rotation at the knee. Note that the XY reference frame is rotated so that tangential forces are oriented in the X direction and normal forces are oriented in the Y direction. (Vectors are not drawn to scale.)

insertion results in a different combination of tangential ($MF_T$) and normal ($MF_N$) force components. The tangential forces create compression or distraction forces at the elbow. By acting with an internal moment arm (IMA), the normal forces also generate an internal torque (i.e., potential rotation) at a joint. As shown in Figure 4–15*A,* a relatively small angle-of-insertion favors a relatively larger tangential force, which directs a larger percentage of the total muscle

force to compress the joint surfaces of the elbow. Because the angle-of-insertion is less than 45 degrees, the tangential force exceeds the normal force. At an angle-of-insertion of 45 degrees, the tangential and normal forces are equal, with each about 71% of the resultant. When the angle-of-insertion of the muscle reaches 90 degrees (Fig. 4–15*B*), 100% of the total force is available to rotate the joint and produce a torque.

As shown in Figure 4–15*C,* the magnitude of the force components continues to change as elbow flexion continues. The 135-degree angle-of-insertion produces equal tangential and normal force components, each about 71% of the resultant. Because the tangential force is now directed away from the joint, it produces a distracting or separating force on the joint. As the angle-of-insertion exceeds 135 degrees (Fig. 4–15*D*), the tangential force component exceeds the normal force component.

In Figure 4–15*A* through *D,* the internal torque is the product of $MF_N$ and the internal moment arm (IMA). Because $MF_N$ changes with angle-of-insertion, the magnitude of an internal torque naturally changes throughout the range of motion. This concept helps explain why people have greater strength at certain locations throughout the joint's range of motion. The torque-generating capabilities of the muscle depend not only on the angle-of-insertion, and subsequent magnitude of $MF_N$, but also on other physiologic factors, discussed in Chapter 3. These include muscle length, activation type (i.e., isometric, concentric, or eccentric), and speed of muscle activation.

Changes in joint angle also affect the external or "resistance" end of the musculoskeletal system. Returning to the example of the isometric knee extension exercise, Figure 4–16 shows how a change in knee joint angle affects the normal component of the external forces. The external torque experienced by the exercising person is equal to the product of the external moment arm (EMA) and the normal component of the external forces ($LW_N$ or $SW_N$). In Figure 4–16*A,* no external torque exists in the sagittal plane because the SW and LW force vectors pass through the axis of rotation and, therefore, have no moment arm. Figure 4–16*B* through *C* shows how a greater external torque is placed against the individual with the knee fully extended compared with the knee flexed 45 degrees. Although the external forces, SW and LW, are the same in all three cases, the external torque is greatest when the knee is in full extension. As a general principle, the external torque applied against a joint is greatest when the resultant external force vector intersects the bone or body segment at a right angle.

## ANALYTIC METHODS OF FORCE ANALYSIS

Thus far, the composition and resolution of forces are primarily described using a graphic method to determine the magnitude of forces. A drawback to this method is that it requires a high degree of precision to accurately represent the forces analyzed. In the solution of problems involving rectangular components, "right-angle trigonometry" provides a more accurate method of force analysis. The trigonometric functions are based on the relationship that exists between the angles and sides of a right triangle. Refer to Appendix IC for a review of this material.

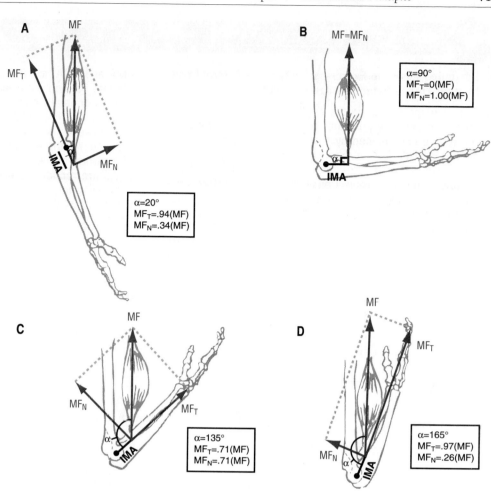

**FIGURE 4–15.** Changing the angle of the elbow joint alters the angle of insertion ($\alpha$) of the muscle into the forearm. These changes, in turn, alter the magnitude of the normal ($MF_N$) and tangential ($MF_T$) components of the biceps muscle force (MF). The proportion of $MF_N$ and $MF_T$ to MF are listed in each of the four boxes: *A*, angle-of-insertion of 20 degrees; *B*, angle-of-insertion of 90 degrees; *C*, angle-of-insertion of 135 degrees; and *D*, angle of insertion of 165 degrees. The internal moment arm (IMA) is drawn as a black line, extending from the axis of rotation to the perpendicular intersection with $MF_N$. The IMA remains constant throughout *A* to *D*. (Modified from LeVeau BF: Williams & Lissner's Biomechanics of Human Motion, 3rd ed. Philadelphia, WB Saunders, 1992.)

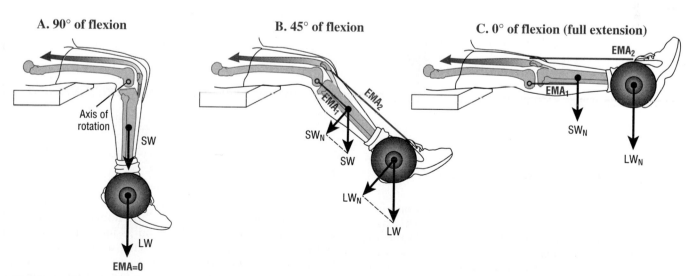

**A. 90° of flexion**

**B. 45° of flexion**

**C. 0° of flexion (full extension)**

**FIGURE 4–16.** A change in knee joint angle affects the magnitude of the normal component of the *external forces* generated by the leg segment weight (SW) and load weight (LW) applied at the ankle. The normal components of LW and SW are indicated as $LW_N$ and $SW_N$, respectively. Different external torques are experienced at different knee angles. The largest external torques are generated when the knee is in full extension (C), since $SW_N$ and $LW_N$ are largest and equal to the full magnitude of SW and LW, respectively. No external torques are produced when the knee is flexed 90 degrees (A), since $SW_N$ and $LW_N$ are zero. ($EMA_1$ is equal to the external moment arm for $SW_N$; $EMA_2$ is equal to the external moment arm for $LW_N$.)

### Designing Resistive Exercises So That the External and Internal Torque Potentials Are Optimally Matched

The concept of altering the angle of a joint is frequently utilized in exercise programs to adjust the magnitude of resistance experienced by the patient or client. It is often desirable to design an exercise program so that *the external torque matches the internal torque potential* of the muscle or muscle group. Consider a person performing a "biceps curl" exercise shown in Figure 4–17A. With the elbow flexed to 90 degrees, both the internal and external torque potentials are greatest, because the product of each resultant force (MF and LW) and their moment arms

(IMA and EMA) are maximal. At this unique elbow position the internal and external torque potentials are maximal as well as optimally matched. As the elbow position is altered in Figure 4–17B, the external torque remains maximal; however, the internal torque potential is significantly reduced. As the elbow approaches extension, the angle-of-insertion of the muscle and the normal muscle force ($MF_N$) are reduced, thereby decreasing the potential for generating internal torque. A person with significant weakness of the elbow flexor muscle may have difficulty holding an object in position *B*, but may have no difficulty holding the same object in position *A*.

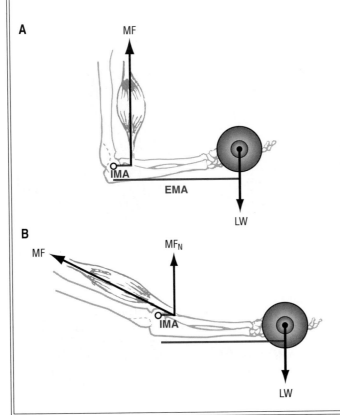

**FIGURE 4–17.** Changing the angle of elbow flexion alters both the internal and external torque potential. *A,* The 90-degree position of the elbow maximizes the potential for both the internal and external torque. *B,* With the elbow closer to extension, the external torque remains maximal, but the internal torque potential (i.e., the product of $MF_N$ and IMA) is reduced. (MF is equal to muscle force; $MF_N$, normal component of muscle force; IMA, internal moment arm; LW, load weight; EMA, external moment arm.) (Modified from LeVeau BF: Williams & Lissner's Biomechanics of Human Motion, 3rd ed. Philadelphia, WB Saunders, 1992.)

### Comparing Two Methods for Determining Torque about a Joint

In the context of kinesiology, a torque is the effect of a force tending to move a body segment about a joint's axis of rotation. *Torque is the rotary equivalent of a force.* Mathematically, torque is the product of a force and its moment arm and has units of Nm. Torque is a vector quantity, having both magnitude and direction.

Two methods for determining torque yield identical mathematical solutions. The methods apply to both internal and external torque, assuming that the system in question is in rotational equilibrium (i.e., the angular acceleration about the joint is zero).

### Internal Torque

The first method for determining internal torque is illustrated in Figure 4–18 (black letters). The internal torque is depicted as the product of $MF_N$ (the normal component of the resultant muscle force (MF) and its internal moment arm ($IMA_1$)). The second method, depicted in red letters in Figure 4–18, does not require the resultant force to be resolved into rectangular components. In this method, internal torque is calculated as the product of the resultant force (MF) and $IMA_2$ (i.e., the internal moment arm that extends between the axis of rotation and a perpendicular intersection with MF). Both methods yield the same internal torque because both satisfy the definition of a torque (i.e., the product of a

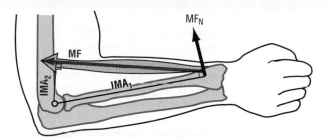

$$\text{Internal Torque: } MF_N \times IMA_1 = MF \times IMA_2$$

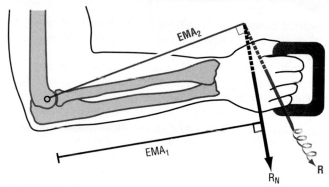

$$\text{External Torque: } R_N \times EMA_1 = R \times EMA_2$$

**FIGURE 4–18.** The internal (muscle-produced) flexion torque at the elbow can be determined using two different methods. The first method (shown in black letters) is expressed as the product of the normal force of the muscle ($MF_N$) times its internal moment arm ($IMA_1$). The second method (shown in red letters) is expressed as the product of the resultant force of the muscle (MF) times its internal moment arm ($IMA_2$). Both expressions yield equivalent internal torques. The axis of rotation is depicted as the open black circle at the elbow.

**FIGURE 4–19.** An external torque is applied to the elbow through a resistance generated by tension in a cable (R). The weight of the body segment is ignored. The external torque can be determined using two different methods. The first method (shown in black letters) is expressed as the product of the normal force of the resistance ($R_N$) times its external moment arm ($EMA_1$). The second method, shown in red letters, is expressed as the product of resultant force of the resistance (R) times its external moment arm ($EMA_2$). Both expressions yield equivalent external torques. The axis of rotation is depicted as the open black circle through the elbow.

force and its associated moment arm). *The associated force and moment arm for any given torque must intersect one another at a 90-degree angle.*

### External Torque

Figure 4–19 shows an external torque applied to the elbow through a resistance produced by a cable (depicted as R). The weight of the body segment is ignored in this example. The first method for determining external torque is shown in black letters. External torque is depicted as the product of $R_N$ (the normal component of the cable's resistive force)

times its external moment arm ($EMA_1$). The second method, shown in red letters, uses the product of the cable's resultant resistive force (R) and its external moment arm ($EMA_2$). As with internal torque, both methods yield the same external torque because both satisfy the definition a torque (i.e., the product of a resistance (external) force and its associated external moment arm).

### A "Shortcut" Method of Estimating Relative Torque Potential

The second method used to measure internal and external torques, depicted in red letters in Figures 4–18 and 4–19, respectively, is considered a "shortcut" because it is not necessary to resolve the resultant forces into their component forces. Consider first *internal torque* (see Fig. 4–18). The relative internal moment arm (depicted as $IMA_2$)—or leverage—of most muscles in the body can be qualitatively assessed by simply visualizing the shortest distance between a given whole muscle and the associated joint's axis of rotation. This experience can be practiced with the aid of a skeletal model and a piece of string that represents the resultant muscle's line-of-force (Fig. 4–20). As apparent in the figure, the moment arm is greater in position *A* than in position *B*; not coincidentally, the maximal internal torque of the elbow flexors is also greater in position *A* than in position *B*. In general, the

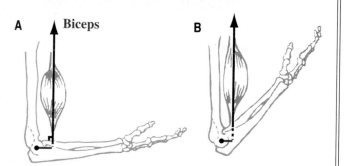

**FIGURE 4–20.** A piece of black string is used to mimic the line-of-force of the resultant force vector of an activated biceps muscle. The internal moment arm is shown as a red line; the axis of rotation at the elbow is shown as a solid black circle. Note that the moment arm is greater when the elbow is in position *A* compared with position *B*. (Modified from LeVeau BF: Williams & Lissner's Biomechanics of Human Motion, 3rd ed. Philadelphia, WB Saunders, 1992.)

*Box continued on following page*

**SPECIAL FOCUS 4 – 6** *Continued*

internal moment arm available to any muscle is greatest when the angle-of-insertion of the muscle is 90 degrees to the bone.

Next consider *external torque.* Clinically, it is often necessary to quickly compare the relative external torque generated by gravity or other external forces applied against a joint. The leverage of an external force, such as $EMA_2$ in Figure 4–19, may need to be adjusted in order to match the internal torque potential of the musculature most effectively. Consider, for example, the external torque at the knee during two squat postures (Fig. 4–21). By visualizing the external moment arm between the knee

and the line-of-force from body weight, it can be readily concluded that the external torque is greater in a deep squat (*A*) compared with a partial squat (*B*). The ability to judge the relative demand placed on the muscles due to the external torque is useful in terms of protecting a joint that is painful or otherwise abnormal. For instance, a person with arthritic pain between the patella and femur is often advised to limit activities that involve lowering and rising from a deep squat position. This activity places large demands on the quadriceps muscle, which increases the compressive forces on the joint surfaces.

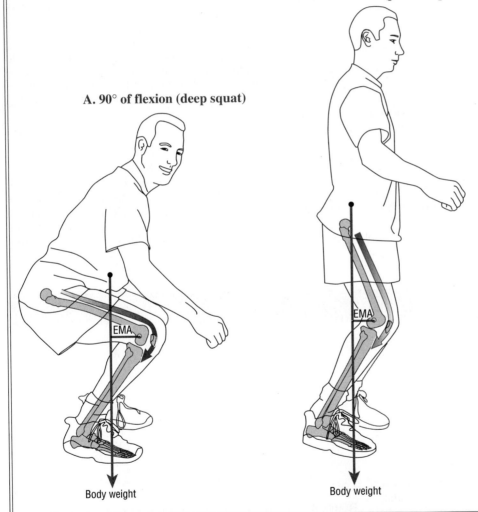

**A. 90° of flexion (deep squat)**

**B. 45° of flexion (partial squat)**

Body weight

Body weight

**FIGURE 4–21.** The depth of a squat significantly affects the magnitude of the external torque produced by body weight at the knee. The relative external torque, within the sagittal plane, can be estimated by comparing the distance that the body weight force vector falls posteriorly to the medial-lateral axis of rotation at the knee. The external moment arm (EMA)—and, thus, the external torque created by body weight—is greater in *A* than in *B*.

### Clinical Issues Related to Joint Force and Torque

*Joint "Protection"*

Some treatments in rehabilitation medicine are directed toward reducing the magnitude of force on joint surfaces during the performance of a physical activity. The purpose of such treatment is to protect a weakened or painful joint

from large and potentially damaging forces. This result can be achieved by reducing the rate of movement (power), providing shock absorption (e.g., cushioned footwear), or limiting the mechanical force demands on the muscle.

Minimizing large muscular-based joint forces may be important for persons with prostheses or artificial joint replacements. A person with a hip replacement, for example, is often advised on ways to minimize unnecessarily large forces produced by the hip abductor muscles.[9,10,12] Figure 4–22 depicts a simple schematic representation of the pelvis and femur while standing on a right lower limb that has a prosthetic hip. The snapshot during the single-limb support phase of gait assumes a condition of static equilibrium (i.e., no acceleration is experienced by the pelvis relative to the femur). In order for equilibrium to be maintained within the frontal plane, the internal (counterclockwise) and external (clockwise) torques about the stance hip must be balanced: the product of hip abductor force (HAF) times its moment arm D must equal body weight (BW) times its moment arm $D_1$, or $HAF \times D = BW \times D_1$. The external moment arm about the hip is almost twice the length of the internal moment arm. The disparity in moment arm lengths requires that the muscle force be almost twice the force of body weight in order to maintain equilibrium. In theory, reducing excessive body weight, carrying lighter loads, or carrying loads in certain fashions can decrease the external moment arm and external torque about the hip.[9] Reduction of unnecessarily large external torques can decrease unnecessarily large force demands on hip abductors and on underlying prosthetic hip joints.

Certain orthopedic procedures illustrate how concepts of joint protection are utilized in rehabilitation practice. Con-sider the case of severe hip osteoarthritis that results in destruction of the femoral head and an associated decrease in the size of the femoral neck and head (Fig. 4–23A). The bony loss shortens the internal moment arm length (D) available to the hip abductor muscles; thus, greater muscle and joint forces are produced to maintain frontal plane equilibrium. A surgical procedure that is an attempt to reduce joint forces on the hip entails the relocation of the greater trochanter to a more lateral position (Fig. 4–23B). This procedure increases the length of the internal moment arm of the hip abductor muscles. An increase in the internal moment arm reduces the force required by the abductor muscles to generate a given torque during single-limb support of gait.

*Manually Applying External Torques During Exercise*

External or resistance torques are often applied manually during an exercise program. For example, if a patient is beginning a knee rehabilitation program to strengthen the quadriceps muscle, the clinician may initially apply manual resistance to the knee extensors at the midtibial region. As the patient's knee strength increases, the clinician can exert a greater force at the midtibial region or the same force near the ankle.

Because external torque is the product of a force (resistance) and an associated external moment arm, an equivalent

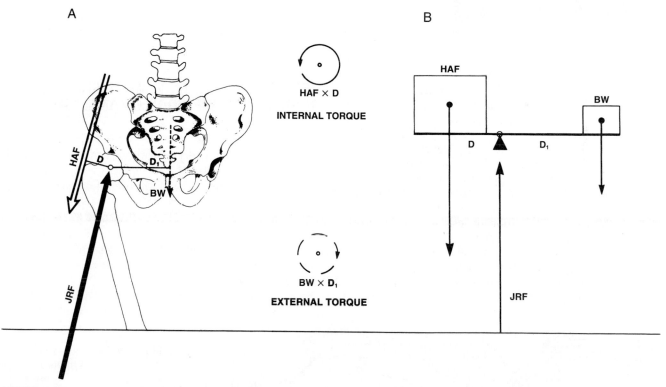

**FIGURE 4–22.** *A,* Hip abductor force (HAF) from the right hip abductor muscles produces a torque necessary for the frontal plane stability of the pelvis during the right single-limb support phase of walking. Rotary stability is established, assuming static equilibrium, when the counterclockwise torque equals the clockwise torque. The counterclockwise torque equals HAF times its moment arm (D), and the clockwise torque equals body weight (BW) times its moment arm ($D_1$). *B,* This first-class lever seesaw model simplifies the model shown in *A.* The joint reaction force (JRF), assuming that all force vectors act vertically, is shown as an upward directed force at a magnitude equal to the sum of the hip abductor force and body weight. (Reprinted and modified with permission from Elsevier Science Publishing Co., Inc., from Neumann DA. Biomechanical analysis of selected principles of hip joint protection. Arthr Care Res 2:146–155, 1989. Copyright 1989 by the Arthritis Health Professions Association.)

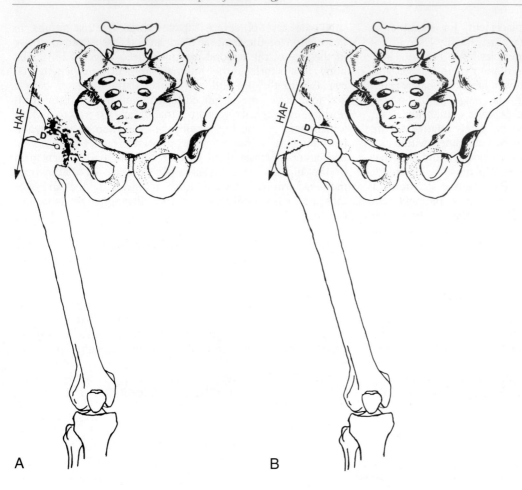

**FIGURE 4–23.** How the internal moment arm used by the hip abductor muscles is altered by disease or surgery. *A,* The right hip is shown with partial degeneration of the femoral head, which decreases the length of the internal moment arm (D) to the hip abductor force (HAF). *B,* A surgical approach is shown in which the greater trochanter is relocated to a more lateral position, thereby increasing the length of the internal moment arm (D) to the hip abductor force. (Adapted and modified from Neumann DA: Biomechanical analysis of selected principles of hip joint protection. Arthr Care Res 2:146–155, 1989. Copyright 1989 by the Arthritis Health Professions Association.)

external torque can be applied by a relatively short external moment arm and a large external force or a long external moment arm and a smaller external force. As depicted in Figure 4–24, the same external torque (15 Nm) applied against the quadriceps muscle can be generated by two different combinations of external forces and moment arms. Note that the resistance *force* applied to the leg is greater in Figure 4–24*A* than in Figure 4–24*B*. The higher contact force may be uncomfortable for the patient and needs to be considered during the application of resistance. A larger external moment arm, shown in Figure 4–24*B,* may be necessary if the clinician chooses to manually challenge a muscle group as potentially forceful as the quadriceps.

## INTRODUCTION TO MOVEMENT ANALYSIS: QUANTITATIVE METHODS OF ANALYSIS

In the previous section, concepts are introduced that provide the framework for performance of quantitative methods of analysis. Many approaches are applied when solving problems in biomechanics. These approaches can be employed to assess (1) the effect of a force at an instant in time (*force-acceleration relationship*); (2) the effect of a force applied over an interval of time (*impulse-momentum relationship*); and (3) the application of a force that causes an object to move through some distance (*work-energy relationship*). The partic-

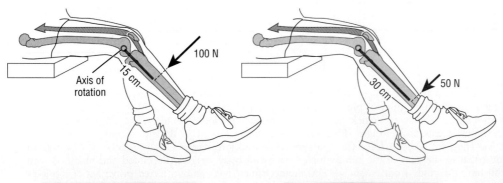

**A** | External Torque = 15 Nm    **B** | External Torque = 15 Nm

**FIGURE 4–24.** The same external torque (15 Nm) is applied against the quadriceps muscle by using a relatively large resistance and small external moment arm (*A*), or a relatively small resistance and large external moment arm (*B*). The external moment arms are indicated by the red lines that extend from the medial-lateral axis of rotation at the knee.

ular approach selected depends on the objective of the analysis. The subsequent sections in this chapter are directed toward the analysis of forces or torques at one instant in time, or the *force (torque)-acceleration approach.*

When considering the effects of a force and the resultant acceleration at an instant in time, two situations can be defined. In the first case, the acceleration has a zero value because the object is either stationary or moving at a constant velocity. This is the branch of mechanics known as *statics.* In the second situation, the acceleration has a nonzero value because the system is subjected to unbalanced forces or torques. This area of study is known as *dynamics.* Static analysis is the simpler approach to problem solving in biomechanics and is the focus in this chapter.

## Static Analysis

Biomechanical studies often induce conditions of static equilibrium in order to simplify the approach to the analysis of human movement. In static analysis, the system is in equilibrium because it is not experiencing acceleration. As a consequence, the sum of the forces or torques acting on the system is zero. The forces or torques in one direction equal the forces or torques in the opposite direction. Because the linear and angular accelerations are equal, the inertial effect of the mass and moment of inertia of the bodies is ignored.

The force equilibrium Equations 4.14 A and B are used for *uniplanar translational motion* and are listed in the box. For *rotational motion,* the forces act together with their moment arms and cause a torque about some axis. In the case of static rotational equilibrium, the sum of the torques about an axis of rotation or another point is zero. The torque equilibrium Equation 4.15 is also included in the box. This equation implies that the sum of the counterclockwise torques must equal the sum of the clockwise torques. The seesaw model of Figure 4–22B provides a simplified example of static rotational equilibrium. The HAF times its moment arm (D) creates a potential counterclockwise (abduction) torque, whereas BW times its moment arm (D₁) creates a potential clockwise (adduction) torque. At any instant, the opposing torques at the hip are assumed to be equal.

---

**Static Analysis: Forces and Torques are Balanced**

**Force Equilibrium Equations**

$$\Sigma F_x = 0 \qquad \text{(Equation 4.14 A)}$$
$$\Sigma F_y = 0 \qquad \text{(Equation 4.14 B)}$$

**Torque Equilibrium Equation**

$$\Sigma T = 0 \qquad \text{(Equation 4.15)}$$

---

## GUIDELINES FOR PROBLEM SOLVING

The guidelines listed in Table 4–4 can help calculate the magnitude and direction of muscle force, torque, and joint reaction force. The following two sample problems illustrate the use of these guidelines for problem solving in a static equilibrium situation.

### Problem 1

Consider the situation in Figure 4–25A, in which a person generates an isometric muscle force at the elbow while hold-

---

**T A B L E  4 – 4. Guidelines for Solving for Muscle Force, Torque, and Joint Reaction Force**

1. Draw the free body diagram and indicate all forces acting on the body or system under consideration. It is necessary to establish an XY reference frame that specifies the desired orientation of the forces. It is often convenient to designate the X axis parallel to the isolated body segment (typically a long bone), and the Y axis perpendicular to the body segment.
2. Resolve all forces into their tangential and normal components.
3. Identify the moment arms associated with each force. The moment arm associated with a given torque is the distance between the axis of rotation and the 90-degree intersection with the force. Note that joint reaction force will not have a moment arm, because it is typically directed through the center of the joint.
4. Use Equations 4–14 and 4–15 as needed to solve the problem.

---

ing an object in the hand. Assuming equilibrium, three unknown variables are to be solved: (1) the internal (muscular-produced) torque, (2) the muscle force, and (3) the joint reaction force at the elbow. To begin, a free body diagram is constructed. The axis of rotation and all moment arm distances are indicated (Figure 4–25B). Although at this point the direction of the joint (reaction) force (JF) is unknown, it is assumed to act in a direction *opposite* to the pull of muscle. This assumption holds true in an analysis in which the mechanical advantage of the system is less than one (i.e., when the muscle forces are greater than the external resistance forces) (see Chapter 1). If after solving the problem the joint force is positive, then this initial assumption is correct.

Because all the resultant forces indicated in this problem act parallel to the Y axis, it is unnecessary to resolve the resultant forces into their component vectors. No forces are acting in the X (horizontal) direction.

*Solving for Internal Torque and Muscle Force*
The external torques originating from the weight of the forearm-hand segment (SW) and the weight of the load (LW) generate a clockwise (extension) torque about the elbow. In order for the system to remain in equilibrium, the elbow flexor muscle has to generate an opposing internal (flexion) torque, acting in a counterclockwise direction. This assumption of rotational equilibrium allows Equation 4.15 to be used to solve for the magnitude of the internal torque and muscle force:

$$\Sigma T = 0 \text{ (Internal torque} + -\text{external torque} = 0)$$

$$\text{Internal torque} = \text{external torque}$$

$$\text{Internal torque} = (SW \times EMA_1) + (LW \times EMA_2)$$

$$\text{Internal torque} = (17N \times 0.15 \text{ m}) + (60 \text{ N} \times 0.35 \text{ m})$$

$$\text{Internal torque} = 23.6 \text{ Nm}$$

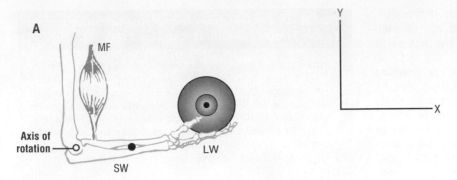

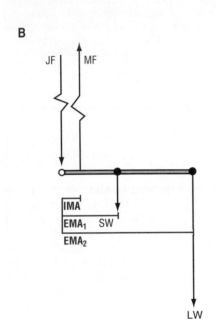

Muscle Force (MF) = unknown
Segment Weight (SW) = 17N
Load Weight (LW) = 60N
Joint Force (JF) at the elbow = unknown
Internal Moment Arm (IMA) to MF = .05m
External Moment Arm to SW (EMA₁) = .15m
External Moment Arm to LW (EMA₂) = .35m

**FIGURE 4–25. Problem 1.** *A,* An isometric elbow flexion exercise is performed against a load weight held in the hand. The forearm is held in the horizontal position, parallel to the X axis. *B,* A free body diagram is shown of the exercise, including a box with the abbreviations and data required to solve the problem. The medial-lateral axis of rotation at the elbow is shown as an open red circle. (*A* modified from LeVeau BF: Williams & Lissner's Biomechanics of Human Motion, 3rd ed. Philadelphia, WB Saunders, 1992.)

The resultant muscle (internal) torque is the net sum of all the muscles that flex the elbow. This type of analysis does not, however, provide information about how the torque is distributed among the various elbow flexor muscles. This requires more sophisticated procedures, such as muscle modeling and optimization techniques, which are beyond the scope of this text.

The muscle force required to maintain the forearm in a static position at a given instant in time is calculated by dividing the external torque by the internal moment arm:

$$MF \times IMA = (SW \times EMA_1) + (LW \times EMA_2)$$

$$\text{Muscle force (MF)} = \frac{(17 \text{ N} \times 0.15 \text{ m}) + (60 \text{ N} \times 0.35 \text{ m})}{0.05 \text{ m}}$$

$$MF = 471.0 \text{ N}$$

The magnitude of the muscle force is over six times greater than the magnitude of the external forces (i.e., forearm-hand segment and load weight). The larger force requirement can be explained by the disparity in moment arm length used by the elbow flexors when compared with the moment arms lengths used by the two external forces. The

disparity in moment arm length is not unique to the elbow flexion model, but it is ubiquitous throughout the muscular-joint systems in the body. For this reason, most muscles of the body routinely generate a force many times greater than the weight of the external load. This principle requires that the bone and articular cartilage absorb large joint forces that result from seemingly nonstressful activities.

*Solving for Joint Force*
Because the joint reaction force (JF) is the only remaining unknown variable depicted in Figure 4–25*B,* this variable is determined by Equation 4.14 B, where downward forces are negative.

$$\Sigma F_y = 0$$

$$MF - SW - LW - JF = 0$$

$$-JF = -MF + SW + LW$$

$$-JF = -471 \text{ N} + 17 \text{ N} + 60 \text{ N}$$

$$-JF = -394.0 \text{ N}$$

$$JF = 394.0 \text{ N}$$

The positive value of the joint reaction force verifies the assumption that the joint force acted downward. Because muscle force is usually the largest force acting about a joint, the direction of the net joint force must oppose the pull of the muscle. Without such a force, for example, the muscle indicated in Figure 4–25 would accelerate the forearm upward, resulting in a unstable joint. In short, the joint force supplied by the humerus against the forearm in this case provides the missing force needed to maintain linear static equilibrium at the elbow. As stated earlier, the joint force does not produce a torque because it is assumed to act through the axis of rotation and, therefore, has a zero moment arm.

### Problem 2

In Problem 1, the forearm is held horizontally, thereby orienting the internal and external forces perpendicular to the forearm. Although this presentation greatly simplifies the calculations, it does not represent a very typical biomechanical situation. Problem 2 shows a more common situation in which the forearm is held at a position other than the horizontal (Fig. 4–26A). As a result of the change in fore-

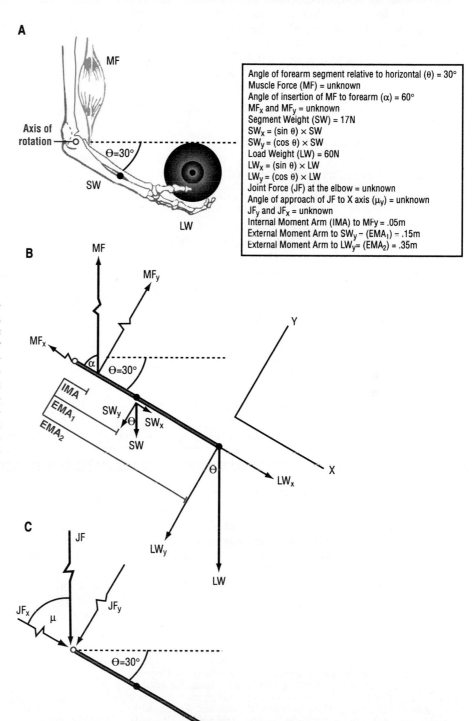

**FIGURE 4–26. Problem 2.** *A*, An isometric elbow flexion exercise is performed against an identical load weight as that depicted in Figure 4–25. The forearm is held 30 degrees below the horizontal position. *B*, A free body diagram is shown including a box with the abbreviations and data required to solve the problem. *C*, The joint reaction force (JF) vectors are shown in response to the biomechanics depicted in *B*. (*A* modified from LeVeau BF: Williams & Lissner's Biomechanics of Human Motion, 3rd ed. Philadelphia, WB Saunders, 1992.)

Angle of forearm segment relative to horizontal $(\theta) = 30°$
Muscle Force (MF) = unknown
Angle of insertion of MF to forearm $(\alpha) = 60°$
$MF_x$ and $MF_y$ = unknown
Segment Weight (SW) = 17N
$SW_x = (\sin \theta) \times SW$
$SW_y = (\cos \theta) \times SW$
Load Weight (LW) = 60N
$LW_x = (\sin \theta) \times LW$
$LW_y = (\cos \theta) \times LW$
Joint Force (JF) at the elbow = unknown
Angle of approach of JF to X axis $(\mu_y)$ = unknown
$JF_y$ and $JF_x$ = unknown
Internal Moment Arm (IMA) to $MF_y$ = .05m
External Moment Arm to $SW_y - (EMA_1)$ = .15m
External Moment Arm to $LW_y = (EMA_2)$ = .35m

arm position, the angle-of-insertion of the elbow flexor muscles and the angle where the external forces intersect the forearm are no longer perpendicular. In principle, all other aspects of this problem are identical to Problem 1, except that the resultant vectors need to be resolved into rectangular (X and Y) components. This requires additional steps and trigonometric calculations. Assuming equilibrium, three unknown variables are once again to be determined: (1) the internal (muscular-produced) torque, (2) the muscle force, and (3) the joint reaction force at the elbow.

Figure 4–26B illustrates the free body diagram of the forearm held at 30 degrees below the horizontal ($\theta$). To simplify calculations, the X-Y reference frame is established, such that the X axis is parallel to the forearm segment. All forces acting on the system are indicated, and each is resolved into their respective tangential (X) and normal (Y) components. The angle-of-insertion of the elbow flexors to the forearm ($\alpha$) is 60 degrees. All numeric data and background information are listed in the box associated with Figure 4–26.

*Solving for Internal Torque and Muscle Force*

$$\Sigma T = 0 \text{ (Internal torque } + \text{ } -\text{external torque} = 0)$$

$$\text{Internal torque} = \text{external torque}$$

$$\text{Internal torque} = (SW_Y \times EMA_1) + (LW_Y \times EMA_2)^*$$

$$\begin{aligned}\text{Internal torque} = &(\cos 30° \times 17 \text{ N} \times 0.15 \text{ m}) \\ &+ (\cos 30° \times 60 \text{ N} \times 0.35 \text{ m})\end{aligned}$$

$$\text{Internal torque} = 20.4 \text{ Nm}$$

The muscle force required to generate the internal flexor torque at the elbow is determined by

$$MF_Y \times IMA = (SW_Y \times EMA_1) + (LW_Y \times EMA_2)$$

$$MF_Y = \frac{(\cos 30° \times 17 \text{ N} \times 0.15 \text{ m}) + (\cos 30° \times 60 \text{ N} \times 0.35 \text{ m})}{.05 \text{ m}}$$

$$MF_Y = 408.0 \text{ N}$$

Because an internal moment arm length of .05 m was used, the last calculation yielded the magnitude of its associated perpendicular vector, $MF_Y$, not MF. The resultant muscle force, or MF, can be determined by

$$MF = MF_Y/\sin 60°$$

$$MF = 408 \text{ N}/.866$$

$$MF = 471.1 \text{ N}$$

The tangential component of the muscle force, $MF_X$, can be solved by

$$MF_X = MF \times \cos 60°$$

$$MF_X = 471.1 \text{ N} \times .5$$

$$MF_X = 235.6 \text{ N}$$

*Solving for Joint Force*
The joint reaction force (JF) and its normal and tangential components ($JF_Y$ and $JF_X$) are shown separately in Figure 4–26C. (This is done to increase the clarity of the illustration.) In reality, the joint forces are acting concurrently on the proximal end of the forearm segment along with the other forces. The directions of $JF_Y$ and $JF_X$ are assumed to act downward (negative) and to the right (positive), respectively. These are directions that oppose the force of the muscle. The rectangular components ($JF_Y$ and $JF_X$) of the joint force (JF) can be readily determined by using Equations 4.14 A and B.

$$\Sigma F_Y = 0$$

$$MF_Y - SW_Y - LW_Y - JF_Y = 0$$

$$-JF_Y = -MF_Y + SW_Y + LW_Y$$

$$-JF_Y = -408 \text{ N} + (\cos 30° \times 17 \text{ N}) + (\cos 30° \times 60 \text{ N})$$

$$-JF_Y = -341.3 \text{ N}$$

$$JF_Y = 341.3 \text{ N}$$

$$\Sigma F_X = 0$$

$$-MF_X + SW_X + LW_X + JF_X = 0$$

$$JF_X = MF_X - SW_X - LW_X$$

$$JF_X = 235.6 \text{ N} - (\sin 30° \times 17 \text{ N}) - (\sin 30° \times 60 \text{ N})$$

$$JF_X = 197.1 \text{ N}$$

As depicted in Figure 4–26C, $JF_Y$ and $JF_X$ act downward and to the right, respectively, in a direction that opposes the force of the muscle. The magnitude of the resultant joint force (JF) can be determined using the Pythagorean theorem:

$$JF = \sqrt{(JF_Y{}^2) + (JF_X{}^2)}$$

$$JF = \sqrt{341.3 \text{ N}^2 + 197.1 \text{ N}^2}$$

$$JF = 394.1 \text{ N}$$

Another characteristic of the joint reaction force that is of interest is the direction of the JF with respect to the axis (X) of the forearm. This is calculated using the relationship:

$$\tan \mu = JF_Y/JF_X$$

$$\mu = \tan^{-1}(341.3\ N/197.1\ N)$$

$$\mu = 60°$$

The resultant joint reaction force has a magnitude of 394.1 N and is directed toward the elbow at an angle of 60 degrees to the forearm segment (i.e., the X axis). The angle is the same as the angle-of-insertion of the muscle, a reminder of the dominant role of muscle in determining both *the magnitude and direction of the joint reaction force.*

## Dynamic Analysis

Static analysis is the most basic approach to kinetic analysis of human movement. This form of analysis is used to evaluate forces on a human when there are little or no significant linear or angular accelerations. In contrast, when linear or angular accelerations occur owing to unbalanced forces, a dynamic analysis must be undertaken. Walking is an example of movement due to unbalanced forces, as the body is in a continual state of losing and regaining balance with each step. Thus, dynamic analysis of gait is a frequently conducted analysis of movement science.

Dynamic forces that act against the body can be measured directly by various instruments, such as a force transducer. Dynamic forces generated from within the body, however, are usually measured indirectly based on Newton's laws of motion. (See Special Focus 4–7 for one such method.) Solving for forces and torques under dynamic conditions requires knowledge of mass or mass moment of inertia and linear or angular acceleration (see Equations 4.16 and 4.17 in the box). Anthropometric data provide the inertial characteristics of body segments (mass, mass moment of inertia), as well as the lengths of body segments and locations of joint centers. Kinematic data, such as displacement, velocity, and accelerations of segments, can be measured through laboratory techniques.

---

**Dynamic Analysis of Force and Torque**

**Force Equations**

$$\Sigma F_x = ma_X \qquad \text{(Equation 4.16 A)}$$

$$\Sigma F_y = ma_Y \qquad \text{(Equation 4.16 B)}$$

**Torque Equation**

$$\Sigma T = I\alpha \qquad \text{(Equation 4.17)}$$

---

## KINEMATIC AND KINETIC MEASUREMENT SYSTEMS

This section introduces common methods and systems used to collect kinematic and kinetic data in the study of human movement.[1,13,14–16] The reader is referred to the Additional Readings at the end of this chapter for further elaboration of the uses, advantages, and disadvantages of these measurement techniques.

### Kinematic Measurement Systems: Electrogoniometer, Accelerometer, Imaging Techniques, and Electromagnetic Tracking Devices

Detailed analysis of movement requires a careful and objective evaluation of the motion of the joints and body as a whole. The analysis most frequently includes an assessment of position, displacement, velocity, and acceleration. Analysis may be used to indirectly measure forces produced by the body or to assess the quality and quantity of motion without regard to forces and torques. Kinematic analysis is performed in a variety of environments, including sport, ergonomics, and rehabilitation.

#### Electrogoniometer

An electrogoniometer measures joint angular displacement during movement. The device typically consists of an electrical potentiometer built into the pivot point (hinge) of two rigid arms. Rotation of a calibrated potentiometer measures the angular position of the joint. The output can be sent to a chart recorder or oscilloscope, or more frequently it is used as input to a computer program. The arms of the electrogoniometer are strapped to the body segments, such that the axis of rotation of the goniometer (potentiometer) is approximately aligned with the joint's axis of rotation (Fig. 4–27). The position data obtained from the electrogoniome-

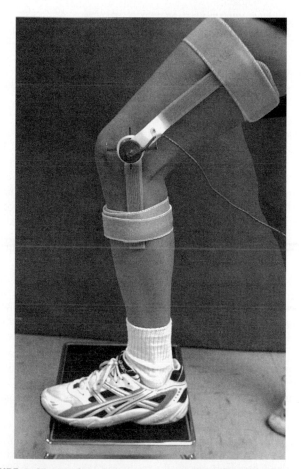

**FIGURE 4–27.** An electrogoniometer is shown strapped to the thigh and leg. The axis of the goniometer contains the potentiometer and is aligned over the medial-lateral axis of rotation at the knee joint. This particular instrument records a single plane of motion only.

ter combined with the time data can be mathematically converted to angular velocity and acceleration. Although the electrogoniometer provides a fairly inexpensive and direct means of capturing joint angular displacement, it encumbers the subject and is difficult to fit and secure over fatty and muscle tissues. A triaxial electrogoniometer measures joint rotation in three planes; however, this system tends to constrain natural movement.

### Accelerometer

An accelerometer is a device that measures acceleration of the segment to which it is attached. Accelerometers are force transducers consisting of a strain gauge or piezoresistive circuit that measures the reaction forces associated with a given acceleration. Based on Newton's second law, acceleration is determined as the ratio of the measured force divided by a known mass.

### Imaging Techniques

Imaging techniques are the most widely used methods for collecting motion data. Many different types of imaging systems are available. This discussion is limited to the systems listed in the box.

---

**Imaging Techniques**
- Photography
- Cinematography
- Videography
- Optoelectronics

---

Unlike the electrogoniometer and accelerometer that measure movement directly from a body, imaging methods typically require additional signal conditioning, processing, and interpreting prior to obtaining meaningful output.

*Photography* is one of the oldest techniques for measuring kinematic data. With the camera shutter held open, light from a flashing strobe can be used to track the location of reflective markers worn on the skin of a moving subject (see Chapter 15 and Fig. 15–3). By knowing the frequency of the strobe light, angular displacement data can be converted to angular velocity and angular acceleration data. In addition to using a strobe as an interrupted light source, a 35-mm camera can use a constant light source and take multiple film exposures of a moving event.

*Cinematography,* the art of movie photography, was once the most popular method of recording motion. High-speed cinematography, using 16-mm film, allowed for the measurement of fast movements. By knowing the shutter speed, a labor-intensive, frame-by-frame digital analysis on the movement in question was performed. Digital analysis was performed on movement of anatomic landmarks or of markers worn by subjects. Two-dimensional movement analysis was performed with the aid of one camera; three-dimensional analysis, however, required two or more cameras.

For the most part, still photography and cinematography analysis are rarely used for the study of human motion. The methods are not practical due to the time required for developing the film and manually analyzing the data. *Videography* has replaced these systems and is one of the most popular methods for collecting kinematic information in both clinical and laboratory settings. The system typically consists of one or more video cameras, a recorder, a monitor, an image

processor or an interface that digitizes the analog signal, a calibration device, and a computer. The procedures involved in video-based systems typically require markers to be attached to a subject at selected anatomic landmarks. Markers are considered passive if they are not connected to another electronic device or power source. Passive markers serve as a light source by reflecting the light back to the camera (Fig. 4–28). Two- and three-dimensional coordinates of markers are identified in space by a computer and are then used to reconstruct the image (or stick figure) for subsequent kinematic analysis.

Video-based systems are quite versatile and are used to analyze activities from swimming to typing. Some systems allow movement to be captured outdoors and processed at a later time. Another desirable feature of the system is that the subject is not encumbered by wires or other electronic devices.

*Optoelectronics* is another popular type of kinematic acquisition system that uses active markers that are pulsed sequentially. The light is detected by special cameras that focus it on a semiconductor diode surface. The system enables collection of data at high sampling rates and can acquire real-time 3D data. The system is limited in its ability to acquire data outside a controlled environment. Subjects may feel hampered by the wires that are connected to the active markers. Telemetry systems enable data to be gathered without the subjects being tethered to a power source, but they are vulnerable to ambient electrical interference.

### Electromagnetic Tracking Devices

*Electromagnetic tracking devices* measure six degrees-of-freedom (three rotational and three translational), providing position and orientation data during both static and dynamic activities. Small receivers are secured to the skin overlying

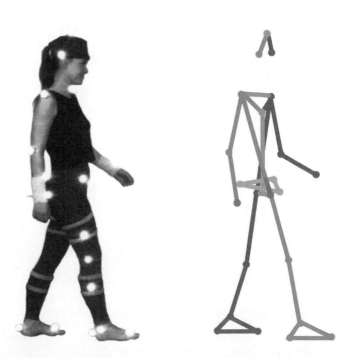

**FIGURE 4–28.** Reflective markers are used to indicate anatomic locations for determination of joint angular displacement of a walking individual. Marker location is acquired using a video-based camera that can operate at variable sampling rates. (Courtesy of Peak Performance Technologies, Inc., Englewood, Colorado.)

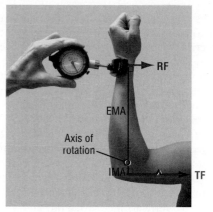

**FIGURE 4–29.** A hand-held dynamometer is used to measure the isometric elbow extension torque produced by the triceps muscle. The product of the resistive force (RF) times its external moment arm (EMA), assuming static equilibrium, is equal to the product of the triceps force (TF) times its internal moment arm (IMA).

anatomic landmarks. Position and orientation data from the receivers located within a specified operating range of the transmitter are sent to the data capture system.

One disadvantage of this system is that the transmitters and receivers are sensitive to metal in their vicinity. The metal distorts the electromagnetic field generated by the transmitters. Although telemetry is available for these systems, most operate with wires that connect the receivers to the data capture system. The wires limit the volume of space from which motion can be recorded.

In any motion analysis system that uses skin sensors to record underlying bony movement, there is the potential for error associated with the extraneous movement of skin and soft tissue.

### Kinetic Measurement Systems: Mechanical Devices, Transducers, and Electromechanical Devices

#### Mechanical Devices

Mechanical devices measure an applied force by the amount of strain or the compression of deformable material. Through purely mechanical means, the strain in the material causes the movement of a dial. The numeric values associated with the dial are calibrated to a known force. Some of the most common mechanical devices for measuring force include a bathroom scale, a grip strength dynamometer, and a hand-held dynamometer. The hand-held dynamometer, for example, provides useful clinical measurement of the internal torque produced by a patient (Fig. 4–29). In the example, the dynamometer measures a resistance force (RF) in response to a maximal effort, isometrically produced elbow extension torque. The triceps force (TF) is determined by dividing the external torque (RF × EMA) by an estimate of the internal moment arm.

**FIGURE 4–30.** Output from a force plate indicates ground reaction forces (GRF) in the vertical (V), medial-lateral (ML), and anterior-posterior (AP) directions during a normal walking trial.

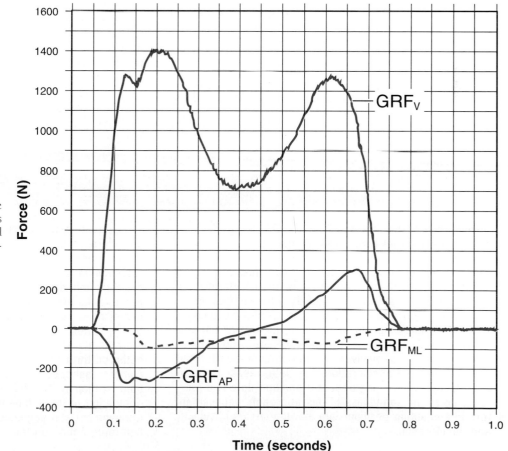

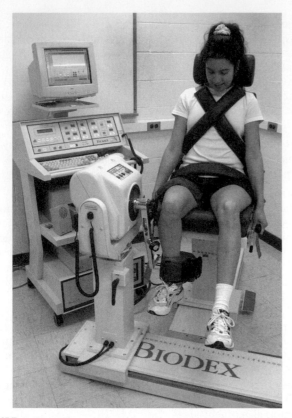

**FIGURE 4–31.** Isokinetic dynamometry. The subject generates maximal-effort knee flexion torque at a joint angular velocity of 60 degrees/sec. The machine is functioning in its "concentric mode," providing resistance against the contracting muscles. Note that the medial-lateral axis of rotation of the right knee is approximately aligned with the axis of rotation of the dynamometer. (Courtesy of Biodex Medical Systems, Inc., Shirley, New York.)

### Transducers

Various types of transducers have been developed and widely used to measure force. Among these are strain gauges and piezoelectric, piezoresistive, and capacitance transducers. Essentially, these transducers operate on the principle that an applied force deforms the transducer, resulting in a change in voltage in a known manner. Output from the transducer is converted to meaningful measures through a calibration process.

One of the most common transducers for collecting kinetic data while a subject is walking, stepping, or running is the *force plate*. Force plates utilize piezoelectric quartz or strain gauge transducers that are sensitive to load in three orthogonal directions. The force plate measures the ground reaction forces in vertical, medial-lateral, and anterior-posterior components (Fig. 4–30). Each component has a characteristic shape and magnitude. The ground reaction force data can be used as input for subsequent dynamic analysis.

### Electromechanical Devices

One of the most popular electromechanical devices for measuring internal torque at a specific joint is the *isokinetic dynamometer*. The device measures the internal torque produced while maintaining a constant angular velocity of the joint. The isokinetic system is adjusted to measure the torque produced by most major muscle groups of the body. The machine measures kinetic data produced by muscles during all three types of activation: concentric, isometric, and eccentric. The angular velocity is determined by the user, varying between 0 degrees/sec (isometric) and up to 500 degrees/sec for nonisometric activation. Figure 4–31 shows a person who is exerting maximal effort, knee flexion torque through a concentric contraction of the right knee flexor musculature. Isokinetic dynamometry provides an objective record of muscular kinetic data, produced during different types of muscle activation at multiple test velocities. The system also provides immediate feedback of kinetic data, which may serve as a source of biofeedback during training or rehabilitation.

## SPECIAL FOCUS 4–7

### Introduction to the "Inverse Dynamic Approach" for Solving for Internal Forces and Torques

Measuring joint reaction forces and muscle-produced net torques during dynamic conditions is often performed indirectly utilizing a technique called the *inverse dynamic approach*.[16] This approach uses data on anthropometry, kinematics, and external forces, such as gravity and contact forces. Accelerations are determined employing the first and second derivatives of position-time data to yield velocity-time and acceleration-time data, respectively. The importance of acquiring accurate position data is a prerequisite to the soundness of this approach, because errors in measuring position data magnify errors in velocity and acceleration.

In the inverse dynamics approach, the system under consideration is often defined as a series of links. Figure 4–32A illustrates the relationship between the anatomic link segment models of the lower limb. In Figure 4–32B, the segments are disarticulated and the individual forces and torques are identified at each segment end point. The center of mass is located for each segment. The analysis on the series of links usually begins with the analysis of the most distal segment, in this case the foot. Information gathered through motion analysis techniques, typically camera-based, serves as input data for the dynamic equations of motion. This information includes the position and orientation of the segment in space, the acceleration of the segment and segment center of mass, and the reaction force acting on the distal end of the segment. From these data, the reaction force and the net muscle torque at the ankle joint are determined. This information is then utilized as input for continued analysis of the next most proximal segment, the leg. Analysis takes place until all segments or links in the model are studied. Several assumptions made during the use of the inverse dynamic approach are included in the box.

> **Assumptions Made During the Inverse Dynamic Approach**
> 1. Each segment or link has a fixed mass that is concentrated at its center of mass.
> 2. The location of each segment's center of mass remains fixed during the movement.
> 3. The joints in this model are considered frictionless hinge joints.
> 4. The mass moment of inertia of each segment is constant during the movement.
> 5. The length of each segment remains constant.

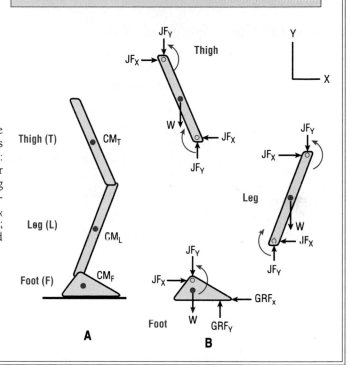

**FIGURE 4–32.** A link model of the lower limb consisting of three segments: thigh (T), leg (L), and foot (F). In *A*, the center of mass (CM) of each segment is represented as a fixed point (red circle): $CM_T$, $CM_L$, and $CM_F$. In *B*, the segments are disarticulated in order for the internal forces and torques to be determined, beginning with the most distal foot segment. The red curved arrows represents torque about the axes of rotation. (W, segment weight; $JF_X$ and $JF_Y$, joint forces in the horizontal (X) vertical (Y) directions; $GRF_X$ and $GRF_Y$, ground reaction forces in the horizontal (X) and vertical directions (Y).)

## REFERENCES

1. Allard P, Stokes IAF, Blanchi JP: Three-Dimensional Analysis of Human Movement. Champaign, Human Kinetics, 1995.
2. Clauser CE, McConville JT, Young JW: Weight, volume, and center of mass segments of the human body. AMRL-TR-69-70, Wright Patterson Air Force Base, 1969.
3. Craik RL, Oatis CA: Gait Analysis: Theory and Application. St. Louis, Mosby-Year Book, 1995.
4. Dempster WT: Space requirements for the seated operator. WADC-TR-55-159, Wright Patterson Air Force Base, 1955.
5. Enoka RM: Neuromechanical Basis of Kinesiology, 2nd ed. Champaign, Human Kinetics, 1994.
6. Hamill J, Knutzen KM: Biomechanical Basis of Human Movement. Baltimore, Williams & Wilkins, 1995.
7. Hatze H: A mathematical model for the computational determination of parameter values of anthropometric segments. J Biomech 13:833–843, 1980.
8. Hindrichs R: Regression equations to predict segmental moments of inertia from anthropometric measurements. J Biomech 18:621–624, 1985.
9. Neumann DA: Biomechanical analysis of selected principles of hip joint protection. Arthritis Care Res 2:146–155, 1989.
10. Neumann DA: Hip abductor muscle activity in persons with a hip prosthesis while walking and carrying loads in one hand. Phys Ther 76: 1320–1330, 1996.
11. Neumann DA: Hip abductor muscle activity in persons who walk with a hip prosthesis with different methods of using a cane. Phys Ther 78: 490–501, 1998.
12. Neumann DA: Arthrokinesiological considerations in the aged adult. In Guccione AA (ed): Geriatric Physical Therapy, 2nd ed. St. Louis, Mosby, 2000.
13. Ozkaya N, Nordin M: Fundamentals of Biomechanics: Equilibrium, Motion and Deformation. New York, Springer-Verlag, 1999.
14. Soderberg GL: Kinesiology: Application to Pathological Motion, 2nd ed. Baltimore, Williams & Wilkins, 1997.
15. Whiting WC, Zernicke RF. Biomechanics of Musculoskeletal Injury. Champaign, Human Kinetics, 1998.
16. Winter DA: Biomechanics and Motor Control of Human Movement, 2nd ed. New York, John Wiley & Sons, 1990.
17. Zatsiorsky VM: Kinematics of Human Motion. Champaign, Human Kinetics, 1998.
18. Zatsiorsky VM, Seluyanov V: Estimation of the mass and inertia characteristics of the human body by means of the best predictive regression equations. In DA Winter, RW Norman, RP Wells, et al (eds): Biomechanics. Champaign, Human Kinetics, 1985.

## ADDITIONAL READINGS

Hall SJ: Basic Biomechanics. St. Louis, Mosby, 1998.
Hay JG: The Biomechanics of Sports Techniques. Englewood Cliffs, Prentice Hall, 1993.
LeVeau BF: Williams & Lissner's Biomechanics of Human Motion. Philadelphia, WB Saunders, 1992.
Low J, Reed A: Basic Biomechanics Explained. Oxford, Butterworth-Heinemann, 1996.
Mow VC, Hayes WC: Basic Orthopaedic Biomechanics. New York, Raven Press, 1991.
Nordin M, Frankel VH: Basic Biomechanics of the Musculoskeletal System. Philadelphia, Lea and Febiger, 1989.

# APPENDIX I

## Appendix IA: Selected Anthropometric Data

Table 1A–1 provides selected anthropometric data on a 670-N man.

## Appendix IB: The "Right-Hand" Rule

As stated in Chapter 1, a torque is defined as a *force multiplied by its moment arm*. Force is a vector quantity that possesses both magnitude and direction. Moment arm length, however, can be treated as a vector or as a scalar quantity. When considering a moment arm as a vector, torque is calculated as the product of two vectors. Multiplying two orthogonal vectors (force and its moment arm) through cross-product multiplication yields a third vector (torque) that is directed perpendicularly to the plane that contains the other two vectors. Using this scheme, the elbow flexors in Figure 1–17, for example, would produce an internal torque vector that is directed either into the page or out of the page. The "right-hand" rule is a convention that can be used to assign a direction to a vector product. The fingers of the right hand are curled in the direction of the rotating segment. The positive direction of the torque is defined by the direction of the extended thumb. In Figure 1–17, the direction of the internal torque is "out of" the page, or in a positive Z direction.

## Appendix IC: Basic Review of Trigonometry

Trigonometric functions are based on the relationship that exists between the angles and sides of a right triangle. The sides of the triangle can represent distances, force magnitude, velocity, and other physical properties. Four of the common trigonometric functions used in quantitative analysis are found in the following table. Each trigonometric function has a specific value for a given angle. If the vectors representing two sides of a right triangle are known, the remaining side of the triangle can be determined by using the *Pythagorean theorem:* $a^2 = b^2 + c^2$, where $a$ is the hypotenuse of the triangle. If one side and one angle other than the right angle are known, the remaining parts of the triangle can be determined by using one of the four trigonometric functions listed in the table.

**Right-Angle Trigonometric Functions Commonly Used in Biomechanical Analysis**

| Trigonometric Function | Definition |
| --- | --- |
| Sine (sin) | Side opposite/hypotenuse |
| Cosine (cos) | Side adjacent/hypotenuse |
| Tangent (tan) | Side opposite/side adjacent |
| Cotangent (cot) | Side adjacent/side opposite |

Figure IC–1 illustrates the use of trigonometry to determine the force components of the posterior deltoid muscle during active isometric activation. The angle-of-insertion ($\alpha$) of the muscle with the bone is 45 degrees. Based on the particular reference frame, the rectangular components of the muscle force (MF) are labeled $MF_Y$ (tangential force) and $MF_X$ (normal force). Given a constant muscle force of 200 N, $MF_Y$ and $MF_X$ can be determined as follows:

$$MF_X = MF \sin 45° = 200\ N \times 0.707 = 141.4\ N$$

$$MF_Y = MF \cos 45° = 200\ N \times 0.707 = 141.4\ N$$

If $MF_X$ and $MF_Y$ are known, MF (hypotenuse) can be determined using the Pythagorean theorem:

$$MF^2 = MF_X^2 + MF_Y^2$$

$$MF = \sqrt{141.4^2 + 141.4^2}$$

$$MF \cong 200\ N$$

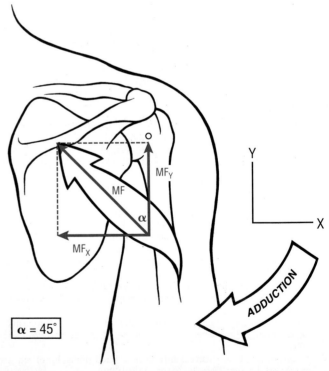

**FIGURE IC–1.** Given an angle-of-insertion of the posterior deltoid ($\alpha = 45$ degrees) and the resultant posterior deltoid muscle force (MF), the two rectangular force components of the muscle force ($MF_X$ and $MF_Y$) are determined using trigonometric relationships. The axis of rotation at the glenohumeral joint is indicated by the open circle at the head of the humerus.

## TABLE IA-1. Selected Anthropometric Data on a 670-N (64.4 kg) Man

| Segment Weight* | Location of Centers of Mass |
|---|---|
| *Head:* 46.2 N (6.9%) | *Head:* In sphenoid sinus, 4 mm beyond anterior inferior margin of sella. (On lateral surface, over temporal fossa on or near nasion-inion line.) |
| *Head and neck:* 52.9 N (7.9%) | *Head and neck:* On inferior surface of basioccipital bone or within bone 23 ± 5 mm from crest of dorsum sellae. (On lateral surface, 10 mm anterior to supratragal notch above head of mandible.) |
| *Head, neck, and trunk:* 395.3 N (59.0%) | *Head, neck, and trunk:* Anterior to eleventh thoracic vertebra. |

| | **Upper Limb** |
|---|---|
| | *Upper limb:* Just above elbow joint. |
| *Arm:* 18.1 N (2.7%) | *Arm:* In medial head of triceps, adjacent to radial groove; 5 mm proximal to distal end of deltoid insertion. |
| *Forearm:* 10.7 N (1.6%) | *Forearm:* 11 mm proximal to most distal part of pronator teres insertion; 9 mm anterior to interosseous membrane. |
| *Hand:* 4.0 N (0.6%) | *Hand (in rest position):* On axis of metacarpal III, usually 2 mm deep to volar skin surface; |
| *Upper limb:* 32.8 N (4.9%) | 2 mm proximal to transverse palmar skin crease, in angle between proximal transverse |
| *Forearm and hand:* 14.7 N (2.2%) | and radial longitudinal crease. |

| | **Lower Limb** |
|---|---|
| | *Lower limb:* Just above knee joint. |
| *Thigh:* 65.0 N (9.7%) | *Thigh:* In adductor brevis muscle (or magnus or vastus medialis) 13 mm medial to linea aspera, deep to adductor canal; 29 mm below apex of femoral triangle and 18 mm proximal to most distal fibers of adductor brevis. |
| *Leg:* 30.2 N (4.5%) | *Leg:* 35 mm below popliteus, at posterior part of posterior tibialis; 16 mm above proximal end of Achilles tendon; 8 mm posterior to interosseous membrane. |
| *Foot:* 9.4 N (1.4%) | *Foot:* In plantar ligaments, or just superficial in adjacent deep foot muscles; below proximal |
| *Lower limb:* 104.5 N (15.6%) | halves of second and third cuneiform bones. On a line between ankle joint center and |
| *Leg and foot:* 40.2 N (6.0%) | ball of foot in plane of metatarsal II. |

| | |
|---|---|
| | *Entire body.* Anterior to second sacral vertebra. |

*Expressed in newtons (N) and percentage of total body weight.

Based on Dempster WT: 1955: Space requirements for the seated operator. WADC-TR-55-159, Wright Patterson Air Force Base. Value for head weight was computed from Braune and Fischer, 1889. Centers of mass loci are from Dempster except those for entire limbs and body.

The normal and tangential components of *external forces,* such as those exerted by a wall pulley, body weight, or by the clinician manually, are determined in a manner similar to that described for the muscle (internal) force.

Trigonometry can also be used to determine the magnitude of the resultant force when one or more components and the angle-of-insertion are known. Consider the same example as given in Figure IC–1, but now consider the goal of the analysis to be determination of the resultant muscle force of the posterior deltoid muscle. The muscle angle-of-insertion is 45 degrees and $MF_X$ is 141.4 N. The resultant muscle force (hypotenuse of the triangle) can be derived using the relationship of the rectangular components:

$$\sin 45° = MF_X/MF$$

$$MF = 141.4 \text{ N}/\sin 45°$$

$$MF \cong 200 \text{ N}$$

If only $MF_Y$ and $MF_X$ are known, the angle-of-insertion of MF can be determined using the inverse $\tan^{-1} \alpha$. Note that the components of the force always have a magnitude less than the magnitude of the resultant vector.

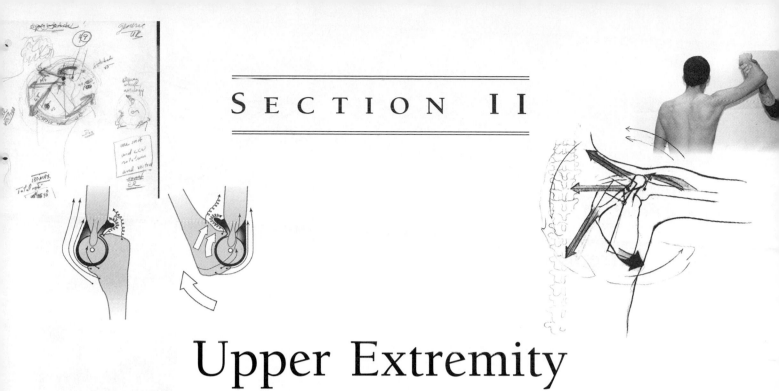

# SECTION II

# Upper Extremity

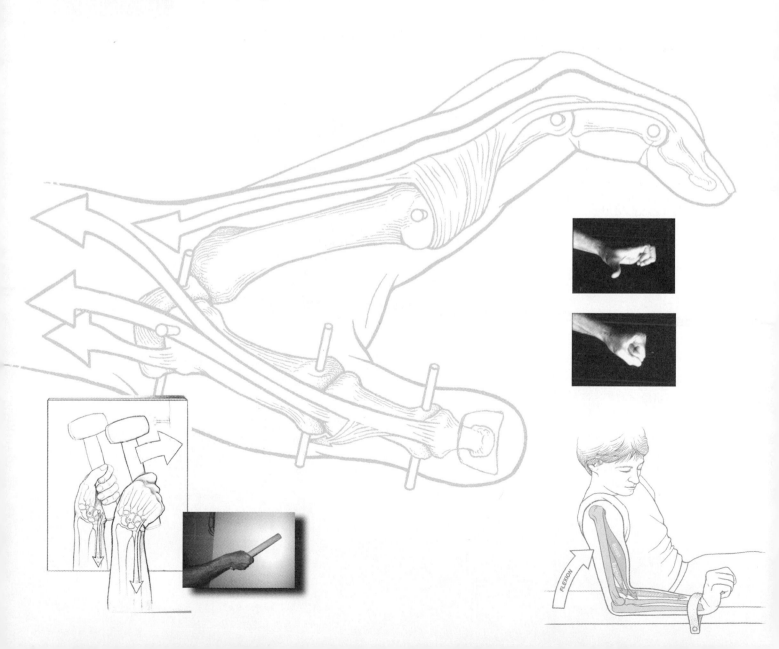

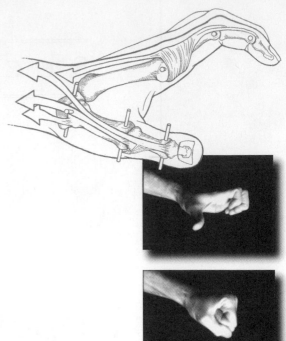
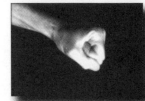

## SECTION II

# Upper Extremity

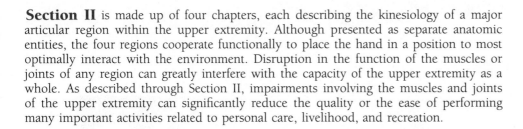

**Section II** is made up of four chapters, each describing the kinesiology of a major articular region within the upper extremity. Although presented as separate anatomic entities, the four regions cooperate functionally to place the hand in a position to most optimally interact with the environment. Disruption in the function of the muscles or joints of any region can greatly interfere with the capacity of the upper extremity as a whole. As described through Section II, impairments involving the muscles and joints of the upper extremity can significantly reduce the quality or the ease of performing many important activities related to personal care, livelihood, and recreation.

# CHAPTER 5

# Shoulder Complex

## DONALD A. NEUMANN, PT, PHD

## TOPICS AT A GLANCE

## INTRODUCTION

Our study of the upper limb begins with the *shoulder complex*, a set of four articulations involving the sternum, clavicle, ribs, scapula, and humerus (Fig. 5–1). This series of joints provides extensive range of motion to the upper extremity, thereby increasing the ability to manipulate objects. Trauma or disease often limits shoulder motion, causing a significant reduction in the effectiveness of the entire upper limb.

Rarely does a single muscle act in isolation at the shoulder complex. Muscles work in "teams" to produce a highly coordinated action that is expressed over multiple joints. The very cooperative nature of shoulder muscles increases the versatility, control, and range of active movements. Because of the nature of this functional relationship among muscles,

paralysis or weakness of *any single muscle* often disrupts the natural kinematic sequencing of the entire shoulder. This chapter describes several of the important muscular synergies that exist at the shoulder complex and how weakness in one muscle can affect the force generation potential in others.

## OSTEOLOGY

### Sternum

The sternum consists of the manubrium, body, and xiphoid process (Fig. 5–2). The *manubrium* possesses a pair of oval-shaped *clavicular facets*, which articulate with the clavicles. The *costal facets*, located on the lateral edge of the manubrium, provide attachment sites for the first two ribs. The

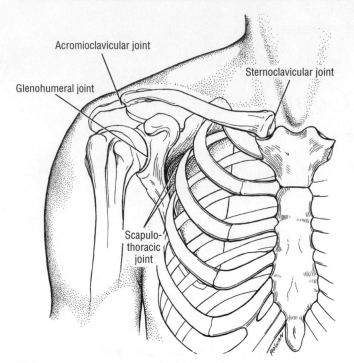

**FIGURE 5–1.** The joints of the right shoulder complex.

*jugular notch* is located at the superior aspect of the manubrium, between the clavicular facets.

> **Osteologic Features of the Sternum**
> • Manubrium
> • Clavicular facets
> • Costal facets
> • Jugular notch

## Clavicle

When looking from above, the *shaft* of the clavicle is curved with its anterior surface being generally convex medially and concave laterally (Fig. 5–3). With the arm in the anatomic position, the long axis of the clavicle is oriented slightly above the horizontal plane and about 20 degrees posterior to the frontal plane (Fig. 5–4; angle A). The rounded and prominent medial or sternal end of the clavicle articulates with the sternum (see Fig. 5–3). The *costal facet* of the clavicle (see Fig. 5–3; inferior surface) rests against the first rib. Lateral and slightly posterior to the costal facet is the distinct *costal tuberosity*, an attachment for the costoclavicular ligament.

> **Osteologic Features of the Clavicle**
> • Shaft
> • Costal facet
> • Costal tuberosity
> • Acromial facet
> • Conoid tubercle
> • Trapezoid line

The lateral or acromial end of the clavicle articulates with the scapula at the oval-shaped *acromial facet* (see Fig. 5–3; inferior surface). The inferior surface of the lateral end of the clavicle is well marked by the *conoid tubercle* and the *trapezoid line*.

## Scapula

The triangular-shaped scapula has *three angles: inferior, superior, and lateral* (Fig. 5–5). Palpation of the inferior angle provides a convenient method for following the movement of the scapula during arm motion. The scapula also has *three borders*. With the arm resting by the side, the *medial or vertebral border* runs almost parallel to the spinal column. The *lateral or axillary border* runs from the inferior angle to the lateral angle of the scapula. The *superior border* extends from the superior angle laterally toward the coracoid process.

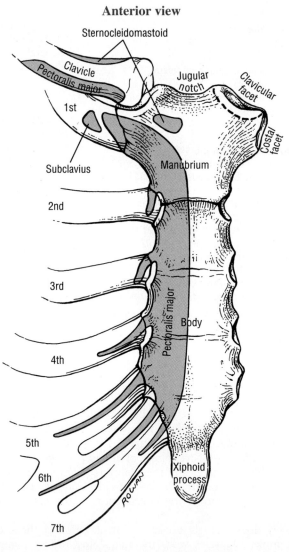

**FIGURE 5–2.** An anterior view of the sternum with left clavicle and ribs removed. The dashed line around the clavicular facet shows the attachments of the capsule at the sternoclavicular joint. Proximal attachments of muscle are shown in red.

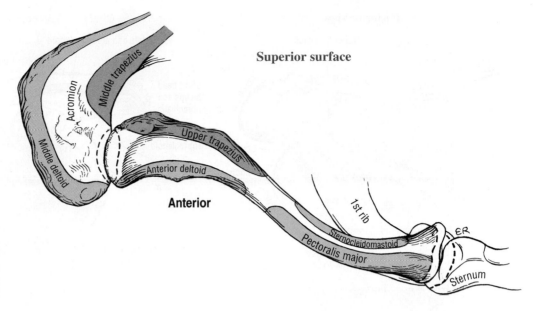

**Superior surface**

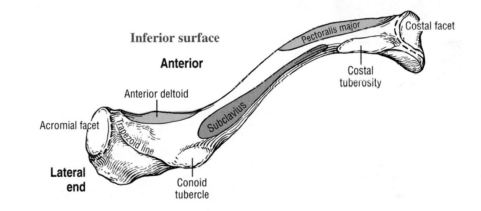

**FIGURE 5–3.** The superior and inferior surfaces of the right clavicle. The dashed line around the ends of the clavicle show attachments of the joint capsule. Proximal attachment of muscles are shown in red, distal attachments in gray.

**Inferior surface**

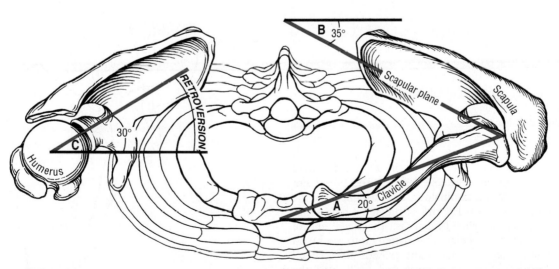

**FIGURE 5–4.** Superior view of both shoulders in the anatomic position. Angle **A:** the orientation of the clavicle deviated about 20 degrees posterior to the frontal plane. Angle **B:** the orientation of the scapula (scapular plane) deviated about 35 degrees anterior to the frontal plane. Angle **C:** retroversion of the humeral head about 30 degrees posterior to the medial-lateral axis at the elbow. The right clavicle and acromion have been removed to expose the top of the right glenohumeral joint.

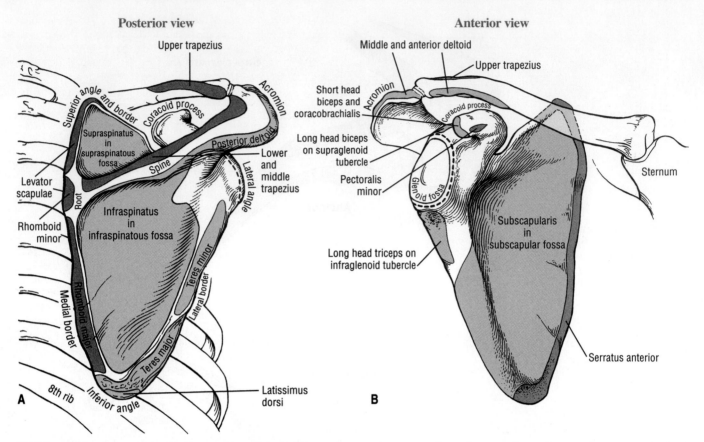

**Posterior view**

Upper trapezius

Superior angle and border

Acromion

Coracoid process

Supraspinatus in supraspinatous fossa

Posterior deltoid

Levator scapulae

Spine

Root

Lower and middle trapezius

Lateral angle

Rhomboid minor

Infraspinatus in infraspinatous fossa

Teres minor

Lateral border

Medial border

Rhomboid major

Teres major

8th rib

Inferior angle

Latissimus dorsi

A

**Anterior view**

Middle and anterior deltoid

Upper trapezius

Short head biceps and coracobrachialis

Acromion

Coracoid process

Long head biceps on supraglenoid tubercle

Pectoralis minor

Glenoid fossa

Sternum

Long head triceps on infraglenoid tubercle

Subscapularis in subscapular fossa

Serratus anterior

B

**FIGURE 5–5.** Posterior (A) and anterior (B) surfaces of the right scapula. Proximal attachment of muscles are shown in red, distal attachments in gray. The dashed lines show the capsular attachments around the glenohumeral joint.

---

**Osteologic Features of the Scapula**
- Angles: inferior, superior, and lateral
- Medial or vertebral border
- Lateral or axillary border
- Superior border
- Supraspinatous fossa
- Infraspinatous fossa
- Spine
- Root of the spine
- Acromion
- Clavicular facet
- Glenoid fossa
- Supraglenoid and infraglenoid tubercles
- Coracoid process
- Subscapular fossa

---

The posterior surface of the scapula is separated into a *supraspinatous fossa* and *infraspinatous fossa* by the prominent *spine*. The depth of the supraspinatous fossa is filled by the supraspinatus muscle. The medial end of the spine diminishes in height at the *root of the spine*. In contrast, the lateral end of the spine gains considerable height and flattens into the broad and prominent *acromion*. The acromion extends in a lateral and anterior direction, forming a horizontal shelf over the glenoid fossa. The *clavicular facet* on the acromion marks the surface of the acromioclavicular joint (see Fig. 5–17B).

The scapula articulates with the head of the humerus at the slightly concave *glenoid fossa* (from the Greek root *glene*;

socket of joint, + *eidos*; resembling) (Fig. 5–5B). The glenoid fossa is tilted upwardly about 5 degrees relative to the scapula's medial border (Fig. 5–6). At rest, the scapula is normally positioned against the posterior-lateral surface of the thorax with the glenoid fossa facing about 35 degrees

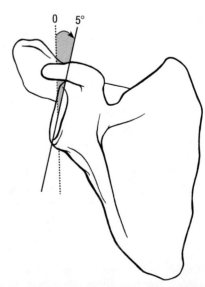

0    5°

**FIGURE 5–6.** Anterior view of the right scapula showing an approximate 5-degree upward tilt of the glenoid fossa relative to the medial border of the scapula.

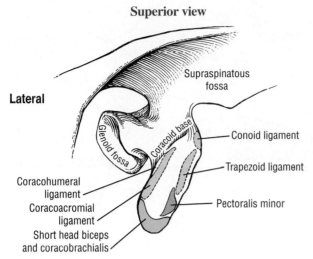

**FIGURE 5–7.** A close-up view of the right coracoid process looking from above. Proximal attachments of muscle are in red, distal attachments in gray. Ligamentous attachment is indicated by light gray area outlined by dashed line.

anterior to the frontal plane (see Fig. 5–4; angle B). This orientation of the scapula is called the *scapular plane*. The scapula and humerus tend to follow this plane when the arm is raised over the head.

Located at the superior and inferior rim of the glenoid fossa are the *supraglenoid* and *infraglenoid tubercles*. These tubercles serve as the proximal attachment for the long head of the biceps and triceps brachii, respectively (see Fig. 5–5B). Near the superior rim of the glenoid fossa is the prominent *coracoid process*, meaning "the shape of a crow's beak." The coracoid process projects sharply from the scapula, providing multiple attachments for ligaments and muscles (Fig. 5–7). The *subscapular fossa* is located on the anterior surface of the scapula. The concavity within the fossa is filled with the thick subscapularis muscle (see Fig. 5–5B).

## Proximal-to-Mid Humerus

The *head of the humerus*, nearly one half of a full sphere, forms the convex component of the glenohumeral joint (Fig. 5–8). The head faces medially and superiorly, forming an approximate 135-degree angle of inclination with the long axis of the humeral shaft (Fig. 5–9A). Relative to a medial-lateral axis through the elbow, the humeral head is rotated posteriorly about 30 degrees within the horizontal plane (Fig. 5–9B). This rotation, known as *retroversion* (from the Latin root *retro;* backward, + *verto;* to turn), orients the humeral head in the scapular plane for articulation with the glenoid fossa (Fig. 5–4; angle C).

The *anatomic neck* of the humerus separates the smooth articular surface of the head from the proximal shaft (Fig. 5–8A). The prominent lesser and greater tubercles surround the anterior and lateral circumference of the extreme proximal end of the humerus (Fig. 5–8B). The *lesser tubercle*

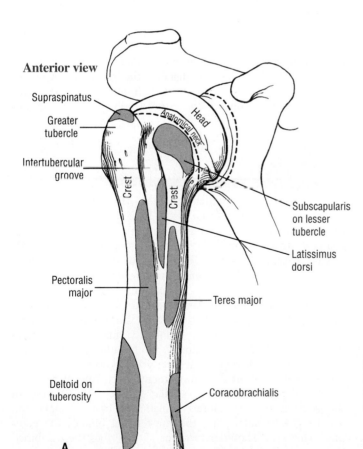

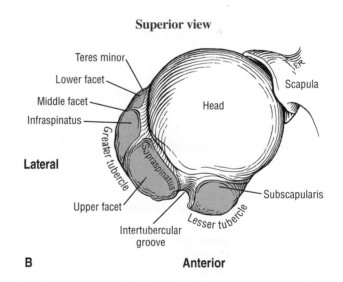

**FIGURE 5–8.** Anterior (*A*) and superior (*B*) aspects of the right humerus. The dashed line in *A* shows the capsular attachments around the glenohumeral joint. Distal attachment of muscles is shown in gray.

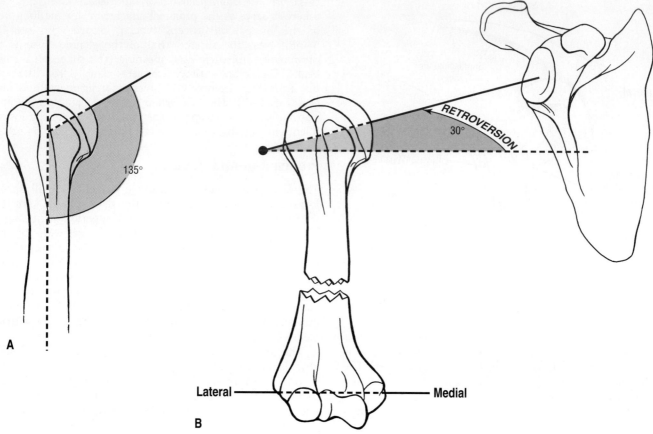

**FIGURE 5–9.** The right humerus showing a 135° "angle of inclination" between the shaft and head of the humerus in the frontal plane (A) and the retroversion of the humeral head relative to the distal humerus (B).

projects rather sharply and anteriorly for attachment of the subscapularis. The large and rounded *greater tubercle* has an *upper, middle, and lower facet,* marking the distal attachment of the supraspinatus, infraspinatus, and teres minor, respectively (Figs. 5–8B and 5–10).

Sharp *crests* extend distally from the anterior side of the greater and lesser tubercles. These crests receive the distal attachments of the pectoralis major and teres major (see Fig. 5–8A). Between these crests is the *intertubercular (bicipital) groove,* which houses the long head of the tendon of the biceps brachii. The latissimus dorsi muscle attaches to the floor of the intertubercular groove, medial to the biceps tendon. Distal and lateral to the termination of the intertubercular groove is the *deltoid tuberosity.*

---

**Osteologic Features of the Proximal-to-Mid Humerus**
- Head of the humerus
- Anatomic neck
- Lesser tubercle and crest
- Greater tubercle and crest
- Upper, middle, and lower facets on the greater tubercle
- Intertubercular (bicipital) groove
- Deltoid tuberosity
- Radial (spiral) groove

---

The *radial (spiral) groove* runs obliquely across the posterior surface of the humerus. The groove separates the proxi-

mal attachments of the lateral and medial head of the triceps (see Fig. 5–10). Traveling distally, the radial nerve spirals around the posterior side of the humerus in the radial groove, heading toward the distal-lateral side of the humerus.

## ARTHROLOGY

The most proximal articulation within the shoulder complex is the *sternoclavicular joint* (see Fig. 5–1). The clavicle, through its attachment to the sternum, functions as a mechanical strut, or prop, holding the scapula at a relatively constant distance from the trunk. Located at the lateral end of the clavicle is the *acromioclavicular joint.* This joint and associated ligaments firmly attach the scapula to the clavicle. The point of contact between the anterior surface of the scapula and the posterior-lateral surface of the thorax is called the *scapulothoracic joint.* In this case, the term does not imply a true anatomic joint, rather an interfacing of two bones. Movement at the scapulothoracic joint is a direct result of individual movements occurring at the sternoclavicular and acromioclavicular joints. The position of the scapula on the thorax provides a base of operation for the *glenohumeral joint,* the most distal link of the complex. The term "shoulder movement" describes the combined motions at both the glenohumeral and the scapulothoracic joint.

## Posterior view

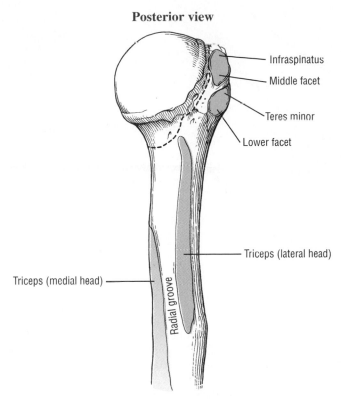

Infraspinatus

Middle facet

Teres minor

Lower facet

Triceps (lateral head)

Triceps (medial head)

Radial groove

**FIGURE 5–10.** Posterior aspect of the right proximal humerus. Proximal attachments of muscles are in red, distal attachments in gray. The dashed line shows the capsular attachments of the glenohumeral joint.

---

**Four Joints Within the Shoulder Complex**
1. Sternoclavicular
2. Acromioclavicular
3. Scapulothoracic
4. Glenohumeral

---

The joints of the shoulder complex function as a series of links, all cooperating to maximize the range of motion available to the upper limb. A weakened, painful, or unstable link anywhere along the chain significantly decreases the effectiveness of the entire complex.

Before discussion of the kinematic analysis of the sternoclavicular and acromioclavicular joints, the movements at the scapulothoracic joint must be defined (Fig. 5–11). The primary movements of the scapulothoracic joint are elevation and depression, protraction and retraction, and upward and downward rotation.

---

**Movements at the Scapulothoracic Joint**
- Elevation and depression
- Protraction and retraction
- Upward and downward rotation

---

**Elevation.** The scapula slides superiorly on the thorax, such as in the shrugging of the shoulders.

**Depression.** From an elevated position, the scapula slides inferiorly on the thorax.

**Protraction.** The medial border of the scapula slides anterior-laterally on the thorax away from the midline.

**Retraction.** The medial border of the scapula slides posterior-medially on the thorax toward the midline, such as occurs during the pinching of the shoulder blades together.

**Upward Rotation.** The inferior angle of the scapula rotates in a superior-lateral direction such that the glenoid fossa faces upward. This rotation occurs as a natural component of the arm reaching upward.

**Downward Rotation.** The inferior angle of the scapula rotates in an inferior-medial direction such that the glenoid fossa faces downward. This motion occurs as a natural com-

---

**Elevation and Depression**          **Retraction and Protraction**          **Downward and Upward Rotation**

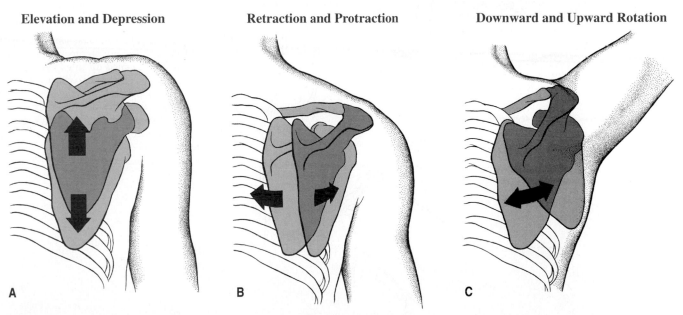

A          B          C

**FIGURE 5–11.** Motions of the right scapula against the posterior-lateral surface of the thorax. *A,* Elevation and depression. *B,* Retraction and protraction. *C,* Downward and upward rotation.

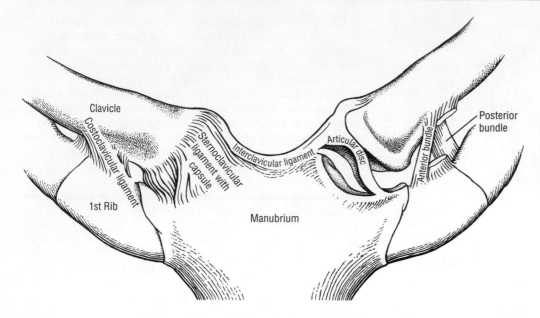

**FIGURE 5–12.** The sternoclavicular joints. The capsule and lateral section of the anterior bundle of the costoclavicular ligament have been removed on the left side.

ponent of the lowering of the arm to the side from the elevated position.

## Sternoclavicular Joint

### GENERAL FEATURES

The sternoclavicular (SC) joint is a complex articulation, involving the medial end of the clavicle, the clavicular facet on the sternum, and the superior border of the cartilage of the first rib (Fig. 5–12). The joint is the basilar joint of the upper extremity, linking the axial skeleton with the appendicular skeleton. As such, the SC joint is subjected to unique functional demands that are met by a complex saddle-shaped articular surface (Fig. 5–13).[68] Although highly variable, the medial end of the clavicle is usually convex along its longitudinal diameter and concave along its transverse

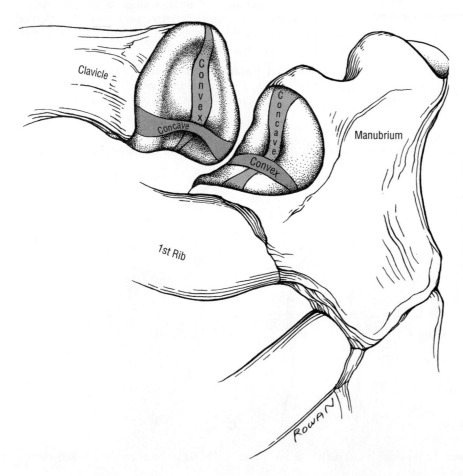

**FIGURE 5–13.** An anterior-lateral view of the articular surfaces of the right sternoclavicular joint. The joint has been opened up to expose its articular surfaces. The longitudinal diameters (red) extend roughly in the frontal plane between superior and inferior points of the articular surfaces. The transverse diameters (gray) extend roughly in the horizontal plane between anterior and posterior points of the articular surfaces.

diameter. The clavicular facet on the sternum typically is reciprocally shaped, with a slightly concave longitudinal diameter and a slightly convex transverse diameter.

The large and exposed articular surface of the clavicle rests against the smaller, sloped, articular surface of the sternum. A prominent articular disc resides within the SC joint, which tends to increase the congruity of otherwise irregular-shaped joint surfaces.

## PERIARTICULAR CONNECTIVE TISSUE

The SC joint is enclosed by a capsule reinforced by *anterior and posterior sternoclavicular ligaments* (Fig. 5–12). The inner surface of the capsule is lined with synovial membrane. In addition, the joint is stabilized anteriorly by the sternal head of the sternocleidomastoid and posteriorly by the sternothyroid and sternohyoid muscles. The *interclavicular ligament* spans the jugular notch, connecting the medial end of the right and left clavicles.

> **Tissues That Stabilize the SC Joint**
> - Anterior and posterior sternoclavicular ligaments
> - Interclavicular ligament
> - Costoclavicular ligament
> - Articular disc
> - Sternocleidomastoid, sternothyroid, and sternohyoid muscles

The *costoclavicular ligament* is a strong structure extending from the cartilage of the first rib to the costal tuberosity on the inferior surface of the clavicle. The ligament has two distinct fiber bundles running perpendicular to each other.[68] The anterior bundle runs obliquely in a superior and lateral direction, and the more posterior bundle runs obliquely in a superior and medial direction (see Fig. 5–12). The costoclavicular ligament firmly stabilizes the SC joint and limits the extremes of all clavicular motion, except for a downward movement of the clavicle (i.e., depression).

The *articular disc* at the SC joint separates the joint into distinct medial and lateral joint cavities (see Fig. 5–12). The disc is a flattened piece of fibrocartilage that attaches inferiorly near the lateral edge of the clavicular facet and superiorly at the head of the clavicle and interclavicular ligament. The remaining outer edge of the disc attaches to the internal surface of the capsule. The disc functions as a shock absorber within the joint by increasing the surface area of joint contact. This absorption mechanism apparently works well since significant age-related degenerative arthritis is relatively rare at this joint.[16]

The tremendous stability at the SC joint is due to the arrangement of the surrounding periarticular connective tissues.[12] Large medially directed forces through the clavicle often cause fracture of the bone's shaft instead of a SC joint dislocation. Clavicular fractures are most common in males under 30 years old. Most often these fractures are the result of contact-sport or road-traffic accidents.[51]

## KINEMATICS

The osteokinematics of the clavicle are defined for 3 degrees of freedom. Each degree of freedom is associated with one of the three cardinal planes: *sagittal, frontal,* and *horizontal.* The clavicle elevates and depresses, protracts and retracts, and rotates about the bone's longitudinal axis (Fig. 5–14). Essentially all functional movement of the shoulder involves at least some movement of the clavicle about the SC joint.

> **Osteokinematics at the SC Joint**
> - Elevation and depression
> - Protraction and retraction
> - Axial rotation of the clavicle

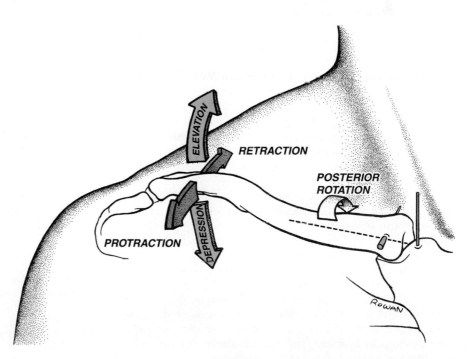

**FIGURE 5–14.** The right sternoclavicular joint showing the osteokinematic motions of the clavicle. The motions are elevation and depression in a near frontal plane (red), protraction and retraction in a near horizontal plane (gray), and posterior clavicular rotation in a near sagittal plane (white). The vertical axis (gray) and anterior-posterior axis (red) are color-coded with the corresponding planes of movement. Longitudinal axis is indicated by the dashed line.

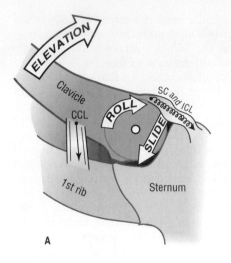

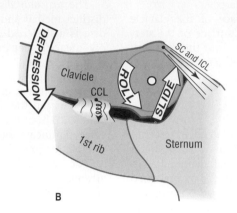

**A**    **B**

**FIGURE 5–15.** Anterior view of a mechanical diagram of the arthrokinematics of roll and slide during elevation (*A*) and depression (*B*) of the clavicle about the right sternoclavicular joint. The axes of rotation are shown in the anterior-posterior direction near the head of the clavicle. Stretched structures are shown as thin elongated arrows, slackened structures are shown as wavy arrows. Note in *A* that the stretched costoclavicular ligament produces a downward force in the direction of the slide. (Costoclavicular ligament = CCL, superior capsule = SC, interclavicular ligament = ICL.)

### Elevation and Depression

Elevation and depression of the clavicle occur approximately parallel to the frontal plane about an anterior-posterior axis of rotation (see Fig. 5–14). A maximum of approximately 45 degrees of elevation and 10 degrees of depression have been reported.[11,38] Elevation and depression of the clavicle are associated with a similar motion of the scapula.

The arthrokinematics for elevation and depression of the clavicle occur along the SC joint's longitudinal diameter (see Fig. 5–13). Elevation of the clavicle occurs as the convex surface of its head rolls superiorly and simultaneously slides inferiorly on the concavity of the sternum (Fig. 5–15A). The stretched costoclavicular ligament helps stabilize the position of the clavicle. Depression of the clavicle occurs by action of its head rolling inferiorly and sliding superiorly (Fig. 5–15B). A fully depressed clavicle elongates and stretches the interclavicular ligament and the superior portion of the capsular ligaments.[4]

### Protraction and Retraction

Protraction and retraction of the clavicle occur nearly parallel to the horizontal plane about a vertical axis of rotation (see Fig. 5–14). The axis is shown in Figure 5–14 intersecting the sternum because, by convention, an axis of rotation always intersects the convex member of a joint for a particular movement. At least 15 to 30 degrees of rotation in each direction have been reported.[11,38,58] The horizontal plane motions of the clavicle are associated with a similar protraction and retraction motion of the scapula.

The arthrokinematics for protraction and retraction of the clavicle occur along the SC joint's transverse diameter (see Fig. 5–13). Retraction occurs as the concave articular surface of the clavicle rolls and slides posteriorly on the convex surface of the sternum (Fig. 5–16). The end ranges of retraction elongate the anterior bundles of the costoclavicular ligament and the anterior capsular ligaments.

The arthrokinematics of protraction about the SC joint are similar to those of retraction, except that they occur in an anterior direction. The extremes of protraction occur during a motion involving maximal forward reach. Excessive tightness in the posterior bundle of the costoclavicular ligament, the posterior capsular ligament, and the scapular retractor muscles may limit the extreme of clavicular protraction.

### Axial (Longitudinal) Rotation of the Clavicle

The 3rd degree of freedom at the SC joint is a rotation of the clavicle about the bone's longitudinal axis (see Fig. 5–14). When the shoulder is abducted or flexed, a point on the superior aspect of the clavicle rotates posteriorly approximately 40 to 50 degrees.[26,63] As the arm is returned to the side, the clavicle rotates back to its original position.

The arthrokinematics of clavicular rotation involve a *spin* of the head of the clavicle about the lateral surface of the articular disc. Full posterior rotation of the clavicle is considered the close-packed position of the SC joint.[68]

## Acromioclavicular Joint

### GENERAL FEATURES

The acromioclavicular (AC) joint is the articulation between the lateral end of the clavicle and the acromion of the scapula (Fig. 5–17A). The clavicular facet on the acromion faces medially and slightly superiorly, providing a fit with the

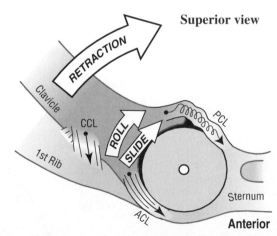

**FIGURE 5–16.** Superior view of a mechanical diagram of the arthrokinematics of roll and slide during retraction of the clavicle about the right sternoclavicular joint. The vertical axis of rotation is shown through the sternum. Stretched structures are shown as thin elongated arrows, slackened structures shown as a wavy arrow. (Costoclavicular ligament = CCL, anterior capsular ligament = ACL, posterior capsular ligaments = PCL.)

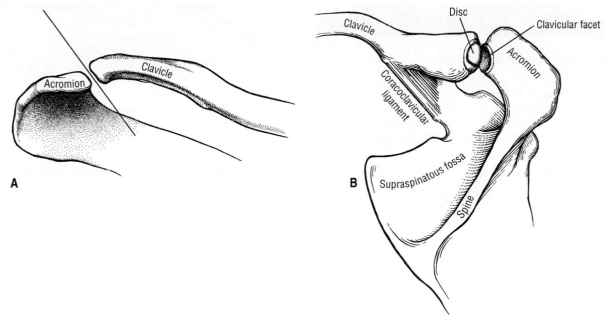

**FIGURE 5–17.** The right acromioclavicular joint. *A,* An anterior view showing the sloping nature of the articulation. *B,* A posterior view of the joint opened up from behind, showing the clavicular facet on the acromion and the disc.

corresponding acromial facet on the clavicle. An articular disc of varying form is present in most AC joints.

The AC joint is most often described as a gliding or plane joint, reflecting the predominantly flat contour of the joint surfaces. Joint surfaces vary, however, from flat to slightly convex or concave (Fig. 5–17B). Because of the predominantly flat joint surfaces, roll-and-slide arthrokinematics are not here described.

## PERIARTICULAR CONNECTIVE TISSUE

The AC joint is surrounded by a capsule that is reinforced by *superior and inferior ligaments* (Fig. 5–18). The superior capsular ligament is reinforced through attachments from the deltoid and trapezius.

| Tissues that Stabilize the AC Joint |
| --- |
| • Superior and inferior AC joint capsular ligaments |
| • Deltoid and upper trapezius |
| • Coracoclavicular ligament |
| • Articular disc |

The *coracoclavicular ligament* provides additional stability to the AC joint (see Fig. 5–18). This extensive ligament consists of the trapezoid and conoid ligaments. The *trapezoid ligament* extends in a superior-lateral direction from the superior surface of the coracoid process to the trapezoid line on the clavicle. The *conoid ligament* extends almost vertically from the proximal base of the coracoid process to the conoid tubercle on the clavicle.

The articular surfaces at the AC joint are lined with a layer of fibrocartilage and often separated by a complete or incomplete *articular disc*. An extensive dissection of 223 sets of AC joints revealed complete discs in only about 10% of the joints.[16] The majority of joints possessed incomplete discs, which appeared fragmented and worn. According to DePalma,[16] the incomplete discs are not structural anomalies, but rather indications of the degeneration that often affects this joint.

## KINEMATICS

Distinct functional differences exist between the SC and AC joints. The SC joint permits relative extensive motion of the clavicle, which guides the general path of the scapula. The

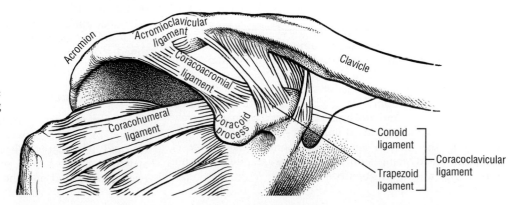

**FIGURE 5–18.** An anterior view of the right acromioclavicular joint including many surrounding ligaments.

### Acromioclavicular Joint Dislocation

The AC joint is inherently susceptible to dislocation due to the sloped nature of the articulation and the high probability of receiving large shearing forces. Consider a person falling and striking the tip of the shoulder abruptly against the ground (Fig. 5–19). The resulting medially directed ground force may displace the acromion medially and under the sloped articular facet of the well-stabilized clavicle. The coracoclavicular ligaments, particularly the trapezoid ligament, naturally resist such an AC joint displacement.[20] On occasion, the force applied to the scapula exceeds the tensile strength of the ligaments, resulting in their rupture and the complete dislocation of the AC joint. Extensive literature exists on the evaluation and treatment of the injured AC joint, especially in athletes.[32]

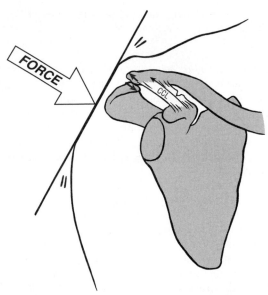

**FIGURE 5–19.** An anterior view of the shoulder striking the ground with the force of the impact directed at the acromion. Note the increased tension and partial tear within the coracoclavicular ligament (CCL).

AC joint, in contrast, permits subtle and often slight movements of the scapula. The slight movements at the AC joint are physiologically important, providing the maximum extent of mobility at the scapulothoracic joint.[63]

The motions of the scapula at the AC joint are described in 3 degrees of freedom (Fig. 5–20A). The primary motions are called upward and downward rotation. Secondary rotational adjustment motions amplify or "fine tune" the final position of the scapula against the thorax.[63] The range of motion at the AC joint is difficult to measure, and this is not done in typical clinical situations.

### Upward and Downward Rotation

Upward rotation of the scapula at the AC joint occurs as the scapula "swings upwardly and outwardly" in relation to the lateral edge of the clavicle (Fig. 5–20A). Reports vary, but up to 30 degrees of upward rotation can occur as the arm is raised over the head.[26,38,63] The motion contributes an extensive component of overall upward rotation at the scapulothoracic joint (Fig. 5–11C). Downward rotation at the AC joint returns the scapula back to its anatomic position, a motion mechanically associated with shoulder adduction or extension. Although Figure 5–20A depicts the upward and downward rotation of the scapula as a pure frontal plane motion, most natural motions occur within the scapular plane.

Complete upward rotation of the scapula at the AC joint is considered the close-packed position.[68] This motion places significant stretch on the inferior AC joint capsule and the coracoclavicular ligament.

### Horizontal and Sagittal Plane "Rotational Adjustments" at the Acromioclavicular Joint

Cineradiographic observations of the AC joint during shoulder movement reveal small pivoting or twisting motions of the scapula about the lateral end of the clavicle (see Fig. 5–20A).[40] These so-called rotational adjustment motions fine tune the position of the scapula or add to the total amount of its motion permitted on the thorax.

Horizontal plane adjustments at the AC joint occur about a vertical axis that causes the medial border of the scapula to pivot away and toward the outer surface of the thorax. Sagittal plane adjustments at the AC joint occur about a medial-lateral axis, which causes the inferior angle to tilt or pivot away or toward the outer surface of the thorax. Rotational adjustments between 10 and 30 degrees have been reported.[6,11,63]

The horizontal and sagittal plane adjustments at the AC joint enhance both the quality and quantity of movement at the scapulothoracic joint. For instance, during protraction of the scapula, small horizontal plane adjustments at the AC joint allow the anterior surface of the scapula to change its position as it follows the curved contour of the thorax (Fig. 5–20B). A similar adjustment occurs in the sagittal plane during elevation of the scapula (Fig. 5–20C). Without these rotational adjustments the scapula is obligated to follow the *exact path* of the moving clavicle, without any ability to fine tune its position relative to the thorax.

## Scapulothoracic Joint

The scapulothoracic joint is not a true joint per se but rather a point of contact between the anterior surface of the scapula and the posterior-lateral wall of the thorax.[67] In the anatomic position, the scapula is typically positioned between the second and the seventh rib, with the medial bor-

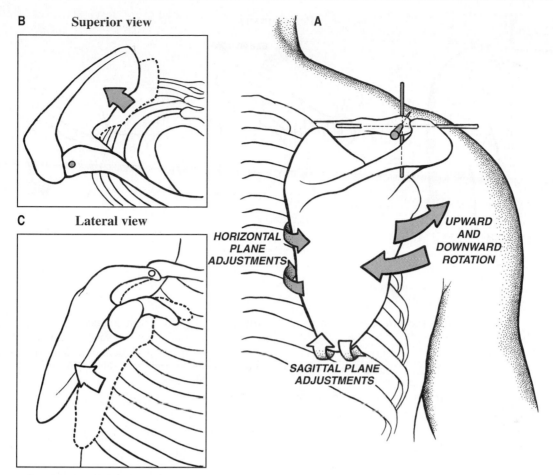

**FIGURE 5–20.** *A,* Posterior view showing the osteokinematics of the right acromioclavicular joint. The primary motions of upward and downward rotation are shown in red. Horizontal and sagittal plane adjustments, considered as secondary motions, are shown in gray and white, respectively. Note that each plane of movement is color-coded with a corresponding axis of rotation. *B* and *C* show examples of the horizontal plane adjustment made during scapulothoracic protraction (*B*) and sagittal plane adjustment made during scapulothoracic elevation (*C*).

der located about 6 cm (2½ in) lateral to the spine. This "resting" posture of the scapula varies considerably from one person to another.

Movements at the scapulothoracic joint are a very important element of shoulder kinesiology. The wide range of motion available to the shoulder is due, in part, to the large movement available to the scapulothoracic joint.

## KINEMATICS

### *Movement of the Scapulothoracic Joint: A Composite of the Sternoclavicular and Acromioclavicular Joint Movements*

The movements that occur between the scapula and the thorax are a result of a cooperation between the SC and the AC joints.

### *Elevation and Depression*

Scapular elevation at the scapulothoracic joint occurs as a composite of SC and AC joint rotations (Fig. 5–21A). For the most part, the motion of shrugging the shoulders occurs as a direct result of the scapula's following the path of the elevating clavicle about the SC joint (Fig. 5–21B). Down-

ward rotation of the scapula at the AC joint allows the scapula to remain nearly vertical throughout the elevation (Fig. 5–21C). Additional adjustments at the AC joint help to keep the scapula flush with the thorax. Depression of the scapula at the scapulothoracic joint occurs as the reverse action described for elevation.

### *Protraction and Retraction*

Protraction of the scapula occurs through a summation of horizontal plane rotations at both the SC and AC joints (Fig. 5–22A). The scapula follows the general path of the protracting clavicle about the SC joint (Fig. 5–22B). The AC joint can amplify or adjust the total amount of scapulothoracic protraction by contributing varying amounts of adjustments within the horizontal plane (Fig. 5–22C). Scapulothoracic protraction increases the extent of forward reach.

Because scapulothoracic protraction occurs as a summation of both the SC and AC joint, a decrease in motion at one joint can be at least partially compensated by an increase at the other. Consider, for example, a case of severe degenerative arthritis and decreased motion at the AC joint. The SC joint may compensate by contributing a greater de-

**Posterior view**

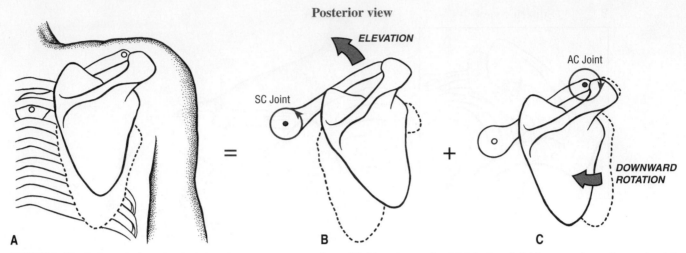

**FIGURE 5–21.** *A*, Scapulothoracic elevation shown as a summation of *B* (elevation at the SC joint) and *C* (downward rotation at the AC joint).

gree of protraction, thereby limiting the extent of loss in the forward reach of the upper limb.

Retraction of the scapula occurs in a similar but reverse fashion as protraction. Retraction of the scapula is often performed in the context of pulling an object toward the body, such as pulling on a wall pulley, climbing a rope, or putting the arm in a coat sleeve.

### *Upward and Downward Rotation*

Upward rotation of the scapulothoracic joint is an integral part of raising the arm over the head (Fig. 5–23A). This motion places the glenoid fossa in a position to support and stabilize the head of the abducted (i.e., raised) humerus. Complete upward rotation of the scapula occurs as a summation of clavicular elevation at the SC joint (Fig. 5–23B) *and* scapular upward rotation at the AC joint (Fig. 5–23C). These dual frontal plane rotations occur about parallel SC and AC joint axes, allowing a total of 60 degrees of scapular rotation. The scapula may rotate upwardly and strictly in the frontal plane as in true abduction, but it usually follows a path closer to its own plane.

Downward rotation of the scapula occurs as the arm is returned to the side from a raised position. The motion is described as similar to upward rotation, except that the clavicle depresses at the SC joint and the scapula downwardly rotates at the AC joint. The motion of downward rotation usually ends when the scapula has returned to the anatomic position.

## Glenohumeral Joint

### GENERAL FEATURES

The glenohumeral (GH) joint is the articulation formed between the large convex head of the humerus and the shallow concavity of the glenoid fossa (Fig. 5–24). This joint operates in conjunction with the moving scapula to produce an extensive range of motion of the shoulder. In the anatomic position, the articular surface of the glenoid fossa is directed anterior-laterally in the scapular plane. In most people, the glenoid fossa is upwardly rotated slightly. This position is dependent on the amount of fixed upward tilt to the fossa (see Fig. 5–6) and to the amount of upward rotation of the scapula in its "resting" posture.

**Superior view**

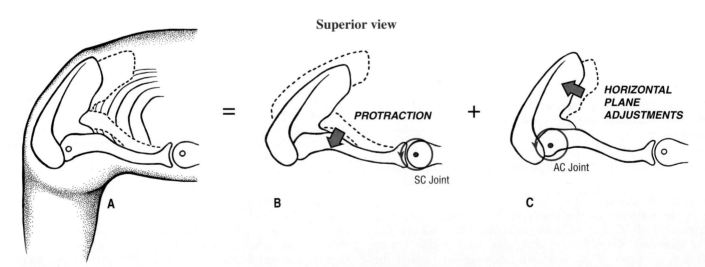

**FIGURE 5–22.** *A*, Scapulothoracic protraction shown as a summation of *B* (protraction at the SC joint) and *C* (slight horizontal plane adjustments at the AC joint).

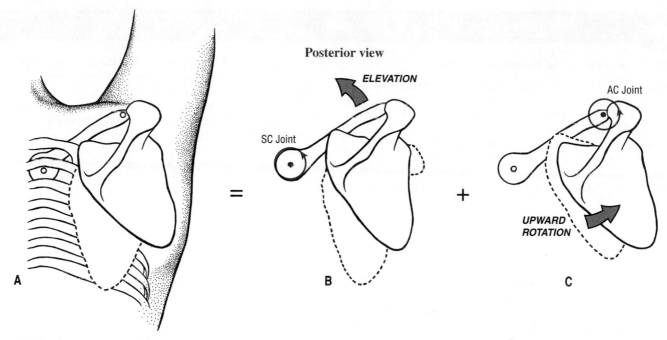

**FIGURE 5–23.** *A,* Scapulothoracic upward rotation shown as a summation of *B* (elevation of the SC joint) and *C* (upward rotation at the AC joint).

In the anatomic position, the articular surface of the humeral head is directed medially and superiorly, as well as posteriorly because of its natural retroversion. This orientation places the head of the humerus directly into the scapular plane and therefore directly against the face of the glenoid fossa (see Fig. 5–4B and 5–4C).

## PERIARTICULAR CONNECTIVE TISSUE

The GH joint is surrounded by a fibrous capsule, which isolates the internal joint cavity from most surrounding tissues (see Fig. 5–24). The capsule attaches along the rim of the glenoid fossa and extends to the anatomic neck of the humerus. A synovial membrane lines the inner wall of the joint capsule. An extension of this synovial membrane lines the intracapsular portion of the tendon of the long head of the biceps brachii. This synovial membrane continues to surround the biceps tendon as it exits the joint capsule and descends into the intertubercular (i.e., bicipital) groove.

The potential volume of space within the GH joint capsule is about twice the size of the humeral head. In conjunction with a loose fitting and expandable capsule, the GH joint allows extensive mobility. This mobility is evident by the amount of passive translation available at the GH joint. The humeral head can be pulled away from the fossa a significant distance without causing pain or trauma to the joint. In the anatomic or adducted position, the inferior portion of the capsule appears as a slackened recess called the *axillary pouch.*

The rotator cuff muscles (subscapularis, supraspinatus, infraspinatus, and teres minor) and the capsular ligaments blend into the fibrous capsule, providing most of the stability to this articulation. The long head of the biceps also contributes stability to the joint.[34]

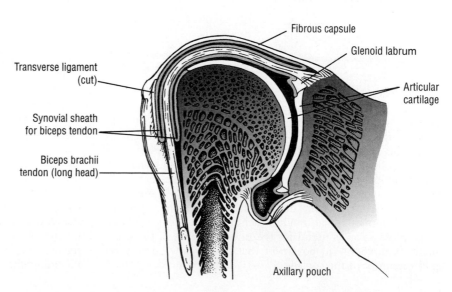

**FIGURE 5–24.** Anterior view of a frontal section through the right glenohumeral joint. Note the fibrous capsule, synovial membrane (red), the long head of the biceps tendon. The axillary pouch is shown as a recess in the inferior capsule.

**SPECIAL FOCUS 5–2**

### The "Loose-Fit" of the Glenohumeral Joint

The articular surface of the glenoid fossa covers only about one third of the articular surface of the humeral head. This size difference allows only a small part of the humeral head to make contact with the glenoid fossa. In a typical adult, the longitudinal diameter of the humeral head is about 1.9 times larger than the same diameter of the glenoid fossa (Fig. 5–25). The transverse diameter of the humeral head is about 2.3 times larger than the op-

posing diameter of the glenoid fossa. By describing the GH joint as a ball-and-socket joint, the erroneous impression is given that the head of the humerus fits *into* the glenoid fossa. The actual structure of the GH joint articulation resembles more that of a golf ball pressed against a coin the size of a quarter. Joint stability is achieved by passive tension produced by periarticular connective tissues and by active forces produced by muscles, not by bony fit.

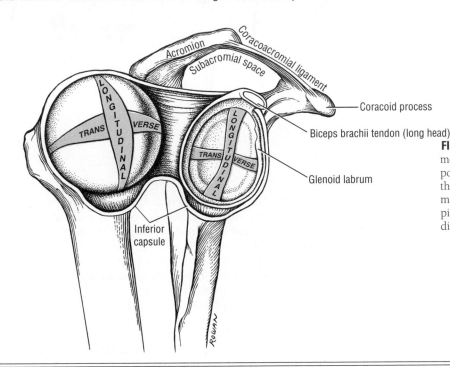

**FIGURE 5–25.** Side view of right glenohumeral joint with the joint opened up to expose the articular surfaces. Note the extent of the subacromial space under the coracoacromial arch. The longitudinal diameter is depicted in the frontal plane and the transverse diameter is depicted in the horizontal plane.

---

**Tissues that Stabilize or Deepen the GH Joint**
- Rotator cuff muscles (subscapularis, supraspinatus, infraspinatus, and teres minor)
- GH joint capsular ligaments
- Coracohumeral ligament
- Long head of the biceps
- Glenoid labrum

The external layers of the anterior and inferior walls of the joint capsule are thickened and strengthened by fibrous connective tissue known simply as the *glenohumeral (capsular) ligaments* (Fig. 5–26). Passive tension in the capsular ligaments limits the extremes of GH joint rotation and translation.

The following discussion provides the essential anatomy and function of the GH joint capsular ligaments. For more detail, refer to additional literature, such as Curl[13] and Bigliani.[5] Table 5–1 lists the distal attachments of the ligaments and the motions that render each capsular ligament taut. This information is useful for the understanding of the cause of the limitations in movement that may follow surgery repair or injury to the capsule.

The GH joint's capsular ligaments consist of complex bands of interlacing collagen fibers, divided into superior, middle, and inferior bands. The ligaments are best visualized from an internal view of the GH joint (Fig. 5–27). The *superior glenohumeral ligament* has its proximal attachment near the supraglenoid tubercle, just anterior to the attachment of the long head of the biceps. The ligament, with associated capsule, attaches distally near the anatomic neck of the humerus above the lesser tubercle. The ligament becomes particularly taut in full adduction or during inferior and posterior translations of the humerus.[53,65]

The *middle glenohumeral ligament* has a wide proximal attachment to the superior and middle aspects of the anterior rim of the glenoid fossa. The ligament blends with the anterior capsule and tendon of the subscapularis muscle, then attaches along the anterior aspect of the anatomic neck. This ligament provides substantial anterior restraint to the GH joint, resisting anterior translation of the humerus and the extremes of external rotation.[41]

The extensive *inferior glenohumeral ligament* attaches proximally along the anterior-inferior rim of the glenoid fossa, including the adjacent glenoid labrum. Distally the inferior

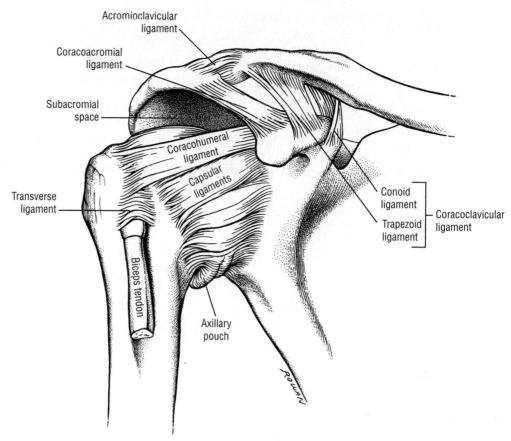

**FIGURE 5–26.** Anterior view of the right glenohumeral joint showing the following external features of the joint capsule: the capsular, coracohumeral, and coracoacromial ligaments. Note the subacromial space located between the top of the humeral head and the underside of the acromion.

glenohumeral ligament attaches as a broad sheet to the anterior-inferior and posterior-inferior margins of the anatomic neck.

This hammock-like inferior capsular ligament has three separate components: an *anterior band,* a *posterior band,* and a sheet of tissue connecting these bands known as an *axillary pouch* (see Fig. 5–27).[41] The axillary pouch and the surrounding inferior capsular ligaments become particularly taut at about 90 degrees of abduction, providing an important element of anterior-posterior stability to the GH joint in this position.[62,65] In the abducted position, the anterior and posterior bands become taut at the extremes of external and internal rotation, respectively.

The GH joint capsule receives additional reinforcement from the *coracohumeral ligament* (see Figs. 5–26 and 5–27). This ligament extends from the lateral border of the coracoid process to the anterior side of the greater tubercle of the humerus. The coracohumeral ligament blends in with the capsule and supraspinatus tendon, becoming taut at the extremes of external rotation, flexion, and extension. The ligament also resists inferior displacement (i.e., translation) of the humeral head.[60]

The GH joint capsule receives significant structural reinforcement through the attachments of the four *rotator cuff muscles* (see Fig. 5–27). The subscapularis lies just anterior to the capsule, and the supraspinatus, infraspinatus, and

## TABLE 5–1. Anatomy and Tissue Mechanics of the Glenohumeral Joint Capsule

| Ligament | Distal Attachments | Motions Drawing Structure Taut |
| --- | --- | --- |
| **Superior** glenohumeral ligament | Anatomic neck, above the lesser tubercle | Full adduction, and/or inferior and posterior translation of the humerus |
| **Middle** glenohumeral ligament | Along the anterior aspect of the anatomic neck | Anterior translation of the humerus and/or external rotation |
| **Inferior** glenohumeral ligament (three parts: anterior band, posterior band, and connecting axillary pouch) | As a broad sheet to the anterior-inferior and posterior-inferior margins of the anatomic neck | *All* fibers: abduction<br>*Anterior band:* abduction and external rotation<br>*Posterior band:* abduction and internal rotation |
| Coracohumeral ligament | Anterior side of the greater tubercle of the humerus | Extremes of external rotation, flexion, and extension; inferior displacement (translation) of the humeral head |

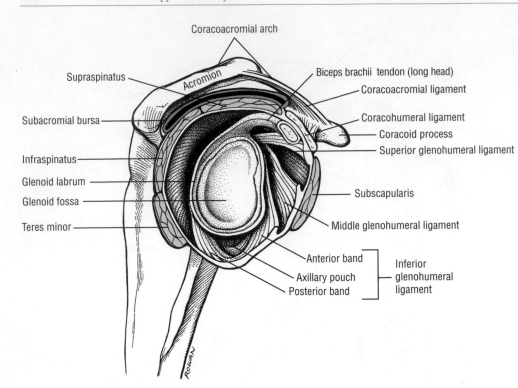

Coracoacromial arch

Supraspinatus

Acromion

Biceps brachii tendon (long head)

Coracoacromial ligament

Subacromial bursa

Coracohumeral ligament

Coracoid process

Superior glenohumeral ligament

Infraspinatus

Glenoid labrum

Glenoid fossa

Teres minor

Subscapularis

Middle glenohumeral ligament

Anterior band

Inferior glenohumeral ligament

Axillary pouch

Posterior band

**FIGURE 5–27.** Lateral aspect of the right glenohumeral joint showing the internal surface of the joint. The humerus has been removed to expose the capsular ligaments and the glenoid fossa. Note the prominent coracoacromial arch and underlying subacromial bursa. The four rotator cuff muscles are shown in pink. Synovial membrane is shown in red.

teres minor lie superior and posterior to the capsule. These muscles provide the majority of the stability to the joint during active motion.

The head of the humerus and the glenoid fossa are both lined with hyaline cartilage. The rim of the glenoid fossa is encircled by a fibrocartilage ring, or lip, known as the *glenoid labrum* (see Fig. 5–27). The long head of the biceps originates as a partial extension of the glenoid labrum. About 50% of the overall depth of the glenoid fossa is attributed to the glenoid labrum.[23] The labrum deepens the concavity of the fossa, providing additional stability to the joint.

## STATIC STABILITY AT THE GLENOHUMERAL JOINT

Normally, when standing at rest with arms at the side, the head of the humerus remains stable against the glenoid fossa. This stability is referred to as *static* since it exists at rest. One mechanism for controlling the static stability at the GH joint is based on the analogy of a ball compressed against an inclined surface (Fig. 5–28A).[3] At rest, the superior capsular structures, including the coracohumeral ligament, provide the primary stabilizing forces between the humeral head and the glenoid fossa. Combining this capsular force vector with the force vector due to gravity yields a

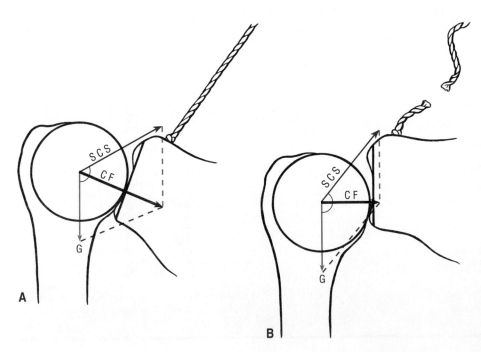

A

B

**FIGURE 5–28.** Static "locking" mechanism at the glenohumeral (GH) joint. *A,* The rope indicates a muscular force that holds the glenoid fossa in a slightly upward rotated position. In this position, the passive tension in the taut superior capsular structure (SCS) is added to the force produced by gravity (G), yielding the compression force (CF). The compression force applied against the slight incline of the glenoid "locks" the joint. *B,* With a loss of upward rotation posture of the scapula (indicated by the cut rope), the change in angle between the SCS and G vectors reduces the magnitude of the compression force across the GH joint. As a consequence, the head of the humerus slides down the now vertically oriented glenoid fossa. The dashed lines indicate the parallelogram method of adding force vectors.

compressive locking force, oriented at right angles to the surface of the glenoid fossa. The compression force pinches the humeral head firmly against the glenoid fossa, thereby resisting any descent of the humerus. The inclined plane of the glenoid also acts as a partial shelf that supports part of the weight of the arm.

Electromyographic (EMG) data suggest that the supraspinatus, and to a lesser extent the posterior deltoid, provides a secondary source of static stability by generating active forces that are directed nearly parallel to the superior capsular force vector. Interestingly, Basmajian and Bazant[3] showed that vertically running muscles, such as the biceps, triceps, and middle deltoid, are generally *not* actively involved in providing static stability, even when significant downward traction is applied to the arm.

An important component of the static locking mechanism is a scapulothoracic posture that maintains the glenoid fossa slightly upwardly rotated. The passive tension within the superior capsular structures is significantly reduced when the scapula loses this upward rotation position (Fig. 5–28*B*). A chronically, downwardly rotated posture may be associated with "poor posture" or may be secondary to paralysis or weakness of certain muscles, such as the upper trapezius. Regardless of cause, loss of the upwardly rotated position increases the angle between the force vectors created by the superior capsular structures and gravity. Vector addition of the forces produced by the superior capsular structures and gravity now yields a reduced compressive force. Gravity can pull the humerus down the face of the glenoid fossa. The GH joint may eventually become mechanically unstable and eventually subluxed completely.

The normally negative intra-articular pressure within the GH joint offers a secondary source of static stability. Experimental release of the pressure within the GH joint capsule by piercing the capsule with a needle has been shown to cause inferior subluxation of the humeral head.[31] The puncturing of the capsule equalizes the pressure on both sides, removing the slight suction force between the head and the fossa.

## CORACOACROMIAL ARCH AND ASSOCIATED BURSA

The *coracoacromial arch* is formed by the coracoacromial ligament and the acromion process of the scapula (see Figs. 5–25 and 5–27). The *coracoacromial ligament* attaches between the anterior margin of the acromion and the lateral border of the coracoid process.

The coracoacromial arch functions as the roof of the GH joint. In the healthy adult, only about 1 cm of distance exists between the undersurface of the arch and the humeral head.[47] This important *subacromial space* contains the supraspinatus muscle and tendon, the subacromial bursa, the long head of the biceps, and part of the superior capsule.

Eight separate *bursa sacs* are located in the shoulder.[68] Some of the sacs are direct extensions of the synovial membrane of the GH joint, such as the subscapular bursa, whereas others are considered separate structures. All are situated in regions where significant frictional forces develop between tendons, capsule and bone, muscle and ligament, or two muscles. Two important bursa are located superior to the humeral head (Fig. 5–29). The *subacromial bursa* lies within the subacromial space above the supraspinatus muscle and below the acromion process. This bursa protects the relatively soft and vulnerable supraspinatus muscle and tendon from the rigid undersurface of the acromion. The *subdeltoid bursa* is a lateral extension of the

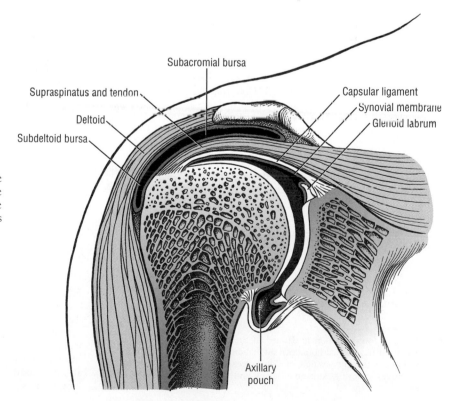

**FIGURE 5–29.** An anterior view of a frontal plane cross-section of the right glenohumeral joint. Note the subacromial and subdeltoid bursa within the subacromial space. The deltoid and supraspinatus muscles are also shown.

Subacromial bursa

Supraspinatus and tendon

Deltoid

Subdeltoid bursa

Capsular ligament

Synovial membrane

Glenoid labrum

Axillary pouch

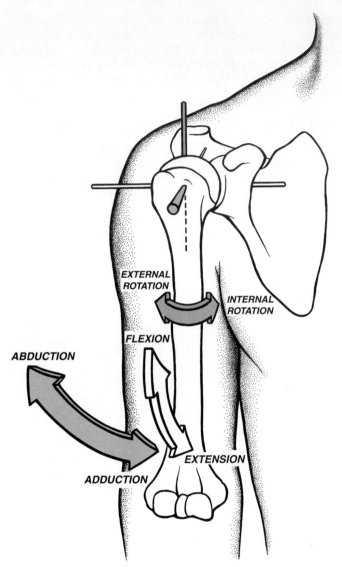

**FIGURE 5–30.** The right glenohumeral joint showing the conventional osteokinematic motions of the humerus. The motions are abduction and adduction (red), flexion and extension (white), and internal and external rotation (gray). Note that each axis of rotation is color-coded with its corresponding plane of movement: medial-lateral axis in white, vertical or longitudinal axis in gray, and anterior-posterior axis in red.

subacromial bursa, limiting frictional forces between the deltoid and the underlying supraspinatus tendon and humeral head.

## KINEMATICS AT THE GLENOHUMERAL JOINT

The GH joint is a universal joint because movement occurs in all 3 degrees of freedom. The primary motions at the GH joint are flexion and extension, abduction and adduction, and internal and external rotation (Fig. 5–30).*

---

*Often, a fourth motion is defined at the GH joint: horizontal flexion and extension (also called horizontal adduction and abduction). The motion occurs from a starting position of 90 degrees of abduction. The humerus moves anteriorly during horizontal flexion and posteriorly during horizontal extension.

Reporting the range of motion at the GH joint uses the anatomic position as the 0-degree or neutral reference point. In the sagittal plane, for example, flexion is described as the rotation of the humerus anterior to the 0-degree position. Extension, in contrast, is described as the rotation of the humerus posterior to the 0-degree position. The term hyperextension is not used to describe normal range of motion at the shoulder.

Virtually any purposeful motion of the GH joint involves motion at the scapulothoracic joint, including the associated movements at the SC and AC joints. The following discussion, however, focuses on the isolated kinematics of the GH joint.

### Abduction and Adduction

Abduction and adduction are traditionally defined as rotation of the humerus in the frontal plane about an axis oriented in the anterior-posterior direction (see Fig. 5–30). This axis remains within 6 mm (about ¼ in) of the humeral head's geometric center throughout full abduction.[48]

The arthrokinematics of abduction involve the convex head of the humerus rolling superiorly while simultaneously sliding inferiorly (Fig. 5–31). These roll-and-slide arthrokinematics occur along, or close to, the longitudinal diameter of the glenoid fossa. The arthrokinematics of adduction are similar to abduction but occur in a reverse direction.

Figure 5–31 shows that part of the supraspinatus muscle attaches to the superior capsule of the GH joint. When the muscle contracts to produce movement, forces are transferred through the capsule, providing dynamic stability to the joint. (Dynamic stability refers to the stability achieved while the joint is moving.) As abduction proceeds, the prominent humeral head unfolds and stretches the axillary pouch of the inferior capsular ligament. The resulting ten-

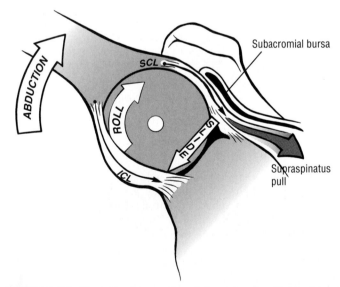

**FIGURE 5–31.** The arthrokinematics of the right glenohumeral joint during active abduction. The supraspinatus is shown contracting to direct the superior roll of the humeral head. The taut inferior capsular ligament (ICL) is shown supporting the head of the humerus like a hammock (see text). Note that the superior capsular ligament (SCL) remains relatively taut owing to the pull from the attached contracting supraspinatus. Stretched tissues are depicted as long black arrows.

sion within the inferior capsule acts as a hammock or sling, which supports the head of the humerus.[41] Excessive stiffness in the inferior capsule due to "adhesive capsulitis" may limit the full extent of the abduction motion.

Approximately 120 degrees of abduction are available at the healthy GH joint. A wide range of values, however, have been reported.[2,19,26,58] Full shoulder abduction requires a simultaneous 60 degrees of upward rotation of the scapula and is discussed further in a subsequent section of this chapter.

### Importance of Roll-and-Slide Arthrokinematics at the Glenohumeral Joint

The roll-and-slide arthrokinematics depicted in Figure 5–31 are essential to the completion of full range abduction. Recall that the longitudinal diameter of the articular surface of the humeral head is almost twice the size as the longitudinal diameter on the glenoid fossa. The arthrokinematics of abduction demonstrate how a simultaneous roll and slide allow a larger convex surface to roll over a much smaller concave surface without running out of articular surface.

Without a sufficient inferior slide during abduction, the superior roll of the humeral head ultimately leads to a jamming or impingement of the head against the coracoacromial arch. An adult-sized humeral head that is rolling up a glenoid fossa *without* a concurrent inferior slide would translate through the 10-mm coracoacromial space after only 22 degrees of abduction (Fig. 5–32A). This situation causes an impingement of the head of the humerus against the supraspinatus muscle, its tendon, and the bursa against the rigid coracoacromial arch. This impingement is painful, blocking further abduction (Fig. 5–32B). In vivo radiographic measurements in the healthy shoulder show that during abduction in the scapular plane, the humeral head remains essentially stationary or may translate superiorly only a negligible distance.[17,43,48] The concurrent inferior slide of the humeral

head offsets most of the inherent superior translation tendency of the humeral head. In healthy persons, the offsetting mechanism provides sufficient space for the supraspinatus tendon and the subacromial bursa.

### Abduction in the Frontal Plane Versus the Scapular Plane

Shoulder abduction in the frontal plane is often used as a representative motion to evaluate overall shoulder function. Despite its common usage, however, this motion is not very natural. Elevating the humerus in the scapular plane (about 35 degrees anterior to the frontal plane) is generally a more functional and natural movement.

The functional differences between abduction in the frontal plane and abduction in the scapular plane can be illustrated by the following example. Attempt to maximally abduct your shoulder in the *pure frontal plane* while consciously avoiding any accompanying external rotation. The difficulty or inability to complete the extremes of this motion is due in part to the greater tubercle of the humerus compressing the contents of the subacromial space against the low point on the coracoacromial arch (Fig. 5–34A). In order to complete full frontal plane abduction, external rotation of the humerus must be combined with the abduction effort. This ensures that the prominent greater tubercle clears the posterior edge of the undersurface of the acromion.

Next, fully abduct your arm in the *scapular plane*. This abduction movement can usually be performed without the need to externally rotate the shoulder.[52] Impingement is avoided since scapular plane abduction places the apex of the greater tubercle under the relatively high point of the coracoacromial arch (Fig. 5–34B). Abduction in the scapular plane also allows the naturally retroverted humeral head to fit more directly into the glenoid fossa. The proximal and distal attachments of the supraspinatus muscle are placed along a straight line. These mechanical differences between

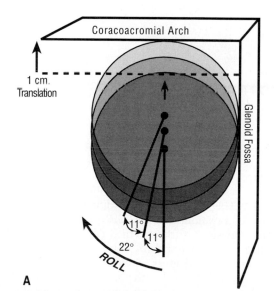
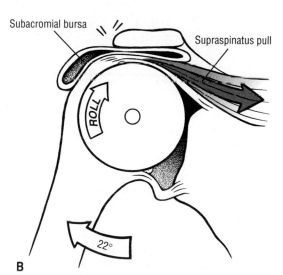

**FIGURE 5–32.** *A*, A model of the glenohumeral joint depicting a ball the size of a typical adult humeral head rolling across a flattened (glenoid) surface. Based on the assumption that the humeral head is a sphere with a circumference of 16.3 cm, the head of the humerus would translate upward 1 cm following a superior roll (abduction) of only 22 degrees. This magnitude of translation would cause the humeral head to impinge against the coracoacromial arch. *B*, Anatomic representation of the model used in *A*. Note that abduction *without* a concurrent inferior slide causes the humeral head to impinge against the arch and block further abduction.

## SPECIAL FOCUS 5–3

### Chronic Impingement Syndrome at the Shoulder

Repeated compression of the humeral head and/or the greater tubercle against the contents of the subacromial space often leads to "chronic impingement syndrome."[27] The syndrome is characterized by the inability to abduct the shoulder in a pain free or natural manner. The condition typically occurs in athletes and laborers who repeatedly abduct their shoulders over 90 degrees, but also occurs in relatively sedentary persons. The impingement of the head of the humerus against the coracoacromial arch can be detected on standard x-ray examination (Fig. 5–33), as well as on magnetic resonance imaging.[56]

Many factors predispose people to shoulder impingement syndrome. One factor is the inability of muscles—such as the rotator cuff or serratus anterior—to optimally coordinate the GH joint arthrokinematics of abduction.[9,17,33] Additional factors include "slouched" thoracic posture,[28]

degeneration of the rotator cuff muscles, instability of the GH joint, tightness or adhesions within the GH joint capsule, and reduced volume in the subacromial space.[46] The last factor may result from the abnormal shape of the acromion, presence of osteophytes around the AC joint, or swelling of structures in and around the subacromial space. Regardless of cause, each time an impingement occurs, the delicate supraspinatus tendon and subacromial bursa become further traumatized. The long head of the biceps and the superior capsule of the GH joint may also be impinged and further traumatized. Therapeutic goals include decreasing inflammation within the subacromial space, conditioning the rotator cuff muscle, improving kinesthetic awareness of the movement, and attempting to restore the natural shoulder arthrokinematics. Ergonomic education is also a factor in goal setting.

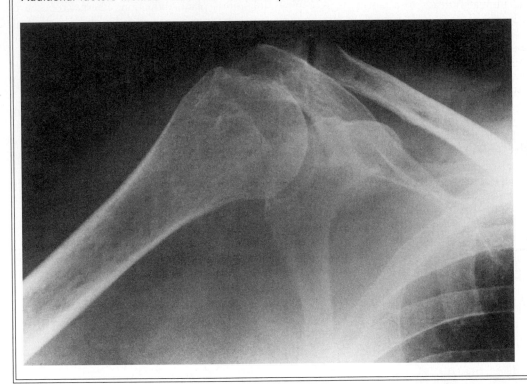

**FIGURE 5–33.** An x-ray of a person with "chronic impingement syndrome" attempting full abduction. Note the position of the humeral head up against the acromion (compare with Fig. 5–32B). (Courtesy of Gary L. Soderberg.)

---

frontal plane and scapular plane abduction should be considered while evaluating and treating patients with shoulder dysfunction, particularly if chronic impingement is suspected.

### Flexion and Extension

Flexion and extension at the GH joint is defined as a rotation of the humerus in the sagittal plane about a medial-lateral axis of rotation (see Fig. 5–30). If the motion occurs strictly in the sagittal plane, the arthrokinematics involve a *spinning* of the humeral head about a somewhat fixed point on the face of the glenoid. No roll or slide is necessary. As shown in Figure 5–35, the spinning action of the humeral head draws most of the surrounding capsular structures taut. Tension within the stretched posterior capsule may cause a slight anterior translation of the humerus at the extremes of flexion.[21]

Direct measurements have shown that flexion at the GH joint is associated with a slight internal rotation of the humerus.[44] This subtle motion is difficult to appreciate through casual observation. As the GH joint is flexed beyond 90 degrees, tension in the stretched coracohumeral ligament may produce a small internal rotation torque on the humerus.

At least 120 degrees of flexion are available to the GH joint. The ability to flex the shoulder to nearly 180 degrees includes the accompanying upward rotation of the scapulothoracic joint.

Full extension of the shoulder occurs to a position of about 45 to 55 degrees behind the frontal plane. The extremes of this motion stretch the anterior capsular ligaments, causing a slight forward tilting of the scapula. This forward tilt may enhance the extent of a backward reach.

**FIGURE 5–34.** Side view of right glenohumeral joint comparing abduction of the humerus in A: the true frontal plane (red arrow) and B: the scapular plane (gray arrow). In both A and B, the glenoid fossa is oriented in the scapular plane. The relative low and high points of the coracoacromial arch are also depicted. The line-of-force of the supraspinatus is shown in B, coursing through the subacromial arch.

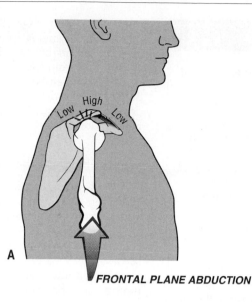
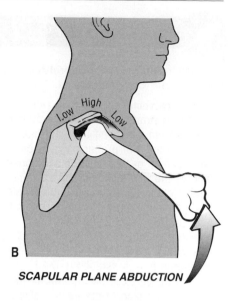

**A**    **FRONTAL PLANE ABDUCTION**

**B**    **SCAPULAR PLANE ABDUCTION**

### Internal and External Rotation

From the anatomic position, internal and external rotation at the GH joint is defined as an axial rotation of the humerus in the horizontal plane (see Fig. 5–30). This rotation occurs about a vertical or longitudinal axis that runs through the shaft of the humerus. The arthrokinematics of external rotation take place over the transverse diameters of the humeral head and the glenoid fossa (see Fig. 5–25). The humeral head simultaneously rolls posteriorly and slides anteriorly on the glenoid fossa (Fig. 5–36). The arthrokinematics for internal rotation are similar, except that the direction of the roll and slide is reversed.

The simultaneous roll and slide of internal and external rotation allows the much larger transverse diameter of the humeral head to roll over a much smaller surface area of the glenoid fossa. The physiologic importance of these anterior and posterior slides is evident by returning to the model of the humeral head shown in Figure 5–32A, but now envision the humeral head rolling over the glenoid fossa's transverse diameter. If, for example, 75 degrees of external rotation occurs by a posterior roll *without* a concurrent anterior slide, the head displaces posteriorly, roughly 38 mm (about 1½ in). This amount of translation completely disarticulates the joint because the *entire* transverse diameter of the glenoid fossa is only about 25 mm (1 in). Normally, however, full external rotation results in only 1 to 2 mm of posterior translation of the humeral head,[21] demonstrating that an "offsetting" anterior slide accompanies the posterior roll.

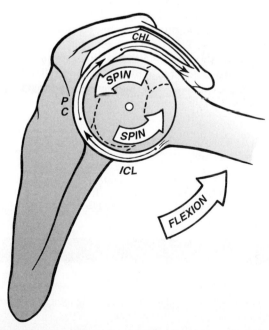

**FIGURE 5–35.** Side view of flexion in the sagittal plane of the right glenohumeral joint. A point on the head of the humerus is shown spinning about a point on the glenoid fossa. Stretched structures are shown as long arrows. (PC = posterior capsule, ICL = inferior capsular ligament, and CHL = coracohumeral ligament.)

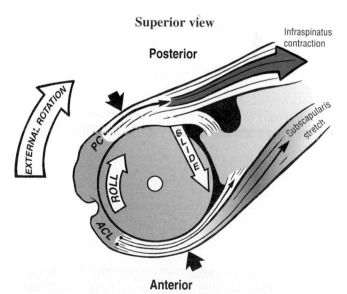

**FIGURE 5–36.** Superior view of the roll-and-slide arthrokinematics during active external rotation of the right glenohumeral joint. The infraspinatus is shown contracting (in dark red) causing the posterior roll of the humerus. The subscapularis muscle and anterior capsular ligament (ACL) generate passive tension from being stretched. The posterior capsule (PC) is held relatively taut due to the pull of the contracting infraspinatus muscle. The two bold black arrows represent forces that centralize and thereby stabilize the humeral head during the external rotation. Stretched tissues are depicted as thin, elongated arrows.

**Centralization of the Humeral Head: Special Function of the Rotator Cuff Muscles**

During all volitional motions at the GH joint, forces from activated rotator cuff muscles combine with the passive forces from stretched capsular ligaments to maintain the humeral head in proper position on the glenoid fossa. As an example of this mechanism, consider Figure 5–36 that shows the infraspinatus muscle contracting to produce active external rotation at the GH joint. Because part of the infraspinatus attaches into the capsule, its contraction prevents the posterior capsule from slackening during the motion. This maintenance of tension in the posterior capsule, combined with the natural rigidity from the activated muscle, stabilizes the posterior side of the joint during active external rotation. In the healthy shoulder, the anterior side of the joint is also well stabilized during active external rotation. Passive tension in the stretched subscapularis muscle, anterior capsule, middle GH capsular ligament, and coracohumeral ligament all add rigidity to the anterior capsule. Forces, therefore, are generated on both sides of the joint during active external rotation, serving to *stabilize* and *centralize* the humeral head against the glenoid fossa. A similar mechanism exists during active internal rotation.

From the anatomic position, about 75 to 85 degrees of internal rotation and 60 to 70 degrees of external rotation are usually possible, but much variation can be expected among people. In a position of 90 degrees of abduction, the external rotation range of motion usually increases to near 90 degrees. Regardless of the position at which these rotations occur, there is usually movement at the scapulothoracic joint. Maximal internal rotation usually includes scapular protraction, and maximal external rotation usually includes scapular retraction.

### Summary of Glenohumoral Joint Arthrokinematics

Table 5–2 shows a summary of the arthrokinematics and osteokinematics at the glenohumeral joint.

## Overall Shoulder Kinematics During Abduction

To this point, this study of shoulder arthrology has focused primarily on the structure and function of the individual

joints. The next discussions focus on the sequencing of motion that occurs *between* the joints. This issue is discussed for the motion of shoulder abduction. The ability to fully abduct in a pain-free and natural fashion is indicative of a healthy shoulder. Knowledge of how the joints of the shoulder interact during this movement is a prerequisite for understanding of shoulder pathology and effective therapeutic intervention.

### SCAPULOHUMERAL RHYTHM

The most widely cited study on the kinematics of shoulder abduction was published by Inman and colleagues in 1944.[26] This classic work focused on shoulder abduction in the frontal plane. Inman wrote that GH joint abduction or flexion occurs simultaneously with scapular upward rotation, an observation referred to as *scapulohumeral rhythm.*

In the healthy shoulder, a natural kinematic rhythm or timing exists between glenohumeral abduction and scapulothoracic upward rotation. Inman reported this rhythm to be remarkably constant throughout most of abduction, occurring at a ratio of 2:1. *For every 3 degrees of shoulder abduction, 2 degrees occurs by GH joint abduction and 1 degree occurs by scapulothoracic joint upward rotation.* Based on this rhythm, a full arc of 180 degree of shoulder abduction is the result of a simultaneous 120 degrees of GH joint abduction and 60 degrees of scapulothoracic upward rotation (Fig. 5–37A).

Since the time of Inman's original work in 1944, additional research has examined the kinematics of shoulder abduction with an emphasis on motion in the scapular plane,[2,19,35,43,48] and on motion while lifting different loads.[36] These studies reported a slightly different, and less consistent, scapulohumeral rhythm. For instance, Bagg and Forrest[2] reported a mean glenohumeral-to-scapular rotation ratio of 3.29:1 between 21 degrees and 82 degrees of abduction; .71:1 between 82 degrees and 139 degrees of abduction; and 1.25:1 between 139 degrees and 170 degrees of abduction. Regardless of the differing ratios reported in the literature, Inman's classic 2:1 ratio still remains a valuable axiom in evaluation of shoulder movement. It is simple to remember and still helps to conceptualize the overall relationship between humeral and scapula motion when considering the full 180 degrees of shoulder abduction.

### STERNOCLAVICULAR AND ACROMIOCLAVICULAR JOINT INTERACTION

Inman's research was the first major study to measure the SC and AC joint contribution to the full 60 degrees of scapulothoracic upward rotation.[26] The following data are

| TABLE 5–2. A Summary of the Arthrokinematics at the GH Joint | | |
|---|---|---|
| **Osteokinematics** | **Plane of Motion/Axis of Rotation** | **Arthrokinematics** |
| Abduction/adduction | Frontal plane/anterior-posterior axis of rotation | *Roll-and-slide* along joint's longitudinal diameter |
| Internal/external rotation | Horizontal plane/vertical axis of rotation | *Roll-and-slide* along joint's transverse diameter |
| Flexion/extension *and* internal/external rotation (in 90 degrees of abduction) | Sagittal plane/medial-lateral axis of rotation | *Spin* between humeral head and glenoid fossa |

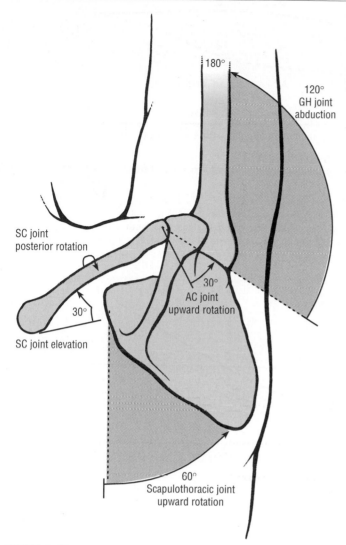

**FIGURE 5–37.** *A*, Posterior view of the right shoulder complex after the arm has abducted to 180 degrees. The 60 degrees of scapulothoracic joint upward rotation and the 120 degrees of glenohumeral (GH) joint abduction are shaded in red. *B*, The scapular upward rotation is depicted as a summation of 30 degrees of elevation at the sternoclavicular (SC) joint and 30 degrees of upward rotation at the acromioclavicular (AC) joint. The posterior rotation of the clavicle at the SC joint is represented by the circular arrow around the middle shaft of the bone.

based on this research. The 180 degrees of abduction has been divided into an early and a late phase.

### Early Phase: Shoulder Abduction to 90 degrees

Assuming a 2:1 scapulohumeral rhythm, shoulder abduction up to about 90 degrees occurs as a summation of 60 degrees of GH abduction and 30 degrees of scapulothoracic upward rotation. The 30 degrees of upward rotation occurs predominantly through a synchronous 20 to 25 degrees of clavicular elevation at the SC joint *and* 5 to 10 degrees of upward rotation at the AC joint (Fig. 5–38; early phase). Other subtle rotational adjustments occur simultaneously at the AC joint.[63]

### Late Phase: Shoulder Abduction from 90 Degrees to 180 Degrees

Shoulder abduction from 90 degrees to 180 degrees occurs as a summation of an additional 60 degrees of GH joint

abduction and an additional 30 degrees of scapulothoracic upward rotation. During this late phase, the clavicle elevates only an additional 5 degrees at the SC joint. The scapula, in contrast, upwardly rotates at the AC joint 20 to 25 degrees (see Fig. 5–38; late phase). By the end of 180 degrees of abduction, the 60 degrees of scapulothoracic upward rotation can be accounted for by 30 degrees of elevation at the SC joint and 30 degrees of upward rotation at the AC joint (Fig. 5–37B).

#### Posterior Rotation of the Clavicle

Inman and fellow researchers were able to demonstrate through in vivo techniques that the clavicle rotates posteriorly about 40 degrees during the late phase of shoulder abduction (Fig. 5–39). Posterior rotation was described during the description of the kinematics at the SC joint. The mechanism that drives this rotation is shown in a highly diagrammatic fashion in Figure 5–40. At the onset of shoulder abduction, the scapula begins to upwardly rotate at the AC joint, stretching the relatively stiff coracoclavicular ligament (Fig. 5–40B). The inability of this ligament to significantly elongate restricts further upward rotation at this joint. According to Inman,[26] tension within the stretched ligament is transferred to the conoid tubercle region of the clavicle, a point posterior to the bone's longitudinal axis. The application of this force rotates the crank-shaped clavicle posteriorly (Fig. 5–40B). This rotation places the clavicular attachment of the coracoclavicular ligament closer to the coracoid process, unloading the ligament slightly and permitting the scapula to continue its final 30 degrees of upward rotation. Inman[26] describes this mechanism as "a fundamental feature of shoulder motion" and without this motion, complete shoulder abduction is not possible.

Table 5–3 summarizes the major kinematic events of the shoulder complex during the late and final phases of shoulder abduction. The data are based on Inman's research, which used a limited sample size. The actual values within the population would certainly vary.

## MUSCLE AND JOINT INTERACTION

### Innervation of the Muscles and Joints of the Shoulder Complex

#### INTRODUCTION TO THE BRACHIAL PLEXUS

The entire upper extremity receives innervation primarily through the *brachial plexus* (Fig. 5–41) The brachial plexus is formed by a consolidation of the ventral nerve roots from mixed spinal nerves $C^5$–$T^1$. Ventral nerve roots $C^5$ and $C^6$ form the *upper trunk*, $C^7$ forms the *middle trunk*, and $C^8$ and $T^1$ form the *lower trunk*. Trunks course a short distance before forming *anterior* or *posterior divisions*. The divisions then reorganize into *three cords* named by their relationship to the axillary artery. The cords branch into *nerves*, which innervate muscles of the upper extremity and lateral trunk.

#### SHOULDER MUSCLE INNERVATION

The majority of the muscles in the shoulder complex receive their motor innervation from two regions of the brachial

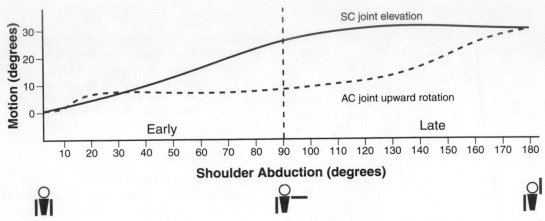

**FIGURE 5–38.** Plot showing the relationship of elevation at the sternoclavicular (SC) joint and upward rotation at the acromioclavicular (AC) joint during full shoulder abduction. The 180 degrees of abduction is divided into early and late phases. (Redrawn from data from Inman VT, Saunders M, Abbott LC: Observations on the function of the shoulder joint. J Bone Joint Surg 26A:1–32, 1944.)

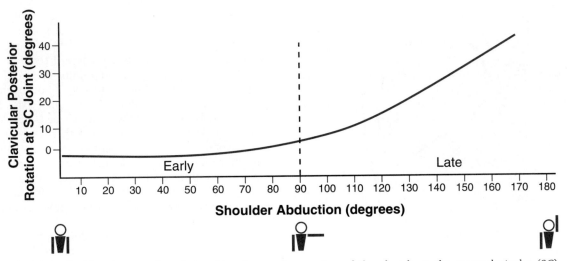

**FIGURE 5–39.** Plot showing the relationship of posterior rotation of the clavicle at the sternoclavicular (SC) joint to full shoulder abduction. (Redrawn from data from Inman VT, Saunders M, Abbott LC: Observations on the function of the shoulder joint. J Bone Joint Surg 26A:1–32, 1944.)

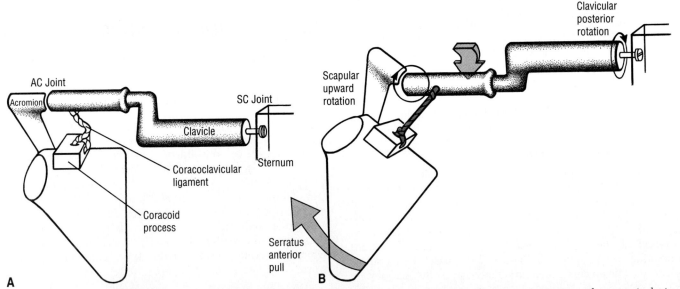

**FIGURE 5–40.** The mechanics of posterior rotation of the right clavicle are shown. *A,* At rest in the anatomic position, the acromioclavicular (AC) and sternoclavicular (SC) joints are shown with the coracoclavicular ligament represented by a slackened rope. *B,* As the serratus anterior muscle rotates the scapula upward, the coracoclavicular ligament is drawn taut. The tension created within the stretched ligament rotates the crank-shaped clavicle in a posterior direction, allowing the AC joint to complete full upward rotation.

116

**TABLE 5-3. Summary of the Major Kinematic Events during Shoulder Abduction*†**

|  | SC Joint | AC Joint | Scapulothoracic Joint | GH Joint |
|---|---|---|---|---|
| Early phase 0 to 90 degrees | 25 degrees of elevation | 5 degrees of upward rotation | 30 degrees of upward rotation | 60 degrees of abduction |
| Late phase 90 to 180 degrees | 5 degrees of elevation and 35 degrees of posterior rotation of the clavicle | 25 degrees of upward rotation | 30 degrees of upward rotation | 60 degrees of abduction |
| Total 0 to 180 degrees | 30 degrees of elevation and 35 degrees of posterior rotation of the clavicle | 30 degrees of upward rotation | 60 degrees of upward rotation | 120 degrees of abduction |

*Data from Inman VT, Saunders M, Abbott LC: Observations on the function of the shoulder joint. J Bone Joint Surg 26A:1–32, 1944. (Some values have been rounded slightly for simplicity but are still close to the original values.)

† External rotation is required if abduction is performed in the frontal plane.

plexus: (1) nerves that branch from the posterior cord, such as the axillary, subscapular, and thoracodorsal nerves, and (2) nerves that branch from more proximal segments of the plexus, such as the dorsal scapular, long thoracic, pectoral, and suprascapular nerves. An exception to this innervation scheme is the trapezius muscle, which is innervated primarily by cranial nerve XI, with lesser motor and sensory innervation from the ventral roots of upper cervical nerves.[68]

The primary motor nerve roots that supply the muscles of the upper extremity are listed in Appendix IIA. Appendix IIB shows key muscles typically used to test the functional status of the C[5]-T[1] ventral nerve roots.

### SENSORY INNERVATION OF THE SHOULDER JOINTS AND SURROUNDING CONNECTIVE TISSUE

The sternoclavicular joint receives sensory (afferent) innervation from the C[3] and C[4] nerve roots from the cervical plexus.[68] Both the acromioclavicular and glenohumeral joints receive sensory innervation via the C[5] and C[6] nerve roots via the suprascapular and axillary nerves.[68]

## Action of the Shoulder Muscles

Most of the muscles of the shoulder complex fall into one of two categories: proximal stabilizers or distal mobilizers. The *proximal stabilizers* consist of muscles that originate on the

**FIGURE 5-41.** The brachial plexus. From Jobe MT, Wright PE: Peripheral nerve injuries: In Canale ST (ed): Campbell's Operative Orthopaedics, 9th ed., vol 4. St. Louis, Mosby, 1998.)

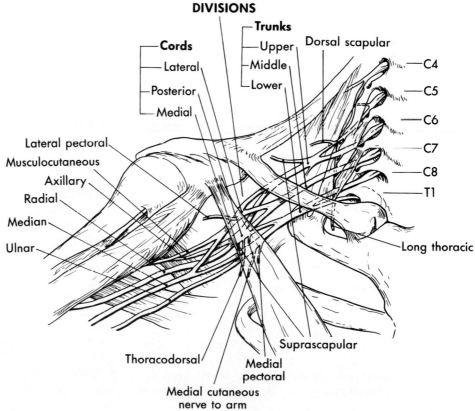

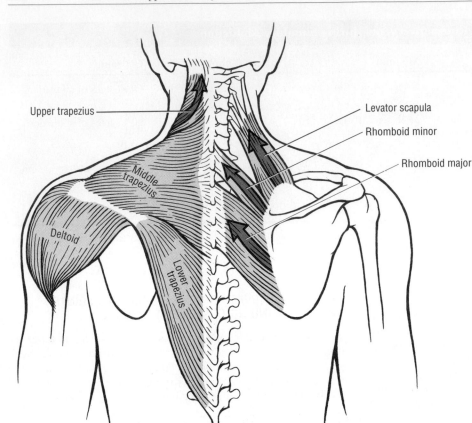

Upper trapezius

Middle trapezius

Deltoid

Lower trapezius

Levator scapula

Rhomboid minor

Rhomboid major

**FIGURE 5–42.** Posterior view showing the upper trapezius, levator scapula, rhomboid major, and rhomboid minor as elevators of the scapulothoracic joint.

spine, ribs, and cranium, and insert on the scapula and clavicle. Examples of these muscles are the serratus anterior and the trapezius. The *distal mobilizers* consist of muscles that originate on the scapula and clavicle and insert on the humerus or forearm. Examples of two distal mobilizers are the deltoid and biceps brachii muscles. As described subsequently, optimal function across the entire shoulder complex is based on a functional interdependence between the proximal stabilizers and the distal mobilizers. For example, in order for the deltoid to generate an effective abduction torque at the glenohumeral joint, the scapula must be firmly stabilized against the thorax by the serratus anterior. In cases of a paralyzed serratus anterior muscle, the deltoid muscle is unable to express its full abduction function. Several examples follow that reinforce this important point. The specific anatomy and nerve supply of the muscles of the shoulder complex can be found in Appendix IIC.

## Muscles of the Scapulothoracic Joint

### ELEVATORS OF THE SCAPULOTHORACIC JOINT

The muscles responsible for elevation of the scapula and clavicle are the *upper trapezius, levator scapulae,* and to a lesser extent, the *rhomboids* (Fig. 5–42).[15] The upper trapezius provides postural support to the shoulder girdle (scapula and clavicle). Ideal posture of the shoulder girdle is often defined as a slightly elevated and retracted scapula, with the glenoid fossa facing slightly upward. The upper trapezius, attaching to the lateral end of the clavicle, provides excellent

---

**SPECIAL FOCUS 5 – 5**

**Paralysis of the Upper Trapezius: Effects on Sternoclavicular and Glenohumeral Joint Stability**

Paralysis of the upper trapezius may result from damage to the spinal accessory nerve (cranial nerve XI). Over time, the scapulothoracic joint may become markedly depressed, protracted, and excessively downwardly rotated owing to the pull of gravity on the arm. A chronically depressed clavicle may eventually result in a *superior* dislocation at the SC joint.[7] As the lateral end of the clavicle is lowered, the medial end is forced upward due to the fulcrum action of the underlying first rib. The depressed shaft of the clavicle may eventually compress the subclavian vessels and part of the brachial plexus.

Perhaps a more common consequence of long-term paralysis of the upper trapezius is an inferior subluxation of the GH joint. Recall from earlier discussion that static stability at the GH joint is partially based on a humeral head that is held against the inclined plane of the glenoid fossa. With long-term paralysis of the trapezius, the glenoid fossa loses its upwardly rotated position, allowing the humerus to slide *inferiorly.* The downward pull imposed by gravity on an unsupported arm may strain the GH joint's capsule and eventually lead to an irreversible subluxation. This complication is often observed following flaccid hemiplegia.

leverage about the SC joint for the maintenance of this posture.

## DEPRESSORS OF THE SCAPULOTHORACIC JOINT

Depression of the scapulothoracic joint is performed by the *lower trapezius, latissimus dorsi, pectoralis minor,* and the *subclavius* (Fig. 5–43).[29,50] The latissimus dorsi depresses the shoulder girdle by pulling the humerus and scapula inferiorly. The force generated by the depressor muscles can be directed through the scapula and upper extremity and applied against some object, such as the spring shown in Figure 5–43A.

If the arm is physically blocked from being depressed, force from the depressor muscles can raise the thorax relative to the fixed scapula and arm. This action can occur only if the scapula is stabilized to a greater extent than the thorax. For example, Figure 5–44 shows a person sitting in a wheelchair using the scapulothoracic depressors to relieve the pressure in the tissues superficial to the ischial tuberosities. With the arm firmly held against the armrest of the wheelchair, contraction of the lower trapezius and latissimus dorsi pulls the thorax and pelvis up toward the fixed scapula. This is a very useful movement especially for persons with quadriplegia who lack sufficient triceps strength to lift body weight through elbow extension.

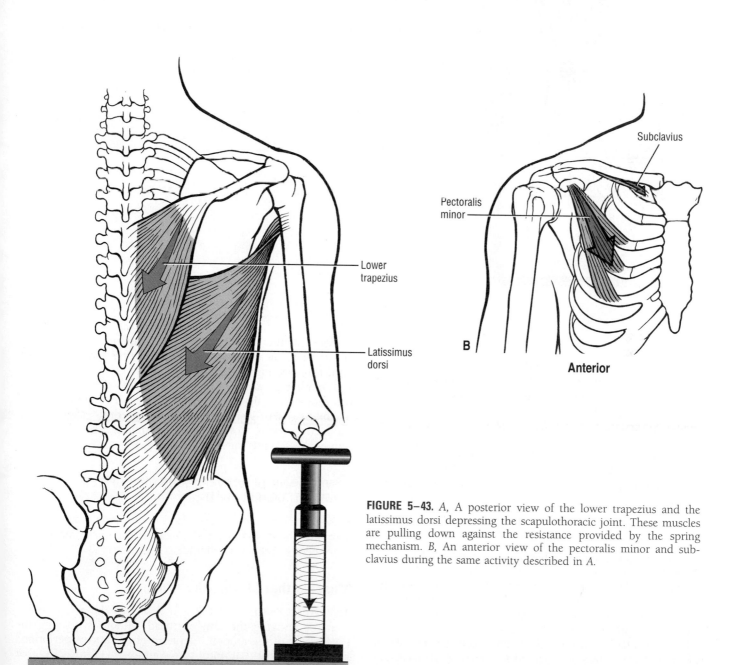

**FIGURE 5–43.** *A,* A posterior view of the lower trapezius and the latissimus dorsi depressing the scapulothoracic joint. These muscles are pulling down against the resistance provided by the spring mechanism. *B,* An anterior view of the pectoralis minor and subclavius during the same activity described in *A.*

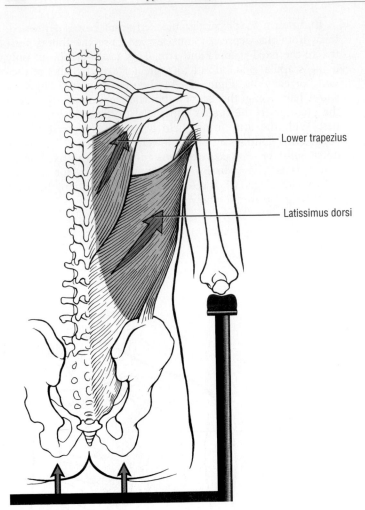

Lower trapezius

Latissimus dorsi

**FIGURE 5–44.** The lower trapezius and latissimus dorsi are shown elevating the ischial tuberosities away from the seat of the wheelchair. The contraction of these muscles lifts the pelvic-and-trunk segment up toward the fixed scapula-and-arm segment.

## PROTRACTORS OF THE SCAPULOTHORACIC JOINT

The *serratus anterior muscle* is the prime protractor at the scapulothoracic joint (Fig. 5–45A). This extensive muscle has excellent leverage for protraction, especially about the SC joint's vertical axis of rotation (Fig. 5–45B). The force of scapular protraction is usually transferred across the GH joint and employed for forward pushing and reaching activities. Persons with serratus anterior weakness have difficulty in performance of forward pushing motions. No other muscle can adequately provide this protraction effect on the scapula.

## RETRACTORS OF THE SCAPULOTHORACIC JOINT

The *middle trapezius muscle* has an optimal line-of-force to retract the scapula (Fig. 5–46). The *rhomboids* and the *lower trapezius muscles* function as secondary retractors. All the retractors are particularly active while using the arms for pulling activities, such as climbing and rowing. The muscles secure the scapula to the axial skeleton.

The secondary retractors show an excellent example of how muscles function as synergists—sharing identical actions. At the same time, however, they function as direct antagonists. During a vigorous retraction effort, the elevation tendency of the rhomboids is neutralized by the depression

tendency of the lower trapezius. A component of each muscles' overall line-of-force summate, however, producing pure retraction (see Fig. 5–46).

Complete paralysis of the trapezius, and to a lesser extent the rhomboids, significantly reduces the retraction potential of the scapula. The scapula tends to "drift" slightly into protraction owing to the partially unopposed protraction action of the serratus anterior muscle.[7]

## UPWARD AND DOWNWARD ROTATORS OF THE SCAPULOTHORACIC JOINT

Muscles that perform upward and downward rotation of the scapulothoracic joint are discussed next in context with movement of the entire shoulder.

### Muscles that Elevate the Arm

The term "elevation" of the arm describes the active movement of bringing the arm overhead without specifying the exact plane of the motion. Elevation of the arm is performed by muscles that fall into three groups: (1) muscles that elevate (i.e., abduct or flex) the humerus at the GH joint; (2) scapular muscles that control the upward rotation and protraction of the scapulothoracic joint; and (3) rotator cuff

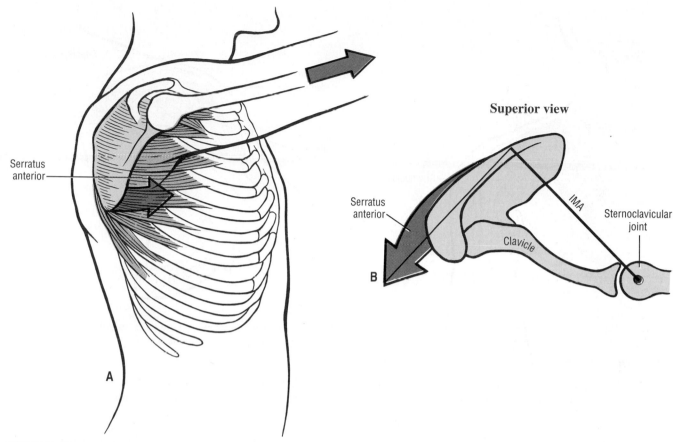

**Superior view**

Serratus
anterior

IMA

Sternoclavicular
joint

Clavicle

B

Serratus
anterior

A

**FIGURE 5–45.** The right serratus anterior muscle. *A,* This expansive muscle passes anterior to the scapula to attach along the entire length of its medial border. The muscle's line-of-force is shown protracting the scapula and arm in a forward pushing or reaching motion. The fibers that attach near the inferior angle may assist with scapulothoracic depression. *B,* A superior view of the right shoulder girdle showing the protraction torque produced by the serratus anterior, i.e., the product of the muscle force multiplied by the associated internal moment arm (IMA). The axis of rotation is shown as the red circle running through the sternoclavicular joint.

muscles that control the dynamic stability and arthrokinematics at the GH joint.

---

**Muscles Responsible for Elevation of the Arm**

1. *GH joint muscles*
   Deltoid
   Supraspinatus
   Coracobrachialis
   Biceps (long head)
2. *Scapulothoracic joint muscles*
   Serratus anterior
   Trapezius
3. *Rotator cuff muscles*

---

## MUSCLES THAT ELEVATE THE ARM AT THE GLENOHUMERAL JOINT

The prime muscles that abduct the GH joint are the anterior deltoid, the middle deltoid, and the supraspinatus muscles (Fig. 5–47). Elevation of the arm through flexion is performed primarily by the anterior deltoid, coracobrachialis,

**SPECIAL FOCUS 5 – 6**

**Serratus Anterior and the "Push-up" Maneuver**

Another important action of the serratus anterior is to exaggerate the final phase of the standard prone "push-up." The early phase of a push-up is performed primarily by the triceps and pectoral musculature. After the elbows are completely extended, however, the chest can be raised farther from the floor by a deliberate protraction of both scapulae. This final component of the push-up is performed primarily by contraction of the serratus anterior. Bilaterally, the muscles raise the thorax toward the fixed stabilized scapulae. This action of the serratus anterior may be visualized by rotating Figure 5–45*A* 90 degrees clockwise and reversing the direction of the arrow overlying the serratus anterior. Exercises designed to strengthen the serratus anterior incorporate this movement.[14]

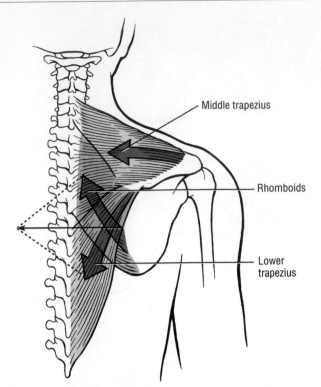

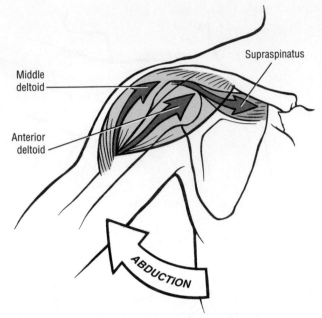

**FIGURE 5–46.** Posterior view of the middle trapezius, lower trapezius, and rhomboids cooperating to retract the scapulothoracic joint. The dashed line-of-force of both the rhomboid and lower trapezius combines to yield a single retraction force shown by the straight arrow.

**FIGURE 5–47.** Anterior view showing the middle deltoid, anterior deltoid, and supraspinatus as abductors of the glenohumeral joint.

and long head of the biceps brachii (Fig. 5–48). The maximal isometric torque generated by the shoulder flexors and the abductors is shown for two joint positions in Table 5–4.

The line-of-force of the middle deltoid and the supraspinatus are similar during shoulder abduction. Both muscles are activated at the onset of elevation, reaching a maximum level near 90 degrees of abduction.[30] Both muscles have a significant internal moment arm that remains essentially constant at about 25 mm (about 1 in) throughout most of abduction.[64]

The deltoid and the supraspinatus muscles contribute about equal shares of the total abduction torque at the GH joint.[22] With the deltoid paralyzed, the supraspinatus muscle is generally capable of fully abducting the GH joint. The torque, however, is reduced. With the supraspinatus paralyzed or ruptured, full abduction is often difficult or not possible due to the altered arthrokinematics at the GH joint. Full active abduction is not possible with a combined deltoid and supraspinatus paralysis.[10]

## UPWARD ROTATORS AT THE SCAPULOTHORACIC JOINT

Upward rotation of the scapula is an essential component of elevation of the arm. To varying degrees, the serratus ante-

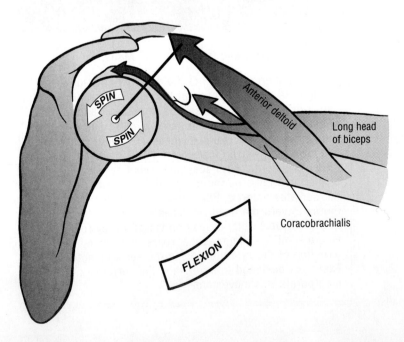

**FIGURE 5–48.** Lateral view of the anterior deltoid, coracobrachialis, and long head of the biceps flexing the glenohumeral joint in the pure sagittal plane. The medial-lateral axis of rotation is shown at the center of the humeral head. An internal moment arm is shown intersecting the line-of-force of the anterior deltoid only.

**TABLE 5-4. Average Maximal Isometric Torques Produced by Shoulder Muscle Groups***

| Muscle Group | Test Position | Torque (kg-cm) |
|---|---|---|
| Flexors | 45° of flexion | 566 ± 24 |
| Extensors | 0° of flexion | 812 ± 40 |
| Abductors | 45° of abduction | 562 ± 23 |
| Adductors | 45° of abduction | 1051 ± 59 |
| Internal rotators | 0° of rotation | 592 ± 27 |
| External rotators | 0° of rotation | 335 ± 15 |

\* Mean ± 1 standard error; data are from 20 young males from two test positions.

Conversion: .098 N-m/kg-cm.

Data from Murray MP, Gore DR, Gardiner GM, et al: Shoulder motion and muscle strength of normal men and women in two age groups. Clin Orthop 182:267–273, 1985.

rior and all parts of the trapezius cooperate during the upward rotation (Fig. 5–49). These muscles drive the scapula through upward rotation and, equally as important, provide stable attachment sites for distal mobilizers, such as the deltoid and supraspinatus.

### Trapezius and Serratus Anterior Interaction

The axis of rotation for scapular upward rotation is depicted in Figure 5–49 as passing in an anterior-posterior direction through the scapula. This axis allows a convenient way to analyze the potential for muscles to rotate the scapula. The axis of rotation of the upwardly rotating scapula is near the root of the spine during the early phase of shoulder abduction, and near the acromion during the late phase of abduction.[2]

The upper and lower fibers of the trapezius and the lower fibers of the serratus anterior form a *force couple* that upwardly rotates the scapula (see Fig. 5–49). All three muscular forces rotate the scapula in the same direction. The upper trapezius upwardly rotates the scapula by attaching to the clavicle. The serratus anterior is the most effective upward rotator due to its larger moment arm for this action.

### SPECIAL FOCUS 5-7

**The Upward Rotation Force Couple: A Familiar Analogy**

The mechanics of the upward rotation force couple are similar to the mechanics of three people walking through a revolving door. As shown in Figure 5–50, three people pushing on the door rail in different linear directions produce torques in the same rotary direction. This form of muscular interaction likely improves the level of control of the movement as well as amplifies the maximal torque potential of the rotating scapula.

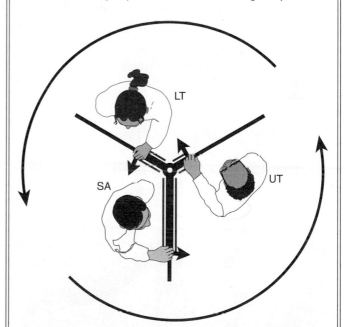

**FIGURE 5–50.** A top view of three people involved in a force couple to rotate a revolving door. The three people are analogous to the three muscles shown in Figure 5–49 upwardly rotating the scapula. (UT = upper trapezius, LT = lower trapezius, SA = serratus anterior.) Each person, or muscle, acts with a different internal moment arm (drawn to actual scale), which combines to cause a substantial torque in a similar rotary direction.

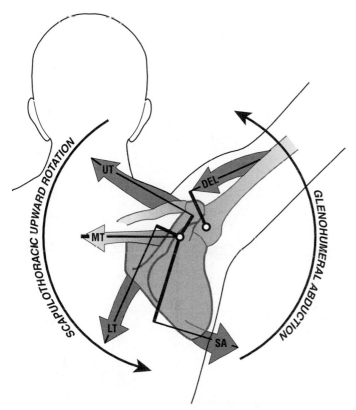

**FIGURE 5–49.** Posterior view of a healthy shoulder showing the muscular interaction between the scapulothoracic upward rotators and the glenohumeral abductors. Shoulder abduction requires a muscular "kinetic arc" between the humerus and the axial skeleton. Note two axes of rotation: the scapular axis located near the acromion, and the glenohumeral joint axis located at the humeral head. Internal moment arms for all muscles are shown as dark black lines. (DEL = deltoid/supraspinatus, UT = upper trapezius, MT = middle trapezius, LT = lower trapezius, and SA = serratus anterior.)

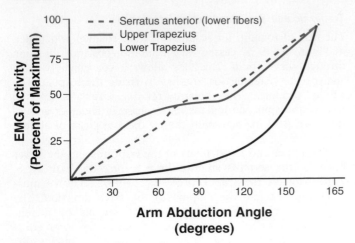

**FIGURE 5–51.** The EMG activation pattern of the upper trapezius and middle trapezius and the lower fibers of the serratus anterior during shoulder abduction in the scapular plane. (Data from Bagg SD, Forrest WJ: Electromyographic study of the scapular rotators during arm abduction in the scapula plane. Am J Phys Med 65: 111–124, 1986.)

The lower trapezius has been shown to be particularly active during the later phase of shoulder abduction (Fig. 5–51).[2] The upper trapezius, by comparison, shows a significant rise in EMG activation level during the initiation of shoulder abduction, then continues a gradual rise in activation throughout the remainder of the range of motion. The upper trapezius must elevate the clavicle throughout the early phase of abduction, while simultaneously balance the inferior pull of the lower trapezius during the late phase of abduction. The serratus anterior muscle shows a gradual increase in amplitude throughout the entire range of shoulder abduction.

Figure 5–49 shows the line-of-force of the middle trapezius running *through* the rotating scapula's axis of rotation. In this case, the middle trapezius is robbed of its leverage to contribute upward rotation torque. This muscle still contributes a needed retraction force on the scapula, which along with the rhomboid muscles helps to balance the formidable protraction effect of the serratus anterior. The net dominance between the middle trapezius and the serratus anterior during elevation of the arm determines the final retraction-protraction position of the upward rotated scapula. Weakness of the middle trapezius or serratus anterior disrupts the resting position of the scapula. The scapula tends to be biased in relative retraction with serratus anterior weakness, and in relative protraction with middle trapezius weakness.

In summary, during elevation of the arm the serratus anterior and trapezius control the mechanics of scapular upward rotation. The serratus anterior has the greater leverage for this motion. Both muscles are synergists in upward rotation, but are agonists and antagonists as they oppose, and thus partially limit, each other's strong protraction and retraction potential.

### Effects of Paralysis of the Upward Rotators of the Scapulothoracic Joint

#### Trapezius Paralysis
Complete paralysis of the trapezius usually causes moderate to marked difficulty in elevating the arm overhead. The task, however, can usually be completed through full range as long as the serratus anterior remains totally innervated. Elevation of the arm in the pure frontal plane is particularly difficult because it requires that the middle trapezius generate a strong retraction force on the scapula.[7]

#### Serratus Anterior Paralysis
Paralysis or weakness of the serratus anterior muscle causes significant disruption in normal shoulder kinesiology. Disability may be slight with partial paralysis, or profound with complete paralysis. Paralysis of the serratus anterior can occur from an overstretching of the long thoracic nerve[66] or from an injury to the cervical spinal cord or nerve roots.

As a rule, persons with complete or marked paralysis

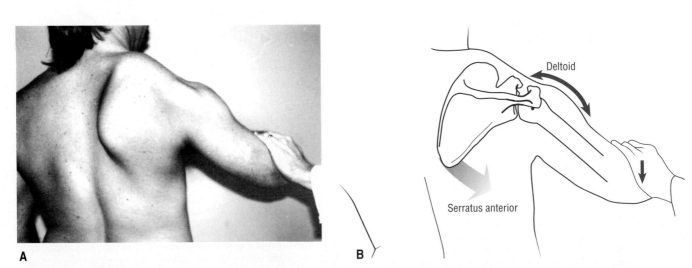

**FIGURE 5–52.** The pathomechanics of "winging" of the scapula. *A,* "Winging" of the right scapula due to marked weakness of the right serratus anterior. The winging is exaggerated when resistance is applied against a shoulder abduction effort. *B,* Kinesiologic analysis of the winging scapula. Without an adequate upward rotation force from the serratus anterior (fading arrow), the scapula becomes unstable and cannot resist the pull of the deltoid. Subsequently, the force of the deltoid (bidirectional arrow) causes the scapula to *downwardly rotate* and the glenohumeral joint to partially abduct.

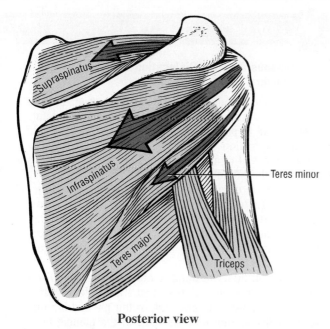

**Posterior view**

**FIGURE 5–53.** Posterior view of the right shoulder showing the supraspinatus, infraspinatus, and teres minor muscles. Note that the distal attachments of these muscles blend into and reinforce the superior and posterior aspects of the joint capsule.

of the serratus anterior cannot elevate their arms above 90 degrees of abduction. This limitation persists even with completely intact trapezius and glenohumeral abductor muscles. Attempts at elevating the arm, especially against resistance, result in a scapula that excessively rotates downwardly with its medial border flaring outwardly. This characteristic posture is often referred to as "winging" of the scapula (Fig. 5–52A). Normally, a fully innervated serratus anterior produces a force that rotates the scapula upward. In the ab-

sence of adequate upward rotation force on the scapula, however, the contracting deltoid and supraspinatus have an overall line-of-force that rotates the scapula *downward* and toward the humerus (Fig. 5–52B). This abnormal motion is associated with a rapid overshortening of the glenohumeral abductor muscles. As predicted by the force-velocity and length-tension relationship of muscle (see Chapter 3), the rapid overshortening of these muscles reduces their maximal force potential. The reduced force output from the overshortened glenohumeral abductors, in conjunction with the downward rotation of the scapula, reduces both the range of motion and torque potential of the elevating arm.

An analysis of the pathomechanics associated with weakness of the serratus anterior provides a valuable lesson in the extreme kinesiologic importance of this muscle. Normally during elevation of the arm, the serratus anterior produces an upward rotation torque on the scapula that exceeds the downward rotation torque produced by the active deltoid and supraspinatus. Interestingly, slight weakness in the serratus anterior can disrupt the normal arthrokinematics of the shoulder. Without the normal range of upward rotation of the scapula, the acromion is more likely to interfere with the arthrokinematics of the abducting humeral head. Indeed, research has shown that persons with chronic impingement syndrome have a reduced upward rotation of the scapula and a reduced relative EMG activity from the serratus anterior during abduction.[33]

## FUNCTION OF THE ROTATOR CUFF MUSCLES DURING ELEVATION OF THE ARM

The rotator cuff group muscles include the subscapularis, supraspinatus, infraspinatus, and teres minor (Figs. 5–53 and 5–54). All these muscles show significant EMG activity when the arm is raised overhead.[30] The EMG activity reflects

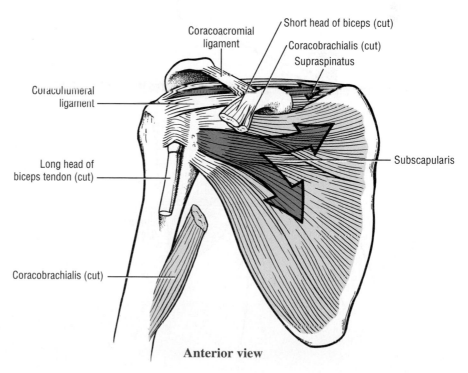

**FIGURE 5–54.** Anterior view of the right shoulder showing the subscapularis muscle blending into the anterior capsule before attaching to the lesser tubercle of the humerus. The subscapularis is shown with diverging arrows, reflecting two main fiber directions. The supraspinatus, coracobrachialis, tendon of the long head of the biceps, and coracohumeral and coracoacromial ligaments are also depicted.

**Anterior view**

the function of these muscles as (1) regulators of the dynamic joint stability and (2) controllers of the arthrokinematics.

### Regulators of Dynamic Stability at the Glenohumeral Joint

The loose fit between the head of the humerus and glenoid fossa permits extensive range of motion at the GH joint. The surrounding joint capsule, therefore, must be free of thick restraining ligaments that otherwise restrict motion. The anatomic design at the glenohumeral joint favors mobility at the expense of stability. An essential function of the rotator cuff group is to compensate for the lack of natural stability at the GH joint. The distal attachment of the rotator cuff muscles blends into the GH joint capsule before attaching to the proximal humerus. The anatomic arrangement forms a protective cuff around the joint (see Figs. 5–53 and 5–54). Nowhere else in the body do so many muscles form such an intimate structural part of a joint's periarticular structure.

Earlier in this chapter the dynamic stabilizing function of the infraspinatus muscle during external rotation is discussed (see Fig. 5–36). This dynamic stabilization is an essential function of all members of the rotator cuff. Forces produced by the rotator cuff not only actively move the humerus, but also stabilize and centralize its head against the glenoid fossa. Dynamic stability at the GH joint, therefore, requires a healthy neuromuscular system and musculoskeletal system.

### Active Controllers of the Arthrokinematics at the Glenohumeral Joint

In the healthy shoulder, the rotator cuff controls much of the active arthrokinematics of the GH joint.[55] Contraction

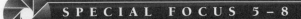

of the horizontally oriented supraspinatus produces a compression force directly into the glenoid fossa. The compression force stabilizes the humeral head firmly against the fossa during its superior roll (Fig. 5–55). Compression

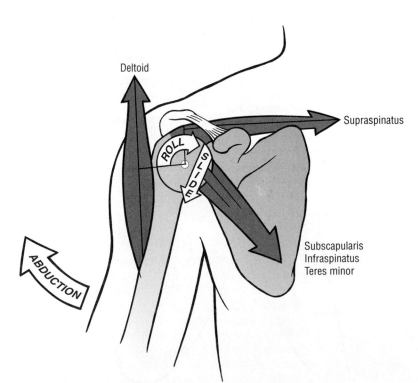

**FIGURE 5–55.** Anterior view of the right shoulder showing the *force couple* between the deltoid and rotator cuff muscles during active shoulder abduction. The deltoid's superior-directed line-of-force rolls the humeral head upward. The supraspinatus rolls the humeral head into abduction, and compresses the joint for added stability. The remaining rotator cuff muscles (subscapularis, infraspinatus, and teres minor) exert a downward translational force on the humeral head to counteract excessive superior translation. Note the internal moment arm used by both the deltoid and supraspinatus.

**The Vulnerability of the Supraspinatus to Excessive Wear**

The supraspinatus muscle may be the most utilized muscle of the entire shoulder complex. In addition to its role in assisting the deltoid during abduction, the muscle also provides dynamic and, at times, static stability to the GH joint. Biomechanically, the supraspinatus is subjected to large internal forces, even during quite routine activities. The supraspinatus has an internal moment arm for shoulder abduction of about 25 mm (about 1 in). Supporting a load by the hand 50 cm (about 20 in) distal to the GH joint creates a mechanical advantage of 1 : 20 (i.e., the ratio of internal moment arm of the muscle to the external moment arm of the load). A 1 : 20 mechanical advantage implies that the supraspinatus must generate a force *20 times greater* than the weight of the load (see Chapter 1). These high forces, generated over many years, may partially tear the muscle tendon as it inserts on the capsule and the humerus. Fortunately, the high force demands are shared by the middle deltoid, but nevertheless the supraspinatus is subjected to substantial force. Persons with a partially torn supraspinatus tendon are advised to hold objects close to the body, thereby minimizing the force demands on the muscle.

Excessive wear on the supraspinatus muscle may be associated with excessive wear on other muscles within the rotator cuff group. This more general condition is often referred to as "rotator cuff syndrome." The condition includes partial tears of the rotator cuff tendons, inflammation and adhesions of the capsule, bursitis, pain, and a generalized feeling of shoulder weakness. The supraspinatus tendon is particularly vulnerable to degeneration if coupled with an age-related compromise in its blood supply.[8] Depending on the severity of the rotator cuff syndrome, the arthrokinematics at the GH joint may be completely disrupted and immobile. This very disabling condition is often referred to as a "frozen shoulder."

---

forces between the joint surfaces increase linearly from 0 to 90 degrees of shoulder abduction, reaching a magnitude of 90% of body weight.[49] The surface area for dissipating joint forces increases to a maximum between 60 degrees and 120 degrees of shoulder elevation.[57] This increase in surface area helps to maintain pressure at tolerable physiologic levels.

> **Functions of the Rotator Cuff Muscles in the Active Control of the Arthrokinematics at the GH Joint**
> - *Supraspinatus:* Compresses the humeral head directly into the glenoid fossa.
> - *Subscapularis, infraspinatus, and teres minor:* Produces an inferior-directed translation force on the humerus head.
> - *Infraspinatus and teres minor:* Rotates the humeral head externally.

Without adequate supraspinatus force, the near vertical line-of-force of a contracting deltoid tends to jam or impinge the humeral head superiorly against the coracoacromial arch, thereby blocking complete abduction. This effect is typically observed following a complete rupture of the supraspinatus tendon. In addition to the compression produced by the supraspinatus, the remaining rotator cuff muscles exert an inferior depression force on the humeral head during abduction (see Fig. 5–55). The inferiorly directed force counteracts much of the tendency for the deltoid muscle to translate the humerus superiorly during abduction.[43] During frontal plane abduction, the infraspinatus and teres minor muscles can rotate the humerus externally in order to increase the clearance between the greater tubercle and the acromion.

## Muscles that Adduct and Extend the Shoulder

Pulling the arm against resistance offered by climbing a rope or propelling through water requires a forceful contraction from the shoulder's powerful adductor and extensor muscles. These muscles are capable of generating the largest isometric torque of any muscle group of the shoulder (Table 5–4).

The *latissimus dorsi* shown in Figure 5–43A and the *sternocostal head of the pectoralis major* shown in Fig. 5–56 are the largest of the adductor and extensor muscles of the shoulder. With the humerus held stable, contraction of the latissimus dorsi can raise the pelvis toward the upper body. Persons with paraplegia often use this action during crutch- and brace-assisted ambulation as a substitute for weakened or paralyzed hip flexors.

The *teres major, long head of the triceps, posterior deltoid, infraspinatus,* and *teres minor* are also primary muscles for shoulder adduction and extension. These muscles have their proximal attachments on the inherently unstable scapula. It is the primary responsibility of the rhomboid muscles to stabilize the scapula during active adduction and extension of the glenohumeral joint. This stabilization function is evident by the downward rotation and retraction movements that naturally occur with shoulder adduction. Figure 5–57 highlights the synergistic relationship between the rhomboids

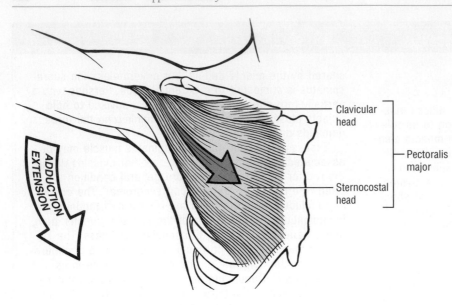

**FIGURE 5–56.** Anterior view of the right pectoralis major showing the adduction/extension function of the sternocostal head. The clavicular head of the pectoralis major is also shown.

and the teres major during a strongly resisted adduction effort of the shoulder. The pectoralis minor (Fig. 5–43B) and the latissimus dorsi fibers that attach to the scapula assist the rhomboids in downward rotation.

The entire rotator cuff group is active during shoulder adduction and extension.[30] Forces produced by these muscles assist with the action directly or stabilize the head of the humerus against the glenoid fossa.[54]

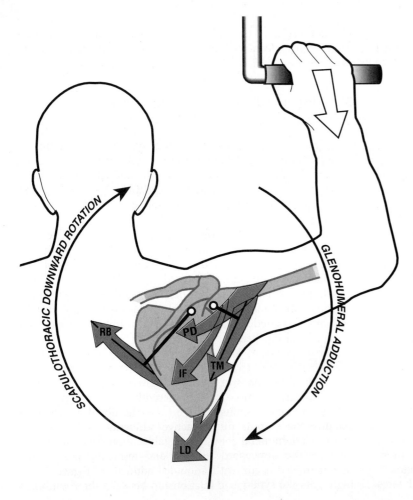

**FIGURE 5–57.** Posterior view of a shoulder showing the muscular interaction between the scapulothoracic downward rotators and the glenohumeral adductors (and extensors) of the right shoulder. For clarity, the long head of the triceps is not shown. The teres major is shown with its internal moment arm (dark line) extending from the glenohumeral joint. The rhomboids are shown with the internal moment extending from the scapula's axis. (See text for further details.) (TM = teres major, LD = latissimus dorsi, IF = infraspinatus and teres minor, PD = posterior deltoid, RB = rhomboids).

### A Closer Look at the Posterior Deltoid

The posterior deltoid is a shoulder extensor and adductor. In addition, this muscle is also the primary *horizontal extensor* at the shoulder. Vigorous contraction of the posterior deltoid during full horizontal extension requires that the scapula is firmly stabilized by the lower trapezius (Fig. 5–58).

Complete paralysis of the posterior deltoid can occur owing to an overstretching of the axillary nerve. Persons with this paralysis frequently report difficulty in combining full shoulder extension and horizontal extension, such as that required to place the arm in the sleeve of a coat.

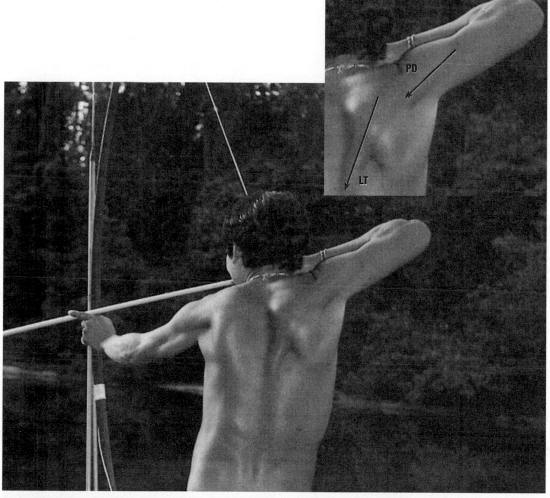

**FIGURE 5–58.** The hypertrophied right posterior deltoid of a Tirio Indian man engaged in bow fishing. Note the strong synergistic action between the right lower trapezius (LT) and right posterior deltoid (PD). The lower trapezius must anchor the scapula to the spine and provide a fixed proximal attachment for the strongly activated posterior deltoid. (Courtesy of Dr. Mark J. Plotkin: Tales of a Shaman's Apprentice. Viking-Penguin, New York, 1993.)

## Muscles that Internally and Externally Rotate the Shoulder

### INTERNAL ROTATOR MUSCLES

The primary muscles that internally rotate the GH joint are the *subscapularis, anterior deltoid, pectoralis major, latissimus*   *dorsi,* and *teres major.* Many of these internal rotators are also powerful extensors and adductors, such as those needed for swimming.

The total muscle mass of the shoulder's internal rotators is much greater than that of the external rotators. This factor explains why the shoulder internal rotators produce about

**Superior view**

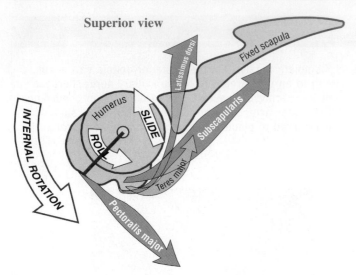

**FIGURE 5–59.** Superior view of the right shoulder showing the group action of the internal rotators about the glenohumeral joint's vertical axis of rotation. In this case, the scapula is fixed and the humerus is free to rotate. The line-of-force of the pectoralis major is shown with its internal moment arm. Note the roll-and-slide arthrokinematics of the convex-on-concave motion. For clarity, the anterior deltoid is not shown.

described as rotators of the humerus relative to a fixed scapula (Fig. 5–59). The arthrokinematics of this motion are based on the convex humeral head rotating on the fixed glenoid fossa. Consider, however, the muscle function and kinematics that occur when the humerus is held in a fixed position and the scapula is free to rotate. As depicted in Figure 5–60, with sufficient muscle force, the scapula and trunk can rotate around a fixed humerus. Note that the arthrokinematics of the scapula-on-humerus rotation involve a concave glenoid fossa rolling and sliding in similar directions on the convex humeral head (Fig. 5–60; insert).

## EXTERNAL ROTATOR MUSCLES

The primary muscles that externally rotate the glenohumeral joint are the *infraspinatus, teres minor,* and *posterior deltoid.* The supraspinatus can assist with external rotation provided the glenohumeral joint is between neutral and full external rotation.[25]

The external rotators are a relatively small percentage of the total muscle mass at the shoulder. Accordingly, maximal effort external rotation produces the smallest isometric torque of any muscle group at the shoulder (see Table 5–4). Regardless of the relatively low maximal torque potential, the external rotators still must generate high-velocity concentric contractions, such as when cocking the arm backward to pitch a ball. Through eccentric activation, these same muscles must decelerate internal rotation of the shoulder at the release phase of pitching: a peak velocity measured at close to 7000 degrees/sec.[18] These large force demands placed on the relatively small infraspinatus and teres minor may cause partial tears within the muscle and capsule, leading to rotator cuff syndrome.[24]

1.75 times greater isometric torque than the external rotators (see Table 5–4).[39] Peak torques of the internal rotators also exceed the external rotators when measured isokinetically, under both concentric and eccentric conditions.[37]

The muscles that internally rotate the GH joint are often

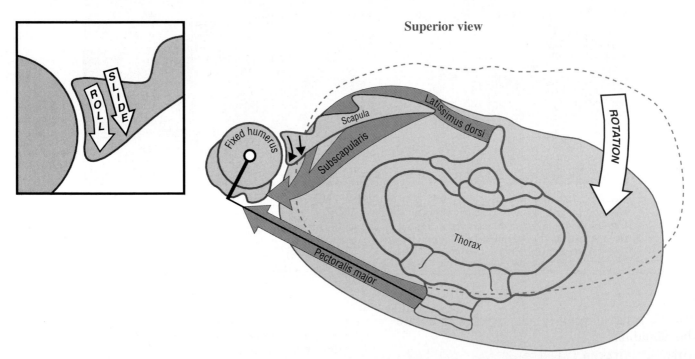

**FIGURE 5–60.** Superior view of the right shoulder showing actions of three internal rotators when the distal (humeral) segment is fixed and the trunk is free to rotate. The line-of-force of the pectoralis major is shown with its internal moment arm originating about the glenohumeral joint's vertical axis. Inset contains the roll-and-slide arthrokinematics during the concave-on-convex motion.

# REFERENCES

1. Bagg SD, Forrest WJ: Electromyographic study of the scapular rotators during arm abduction in the scapula plane. Am J Phys Med 65:111–124, 1986.
2. Bagg SD, Forrest WJ: A biomechanical analysis of scapula rotation during arm abduction in the scapula plane. Am J Phys Rehabil 7:238–245, 1988.
3. Basmajian JV, Bazant FJ: Factors preventing downward dislocation of the adducted shoulder joint. J Bone Joint Surg 41A:1182–1186, 1959.
4. Bearn JG: Direct observations on the function of the capsule of the sternoclavicular joint in clavicular support. J Anat 101:159–170, 1967.
5. Bigliani LU, Kelkar R, Flatow EL, et al: Glenohumeral stability: Biomechanical properties of passive and active stabilizers. Clin Orthop (S15)330:13–30, 1996.
6. Branch TP, Burdette HL, Shahriari AS, et al: The role of the acromioclavicular ligaments and the effect of distal clavicle resection. Am J Sports Med (S8)24:293–297, 1996.
7. Brunnstrom S: Muscle testing around the shoulder girdle. J Bone Joint Surg 23A:263–272, 1941.
8. Chansky HA, Iannotti JP: The vascularity of the rotator cuff. Clin Sports Med 10:807–822, 1991.
9. Chen SK, Simonian PT, Wickiewicz TL, et al: Radiographic evaluation of glenohumeral kinematics: A muscle fatigue model. J Shoulder Elbow Surg (S2)8:49–52, 1999.
10. Colachis SC, Strohm BR: Effect of suprascapular and axillary nerve blocks on muscle force in upper extremity. Arch Phys Med Rehabil 52:22–29, 1971.
11. Conway AM: Movements at the sternoclavicular and acromioclavicular joints. Phys Ther 41:421–432, 1961.
12. Cope R: Dislocations of the sternoclavicular joint. Skeletal Radiol 22:233–238, 1993.
13. Curl LA, Warren RF: Glenohumeral joint stability: Selective cutting studies on the static capsular restraints. Clin Orthop (S15)330:54–65, 1996.
14. Decker MJ, Hintermeister RA, Faber KL, et al: Serratus anterior muscle activity during selected rehabilitation exercises. Am J Sports Med (S26)27:784–791, 1999.
15. DeFreitas V, Vitti M, Furlani J: Electromyographic analysis of the levator scapulae and rhomboideus major muscle in movements of the shoulder. Electromyogr Clin Neurophysiol 19:335–342, 1979.
16. DePalma AF: Degenerative changes in sternoclavicular and acromioclavicular joints in various decades. Springfield, Ill, Charles C Thomas, 1957.
17. Deutsch A, Altchek DW, Schwartz E, et al: Radiologic measurement of superior displacement of the humeral head in the impingement syndrome. J Shoulder Elbow Surg 5:186–193, 1996.
18. Dillman CJ, Fleisig GS, Andrews JR: Biomechanics of pitching with emphasis upon shoulder kinematics. J Orthop Sports Phys Ther 18:402–408, 1993.
19. Freedman L, Munroe RR: Abduction of the arm in the scapular plane: Scapular and glenohumeral movements. J Bone Joint Surg 48A:1503–1510, 1966.
20. Fukuda K, Craig EV, An KN, et al: Biomechanical study of the ligamentous system of the acromioclavicular joint. J Bone Joint Surg 68A:434–440, 1986.
21. Harryman DT, Sidles JA, Clark JM, et al: Translation of the humeral head on the glenoid with passive glenohumeral motion. J Bone Joint Surg 72A:1334–1343, 1990.
22. Howell SM, Imobersteg AM, Seger DH, et al: Clarification of the role of the supraspinatus muscle in shoulder function. J Bone Joint Surg 68A:398–404, 1986.
23. Howell SM, Galinat BJ: The glenoid-labral socket. Clin Orthop 243:122–125, 1989.
24. Hughes RE, An KN: Force analysis of rotator cuff muscles. Clin Orthop (S15)330:75–83, 1996.
25. Ihashi K, Matsushita N, Yagi R, et al: Rotational action of the supraspinatus muscle on the shoulder joint. J Electromyogr Kinesiol 8:337–346, 1998.
26. Inman VT, Saunders M, Abbott LC: Observations on the function of the shoulder joint. J Bone Joint Surg 26A:1–32, 1944.
27. Jobe CM: Superior glenoid impingement: Current concepts. Clin Orthop 330:98–107, 1996.
28. Kebaetse M, McClure P, Pratt NA: Thoracic position effect on shoulder range of motion, strength, and three-dimensional scapular kinematics. Arch Phys Med Rehab 80(S10):945–950, 1999.
29. Kendall FP, McCreary AK, Provance PG: Muscles: Testing and Function, 4th ed. Baltimore, Williams & Wilkins, 1993.
30. Kronberg M, Nemeth G, Brostrom LA: Muscle activity and coordination in the normal shoulder. Clin Orthop Res 257:76–85, 1990.
31. Kumar VP, Balasubramaniam P: The role of atmospheric pressure in stabilising the shoulder: An experimental study. J Bone Joint Surg 67B:719–721, 1985.
32. Lemos ML: The evaluation and treatment of the injured acromioclavicular joint in athletes. Am J Sports Med (S8)26:137–144, 1998.
33. Ludewig PM, Cook TM: Alterations in shoulder kinematics and associated muscle activity in people with symptoms of shoulder impingement. Phys Ther 80(S12B):276–291, 2000.
34. Malicky DM, Soslowsky LJ, Blasier RP, et al: Anterior glenohumeral stabilization factors: Progressive effects in a biomechanical model. J Orthop Res (S15)14:282–288, 1996.
35. Mandalidis DG, McGlone BS, Quigley RF, et al: Digital fluoroscopic assessment of the scapulohumeral rhythm. Surg Radiol Anat (S10)21:241–246, 1999.
36. McQuade KJ, Smidt GL: Dynamic scapulohumeral rhythm: The effects of external resistance during elevation of the arm in the scapular plane. J Orthop Sports Phys Ther (S10)27:125–133, 1998.
37. Mikesky AE, Edwards JE, Wigglesworth JK, et al: Eccentric and concentric strength of the shoulder and arm musculature in collegiate baseball pitchers. Am J Sports Med 23:638–642, 1995.
38. Moseley HF: The clavicle: Its anatomy and function. Clin Orthop 58:17–27, 1968.
39. Murray MP, Gore DR, Gardiner GM, et al: Shoulder motion and muscle strength of normal men and women in two age groups. Clin Orthop 182:267–273, 1985.
40. Neumann DA, Seeds R: Observations from cineradiography analysis. Marquette University, Milwaukee, WI, 1999.
41. O'Brien SJ, Neves MC, Arnoczky SP, et al: The anatomy and histology of the inferior glenohumeral ligament complex of the shoulder. Am J Sports Med 18:449–456, 1990.
42. O'Connell PW, Nuber GW, Mileski RA, et al: The contribution of the glenohumeral ligaments to anterior stability of the shoulder joint. Am J Sports Med 18:579–584, 1990.
43. Paletta GA, Warner JJP, Warren RF, et al: Shoulder kinematics with two-plane x-ray evaluation in patients with anterior instability or rotator cuff tearing. J Should Elbow Surg 6:516–527, 1997.
44. Palmer ML, Blakely RL: Documentation of medial rotation accompanying shoulder flexion. Phys Ther 66:55–58, 1986.
45. Palmer WE, Caslowitz PL: Anterior shoulder instability: Diagnostic criteria determined from prospective analysis of 121 MR arthrograms. Radiology 197:819–825, 1995.
46. Payne LZ, Deng XH, Craig EV, et al: The combined dynamic and static contributions to subacromial impingement. Am J Sports Med 25:801–808, 1997.
47. Petersson CJ, Redlund-Johnell I: The subacromial space in normal shoulder radiographs. Acta Orthop Scand 55:57–58, 1984.
48. Poppen NK, Walker PS: Normal and abnormal motion of the shoulder. J Bone Joint Surg Am 58A:195–201, 1976.
49. Poppen NK, Walker PS: Forces at the glenohumeral joint in abduction. Clin Orthop 135:165–170, 1978.
50. Reis FP, deCamargo AM, Vitti M, deCarvalho CA: Electromyographic study of the subclavius. Acta Anat 105:284–290, 1979.
51. Robinson CM: Fractures of the clavicle in the adult. J Bone Joint Surg 80B:476–484, 1998.
52. Saha AK: Mechanism of shoulder movements and a plea for the recognition of "zero position" of glenohumeral joint. Clin Orthop 173:3–10, 1983.
53. Schwartz E, Warren RF, O'Brien SJ, et al: Posterior shoulder instability. Orthop Clin North Am 18:409–419, 1987.
54. Sharkey NA, Marder RA, Hanson PB: The entire rotator cuff contributes to elevation of the arm. J Orthop Res 12:699–708, 1994.
55. Sharkey NA, Marder RA: The rotator cuff opposes superior translation of the humeral head. Am J Sports Med 23:270–275, 1995.
56. Shibuta H, Tamai K, Tabuchi KI: Magnetic resonance imaging of the shoulder in abduction. Clin Orthop 348:107–113, 1998.
57. Soslowsky LJ, Flatow EI, Bigliani LU, et al: Quantification of in situ contact areas at the glenohumeral joint: A biomechanical study. J Orthop Res 10:524–534, 1992.
58. Steindler A: Kinesiology of the Human Body, Springfield, Ill, Charles C Thomas, 1955.

59. Stevens KJ, Preston BJ, Wallace WA, et al: CT imaging and three-dimensional reconstructions of shoulders with anterior glenohumeral instability. Clin Anat 12:326–336, 1999.
60. Terry GC, Hammon D, France P, et al: The stabilizing function of passive shoulder restraints. Am J Sports Med 19:26–34, 1991.
61. Thomas CB, Friedman RJ: Ipsilateral sternoclavicular dislocation and clavicle fracture. J Orthop Trauma 3:355–357, 1989.
62. Ticker JB, Bigliani LU, Soslowsky LJ, et al: Inferior glenohumeral ligament: geometric and strain-rate dependent properties. J Shoulder Elbow Surg 5:269–279, 1996.
63. Van Der Helm FCT, Pronk GM: Three-dimensional recording and descriptions of motions of the shoulder mechanism. J Biomech Eng 117:27–40, 1995.
64. Walker PS, Poppen NK: Biomechanics of the shoulder joint abduction in the plane of the scapula. Bull Hosp Joint Dis 38:107–111, 1977.
65. Warner JJ, Deng XH, Russell WF, et al: Static capsuloligamentous restraints to superior-inferior translation of the glenohumeral joint. Am J Sports Med 20:675–685, 1992.
66. Watson CJ, Schenkman M: Physical therapy management of isolated serratus anterior muscle paralysis. Phys Ther 75:194–202, 1995.
67. Williams GR, Shakil M, Klimkiewicz J, et al: Anatomy of the scapulothoracic articulation. Clin Orthop 359:237–246, 1999.
68. Williams PL, Bannister LH, Berry M, Collins P, et al: Gray's Anatomy, 38th ed, New York, Churchill Livingstone, 1995.

## ADDITIONAL READINGS

Basmajian JV: *Muscles Alive*. Their Functions Revealed by Electromyography, 4th ed. Baltimore, Williams & Wilkins, 1978.
Bey MJ, Huston LJ, Blasier RB, et al: Ligamentous restraints to external rotation of the humerus in the late-cocking phase of throwing: A cadaveric biomechanical investigation. Am J Sports Med 28:200–205, 2000.
Codman EA: The Shoulder. Boston, Thomas Todd Company, 1934.

Ferrari DA: Capsular ligaments of the shoulder: Anatomical and functional study of the anterior superior capsule. Am J Sports Med 18:20–24, 1990.
Friedman RJ, Blocker ER, Morrow DL: Glenohumeral Instability. J South Orthop Assoc 4:182–199, 1995.
Guttmann D, Paksima NE, Zuckerman JD: Complications of treatment of complete acromioclavicular joint dislocations. Instr Course Lect 49:407–413, 2000.
Halder AM, Itoi E, An KN: Anatomy and biomechanics of the shoulder. Orthop Clin N Am 31:159–176, 2000.
Johnson G, Bogduk N, Nowitzke A, et al: Anatomy and actions of the trapezius. Clin Biomech 9:44–50, 1994.
Johnson GR, Spalding D, Nowitzke A, et al: Modelling the muscles of the scapula: Morphometric and coordinate data and functional implications. J Biomech 29:1039–1051, 1996.
Mayer F, Horstmann T, Rocker K, et al: Normal values of isokinetic maximum strength, the strength/velocity curve, and the angle at peak torque of all degrees of freedom in the shoulder. Int J Sports Med 15:19–25, 1994.
Medvecky MJ, Zuckerman JD: Sternoclavicular joint injuries and disorders. Instr Course Lect 49:397–406, 2000.
Otis JC, Jiang CC, Wickiewicz TL, et al: Changes of moment arms in the rotator cuff and deltoid muscles with abduction and rotation. J Bone Joint Surg 76A:667–676, 1994.
Placzek JD, Roubal PJ, Freeman DC, et al: Long-term effectiveness of translational manipulation for adhesive capsulitis. Clin Orthop 356:181–191, 1998.
Saha AK: Dynamic stability of the glenohumeral joint. Acta Orthop Scand 42:491–505, 1971.
Sanders TG, Morrison WB, Miller MD. Imaging techniques for the evaluation of glenohumeral instability. Am J Sports Med 28:414–434, 2000.
Wuelker N, Wolfgang P, Roetman B, et al: Function of the supraspinatus muscle. Acta Orthop Scand 65:442–446, 1994.
Wuelker N, Schmotzer H, Thren K, et al: Translation of the glenohumeral joint with simulated active elevation. Clin Orthop 309:193–200, 1994.

# CHAPTER 6

# Elbow and Forearm Complex

### DONALD A. NEUMANN, PT, PHD

## TOPICS AT A GLANCE

## INTRODUCTION

The elbow and forearm complex consists of three bones and four joints (Fig. 6–1). The *humeroulnar* and *humeroradial joints* form the elbow. The motions of flexion and extension of the elbow provide a means to adjust the overall functional length of the upper limb. This function is used for many important activities, such as feeding, reaching, and throwing, and personal hygiene.

The radius and ulna articulate with one another within the forearm at the *proximal* and *distal radioulnar joints*. This set of articulations allows the palm of the hand to be turned up (supinated) or down (pronated), without requiring motion of the shoulder. Pronation and supination can be performed in conjunction with, or independent from, elbow flexion and extension. The interaction between the elbow and forearm joints greatly increases the range of effective hand placement.

> **Four Articulations Within the Elbow and Forearm Complex**
> 1. Humeroulnar joint
> 2. Humeroradial joint
> 3. Proximal radioulnar joint
> 4. Distal radioulnar joint

## OSTEOLOGY

### Mid-to-Distal Humerus

The anterior and posterior surfaces of the mid-to-distal humerus provide proximal attachments for the brachialis and the medial head of the triceps brachii (Figs. 6–2 and 6–3). The distal end of the shaft of the humerus terminates medially as the trochlea and the medial epicondyle, and laterally

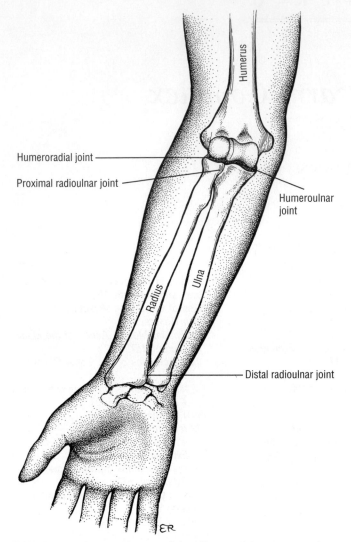

**FIGURE 6–1.** The articulations of the elbow and forearm complex.

Directly lateral to the trochlea is the rounded *capitulum*. The capitulum forms nearly one half of a sphere. A small *radial fossa* is located just proximal to the anterior side of the capitulum.

The *medial epicondyle* of the humerus projects medially from the trochlea (see Figs. 6–2 and 6–4). This prominent and easily palpable structure serves as the proximal attach-

as the capitulum and lateral epicondyle. The *trochlea* resembles a rounded, empty spool of thread. On either side of the trochlea are its *medial and lateral lips*. The medial lip is prominent and extends farther distally than the adjacent lateral lip. Midway between the medial and lateral lips is the *trochlear groove* which, when looking from posterior to anterior, spirals slightly toward the medial direction (Fig. 6–4). The *coronoid fossa* is located just proximal to the anterior side of the trochlea (see Fig. 6–2).

---

**Osteologic Features of the Mid-to-Distal Humerus**

- Trochlea including groove and medial and lateral lips
- Coronoid fossa
- Capitulum
- Radial fossa
- Medial and lateral epicondyles
- Medial and lateral supracondylar ridges
- Olecranon fossa

---

**Anterior view**

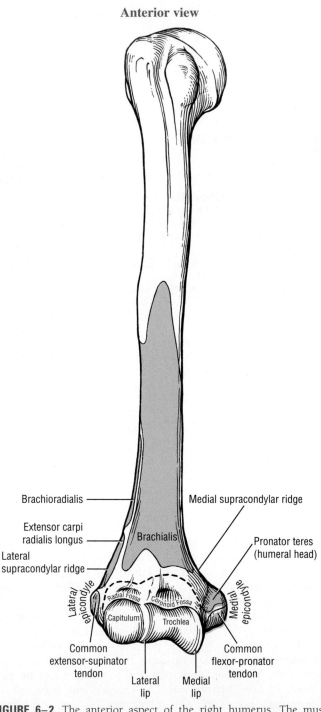

**FIGURE 6–2.** The anterior aspect of the right humerus. The muscle's proximal attachments are shown in red. The dotted lines show the capsular attachments of the elbow joint.

**Posterior view**

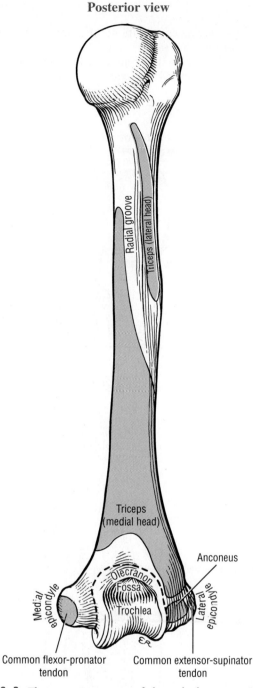

**FIGURE 6–3.** The posterior aspect of the right humerus. The muscle's proximal attachments are shown in red. The dashed lines show the capsular attachments around the elbow joint.

ment of the medial collateral ligament of the elbow as well as the forearm pronator and wrist flexor muscles.

The *lateral epicondyle* of the humerus, less prominent than the medial epicondyle, serves as the proximal attachment for the lateral collateral ligament of the elbow as well as the forearm supinator and wrist extensor muscles. Immediately proximal to both epicondyles are the *medial* and *lateral supracondylar ridges*.

On the posterior side of the humerus, just proximal to the trochlea, is the very deep and broad *olecranon fossa*. Only a thin sheet of bone or membrane separates the olecranon fossa from the coronoid fossa.

## Ulna

The ulna has a very thick proximal end with distinct processes (Figs. 6–5 and 6–6). The *olecranon process* forms the large, blunt, proximal tip of the ulna, making up the "point" of the elbow (Fig. 6–7). The roughened posterior surface of the olecranon process accepts the attachment of the triceps brachii. The *coronoid process* projects sharply from the anterior body of the proximal ulna.

---

**Osteologic Features of the Ulna**
- Olecranon process
- Coronoid process
- Trochlear notch and longitudinal crest
- Radial notch
- Supinator crest
- Tuberosity of the ulna
- Ulnar head
- Styloid process

---

The *trochlear notch* of the ulna is the large jawlike process located between the anterior tips of the olecranon and coronoid processes. This concave notch articulates firmly with the reciprocally shaped trochlea of the humerus, forming the humeroulnar joint. A thin raised *longitudinal crest* divides the trochlear notch down its midline.

The *radial notch* of the ulna is an articular depression just lateral to the inferior aspect of the trochlear notch (see Fig. 6–7). Extending distally, and slightly dorsally, from the radial notch is the *supinator crest,* marking the distal attachments for part of the lateral collateral ligament and the supinator muscle. The *tuberosity of the ulna* is a roughened impression just distal to the coronoid process, formed by the attachment of the brachialis muscle (see Fig. 6–5).

**Right humerus: Inferior view**

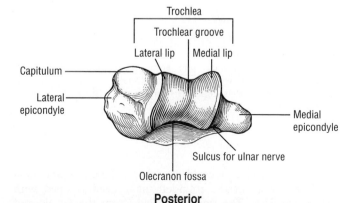

**Posterior**

**FIGURE 6–4.** The distal end of the right humerus, inferior view.

## Anterior view

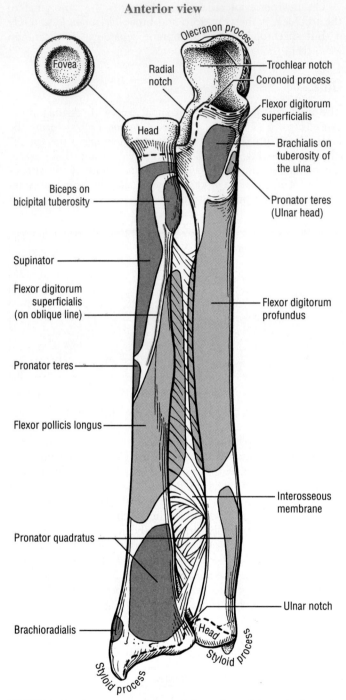

**FIGURE 6–5.** The anterior aspect of the right radius and ulna. The muscle's proximal attachments are shown in red and distal attachments in gray. The dashed lines show the capsular attachments around the elbow and wrist and the proximal and distal radioulnar joints. The radial head is depicted from above to show the concavity of the fovea.

The *ulnar head* is located at the distal end of the ulna (Fig. 6–8). Most of the rounded ulnar head is lined with articular cartilage. The pointed *styloid* (from the Greek root *stylos;* pillar, + *eidos;* resembling) *process* projects distally from the posterior-medial region of the extreme distal ulna.

## Radius

In the fully supinated position, the radius lies parallel and lateral to the ulna (see Figs. 6–5 and 6–6). The proximal end of the radius is small and as such constitutes a relatively small structural component of the elbow. Its distal

## Posterior view

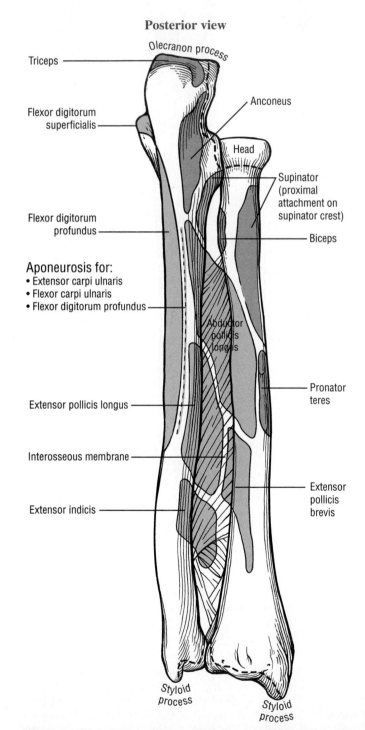

**FIGURE 6–6.** The posterior aspect of the right radius and ulna. The muscle's proximal attachments are shown in red and distal attachments in gray. The dashed lines show the capsular attachments around the elbow and wrist and the proximal and distal radioulnar joints.

**Lateral view**

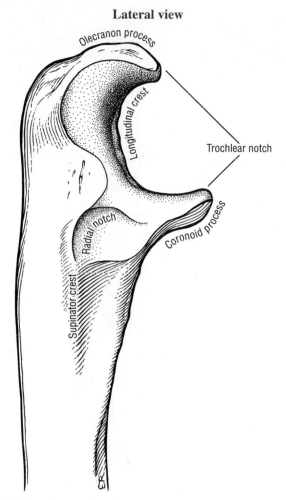

**FIGURE 6–7.** A lateral (radial) view of the right proximal ulna, with the radius removed. Note the jawlike shape of the trochlear notch.

end, however, is enlarged, forming a major part of the wrist joint.

---

**Osteologic Features of the Radius**
- Radial head
- Fovea
- Bicipital tuberosity
- Ulnar notch
- Styloid process

---

The *radial head* is a disclike structure located at the extreme proximal end of the radius. Most of the outer rim of the radial head is covered with a layer of articular cartilage. The rim of the radial head contacts the radial notch of the ulna, forming the proximal radioulnar joint.

The superior surface of the radial head consists of a shallow, cup-shaped depression known as the *fovea*. This cartilage-lined concavity articulates with the capitulum of the humerus, forming the humeroradial joint. The biceps brachii muscle attaches to the radius at the *bicipital tuberosity,* a roughened region located at the anterior-medial edge of the proximal radius.

The distal end of the radius articulates with carpal bones to form the radiocarpal joint at the wrist (see Fig. 6–8). The *ulnar notch* of the distal radius accepts the ulnar head at the distal radioulnar joint. The prominent *styloid process* projects from the lateral surface of the distal radius.

## ARTHROLOGY

### Part 1: Joints of the Elbow

#### GENERAL FEATURES OF THE HUMEROULNAR AND HUMERORADIAL JOINTS

The elbow joint consists of the humeroulnar and humeroradial articulations. The tight fit between the trochlea and trochlear notch at the humeroulnar joint provides most of the elbow's structural stability.

Early anatomists classified the elbow as a *ginglymus* or *hinged joint* owing to its predominant uniplanar motion of flexion and extension. The term *modified hinge joint* is actually more appropriate since the ulna experiences a slight amount of axial rotation (i.e., rotation about its own longitudinal axis) and side-to-side motion as it flexes and extends.[29] Bioengineers must account for these relatively small "extra-sagittal" accessory motions in the design of elbow joint prostheses. Without attention to this detail, the prosthetic implants are more likely to demonstrate premature loosening.[2]

#### *Normal "Valgus Angle" of the Elbow*

Elbow flexion and extension occur about a medial-lateral axis of rotation, passing through the vicinity of the lateral epicondyle (Fig. 6–9A).[45] From medial to lateral, the axis courses slightly superiorly owing in part to the distal pro-

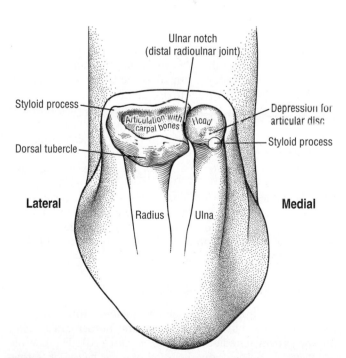

**FIGURE 6–8.** The distal end of the right radius and ulna with carpal bones removed. The forearm is in full supination. Note the prominent ulnar head and nearby styloid process of the ulna.

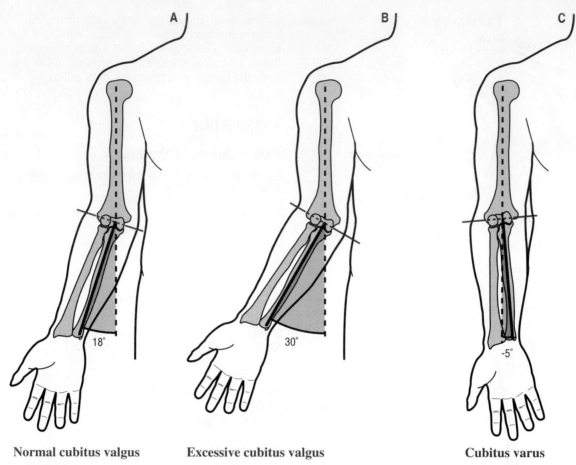

**Normal cubitus valgus**      **Excessive cubitus valgus**                    **Cubitus varus**

**FIGURE 6–9.** *A,* The elbow's axis of rotation (shown as red line) extends slightly obliquely in a medial-lateral direction through the capitulum and the trochlea. *Normal cubitus valgus* of the elbow is shown with the forearm deviated laterally from the longitudinal axis of the humerus axis about 18 degrees. *B, Excessive cubitus valgus* deformity is shown with the forearm deviated laterally 30 degrees. *C, Cubitus varus* deformity is depicted with the forearm deviated medially 5 degrees.

longation of the medial lip of the trochlea. The asymmetry in the trochlea causes the ulna to deviate laterally relative to the humerus. The natural frontal plane angle made by the extended elbow is referred to as *cubitus valgus.* (The term "carrying angle" is often used, reflecting the fact that the valgus angle tends to keep carried objects away from the side of the thigh while walking.) In full elbow extension, the normal carrying angle is about 15 degrees.[45]

Occasionally, the extended elbow may show an excessive cubitus valgus greater than 20 degrees (Fig. 6–9B). In contrast, the forearm may less commonly show a *cubitus varus* deformity, where the forearm is deviated toward the midline (Fig. 6–9C). Valgus and varus are terms derived from the Latin *turned outward* (abducted) and *turned inward* (adducted), respectively.

## PERIARTICULAR CONNECTIVE TISSUE

The *articular capsule* of the elbow encloses three different articulations: the humeroulnar joint, the humeroradial joint, and the proximal radioulnar joint (Fig. 6–10). The capsule is thin and reinforced anteriorly by oblique bands of fibrous tissue. A *synovial membrane* lines the internal surface of the capsule (Fig. 6–11).

The articular capsule of the elbow is strengthened by an extensive set of collateral ligaments (Table 6–1). These ligaments provide an important source of stability to the elbow joint. The *medial collateral ligament* consists of anterior, posterior, and transverse fiber bundles (Fig. 6–12). The *anterior fibers* are the strongest and stiffest of the medial collateral ligament.[41] As such, these fibers provide the most significant resistance against a valgus (abduction) force at the elbow. The anterior fibers arise from the anterior part of the medial epicondyle and insert on the medial part of the coronoid process of the ulna. The majority of the anterior fibers become taut near full extension.[13] A few fibers, however, become taut at full flexion. The anterior fiber bundle as a whole, therefore, provides articular stability throughout the entire range of motion.[8]

The *posterior fibers* of the medial collateral ligament attach on the posterior part of the medial epicondyle and insert on the medial margin of the olecranon process. The posterior fibers become taut in the extremes of elbow flexion.[13,41] A third and poorly developed set of *transverse fibers* of the medial collateral ligament cross from the olecranon to the coronoid process of the ulna. Because these fibers originate and insert on the same bone, they do not provide significant articular stability.

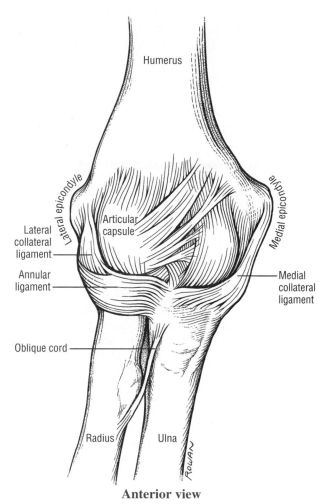

**Anterior view**

**FIGURE 6–10.** An anterior view of the right elbow showing the capsule and collateral ligaments.

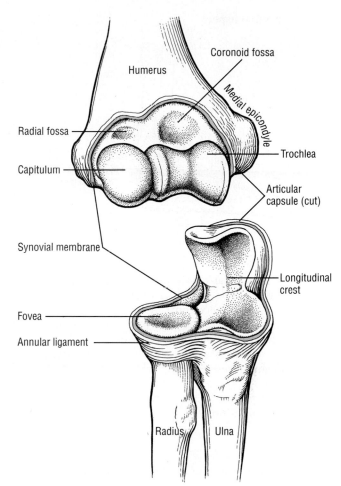

**FIGURE 6–11.** Anterior view of the right elbow disarticulated to expose the humeroulnar and humeroradial joints. The margin of the proximal radioulnar joint is shown within the elbow's capsule. Note the small area on the trochlear notch lacking articular cartilage. The synovial membrane lining the internal side of the capsule is shown in red.

The *lateral collateral ligament* of the elbow is less defined and more variable in form than the medial collateral ligament (Fig. 6–13).[27] The ligament originates on the lateral epicondyle and immediately splits into two fiber bundles. One fiber bundle, traditionally known as the *radial collateral ligament*, fans out to blend with the annular ligament. A second fiber bundle, called the *lateral (ulnar) collateral ligament*, attaches distally to the supinator crest of the ulna. These fibers become taut at full flexion.[41]

All the fibers of the lateral collateral ligament and the posterior-lateral aspect of the capsule stabilize the elbow against a varus-directed force.[36] By attaching to the ulna, the lateral (ulnar) collateral ligament and the anterior fibers of the medial collateral ligament function as collateral "guy-wires" to the elbow, stabilizing the path of the ulna during sagittal plane motion.

The ligaments around the elbow are endowed with mechanoreceptors, consisting of Golgi organs, Ruffini terminals, Pacini corpuscles, and free nerve endings.[38] These receptors may supply important information to the nervous system for augmenting proprioception and detecting safe limits of passive tension in the structures around the elbow.

**TABLE 6–1. Ligaments of the Elbow and Motions that Increase Tension**

| Ligaments | Motions that Increase Tension |
|---|---|
| Medial collateral ligament (anterior fibers*) | Valgus<br>Extension and to a lesser extent flexion |
| Medial collateral ligament (posterior fibers) | Valgus<br>Flexion |
| Lateral collateral ligament (radial collateral component) | Varus |
| Lateral collateral ligament (lateral (ulnar) collateral component*) | Varus<br>Flexion |
| Annular ligament | Distraction of the radius |

* Primary valgus or varus stabilizers.

**Medial aspect**

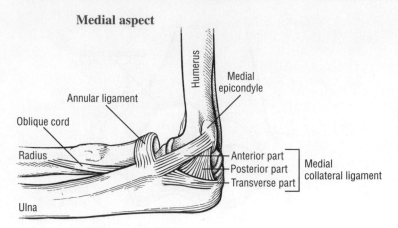

**FIGURE 6–12.** The components of the medial collateral ligament of the right elbow.

As in all joints, the elbow joint has an intracapsular air pressure. This pressure, which is determined by the ratio of the volume of air to the volume of space, is lowest when the capsule is most compliant, or less stiff. The intracapsular air pressure is lowest at about 80 degrees of flexion.[15] This joint position is often a "position of comfort" for persons with joint inflammation and swelling.[26] Maintaining a swollen elbow in a flexed position may improve comfort but may also predispose the person to an elbow flexion *contracture* (from the Latin root *contractura;* to draw together).

## KINEMATICS

### *Functional Considerations of Flexion and Extension*

Elbow flexion provides several important physiologic functions, such as pulling, lifting, feeding, and grooming. The inability to actively bring the hand to the mouth for feeding, for example, significantly limits the level of functional independence. Persons with a spinal cord injury above the $C^5$ nerve root have this profound disability due to total paralysis of elbow flexor muscles.

Elbow extension occurs with activities such as throwing, pushing, and reaching. Loss of complete extension due to an elbow flexion contracture is often caused by marked stiffness in the elbow flexor muscles. The muscles become abnormally stiff after long periods of immobilization in a flexed and shortened position. Long-term flexion may be the result of casting following a fractured bone, an elbow joint inflammation, an elbow flexor muscle spasticity, a paralysis of the triceps muscle, or a scarring of the skin over the anterior elbow. In addition to the tightness in the flexor muscles, increased stiffness may occur in the anterior capsule and anterior parts of the collateral ligaments.

The maximal range of passive motion generally available to the elbow is from 5 degrees of hyperextension through 145 degrees of flexion (Fig. 6–15A and B). Research indicates, however, that several common activities of daily living use only a limited arc of motion, usually between 30 and 130 degrees of flexion.[28] Unlike lower extremity joints, such as in the knee, the loss of the *extremes of motion* at the elbow usually results in only minimal functional impairment.

### *Arthrokinematics at the Humeroulnar Joint*

The humeroulnar joint is the articulation of the concave trochlear notch of the ulna around the convex trochlea of the humerus (Fig. 6–16). From a sagittal section, the humeroulnar joint resembles a ball-and-socket joint. The firm mechanical link between the trochlea and trochlear notch, however, limits the motion to essentially the sagittal plane.

**Lateral aspect**

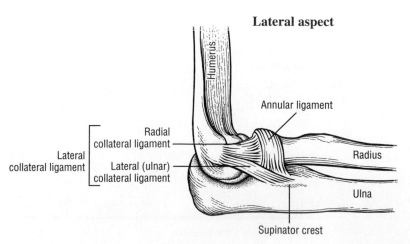

**FIGURE 6–13.** The components of the lateral collateral ligament of the right elbow.

**SPECIAL FOCUS 6 – 1**

### Elbow Flexion Contracture and Loss of Forward Reach

One of the most disabling consequences of an elbow flexion contracture is reduced reaching capacity. The loss of forward reach varies with the degree of elbow flexion contracture. As shown in Figure 6–14, a fully extendable elbow (i.e., with a 0-degree contracture) demonstrates a 0-degree loss in area of forward reach. The area of forward reach diminishes only slightly (less than 6%) with a flexion contracture of less than 30 degrees. A flexion contracture that exceeds 30 degrees, however, results in a much greater loss of forward reach. As noted in the graph, a flexion contracture of 90 degrees reduces total reach by almost 50%. Minimizing a flexion contracture to less than 30 degrees is therefore an important functional goal for patients following elbow trauma, prolonged immobilization, or joint replacement.

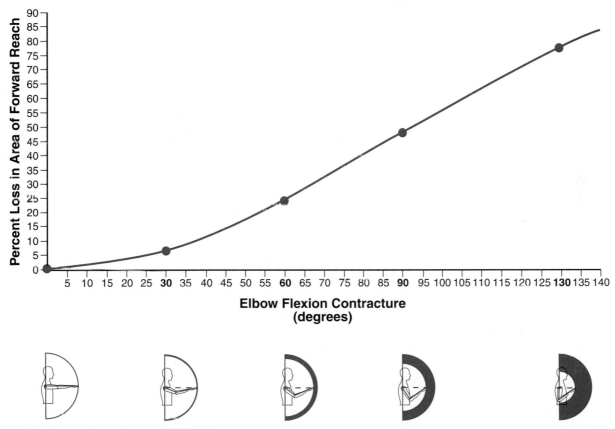

**FIGURE 6–14.** A graph showing the percent loss in area of forward reach of the arm—from the shoulder to finger—as a function of the severity of an elbow flexion contracture in the horizontal axis. Note the sharp increase in the reduction in reach as the flexion contracture exceeds 30 degrees. The figures across the bottom of the graph depict the progressive loss of reach indicated by the increased semicircle area, as the flexion contracture becomes more severe.

Hyaline cartilage covers about 300 degrees of articular surface on the trochlea compared with only 180 degrees on the trochlear notch. In order for the humeroulnar joint to be fully, passively extended, sufficient extensibility is required in the dermis, flexor muscles, anterior capsule, and anterior fibers of the medial collateral ligament (Fig. 6–17A). Once in full extension, the humeroulnar joint is stabilized by the increased tension in most of the anterior fibers of the medial collateral ligament, anterior capsule, and flexor muscles, particularly the broad tendon of the brachialis. The prominent tip of the olecranon process becomes wedged into the olecranon fossa. Excessive ectopic (from the Greek root *ecto*; outside, + *topos*; place) bone formation around the olecranon fossa can limit full passive extension.

During flexion at the humeroulnar joint, the concave surface of the trochlear notch rolls and slides on the convex trochlea (see Fig. 6–17B). Full passive elbow flexion requires elongation of the posterior capsule, extensor muscles, ulnar nerve,[44] and certain collateral ligaments, especially the posterior fibers of the medial collateral ligament.

### Arthrokinematics at the Humeroradial Joint

The humeroradial joint is an articulation between the cup-like fovea of the radial head and the reciprocally shaped

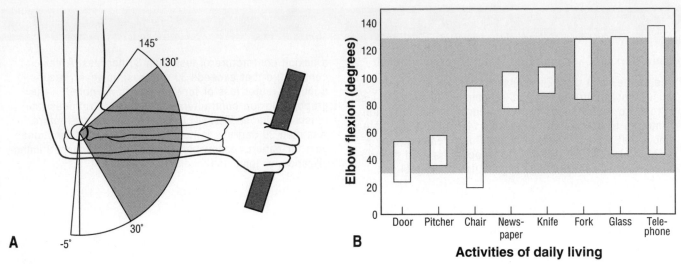

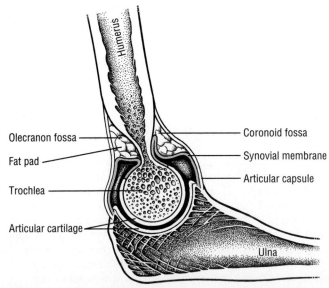

**FIGURE 6–15.** Range of motion at the elbow. *A,* Typical healthy elbow showing the extent of range of motion from 5 degrees beyond extension (hyperextension) through 145 degrees of flexion. The 100-degree "functional arc" from 30 to 130 degrees of flexion in red based on the histogram. *B,* The histogram shows the range of motion at the elbow typically needed to perform the following activities of daily living: opening a *door,* pouring from a *pitcher,* rising from a *chair,* holding a *newspaper,* cutting with a *knife,* bringing a *fork* to the mouth, bringing a *glass* to the mouth, and holding a *telephone.* (Modified with permission from Morrey BF, Askew LJ, An KN, et al: A biomechanical study of normal functional elbow motion. J Bone Joint Surg 63A:872–876, 1981.)

rounded capitulum. At rest in full extension, little if any physical contact exists at the humeroradial joint.[17] During *active flexion,* however, muscle contraction pulls the radial fovea against the capitulum.[30] The arthrokinematics of flexion and extension consist of the fovea of the radius rolling and sliding across the convexity of the capitulum (Fig. 6–18).

Compared with the humeroulnar joint, the humeroradial joint provides minimal structural stability to the elbow. The humeroradial joint does, however, provide an important bony resistance against a valgus force.[31]

### Force Transmission Through the Interosseous Membrane of the Forearm

Most of the fibers of the *interosseous membrane* of the forearm are directed away from the radius in an oblique medial and distal direction (Fig. 6–19). A few separate sparse and poorly defined bands flow perpendicular to the membrane's main fiber direction. One of these bands, the *oblique cord,* runs from the lateral side of the tuberosity of the ulna to just distal to the bicipital tuberosity. Another unnamed band is located at the extreme distal end of the interosseous membrane.

The interosseous membrane has several functions related to force transmission through the upper limb. As illustrated in Figure 6–20, about 80% of the compression force due to bearing weight through the forearm crosses the wrist between the lateral side of the carpus and the radius. The remaining 20% of the compression force passes across the medial side of the carpus and the ulna, at the "ulnocarpal space."[37] Because of the fiber direction of the interosseous membrane, part of the proximal directed force through the radius is transferred across the membrane to the ulna.[39] This mechanism allows a share of the compression force at the wrist to cross the elbow via the humeroulnar joint, thereby reducing the amount of force that must cross the limited surface area of the humeroradial joint.[30] The periarticular

tissues at the proximal and distal radioulnar joints also transfer a portion of the compression force from the radius to the ulna.

Most elbow flexors, and essentially all the major supinator and pronator muscles, have their distal attachments on the radius. Contraction of these muscles, therefore, pulls the radius proximally against the humeroradial joint.[44] An additional function of the interosseous membrane, therefore, is to

**FIGURE 6–16.** A sagittal section through the humeroulnar joint showing the well-fitting joint surfaces between the trochlear notch and trochlea. The synovial membrane lining the internal side of the capsule is shown in red.

**FIGURE 6–17.** A sagittal section through the humeroulnar joint. *A,* The joint is resting in full extension. *B,* The joint is passively flexed through full flexion. Note that in full flexion, the coronoid process of the ulna fits into the coronoid fossa of the humerus. The medial-lateral axis of rotation is shown through the center of the trochlea. The stretched (taut) structures are shown as thin elongated arrows, and slackened structures are shown as wavy arrows. AC = anterior capsule, PC = posterior capsule, MCL-Anterior = anterior fibers of the medial collateral ligament, MCL-Posterior = posterior fibers of the medial collateral ligament.) See text for further details.

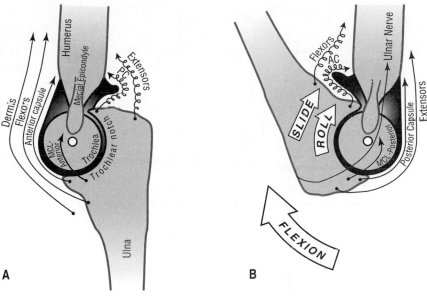

**Resting in Extension**

transfer a component of the muscle force applied to the radius to the ulna. This occurs through a mechanism similar to that during weight bearing through the forearm. A mechanism that permits two joints to "share" these compression forces reduces each individual joint's long-term wear and tear. Failure of the integrity of this mechanism may lead to joint deterioration and possible osteoarthritis.

The predominant fiber direction of the interosseous membrane is not aligned to resist *distally applied forces* on the radius. For example, holding a heavy suitcase with the elbow extended causes a distracting force almost entirely through the radius (Fig. 6–21). The distal pull on the radius slackens rather than tenses the interosseous membrane, thereby necessitating other less capable tissues, such as the oblique cord and annular ligament, to accept the weight of the load. Contraction of the brachioradialis or other muscles normally

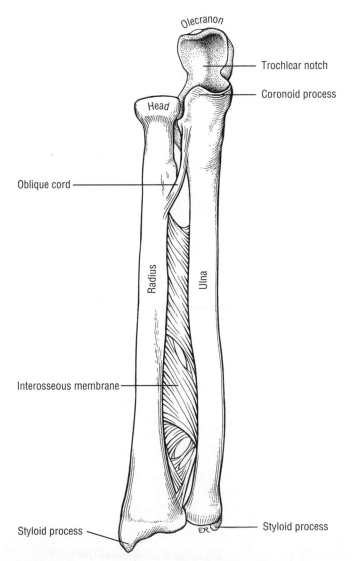

**FIGURE 6–19.** An anterior view of the interosseous membrane of the right forearm. Note the contrasting fiber direction of the oblique cord.

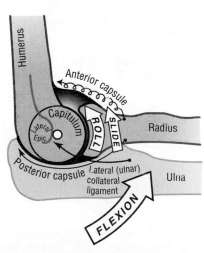

**FIGURE 6–18.** A sagittal section through the humeroradial joint during flexion. Note the medial-lateral axis of rotation in the center of the capitulum. The stretched (taut) structures are shown as thin elongated arrows, and slackened structures are shown as wavy arrows. Note the elongation of the lateral (ulnar) collateral ligament during flexion.

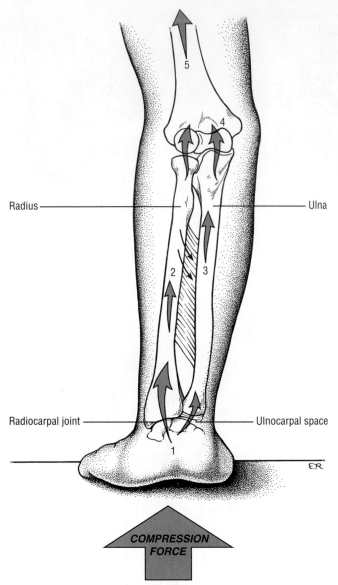

susceptible to injury when the fully extended elbow receives a violent valgus force, often from a fall (Fig. 6–22). The anterior capsule may be involved with the valgus injury if the joint is also forced into hyperextension. The medial collateral ligament is also susceptible to injury from repetitive valgus forces in non-weight-bearing activities, such as pitching a baseball and spiking a volleyball.[25]

In severe elbow injuries, the trochlear notch of the ulna may dislocate posterior to the trochlea of the humerus (Fig.

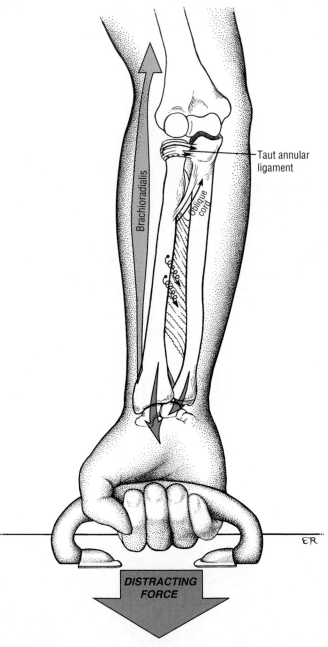

**FIGURE 6–20.** A *compression force* through the hand is transmitted primarily through the wrist (#1) at the radiocarpal joint and to the radius (#2). This force stretches the interosseous membrane (shown by double taut arrows) that transfers a part of the compression force to the ulna (#3) and across the elbow at the humeroulnar joint (#4). The compression forces that cross the elbow are finally directed toward the shoulder (#5). The stretched (taut) structures are shown as thin elongated arrows.

involved with grasp can assist with holding the radius and load against the humeroradial joint. Complaints of a deep aching in the forearm from persons who carry heavy loads for extended periods may be from fatigue in these muscles. Supporting loads through the forearm at shoulder level, for example, like a waiter carrying a tray of food, directs the weight proximally through the radius where the interosseous membrane can assist with dispersing these loads more evenly through the forearm.

## TRAUMATIC CAUSES OF ELBOW JOINT INSTABILITY

Injury to the collateral ligaments of the elbow can result in marked elbow instability. The medial collateral ligament is

**FIGURE 6–21.** Holding a load, such as a suitcase, places a distal-directed *distracting force* predominantly through the radius. This distraction slackens the interosseous membrane shown by wavy arrows over the membrane. Other structures, such as the oblique cord, the annular ligament, and the brachioradialis, must assist with the support of the load. The stretched (taut) structures are shown as thin elongated arrows, and the slackened structures are shown as wavy arrows.

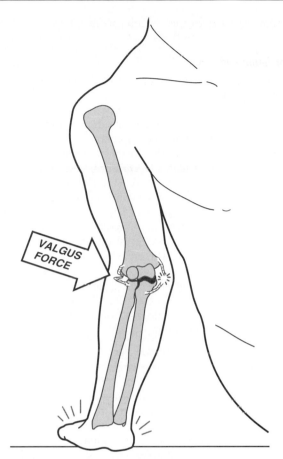

**FIGURE 6–22.** Attempts at catching oneself from a fall may induce a severe valgus force, overstretching or rupturing the medial collateral ligament.

6–23). This dislocation is frequently caused from a fall onto an outstretched arm and hand and, thus, may be associated with a fracture of the proximal radius and humeral capitulum.

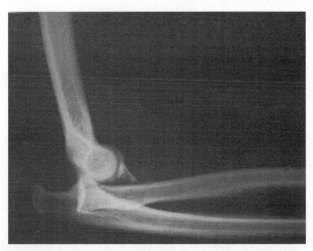

**FIGURE 6–23.** A posterior dislocation of the humeroulnar joint. (From O'Driscoll SW: Elbow dislocations. In Morrey BF (ed): The Elbow and Its Disorders, 3rd ed. Philadelphia, WB Saunders, 2000, p 410. By permission of the Mayo Foundation for Medical Education and Research.)

## Part II: Joints of the Forearm

### GENERAL FEATURES OF THE PROXIMAL AND DISTAL RADIOULNAR JOINTS

The radius and ulna are bound together by the interosseous membrane and the proximal and distal radioulnar joints. This set of joints, situated at either end of the forearm, allows the forearm to rotate into pronation and supination. Forearm supination places the palm up, or supine, and pronation places the palm down, or prone. This forearm rotation occurs about an axis of rotation that extends from the radial head through the head of the ulna—an axis that intersects and connects both radioulnar joints (Fig. 6–24).[53]

As is apparent in Figure 6–24, pronation and supination provide a mechanism that allows independent "rotation" of the hand without an obligatory rotation of the ulna or humerus. A person with limited pronation or supination range of motion must rely on greater internal or external rotation of the shoulder to perform activities such as tightening a screw and turning a doorknob.

The kinematics of forearm rotation are more complicated than those implied by the simple "palm-up and palm-down" terminology. The palm does indeed rotate, but only because the hand and wrist connect to the radius and *not to the ulna.* The space between the distal ulna and the medial side of the carpus allows the carpal bones to rotate freely—along with the radius—without interference from the distal ulna.

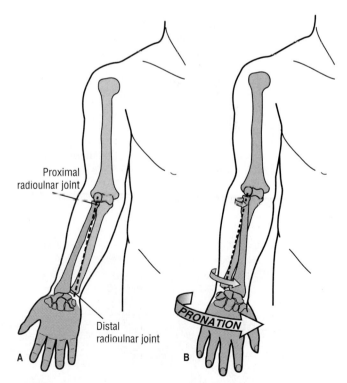

**FIGURE 6–24.** Anterior view of the right forearm. *A,* In full supination with the radius and ulna parallel. *B,* Moving into full pronation with the radius crossing over the ulna. The axis of rotation (shown by dashed line) extends obliquely across the forearm from the radial head to the ulnar head. The radius and hand (shown in red) is the distal segment of the forearm complex. The humerus and ulna (shown in gray) is the proximal segment of the forearm complex. Note that the thumb stays with the radius during pronation.

In the anatomic position, the forearm is fully supinated when the ulna and radius lie parallel to one another (Fig. 6–24A). During pronation, the distal segment of the forearm complex (i.e., the radius and hand) rotates and crosses over an essentially fixed ulna (Fig. 6–24B). The ulna, through its firm attachment to the humerus at the humeroulnar joint, remains essentially stationary during pronation and supination movements. A stable ulna provides an important rigid link that the radius, wrist, and hand can pivot upon. Only very slight motion occurs in the ulna during supination and pronation.[3] The ulna tends to rotate slightly in the frontal plane during active pronation and supination; toward abduction (valgus) during pronation, and toward adduction (varus) during supination. Other than design of an elbow prosthesis, this slight accessory movement of the ulnar is clinically insignificant.

## JOINT STRUCTURE AND PERIARTICULAR CONNECTIVE TISSUE

### Proximal Radioulnar Joint

The proximal radioulnar joint, the humeroulnar joint, and the humeroradial joint all share one articular capsule. Within this capsule, the radial head is held against the proximal ulna by a fibro-osseous ring. This ring is formed by the radial notch of the ulna and the annular ligament (Fig. 6–25A). About 75% of the ring is formed by the annular ligament and 25% by the radial notch of the ulna.

The *annular* (from the Latin *annulus;* ring) *ligament* is a thick circular band of connective tissue, attaching to the ulna on either side of the radial notch (Fig. 6–25B). The ligament fits snugly around the radial head, holding the proximal radius against the ulna. The internal circumference of the annular ligament is lined with cartilage to reduce the friction against the radial head during pronation and supination. The external surface of the ligament receives attachments from the elbow capsule, the radial collateral ligament, and the supinator muscle. The *quadrate ligament* is a short, stout ligament that arises just below the radial notch of the ulna and attaches to the medial surface of the neck of the radius (Fig. 6–25B). This ligament lends structural support to the capsule of the proximal radioulnar joint.

### Distal Radioulnar Joint

The distal radioulnar joint consists of the convex head of the ulna fitting into a shallow concavity formed by the ulnar notch on the radius and the proximal surface of an articular disc (Fig. 6–27A). This important joint stabilizes the distal forearm during pronation and supination.

The articular disc at the distal radioulnar joint is also known as the *triangular fibrocartilage,* indicating its shape and predominant tissue type. As depicted in Figure 6–27A, the lateral side of the disc attaches along the entire rim of the ulnar notch of the radius. The main body of the disc fans out horizontally into a triangular shape, with its apex attaching medially into the depression on the ulna head and adjacent styloid process. The anterior and posterior edges of the disc are continuous with the *palmar (anterior) and dorsal (posterior) radioulnar joint capsular ligaments* (Fig. 6–27A and B). The proximal surface of the disc, along with the attached capsular ligaments, holds the head of the ulna snugly against the ulnar notch of the radius.[33]

### Introduction to the Ulnocarpal Complex

The articular disc is part of a larger set of connective tissue known as the *ulnocarpal complex.*[37,42] This complex is often referred to as the *triangular fibrocartilage complex.* The ulnocarpal complex occupies most of the space between the distal end of the ulna and the ulnar side of the carpal bones. Several wrist ligaments, such as the ulnar collateral ligament, are included with this complex (see Fig. 6–27B). The ulnocarpal complex is the primary stabilizer of the distal radioulnar joint, particularly important during the dynamics of pronation and supination. Other structures that provide joint stability are the pronator quadratus, joint capsule, tendon of the extensor carpi ulnaris, and interosseous membrane. Tears or disruptions of the ulnocarpal complex, especially the disc,[23] may cause complete dislocation or generalized instability of the distal radioulnar joint, making pronation and supination motions, as well as motions of the wrist, painful and difficult to perform.[11] (The ulnocarpal complex is discussed further in Chapter 7).

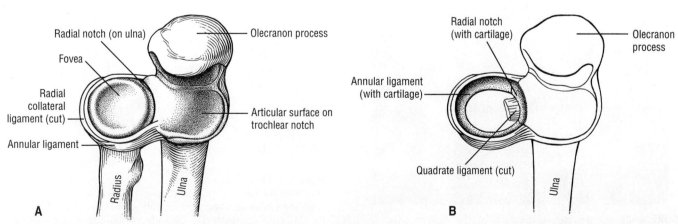

**FIGURE 6–25.** The right proximal radioulnar joint as viewed from above. *A,* The radius is held against the radial notch of the ulna by the annular ligament. *B,* The radius is removed, exposing the internal surface of the concave component of the proximal radioulnar joint. Note the cartilage lining the entire fibro-osseous ring. The quadrate ligament is cut near its attachment to the neck of the radius.

## SPECIAL FOCUS 6–2

### Dislocations of the Proximal Radioulnar Joint: The "Pulled-Elbow" Syndrome

A strenuous pull on the forearm through the hand can cause the radial head to slip through the distal side of the annular ligament. Children are particularly susceptible to this "pulled-elbow" syndrome due to ligamentous laxity and increased likelihood of others pulling on their arms (Fig. 6–26). One of the best ways to prevent this dislocation is to explain to parents how a sharp pull on the child's hand can cause such a dislocation.

**Causes of "pulled" elbow**

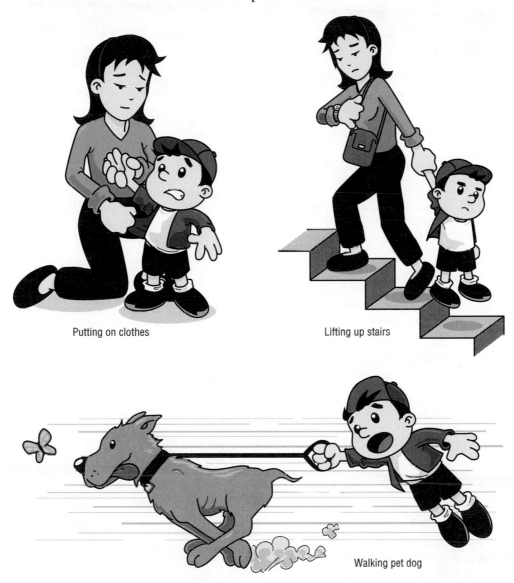

Putting on clothes

Lifting up stairs

Walking pet dog

**FIGURE 6–26.** Three examples of causes of "pulled elbow syndrome." (Redrawn with permission from Letts RM: Dislocations of the child's elbow. In Morrey BF (ed): The Elbow and Its Disorders, 3rd ed. Philadelphia, WB Saunders, 2000. By permission of the Mayo Foundation for Medical Education and Research.)

---

**Stabilizers of the Distal Radioulnar Joint**
- Ulnocarpal complex (triangular fibrocartilage complex)
- Joint capsule
- Pronator quadratus
- Tendon of the extensor carpi ulnaris
- Interosseous membrane

## KINEMATICS

### *Functional Considerations of Pronation and Supination*

Forearm supination occurs during many activities that involve rotating the palmar surface of the hand toward the face, such as feeding, washing, and shaving. Forearm pronation, in contrast, is used to place the palmar surface of the

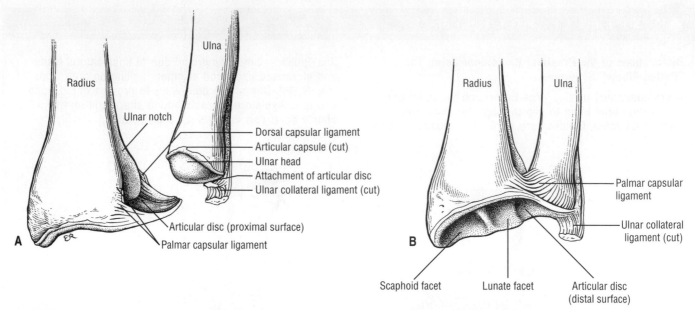

**FIGURE 6-27.** An anterior view of the right distal radioulnar joint. *A,* The ulnar head has been pulled away from the concavity formed by the proximal surface of the articular disc and the ulnar notch of the radius. *B,* The distal forearm has been tilted slightly to expose part of the distal surface of the articular disc and its connections with the palmar capsular ligament of the distal radioulnar joint. The articular disc (also called the triangular fibrocartilage), the capsular ligaments, and the ulnar collateral ligament are collectively referred to as the ulnocarpal complex. See text for further descriptions. The scaphoid and lunate facets on the distal radius show impressions made by these carpal bones at the radiocarpal joint of the wrist.

hand down on an object, such as grasping a coin or pushing up from a chair.

The neutral or zero reference position of forearm rotation is the "thumb-up" position, midway between complete pro-

nation and supination. On average, the forearm rotates through about 75 degrees of pronation and 85 degrees of supination (Fig. 6-28A). As shown in Figure 6-28B, several activities of daily living require only about 100 degrees of

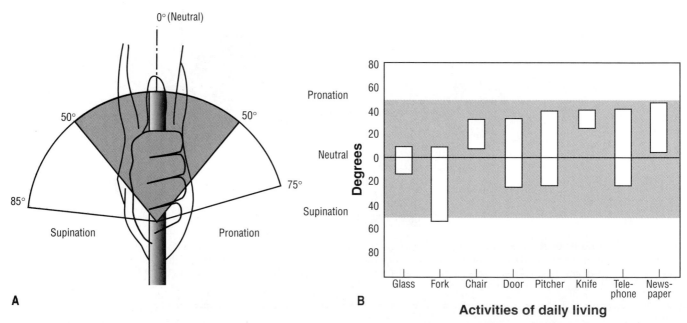

**FIGURE 6-28.** Range of motion at the forearm complex. *A,* Typical healthy forearm showing range of motion: 0 to 85 degrees of supination and 0 to 75 degrees of pronation. The 0-degree neutral position is shown with the thumb pointing straight up. As with the elbow, a 100-degree "functional arc" exists (shown in red). This arc is derived from the histogram in *B. B,* Histogram showing the amount of forearm rotation usually required for healthy persons to perform the following activities of daily living: bringing a *glass* to the mouth, bringing a *fork* to the mouth, rising from a *chair,* opening a *door,* pouring from a *pitcher,* cutting with a *knife,* holding a *telephone,* and reading a *newspaper.* (Modified with permission from Morrey BF, Askew LJ, An KN, et al: A biomechanical study of normal functional elbow motion. J Bone Joint Surg 63A:872-876, 1981.)

forearm rotation—from about 50 degrees of pronation through 50 degrees of supination.[28] Similar to the elbow joint, a 100 degree functional arc exists—an arc that does not include the terminal ranges of motion. Persons who lack the last 30 degrees of complete forearm rotation are still capable of performing many routine activities of daily living.

### Arthrokinematics at the Proximal and Distal Radioulnar Joints

Pronation and supination require simultaneous joint movement at both proximal and distal radioulnar joints. A restriction at one joint limits motion at the other.

#### Supination

Supination at the proximal radioulnar joint occurs as a spinning of the radial head within the fibro-osseous ring formed by the annular ligament and radial notch of the ulna (Fig. 6–29, bottom inset). Supination at the distal radioulnar joint occurs as the concave ulnar notch of the radius rolls and slides in similar directions on the head of the ulna (Fig. 6–29, top inset). During supination, the proximal surface of the articular disc remains in contact with the ulna head. At the end range of supination, the palmar capsular ligament is stretched to its maximal length, creating a stiffness that naturally stabilizes the joint.[12,50]

#### Pronation

The arthrokinematics of pronation at the proximal and distal radioulnar joints occur by mechanisms similar to those described for supination (Fig. 6–30). As depicted in the top inset of Figure 6–30, full pronation maximally elongates the dorsal capsular ligament at the distal radioulnar joint, as the palmar capsular ligament slackens to about 70% of its original length.[44] Full pronation exposes the articular surface of

the ulnar head (see the asterisk in Fig. 6–30, top inset), making it readily palpable.

### Restrictions in Passive Range of Pronation and Supination Motions

Restrictions in passive range of pronation and supination motions can occur from tightness in muscle and/or con-

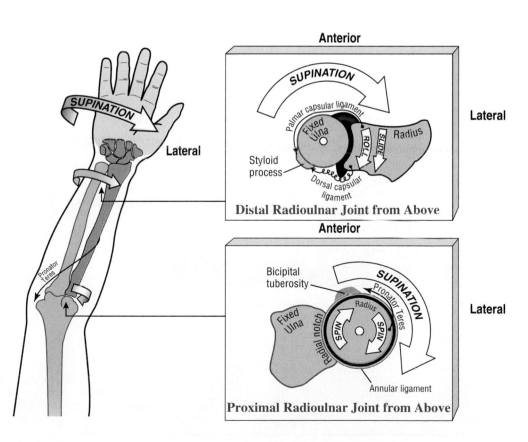

**FIGURE 6–29.** Illustration on the left shows the anterior aspect of a right forearm after completing full *supination*. During supination, the radius and hand (shown in red) rotate around the fixed humerus and ulna (shown in gray). The inactive but stretched pronator teres is also shown. Viewed as though looking down at the right forearm, the two insets depict the arthrokinematics at the proximal and distal radioulnar joints. The stretched (taut) structures are shown as thin elongated arrows, and slackened structures are shown as wavy arrows. See text for further details.

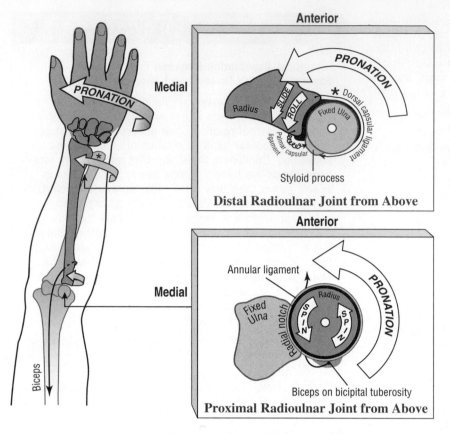

**Distal Radioulnar Joint from Above**

**Proximal Radioulnar Joint from Above**

**FIGURE 6–30.** Illustration on the left shows the right forearm after completing full *pronation*. During pronation, the radius and hand (shown in red) rotates around the fixed humerus and ulna (shown in gray). The inactive but stretched biceps muscle is also shown. As viewed in Figure 6–29, the two insets show a superior view of the arthrokinematics at the proximal and distal radioulnar joints. The stretched (taut) structures are shown as thin elongated arrows, and slackened structures are shown as wavy arrows. The asterisks mark the exposed point on the anterior aspect of the ulna head, which is apparent once the radius rotates fully around the ulna into complete pronation. See text for further details.

nective tissues. Samples of these tissues are listed in Table 6–2.

### Humeroradial Joint: A "Shared" Joint Between the Elbow and the Forearm

During active pronation and supination, the extreme proximal end of the radius articulates with the ulna or humerus in two locations. First, as described in Figures 6–29 and 6–30, the circumference of the radial head articulates with the fibro-osseous ring at the proximal radioulnar joint. Second, the fovea of the radial head makes contact with the capitulum of the humerus at the humeroradial joint. During pronation, for instance, the fovea of the radial head spins against the rounded capitulum of the humerus (Fig. 6–31). Any motion at the elbow-and-forearm complex involves motion at the humeroradial joint. A limitation of motion at the humeroradial joint can therefore disrupt both flexion and extension and pronation and supination.

### Pronation and Supination with the Radius and Hand Held Fixed

Up to this point, the kinematics of pronation and supination are described as a rotation of the *radius and hand* relative to

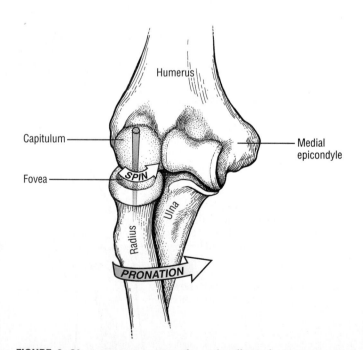

**FIGURE 6–31.** An anterior view of a right elbow during pronation of the forearm. During pronation, the fovea of the radial head must spin against the capitulum. The rotation occurs about an axis that is coincident with the axis of rotation through the proximal radioulnar joint.

| TABLE 6–2. Structures that can Restrict Supination and Pronation | |
| --- | --- |
| **Limit Supination** | **Limit Pronation** |
| Pronator teres, pronator quadratus | Biceps or supinator muscles |
| Palmar capsular ligament at the distal radioulnar joint[20] | Dorsal capsular ligament at the distal radioulnar joint |
| Oblique cord, interosseous membrane, and quadrate ligament[7,19] | |
| Ulnocarpal complex | Ulnocarpal complex |

a stationary, or fixed, humerus and ulna (see Figs. 6–29 and 6–30). The rotation of the forearm occurs when the upper limb is assumed to be in a *non-weight-bearing position*. Pronation and supination are next described when the upper limb is assumed to be in a weight-bearing position. In this case, the humerus and ulna rotate relative to a stationary, or fixed, radius and hand.

Consider a person bearing weight through an upper extremity with elbow and wrist extended (Fig. 6–32A). The person's right glenohumeral joint is held partially internally rotated. The ulna and radius are positioned parallel in full supination. (The "rod" placed through the epicondyles of the humerus helps with the orientation of this position.) With the radius and hand held firmly fixed with the ground, pronation of the forearm occurs by an *external rotation* of the humerus and ulna (Fig. 6–32B). Because of the tight structural fit of the humeroulnar joint, rotation of the humerus is transferred, almost degree for degree, to the rotating ulna. Return to the fully supinated position involves internal rotation of the humerus and ulna, relative to the fixed radius and hand.

Figure 6–32B depicts an interesting muscle "force-couple" used to pronate the forearm from the weight-bearing position. The infraspinatus rotates the humerus relative to a fixed scapula, while the pronator quadratus rotates the ulna relative to a fixed radius. Both muscles, acting at either end of the upper extremity, produce forces that contribute to a pronation torque at the forearm. From a therapeutic perspective, an understanding of the muscular mechanics of pronation and supination from both a non-weight-bearing and weight-bearing perspective provides additional exercise strategies for strengthening or stretching muscles of the forearm and shoulder.

The right side of Figure 6–32B illustrates the arthrokinematics at the radioulnar joints during pronation while the radius and hand are stationary. At the proximal radioulnar joint, the annular ligament and radial notch of the ulna spin around the fixed radial head (see Fig. 6–32B, top inset). At the distal radioulnar joint, the head of the ulna rotates around the fixed ulnar notch of the radius (see Fig. 6–32B, bottom inset). Table 6–3 summarizes and compares the active arthrokinematics at the radioulnar joints for both weight-bearing and non-weight-bearing conditions of the upper limb.

## MUSCLE AND JOINT INTERACTION

### Neuroanatomy Overview

#### Paths of the Musculocutaneous, Radial, Median, and Ulnar Nerves Throughout the Elbow, Forearm, Wrist, and Hand

The musculocutaneous, radial, median, and ulnar nerves provide motor and sensory innervation to the muscles and connective tissues of the elbow, forearm, wrist, and hand

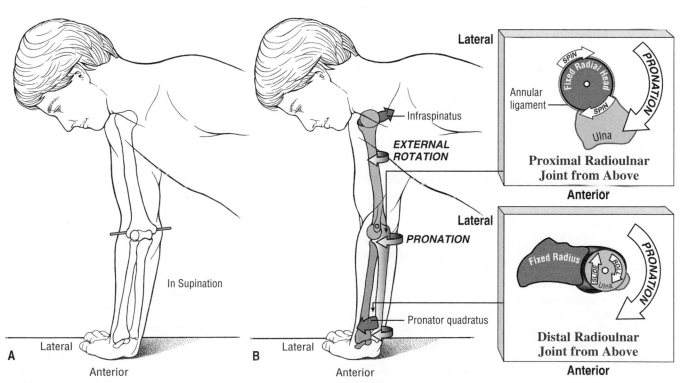

**FIGURE 6–32.** *A,* A person is shown supporting his upper body weight through his right forearm, which is in full supination (i.e., the bones of the forearm are parallel). The radius is held fixed to the ground through the wrist; however, the humerus and ulna are free to rotate. *B,* The humerus and ulna have rotated about 80 to 90 degrees externally from the initial position shown in *A.* This rotation produces pronation at the forearm as the ulna rotates around the fixed radius. Note the activity depicted in the infraspinatus and pronator quadratus muscles. The two insets each show a superior view of the arthrokinematics at the proximal and distal radioulnar joints.

## TABLE 6-3. Arthrokinematics of Pronation and Supination

| | Weight-Bearing (Radius and Hand Fixed) | Non-weight-bearing (Radius and Hand Free to Rotate) |
|---|---|---|
| **Proximal Radioulnar Joint** | Annular ligament *and* radial notch of the ulna spin around a fixed radial head. | Radial head spins within a ring formed by the annular ligament *and* the radial notch of the ulna. |
| **Distal Radioulnar Joint** | Convex ulnar head rolls and slides in opposite directions on the concave ulnar notch of the radius. | Concavity of the ulnar notch of the radius rolls and slides in similar directions on the convex ulna head. |

The anatomic path of these nerves is described as a foundation for this chapter and the following two chapters on the wrist and the hand.

The *musculocutaneous nerve,* formed from the $C^{5-7}$ nerve roots, innervates the biceps brachii, coracobrachialis, and brachialis muscles (Fig. 6–33A). As its name implies, the musculocutaneous nerve innervates muscle, then continues distally as a sensory nerve to the skin, supplying the lateral forearm.

The *radial nerve,* formed from $C^5–T^1$ nerve roots, is a direct continuation of the posterior cord of the brachial plexus (Fig. 6–33B). This large nerve courses within the radial groove of the humerus to innervate the triceps and the anconeus. The radial nerve then emerges laterally at the distal humerus to innervate muscles that attach on or near the lateral epicondyle. Proximal to the elbow, the radial nerve innervates the brachioradialis, a small lateral part of the brachialis, and the extensor carpi radialis longus. Distal to the elbow, the radial nerve consists of superficial and deep branches. The *superficial branch* is purely sensory, supplying the posterior-lateral aspects of the extreme distal forearm and hand, especially concentrated at the dorsal "web space" of the thumb. The *deep branch* contains the remaining motor fibers of the radial nerve. This motor branch supplies the extensor carpi radialis brevis and the supinator muscle. After piercing through an intramuscular tunnel in the supinator muscle, the final section of the radial nerve courses toward the posterior side of the forearm. This terminal branch, often referred to as the posterior interosseous nerve, supplies the extensor carpi ulnaris and several muscles of the forearm, which function in extension of the digits.

The *median nerve,* formed from $C^6–T^1$ nerve roots, courses toward the elbow to innervate most muscles attaching on or near the medial epicondyle of the humerus. These muscles include the wrist flexors and forearm pronators (pronator teres, flexor carpi radialis, and palmaris longus), and the deeper flexor digitorum superficialis (Fig. 6–33C). A deep branch of the median nerve, often referred to as the anterior interosseous nerve, innervates the deep muscles of the forearm: the lateral half of the flexor digitorum profundus, the flexor pollicis longus, and the pronator quadratus. The main part of the median nerve continues distally to cross the wrist through the carpal tunnel, under the cover of the transverse carpal ligament. The nerve then innervates several of the intrinsic muscles of the thumb and the lateral fingers. The median nerve provides a source of sensory fibers to the lateral palm, palmar surface of the thumb, and lateral two and one-half fingers (Fig. 6–33C, see inset on median nerve sensory distribution). This sensory supply is especially rich and concentrated about the distal ends of the index and middle fingers.

The *ulnar nerve,* formed from nerve roots $C^8–T^1$, is formed by a direct branch of the medial cord of the brachial plexus (Fig. 6–33D). After passing posteriorly to the medial epicondyle, the ulnar nerve innervates the flexor carpi ulnaris and the medial half of the flexor digitorum profundus. The nerve then crosses the wrist external to the carpal tunnel and supplies motor innervation to many of the intrinsic muscles of the hand. The ulnar nerve supplies sensory structures to the skin on the ulnar side of the hand, including the medial side of the ring finger and entire little finger. This sensory supply is especially concentrated about the little finger and ulnar border of the hand.

## Innervation of Muscles and Joints of the Elbow and Forearm

Knowledge of the innervation to the muscle, skin, and joints is useful clinical information in the treatment of injury to the peripheral nerves or nerve roots. The informed clinician can anticipate the extent of the sensory and motor involvement following an acute injury. Therapeutic activities, such as splinting, selective strengthening, range of motion exercise, and patient education, can be initiated almost immediately following injury. This proactive approach minimizes the potential for deformity and damage to insensitive skin and joints, thereby limiting the amount of permanent disability.

### INNERVATION TO MUSCLE

The *elbow flexors* have three different sources of peripheral nerve supply: the musculocutaneous nerve to the biceps brachii and brachialis, the radial nerve to the brachioradialis and lateral part of the brachialis, and the median nerve to the pronator teres, which is a secondary flexor. In contrast the *elbow extensors,* the triceps brachii and anconeus, have a single source of nerve supply through the radial nerve. Injury to this nerve can result in complete paralysis of the elbow extensors. In contrast three different nerves must be affected to paralyze all elbow flexors. Fortunately, redundant innervation to the elbow flexor muscles helps preserve the important hand-to-mouth function required for essential activities such as feeding.

The muscles that *pronate the forearm* (pronator teres, pronator quadratus, and other secondary muscles that originate from the medial epicondyle) are innervated through the median nerve. *Supination of the forearm* is driven by the biceps

## A MUSCULOCUTANEOUS NERVE (C⁵⁻⁷)

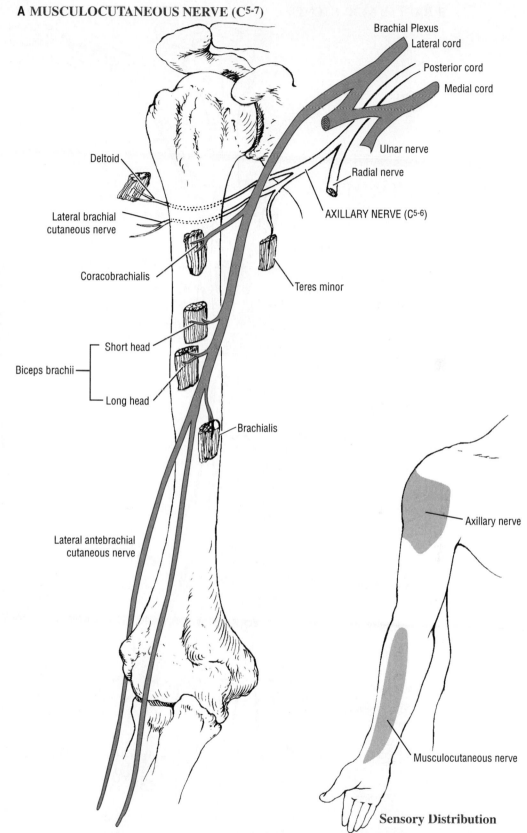

**FIGURE 6–33.** Paths of the peripheral nerves throughout the elbow, wrist, and hand. The following illustrate the path and general proximal-to-distal order of muscle innervation. The location of some muscles is altered slightly for illustration purposes. The primary roots for each nerve are shown in parentheses. (*A* to *D* modified with permission from deGroot J: Correlative Neuroanatomy, 21st ed. Norwalk, Appleton & Lange, 1991. Photograph by Donald A. Neumann.) *A,* The path of the right musculocutaneous nerve is shown as it innervates the coracobrachialis, biceps brachii, and brachialis muscles. The sensory distribution is shown along the lateral forearm. The motor and sensory components of the axillary nerve are also shown.

**Sensory Distribution**

*Illustration continued on following page*

## B RADIAL NERVE (C⁵-T¹)

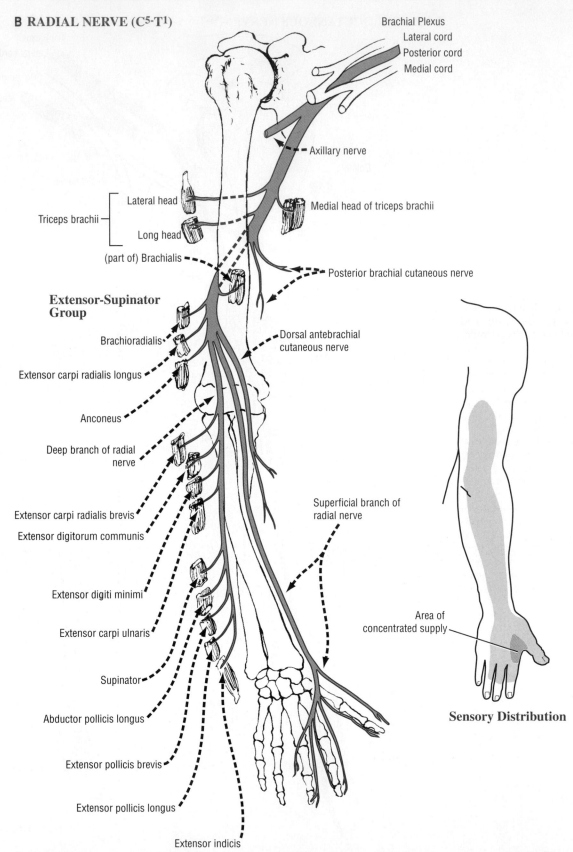

**Brachial Plexus**
Lateral cord
Posterior cord
Medial cord

Axillary nerve

Triceps brachii — { Lateral head

Long head

Medial head of triceps brachii

(part of) Brachialis

Posterior brachial cutaneous nerve

**Extensor-Supinator Group**

Brachioradialis

Dorsal antebrachial cutaneous nerve

Extensor carpi radialis longus

Anconeus

Deep branch of radial nerve

Extensor carpi radialis brevis

Extensor digitorum communis

Superficial branch of radial nerve

Extensor digiti minimi

Extensor carpi ulnaris

Supinator

Abductor pollicis longus

Area of concentrated supply

**Sensory Distribution**

Extensor pollicis brevis

Extensor pollicis longus

Extensor indicis

**FIGURE 6–33** *Continued. B,* The general path of the right radial nerve is shown as it innervates most of the extensors of the arm, forearm, wrist, and digits. See text for more detail on the proximal-to-distal order of muscle innervation. The sensory distribution of the radial nerve is shown with its area of concentrated supply at the dorsal "web space" of the hand.

*Illustration continued on opposite page*

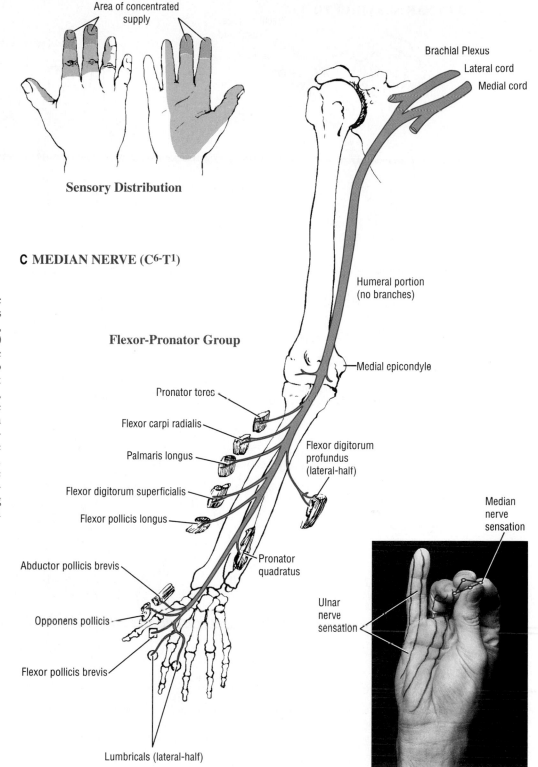

Area of concentrated supply

**Sensory Distribution**

**C MEDIAN NERVE (C⁶-T¹)**

Brachial Plexus
Lateral cord
Medial cord

Humeral portion
(no branches)

Medial epicondyle

**Flexor-Pronator Group**

Pronator teres

Flexor carpi radialis

Palmaris longus

Flexor digitorum profundus
(lateral-half)

Flexor digitorum superficialis

Flexor pollicis longus

Pronator quadratus

Abductor pollicis brevis

Opponens pollicis

Flexor pollicis brevis

Median nerve sensation

Ulnar nerve sensation

Lumbricals (lateral-half)

**FIGURE 6–33** *Continued. C,* The path of the right median nerve is shown supplying the pronators, wrist flexors, long (extrinsic) flexors of the digits (except the flexor digitorum profundus to the ring and little finger), most intrinsic muscles to the thumb, and two lateral lumbricals. The sensory distribution is shown with its area of concentrated supply along the distal end of the index and middle fingers. *Inset,* The median nerve supplies the sensation of the skin that naturally makes contact in a pinching motion between the thumb and fingers.

*Illustration continued on following page*

brachii via the musculocutaneous nerve and the supinator muscle, plus other secondary muscles that arise from the lateral epicondyle and dorsal forearm, via the radial nerve. Table 6–4 summarizes the peripheral nerve and primary nerve root innervation to the muscles of the elbow and forearm. This table was derived from Appendix IIA, which lists the primary motor nerve roots for all the muscles of the upper extremity. Appendix IIB shows key muscles typically used to test the functional status of the C⁵-T¹ ventral nerve roots.

## D ULNAR NERVE (C⁸-T¹)

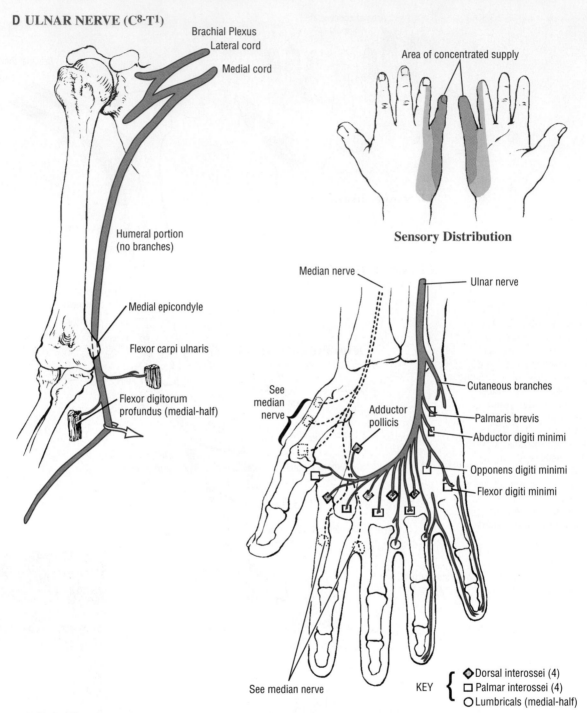

Brachial Plexus
Lateral cord
Medial cord

Humeral portion
(no branches)

Medial epicondyle

Flexor carpi ulnaris

Flexor digitorum
profundus (medial-half)

Area of concentrated supply

**Sensory Distribution**

Median nerve

Ulnar nerve

See
median
nerve

Adductor
pollicis

Cutaneous branches

Palmaris brevis

Abductor digiti minimi

Opponens digiti minimi

Flexor digiti minimi

See median nerve

KEY
◆ Dorsal interossei (4)
□ Palmar interossei (4)
○ Lumbricals (medial-half)

**FIGURE 6–33** *Continued. D,* The path of the right ulnar nerve is shown supplying most of the intrinsic muscles of the hand, including the two medial lumbricals. The sensory distribution is shown with its area of concentrated supply along the entire region of the small finger and ulnar aspect of the hand.

## SENSORY INNERVATION TO JOINTS

### *Humeroulnar Joint and Humeroradial Joint*

The humeroulnar and humeroradial joints and the surrounding connective tissues receive their sensory innervation from the C⁶⁻⁸ nerve roots.[18] These afferent nerve roots are carried

primarily by the musculocutaneous and radial nerves and by the ulnar and median nerves.[51]

### *Proximal and Distal Radioulnar Joints*

The proximal radioulnar joint and surrounding elbow capsule receive sensory innervation from C⁶⁻⁷ nerve roots within

TABLE 6-4. Motor Innervation to the Muscles of the Elbow and Forearm

| Muscle | Innervation |
|--------|-------------|
| **Elbow flexors** | |
| Brachialis | Musculocutaneous nerve ($C^{5,6}$) |
| Biceps brachii | Musculocutaneous nerve ($C^{5,6}$) |
| Brachioradialis | Radial nerve ($C^{5,6}$) |
| Pronator teres | Median nerve ($C^{6,7}$) |
| **Elbow extensors** | |
| Triceps brachii | Radial nerve ($C^{7,8}$) |
| Anconeus | Radial nerve ($C^{7,8}$) |
| **Forearm supinators** | |
| Biceps brachii | Musculocutaneous nerve ($C^{5,6}$) |
| Supinator | Radial nerve ($C^6$) |
| **Forearm pronators** | |
| Pronator quadratus | Median nerve ($C^8$, $T^1$) |
| Pronator teres | Median nerve ($C^{6,7}$) |

The primary nerve root innervation of the muscles are in parentheses.

the median nerve.[51] The distal radioulnar joint receives most of its sensory innervation from the $C^8$ nerve root within the ulnar nerve.[18]

## Function of the Elbow Muscles

Muscles that attach distally on the ulna flex or extend the elbow, with no ability to pronate or supinate the forearm. In contrast, muscles that attach distally on the radius may, in theory, flex or extend the elbow, but also have a potential to pronate or supinate the forearm. This basic concept serves as the underlying theme through much of the remainder of this chapter.

Muscles that act primarily on the wrist also cross the elbow joint. For this reason, many of the wrist muscles have a potential to flex or extend the elbow.[3] This potential is relatively minimal and is not discussed further. The anatomy and nerve supply of the muscles of the elbow and forearm can be found in Appendix IIC.

## ELBOW FLEXORS

The biceps brachii, brachialis, brachioradialis, and pronator teres are primary elbow flexors. Each of these muscles produces a force that passes anterior to the medial-lateral axis of rotation at the elbow. Structural and related biomechanical variables of these muscles are included in Table 6-5.

### Individual Muscle Action of the Elbow Flexors

The *biceps brachii* attaches proximally on the scapula and distally on the bicipital tuberosity on the radius (Fig. 6-34). Secondary distal attachments are made into the deep fascia of the forearm through an aponeurotic sheet known as the *fibrous lacertus*.

The biceps produces its maximal electromyography (EMG) levels when performing both flexion and supination simultaneously,[5] such as bringing a spoon to the mouth. The biceps exhibits relatively low levels of EMG activity when flexion is performed with the forearm deliberately held in pronation. This lack of muscle activation can be verified by self-palpation.

The *brachialis* muscle lies deep to the biceps, originating on the anterior humerus and attaching distally on the extreme proximal ulna (Fig. 6-35). According to Table 6-5, the brachialis has an average physiologic cross-section of 7 cm², the largest of any muscle crossing the elbow. For comparison, the long head of the biceps has a cross-sectional area of only 2.5 cm². Based on its large physiologic cross-section, the brachialis is expected to generate the greatest force of any muscle crossing the elbow.

The *brachioradialis* is the longest of all elbow muscles, attaching proximally on the lateral supracondylar ridge

TABLE 6-5. Structural and Related Biomechanical Variables of the Primary Elbow Flexor Muscles*

| Muscle | Work Capacity Volume (cm³) | Contraction Excursion Length (cm)† | Peak Force Physiologic Cross-sectional Area (cm²) | Leverage Internal Moment Arm (cm)‡ |
|--------|------------------------------|-------------------------------------|-----------------------------------------------------|--------------------------------------|
| Biceps brachii (long head) | 33.4 | 13.6 | 2.5 | 3.20 |
| Biceps brachii (short head) | 30.8 | 15.0 | 2.1 | 3.20 |
| Brachialis | 59.3 | 9.0 | 7.0 | 1.98 |
| Brachioradialis | 21.9 | 16.4 | 1.5 | 5.19 |
| Pronator teres | 18.7 | 5.6 | 3.4 | 2.01 |

* Structural properties are indicated by italics. The related biomechanical variables are indicated above in bold.
† Muscle belly length measured at 70 degrees of flexion.
‡ Internal moment arm measured with elbow flexed to 100 degrees and forearm fully supinated.
(Data from An KN, Hui FC, Morrey BF, et al: Muscles across the elbow joint: A biomechanical analysis. J Biomech 14:659–669, 1981.)

The brachioradialis muscle can be readily palpated on the anterior-lateral aspect of the forearm. Resisted elbow flexion, from a position of about 90 degrees of flexion and neutral forearm rotation, causes the muscle to stand out or "bowstring" sharply across the elbow (Fig. 6–36). The bowstringing of this muscle increases its flexion moment arm to a length that exceeds all other flexors (see Table 6–5).

### Biomechanics of the Elbow Flexors

#### Maximal Torque Production of the Elbow Flexor Muscles

Figure 6–37 shows the line-of-force of three primary elbow flexors. The strength of the flexion torque varies considerably based on age,[14] gender, "weightlifting" experience,[49] speed of muscle contraction, and position of the joints across the upper extremity.[52] According to a study reported by Gallagher and colleagues,[14] the dominant side produced

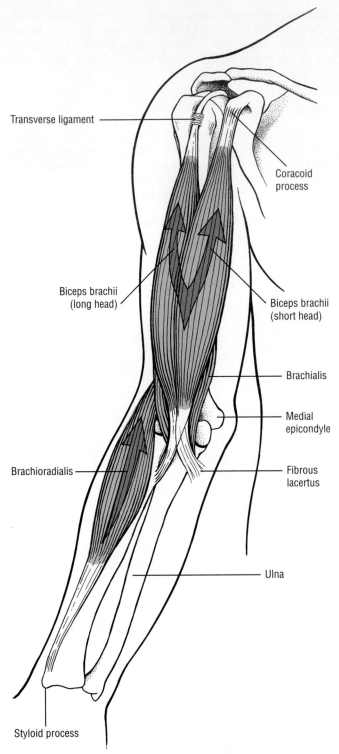

**FIGURE 6–34.** Anterior view of the right biceps brachii and brachioradialis muscles. The brachialis is deep to the biceps.

of the humerus and distally near the styloid process of the radius (see Fig. 6–34). Maximal shortening of the brachioradialis causes full elbow flexion and rotation of the forearm to the near neutral position. EMG studies suggest that the brachioradialis is a primary elbow flexor, especially during rapid movements against a high resistance.[5,10,12]

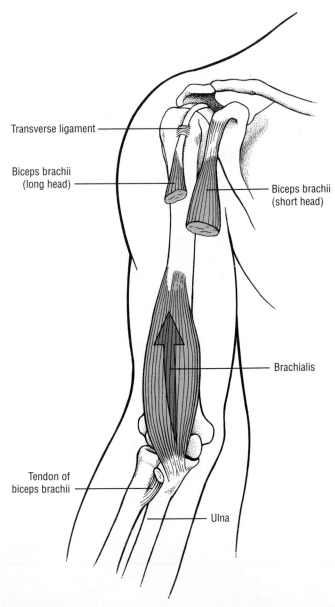

**FIGURE 6–35.** Anterior view of the right brachialis shown deep to the biceps muscle.

**Brachialis: The "Work-horse" of the Elbow Flexors**

In addition to a large cross-sectional area, the brachialis muscle also has the largest volume of all elbow flexors (see Table 6–5). Muscle volume can be measured by recording the volume of water displaced by the muscle.[3] Large muscle volume suggests that the muscle has a large *work capacity*. For this reason, the brachialis has been called the "work-horse" of the elbow flexors.[5] This name is due in part to its large work capacity, but also to its active involvement in all types of elbow flexion activities, whether performed fast or slow, or combined with pronation or supination. Since the brachialis attaches distally to the ulna, the motion of pronation or supination has no influence on its length, line-of-force, or internal moment arm.

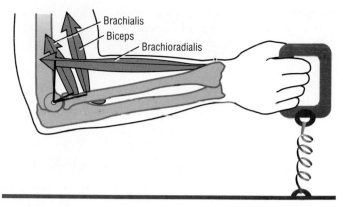

**FIGURE 6–37.** A lateral view showing the line-of-force of three primary elbow flexors. The internal moment arm (shown as dark lines) for each muscle is drawn to approximate scale. Note that the elbow has been flexed about 100 degrees, placing the biceps tendon at 90 degrees of insertion with the radius. See text for further details. The elbow's medial-lateral axis of rotation is shown piercing the capitulum.

significantly higher levels of flexion torque, work, and power. No significant differences were found across sides, however, for elbow extension and forearm pronation and supination.

Maximal effort flexion torques of 725 kg-cm for men and 336 kg-cm for women have been reported for healthy middle-aged persons. (Table 6–6).[4] As noted in Table 6–6, flexion torques are about 70% greater than elbow extensor torques. Furthermore, elbow flexor torques produced with the forearm supinated are about 20 to 25% greater than those produced with the forearm fully pronated.[40] This difference is due to the increased flexor moment arm of the biceps[32] and the brachioradialis muscles when the forearm is in or near full supination.

Biomechanical and physiologic data can be used to predict the maximal flexion torque produced by the major elbow flexor muscles across a full range of motion (Fig.

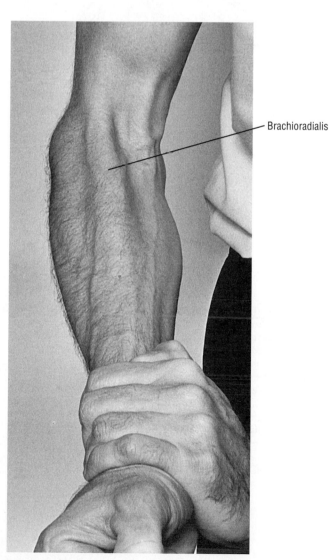

**FIGURE 6–36.** The right brachioradialis muscle is shown "bowstringing" over the elbow during a maximal effort isometric activation.

| TABLE 6–6. Average Maximal Isometric Internal Torques* | | |
|---|---|---|
| **Movement** | **Torque (kg-cm)** | **Torque (kg-cm)** |
| | *Males* | *Females* |
| Flexion | 725 (154) | 336 (80) |
| Extension | 421 (109) | 210 (61) |
| Pronation | 73 (18) | 36 (8) |
| Supination | 91 (23) | 44 (12) |

*These are reported for the major movements of the elbow and forearm. Standard deviations are in parentheses. Data are from 104 healthy subjects; $\overline{X}$ age male = 41 yrs, $\overline{X}$ age female = 45.1 yrs. The elbow is maintained in 90 degrees of flexion with neutral forearm rotation. Data are shown for dominant limb only.

Conversions: .098 N-m/kg-cm.

(Data from Askew LJ, An KN, Morrey BF, et al: Isometric elbow strength in normal individuals. Clin Orthop 222:261–266, 1987.)

6–38*A*). The predicted maximal torque for all muscles occurs at about 90 degrees of flexion, which agrees in general with actual torque measurements made on healthy persons.[40,49]

The two primary factors responsible for the overall shape of the maximal torque-angle curve of the elbow flexors are (1) the muscle's maximal flexion *force* potential and (2) the internal *moment arm* length. The data plotted in Figure 6–38*B* predict that the maximal force of all muscles occurs at a muscle length that corresponds with about 80 degrees of flexion. The data plotted in Figure 6–38*C* predict that the average maximal internal moment arm of all muscles occurs at about 100 degrees of flexion. At this joint angle, insertion of the biceps tendon to the radius is about

90 degrees (see Fig. 6–37). This mechanical condition maximizes the internal moment arm of a muscle and thereby maximizes the conversion of a muscle force to a joint torque. It is interesting that the data presented in Figures 6–38*B* and *C* predict peak torques across generally similar joint angles.

### Polyarticular Biceps Brachii: A Physiologic Advantage of Combining Elbow Flexion with Shoulder Extension

The biceps is a polyarticular muscle that can produce forces across multiple joints. As subsequently described, combining active elbow flexion with shoulder extension is a natural and effective way for producing biceps-generated elbow flexor torque.

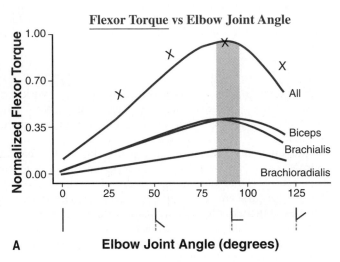

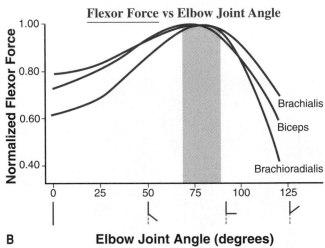

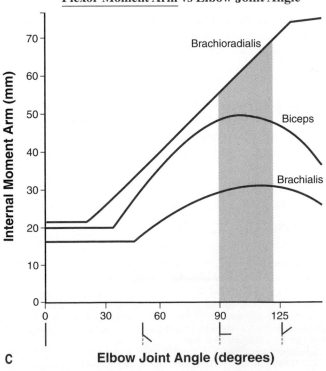

**FIGURE 6–38.** *A*, Predicted maximal isometric torque-angle curves for three primary elbow flexors based on a theoretical model that incorporates each muscle's architecture, length-tension relationship, and internal moment arm. *B*, The length-tension relationships of the three muscles are shown as a normalized flexor force plotted against elbow joint angle. Note that muscle length decreases as joint angle increases. *C*, The length of each muscle's internal moment arm is plotted against the elbow joint angle. The joint angle of each maximal predicted variable is highlighted in red. (Data for *A* and *B* from An KN, Kaufman KR, Chao EYS: Physiological considerations of muscle force through the elbow joint. J Biomechanics 22: 1249–1256, 1989. Data for *C* from Amis AA, Dowson D, Wright V: Muscle strengths and musculoskeletal geometry of the upper limb. Engng Med 8:41–48, 1979.)

For the sake of discussion, assume that at rest in the anatomic position the biceps is about 30 cm long (Fig. 6–39A). The biceps shortens to about 23 cm after an active motion that combines 45 degrees of shoulder flexion and 90 degrees of elbow flexion (Fig. 6–39B). If the motion took 1 second to perform, the muscle experiences an average contraction velocity of 7cm/sec. In contrast, consider a more natural but effective method of biceps activation that combines *elbow flexion* with *shoulder extension* (Fig. 6–39C). During an activity such as pulling a heavy load up toward the side, for example, the biceps produces elbow flexion while, at the same time, is elongated across the extending shoulder. In effect, the contraction of the posterior deltoid reduces the net shortening of the biceps. Based on the example in Figure 6–39C, combining elbow flexion with shoulder extension reduces the average contraction velocity of the biceps to 5cm/sec. This is 2cm/sec slower than combining elbow flexion with shoulder flexion. As described in Chapter 3, the maximal force output of a muscle is greater when its contraction velocity is closer to zero, or isometric.

The simple model described here illustrates one of many examples in which a one-joint muscle, such as the posterior deltoid, can enhance the force potential of another muscle. In the example, the posterior deltoid serves as a powerful shoulder extensor for a vigorous pulling motion. In addition, the posterior deltoid assists in controlling the optimal contraction velocity and operational length of the biceps throughout the elbow flexion motion. The posterior deltoid, especially during high power activities, is a very important synergist to the elbow flexors. Consider the consequences of performing the lift described in Figure 6–39C with total paralysis of the posterior deltoid.

## ELBOW EXTENSORS

### *Muscular Components*

The primary elbow extensors are the *triceps brachii* and the *anconeus*. These muscles converge to a common tendon attaching to the olecranon process of the ulna (Figs. 6–41 and 6–42).

The triceps brachii has three heads: long, lateral, and medial. The *long head* has its proximal attachment on the infraglenoid tubercle of the scapula, thereby allowing the muscle to extend and adduct the shoulder. The long head has an extensive volume, exceeding all other muscles of the elbow (Table 6–7).

The *lateral and medial heads* of the triceps muscle have their proximal attachments on the humerus, on either side and along the radial groove. The medial head has an extensive proximal attachment on the posterior side of the humerus, occupying a location relatively similar to that of the brachialis on the bone's anterior side.

The *anconeus* muscle is a small triangular muscle spanning the posterior side of the elbow. The muscle is located between the lateral epicondyle of the humerus and a strip along the posterior aspect of the proximal ulna (see Fig. 6–41). The anconeus appears as a fourth head of the extensor mechanism, similar to the quadriceps at the knee.

The triceps brachii produces the majority of the total extensor torque at the elbow. Compared with the triceps muscle, the anconeus has a relatively small cross-sectional area and a small moment arm for extension (see Table 6–7).

### *Electromyographic Analysis of Elbow Extension*

Maximal effort elbow extension generates maximum levels of EMG from all components of the elbow extensor group. During submaximal efforts of elbow extension, however, different muscles are recruited only at certain levels of effort.[48] The anconeus is usually the first muscle to initiate and maintain low levels of elbow extension force.[21] As extensor effort gradually increases, the medial head of the triceps is usually next in line to join the anconeus.[48] The medial head remains active for most elbow extension movements.[12] The medial head has been termed "the workhorse" of the extensors, functioning as the extensor counterpart to the brachialis.[48]

Only after extensor demands at the elbow increase to moderate-to-high levels does the nervous system recruit the lateral head of the triceps, followed closely by the long head.

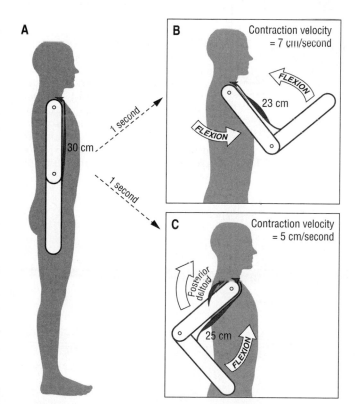

**FIGURE 6–39.** *A,* This model is showing a person standing in the anatomic position with a 30-cm long biceps muscle. *B,* After a 1-sec contraction, the biceps has contracted to a length of 23 cm, causing a simultaneous motion of 90 degrees of *elbow flexion* and 45 degrees of *shoulder flexion.* The biceps has shortened at a contraction velocity of 7 cm/sec. *C,* The biceps *and* posterior deltoid are shown active in a typical pulling motion. The contraction lasts 1 sec and causes a simultaneous motion of 90 degrees of elbow *flexion* and 45 degrees of shoulder *extension.* Because of the contraction of the posterior deltoid, the biceps shortened only 5 cm, at a contraction velocity of only 5 cm/sec.

### "Reverse Action" of the Elbow Flexor Muscles: A Clinical Example

Contraction of the elbow flexor muscles is typically performed to rotate the forearm to the arm. Contraction of the same muscles, however, can rotate the arm to the forearm, provided that the distal aspect of the upper extremity is well fixed. A clinical example of the usefulness of such a "reverse contraction" of the elbow flexors is shown for a person with C⁶ quadriplegia (Fig. 6–40). The person has complete paralysis of the trunk and lower extremity muscles, but near normal strength of the shoulder, elbow flexor, and wrist extensor muscles. With the distal aspect of the upper limb well fixed by action of the wrist extensor muscles, the elbow flexor muscles can generate sufficient force to rotate the arm toward the forearm. This maneuver allows the elbow flexor muscles to assist the person while moving up to a sitting position. Interestingly, the arthrokinematics at the humeroulnar joint during this action involve a roll and slide in *opposite* directions.

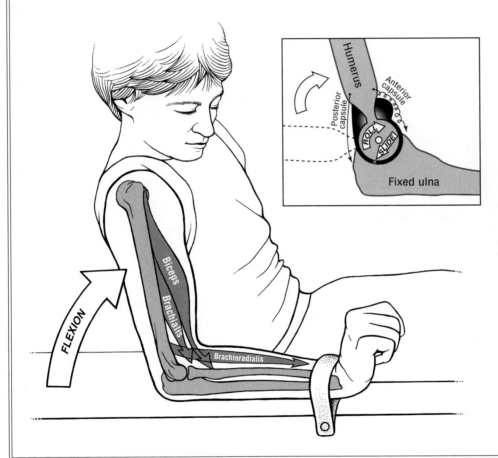

**FIGURE  6–40.** A person with mid-level (cervical) quadriplegia using his muscles to flex the elbow and bring his trunk off the mat. Note that the distal forearm is held fixed by the action of the wrist extensors. *Inset,* The arthrokinematics at the humeroulnar joint are shown during this movement. The anterior capsule is in a slackened position, and the posterior capsule is taut.

The long head functions as a "reserve" elbow extensor, equipped with a large volume suited for tasks that require high work performance.

### Torque Demands on the Elbow Extensors

The elbow extensor muscles provide static stability to the elbow, similar to the way the quadriceps are often used to stabilize the knee. Consider the common posture of bearing weight through the upper limb with elbows held partially flexed. The extensors stabilize the flexed elbow through isometric contraction or very low-velocity eccentric activation. In contrast, these same muscles are required to generate very large and dynamic extensor torques through high-velocity concentric or eccentric activations. Consider activities such as throwing a ball, pushing up from a low chair or rapidly pushing open a door. As with many explosive pushing activities, elbow extension is typically combined with some degree of shoulder flexion (Fig. 6–43). The shoulder flexion function of the anterior deltoid is an important synergistic component of the forward push. The an-

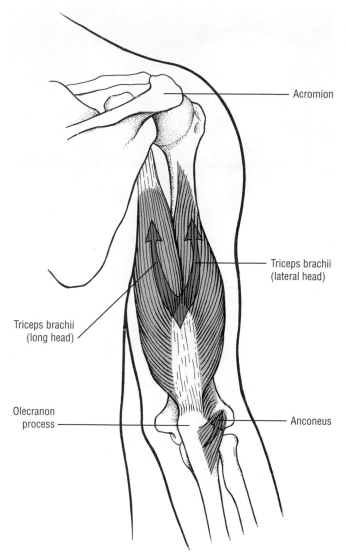

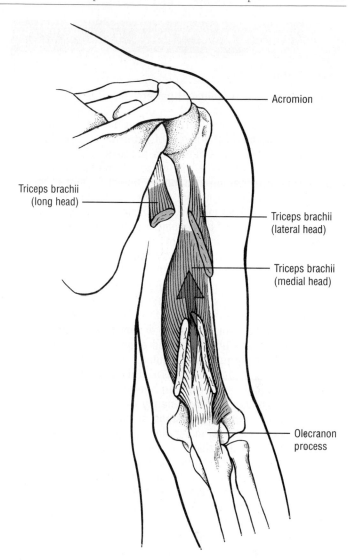

**FIGURE 6–41.** A posterior view of the right triceps brachii and anconeus muscles. The medial head of the triceps is deep to the long and lateral heads and therefore not visible.

**FIGURE 6–42.** A posterior view shows the right medial head of the triceps brachii. The long head and lateral head of the triceps are partially removed to expose the deeper medial head.

**TABLE 6–7. Structural and Related Biomechanical Variables of the Primary Elbow Extensor Muscles***

| | Work Capacity | Contraction Excursion | Peak Force | Leverage |
|---|---|---|---|---|
| *Muscle* | *Volume (cm³)* | *Length (cm)†* | *Physiologic Cross-sectional Area (cm²)* | *Internal Moment Arm (cm)‡* |
| Triceps brachii (long head) | 66.6 | 10.2 | 6.7 | 1.87 |
| Triceps brachii (medial head) | 38.7 | 6.3 | 6.1 | 1.87 |
| Triceps brachii (lateral head) | 47.3 | 8.4 | 6.0 | 1.87 |
| Anconeus | 6.7 | 2.7 | 2.5 | .72 |

* Structural properties are indicated by italics. The related biomechanical variables are indicated above in bold.
† Muscle belly length measured at 70 degrees of flexion.
‡ Internal moment arm measured with elbow flexed to 100 degrees.
(Data from An KN, Hui FC, Morrey BF, et al: Muscles across the elbow joint: A biomechanical analysis. J Biomechan 14:659–669, 1981.)

**Law of Parsimony**

The hierarchical recruitment pattern described by the actions of the various members of the elbow extensors is certainly not the only strategy used by the nervous system to modulate the levels of extensor torque. As with most active movements, the process of muscle activation varies greatly from muscle to muscle and from person to person. It appears, however, that a general hierarchical recruitment pattern exists for the elbow extensors. This method of muscle group activation illustrates the *law of parsimony,* a principle eluded to in other works.[24,35] In the present context, the law of parsimony states that the nervous system tends to activate the fewest muscles or muscle fibers possible for the control of a given joint action. Recall that it is the responsibility of the small anconeus and medial head of the triceps to control activities that require lower level extensor torque. Not until more dynamic or highly resisted extensor torque is needed does the nervous system select the larger, polyarticular, long head of the triceps. This hierarchical pattern of muscle recruitment makes practical sense from an energy perspective. Consider, for example, the inefficiency of having only the long head of the triceps, instead of the anconeus, performing very low level maintenance types of stabilization functions at the elbow. Additional muscular forces would be required from shoulder flexors, assuming gravitation forces are inadequate, to neutralize the undesired shoulder extension potential of the long head of the triceps. A simple task would require greater muscle activity than what is absolutely necessary. As EMG evidence and general intuition suggests, tasks with low level force demands are often accomplished by one-joint muscles. As force demands increase, larger polyarticular muscles are recruited, along with the necessary neutralizer muscles.

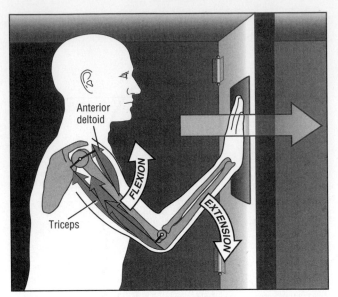

**FIGURE 6–43.** The triceps is shown generating an extensor torque across the elbow to rapidly push open a door. Note that the elbow is extending as the anterior deltoid is flexing the shoulder. The anterior deltoid must oppose and exceed the shoulder extensor torque produced by the long head of the triceps. See text for further description. The internal moment arms are shown as bold lines originating at the joints' axis of rotation.

the triceps (Fig. 6–44). The fact that peak elbow extensor torque occurs near 90 degrees of flexion, instead of near extension, suggests that muscle length, not leverage, is very influential in determining the point in the range of motion where elbow extension torque naturally occurs.

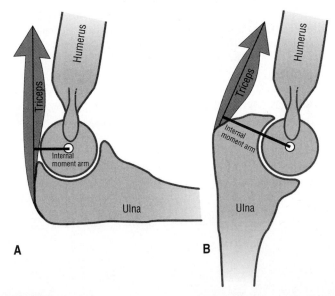

**FIGURE 6–44.** The internal moment arm of the triceps is shown with the elbow flexed to 90 degrees (*A*) and fully extended to near 0 degrees (*B*). The moment arm is increased in extension since the olecranon process extends the distance between the axis of rotation and the perpendicular intersection with the line-of-force of the triceps.

terior deltoid produces a shoulder flexion torque that drives the limb forward and neutralizes the shoulder extension tendency of the long head of the triceps. From a physiologic perspective, combining shoulder flexion with elbow extension minimizes the rate and amount of shortening required by the long head of the triceps to completely extend the elbow.

*Biomechanical Factors Influencing the Magnitude of Elbow Extensor Torque*

Similar to the elbow flexors, the elbow extensors produce maximal level torque when the elbow is flexed to about 90 degrees.[9,40] Unlike the elbow flexors, the peak torque of the extensors does *not* occur when the muscle has its greatest extensor moment arm. In contrast, the internal moment arm of the elbow extensor is greatest near full extension.[3] This position places the thick olecranon process between the joint's axis of rotation and the line-of-force of the tendon of

**SPECIAL FOCUS 6–7**

### Using Shoulder Muscles to Substitute for Triceps Paralysis

Fractures of the cervical spine may result in $C^6$ quadriplegia, with loss of motor and sensory function below the $C^6$ nerve root level. Symptoms include total paralysis of the trunk and lower extremity muscles with partial paralysis of the upper extremity muscles. Because of the sparing of certain muscles innervated by $C^6$ and above, persons with this level of quadriplegia may still be able to perform many independent functional activities. Examples are moving up to the sitting position, dressing, and transferring between a wheelchair and bed. Therapists and physicians who specialize in mobility training for persons with quadriplegia develop movement strategies that allow an innervated muscle to substitute for part of the functional loss imposed by a paralyzed muscle.[34] This art of "muscle substitution" is an essential component to maximizing the movement efficiency in a person with paralysis.

Persons with $C^6$ quadriplegia have marked or total paralysis of elbow extensors, since these muscles receive most of the nerve root innervation below $C^6$. Loss of elbow extension reduces the ability to reach away from the body. Activities such as moving up to sit or transferring from a wheelchair become very difficult and labor intensive. A valuable method of muscle substitution uses innervated proximal shoulder muscles, such as the clavicular head of the pectoralis major and/or the anterior deltoid to actively extend and lock the elbow (Fig. 6–45).[16] This ability of a proximal muscle to extend the elbow requires that the hand is firmly fixed to some object. Under these circumstances, contraction of the shoulder musculature adducts, and/or horizontally flexes, the glenohumeral joint, pulling the humerus toward the midline. Controlling the stability of the elbow

by using more proximal musculature is a very useful clinical concept. This concept also applies to the lower limb, since the hip extensors are able to extend the knee even in the absence of the quadriceps muscle, as long as the foot is fixed to the ground.

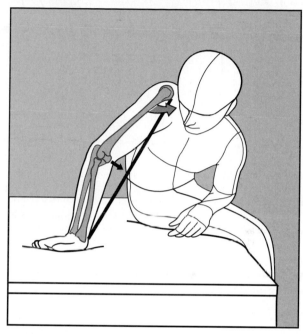

**FIGURE 6–45.** A depiction of a person with $C^6$ quadriplegia using the innervated clavicular portion of the pectoralis major and anterior deltoid (red arrow) to pull the humerus toward the midline. With the wrist fixed to the bed, the muscles rotate the elbow into extension. Once locked into extension, the stable elbow allows the entire limb to accept weight without buckling at its middle link. The model in the illustration is assumed to have total paralysis of the triceps.

---

## Function of the Supinator and Pronator Muscles

The lines-of-force of most pronator and supinator muscles of the forearm are shown in Figure 6–46. In order to pronate or supinate, a muscle must possess two biomechanical features. *First,* the muscle must have one attachment on the humerus and ulna, and the other on the radius and hand. (See the supinator muscle in Fig. 6–46A or the pronator teres in Fig. 6–46B.) Muscles such as the brachialis or extensor pollicis brevis, therefore, cannot pronate or supinate the forearm. *Second,* the muscle must have a line-of-force that intersects the axis of rotation for pronation and supination. As a general rule, the closer the line-of-force of a muscle is to a perpendicular intersection with the axis of rotation, the more likely the muscle is a significant torque generator. (See the pronator quadratus in Fig. 6–46B, for example.) A muscle with a line-of-force that

runs parallel to the axis of rotation has a 0 degree angle of intersection and, therefore, has no moment arm to pronate or supinate.

### SUPINATOR MUSCLES

The primary supinator muscles are the *supinator* and *biceps brachii.* Secondary muscles with a limited potential to supinate are the radial wrist extensors, which attach near the lateral epicondyle, the extensor pollicis longus, and the extensor indicis (see Fig. 6–46A). The brachioradialis may also be considered as a secondary supinator and pronator, but its potential is slight.[5,10,12] Contraction of the brachioradialis can help to supinate to the neutral position from a fully pronated position, and pronate to the neutral position from a fully supinated position.[32] An EMG study shows limited activity only during short-arc, high-power pronation and supination.[5]

**Supinators**

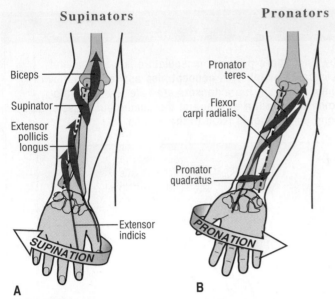

**Pronators**

Biceps

Supinator

Extensor
pollicis
longus

SUPINATION

Extensor
indicis

Pronator
teres

Flexor
carpi radialis

Pronator
quadratus

PRONATION

**A**

**B**

**FIGURE 6–46.** The line-of-force of the supinators (*A*) and the pronators (*B*) of the forearm during an active motion. Note the degree to which all muscles intersect the forearm's axis of rotation (shown as dashed line). For clarity, not all the secondary supinators and pronators are depicted.

---

**Primary Supinator Muscles**

• Supinator
• Biceps brachii

**Secondary Supinator Muscles**

• Radial wrist extensors
• Extensor pollicis longus
• Extensor indicis
• Brachioradialis

---

### Supinator versus Biceps Brachii

The *supinator muscle* has a complex proximal muscle attachment (Fig. 6–47). A superficial set of fibers arises from the lateral epicondyle of the humerus and the radial collateral and annular ligaments. A deeper set of fibers arises from the ulna near and along the supinator crest. Both sets of muscle fibers attach along the proximal one third of the radius. From a pronated view (Fig. 6–47), the supinator is elongated and in excellent position to rotate the radius into supination. The supinator has only minimal attachments to the humerus and passes too close to the medial-lateral axis of rotation at the elbow to produce significant torque.

The supinator muscle is a relentless forearm supinator, similar to the brachialis during elbow flexion. The supinator muscle generates significant EMG activity during forearm supination, regardless of the elbow angle or the speed or power of the action.[47] The biceps muscle, also a primary supinator, is normally recruited during higher power supination activities, especially those associated with elbow flexion.

The nervous system usually recruits the supinator muscle for low-power tasks that require a supination motion only, while the biceps remains relatively inactive. (This is in accord with the law of parsimony described earlier in this chapter.) Only during moderate or high-power supination

motions does the biceps show significant EMG activity (Fig. 6–48). Using the large polyarticular biceps to perform a simple, low-power supination task is not an efficient motor response. Additional muscles, such as the triceps and posterior deltoid, are required to neutralize any undesired biceps action at the shoulder and elbow. A simple movement then becomes increasingly more complicated and more energy consuming than absolutely necessary.

The *biceps brachii* is a powerful supinator muscle of the forearm. The biceps has about three times the physiologic cross-section area as the supinator muscle.[22] The dominant role of the biceps as a supinator can be verified by palpating the biceps during a series of rapid and forceful pronation-to-supination motions, especially with the elbow flexed to 90 degrees. As the forearm is pronated, the biceps tendon wraps around the proximal radius. From a fully pronated position, active contraction of the biceps can "spin" the radius sharply into supination.

The effectiveness of the biceps as a supinator is greatest when the elbow is flexed to about 90 degrees. Supination torque performed with the elbow flexed to 90 degrees may produce twice the torque than with the elbow held near full extension. At a 90-degree elbow angle, the tendon of the biceps approaches a 90-degree angle-of-insertion into the radius (Fig. 6–49, *top*). This biomechanical situation allows the entire magnitude of a maximal effort biceps force, shown

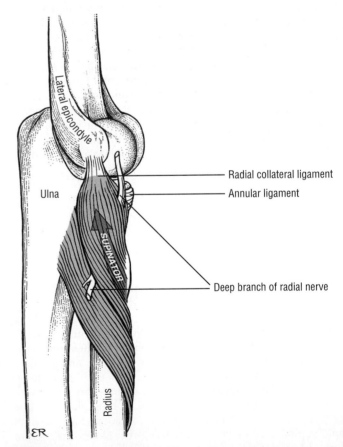

Lateral epicondyle

Ulna

Radial collateral ligament

Annular ligament

SUPINATOR

Deep branch of radial nerve

Radius

**FIGURE 6–47.** A lateral view of the right supinator muscle. The deep branch of the radial nerve is shown exiting between the superficial and deep fibers of the muscle. The radial nerve is coursing distally, as the dorsal interosseous nerve, to innervate the finger and thumb extensors.

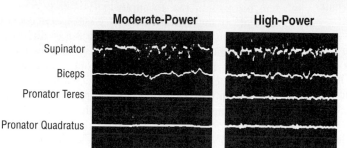

**Active Supination**

**Low-Power**

Supinator

Biceps

Pronator Teres

Pronator Quadratus

**Moderate-Power**          **High-Power**

Supinator

Biceps

Pronator Teres

Pronator Quadratus

**FIGURE 6–48.** The EMG signal from four muscles during three levels of active supination. The minimal EMG activity shown by the pronator muscles during high-power supination may reflect low level eccentric activity from these muscles. (Modified from Basmajian JV: Muscles Alive. Their Functions Revealed by Electromyography, 4th ed. Baltimore, Williams & Wilkins, 1978.)

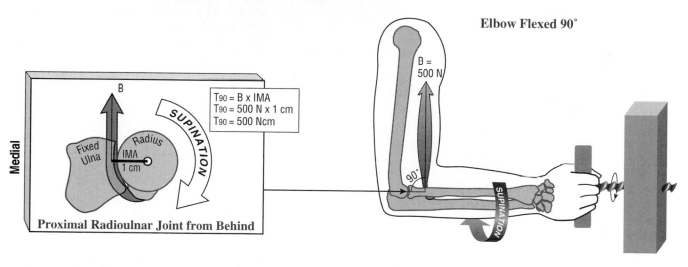

**Elbow Flexed 90°**

B = 500 N

Medial

B

SUPINATION

Fixed Ulna    Radius

IMA 1 cm

$T_{90} = B \times IMA$
$T_{90} = 500 \text{ N} \times 1 \text{ cm}$
$T_{90} = 500 \text{ Ncm}$

**Proximal Radioulnar Joint from Behind**

90°

SUPINATION

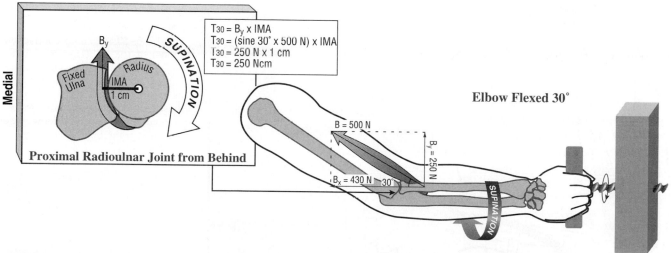

Medial

$B_y$

SUPINATION

Fixed Ulna    Radius

IMA 1 cm

$T_{30} = B_y \times IMA$
$T_{30} = (\text{sine } 30° \times 500 \text{ N}) \times IMA$
$T_{30} = 250 \text{ N} \times 1 \text{ cm}$
$T_{30} = 250 \text{ Ncm}$

**Proximal Radioulnar Joint from Behind**

**Elbow Flexed 30°**

B = 500 N

$B_y$ = 250 N

$B_x$ = 430 N    30°

SUPINATION

**FIGURE 6–49.** The difference in the ability of the biceps to produce a supination torque is illustrated when the elbow is flexed 90 degrees, and the elbow is flexed 30 degrees. *Top,* lateral view shows the biceps attaching to the radius at a 90-degree angle. The muscle (B) is contracting to supinate the forearm with a maximal effort force of 500 N. The calculations show that the maximum supination torque at a 90-degree elbow angle ($T_{90}$) is 500 Ncm (the product of the maximal force (B) times the 1-cm internal moment arm (IMA)). *Bottom,* the angle of the insertion of the biceps to the radius is 30 degrees. The biceps force of 500 N (B) must be trigonometrically resolved into that which supinates ($B_y$) and that which runs parallel to the radius ($B_x$). The calculations show that the maximum supination torque with the elbow flexed 30 degrees is reduced to 250 Ncm (sine 30 degrees = .5, and cosine 30 degrees = .86).

## SPECIAL FOCUS 6 – 8

### Supination vs. Pronation Torque Potential

As a group, the supinators produce about 25% greater isometric torque than the pronators (see Table 6–6). This difference may be partially explained by the fact that the supinator muscles possess about twice the physiologic cross-sectional area than the pronator muscles.[22] Many functional activities rely on the greater strength of supination. Consider the activity of using a screwdriver to tighten a screw. When performed by the right hand, a clockwise tightening motion is driven by a concentric contraction of the supinator muscles. The direction of the threads on a standard screw reflects the dominance in strength of the supinator muscles. Unfortunately for the left-hand dominant, a clockwise rotation of the left forearm must be performed by the pronators. A left-handed person often uses the right hand for this activity, explaining why so many are somewhat ambidextrous.

as 500 N in Figure 6–49, *top,* to be generated at near right angles to the axis of rotation of the forearm. Subsequently, all of the biceps force is multiplied by the estimated 1-cm internal moment arm available for supination, producing 500 Ncm of torque. As a contrast, consider the reduced effectiveness of the biceps as a supinator when the elbow is flexed to 30 degrees (Fig. 6–49, *bottom*). This elbow angle changes the angle that the biceps tendon inserts onto the radius to about 30 degrees. This insertion angle reduces the force that the biceps can use to supinate (i.e., that generated perpendicular to the radius) to 250 N ($B_y$). An even larger force component of the biceps, labeled $B_x$, is directed proximally through the radius in a direction parallel with the forearm's axis of rotation. This force component has no moment arm to supinate. As shown by the calculations in Figure 6–49, *bottom,* the effective supination torque from a maximal effort muscle contraction yields 250 Ncm.

The aforementioned sample problem shows that with an equivalent maximal effort muscle force, the supination torque is reduced by 50% owing to the change in elbow angle. Clinically, this difference is important when evaluating the torque output from a strength-testing apparatus, or when providing advice about ergonomics.

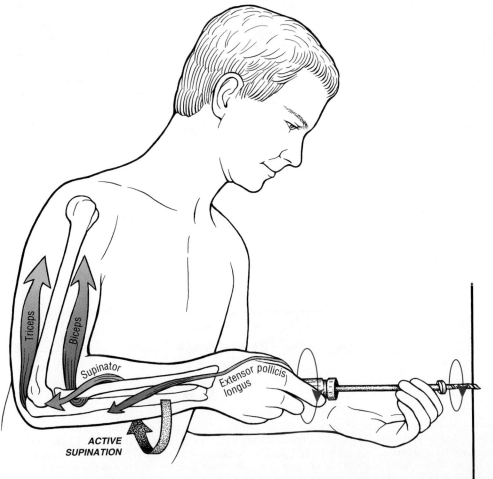

**FIGURE 6–50.** Vigorous contraction is shown of the right biceps, supinator, and extensor pollicis longus muscles to tighten a screw using a clockwise rotation with a screwdriver. The triceps muscle is activated isometrically to neutralize the strong elbow flexion tendency of the biceps.

## PRONATOR MUSCLES

The primary muscles for pronation are the *pronator quadratus* and the *pronator teres* (Fig. 6–51). The flexor carpi radialis and the palmaris longus are secondary pronators, both attaching to the medial epicondyle of the humerus (see Fig. 6–46*B*).

---

**Primary Pronator Muscles**
- Pronator teres
- Pronator quadratus

**Secondary Pronator Muscles**
- Flexor carpi radialis
- Palmaris longus

---

### Pronator Quadratus vs. Pronator Teres

The *pronator quadratus* is located at the extreme distal end of the anterior forearm, deep to all the wrist flexors and extrinsic finger flexors. This flat, quadrilateral muscle attaches between the anterior surfaces of the distal one quarter of the ulna and the radius. Overall, from proximal to distal, the pronator quadratus has a slight obliquity in fiber direction, similar to, but not quite as angled as, the pronator teres.

The pronator quadratus is the most active and consistently used pronator muscle, involved during all pronation movements, regardless of the power demands or the amount of associated elbow flexion.[6]

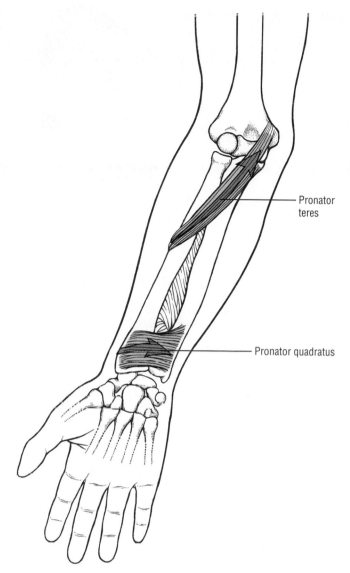

**FIGURE 6–51.** Anterior view of the right pronator teres and pronator quadratus.

When high-power supination torques are needed to vigorously turn a screw, the biceps is used to assist other muscles, such as the supinator muscle and extensor pollicis longus (Fig. 6–50). The elbow is usually held flexed to about 90 degrees in order to augment the supination torque potential of the biceps. The maintenance of this elbow posture during the task requires that the triceps muscle co-contract synchronously with the biceps muscle. The triceps supply an essential force during this activity since it prevents the biceps from actually flexing the elbow and shoulder during every supination effort. Unopposed biceps action causes the screwdriver to be pulled away from the screw on every effort—hardly effective. By attaching to the ulna versus the radius, the triceps is able to neutralize the elbow flexion tendency of the biceps *without* interfering with the supination task. This muscular cooperation is an excellent example of how two muscles can function as synergists for one activity, while at the same time remain as direct antagonists.

## SPECIAL FOCUS 6 – 9

### A Return to the Law of Parsimony

Low-power activities that involve isolated pronation are generally initiated and controlled by the pronator quadratus. Throughout this chapter, a theme has developed between the function of a usually smaller one-joint muscle and an associated larger polyarticular muscle. In all cases, the hierarchical recruitment of the muscles followed the law of parsimony. At the elbow, low-power flexion or extension activities tend to be controlled or initiated by the brachialis, the anconeus, or the medial head of the triceps. Only when relatively high-power actions are required does the nervous system recruit the larger polyarticular biceps and long head of the triceps. At the forearm, low-power supination and pronation activities are controlled by the small supinator or the pronator quadratus; high-power actions require assistance from the biceps and pronator teres. Each time the polyarticular muscles are recruited, however, additional muscles are needed to stabilize their undesired actions. Increasing the power of any action at the elbow and forearm creates a sharp disproportionate rise in overall muscle activity. Not only do the one-joint muscles increase their activity, but so do the polyarticular "reserve" muscles and a host of other neutralizer muscles.

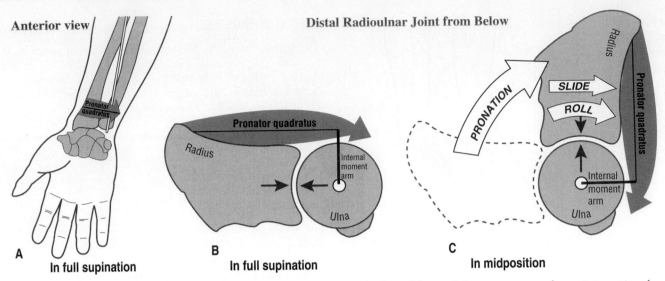

**Anterior view**

**Distal Radioulnar Joint from Below**

A **In full supination**

B **In full supination**

C **In midposition**

**FIGURE 6–52.** *A,* Anterior view of the distal radioulnar joint shows the line-of-force of the pronator quadratus intersecting the forearm's axis of rotation (white rod) at a right angle. *B,* The line-of-force of the pronator quadratus, with its internal moment arm, is shown with the wrist removed and forearm in full supination. The pronator quadratus produces a pronation torque, which is the product of pronator muscle's force times the internal moment arm, *and* a compression force between the joint surfaces (opposing arrows). *C,* This dual function of the pronator quadratus is shown as the muscle pronates the forearm to the midposition. The roll-and-slide arthrokinematics are also indicated.

The *pronator teres* has two heads: humeral and ulnar. The median nerve passes between these two heads. The pronator teres functions as a primary forearm pronator, in addition to a secondary elbow flexor. This pronator teres produces its greatest EMG activity during higher power pronation actions,[6] such as attempting to unscrew an overtightened screw with the right hand or pitching a baseball. The triceps is an important synergist to the pronator teres, often required to neutralize the tendency of the pronator teres to flex the elbow.

In cases of median nerve injury proximal to the elbow, all pronator muscles are paralyzed, and active pronation is essentially lost. The forearm tends to remain chronically supinated owing to the unopposed action of the innervated supinator and biceps muscles.

### *Pronator Quadratus: Dual Role as Torque Producer and Stabilizer of Distal Radioulnar Joint*

The pronator quadratus is well designed biomechanically as an effective torque producer and a stabilizer at the distal radioulnar joint.[46] The pronator quadratus has a line-of-force oriented almost perpendicular to the forearm's axis of rotation (Fig. 6–52A). This design maximizes the potential of the muscle to produce a torque. The force produced by the pronator quadratus causes a pronation torque. At the same time, it compresses the ulnar notch of the radius directly against the ulna head (Fig. 6–52B). This compression force provides an important element of stabilization to the distal radioulnar joint, which continues throughout pronation (Fig. 6–52C). The force of the pronator quadratus also guides the joint through its natural arthrokinematics.

In the healthy joint, the compression force from the pronator quadratus and other muscles is absorbed by the joint without difficulty. In cases of severe rheumatoid arthritis, the articular cartilage, bone, and periarticular connective tissue lose their ability to adequately absorb joint forces. These myo-

genic (from the Greek root *myo;* muscle + *genesis;* generation) compressive forces can become detrimental to joint stability. The same forces that help stabilize the joint in the healthy state may cause joint destruction in the diseased state.

### REFERENCES

1. An KN, Morrey BF: Biomechanics of the elbow. In Morrey BF (ed): The Elbow and Its Disorders. Philadelphia, WB Saunders, 1993.
2. An KN, Morrey BF: Biomechanics. In Morrey BF (ed): Joint Replacement Arthroplasty. New York, Churchill Livingstone, 1991.
3. An KN, Hui FC, Morrey BF, et al: Muscles across the elbow joint: A biomechanical analysis. J Biomech 14:659–669, 1981.
4. Askew LJ, An KN, Morrey BF, et al: Isometric elbow strength in normal individuals. Clin Orthop 222:261–266, 1987.
5. Basmajian JV, Latif A: Integrated actions and functions of the chief flexors of the elbow. J Bone Joint Surg 39A:1106–1118, 1957.
6. Basmajian JV, Travill A: Electromyography of the pronator muscles of the forearm. Anat Rec 139:45–49, 1961.
7. Bert JM, Linscheid RL, McElfresh EC: Rotary contracture of the forearm. J Bone Joint Surg 62A:1163–1168, 1980.
8. Callaway GH, Field LD, Deng XH, et al: Biomechanical evaluation of the medial collateral ligament of the elbow. J Bone Joint Surg 79A:1223–1231, 1997.
9. Currier DP: Maximal isometric tension of the elbow extensors at varied positions. Phys Ther 52:1043–1049, 1972.
10. De Sousa OM, De Moraes JL, Viera FLD: Electromyographic study of the brachioradialis muscle. Anat Rec 139:125–131, 1961.
11. Drobner WS, Hausman MR: The distal radioulnar joint. Hand Clin 8:631–644, 1992.
12. Funk DA, An KN, Morrey BF, et al: Electromyographic analysis of muscles across the elbow joint. J Orthop Res 5:529–538, 1987.
13. Fuss FK: The ulnar collateral ligament of the human elbow joint. Anatomy, function and biomechanics. J Anat 175:203–212, 1991.
14. Gallagher MA, Cuomo F, Polonsky L, et al: Effects of age, testing speed, and arm dominance on isokinetic strength of the elbow. J Shoulder Elbow Surg 6:340–346, 1997.
15. Galley SH, Richards RR, O'Driscoll SW: Intraarticular capacity and compliance of stiff and normal elbows. J Arthroscop Rel Surg 9:9–13, 1993.
16. Gefen JY, Gelmann AS, Herbison GJ, et al: Use of shoulder flexors to achieve isometric elbow extension in C[6] tetraplegia patients during weight shift. Spinal Cord 35:308–313, 1997.

17. Goel VK, Singh D, Bijlani V: Contact areas in human elbow joints. J Biomech Eng 104:169–175, 1982.

18. Inman VT, Saunders JB: Referred pain from skeletal structures. J Nerv Ment Dis 99:660–667, 1944.

19. Kapandji IA: The Physiology of the Joints, vol 1, 5th ed. Edinburgh, Churchill Livingstone, 1982.

20. Kleinman WB, Graham TJ: The distal radioulnar joint capsule: Clinical anatomy and role in post-traumatic limitation of forearm rotation. J Hand Surg 23A:588–599, 1998.

21. Le Bozec S, Maton B, Cnockaert JC: The synergy of elbow extensor muscles during static work in man. Eur J Appl Physiol 43:57–68, 1980.

22. Lehmkuhl LD, Smith LK: Brunnstrom's Clinical Kinesiology, 4th ed. Philadelphia, FA Davis, 1983.

23. Lindau T, Adlercreutz C, Aspendberg P: Peripheral tears of the triangular fibrocartilage complex cause distal radioulnar joint instability after distal radial fractures. J Hand Surg 25A:464–468, 2000.

24. MacConaill MA, Basmajian JV: Muscles and Movements: A Basis for Human Kinesiology. New York, Robert E. Krieger, 1977.

25. Maloney MD, Mohr KJ, El Attrache NS: Elbow injures in the throwing athlete. Clin Sports Med 18:795–809, 1999.

26. Morrey BF: Post-traumatic contracture of the elbow: Operative treatment including distraction arthroplasty. J Bone Joint Surg 72A:601–618, 1990.

27. Morrey BF, An KN: Functional anatomy of the ligaments of the elbow. Clin Orthop 201:84–90, 1985.

28. Morrey BF, Askew LJ, An KN, et al: A biomechanical study of normal functional elbow motion. J Bone Joint Surg 63A:872–876, 1981.

29. Morrey BF, Chao EY: Passive motion of the elbow joint. J Bone Joint Surg 58A:501–508, 1976.

30. Morrey BF, An KN, Stormont TJ: Force transmission through the radial head. J Bone Joint Surg 70A:250–256, 1988.

31. Morrey BF, Tanaka S, An KN: Valgus stability of the elbow. Clin Orthop 265:187–195, 1991.

32. Murray WM, Delp SL, Buchanan TS: Variation of muscle moment arms with elbow and forearm positions. J Biomech 28:513–525, 1995.

33. Nakamura T, Yabe Y, Horiuchi Y: Dynamic changes in the shape of the triangular fibrocartilage during rotation demonstrated with high resolution magnetic resonance imaging. J Hand Surg 24B:338–341, 1999.

34. Neumann DA: Use of the diaphragm to assist in rolling in the patient with quadriplegia. Phys Ther 59:39, 1979.

35. Neumann DA, Soderberg GL, Cook TM: Electromyographic analysis of hip abductor musculature in healthy right-handed persons. Phys Ther 69:431–440, 1989.

36. Olsen BS, Sojbjerg JO, Dalstra M, et al: Kinematics of the lateral ligamentous constraints of the elbow joint. J Shoulder Elbow Surg 5:333–341, 1996.

37. Palmer AK, Werner FW: Biomechanics of the distal radioulnar joint. Clin Orthop 187:26–35, 1984.

38. Petrie S, Collins JG, Solomonow M, et al: Mechanoreceptors in the human elbow ligaments. J Hand Surg 23A:512–518, 1998.

39. Pfaeffle HJ, Fischer KJ, Manson TT, et al: Role of the forearm interosseous ligament: Is it more than just longitudinal load transfer? J Hand Surg 25A:683–688, 2000.

40. Provins KA, Salters N: Maximum torque exerted about the elbow joint. J Appl Phys 7:393–398, 1955.

41. Regan WD, Korinek SL, Morrey BF, et al: Biomechanical study of ligaments around the elbow joint. Clin Orthop 271:170–179, 1991.

42. Schuind FA, An KN, Berglund L, et al: The distal radioulnar joint ligaments: A biomechanical study. J Hand Surg 16A:1106–1114, 1991.

43. Schuind FA, Linscheid RL, An KN, et al: Changes in wrist and forearm configuration with grasp and isometric contraction of elbow flexors. J Hand Surg 17A:698–703, 1992.

44. Schuind FA, Goldschmidt D, Bastin C, et al: A biomechanical study of the ulnar nerve at the elbow. J Hand Surg 20B:623–627, 1995.

45. Stokdijk M, Meskers CGM, Veeger HEJ, et al: Determination of the optimal elbow axis for evaluation of placement of prosthesis. Clin Biomech 14:177–184, 1999.

46. Stuart PR: Pronator quadratus revisited. J Hand Surg 21B:714–722, 1996.

47. Travill A, Basmajian JV: Electromyography of the supinators of the forearm. Anat Rec 130:557–560, 1961.

48. Travill AA: Electromyographic study of the extensor apparatus. Anat Rec 144:373–376, 1962.

49. Tsunoda N, O'Hagan F, MacDougall JD: Elbow flexion strength curves in untrained men and women and male bodybuilders. Eur J Appl Physiol 66:235–239, 1993.

50. Van der Heijden EP, Hillen B: A two-dimensional kinematic analysis of the distal radioulnar joint. J Hand Surg. 21B:824–829, 1996.

51. Williams PL, Bannister LH, Berry M, et al: Gray's Anatomy, 38th ed. New York, Churchill Livingstone, 1995.

52. Winters JM, Kleweno DG: Effect of initial upper-limb alignment on muscle contributions to isometric strength curves. J Biomech 26:143–153, 1993.

53. Youm Y, Dryer RF, Thambyrajah K, et al: Biomechanical analysis of forearm pronation-supination and elbow flexion-extension. J Biomech 12:245–255, 1979.

## ADDITIONAL READINGS

Bade H, Koebke J, Schluter M: Morphology of the articular surfaces of the distal radio-ulnar joint. Anat Rec 246:410–414, 1996.

Davidson PA, Pink M, Perry J, et al: Functional anatomy of the flexor pronator muscle group in relation to the medial collateral ligament of the elbow. Am J Sports Med 23:245–250, 1995.

Eckstein F, Lohe F, Hillebrand S, et al: Morphomechanics of the humeroulnar joint: I. Joint space width and contact areas as a function of load and flexion angle. Anat Rec 243:318–326, 1995.

Fleisig GS, Andrews JR, Dillman CJ, et al: Kinetics of baseball pitching with implications about injury mechanisms. Am J Sports Med 23:233–239, 1995.

Kihara H, Short WH, Werner FW, et al: The stabilizing mechanism of the distal radioulnar joint during pronation and supination. J Hand Surg 20A:930–936, 1995.

London JT: Kinematics of the elbow. J Bone Joint Surg 63A:529–535, 1981.

O'Driscoll SW, Horii E, Morrey BF, et al: Anatomy of the ulnar part of the lateral collateral ligament of the elbow. Clin Anat 5:296–303, 1992.

Palmer AK, Werner FW: The triangular fibrocartilage complex of the wrist: Anatomy and function. J Hand Surg 6:153–161, 1981.

Pauly JE, Rushing JL, Scheving LE: An electromyographic study of some muscles crossing the elbow joint. Anat Rec 159:47–53, 1967.

Sojbjerg JO: The stiff elbow. Acta Orthop Scand 67:626–631, 1996.

Totterman SMS, Miller RJ: Triangular fibrocartilage complex: Normal appearance on coronal three-dimensional gradient-recalled-echo MR images. Radiology 195:521–527, 1995.

# Wrist

## DONALD A. NEUMANN, PhD, PT

### TOPICS AT A GLANCE

## INTRODUCTION

The wrist contains eight small carpal bones, which as a group act as a flexible "spacer" between the forearm and hand (Fig. 7–1). In addition to several small intercarpal joints, the wrist or carpus functions as two major articulations. The *radiocarpal joint* is located between the distal end of the radius and the proximal row of carpal bones. Just distal to this joint is the *midcarpal joint,* located between the proximal and distal row of carpal bones. These two joints allow the wrist to flex and extend and to move from side to side in a motion called radial and ulnar deviation. The distal radioulnar joint is considered part of the forearm complex, rather than the wrist, due to its role in pronation and supination.

The position of the wrist significantly affects the function of the hand. Many muscles that control the fingers originate extrinsic to the hand, with their proximal attachments located in the forearm. The position of the wrist, therefore, is critical in setting the length-tension relationship of the extrinsic finger muscles. A fused, painful, or weak wrist often assumes a posture that interferes with the optimal length of the extrinsic musculature. The kinesiology of the wrist is very much linked to the kinesiology of the hand.

Several new terms are introduced here to describe the relative position, or topography, within the wrist and the hand. *Palmar* and *volar* are synonymous with *anterior; dorsal* is synonymous with *posterior.* These terms are used interchangeably throughout this chapter and the next chapter on the hand.

## OSTEOLOGY

### Distal Forearm

The dorsal surface of the distal radius has several grooves and raised areas that help guide many tendons of extrinsic muscles (Fig. 7–2). For example, the palpable *dorsal (or Lister's) tubercle* separates the tendons of the extensor carpi radialis brevis from the extensor pollicis longus.

---

**Osteologic Features of the Distal Forearm**
- Dorsal or Lister's tubercle of the radius
- Styloid process of the radius
- Styloid process of the ulna
- Distal articular surface of the radius

---

The palmar surface of the distal radius is the location of the proximal attachments of the wrist capsule and the thick palmar radiocarpal ligaments (Fig. 7–3). The *styloid process of the radius* projects distally from the lateral side of the radius. The *styloid process of the ulna,* much sharper than its radial counterpart, extends distally from the posterior-medial surface of the ulna.

The *distal articular surface of the radius* is concave in both medial-lateral and anterior-posterior directions (see Fig. 6–27B). Facets are formed in the articular cartilage from

angles about 25 degrees toward the ulnar (medial) direction (Fig. 7–4A). This *ulnar tilt* allows the wrist and hand to rotate farther into ulnar deviation than into radial deviation. As a result of this tilt, radial deviation of the wrist is limited by impingement of the lateral side of the carpus against the styloid process of the radius. Second, the distal articular surface of the radius is angled about 10 degrees in the palmar direction (Fig. 7–4B). This *palmar tilt* accounts, in part, for the greater amounts of flexion than extension at the wrist.

## Carpal Bones

From a radial (lateral) to ulnar direction, the proximal row of carpal bones includes the scaphoid, lunate, triquetrum, and pisiform. The distal row includes the trapezium, trapezoid, capitate, and hamate (Figs. 7–2, 7–3, 7–5, and 7–6).

---

**Proximal Row of Carpal Bones**
- Scaphoid
- Lunate
- Triquetrum
- Pisiform

**Distal Row of Carpal Bones**
- Trapezium
- Trapezoid
- Capitate
- Hamate

---

The proximal row of carpal bones is joined in a relatively loose fashion. In contrast, the distal row of carpal bones is bound tightly by strong ligaments, providing a rigid and stable base for articulation with the metacarpal bones.

The following section presents a general anatomic description of each carpal bone. The ability to visualize each

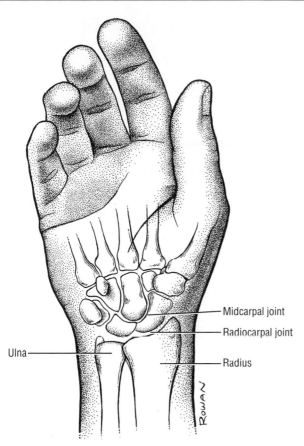

**FIGURE 7–1.** The bones and major articulations of the wrist.

Ulna

Midcarpal joint
Radiocarpal joint
Radius

indentations made by the scaphoid and lunate bones of the wrist.

The distal end of the radius has two configurations of biomechanical importance. First, the distal end of the radius

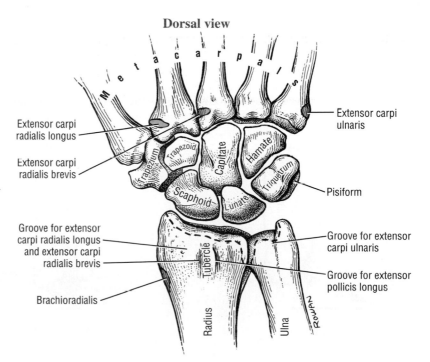

**FIGURE 7–2.** The dorsal aspect of the bones of the right carpus. The muscle's distal attachments are shown in gray. The dashed lines show the proximal attachment of the dorsal capsule of the wrist.

**Dorsal view**

Metacarpals

Extensor carpi radialis longus
Extensor carpi radialis brevis
Groove for extensor carpi radialis longus and extensor carpi radialis brevis
Brachioradialis

Trapezium
Trapezoid
Capitate
Hamate
Scaphoid
Lunate
Triquetrum
Tubercle
Radius
Ulna

Extensor carpi ulnaris
Pisiform
Groove for extensor carpi ulnaris
Groove for extensor pollicis longus

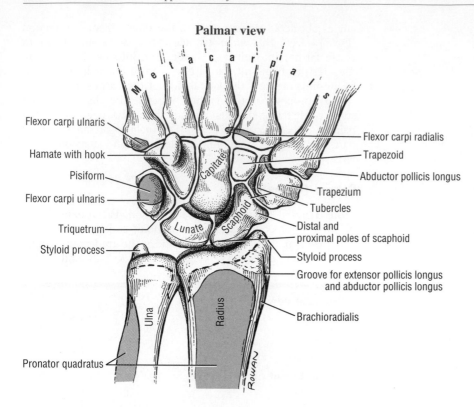

**Palmar view**

Flexor carpi ulnaris
Hamate with hook
Pisiform
Flexor carpi ulnaris
Triquetrum
Styloid process
Pronator quadratus

Flexor carpi radialis
Trapezoid
Abductor pollicis longus
Trapezium
Tubercles
Distal and proximal poles of scaphoid
Styloid process
Groove for extensor pollicis longus and abductor pollicis longus
Brachioradialis

**FIGURE 7–3.** The palmar aspect of the bones of the right carpus. The muscle's proximal attachments are shown in red and distal attachments in gray. The dashed lines show the proximal attachment of the palmar capsule of the wrist.

bone's relative position and shape is helpful in an understanding of the ligamentous anatomy and wrist kinematics.

## SCAPHOID

The scaphoid, or navicular, is named based on its vague resemblance to a boat (navicular: from the Latin *navicularis;* pertaining to shipping). Most of the "hull" or bottom of the boat rides on the radius; the cargo area of the "boat" is filled with the head of the capitate (see Fig. 7–3). The scaphoid contacts four carpal bones and the radius.

The scaphoid has two convex surfaces called poles. The *proximal pole* articulates with the scaphoid facet of the radius (see Fig. 6–27). The *distal pole* of the scaphoid is a slightly rounded surface, which articulates the trapezium and trapezoid. The scaphoid has a rather large and blunt *tubercle,* which projects palmarly from the distal pole. The scaphoid

tubercle can be palpated at the radial side of the base of the palm.

The distal-medial surface is deeply concave to accept the lateral half of the prominent head of the capitate bone (see Fig. 7–3). A small facet on the medial side contacts the lunate. The scaphoid and radius are located in the direct path of most of the force transmission through the wrist. Injury from falling on an extended and radially deviated wrist often results in fracture to the scaphoid. Fracture of the scaphoid occurs more frequently than any other fracture of the carpal bones. Healing is often hindered if the fracture is at the scaphoid's proximal pole because blood supply is often absent or minimal in this region. Seventeen percent of all scaphoid fractures are associated with other injuries along the weight-bearing path of the wrist and hand.[39] Associated injuries often involve fracture and/or dislocation of the lunate and fracture of the trapezium and distal radius.

**A**  **Anterior view**

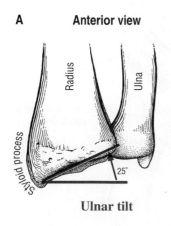

**Ulnar tilt**

**B**  **Medial view**

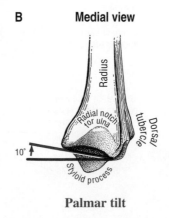

**Palmar tilt**

**FIGURE 7–4.** *A,* Anterior view of the distal radius showing an ulnar tilt of about 25 degrees. *B,* A medial view of the distal radius showing a palmar tilt of about 10 degrees.

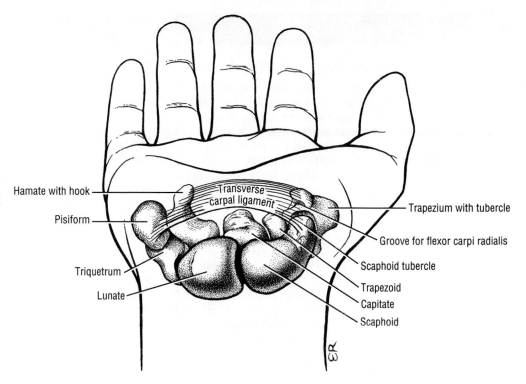

**FIGURE 7–5.** A view through the carpal tunnel of the right wrist with all contents removed. The transverse carpal ligament is shown as the roof of the tunnel.

Hamate with hook

Pisiform

Triquetrum

Lunate

Transverse carpal ligament

Trapezium with tubercle

Groove for flexor carpi radialis

Scaphoid tubercle

Trapezoid

Capitate

Scaphoid

## LUNATE

The lunate (from the Latin *luna,* moon) bone is the central bone of the proximal row, wedged between the scaphoid and triquetrum. Like the scaphoid, the lunate's proximal surface is convex to fit into the concave facet on the radius (Fig. 6–27B). The distal surface of the lunate is deeply concave, giving the bone its crescent moon–shaped appearance (see Fig. 7–3). This articular surface accepts two convexities: the medial half of the head of the capitate and part of the apex of the hamate.

## TRIQUETRUM

The triquetrum, or triangular bone, occupies the most ulnar position in the wrist, just medial to the lunate. The lateral surface of the triquetrum is long and flat for articulation with a similarly shaped surface on the hamate.

## PISIFORM

The pisiform, meaning "shaped like a pea," articulates loosely with the palmar surface of the triquetrum. The pisi-

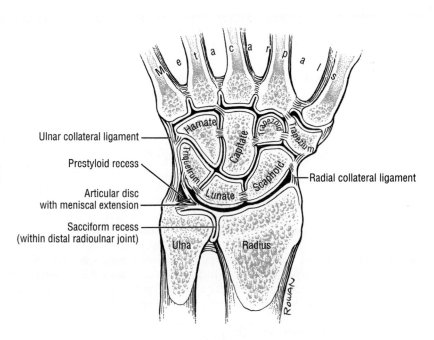

**FIGURE 7–6.** A frontal plane cross-section through the right wrist and distal forearm showing the shape of the bones and connective tissues.

Ulnar collateral ligament

Prestyloid recess

Articular disc with meniscal extension

Sacciform recess (within distal radioulnar joint)

Radial collateral ligament

Metacarpals

Hamate

Capitate

Trapezoid

Trapezium

Triquetrum

Lunate

Scaphoid

Ulna

Radius

**Kienböck's Disease: Avascular Necrosis of the Lunate**

Kienböck's disease is a painful orthopedic disorder of unknown etiology, characterized by avascular necrosis of the lunate.[39] Without adequate blood supply, the lunate may become fragmented and shortened, significantly altering the relative position of the other carpal bones. In severe cases, the lunate may totally collapse, disrupting the normal kinematics of the entire wrist. This tends to occur more often in those involved in manual labor.

Treatment of Kienböck's disease may be conservative or radical, depending on the severity. In relatively mild or early forms of the disease—before the lunate fragments and becomes sclerotic—treatment may involve immobilization by casting. In more advanced cases, the ulna may be surgically lengthened in order to reduce the compression at the radiocarpal joint. Alternatively, the radius may be surgically shortened to accomplish the same unloading effect.[28] The scaphoid, trapezium, and trapezoid may also be fused to add stability to the radial side of the wrist.

form bone rests upon the triquetrum's palmar surface This easily mobile and palpable bone is the attachment site for several muscles and ligaments. Otherwise, the pisiform has little functional significance in the kinematics of the wrist.

### CAPITATE

The capitate is the largest of all carpal bones, occupying a central location within the wrist. The word capitate is derived from the Latin root meaning *head,* which describes the shape of the bone's proximal surface. The large head articulates with the deep concavity provided by the scaphoid and lunate. The axis of rotation for all wrist motion passes through the capitate. The capitate is well stabilized between the hamate and trapezoid by short strong ligaments.

The capitate's distal surface is rigidly joined to the base of the third and, to a lesser extent, the second and fourth metacarpal bones. This rigid articulation allows the capitate and the third metacarpal to function as a single column, providing significant longitudinal stability to the entire wrist and hand.

### TRAPEZIUM

The trapezium, or greater multangular bone, has an asymmetric shape. The proximal surface is slightly concave for articulation with the scaphoid. Of particular importance is the distal saddle-shaped surface, which articulates with the base of the first metacarpal. The carpometacarpal joint is a highly specialized articulation allowing a wide range of motion to the human thumb.

A slender and sharp *tubercle* projects from the palmar

surface of the trapezium. This tubercle and palmar tubercle of the scaphoid provide attachment for the lateral side of the transverse carpal ligament (see Fig. 7–5). Immediately medial to the palmar tubercle is a distinct groove for the tendon of the flexor carpi radialis.

### TRAPEZOID

The trapezoid, or lesser multangular, is a small bone wedged tightly between the capitate and the trapezium. The trapezoid, like the trapezium, has a proximal surface that is slightly concave for articulation with the scaphoid. The bone makes a relatively firm articulation with the base of the second metacarpal bone.

### HAMATE

The hamate is named after the large hooklike process that projects from its palmar surface. The hamate has a general shape of a pyramid. Its base, or distal surface, articulates with the bases of the fourth and fifth metacarpals. This articulation provides mobility to the ulnar aspect of the hand, most noticeably when cupping the hand.

The apex of the hamate, its proximal surface, projects toward the concave surfaces of the lunate. The hook of the hamate and the pisiform bone provides attachment for the medial side of the transverse carpal ligament (see Fig. 7–5).

## Carpal Tunnel

As illustrated in Figure 7–5, the palmar side of the carpal bones forms a concavity. Arching over this concavity is a thick fibrous band of connective tissue known as the *transverse carpal ligament*. This ligament is connected to four raised points on the palmar carpus, namely, the pisiform and the hook of the hamate on the ulnar side and the tubercles of the scaphoid and the trapezium on the radial side. The transverse carpal ligament serves as a primary attachment site for many muscles located within the hand and the palmaris longus, a wrist flexor muscle.

The transverse carpal ligament converts the palmar concavity made by the carpal bones into a *carpal tunnel*. The tunnel serves as a passageway for the median nerve and tendons of extrinsic digital flexor muscles.

## ARTHROLOGY

### Joint Structure and Ligaments of the Wrist

#### JOINT STRUCTURE

The primary joints of the wrist are the *radiocarpal joint* and the *midcarpal joint* (see Fig. 7–1). Many less significant *intercarpal joints* exist between adjacent carpal bones (see Fig. 7–6). Intercarpal joints contribute to wrist motion through small gliding motions. Compared with the large range of motion permitted at the radiocarpal and midcarpal joints, motion at the intercarpal joints is relatively small. Nevertheless, it is important to the completion of full range of wrist motion.

### Joints of the Wrist
  * Radiocarpal joint
  * Midcarpal joint
    Medial compartment
    Lateral compartment
  * Intercarpal joints

### Radiocarpal Joint

The proximal components of the radiocarpal joint are the concave surfaces of the radius and the adjacent articular disc (Fig. 7–7A). The distal components of this joint are the convex proximal surfaces of the scaphoid and the lunate. The triquetrum is also considered part of the radiocarpal joint because at full ulnar deviation its medial surface makes contact with the articular disc (see Fig. 7–6).

The thick articular surface of the distal radius and the articular disc accept and disperse the forces that pass from the carpus to the forearm. Approximately 20% of the total compression force that crosses the wrist passes through the disc. The remaining 80% passes directly through the scaphoid and lunate to the radius.[20] The contact areas at the radiocarpal joint tend to be greatest when the wrist is extended and ulnarly deviated.[14] This is a wrist position where maximal grip strength is obtained.

### Midcarpal Joint

The midcarpal joint is the articulation between the proximal and distal row of carpal bones (see Fig. 7–7). The capsule that surrounds the midcarpal joint is continuous with each of the intercarpal joints.

The midcarpal joint can be divided into medial and lateral joint compartments.[38] The larger *medial compartment* is formed by the convex head of the capitate and apex of the hamate, fitting into the concave recess formed by the distal surfaces of the scaphoid, lunate, and triquetrum (Fig. 7–7B). The head of the capitate fits into this concave recess much like a ball-in-socket joint.

The *lateral compartment* of the midcarpal joint is formed by the junction of the slightly convex distal pole of the scaphoid with the slightly concave proximal surfaces of the trapezium and the trapezoid. The lateral compartment lacks the pronounced ovoid shape of the medial compartment. Cineradiography of wrist motion shows less movement at the lateral than the medial compartment.[17] For this reason, subsequent arthrokinematic analysis of the midcarpal joint focuses on the medial compartment.

## WRIST LIGAMENTS

Many of the ligaments of the wrist are small and difficult to isolate. Their inconspicuous nature does not, however, indicate their kinesiologic importance. Wrist ligaments are essential to maintaining natural intercarpal alignment and transferring forces through and across the carpus.[2] Muscles supply the forces for active wrist motion, and ligaments supply the control and guidance to arthrokinematics. Ligaments that are damaged through injury and disease leave the wrist vulnerable to deformation and instability.

Wrist ligaments are classified as extrinsic or intrinsic.[33] Extrinsic ligaments have their proximal attachments outside the carpal bones, but attach distally to the carpal bones. Intrinsic ligaments, in contrast, have both their proximal and distal attachments on carpal bones (Table 7–1).

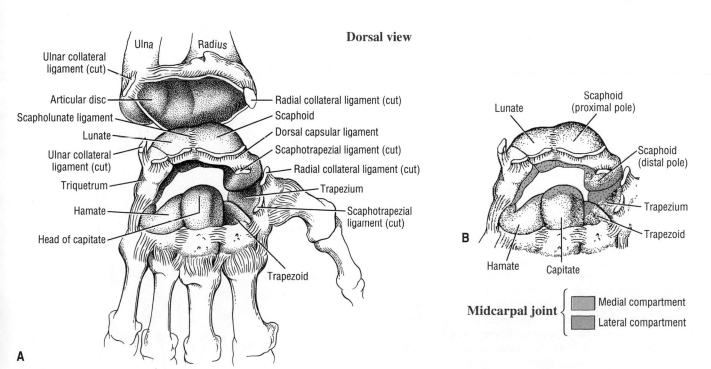

**Dorsal view**

Ulna — Radius
Ulnar collateral ligament (cut)
Articular disc
Scapholunate ligament
Lunate
Ulnar collateral ligament (cut)
Triquetrum
Hamate
Head of capitate
Radial collateral ligament (cut)
Scaphoid
Dorsal capsular ligament
Scaphotrapezial ligament (cut)
Radial collateral ligament (cut)
Trapezium
Scaphotrapezial ligament (cut)
Trapezoid

**A**

Lunate — Scaphoid (proximal pole)
Scaphoid (distal pole)
Trapezium
Trapezoid
Hamate    Capitate

**B**

**Midcarpal joint** { ▨ Medial compartment  ▨ Lateral compartment

**FIGURE 7–7.** *A*, Dissected right wrist showing a dorsal view of the radiocarpal and midcarpal joints. Refer to text for description of ligaments and other soft tissues. *B*, Red and gray highlight the lateral and medial compartments of the midcarpal joint.

---

### TABLE 7–1. Extrinsic and Intrinsic Ligaments of the Wrist

**Extrinsic Ligaments**

**Dorsal radiocarpal ligament**

**Radial collateral ligament**

**Palmar radiocarpal ligaments**
- Radiocapitate
- Radiolunate
- Radioscapholunate

**Ulnocarpal complex**
- Articular disc
- Ulnar collateral ligament
- Palmar ulnocarpal ligament

**Intrinsic Ligaments**

**Short ligaments** of the distal row

**Intermediate ligaments**
- Lunotriquetral
- Scapholunate
- Scaphotrapezial

**Long ligaments**
- Palmar intercarpal
  *Lateral leg:* fibers between the capitate and the scaphoid
  *Medial leg:* fibers between the capitate and the triquetrum
- Dorsal intercarpal: fibers between the scaphoid and triquetrum

---

### Extrinsic Ligaments

A fibrous capsule surrounds the external surface of the wrist and the distal radioulnar joint. Dorsally, the capsule thickens slightly to form ligamentous bands known as the *dorsal radiocarpal ligaments* (Fig. 7–8). The ligaments are thin and very difficult to distinguish from the capsule itself.

In general, the dorsal radiocarpal ligaments travel distally in an ulnarly direction, from the distal radius to the dorsal surfaces of the scaphoid and the lunate. A larger discrete set of fibers extends to the triquetrum. The dorsal radiocarpal ligaments reinforce the posterior side of the radiocarpal joint, becoming taut in full flexion.[30]

The lateral part of the wrist capsule is strengthened by fibers called the *radial collateral ligament*. These fibers attach proximally to the styloid process, and distally at the scaphoid tubercle, trapezium, and adjacent transverse carpal ligament (see Figs. 7–6 and 7–8). This ligament provides only part of the lateral stability to the wrist. A major portion is furnished by extrinsic muscles, such as the abductor pollicis longus and the extensor pollicis brevis. The radial collateral ligament is more developed palmar-laterally than dorsal-laterally. These fibers, therefore, become maximally taut when ulnar deviation of the wrist is combined with extension.

Deep and separate from the palmar capsule of the wrist are several stout and extensive ligaments known collectively as the *palmar radiocarpal ligaments*. These include the *radiocapitate ligament,* the *radiolunate ligament,* and, in a deeper plane, the *radioscapholunate ligament* (Fig. 7–9). Each ligament arises from a roughened area on the distal radius, travels distally in an ulnar direction, and attaches to the

palmar surface of several carpal bones. The palmar radiocarpal ligaments are much stronger and thicker than the dorsal radiocarpal ligaments. Significant tension exists in these ligaments even in the relaxed neutral wrist position.[36] In general, the palmar radiocarpal ligaments become maximally taut at full wrist extension.[30]

A complex set of connective tissues exists near the ulnar border of the wrist known as the *ulnocarpal complex*. This group of connective tissue is often referred to as the triangular fibrocartilage complex (TFCC).[20] The ulnocarpal complex includes the articular disc, the ulnar collateral ligament, and the palmar ulnocarpal ligament (see Fig. 7–9). This complex set of tissues fills most of the *ulnocarpal space* between the distal ulna and the carpal bones (Fig. 7–10). The ulnocarpal space allows the carpal bones to pronate and supinate with the radius, without interference from the distal end of the ulna.

The *articular disc,* the main feature of the ulnocarpal complex, attaches from the ulnar notch of the radius to near the styloid process of the ulna (see Fig. 6–27). This disc is an important structural component of both the distal radioulnar joint and the radiocarpal joint. Figure 7–6 shows a frontal plane cross-section through the ulnocarpal space, illustrating a poorly defined meniscal extension of the articular disc.[33] The meniscal extension of the disc is often called the ulnocarpal meniscal homologue, indicating its vestigial function of once connecting the carpus to the triquetrum. Between the meniscal extension of the disc and the ulnar collateral ligament is the small *prestyloid recess,* a space filled with synovial fluid. This space often becomes distended and painful with rheumatoid arthritis. Tears in the articular disc may permit synovial fluid to spread from the radiocarpal joint to the distal radioulnar joint.

The *ulnar collateral ligament* is a thickening of the ulnar side of the wrist capsule (Figs. 7–6 and 7–8). The ligament originates from the styloid process of the ulna, crosses the ulnocarpal space, and attaches distally to the ulnar side of

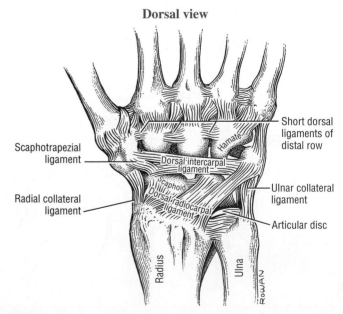

**Dorsal view**

Scaphotrapezial ligament

Radial collateral ligament

Short dorsal ligaments of distal row

Dorsal intercarpal ligament

Hamate

Scaphoid

Dorsal radiocarpal ligament

Ulnar collateral ligament

Articular disc

Radius

Ulna

**FIGURE 7–8.** The dorsal ligaments of the right wrist.

**Palmar view**

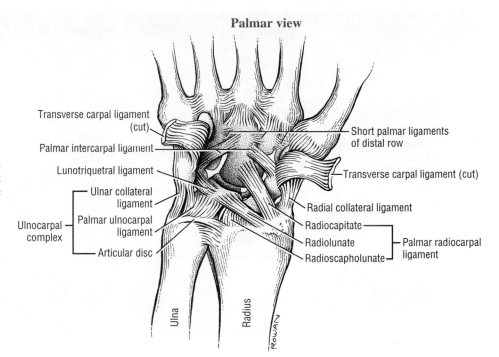

**FIGURE 7–9.** The palmar ligaments of the right wrist. The transverse carpal ligament has been cut and reflected to show the underlying ligaments.

the triquetrum and as far distal as the base of the fifth metacarpal. Full radial deviation of the wrist elongates the ulnar collateral ligament and surrounding capsule. The extensor carpi ulnaris assists the ulnar collateral ligament in reinforcing the ulnar margin of the wrist.[1]

The *palmar ulnocarpal ligament* is a thickened band of connective tissue that originates from the anterior margin of the articular disc (see Fig. 7–9). The ligament attaches distally to the palmar surfaces of the lunate and, to a lesser degree, the triquetrum.[16] It becomes taut in full wrist extension and full ulnar deviation.[36]

### Intrinsic Ligaments

The intrinsic ligaments of the wrist are classified as short, intermediate, or long (see Table 7–1).[33] *Short ligaments* within the wrist connect the bones of the distal row by their palmar, dorsal, or interosseous surfaces (Figs. 7–8 and 7–9). The short ligaments firmly stabilize and unite the row of bones, permitting them to function as a single mechanical unit. Three *intermediate ligaments* exist within the wrist. The *lunotriquetral ligament* is a fibrous continuation of the palmar radiolunate ligament (see Fig. 7–9). The *scapholunate ligament* is a broad collection of fibers that links the scaphoid with the lunate (see Fig. 7–7A). Several *scaphotrapezial ligaments* reinforce the articulation between the scaphoid and the trapezium (see Figs. 7–7A and 7–8).

Two relatively *long ligaments* are present within the wrist. The *palmar intercarpal ligament* is firmly attached to the palmar surface of the capitate bone (see Fig. 7–9). The ligament bifurcates proximally into two fiber groups that form an inverted **V** shape. The lateral leg of the inverted **V** is formed by fibers from the capitate to the scaphoid; the medial leg is formed by fibers between the capitate and triquetrum. A thin ligament, the *dorsal intercarpal ligament,* provides transverse stability to the wrist by binding the scaphoid to the triquetrum (see Fig. 7–8).

## Kinematics of Wrist Motion

### OSTEOKINEMATICS

The osteokinematics of the wrist are limited to 2 degrees of freedom: flexion-and-extension and ulnar-and-radial deviation (Fig. 7–11). Wrist circumduction—a full circular motion made by the wrist—is a combination of the aforementioned movements, not a third degree of freedom.

Except for minimal passive accessory motions, the wrist does not rotate about an axis running longitudinally through the radius. This motion is blocked by the bony fit of the radiocarpal joint and the fiber direction of many radiocarpal ligaments.[25] The apparent axial rotation of the palm—called pronation and supination—occurs at the proximal and distal

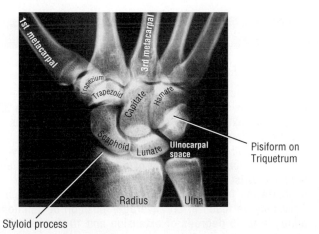

**FIGURE 7–10.** An x-ray of the right wrist showing the carpal bones and ulnocarpal space.

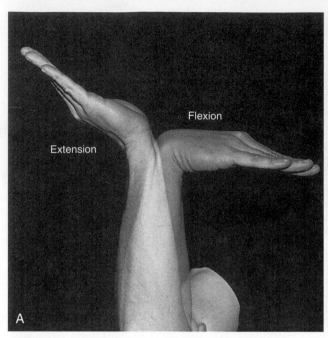
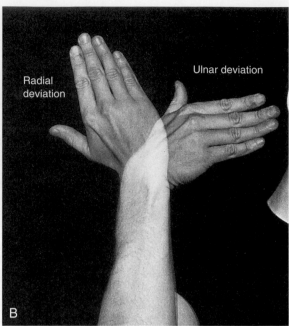

**FIGURE 7–11.** Osteokinematics of the wrist. *A,* Flexion and extension. *B,* Ulnar and radial deviation. Note that flexion exceeds extension and ulnar deviation exceeds radial deviation.

radioulnar joints of the forearm. Forearm motions require that the hand moves with the radius, not separately from it. The lack of this third degree of freedom at the radiocarpal joint allows the pronator and supinator muscles to transfer torques across the wrist to the working hand.

The wrist rotates in the sagittal plane about 130 to 140 degrees (Fig. 7–11A). On average, the wrist flexes from 0 degrees to about 65 to 80 degrees and extends from 0 degrees to about 55 to 70 degrees.[18,22,29] As with any diarthrodial joint, wrist range of motion varies with age and state of health and whether the motion is performed actively or passively. Total flexion normally exceeds extension by about 10 to 15 degrees. End-range extension can be limited by stiffness in the thick palmar radiocarpal ligaments. In some persons, a greater than average palmar tilt of the distal radius may limit the extension range (see Fig. 7–4B).

The wrist rotates in the frontal plane approximately 45 to 55 degrees (Fig. 7–11B).[18,22,41] Radial and ulnar deviation is measured as the angle between the radius and the shaft of the third metacarpal. Ulnar deviation of the wrist occurs from 0 degrees to about 30 degrees. Radial deviation occurs from 0 degrees to about 15 degrees. Because of the ulnar tilt of the distal radius (see Fig. 7–4A), maximum ulnar deviation normally is double that of radial deviation.

Most natural movements of the wrist use a combination of frontal and sagittal plane motions. The greatest continuous arc of motion at the wrist exists between full extension/radial deviation and full flexion/ulnar deviation.

## ARTHROKINEMATICS

Studies have quantified carpal bone kinematics using various technical methods, often as a prerequisite to the design of wrist joint prostheses.[23] These methodologies include the following:

- X-ray
- Anatomic dissection
- Placement of pins in bones
- Three-dimensional computer imaging
- Sonic digitizing
- Cineradiography
- Stereophotography
- Optoelectric systems
- Magnetic tracking devices

Despite many studies, several explanations exist on the precise detail of these kinematics.

The axis of rotation for wrist movement is assumed to pass through the head of the capitate.[40] The axis runs in a medial-lateral direction for flexion and extension, and in an anterior-posterior direction for radial and ulnar deviation

---

**S P E C I A L   F O C U S   7 – 2**

### "Position of Function" of the Wrist

Many daily activities require 45 degrees of sagittal plane motion: from 5 to 10 degrees of flexion to 30 to 35 degrees of extension. In addition, many daily activities require 25 degrees of frontal plane motion: from 15 degrees of ulnar deviation to 10 degrees of radial deviation.[5,21] Medical management of a severely painful or an unstable wrist sometimes requires surgical fusion. To minimize the functional impairment of this procedure, a wrist may be fused in an "average" position of function: about 10 to 15 degrees of extension and 10 degrees of ulnar deviation.[5,27]

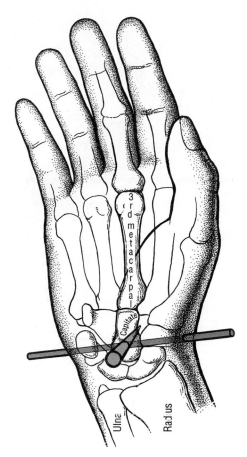

**FIGURE 7–12.** The medial-lateral (gray) and anterior-posterior (red) axes of rotation for wrist movement are shown piercing the head of the capitate bone.

(Fig. 7–12). Although the axes are depicted as stationary, in reality they migrate slightly throughout the full range of motion.[23] The firm articulation between the capitate and the base of the third metacarpal bone causes the rotation of the capitate to direct the osteokinematic path of the entire hand.

The wrist is a double-joint system with motion occurring simultaneously at both the radiocarpal and midcarpal joints. The next discussion on arthrokinematics focuses on the dynamic relationship between these two joints.

### Wrist Extension and Flexion

Several models have been created to attempt to define the individual angular contributions of the radiocarpal and midcarpal joints to the total sagittal plane motion of the wrist.[10,12,23,26,29,41] The essential kinematics of the sagittal plane involve movements that occur within the *central column* of the wrist (i.e., that formed by the series of articulations among the radius, lunate, capitate, and third metacarpal bone) (Fig. 7–13). Within this column, the radiocarpal joint is represented by the articulation between the radius and lunate, and the medial compartment of the midcarpal joint is represented by the articulation between the lunate and the capitate. The carpometacarpal joint is assumed to be a rigid articulation between the capitate and the base of the third metacarpal. Although this mechanical depiction of the wrist represents an oversimplification of very complex ar-

thrology, it does show many of the paramount features of sagittal plane wrist arthrokinematics.

### *Dynamic Interaction Within the Joints of the Central Column of the Wrist*

The arthrokinematics of wrist extension are based on synchronous convex-on-concave rotations at the radiocarpal and midcarpal joints. At the radiocarpal joint shown in red in Figure 7–14, extension occurs as the convex surface of the lunate rolls dorsally on the radius and simultaneously slides palmarly. Rotation directs the lunate's distal surface in an extended, dorsal direction. At the midcarpal joint shown in gray in Figure 7–14, the head of the capitate rolls dorsally on the lunate and simultaneously slides in a palmar direction. Combining the arthrokinematics over both joints produces about 60 degrees of total wrist extension. An advantage of two joints contributing to a motion is that a significant total range of motion is produced by only moderate rotations at each individual joint. Mechanically, this combination allows each joint to move within a more restricted and more stable arc of motion.

Full wrist extension elongates the palmar radiocarpal ligaments (see Fig. 7–14) and the palmar capsule and the wrist and finger flexor muscles. Tension within these structures stabilizes the wrist in its close-packed position of extension.[15] Stability in wrist extension is useful when weight is borne through the upper extremity during activities such as crawling on the hands and knees, and pushing up—when transferring from a wheelchair to a bed.

The arthrokinematics of wrist flexion are similar to those described for extension, but occur in a reverse fashion (see Fig. 7–14). The wrist is not very stable in full flexion and is poorly suited to accept weight-bearing forces through the upper extremity.

Describing flexion and extension of the wrist using the central column concept allows an excellent conceptualization of a rather complex event. A limitation of the model, however, is that it does not account for all the carpal bones that participate in the motion. For instance, the model ignores

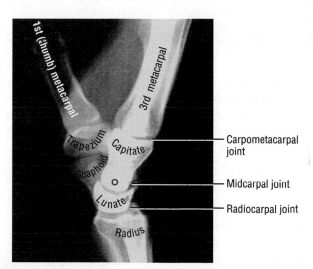

**FIGURE 7–13.** A lateral view of the central column through the wrist. The axis of rotation for flexion and extension is shown as a small circle through the capitate.

**Lateral view**

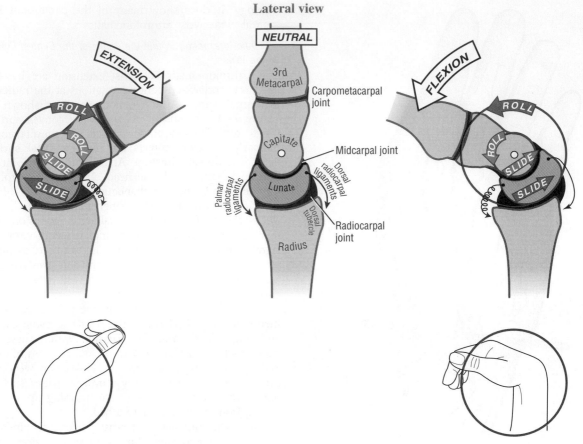

**FIGURE 7–14.** A model of the central column of the right wrist showing flexion and extension. The wrist in the center is shown at rest, in a neutral position. The roll-and-slide arthrokinematics are shown in red for the radiocarpal joint and in light gray for the midcarpal joint. During wrist extension (*left*), the dorsal radiocarpal ligaments become slackened and the palmar radiocarpal ligaments taut. The reverse arthrokinematics occur during wrist flexion (*right*).

the kinematics of the scaphoid bone at the radiocarpal joint. In brief, the arthrokinematics of the scaphoid on the radius are similar to those of the lunate during flexion and extension, except for one feature. Based on the different size and curvature of the two bones, the scaphoid rolls on the radius at a different speed than the lunate.[26] This difference causes a slight displacement between the scaphoid and lunate by the end of full motion. Normally, in the healthy wrist, the amount of displacement is minimized by the action of ligaments, especially the scapholunate ligament (see Fig. 7–7A). Damage to this ligament can occur through traumatic scapholunate dislocation, chronic synovitis from rheumatoid arthritis, and even from surgical removal of a ganglion cyst. A torn scapholunate ligament may predispose a person to scapholunate joint instability, which interferes with the natural kinematics at the wrist.[3]

### Ulnar and Radial Deviation of the Wrist

#### Dynamic Interaction Between the Radiocarpal Joint and the Midcarpal Joint

Like flexion and extension, ulnar and radial deviation occur through synchronous convex-on-concave rotations at both the radiocarpal joint and the midcarpal joint. The arthrokinematics of ulnar and radial deviation, however, are slightly more complicated than those of flexion and extension.

During ulnar deviation, the radiocarpal and midcarpal joints contribute fairly equally to overall wrist motion (Fig. 7–15). At the radiocarpal joint shown in red in Figure 7–15, the scaphoid, lunate, and triquetrum roll ulnarly and slide a significant distance radially. The extent of this radial slide is evident by noting the final position of the lunate relative to the radius at full ulnar deviation.

Ulnar deviation at the midcarpal joint occurs primarily from the capitate rolling ulnarly and sliding slightly radially. Full range of ulnar deviation causes the triquetrum to contact the articular disc. Compression of the hamate against the triquetrum pushes the proximal row of carpal bones radially against the styloid process of the radius. This compression helps stabilize the wrist for activities that require large gripping forces.

Radial deviation at the wrist occurs through similar arthrokinematics as described for ulnar deviation (see Fig. 7–15). The amount of radial deviation at the radiocarpal joint is limited as the radial side of the carpus impinges against the styloid process of the radius. Most radial deviation of the wrist, therefore, occurs at the midcarpal joint. The hamate and triquetrum separate by the end of full radial deviation.

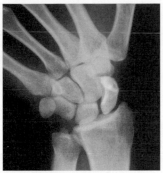

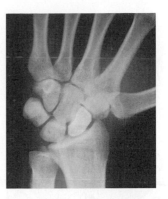

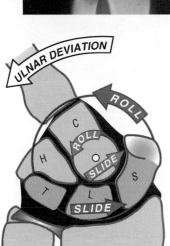

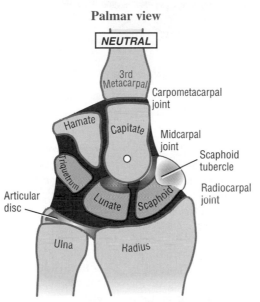

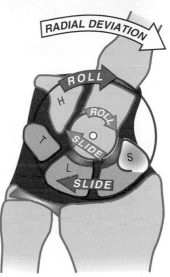

**Palmar view**

NEUTRAL

ULNAR DEVIATION

ROLL

ROLL

SLIDE

SLIDE

RADIAL DEVIATION

ROLL

ROLL

SLIDE

SLIDE

3rd Metacarpal

Carpometacarpal joint

Hamate

Capitate

Midcarpal joint

Scaphoid tubercle

Triquetrum

Radiocarpal joint

Articular disc

Lunate    Scaphoid

Ulna    Radius

**FIGURE 7–15.** X-rays and mechanical depiction of the arthrokinematics of ulnar and radial deviation for the right wrist. The roll-and-slide arthrokinematics are shown in red for the radiocarpal joint and in light gray for the midcarpal joint. (Arthrokinematics are based on observations made from cineradiography conducted at Marquette University, Milwaukee, WI, in 1999.)

*Tension in the "Double V" System of Ligaments During Radial and Ulnar Deviation*

The arthrokinematics of wrist motion are actively driven by muscle, but controlled by the passive tension action of liga-ments. A *double V* system of ligaments illustrates one way in which ligaments help control ulnar and radial deviation (Fig. 7–16).[33] In the neutral position, the four ligaments of the double V system appear as two inverted Vs. The distal in-

## SPECIAL FOCUS 7–3

### Additional Arthrokinematics Involving the Proximal Row of Carpal Bones

Careful observation of ulnar and radial deviation on cine-radiography or serial static x-rays reveals more compli-cated arthrokinematics than previously described. During motion, the proximal row of carpal bones "rock" slightly into flexion and extension and, to a much less extent, "twist." The rocking motion is most noticeable in the scaphoid and, to a lesser extent, the lunate. During radial deviation the proximal row flexes slightly; during ulnar deviation the proximal row extends slightly.[11] Note that in Figure 7–15, especially on x-ray, the change in position of the scaphoid tubercle between the extremes of ulnar and radial deviation. At full ulnar deviation, the scaphoid is rotated about 20 degrees into extension,

relative to the radius. The scaphoid appears to "stand up" or to lengthen, which projects its tubercle distally. At full radial deviation, the scaphoid flexes beyond neutral about 20 degrees, taking on a shortened stature with its tubercle having approached the radius. A functional shortening of the scaphoid allows a few more degrees of radial devia-tion before complete blockage against the styloid process of the radius. The exact mechanism responsible for the slight flexion and extension of the proximal carpal row during ulnar and radial deviation is not fully understood, but many explanations have been offered.[26,37] Most likely, the mechanism is driven by forces generated by stretched ligaments and compressions that occur between the mov-ing carpal bones.

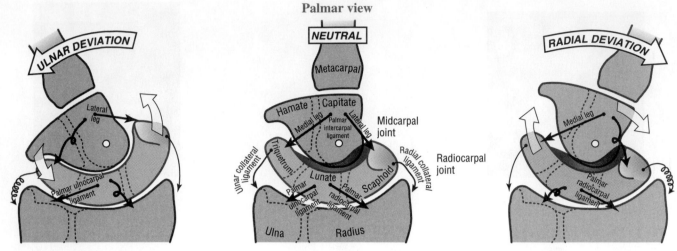

**Palmar view**

**FIGURE 7–16.** The tensing and slackening of the "double V" system ligaments of the wrist are illustrated. The collateral ligaments are also shown. The bones have been blocked together for simplicity. Taut lines represent ligaments under increased tension.

verted V represents the medial and lateral legs of the palmar intercarpal ligament (see Fig. 7–9). The proximal inverted V is formed by fibers of the palmar ulnocarpal and palmar radiocarpal ligaments. All four legs of the ligamentous mechanism are under slight tension even in the neutral position. During ulnar deviation, passive tension rises diagonally across the wrist by the stretch placed in the lateral leg of the palmar intercarpal ligament and fibers of the palmar ulnocarpal ligament.[36] During radial deviation, tension is created in the opposite diagonal by a stretch in the medial leg of the palmar intercarpal ligament and fibers of the palmar radiocarpal ligament. A gradual increase in tension within these ligaments provides an important source of control to the movement, as well as dynamic stability to the carpal bones.

---

**Tensions Created within the "Double V" System of Ligaments during Frontal Plane Movement**

During *ulnar deviation,* tension rises in the
Lateral leg of the palmar intercarpal ligament
Palmar ulnocarpal ligament.
During *radial deviation,* tension rises in the
Medial leg of the palmar intercarpal ligament
Palmar radiocarpal ligament.

---

Tension in stretched collateral ligaments of the double V system helps determine the end range of motion of radial and ulnar deviation. Passive ulnar deviation is limited by tension in the stretched radial collateral and palmar ulnocarpal ligaments. Radial deviation, in contrast, is limited by tension in the stretched ulnar collateral and palmar radiocarpal ligaments.

## Carpal Instability

The pathomechanics of carpal instability occur in many forms.[32] Essentially all types of carpal instability lead to a loss of function due to a loss of normal anatomic alignment. The following examples describe two common types of carpal instability.

---

**Two Common Types of Carpal Instability**

1. *Rotational collapse of wrist:* The "zig-zag" deformity
    Volar intercalated segment instability (VISI)
    Dorsal intercalated segment instability (DISI)
2. *Translocation of the carpus*

---

**Rotational Collapse of Wrist.** Mechanically, the wrist consists of a mobile proximal row of carpal bones intercalated or interposed between two rigid structures: the forearm and the distal row of carpal bones.[14] Like derailed cars of a freight train, the proximal row of carpal bones is prone to a rotational collapse in a zig-zag fashion when compressed from both ends (Fig. 7–17). The compression forces that

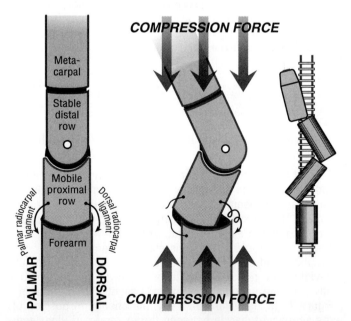

**FIGURE 7–17.** A highly diagrammatic depiction of a "zig-zag" collapse of the central column of the wrist following large compression force.

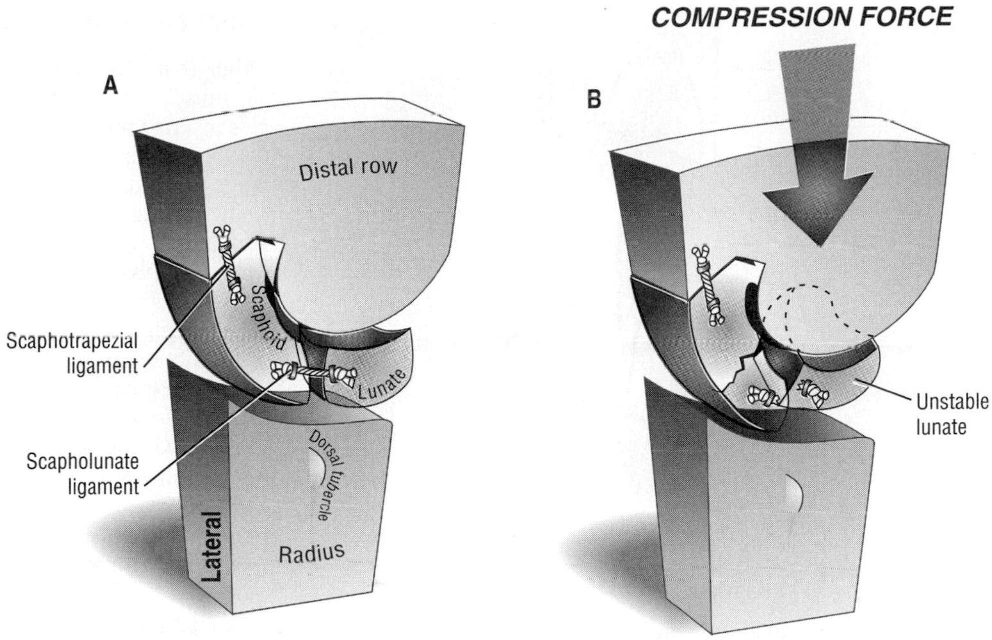

**COMPRESSION FORCE**

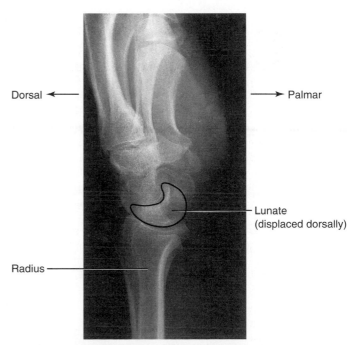

**FIGURE 7–18.** *A,* Acting through ligaments, the scaphoid provides a mechanical linkage between the relatively mobile lunate and the rigid distal row of carpal bones. *B,* Compression forces through the wrist from a fall may fracture the scaphoid and tear the scapholunate ligament. Loss of the mechanical link provided by the scaphoid often leads to lunate instability and/or dislocation.

cross the wrist are due to muscle activation and contact with the surrounding environment. In most healthy persons, the wrist remains perfectly stable throughout life. Collapse and subsequent joint dislocation are prevented by resistance from ligaments, tendons, and intercarpal articulations.

The lunate is the most frequently dislocated carpal bone.[39] Because no muscles attach to the lunate, stability must be provided by ligaments and contact with adjacent bones, most notably the scaphoid (Fig. 7–18A). The scaphoid functions as a mechanical link between the lunate and the rigid, distal row of carpal bones. The continuity of this link requires that the scaphoid is well stabilized by intrinsic ligaments. Consider, for example, a fall over an outstretched hand with a resulting fracture of the scaphoid and tearing of the scapholunate ligament (Fig. 7–18B). Disruption of the mechanical link provided by the scaphoid often leads to lunate dislocation. As shown in Figure 7–18B, the lunate most often dislocates so its distal articular surface faces dorsally. This condition is referred to clinically as *dorsal intercalated segment instability (DISI)* (Fig. 7–19). Injury to other ligaments, such as the lunotriquetral ligament, may cause a lunate dissociation with its distal articular surfaces, facing volarly (palmarly). This condition is referred to as *volar (palmar) intercalated segment instability (VISI).*[31] Regardless of the type of rotational collapse, the consequences can be painful and disabling. Changes in the natural arthrokinematics may create regions of high stress, eventually leading to joint destruction and carpal morphology changes. A painful and arthritic wrist may fail to provide a stable platform for the hand. A collapsed wrist may shorten its length, thereby altering the length-tension relationship and moment arms of the muscles that cross the wrist.[34]

**Ulnar Translocation of the Carpus.** As pointed out earlier, the distal end of the radius is angled from side to side so that its articular surface is sloped ulnarly about 25 degrees (see Fig. 7–4A). Ulnar tilt of the radius creates a natural tendency for the carpus to slide (translate) in an ulnar direction. Figure 7–20 shows that a wrist with an ulnar tilt of 25 degrees has an ulnar translation force of 42% of the total compression force that crosses the wrist. This translational force is naturally resisted by passive forces from various extrinsic ligaments, such as palmar radiocarpal ligament. A disease like rheumatoid arthritis significantly weakens wrist ligaments. Over time, the carpus may migrate ulnarly. An excessive ulnar translocation can significantly alter the biomechanics of the entire wrist and hand.

**FIGURE 7–19.** Lateral x-ray showing the dislocation and subsequent rotational deformity of the lunate in the dorsal direction. Compare with Figure 7–18B. (Courtesy of Jon Marion, CHT, OTR, and Thomas Hitchcock, MD. Marshfield Clinic, Marshfield, WI.)

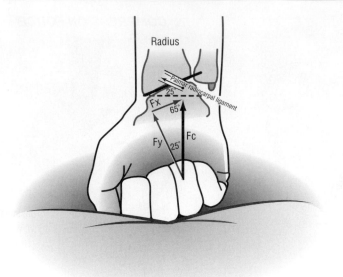

**FIGURE 7–20.** This shows how the ulnar tilt of the distal radius can predispose an individual to ulnar translocation of the carpus. Compression forces ($F_C$) that cross the wrist are resolved into (1) a force vector acting perpendicularly to the radiocarpal joint ($F_y$) and (2) a force vector ($F_x$) running parallel to the radiocarpal joint. The $F_y$ force compresses and stabilizes the radiocarpal joint with a magnitude of about 90% of $F_C$ (cosine 25 degrees × $F_C$). The $F_x$ force tends to translate the carpus in an ulnar direction, however, with a magnitude of 42% of $F_C$ (sine 25 degrees × $F_C$). Note that the fiber direction of the palmar radiocarpal ligaments resists this natural ulnar translation of the carpus. The greater the ulnar tilt and/or the greater the compression force across the wrist, the greater the potential for the ulnar translation.

## MUSCLE AND JOINT INTERACTION

### Innervation of the Wrist Muscles and Joints

#### MOTOR INNERVATION TO MUSCLE

The *radial nerve* supplies all the muscles that cross the dorsal side of the wrist (see Fig. 6–33B). Muscles with prime action at the wrist are the extensor carpi radialis longus, extensor carpi radialis brevis, and extensor carpi ulnaris. The *median and ulnar nerves* innervate all muscles that cross the palmar side of the wrist, including the primary wrist flexors (Fig. 6–33C and D). The flexor carpi radialis and palmaris longus are innervated by the median nerve; the flexor carpi ulnaris is innervated by the ulnar nerve. The motor nerve roots that supply all the muscles of the upper limb are listed in Appendix IIA. Appendix IIB shows the key muscles typically used to test the functional status of the $C^5$-$T^1$ ventral nerve roots.

#### SENSORY INNERVATION TO THE JOINTS

The radiocarpal and midcarpal joints receive sensory fibers from the $C^{6,7}$ nerve roots carried in the median and radial nerves.[7,8] The midcarpal joint is also innervated by sensory nerves traveling to the $C^8$ nerve root via the deep branch of the ulnar nerve.[7]

## Function of the Muscles at the Wrist

Other than the flexor carpi ulnaris, no tendon of any extrinsic muscle attaches directly to the carpal bones. Most muscles exert their primary action at the wrist through their distal attachments to the base of the metacarpals and phalanges. Extrinsic muscles to the hand, such as the extensor pollicis longus and the flexor digitorum superficialis, are considered in detail in Chapter 8. The attachments and nerve supply of the muscles of the wrist can be found in Appendix IIC.

As depicted in Figure 7–12, the axis of rotation for all wrist motion is located at the base of the capitate. No wrist muscle actually crosses the wrist directly anterior-posterior or medial-lateral to this axis of rotation. All muscles, therefore, have moment arms of varying lengths to produce torques in both the sagittal and frontal planes. The extensor carpi radialis brevis, for example, passes dorsally to the wrist's medial-lateral axis of rotation and laterally to the wrist's anterior-posterior axis of rotation. This muscle has a moment arm for wrist extension as well as radial deviation.

Table 7–2 lists the cross-sectional areas of most muscles that cross the wrist. This information helps predict a muscle's relative force potential.[13] Some research describes the position and length of moment arms for most wrist muscles as they cross the head of the capitate.[35] Combining these data provides a useful method for estimating the action and relative torque potential of wrist muscles (Fig. 7–21). Consider, for instance, the extensor carpi ulnaris and the flexor carpi ulnaris. By noting the location of each muscle from the axis of rotation, it is evident that the extensor carpi ulnaris is an extensor and ulnar deviator, and the flexor carpi ulnaris is a flexor and ulnar deviator. Because both muscles have similar cross-sectional areas, they likely produce comparable levels of maximal force. In order to estimate the relative

| TABLE 7–2. Cross-sectional Area of Most Muscles that Cross the Wrist | |
|---|---|
| **Potential Wrist *Flexor*** | **Cross-sectional Area (cm²)** |
| Flexor digitorum profundus | 10.8 |
| Flexor digitorum superficialis | 10.7 |
| Flexor carpi ulnaris | 5.0 |
| Flexor pollicis longus | 2.9 |
| Flexor carpi radialis | 2.16 |
| Abductor pollicis longus | 1.84 |
| Extensor pollicis brevis* | .40 |
| All flexor muscles | 33.8 |
| **Potential Wrist *Extensor*** | **Cross-sectional Area (cm²)** |
| Extensor carpi ulnaris | 5.30 |
| Extensor digitorum communis | 4.30 |
| Extensor carpi radialis longus | 3.14 |
| Extensor carpi radialis brevis | 2.22 |
| Extensor pollicis longus | .56 |
| All extensor muscles† | 15.5 |

\* Estimated.
† Excluding the extensor indicis and extensor digiti minimi.
(Data from Fick R: Lehmkuhl LD, Smith LK: Brunnstrom's Clinical Kinesiology, 4th ed. Philadelphia, FA Davis, 1983.)

**FIGURE 7–21.** A distal perspective through the right carpal tunnel similar to that in Figure 7–5. The plot shows the *cross-sectional area* and the *internal moment arm* for most muscles that cross the wrist at the level of the head of the capitate. The area each muscle occupies on the grid is proportional to its cross-section area and, therefore, is indicative of relative maximal force production. The wrist's medial-lateral (ML) axis of rotation (gray) and anterior-posterior (AP) axis of rotation (red) intersect at the capitate bone. Each muscle's internal moment arm for a particular action is equal to the linear distance each muscle lies from either axis. The length of each internal moment arm (expressed in cm) is indicated by the major tic marks. Assume that the wrist is held in a neutral position.

**Dorsal view**

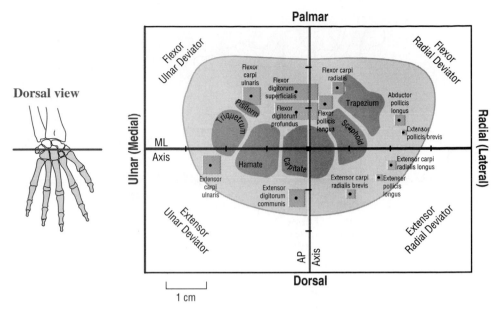

torque production, however, each muscle's cross-sectional area must be multiplied by the appropriate internal moment arm. The extensor carpi ulnaris, therefore, is considered a more potent ulnar deviator than an extensor; the flexor carpi ulnaris is considered both a potent flexor and a potent ulnar deviator.

## FUNCTION OF THE WRIST EXTENSORS

### Muscular Anatomy

The three primary wrist extensors are the *extensor carpi radialis longus,* the *extensor carpi radialis brevis,* and the *extensor carpi ulnaris* (Fig. 7–22). The extensor digitorum communis is capable of generating significant wrist extension torque, but is primarily involved with finger extension. Other secondary wrist extensors are the extensor indicis, extensor digiti minimi, and extensor pollicis longus. The function of these muscles is studied in greater detail in Chapter 8.

---

**Wrist Extensor Muscles**

*Primary*
- Extensor carpi radialis longus
- Extensor carpi radialis brevis
- Extensor carpi ulnaris

*Secondary*
- Extensor digitorum communis
- Extensor indicis
- Extensor digiti minimi
- Extensor pollicis longus

---

The proximal attachments of the primary wrist extensors are located on and near the lateral ("extensor-supinator") epicondyle of the humerus and dorsal border of the ulna (see Figs. 6–2 and 6–6). Distally, the extensor carpi radialis longus and brevis attach side by side to the dorsal bases of the second and third metacarpals; the extensor carpi ulnaris attaches to the dorsal base of the fifth metacarpal.

**Posterior view**

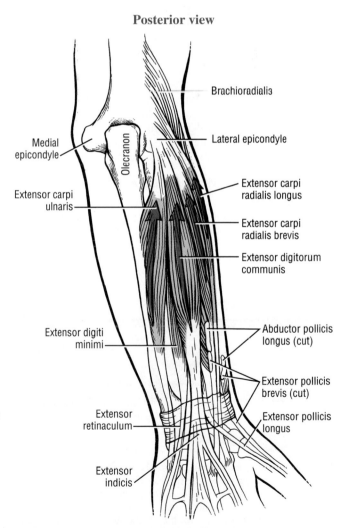

**FIGURE 7–22.** A posterior view of the right forearm showing the primary wrist extensor muscles: extensor carpi radialis longus, extensor carpi radialis brevis, and extensor carpi ulnaris. The extensor digitorum communis is depicted as a wrist extensor because of its large potential to assist with this action. Many of the secondary wrist extensors are also shown.

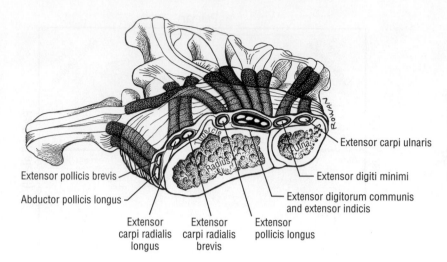

**FIGURE 7–23.** A dorsal oblique view shows a cross-section of the tendons of the extensor muscles of the wrist and digits passing through the extensor retinaculum of the wrist. All muscles that cross the dorsal aspect of the wrist travel within one of six fibrous tunnels embedded within the extensor retinaculum. Synovial lining is indicated by red.

The tendons of the muscles that cross the dorsal and dorsal-radial side of the wrist are secured in place across the wrist by the *extensor retinaculum* (Fig. 7–23). The extensor retinaculum wraps around the styloid process of the ulna to attach palmarly to the flexor carpi ulnaris, pisiform, and pisometacarpal ligament. The retinaculum attaches to the styloid process of the radius and the radial collateral ligament. Between the extensor retinaculum and the dorsal surface of the wrist are six fibro-osseus tunnels that house the tendons along with their synovial sheaths. The extensor retinaculum prevents the tendons from "bowstringing" up and away from the radiocarpal joint during active extension. The retinaculum and associated tendons also assist the dorsal capsular ligaments in stabilizing the dorsal side of the wrist.

### Wrist Extensor Activity While Making a Fist

The main function of the wrist extensors is to position and stabilize the wrist for activities involving the fingers. Of particular importance is the role of the wrist extensor muscles in making a fist. To demonstrate this, rapidly tighten and release the fist and note the strong synchronous activity from the wrist extensors. The extrinsic finger flexor muscles, namely the flexor digitorum profundus and flexor digitorum superficialis, pass a significant distance palmar to the wrist's medial-lateral axis of rotation (see Fig. 7–21). Their contraction as primary finger flexors generates a significant flexion torque at the wrist that must be counterbalanced by the extensor muscles (Fig. 7–24). As a strong grip is applied to an object, the wrist extensors hold the wrist in about 35 degrees of extension and about 5 degrees of ulnar deviation.[19] This position optimizes the length-tension relationship of the extrinsic finger flexors, thereby facilitating maximal grip strength (Fig. 7–25).

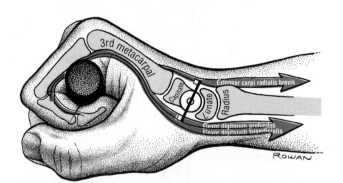

**FIGURE 7–24.** Muscle mechanics are shown that are involved with the application of a strong grip. Contraction of the long finger flexors flex the fingers but also cause a simultaneous *wrist flexion torque.* Activation of the wrist extensors, such as the extensor carpi radialis brevis, is necessary to block the wrist flexion tendency caused by activated finger flexors. In this manner, the wrist extensors are able to maintain the optimal length of the finger flexors to effectively flex the fingers. The internal moment arms for the extensor carpi radialis brevis and finger flexors are shown in dark bold lines.

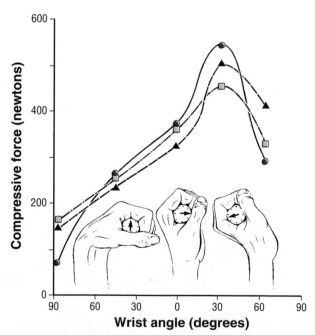

**FIGURE 7–25.** The compression forces produced by a maximal effort grip are shown for different wrist positions. Maximal grip force occurs at about 30 degrees of extension. (Data are from three subjects. With permission from Inman VT, Ralston HJ, Todd F: Human Walking. Baltimore, Williams & Wilkins, 1981.)

The most active wrist extensor muscle during light closure of the fist is the extensor carpi radialis brevis. As grip force increases, the extensor carpi ulnaris, followed closely by the extensor carpi radialis longus, joins the activated extensor brevis.[24] Activities that require repetitive forceful grasp, such as hammering or playing tennis, may overwork the wrist extensors, especially the highly active extensor carpi radialis brevis. A condition known as lateral epicondylitis, or "tennis elbow," occurs from stress and resultant inflammation of the proximal attachment of the wrist extensors.[4]

As evident in Figure 7–25, grip strength is significantly reduced when the wrist is fully flexed. The decreased grip strength is caused by a combination of two factors. First, and likely foremost, the finger flexors cannot generate adequate force because they are functioning at an extremely shortened (slackened) length on their length-tension curve. Second, the overstretched finger extensors, particularly the extensor digitorum communis, create a passive extensor torque at the fingers, which further reduces effective grip force. This combination of physiologic events explains why a person with paralyzed wrist extensors has difficulty producing an effective grip even though the finger flexors remain fully innervated. Attempts at producing a maximal-effort grip when the wrist extensors are paralyzed results in a posture of finger flexion with wrist flexion (Fig. 7–26A). Stabilizing the wrist in greater extension enables the finger flexor muscles to nearly triple their grip force (Fig. 7–26B). Manually or orthotically preventing the wrist from flexing maintains the extrinsic finger flexors at an elongated length more conducive to the higher force production.

Ordinarily, the person depicted in Figure 7–26 wears a splint that holds the wrist in 10 to 20 degrees of extension. When the radial nerve fails to re-innervate the wrist extensor muscles, a tendon from another muscle is often surgically transferred to provide wrist extension torque. Often, the pronator teres muscle, innervated by the median nerve, is connected to the tendon of the extensor carpi radialis brevis. Of the three primary wrist extensors, the extensor carpi radialis brevis is located most centrally at the wrist and has the greatest moment arm for extension (see Fig. 7–21).

---

**Wrist Flexor Muscles**

*Primary*
- Flexor carpi radialis
- Flexor carpi ulnaris
- Palmaris longus

*Secondary*
- Flexor digitorum profundus
- Flexor digitorum superficialis
- Flexor pollicis longus

---

## FUNCTION OF THE WRIST FLEXORS

### Muscular Anatomy

The three primary wrist flexors are the *flexor carpi radialis,* the *flexor carpi ulnaris,* and, when present and fully formed, the *palmaris longus* (Fig. 7–27). The palmaris longus is missing in about 10% of people, however. When present, it is extremely variable and may have several small tendons. Tendons of these muscles are easily identified on the anterior distal wrist, especially during strong isometric activation. The palmar carpal ligament, not easily identified by palpation, is located proximal to the transverse carpal ligament. This structure, analogous to the extensor retinaculum, stabilizes the tendons of the wrist flexors and prevents excessive bowstringing during flexion.

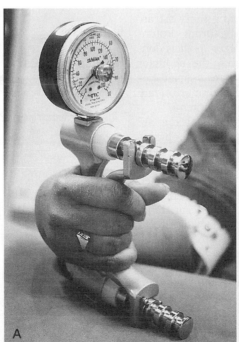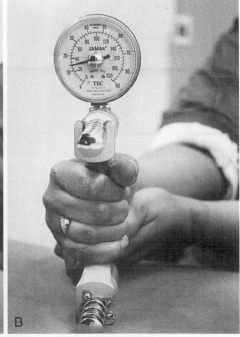

**FIGURE 7–26.** A person with paralysis of the right wrist extensor muscles, following a radial nerve injury, is performing a maximal effort grip using a dynamometer. *A,* Despite normally innervated finger flexor muscles, maximal grip strength measures only about 10 pounds. *B,* The same person is shown stabilizing her wrist in order to prevent it from flexing during the grip effort. Note that the grip force has nearly tripled.

**Anterior view**

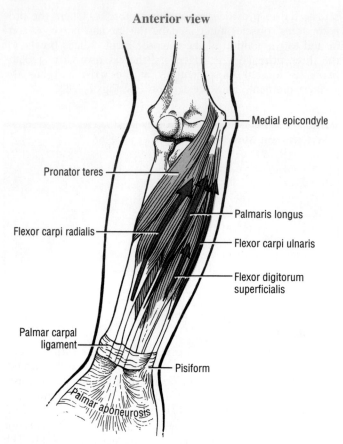

Medial epicondyle

Pronator teres

Palmaris longus

Flexor carpi radialis

Flexor carpi ulnaris

Flexor digitorum superficialis

Palmar carpal ligament

Pisiform

Palmar aponeurosis

**FIGURE 7–27.** Anterior view of the right forearm showing the primary wrist flexors muscles: flexor carpi radialis, palmaris longus, and flexor carpi ulnaris. The flexor digitorum superficialis is shown as a wrist flexor because of its large potential to assist with this action. The pronator teres muscle is shown but does not flex the wrist.

*Functional Considerations of the Wrist Flexors*

Based on internal moment arm and cross-sectional area (see Fig. 7–21 and Table 7–2), the flexor carpi ulnaris produces the greatest flexor torque of the three primary wrist flexor muscles.

In addition to the primary wrist flexors, the extensor carpi ulnaris demonstrates significant electromyographic (EMG) activity during active wrist flexion.[1] This EMG activity reflects eccentric activity from the muscle, as it produces a force to assist the ulnar collateral ligament with stability of the ulnar side of the wrist. The ulnocarpal space is inherently fragile due to its lack of bony reinforcement (see Fig. 7–10).

The flexor carpi radialis and ulnaris function synergistically to flex the wrist; however, they oppose each other's radial and ulnar deviation ability (see Fig. 7–21). Depending on the relative activation level of the two muscles, a posture of wrist flexion is combined with varying degrees of radial or ulnar deviation.

Table 7–2 shows that muscles that flex the wrist have a total cross-sectional area twice that of the muscles that extend the wrist. A similar disparity is observed in the strength dominance of the flexors over the extensors (Table 7–3). Of particular interest are the extrinsic finger flexors (flexors digitorum superficialis and profundus) that account for about two thirds of the total cross-sectional area of the wrist flexors. Many activities that require a powerful grip, such as lifting and pulling heavy objects, also require large isometric wrist flexor torques. Co-activation of the wrist extensors is usually required to position the wrist toward extension in

Other secondary muscles capable of flexing the wrist are the extrinsic flexors of the digits (flexor digitorum profundus, flexor digitorum superficialis, and flexor pollicis longus). With the wrist in a neutral position, the abductor pollicis longus and extensor pollicis brevis have a small moment arm for wrist flexion (see Fig. 7–21). These secondary wrist muscles are studied in greater detail in Chapter 8.

The proximal attachments of the primary wrist flexors are located on and near the medial ("flexor-pronator") epicondyle of the humerus and dorsal border of the ulna (see Figs. 6–2, 6–3, and 6–6). Technically, the tendon of the flexor carpi radialis does not cross the wrist in the carpal tunnel; rather, the tendon passes in a separate tunnel formed by a groove in the trapezium and fascia from the adjacent transverse carpal ligament (Fig. 7–28). The tendon of the flexor carpi radialis attaches distally to the palmar base of the second and, sometimes, the third metacarpal. The palmaris longus has an extensive distal attachment primarily into the thick aponeurosis of the palm of the hand. The tendon of the flexor carpi ulnaris courses distally to attach to the pisiform bone and, in a plane superficial to the transverse carpal ligament, into the pisohamate and pisometacarpal ligaments and the palmar base of the fifth metacarpal bone.

**Palmar view**

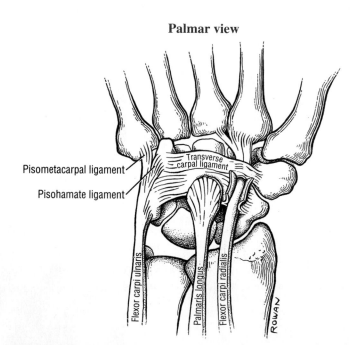

Pisometacarpal ligament

Transverse carpal ligament

Pisohamate ligament

Flexor carpi ulnaris

Palmaris longus

Flexor carpi radialis

ROWAN

**FIGURE 7–28.** The palmar aspect of the right wrist showing the distal attachments of the primary wrist flexors. Note that the tendon of the flexor carpi radialis courses through a sheath located within the superficial fibers of the transverse carpal ligament. Most of the distal attachment of the palmaris longus has been removed with the palmar aponeurosis.

| TABLE 7–3. Magnitude and Joint Position of Peak Isometric Torque for Wrist Movements | | |
|---|---|---|
| **Wrist Movement** | **Mean Peak Torque (Nm)** | **Angles of Peak Torque** |
| Flexion | 12.2 (3.7) | 40° of flexion |
| Extension | 7.1 (2.1) | From 30° of flexion to 70° of extension |
| Radial deviation | 11 (2) | 0° (neutral) |
| Ulnar deviation | 9.5 (2.2) | 0° (neutral) |

Standard deviations in parenthesis. Results from study of ten healthy adult males.

Conversions: 1.36 N-m/ft-lb.

(Data from Delp SL, Grierson AE, Buchanan TS: Maximum isometric moments generated by the wrist muscles in flexion-extension and radial-ulnar deviation. J Biomechan 29:1371–1375, 1996.)

order to maintain favorable activation length of the finger flexors.

## FUNCTION OF THE RADIAL AND ULNAR DEVIATORS

Muscles capable of producing radial deviation of the wrist are the extensor carpi radialis brevis and longus, extensor pollicis longus and brevis, flexor carpi radialis, abductor pollicis longus, and flexor pollicis longus (see Fig. 7–21). In the neutral wrist position, the extensor carpi radialis longus possesses the largest product of cross-sectional area and the moment arm for radial deviation torque, followed by the abductor pollicis longus and the extensor carpi radialis brevis. The extensor pollicis brevis has the greatest moment arm of all radial deviators; however, because of a very small cross-sectional area, this muscle's torque production is likely small. The abductor pollicis longus and extensor pollicis brevis provide important stability to the radial side of the wrist along with the radial collateral ligament. As shown in

Table 7–3, the radial deviator muscles generate about 15% greater isometric torque than the ulnar deviator muscles.[6]

| Radial Deviators of the Wrist |
|---|
| • Extensor carpi radialis longus |
| • Extensor carpi radialis brevis |
| • Extensor pollicis longus |
| • Extensor pollicis brevis |
| • Flexor carpi radialis |
| • Abductor pollicis longus |
| • Flexor pollicis longus |

Figure 7–29 shows the radial deviator muscles contracting while using a hammer. All these muscles pass laterally to the wrist's anterior-posterior axis of rotation. The action of the extensor carpi radialis longus and the flexor carpi radialis, shown with moment arms, illustrates a fine example of two muscles cooperating as synergists for one action and acting as antagonists in another. By opposing each other's flexion and extension potential, these muscles stabilize the wrist in an extended position necessary to grasp the hammer effectively.

The primary muscles capable of ulnar deviation of the wrist are the extensor carpi ulnaris and the flexor carpi ulnaris. Figure 7–30 shows both ulnar deviator muscles contracting to drive a nail with a hammer. Both the flexor and extensor carpi ulnaris contract synergistically to perform the ulnar deviation, but also stabilize the wrist in a slightly extended position. Because of the strong functional association between the flexor and extensor carpi ulnaris muscles, injury to either muscle can incapacitate the overall kinetics of ulnar deviation. For example, rheumatoid arthritis often causes inflammation and pain in the extensor carpi ulnaris tendon near its distal attachment. Attempts at active ulnar deviation with minimal to no activation in the painful extensor carpi ulnaris causes the action of the flexor carpi ulnaris

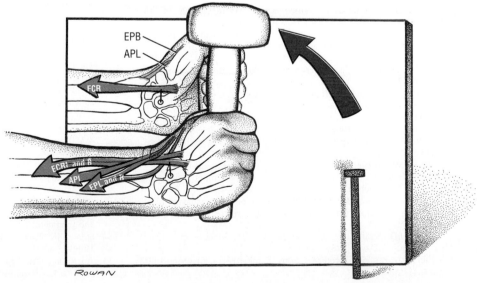

**FIGURE 7–29.** The muscles that perform radial deviation of the wrist are shown preparing to strike a nail with a hammer. Images in the background are mirror reflections of objects in the foreground. The axis of rotation is through the capitate with the internal moment arms shown for the extensor carpi radialis brevis (ECRB) and the flexor carpi radialis (FCR) only. The flexor pollicis longus is not shown. (ECRL and B = extensor carpi radialis longus and brevis; APL = abductor pollicis longus; and EPL and B = extensor pollicis longus and brevis.)

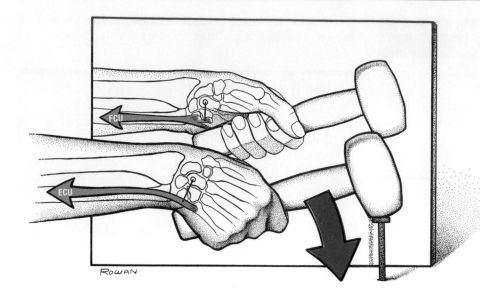

**FIGURE 7–30.** The muscles that perform ulnar deviation are shown striking a nail with a hammer. The images in the background are a mirror reflection of the objects in the foreground. The axis of rotation is shown through the capitate with internal moment arms shown for the flexor carpi ulnaris (FCU) and the extensor carpi ulnaris (ECU).

to remain unopposed. The resulting flexed posture of the wrist is thereby not suitable for an effective grasp.

---

**Ulnar Deviators of the Wrist**

- Extensor carpi ulnaris
- Flexor carpi ulnaris

---

## REFERENCES

1. Backdahl M, Carlsoo S: Distribution of activity in muscles acting on the wrist. Acta Morph. Neerl Scand 4:136–144, 1961.
2. Berger RA: The ligaments of the wrist: A current overview of anatomy with consideration of their potential functions. Hand Clin 13:63–82, 1997.
3. Berger RA, Imeada T, Berglund L, et al: Constraint and material properties of the subregions of the scapholunate interosseous ligament. J Hand Surg 24:953–962, 1999.
4. Blackwell JR, Cole KJ: Wrist kinematics differ in expert and novice tennis players performing the backhand stroke: Implications for tennis elbow. J Biomech 27:509–516, 1994.
5. Brumfield RH, Champoux JA: A biomechanical study of normal functional wrist motion. Clin Orthop 187:23–25, 1984.
6. Delp SL, Grierson AE, Buchanan TS: Maximum isometric moments generated by the wrist muscles in flexion-extension and radial-ulnar deviation. J Biomechan 29:1371–1375, 1996.
7. Gray DJ, Gardner E: The innervation of the joints of the wrist and hand. Anat Rec 151:261–266, 1965.
8. Inman VT, Saunders JB: Referred pain from skeletal structures. J Nerv Ment Dis 99:660–667, 1944.
9. Kapandji IA: The Physiology of the Joints, vol. 1, 5th ed. Edinburgh, Churchill Livingstone, 1982.
10. Kauer JMG. The mechanism of the carpal joint. Clin Orthop 202:16–26, 1986.
11. Kobayashi MK, Berger RA, Nagy L, et al: Normal kinematics of carpal bones: A three-dimensional analysis of carpal bone motion relative to the radius. J Biomechan 30:787–793, 1997.
12. Lange A de, Kauer JMG, Huiskes R: The kinematic behavior of the human wrist joint: A roentgen-stereophotogrammetric analysis. Orthop Res 3:56–64, 1985.
13. Lehmkuhl LD, Smith LK: Brunnstrom's Clinical Kinesiology, 4th ed. Philadelphia, FA Davis, 1983.
14. Linscheid RL: Kinematic considerations of the wrist. Clin Orthop 202:27–39, 1986.
15. MacConaill MA, Basmajian JV: Muscles and Movements: A Basis for Human Kinesiology. New York, Robert E. Krieger, 1977.
16. Mayfield JK, Johnson RP, Kilcoyne RF: The ligaments of the human wrist and their functional significance. Anat Rec 186:417–428, 1976.
17. Neumann DA: Observations from cineradiography analysis. Marquette University, Milwaukee, WI, 2000.
18. Norkin CC, White DJ: Measurement of Joint Motion: A Guide to Goniometry, 2nd ed. Philadelphia, FA Davis, 1995.
19. O'Driscoll SW, Horii E, Ness R, et al: The relationship between wrist position, grasp size, and grip strength. J Hand Surg 17A:169–177, 1992.
20. Palmer AK, Werner FW: Biomechanics of the distal radioulnar joint. Clin Orthop 187:26–35, 1984.
21. Palmer AK, Werner FW, Murphy D, et al: Functional wrist motion: A biomechanical study. J Hand Surg 10A:39–46, 1985
22. Palmer AK, Skahen JR, Werner FW, et al: The extensor retinaculum of the wrist: An anatomical and biomechanical study. J Hand Surg 10B:11–16, 1985.
23. Patterson RM, Nicodemus CL, Viegas SF, et al: High-speed, three-dimensional kinematic analysis of the normal wrist. J Hand Surg 23A:446–453, 1998.
24. Radonjic D, Long C: Kinesiology of the wrist. Am J Phys Med 50:57–71, 1971.
25. Ritt MJ, Stuart PR, Berglund LJ, et al: Rotational stability of the carpus relative to the forearm. J Hand Surg 20A:305–311, 1995.
26. Ruby LK, Cooney WP, An KN, et al: Relative motion of selected carpal bones: A kinematic analysis of the normal wrist. J Hand Surg 13A:1–10, 1988.
27. Safaee-Rad R, Shwedyk E, Quanbury AO, et al: Normal functional range of motion of upper limb joints during performance of three feeding activities. Arch Phys Med Rehabili 71:505–509, 1990.
28. Salmon J, Stanley JK, Trail IA: Kienbock's disease: Conservative management versus radial shortening. J Bone Joint Surg 82B:820–823, 2000.
29. Sarrafian SK, Melamed JL, Goshgarian GM: Study of wrist motion in flexion and extension. Clin Orthop 126:153–159, 1977.
30. Savelberg HHCM, Kooloos JGM, Huiskes R, et al: Strains and forces in selected carpal ligaments during in vitro flexion and deviation movements of the hand. J Orthop Res 10:901–910, 1992.
31. Shin AY, Battaglia MJ, Bishop AT: Lunotriquetral instability: Diagnosis and treatment. J Am Acad Orthop Surg 8:170–179, 2000
32. Stanley JK, Trail IA: Carpal instability. J Bone Joint Surg 76B:691–700, 1994.
33. Taleisnik J: The ligaments of the wrist. In Taleisnik J (ed): The Wrist. New York, Churchill Livingstone, 1985.

34. Tang JB, Ryu J, Han JS, et al: Biomechanical changes of the wrist flexor and extensor tendons following loss of scaphoid integrity. J Orthop Res 15:69–75, 1997.

35. Tolbert JR, Blair, WF, Andrews JG, et al: The kinetics of normal and prosthetic wrists. J Biomech 18:887–897, 1985.

36. Weaver L, Tencer AF, Trumble TE: Tensions in the palmar ligaments of the wrist. The normal wrist. J Hand Surg 19A:464–474, 1994.

37. Weber ER: Concepts governing the rotational shift of the intercalated segment of the carpus. Orthop Clin North Am 15:193–207, 1984.

38. Williams PL, Bannister IH, Berry M, et al: Gray's Anatomy, 38th ed, New York, Churchill Livingstone, 1995.

39. Wright PE: Wrist. In Crenshaw AH (ed): Campbells's Operative Orthopaedics, vol 5, 8th ed. St. Louis, Mosby, 1992.

40. Youm Y, McMurty RY, Flatt AE, et al: Kinematics of the wrist. I: An experimental study of radial-ulnar deviation and flexion-extension. J Bone Joint Surg 60A:423–431, 1978.

41. Youm Y, Flatt AE: Kinematics of the wrist. Clin Orthop 149:21–32, 1980.

## ADDITIONAL READINGS

Berger RA: The anatomy and the basic biomechanics of the wrist joint. J Hand Surg 9:84–93, 1996.

Green DP: Carpal dislocations and instabilities. In Green DP (ed): Operative Hand Surgery, vol 1, 3rd ed. New York, Churchill Livingstone, 1993.

Jackson WT, Hefzy, Guo H: Determination of wrist kinematics using a magnetic tracking device. Med Eng Phys 16:123–133, 1994.

Kauer JMG. Functional anatomy of the wrist. Clin Orthop 149:9–20, 1980.

Kobayashi M, Berger RA, Linscheid RL, et al: Intercarpal kinematics during wrist motion. Hand Clin 13:143–149, 1997.

Schubert HE: Scaphoid fracture. Review of diagnostic tests and treatment. Can Fam Physician. 46:1825–1832, 2000.

Short WH, Werner FW, Fortino MD, et al: A dynamic biomechanical study of scapholunate ligament sectioning. J Hand Surg 20A:986–999, 1995.

Simoneau GG, Marklin RW, Monroe JF: Wrist and forearm postures of users of conventional computer keyboards. Hum Factors 41:413–424, 1999.

Stanley JK, Trail IA: Carpal instability. J Bone Joint Surg 76B:691–699, 1995.

Stuchin SA: Wrist anatomy. Hand Clin 8:603–609, 1992.

Sun JS, Shih TT, Ko CM, et al: In vivo kinematic study of normal wrist motion: An ultrafast computed topographic study. Clin Biomech 15:212–216, 2000.

Timins ME, Jahnke JP, Krah SF, et al: MR imaging of the major carpal stabilizing ligaments: Normal anatomy and clinical examples. Radiographics 15:575–587, 1995.

Wolfe SW, Crisco JJ, Katz LD: A noninvasive method for studying in vivo carpal kinematics. J Hand Surg 22B:147–152, 1997.

# CHAPTER 8

# *Hand*

DONALD A. NEUMANN, PT, PHD

## TOPICS AT A GLANCE

## INTRODUCTION

### Background

Just as our eyes and skin do, the hand serves as an important sensory organ for the perception of our surroundings (Fig. 8–1). The hand is also the primary effector organ for our most complex motor behaviors. And, the hands help to express emotions through gesture, touch, craft, and art.

The 19 bones and 19 articulations within the hand are driven by 29 muscles. Biomechanically, these structures interact with superb proficiency. The hand may be used in a very primitive fashion, such as a hook or a club. More often, however, the hand functions as a highly specialized instrument performing very complex manipulations, requiring infinite levels of force and precision.

Because of its enormous biomechanical complexity, the function of the hand involves a disproportionately large re-

gion of the cortex of the brain (Fig. 8–2). Diseases or injuries affecting the hand often create equally disproportionate disabilities. A hand totally incapacitated by rheumatoid arthritis or nerve injury, for instance, can dramatically reduce the functional importance of the remaining joints of the upper limb. This chapter describes the kinesiologic principles behind many of the musculoskeletal problems encountered in medical and rehabilitation settings.

## TERMINOLOGY

The wrist, or carpus, has eight carpal bones. The hand has five metacarpals, often referred to collectively as the "metacarpus." Each of the five digits contains a set of phalanges. The digits are designated numerically from one to five, or as the thumb and the index, middle, ring, and little fingers

194

security of grasp. The location of the creases serves as useful clinical references for the underlying anatomy. The distal and middle *digital creases* are superficial to the DIP and PIP joints. The proximal digital creases are located distal to the actual joint line of the MCP joints. The proximal and distal palmar creases are enhanced by the folding of the dermis during flexion of the MCP joints of the fingers. The *thenar crease* is formed by the folding of the dermis as the thumb is moved across the palm. On the palmar (anterior) side of the wrist are the proximal and distal *wrist creases*.

## OSTEOLOGY

### Metacarpals

The metacarpals, like the digits, are designated numerically as one through five, beginning on the radial (lateral) side.

The morphology of each metacarpal is generally similar (Figs. 8–4 and 8–5). The first (thumb) metacarpal is the shortest and stoutest. Observe that the second metacarpal is usually the longest, and the length of the remaining three bones decreases from the radial to ulnar (medial) direction.

> **Osteologic Features of a Metacarpal**
> * Shaft
> * Base
> * Head
> * Posterior tubercles

Each metacarpal has an elongated *shaft* with articular surfaces at each end (Fig. 8–6). The palmar surface of the shaft is slightly concave longitudinally to accommodate many muscles and tendons in this region. Its proximal end, or *base,* articulates with one or more of the carpal bones. The bases of the second through the fifth metacarpal possess small facets for articulation with adjacent metacarpal bases.

The distal end of each metacarpal has a large convex *head* which, as a group, is evident as the "knuckles" on the dorsal side of a clenched fist. A pair of *posterior tubercles* marks the attachment sites for the collateral ligaments at the MCP joints.

With the hand at rest in the anatomic position, the thumb's metacarpal is oriented in a different plane from the other digits. The second through the fifth metacarpals are aligned generally side-by-side, with their palmar surfaces facing anteriorly. The position of the thumb's metacarpal, however, is rotated almost 90 degrees medially (i.e., internally), relative to the other digits (see Fig. 8–3A). Rotation places the sensitive palmar surface of the thumb toward the midline of the hand. Optimum prehension depends on flexion of the thumb occurring in a plane that intersects, versus parallels, the plane of the flexing fingers. In addition, the thumb's metacarpal is positioned well anterior, or palmar, to the other metacarpals (Fig. 8–7). This position of the metacarpal and trapezium is caused by the palmar projection of the distal pole of the scaphoid.

The location of the first metacarpal allows the entire thumb to sweep freely across the palm toward the fingers. Virtually all prehensile motions, from pinch to precision

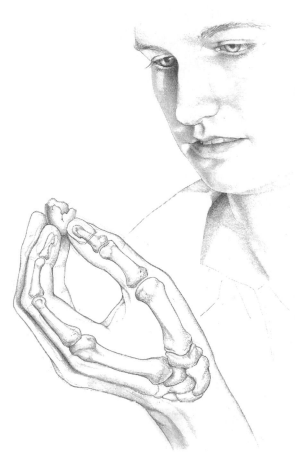

**FIGURE 8–1.** A very strong functional relationship exists between the hand and the eyes.

(Fig. 8–3A). A *ray* describes one metacarpal bone and its associated phalanges.

Each finger has two *interphalangeal joints:* a proximal interphalangeal (PIP) and a distal interphalangeal (DIP) joint (see Fig. 8–3A). The thumb has only two phalanges and, therefore, only one interphalangeal (IP) joint. The articulations between the metacarpals and the proximal phalanges are called the *metacarpophalangeal (MCP) joints.* The articulations between the proximal end of the metacarpals and the distal row of carpal bones are called the *carpometacarpal (CMC) joints.*

> **Articulations Common to Each "Ray" of the Hand**
> * Carpometacarpal (CMC) joint
> * Metacarpophalangeal (MCP) joint
> * Interphalangeal (IP) joints
>   Thumb has one IP joint
>   Fingers have a proximal interphalangeal (PIP) joint and a distal interphalangeal (DIP) joint

Figure 8–3B shows several features of the external anatomy of the hand. Observe the *palmar creases,* or folds, that exist in the skin of the palm. They function both as dermal "hinges," marking where the skin folds upon itself during movement, and to increase palmar friction to enhance the

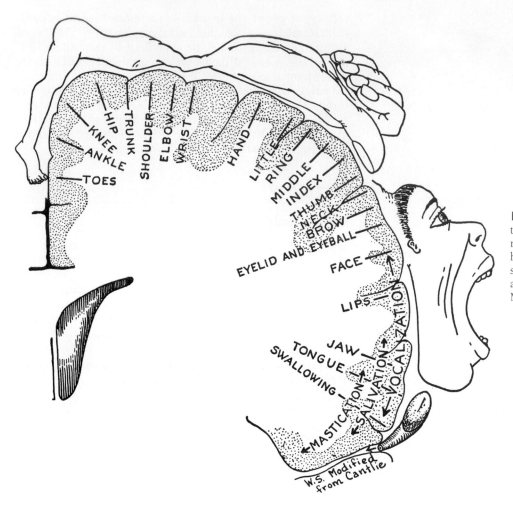

**FIGURE 8–2.** A motor homunculus of the brain showing the somatotopic representation of body parts. The sensory homunculus of the human brain has a similar representation. (After Penfield and Rosnussen: Cerebral Cortex of Man. The Macmillan Co., 1950.)

handling, require the thumb to interact with the fingers. Without a healthy and mobile thumb, the overall function of the hand is substantially reduced.

The medially rotated thumb requires unique terminology to describe its movement as well as position. In the anatomic position, the dorsal surface of the bones of the thumb (i.e., the surface where the thumbnail resides) faces laterally (Fig. 8–8). The palmar surface, therefore, faces medially, the radial surface anteriorly, and the ulnar surface posteriorly. The terminology to describe the surfaces of the carpal bones and all other digital bones is standard: a palmar surface faces anteriorly, radial surface faces laterally, and so forth.

## Phalanges

The hand has 14 phalanges (the Greek root *phalanx;* a line of soldiers). The phalanges within each finger are referred to as proximal, middle, and distal (Fig. 8–3A). The thumb has only a proximal and a distal phalanx.

---

**Osteologic Features of a Phalanx**
- Base
- Shaft
- Head
- Tuberosity (distal phalanx only)

---

Except for differences in sizes, all phalanges within a particular digit have similar morphology (see Figs. 8–4 and 8–5). The proximal and middle phalanges of each finger have a *concave base, shaft,* and *convex head.* Like the metacarpals, their palmar surfaces are slightly concave longitudinally (see Fig. 8–6). The distal phalanx of each digit has a concave base. At its distal end is a rounded *tuberosity* that anchors the fleshy pulp of soft tissue to the terminus of each digit.

## Arches of the Hand

Observe the natural concavity to the palmar surface of your relaxed hand. Control of this concavity allows the human hand to securely hold and manipulate objects of many and varied shapes and sizes. The natural palmar concavity of the hand is supported by three integrated arch systems: two transverse and one longitudinal (Fig. 8–9). The *proximal transverse arch* is formed by the distal row of carpal bones. This carpal arch is a static, rigid structure that forms the carpal tunnel. Like most arches in buildings and bridges, the arches of the hand are supported by a central keystone structure. The capitate bone is the keystone of the proximal transverse arch, reinforced by strong intercarpal ligaments.

The *distal transverse arch* passes through the MCP joints. In contrast to the rigidity of the proximal arch, the sides of

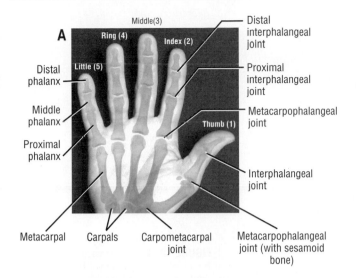

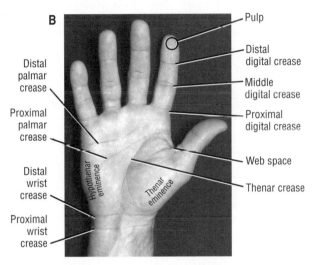

**FIGURE 8-3.** A palmar view of the basic anatomy of the hand. *A,* Major bones and joints. *B,* External landmarks.

the distal arch are mobile. To appreciate this mobility, imagine transforming your completely flat hand into a cup-shaped hand that surrounds a baseball. Transverse flexibility within the hand occurs by action of the peripheral metacarpals (first, fourth, and fifth) "collapsing" around the more stable central (second and third) metacarpals. The keystone of the distal transverse arch is formed by the MCP joints of these central metacarpals.

The *longitudinal arch* of the hand follows the general shape of the second and third rays. The metacarpal or proximal end of this arch is firmly linked to the carpus by the carpometacarpal (CMC) joints. These rigid articulations provide an important element of longitudinal stability to the hand. The phalangeal or distal end of the arch is very mobile. The mobility is exhibited by flexing and extending the fingers. The keystone of the longitudinal arch is provided by the second and third MCP joints. Note that the MCP joints serve as keystones to both the longitudinal and distal transverse arches.

As depicted in Figure 8-9, all three arches of the hand are mechanically interlinked. Both transverse arches are

joined together by the "rigid tie-beam" provided by the second and third metacarpals.[19] In the healthy hand, this mechanical linkage reinforces the entire arch system. In the hand with joint disease, however, a structural failure at any arch may weaken another. A classic example is the destruction of the MCP joints from severe rheumatoid arthritis. Because this joint is the common keystone for both the longitudinal and the distal transverse arches, its destruction has devastating effects on the entire arch system. This partially explains why a hand with severe rheumatoid arthritis often appears flat.

## ARTHROLOGY

The terminology that describes the movement of the fingers and thumb must be defined. The following descriptions assume that a particular movement starts from the anatomic position, with the elbow extended, forearm fully supinated, and wrist in a neutral position. Movement of the fingers is described in the standard fashion using the cardinal planes of the body: *flexion and extension* occur in the sagittal plane, and *abduction and adduction* occur in the frontal plane (Fig. 8-10A-D). The middle finger is the reference digit for the naming of abduction and adduction. The side-to-side movement of the middle finger is called radial and ulnar deviation.

Because the entire thumb is rotated almost 90 degrees in relation to the fingers, the terminology used to describe thumb movement is different from that for the fingers. *Flexion* is the movement of the palmar surface of the thumb in the frontal plane across the palm. *Extension* returns the thumb to its anatomic position. *Abduction* is the forward movement of the thumb away from the palm in a near sagittal plane. *Adduction* returns the thumb to the plane of the hand. Other terms frequently used to describe the movements of the thumb include ulnar adduction for flexion, radial abduction for extension, and palmar abduction for abduction.[55] *Opposition* is a special term describing the movement of the thumb across the palm, making direct contact with the tip of any of the fingers. *Reposition* is a movement from full opposition back to the anatomic position.

### Carpometacarpal Joints

#### OVERVIEW

The CMC joints of the hand form the articulation between the distal row of the carpal bones and the bases of the five metacarpal bones. The CMC joints are located at the very proximal end of the hand.

Figure 8-11 shows a mechanical illustration of the relative mobility at the CMC joints. The joints of the second and third digits shown in gray are rigidly joined to the distal carpus, forming a stable *central pillar* throughout the hand. In contrast, the more peripheral CMC joints shown in red form mobile radial and ulnar borders, which are capable of folding around the hand's central pillar, thereby altering the shape of the palm. The contrast in mobility at these two sets of joints accounts for the dynamics described earlier for the distal transverse arch.

**Palmar view**

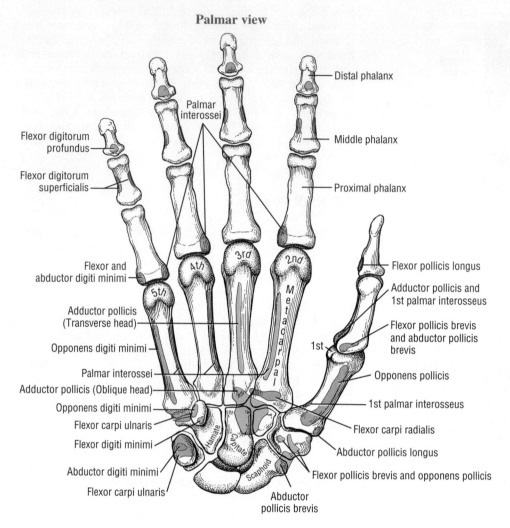

Flexor digitorum profundus

Flexor digitorum superficialis

Palmar interossei

Distal phalanx

Middle phalanx

Proximal phalanx

Flexor and abductor digiti minimi

Adductor pollicis (Transverse head)

Opponens digiti minimi

Palmar interossei

Adductor pollicis (Oblique head)

Opponens digiti minimi

Flexor carpi ulnaris

Flexor digiti minimi

Abductor digiti minimi

Flexor carpi ulnaris

Abductor pollicis brevis

Flexor pollicis longus

Adductor pollicis and 1st palmar interosseus

Flexor pollicis brevis and abductor pollicis brevis

Opponens pollicis

1st palmar interosseus

Flexor carpi radialis

Abductor pollicis longus

Flexor pollicis brevis and opponens pollicis

**FIGURE 8–4.** A palmar view of the bones of the right wrist and hand. Proximal attachments of muscle are indicated in red and distal attachments in gray.

The function of the CMC joints allows the concavity of the palm to fit around many objects. This feature is one of the most impressive functions of the human hand. Cylindric objects, for example, can fit snugly into the palm, with the index and middle digits positioned to reinforce the security of the grasp (Fig. 8–12). Without this ability, the dexterity of the hand is reduced to a primitive hingelike grasping motion.

## SECOND THROUGH FIFTH CARPOMETACARPAL JOINTS

### General Features and Ligamentous Support

The second CMC joint is formed through the articulation between the enlarged base of the second metacarpal and the distal surface of the trapezoid, and, to a lesser extent, the capitate and trapezium (see Figs. 8–4 and 8–5). The third CMC joint is formed primarily by the articulation between the base of the third metacarpal and the distal surface of the capitate. The fourth CMC joint is formed by the articulation of the base of the fourth metacarpal and the distal surface of the hamate and, to lesser extent, the capitate. The fifth CMC

joint consists of the articulation between the base of the fifth metacarpal and the distal surface of the hamate only. The bases of the second through fifth metacarpals have small facets for attachments to one another through intermetacarpal joints. These joints help stabilize the bases of the second through fifth metacarpals, thereby reinforcing the carpometacarpal joints.

All CMC joints of the fingers are surrounded by articular capsules and strengthened by dorsal, palmar, and interosseous ligaments. The dorsal ligaments are particularly well developed, especially around the middle CMC joint (Fig. 8–13).

### Joint Structure and Kinematics

The CMC joints of the second and third digits are classified as complex saddle joints (Fig. 8–14).[55] Their jagged interlocking articular surfaces provide very little movement. As mentioned earlier, stability at these joints allows the second and third metacarpals to provide the central pillar of the hand.

The flat to slightly convex base of the fourth and fifth metacarpals articulates with a slightly concave articular surface formed by the hamate (see Fig. 8–14).[17] Two ulnar

**Dorsal view**

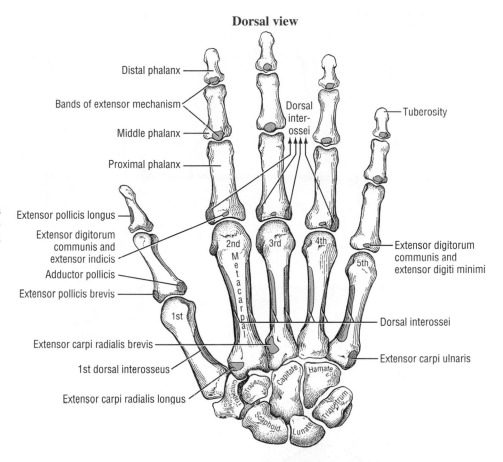

**FIGURE 8-5.** A dorsal view of the bones of the right wrist and hand. Proximal attachments of muscle are indicated in red and distal attachments in gray.

Labels on figure:
Distal phalanx
Bands of extensor mechanism
Middle phalanx
Proximal phalanx
Dorsal interossei
Tuberosity
Extensor pollicis longus
Extensor digitorum communis and extensor indicis
Adductor pollicis
Extensor pollicis brevis
Extensor carpi radialis brevis
1st dorsal interosseus
Extensor carpi radialis longus
Extensor digitorum communis and extensor digiti minimi
Dorsal interossei
Extensor carpi ulnaris
2nd Metacarpal
3rd
4th
5th
1st
Capitate
Hamate
Trapezoid
Trapezium
Scaphoid
Lunate

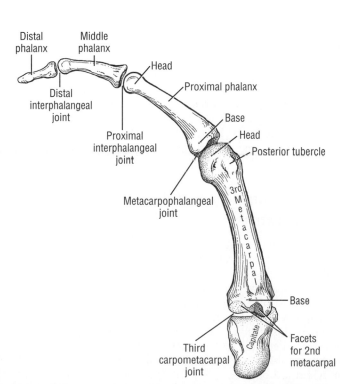

**FIGURE 8-6.** A radial view of the bones of the third ray (metacarpal and associated phalanges), including the capitate bone of the wrist.

Labels on figure:
Distal phalanx
Middle phalanx
Head
Proximal phalanx
Distal interphalangeal joint
Base
Head
Posterior tubercle
Proximal interphalangeal joint
Metacarpophalangeal joint
3rd Metacarpal
Base
Capitate
Third carpometacarpal joint
Facets for 2nd metacarpal

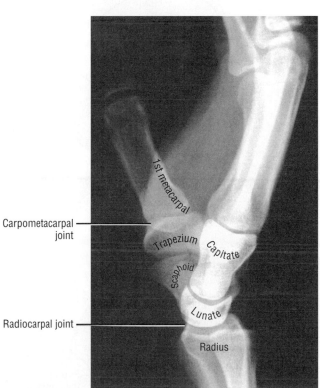

**FIGURE 8-7.** A lateral x-ray with an emphasis on the palmar projection of the thumb (first metacarpal), scaphoid, and trapezium. Note the contrast in the spatial orientation of the capitate and other metacarpal bones.

Labels on figure:
1st metacarpal
Carpometacarpal joint
Trapezium
Capitate
Scaphoid
Radiocarpal joint
Lunate
Radius

**Palmar view**

**Lateral view**

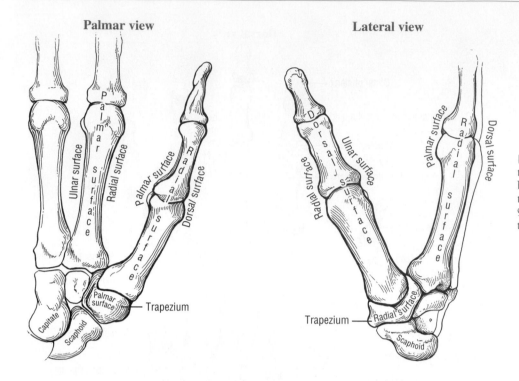

**FIGURE 8–8.** Palmar and lateral views of the hand showing the orientation of the bony surfaces of the right thumb. Note that the bones of the thumb are rotated 90 degrees relative to the other bones of the wrist and the hand.

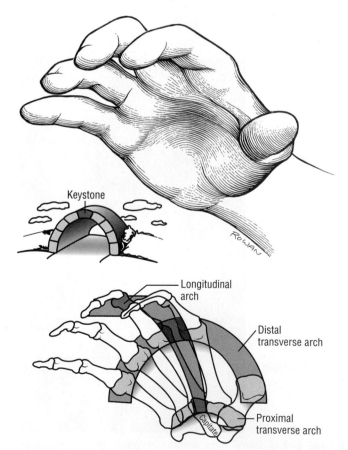

**FIGURE 8–9.** The natural concavity of the palm of the hand is supported by three integrated arch systems: one longitudinal and two transverse.

CMC joints contribute a subtle but important element of mobility to the hand.[3] As depicted in Figure 8–11, the articulations at the fourth and fifth CMC joints allow the ulnar border of the hand to fold slightly toward the center of the hand, thereby deepening the palmar concavity. Ulnar mobility, often referred to as a cupping motion, occurs by forward flexion and slight rotation of the ulnar metacarpals toward the middle digit. The fourth metacarpal flexes about 10 degrees, and the more mobile fifth metacarpal flexes about 20 to 25 degrees. The irregular and varied shapes of these joint surfaces prohibit standard arthrokinematic description. The mobility at these ulnar CMC joints can be appreciated by observing the movement of the fourth and fifth metacarpal heads while clenching a fist (Fig. 8–15).

## Carpometacarpal Joint of the Thumb

### GENERAL FEATURES

The CMC joint of the thumb is located between the base of the thumb metacarpal and the trapezium (see Fig. 8–4). This joint is by far the most complex of the CMC joints, enabling extensive movements of the thumb. The unique saddle shape of this joint allows the thumb to fully oppose, thereby easily contacting the tips of the other digits. Through this action, the thumb is able to encircle objects placed in the palm. Opposition greatly enhances the security of grasp, which is especially useful when holding spherical or cylindrical objects.

The large functional demands placed on the CMC joint of the thumb often result in a painful condition called "basilar" joint arthritis. The term basilar refers to the CMC joint being

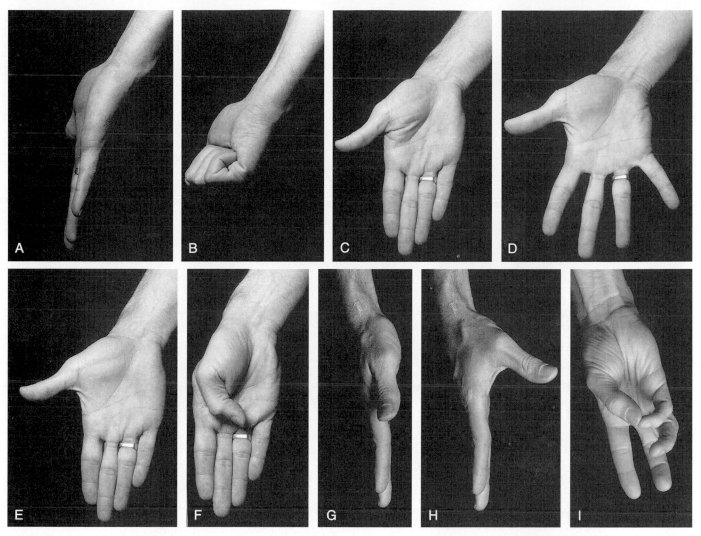

**FIGURE 8–10.** The system for naming the movements within the hand. *A* to *D*, Finger motion. *E* to *I*, Thumb motion. (*A*, finger extension; *B*, finger flexion; *C*, finger adduction; *D*, finger abduction; *E*, thumb extension; *F*, thumb flexion; *G*, thumb adduction; *H*, thumb abduction; and *I*, thumb opposition.)

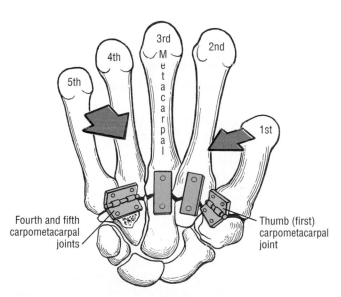

**FIGURE 8–11.** Palmar view of the right hand showing a highly mechanical depiction of the mobility across the five carpometacarpal joints. The peripheral joints—the first, fourth, and fifth (red)—are much more mobile than the central two joints (gray).

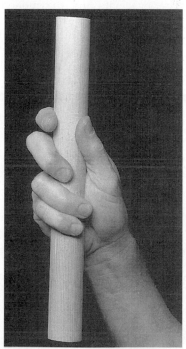

**FIGURE 8–12.** The mobility of the carpometacarpal joints of the hand enhances the security of grasping objects, such as this cylindric pole.

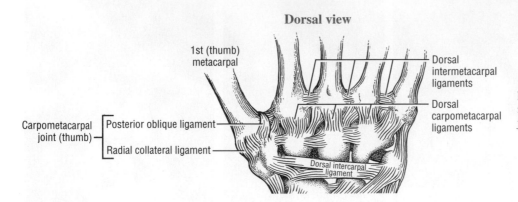

**Dorsal view**

1st (thumb) metacarpal

Dorsal intermetacarpal ligaments

Dorsal carpometacarpal ligaments

Carpometacarpal joint (thumb) — Posterior oblique ligament

Radial collateral ligament

Dorsal intercarpal ligament

**FIGURE 8–13.** Dorsal side of the right hand showing the capsule and ligaments that stabilize the carpometacarpal joints.

the base joint of the entire thumb. Basilar joint arthritis can be very incapacitating, often affecting women in the fifth to sixth decades of life.[41]

## CAPSULE AND LIGAMENTS OF THE THUMB CARPOMETACARPAL JOINT

The capsule at the CMC joint of the thumb is naturally loose to accommodate to a large range of motion. The capsule is, however, thickened by ligaments and reinforced by active muscular contraction.

Many names have been used to describe the ligaments at the CMC joint of the thumb.[4,16,42] This text incorporates the scheme of naming ligaments based on their attachments to the trapezium, not to the thumb metacarpal (see Fig. 8–8). The terminology to describe the ligaments of the CMC joints is not well established and, therefore, may differ in other sources.

The CMC joint of the thumb is surrounded by five ligaments (Fig. 8–16).[2] Table 8–1 summarizes the major attachments of these ligaments and the motions that cause them to become taut. In general, extension, abduction, and opposition of the thumb elongate most of the ligaments. All five ligaments listed in Table 8–1 are important stabiliz-

ers at the CMC joint of the thumb.[4,16,23,37,41] As a group, they resist the tendency for the CMC joint to dislocate. When the ligaments are weakened by arthritis, the joint often dislocates laterally relative to the trapezium.

## SADDLE JOINT STRUCTURE

The CMC joint of the thumb is the classic saddle joint of the body (Fig. 8–17). The characteristic feature of a saddle joint is that each articular surface is convex in one dimension and concave in the other.[55,58] The *longitudinal diameter* of the articular surface of the *trapezium* (see Fig. 8–17) is generally concave from a palmar-to-dorsal direction. This surface is analogous to the contour of the front-to-rear diameter of a horse's saddle. The corresponding *transverse diameter* on the articular surface of the *trapezium* is generally convex along a medial-to-lateral direction.[30] The convexity of the transverse diameter is analogous to the side-to-side convex contour of a horse's saddle. The contour of the proximal articular surface of the thumb metacarpal has the reciprocal shape of that described for the trapezium (see Fig. 8–17). The longitudinal diameter along the articular surface of the metacarpal is convex from a palmar to dorsal direction. Its transverse diameter is concave from a medial to lateral direction.

## TABLE 8–1. Ligaments of the Carpometacarpal Joint of the Thumb*

| Name | Proximal Attachment | Distal Attachment | Most Taut Positions |
|---|---|---|---|
| Anterior oblique | Palmar tubercle on trapezium | Palmar base of thumb metacarpal | Abduction, extension, and opposition |
| Ulnar collateral† | Transverse carpal ligament | Palmar-ulnar base of thumb metacarpal | Abduction, extension, and opposition |
| First intermetacarpal | Dorsal side of base of second metacarpal | Palmar-ulnar base of thumb metacarpal with ulnar collateral | Abduction and opposition |
| Posterior oblique | Posterior surface of trapezium | Palmar-ulnar base of thumb metacarpal | Abduction and opposition |
| Radial collateral‡ | Radial surface of trapezium | Dorsal surface of thumb metacarpal | All movements to varying degrees except extension |

* Ligament names are based on attachment to trapezium surfaces *not* the thumb metacarpal.
† Also called "palmar oblique" ligament based on attachment to the metacarpal.
‡ Also called "dorsal-radial" ligament.

## Palmar view

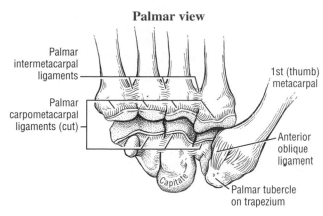

Palmar intermetacarpal ligaments

Palmar carpometacarpal ligaments (cut)

1st (thumb) metacarpal

Anterior oblique ligament

Palmar tubercle on trapezium

Capitate

**FIGURE 8–14.** The palmar side of the right hand showing internal surfaces of the second through the fifth carpometacarpal joints. The capsule and palmar carpometacarpal ligaments of digits 2 to 5 have been cut.

## KINEMATICS

The primary motions at the CMC joint occur in 2 degrees of freedom. As depicted in Figure 8–18, abduction and adduction occur generally in the sagittal plane, and flexion and extension occur generally in the frontal plane. Being a saddle joint, each of the two axes of rotation passes through a different convex articular surface.[23]

Opposition and reposition of the thumb are mechanically derived from the two primary planes of motion at the CMC joint. The kinematics of opposition and reposition are discussed following the description of the two primary motions.

### Abduction and Adduction at the Thumb Carpometacarpal Joint

In the position of adduction of the CMC joint, the thumb lies within the plane of the hand. Maximum abduction, in contrast, positions the thumb metacarpal about 45 degrees

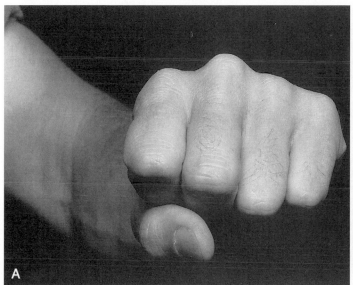

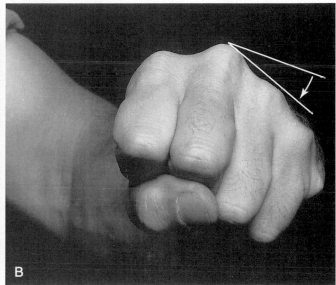

**FIGURE 8–15.** Mobility of the ulnar (fourth and fifth) carpometacarpal joints of the left hand. *A,* Hand closed but relaxed. *B,* With a firm grip, the finger flexor muscles flex and rotate the ulnar metacarpals.

**FIGURE 8–16.** Palmar and lateral views of the ligaments of the carpometacarpal joint of the right thumb. Note the distal attachment of the abductor pollicis longus into the capsule of the carpometacarpal joint of the thumb.

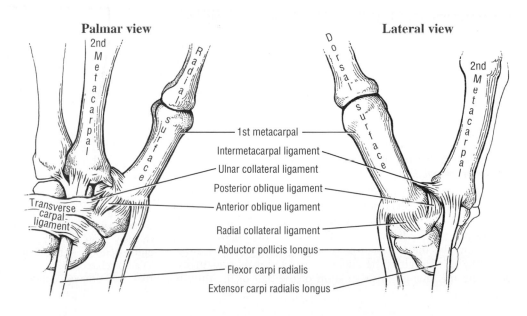

**Palmar view**

2nd Metacarpal

Radial Surface

Transverse carpal ligament

**Lateral view**

Dorsal Surface

2nd Metacarpal

1st metacarpal

Intermetacarpal ligament

Ulnar collateral ligament

Posterior oblique ligament

Anterior oblique ligament

Radial collateral ligament

Abductor pollicis longus

Flexor carpi radialis

Extensor carpi radialis longus

**Palmar view**

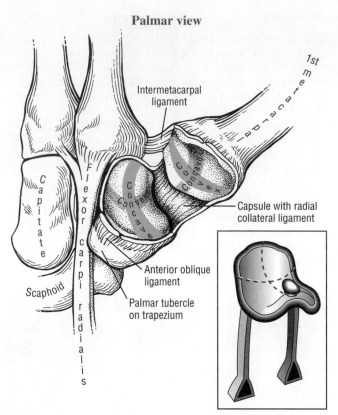

**FIGURE 8–17.** The carpometacarpal of the right thumb is opened to expose the saddle shape of the joint. The longitudinal diameters are shown in gray and the transverse diameters in red.

anterior to the plane of the palm.[11] Full abduction opens the web space of the thumb, forming a wide concave curvature useful for grasping large objects (Fig. 8–19A). Varying degrees of abduction at the CMC joint are also used while holding and/or manipulating small objects between the index finger and thumb (Fig. 8–19B).

The arthrokinematics of abduction and adduction are based on the convex articular surface of the thumb metacarpal moving on the fixed concave (longitudinal) diameter of the trapezium (see Fig. 8–17).[23,30] During *abduction,* the convex articular surface of the metacarpal rolls palmarly and slides dorsally on the concave surface of the trapezium (Fig. 8–20). Full abduction at the CMC joint elongates the adductor pollicis muscle and most ligaments at the CMC joint, especially those imbedded around the posterior aspect of the joint capsule. The arthrokinematics of *adduction* occur in the reverse order from that described for abduction.

### Flexion and Extension at the Thumb Carpometacarpal Joint

Actively performing flexion and extension of the CMC joint of the thumb is associated with varying amounts of axial rotation of the metacarpal. During flexion, the metacarpal rotates slightly medially (i.e., toward the third digit); during extension, the metacarpal rotates slightly laterally (i.e., away from the third digit). The slight axial rotation is evident by watching the change in orientation of the nail of the thumb

between full extension and full flexion. This rotation is not considered a third degree of freedom because it cannot be executed independently of the other motions.

In the anatomic position, the thumb metacarpal assumes a position of nearly full extension. From this position, the CMC joint can be extended only an additional 10 to 15 degrees.[11] From full extension, the thumb metacarpal flexes across the palm about 45 to 50 degrees.

The arthrokinematics of flexion and extension at the CMC joint are based on the concave articular surface of the metacarpal moving across the convex (transverse) diameter on the trapezium (see Fig. 8–17). During *flexion,* the concave surface of metacarpal rolls and slides in an ulnar (medial) direction (Fig. 8–21A).[23] A shallow groove in the transverse diameter of the trapezium helps guide the slight medial rotation of the metacarpal. Full flexion elongates tissues such as the radial collateral ligament.[58]

During *extension* of the CMC joint, the concave metacarpal rolls and slides in a lateral (radial) direction across the

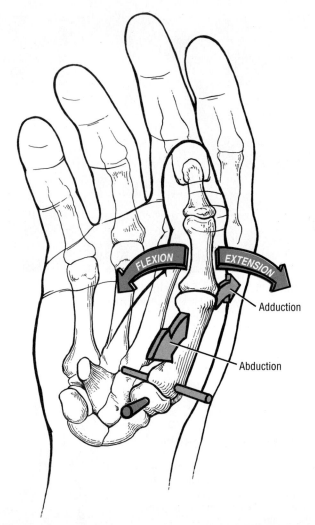

**FIGURE 8–18.** The primary biplanar osteokinematics at the carpometacarpal joint of the right thumb. Note that abduction and adduction occur about a medial-lateral axis of rotation (gray); flexion and extension occur about an anterior-posterior axis of rotation. The more complex motion of opposition requires a combination of these two primary motions. (See text for further details.)

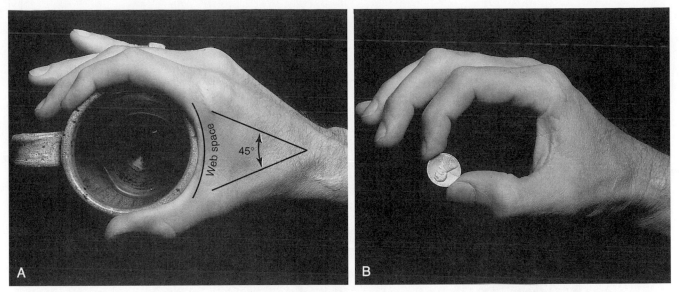

**FIGURE 8–19.** Abduction of the carpometacarpal joint of the thumb. *A,* Maximum abduction of 45 degrees opens the web space of the thumb. *B,* Moderate abduction for fine manipulation with the index finger.

transverse diameter of the joint (Fig. 8–21B). The groove on the articular surface of the trapezium guides the metacarpal into slight lateral rotation.[11,30] Full extension requires elongation of the anterior oblique ligament. Table 8–2 shows a summary of the kinematics for flexion-extension and abduction-adduction at the CMC joint of the thumb.

### Opposition of the Thumb Carpometacarpal Joint

For ease of discussion, Fig. 8–22A shows the full arc of *opposition* divided into two phases. In *phase one,* the thumb metacarpal abducts. In *phase two,* the abducted metacarpal flexes and medially rotates across the palm toward the little finger. Figure 8–22B shows the detail of the kinematics of this complex movement. During abduction, the base of the thumb metacarpal takes a path in a palmar direction across the surface of the trapezium. During flexion-medial rotation, the base of this metacarpal turns slightly medially, led by the groove on the surface of the trapezium.[58] Muscle force, especially from the opponens pollicis, helps guide the metacarpal to the extreme medial side of the transverse articular surface of the trapezium. The partially abducted CMC joint increases the passive tension in certain connective tissues. For example, increased tension in the stretched posterior oblique ligament promotes the medial rotation (spin) of the metacarpal shaft.[58]

As evident by the change in orientation of the thumbnail, full opposition incorporates at least 45 to 60 degrees of medial rotation of the thumb. The CMC joint of the thumb cannot account for all of this rotation. Lesser amounts of axial rotation, in the form of accessory motions, occur at the MCP and IP joints of the thumb. The body of the trapezium also medially rotates slightly against the scaphoid and the trapezoid.[40] Trapezial rotation, likely the result of passive tension in taut ligaments, amplifies the final magnitude of the metacarpal rotation. The little finger contributes to opposition through a cupping motion at the fifth CMC joint. This motion allows the tip of the thumb to make firm contact with the tip of the little finger.

Full opposition is the close-packed position of the thumb CMC joint.[55] In this position, the CMC joint is usually under active control of muscle. Many of the ligaments are

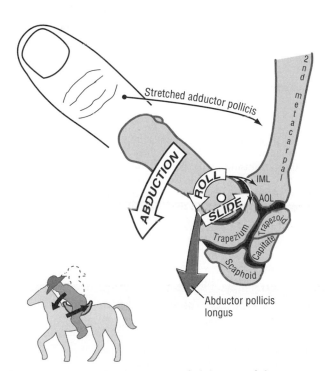

**FIGURE 8–20.** The arthrokinematics of abduction of the carpometacarpal joint of the thumb. Full abduction stretches the anterior oblique ligament (AOL), the intermetacarpal ligament (IML), and the adductor pollicis muscle. A muscle responsible for the active roll at the joint is the abductor pollicis longus. Note the analogy shown between the arthrokinematics of abduction and a cowboy falling forward on the horse's saddle: As the cowboy falls forward (toward abduction), a point on his chest "rolls" anteriorly, but a point on his rear end "slides" posteriorly.

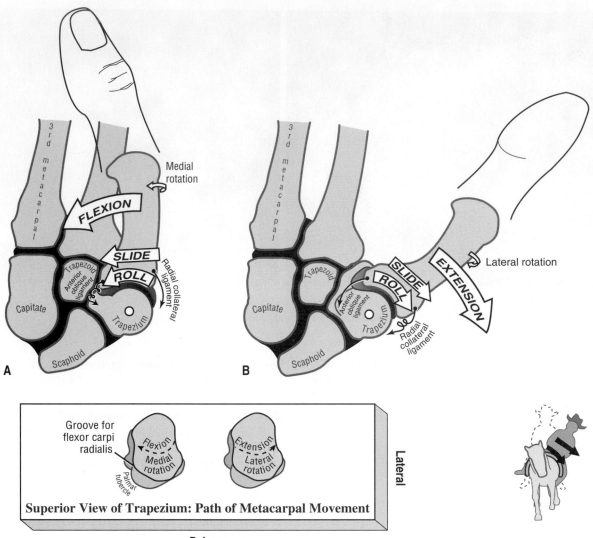

**FIGURE 8–21.** The arthrokinematics of flexion and extension at the carpometacarpal joint of the thumb. *A*, Flexion is associated with a slight medial rotation, causing elongation in the radial collateral ligament. The anterior oblique ligament is slack. *B*, Extension is associated with slight lateral rotation, causing elongation of the anterior oblique ligament. The approximate path of motion of the metacarpal on the trapezium is shown in the insert. Note the analogy shown between the arthrokinematics of extension and a cowboy falling sideways on the horse's saddle: As the cowboy falls sideways (toward extension), points on his chest and rear end both "roll and slide" in the same lateral direction.

TABLE **8 – 2.** **Factors Associated with Kinematics of the Primary Motions of the CMC Joint of the Thumb***

| Motion | Osteokinematics | Joint Geometry | Arthrokinematics |
|---|---|---|---|
| Abduction and adduction | Sagittal plane movement about a medial-lateral axis of rotation through the metacarpal | Convex (longitudinal diameter) of metacarpal moving on a concave surface of the trapezium | Abduction: palmar roll and dorsal slide<br>Adduction: dorsal roll and palmar slide |
| Flexion and extension | Frontal plane movement about an anterior-posterior axis of rotation through the trapezium | Concave (transverse) diameter of the metacarpal moving on a convex surface of the trapezium | Flexion: medial roll and slide<br>Extension: lateral roll and slide |

* Opposition and reposition are not shown because they are derived from the two primary planes of motions (see text for further explanation).

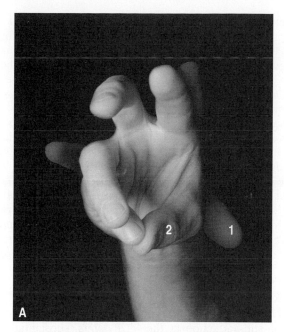

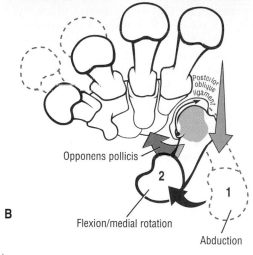

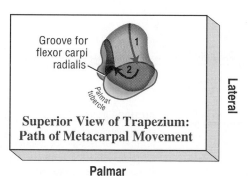

**FIGURE 8–22.** The kinematics of opposition of the carpometacarpal joint of the thumb. *A,* Two phases of opposition are shown: (1) abduction and (2) flexion with medial rotation *B,* The detailed kinematics of the two phases of opposition: the posterior oblique ligament is shown taut; the opponens pollicis is shown contracting (red).

twisted taut. *Reposition* of the CMC joint returns the metacarpal from full opposition back to the anatomic position. This motion involves arthrokinematics of both adduction and extension-lateral rotation of the thumb metacarpal.

## Metacarpophalangeal Joints

### FINGERS

#### General Features and Ligaments

The MCP joints of the fingers are relatively large, ovoid articulations between the convex heads of the metacarpals and the shallow concave proximal surfaces of the proximal phalanges (Fig. 8–23). Motion at the MCP joint occurs predominantly in two planes: flexion and extension in the sagittal plane, and abduction and adduction in the frontal plane.

Mechanical stability at the MCP joint is critical to the overall biomechanics of the hand. As discussed earlier, the MCP joints serve as keystones for support of the mobile arches of the hand. In the healthy hand, stability at the MCP joints is achieved by an elaborate set of interconnecting connective tissues. Imbedded within the capsule of each MCP joint is a pair of radial and ulnar collateral ligaments and one palmar ligament or plate (Fig. 8–24). Each *collateral ligament* has its proximal attachment on the posterior tubercles of the metacarpal head. Crossing the MCP joint in an oblique palmar direction, the ligament forms two distinct parts. The *cord part* of the ligament is thick and strong,

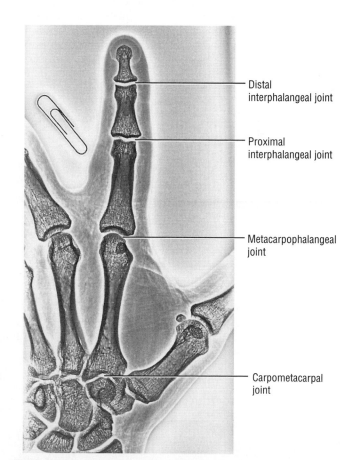

**FIGURE 8–23.** The joints of the index finger.

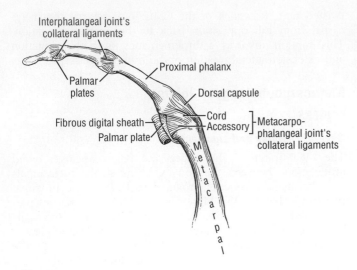

**FIGURE 8–24.** A lateral view of the collateral ligaments and associated connective tissues of the metacarpophalangeal, proximal interphalangeal, and distal interphalangeal joints of the finger.

attaching distally to the palmar aspect of the proximal end of the phalanx. The *accessory part* consists of fanshaped fibers, which attach distally along the edge of each palmar plate.

Located palmar to each MCP joint are ligamentous-like structures called *palmar (or volar) plates* (see Fig. 8–24). The term plate describes a composition of dense, thick discs of fibrocartilage. The distal end of each plate attaches to the base of each proximal phalanx. At this region, the plates are relatively thick and stiff. The thinner and more elastic proxi-

mal ends of the palmar plates attach to the metacarpal bone, just proximal to the head. *Fibrous digital sheaths,* which form tunnels or pulleys for the extrinsic finger flexors, are anchored immediately anterior to the palmar plates. The primary function of the palmar plates is to strengthen the MCP joint and resist hyperextension (i.e., the range of posterior motion beyond the 0° position).

Figure 8–25 illustrates anatomic aspects of the MCP joints. The concave component of the MCP joint is formed by the articular surface of the proximal phalanx, the collateral ligaments, and the dorsal surface of the palmar plate. These tissues form a three-sided receptacle aptly suited to accept the heads of the metacarpals. This structure adds joint stability and increases the area of articular contact. Attaching between the palmar plates are three *deep transverse metacarpal ligaments* (see Fig. 8–25). The wide, flat structure helps to interconnect the second through fifth metacarpals.

### Metacarpophalangeal Joint Kinematics

#### Osteokinematics

In addition to the motions of flexion-and-extension and abduction-and-adduction at the MCP joints, substantial accessory motions occur. On the relaxed and nearly extended MCP joint, it is possible to feel significant passive translation in an anterior-to-posterior direction, side-to-side direction, and distraction. Note also the passive axial rotation of the proximal phalanx against the metacarpal head. Although limited, these accessory motions at the MCP joint permit the fingers to better conform to the shapes of objects, thereby increasing security and control of the grasp (Fig. 8–26). The range of this passive axial rotation at the MCP joints is greatest at the ring and little fingers, with average rotations of about 30 to 40 degrees.[29]

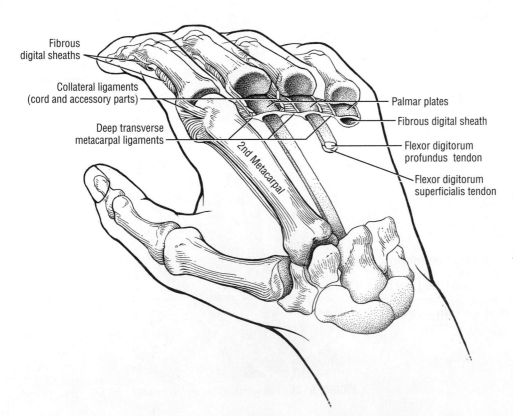

**FIGURE 8–25.** A dorsal view of the hand with emphasis on the periarticular connective tissues at the metacarpophalangeal joints. Several metacarpal bones have been removed to expose various joint structures.

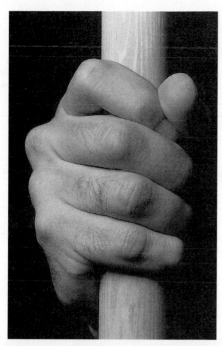

**FIGURE 8–26.** The passive accessory motions at the metacarpophalangeal joints during the grasp of a cylinder. Axial rotation of the index finger is most notable.

---

> ## The MCP Joint of the Finger Allows Movement Primarily in 2 Degrees of Freedom
> - *Flexion and extension* occur in the sagittal plane about a medial-lateral axis of rotation.
> - *Abduction and adduction* occur in the frontal plane about an anterior-posterior axis of rotation.
>
> Both axes of rotation pass through the head of the metacarpal

The overall range of flexion and extension at the MCP joints increases gradually from the second to the fifth digit.[3] About 90 degrees of flexion is available at the second (index) MCP joint and about 110 to 115 degrees is available at the fifth. The greater mobility allowed at the more ulnar MCP joints is similar to that at the CMC joints. The MCP joints can be passively hyperextended beyond the neutral position for a considerable range of 30 to 45 degrees.

Abduction and adduction at the MCP joints occurs to about 20 degrees on either side of the midline reference formed by the third metacarpal. Mobility is greatest in the second and fifth digits where adjacent fingers do not limit motion.[3]

### Arthrokinematics

Each metacarpal head has a slightly different shape, but in general each is rounded at the apex and nearly flat on the palmar surface (see Fig. 8–6). Articular cartilage covers the entire head and most of the palmar surface. The convex-concave relationship of the joint surfaces is readily apparent (Fig. 8–27). The longitudinal diameter of the joint follows the sagittal plane; the shorter transverse diameter follows the frontal plane.

The arthrokinematics at the MCP joint are based on the concave articular surface of the phalanx moving on the convex metacarpal head. During active extension, the base of the proximal phalanx rolls and slides in a dorsal direction under the power of the extensor digitorum communis muscle (Fig. 8–28A). At about 60 to 70 degrees of flexion, the cord portion of the collateral ligaments is maximally taut. The eccentric or "out-of-round" cam-shape of the metacarpal head is responsible for the stretch in the collateral ligaments.[19] At 0 degrees of extension (Fig. 8–28B), the collateral ligaments slacken while the palmar plate unfolds and makes total contact with the head of the metacarpal. Full hyperextension is limited by the stretch placed in the palmar plate (Fig. 8–28C). The arthrokinematics of MCP flexion are similar to those described for extension except that the roll and slide of the metacarpal occur toward the palmar direction (see Fig. 8–29).

The *close-packed position* at the MCP joint is about 70 degrees of flexion.[19] In this position, accessory motion is minimal. Most fibers of the cord portion of the collateral ligaments are pulled taut. The flexed position, therefore, offers substantial stability to the base of the fingers. At near extension, the collateral ligaments slacken, allowing maximal accessory motions.

The arthrokinematics of abduction and adduction of the MCP joints are similar to those described for flexion and extension. During abduction of the index MCP joint, for instance, the proximal phalanx rolls and slides in a radial direction (Fig. 8–30). The first dorsal interosseus muscle directs both the roll and the slide arthrokinematics.

The amount of active abduction and adduction at the MCP joints is significantly less in full flexion compared with full extension. Two factors can account for this difference. First, the collateral ligaments are taut near full flexion.

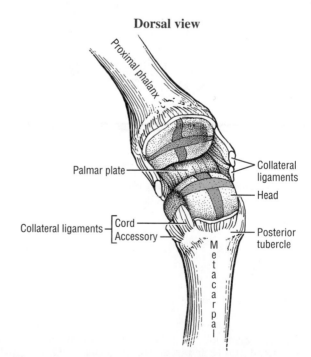

**FIGURE 8–27.** A dorsal view of the metacarpophalangeal joint opened to expose the shape of the articular surfaces. The longitudinal diameter of the joint is shown in gray; the transverse diameter in red.

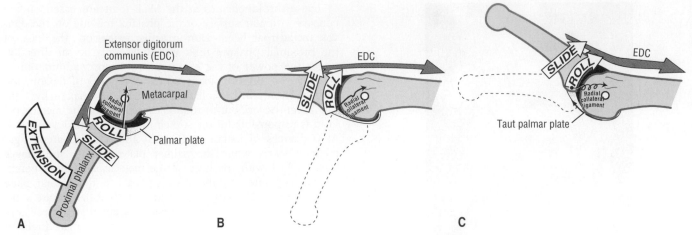

**FIGURE 8–28.** The arthrokinematics of active extension of the metacarpophalangeal joint. *A,* Active extension starting from a position of 70 degrees of flexion. The extensor digitorum communis (EDC) is shown contracting and then starting to drive the roll-and-slide kinematics. The radial collateral ligament is pulled taut in flexion. *B,* At 0 degrees of extension, the radial collateral ligament is relatively slack. *C,* Hyperextension further slackens the radial collateral ligament but maximally stretches the palmar plate. Note that the axis of rotation for this motion is in the medial-lateral direction, through the head of the metacarpal.

Stored passive tension in these ligaments theoretically increases the compression force between the joint surfaces, thereby reducing active motion. Second, in the position of about 70 degrees of flexion, the articular surface of the

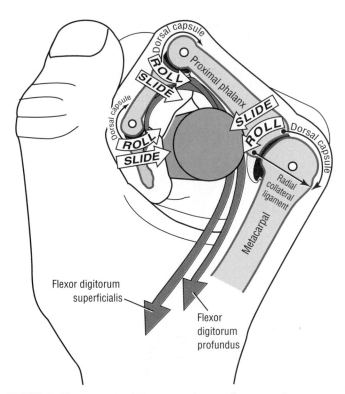

**FIGURE 8–29.** The arthrokinematics of active flexion at the metacarpophalangeal, proximal interphalangeal, and distal interphalangeal joints of the index finger. The radial collateral ligament at the metacarpophalangeal joint is pulled taut in flexion. Flexion elongates the dorsal capsule and other associated connective tissues. The joints are shown flexing under the power of the flexor digitorum superficialis and the flexor digitorum profundus. The axis of rotation for flexion and extension at all three finger joints is in the medial-lateral direction, through the convex member of the joint.

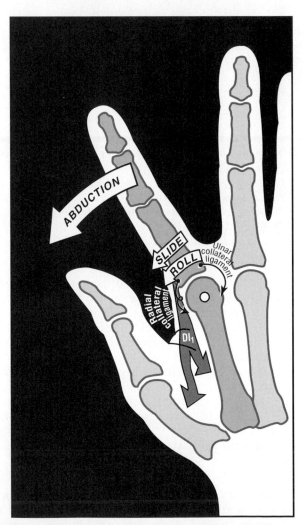

**FIGURE 8–30.** The arthrokinematics of active abduction at the metacarpophalangeal joint. Abduction is shown powered by the first dorsal interosseus muscle ($DI_1$). At full abduction, the ulnar collateral ligament is taut and the radial collateral ligament is slack. Note that the axis of rotation for this motion is in an anterior-posterior direction, through the head of the metacarpal.

**Clinical Relevance of the Close-Packed Position at the Metacarpophalangeal Joints**

Following surgery or trauma, the hand is often temporarily immobilized to promote healing and relieve pain. During a prolonged period, connective tissues immobilized at a shortened length are likely to become increasingly stiff and resistant to elongation. To reduce the likelihood of tightness within the collateral ligaments at the MCP joints, the hand is often splinted with the MCP joints flexed to 60 to 70 degrees (Fig. 8–31). This close-packed position of the joints places both the collateral ligaments[36] and extrinsic extensor muscles in a relatively elongated and taut position. This position may prevent subsequent shortening of these tissues.

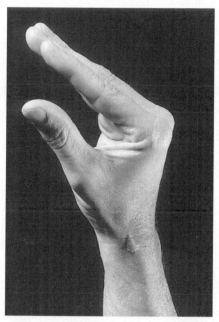

**FIGURE 8–31.** Common position used for long-term immobilization of the hand. The flexed position of the metacarpophalangeal joints elongates the collateral ligaments and the extensor digitorum communis muscle. The proximal interphalangeal and distal interphalangeal joints are immobilized near full extension to prevent flexion contractures at these joints. (See text for further details.)

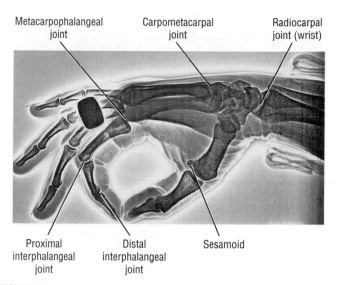

Metacarpophalangeal joint    Carpometacarpal joint    Radiocarpal joint (wrist)

Proximal interphalangeal joint    Distal interphalangeal joint    Sesamoid

**FIGURE 8–32.** A side view showing the shape of many joint surfaces in the wrist and hand. Note the sesamoid bone on the palmar side of the metacarpophalangeal joint of the thumb.

thumb (Fig. 8–32). A pair of sesamoid bones is usually located within the palmar side of the joint capsule.

The basic structure and arthrokinematics of the MCP joint of the thumb are similar to those of the fingers. Marked differences exist, however, in osteokinematics. Active and passive motions at the MCP joint of the thumb are significantly less than those at the MCP joints of the fingers. For all practical purposes, the MCP joint of the thumb allows only 1 degree of freedom: flexion and extension within the frontal plane.[17] From full extension, the proximal phalanx of the thumb can actively flex about 60 degrees across the palm toward the middle digit. Figure 8–33 depicts the arthrokinematics at the MCP joint during active flexion under the power of the intrinsic and extrinsic flexor muscles. Unlike the MCP joints of the fingers, hyperextension of the thumb MCP joint is usually limited to just a few degrees.

Active abduction and adduction of the thumb MCP joint is very limited and, therefore, considered as an accessory motion. This can be observed on the hand by attempting to actively abduct or adduct the proximal phalanx while firmly stabilizing the thumb metacarpal. Collateral ligaments at this joint markedly restrict this motion. The paucity of this motion lends longitudinal stability throughout the entire ray of the thumb. Abduction and adduction torques that cross the MCP joint of the thumb are transferred proximally across the CMC joint.

## Interphalangeal Joints

### FINGERS

The proximal and distal interphalangeal joints of the fingers allow only 1 degree of freedom: flexion and extension. From both a structural and functional perspective, these joints are simpler than the MCP joints.

### General Features and Ligaments

The *proximal interphalangeal (PIP) joints* are formed by the articulation between the heads of the proximal phalanges

proximal phalanges contacts the flattened palmar part of the metacarpal heads (see Fig. 8–28A). This relatively flat surface blocks the natural arthrokinematics required for maximal abduction and adduction range of motion.

## THUMB

### General Features and Ligaments

The MCP joint of the thumb consists of the articulation between the convex head of the first metacarpal and the concave proximal surface of the proximal phalanx of the

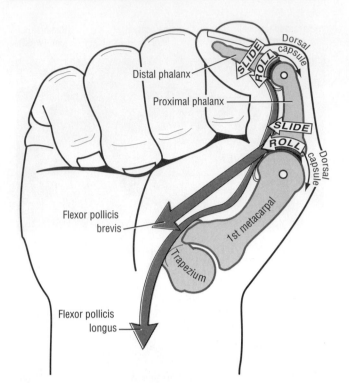

**FIGURE 8–33.** The arthrokinematics of active flexion at the metacarpophalangeal and interphalangeal joints of the thumb. Flexion is shown powered by the flexor pollicis longus and the flexor pollicis brevis. The axis of rotation for flexion and extension at the these joints is in the anterior-posterior direction, through the convex member of the joints.

tissue are essentially the same as that of the PIP joint, except for the absence of the check-rein ligaments.

### Proximal Interphalangeal and Distal Interphalangeal Joint Kinematics

The PIP joints flex to about 100 to 120 degrees. The DIP joints show less flexion, to about 70 to 90 degrees. Like the MCP joints, flexion at the IP joints is greater in the more ulnar digits. Minimal hyperextension is usually available at the PIP joints. The DIP joints, however, normally allow up to 30 degrees of hyperextension.

Flexion range of motion is greater at the PIP joints than at the DIP joints. Flexion and extension of IP joints of the ring and little fingers occur in conjunction with slight axial rotation. During flexion, this rotation turns the pulp of the fingertips toward the base of the thumb. Axial rotation allows these fingers to contact the opposing thumb more effectively.[27]

Similarities in joint structure cause similar arthrokinematics at the PIP and DIP joints. During active flexion at the PIP joint, for instance, the concave base of the middle phalanx rolls and slides in a palmar direction by the pull of the extrinsic finger flexors (see Fig. 8–29). During flexion, the passive tension created in the stretched connective tissues on the dorsal side of the joint help guide and stabilize the roll-and-slide arthrokinematics.

In contrast to the MCP joints, passive tension in the collateral ligaments at the IP joints remains relatively con-

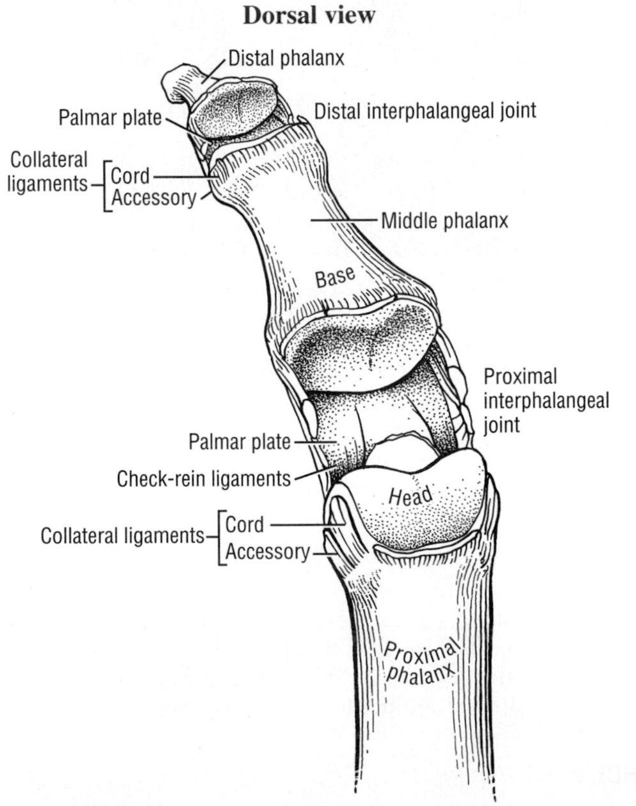

and the bases of the middle phalanges (see Fig. 8–34). The articular surface of a PIP joint appears as a tongue-in-groove articulation similar to that used in carpentry to join planks of wood. The head of the proximal phalanx has two rounded condyles, separated by a shallow central groove. The opposing surface of the middle phalanx has two shallow concave facets separated by a central ridge. Tongue-in-groove articulation helps guide the motion of flexion and extension and restricts axial rotation.

The PIP joints are surrounded by a capsule that is reinforced by radial and ulnar *collateral ligaments*. The cord portion of the collateral ligament at the PIP joint significantly limits abduction and adduction motion. As with the MCP joint, the accessory portion of the collateral ligament blends with and reinforces the palmar plate (see Fig. 8–34). The anatomic connections between the collateral ligaments and palmar plate form a secure seat for the head of the proximal phalanx. Palmar *check-rein ligaments* at the PIP joint strengthen the connection between the palmar plate and the middle phalanx. Similar to the palmar plates, these ligaments resist hyperextension of the PIP joint.[6,14] Severe hyperextension of the PIP joint is a common athletic injury, with tearing of both the palmar plate and the check-rein ligaments.

The *distal interphalangeal (DIP) joints* are formed through the articulation between the heads of the middle phalanges and the bases of the distal phalanges (see Fig. 8–34). The structure of the DIP joint and the surrounding connective

**Dorsal view**

**FIGURE 8–34.** A dorsal view of the proximal interphalangeal and distal interphalangeal joints opened to expose the shape of the articular surfaces.

stant throughout the range of motion. Perhaps the more concentric shape of the head of the phalanges prevents a large change in length in these collateral ligaments. The close-packed position of the PIP and DIP joints is near full extension,[55] most likely caused by the stretch placed on the palmar plates. During periods of immobilization of the hand, the IP joints are often splinted in near or full extension (see Fig. 8–31). This position places a stretch on the palmar plates, collateral ligaments, and extrinsic finger flexor muscles, reducing the likelihood of flexion contracture of these joints.

## THUMB

The structure and function of the IP joint of the thumb is similar to those of the IP joints of the fingers (see Fig. 8–33). Motion is limited primarily to 1 degree of freedom, allowing active flexion to about 70 degrees. The IP joint can be passively hyperextended beyond neutral to about 20 de-

grees. This motion is often employed to apply a force between the pad of the thumb and an object, such as pushing a tack into a wall. The amount of passive hyperextension often increases throughout life owing to years of stretch placed on palmar structures, including the palmar plate.

## MUSCLE AND JOINT INTERACTION

### Innervation of Muscles, Skin, and Joints of the Hand

#### MUSCLE AND SKIN INNERVATION

Innervation to the muscles and skin of the hand is illustrated in Figure 6–33. The *radial nerve* innervates the extrinsic extensor muscles of the digits. These muscles, located on the dorsal aspect of the forearm, are the extensor digitorum communis, extensor digiti minimi, extensor indicis, extensor pollicis longus, extensor pollicis brevis, and abductor pollicis longus. The radial nerve is responsible for the sensation on the dorsal aspect of the wrist and hand, especially around the dorsal region of the thenar web space.

The *median nerve* innervates most of the extrinsic flexors of the digits. In the forearm, the median nerve innervates the flexor digitorum superficialis. A branch of the median nerve (anterior interosseous nerve) then innervates the lateral half of the flexor digitorum profundus, the flexor pollicis longus, and the pronator quadratus.

The median nerve enters the hand through the carpal tunnel, deep to the transverse carpal ligament. Once in the hand, the median nerve innervates the muscles that form the thenar eminence (flexor pollicis brevis, abductor pollicis brevis, and opponens pollicis) and the lateral two lumbricals. The median nerve is responsible for the sensation on the palmar-lateral aspect of the hand, including the tips and the palmar aspect of the lateral three and one-half digits.

The *ulnar nerve* innervates the medial half of the flexor digitorum profundus. Distally, the ulnar nerve crosses the wrist superficial to the carpal tunnel. In the hand, the deep motor branch of the ulnar nerve innervates the hypothenar muscles (flexor digiti minimi, abductor digiti minimi, opponens digiti minimi, and palmaris brevis) and the medial two lumbricals. The deep motor branch continues laterally, deep in the hand, to innervate the palmar and dorsal interossei muscles, and finally the adductor pollicis. The ulnar nerve is responsible for the sensation on the ulnar border of the hand, including most of the skin of the ulnar one and one-half digits.

The motor nerve roots that supply all the muscles of the upper extremity are listed in Appendix IIA. Appendix IIB shows key muscles typically used to test the functional status of the $C^5$-$T^1$ ventral nerve roots.

#### SENSORY INNERVATION TO THE JOINTS

The periarticular connective tissue of the digits has a rich sensory nerve supply. Ample neural feedback is necessary to control the fine and complex movements. For the most part, the joints of the hand receive sensation from similar nerve roots that supply the overlying dermatomes. These nerve roots are carried in the radial, median, and ulnar nerves as

### SPECIAL FOCUS 8–2

#### "Position of Function" of the Wrist and Hand

Some medical conditions, such as a severe "stroke" or high-level quadriplegia, often result in a permanent deformity of the digits. The deformity is often inevitable, regardless of the quality or timing of the therapeutic intervention. Clinicians, therefore, often use splints that favor a position of the hand that maximally preserves its functional potential. This position, often called the *position of function* is shown in Figure 8–35. The highlights of this position are: *wrist:* 20 to 30 degrees of extension with slight ulnar deviation; *fingers:* 45 degrees of MCP joint flexion and 15 degrees of PIP and DIP joint flexion; and *thumb:* 45 degrees of abduction. This position of function provides a slightly cupped hand, with a wrist in position to maintain optimal length of the finger flexor muscles.

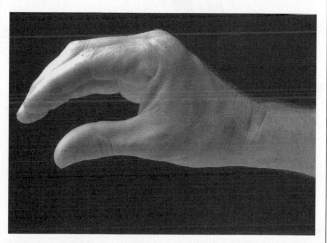

**FIGURE 8–35.** The "position of function" of the wrist and hand.

## TABLE 8-3. Extrinsic and Intrinsic Muscles of the Hand

| Extrinsic Muscles | Intrinsic Muscles |
|---|---|
| **Flexors of the digits**<br>Flexor digitorum superficialis<br>Flexor digitorum profundus<br>Flexor pollicis longus | **Thenar eminence**<br>Abductor pollicis brevis<br>Flexor pollicis brevis<br>Opponens pollicis |
| **Extensors of the fingers**<br>Extensor digitorum communis<br>Extensor indicis<br>Extensor digiti minimi | **Hypothenar eminence**<br>Abductor digiti minimi<br>Flexor digiti minimi<br>Opponens digiti minimi<br>Palmaris brevis |
| **Extensors of the thumb**<br>Extensor pollicis longus<br>Extensor pollicis brevis<br>Abductor pollicis longus | **Adductor pollicis** (two heads)<br><br>**Lumbricals (four)**<br>**Interossei**<br>Palmar (four)<br>Dorsal (four) |

## Muscular Function in the Hand

Muscles that operate the digits are classified as either *extrinsic* or *intrinsic* to the hand (Table 8–3). Extrinsic muscles have their proximal attachment in the forearm or, in some cases, as far proximal as the epicondyles of the humerus. Intrinsic muscles, in contrast, have both their proximal and distal attachments within the hand. As a summary and reference, the detailed anatomy and nerve supply of the muscles of the hand is in Appendix IIC.

Most active movements of the hand, such as opening and closing the fingers, require a precise cooperation between the extrinsic and the intrinsic muscles of the hand and the muscles of the wrist.

### EXTRINSIC FLEXORS OF THE DIGITS

#### Anatomy and Joint Action of the Extrinsic Flexors of the Digits

The extrinsic flexor muscles of the digits are the flexor digitorum superficialis, flexor digitorum profundus, and flexor pollicis longus (Figs. 8–36 and 8–37). These muscles have

follows: $C^6$ supplying the thumb and index finger, $C^7$ supplying the middle finger, and $C^8$ supplying the ring and little fingers.[20,24] The CMC joints are also innervated by sensory nerves of the $C^8$ nerve root via the deep branch of the ulnar nerve.[20]

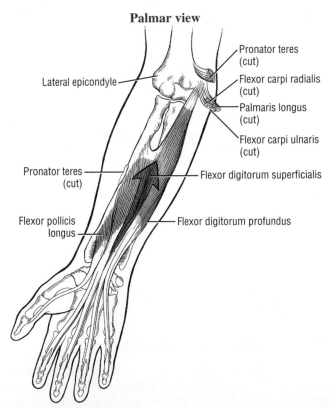

**FIGURE 8–36.** An anterior view of the right forearm highlighting the flexor digitorum superficialis muscle. Note the cut proximal ends of the wrist flexors and pronator teres muscles.

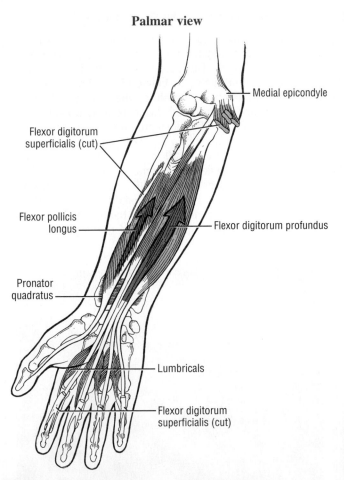

**FIGURE 8–37.** An anterior view of the right forearm highlighting the flexor digitorum profundus and the flexor pollicis longus muscles. The lumbrical muscles are shown attaching to the tendons of the flexor profundus. Note the cut proximal and distal ends of the flexor digitorum superficialis muscle.

extensive proximal attachments from the medial epicondyle of the humerus and from the regions of the forearm.

The muscle belly of the *flexor digitorum superficialis* is located in the anterior forearm, just deep to the three primary wrist flexors and the pronator teres muscle (see Fig. 8–36). The four tendons cross the wrist and enter the palmar side of the hand. At the level of the proximal phalanx, each tendon splits to allow passage of the tendon of the flexor digitorum profundus (Fig. 8–38). The two split parts of each tendon partially reunite, cross the PIP joint, and attach on the sides of the palmar aspect of the middle phalanx.[48]

The primary action of the flexor digitorum superficialis is to flex the PIP joints. This muscle, however, can flex all joints it crosses. In general, with the exception of the little finger, each tendon of the superficialis can be controlled relatively independently of the other. This independence of function is especially evident at the index finger.

The muscle belly of the *flexor digitorum profundus* is lo- cated in the deepest muscular plane of the forearm, deep to the flexor digitorum superficialis muscle (see Fig. 8–37). Once in the hand, each tendon passes through the split tendon of the superficialis. Each profundus tendon then continues distally to attach to the palmar side of the base of the distal phalanx (see Fig. 8–38, index finger). The profundus is the sole flexor of the DIP joint, but like the superficialis can assist in flexing every joint it crosses.

The flexor digitorum profundus to the index finger can be controlled relatively independently of the other profundus tendons. The remaining three tendons, however, are interconnected through various muscular fasciculi, which usually prohibit isolated DIP joint flexion of a single finger. To appreciate this interconnection, grasp the middle finger and maximally extend all of its joints. While holding this position, attempt to actively flex *only* the DIP joint of the ring finger. The inability or difficulty in performing this motion is due to the excessive elongation placed on the entire muscle belly of the profundus by the extension of the

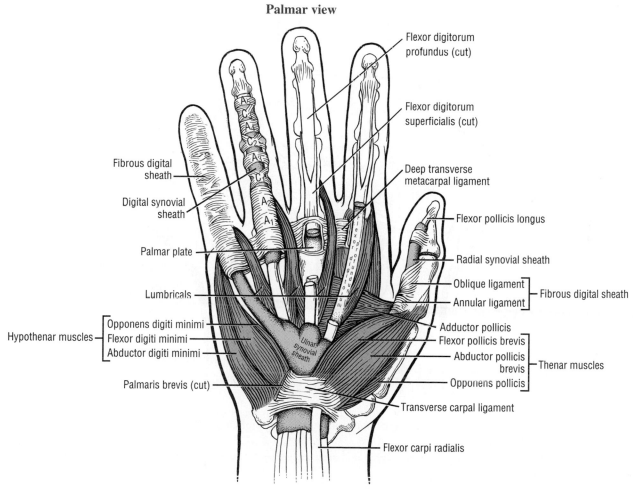

**Palmar view**

Flexor digitorum profundus (cut)

Flexor digitorum superficialis (cut)

Deep transverse metacarpal ligament

Flexor pollicis longus

Radial synovial sheath

Oblique ligament ⎤
Annular ligament ⎦ Fibrous digital sheath

Adductor pollicis

Flexor pollicis brevis ⎤
Abductor pollicis brevis ⎥ Thenar muscles
Opponens pollicis ⎦

Transverse carpal ligament

Flexor carpi radialis

Fibrous digital sheath

Digital synovial sheath

Palmar plate

Lumbricals

Opponens digiti minimi ⎤
Hypothenar muscles — Flexor digiti minimi ⎥
Abductor digiti minimi ⎦

Palmaris brevis (cut)

**FIGURE 8–38.** A palmar view illustrates several important structures of the hand. Note the *little finger* showing the fibrous digital sheath and ulnar synovial sheath encasing the extrinsic flexor tendons. The *ring finger* has the digital sheath removed, thereby highlighting the digital synovial sheath (red) and the annular ($A_{1-5}$) and cruciate ($C_{1-3}$) pulleys. The *middle finger* shows the pulleys removed to expose the distal attachments of the flexor digitorum superficialis and profundus. The *index finger* has a portion of flexor digitorum superficialis tendon removed, thereby exposing the deeper tendon of the flexor digitorum profundus and attached lumbrical. The *thumb* highlights the oblique and annular pulleys along with the radial synovial sheath, surrounding the tendon of the flexor pollicis longus.

## SPECIAL FOCUS 8–3

### Anatomical Basis for "Carpal Tunnel Syndrome"

All nine extrinsic flexor tendons of the digits travel with the median nerve through the carpal tunnel (Fig. 8–39). The tendons are surrounded by two separate synovial sheaths that reduce friction between the structures. An *ulnar synovial sheath* surrounds the eight tendons of the flexors digitorum superficialis and profundus, and a separate *radial synovial sheath* surrounds the tendon of the flexor pollicis longus. Hand activities that require prolonged and extreme wrist positions can irritate these tendons. Because of the closed and relatively small compartment of the carpal tunnel, swelling of the synovial membranes may increase the pressure on the median nerve. *Carpal tunnel syndrome* may result, which is

characterized by pain and/or paresthesia over the sensory distribution of the median nerve. With progression of the syndrome, muscular weakness and atrophy may occur in the thenar eminence. Pressures within the carpal tunnel in persons with carpal tunnel syndrome increase significantly during many activities that involve the hand.[46] Pressures increase most significantly during the extremes of all wrist motions, including the action of making a fist. Carpal tunnel syndrome may be associated with prolonged use of a computer keyboard. Alternative design of the standard computer keyboard may reduce the extremes of motions used during typing and thereby reduce the severity of this painful condition.[35]

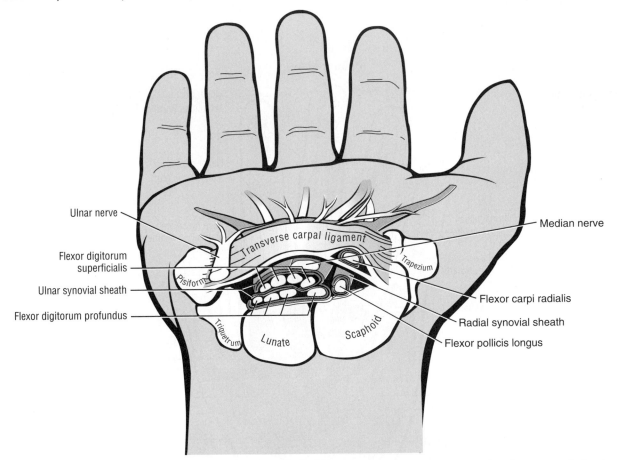

**FIGURE 8–39.** A transverse view through the entrance of the carpal tunnel of the right wrist. The ulnar synovial sheath (red) surrounds the tendons of the flexors digitorum superficialis and profundus. The radial synovial sheath surrounds the tendon of the flexor pollicis longus.

middle finger. This maneuver is often used to inhibit profundus action, thereby isolating the PIP joint flexor action of the superficialis.

The *flexor pollicis longus* resides in the deepest muscular plane of the forearm, just lateral to the profundus (see Fig. 8–37). This muscle crosses the wrist to attach distally to the

palmar side of the base of the distal phalanx of the thumb. The flexor pollicis longus is the sole flexor at the IP joint of the thumb and exerts a flexion torque at the MCP and CMC joints of the thumb and at the wrist joint.

Distal to the carpal tunnel, the *ulnar synovial sheath* surrounds the flexor digitorum superficialis and profundus tendons. This sheath ends in the proximal palm, except for a distal continuation around the tendons of fifth digit (see Fig. 8–38). The *radial synovial sheath* remains in contact with the tendon of the flexor pollicis longus to its distal insertion on the thumb.

The extrinsic flexor tendons of the digits are guided to their distal attachment in protective fibro-osseous tunnels known as *fibrous digital sheaths* (see Fig. 8–38, fifth finger). Sheaths start proximally as a continuation of the thick apo neurosis just under the skin of the palm. Throughout the length of each digit, the sheaths are anchored to the phalanges and the palmar plates (see Fig. 8–24). Embedded within each digital sheath are discrete bands of tissue called *flexor pulleys* (see Fig. 8–38, A1–5, C1–3 in ring finger). Deep to these pulleys is a *digital synovial sheath*, surrounding the flexor tendons from the distal palmar crease to the DIP joint. This sheath serves as a nutritional source for the enclosed tendons. The synovial fluid secreted from the sheath reduces the friction between the flexor digitorum superficialis and profundus tendons. A lacerated tendon within the digital sheath may heal with adhesions to the digital sheaths or adjacent tendons. Splinting and exercise are usually initiated after surgery to facilitate the free gliding of the tendons within the sheath.

### Anatomy and Function of the Flexor Pulleys

Figure 8–38 shows the flexor pulleys that are embedded within the fibrous digital sheath. Five *annular pulleys* have been described, designated as A1 to A5.[13] The major pulleys (A2 and A4) attach to the shaft of the proximal and middle phalanges. The minor pulleys (A1, A3, and A5) attach directly to the palmar plate at each of the three joints within a finger. Three less distinct *cruciate pulleys* (C1 to C3) have also been described. The cruciate pulleys are made of thin, flexible fibers that crisscross over the tendons at regions where the digital sheaths bend during flexion.

---

## SPECIAL FOCUS 8–4

### Biomechanics of a Ruptured Flexor Pulley

As previously stated, a function of the flexor pulleys is to maintain a near constant moment arm length of the flexor tendons. In a damaged or ruptured pulley, the force of the contracting muscle causes the tendon to "pull away" from the joint's axis of rotation, a phenomenon called "bowstringing" of the tendon. Bowstringing of a tendon significantly increases the internal moment arm of the tendon and, in turn, increases the mechanical advantage of the muscle. As described in Chapter 1, increasing a muscle's mechanical advantage has two effects on joint mechanics: (1) amplification of the torque produced per level muscle force, and (2) reduction of the angular rotation of the joint per linear distance of muscle shortening. The negative clinical implications of a ruptured flexor pulley primarily involve the second factor. To illustrate this effect on grasping, as-sume that with intact A2, A3, and A4 pulleys, the moment arm of the flexor digitorum profundus tendon is about .75 cm at the PIP joint (Fig. 8–40A). A muscle contraction of 1.5 cm would theoretically produce about 115 degrees of PIP joint flexion.[7] A finger with ruptured pulleys, as shown in Figure 8–40B, may cause a two-fold increase in the moment arm of the flexor digitorum profundus across the PIP joint. Consequently, a muscle contraction of 1.5 cm, in theory, produces only about 58 degrees of joint rotation—about half the motion produced with intact pulleys. Asssuming that the maximal shortening range of the flexor digitorum profundus is about 2.0 cm,[1] the finger with a ruptured pulley fails to flex fully, regardless of effort. This loss in contraction-to-rotation efficiency tends to be most profound in rupture of the A4 pulley.[45] A ruptured pulley often requires surgical correction.

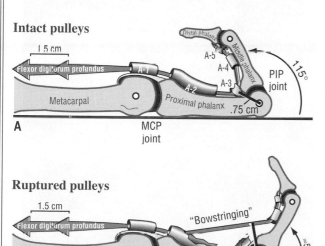

**FIGURE 8–40.** The pathomechanics of ruptured flexor pulleys. *A,* With intact pulleys, the moment arm of the finger flexors across the proximal interphalangeal (PIP) joint is about .75 cm. With this moment arm length, a 1.5-cm contraction excursion of the flexor digitorum profundus would in theory produce about 115 degrees flexion at the proximal interphalangeal joint. *B,* With a rupture of the A-2 and A-3 pulleys, the bowstringing of the tendon across the proximal interphalangeal joint would double the length of the moment arm to 1.5 cm. In this case, a 1.5-cm contraction excursion of the flexor digitorum profundus would produce only about 58 degrees of proximal interphalangeal joint flexion.

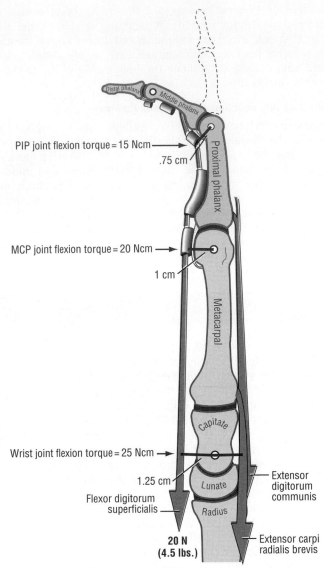

PIP joint flexion torque = 15 Ncm

.75 cm

Distal phalanx

Middle phalanx

Proximal phalanx

MCP joint flexion torque = 20 Ncm

1 cm

Metacarpal

Capitate

Wrist joint flexion torque = 25 Ncm

1.25 cm

Lunate

Flexor digitorum superficialis

Radius

Extensor digitorum communis

**20 N (4.5 lbs.)**

Extensor carpi radialis brevis

**FIGURE 8–41.** The muscle activation required to produce the simple motion of proximal interphalangeal joint flexion. A 20 N (4.5 pound) force produced by the flexor digitorum superficialis creates a flexion torque across every joint it crosses. Because of the progressively larger moment arms in the more proximal joints, the flexor torques progressively increase in a proximal direction from 15 to 25 Ncm. To isolate only proximal interphalangeal joint flexion, the extensor digitorum communis and the extensor carpi radialis brevis must resist the flexion effect of the flexor digitorum superficialis across the wrist and metacarpophalangeal joints.

Flexor pulleys, palmar aponeurosis, and skin share a similar function of holding the underlying tendons at a relatively fixed distance from the joints.[1,7] Without this function, the force produced by contraction of the extrinsic finger flexor muscles pulls the tendons away from the axis of rotation at the joint.

### Role of Proximal Stabilizer Muscles during Active Finger Flexion

The extrinsic digital flexors are mechanically capable of flexing multiple joints, from the DIP joint to, at least theoreti-

cally, the elbow. In order for these muscles to isolate their flexion potential across a single joint in the hand requires additional muscles to act synergistically with the extrinsic digital flexors. Consider the flexor digitorum superficialis performing isolated PIP joint flexion (Fig. 8–41). At the onset of contraction, the extensor digitorum communis must act as a proximal stabilizer to prevent the flexor digitorum superficialis from flexing the MCP joint and the wrist. Because the flexor moment arm length of the flexor digitorum superficialis progressively increases at the more proximal joints, a relatively small force at a distal joint is amplified to a greater torque at the more proximal joints. Figure 8–41 shows that a 20 N (4.5 lb) force within the superficialis tendon produces a 15 Ncm torque at the PIP joint, a 20 Ncm torque at the MCP joint, and a 25 Ncm torque at the midcarpal joint of the wrist. The greater the force produced by the flexor digitorum superficialis, the greater the force demands placed on the proximal stabilizers. The proximal stabilizers include the extensor digitorum and, if needed, the wrist extensors. The amount of muscle force and muscular interaction required for a simple action of PIP joint flexion is actually more than what it first appears to be.

### Passive Finger Flexion via Tenodesis Action of the Digital Flexors

The position of the wrist significantly alters the length of the extrinsic digital flexors. One implication of this arrangement can be appreciated by actively extending the wrist and observing the *passive flexion* of the fingers and thumb (Fig. 8–42). The force responsible for the digital flexion is generated by the stretch placed on the extrinsic digital flexors, such as the flexor digitorum profundus. The stretching of a polyarticular muscle across one joint, which generates a passive movement at the other, is referred to as a *tenodesis action* of a muscle. Figure 8–42 demonstrates that in the position

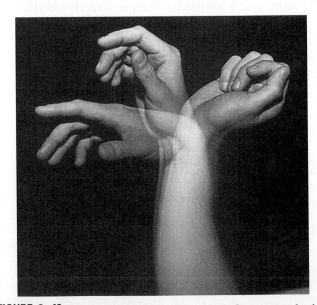

**FIGURE 8–42.** "Tenodesis action" of the finger flexors in a healthy person. As the wrist is extended, the thumb and fingers automatically flex due to the stretch placed on the extrinsic digital flexors. The flexion occurs passively, without effort from the subject.

**SPECIAL FOCUS 8-5**

**Clinical Implications of Tenodesis in Persons with Quadriplegia**

The natural tenodesis action of the extrinsic digital flexors has important clinical implications. One example involves a person with C[6] quadriplegia who has paralyzed finger flexors and extensors, but innervated wrist extensors. Those with this level of spinal injury often employ a tenodesis action for many functions, such as holding a cup of water. In order to open the hand to grasp a cup of water, the person allows gravity to flex the wrist. This, in turn, stretches the partially paralyzed extensor digitorum communis (Fig. 8–43*A*). In Figure 8–43*B*, *active extension* of the wrist stretches the paralyzed finger flexors, such as the flexor digitorum profundus, which creates enough passive force in these muscles to grasp the cup. The amount of passive force in the finger flexors is controlled by the degree of active wrist extension.

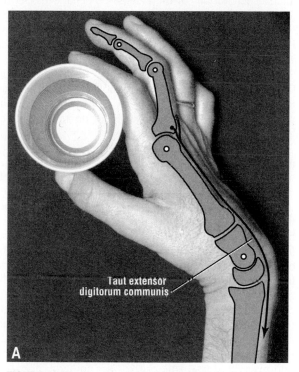

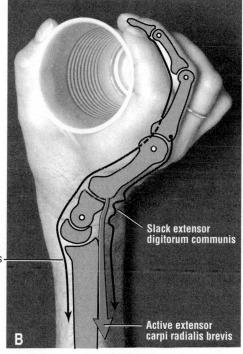

**FIGURE 8–43.** A person with C[6]-level quadriplegia using "tenodesis action" to grasp a cup of water. *A*, To prepare for grasp, the hand is opened by gravity flexing the wrist. The stretched (taut) extensor digitorum communis generates passive force that partially extends the fingers. *B*, By actively extending the wrist by the innervated extensor carpi radialis brevis (red), the stretched finger flexors—such as the flexor digitorum profundus—create a passive force to assist with grasping the cup.

of full wrist flexion, the fingers—most notably the index—are passively extended owing to a similar tenodesis action caused by the stretched extrinsic digital extensors. Tenodesis occurs to varying degrees in essentially all polyarticular muscles in the body.

## EXTRINSIC EXTENSORS OF THE FINGERS

### *Muscular Anatomy*

The extrinsic extensors of the fingers are the extensor digitorum communis, the extensor indicis, and the extensor digiti minimi (see Fig. 7–22). The extensor digitorum communis and the extensor digiti minimi originate by a common tendon from the lateral epicondyle of the humerus. The exten-

sor indicis has its proximal attachment on the dorsal region of the forearm. The *extensor digitorum communis*, in terms of cross-sectional area, is by far the predominant digital extensor. The name communis refers to the set of usually four extensor tendons that supply the four fingers. In addition to functioning as finger extensors, the extensor digitorum has an excellent moment arm as a wrist extensor (see Fig. 7–21).

The *extensor digiti minimi* is a small fusiform muscle often interconnected with the extensor digitorum. With the extensor digitorum and extensor minimi removed, the deeper extensor indicis, and the extrinsic extensor muscles of the thumb become fully exposed (Fig. 8–44). The *extensor indicis* muscle has only one tendon that serves the index finger.

**Dorsal view**

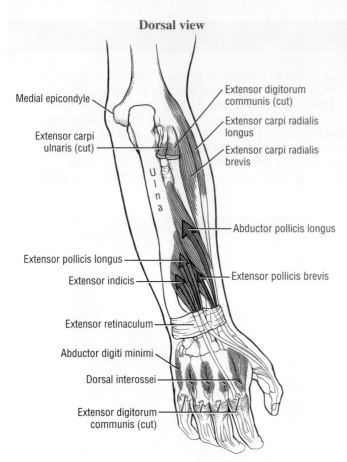

Medial epicondyle

Extensor carpi ulnaris (cut)

U l n a

Extensor pollicis longus

Extensor indicis

Extensor retinaculum

Abductor digiti minimi

Dorsal interossei

Extensor digitorum communis (cut)

Extensor digitorum communis (cut)

Extensor carpi radialis longus

Extensor carpi radialis brevis

Abductor pollicis longus

Extensor pollicis brevis

**FIGURE 8–44.** A dorsal view of the right upper extremity highlighting the group of extensors of the digits: the extensor indicis, extensor pollicis longus, extensor pollicis brevis, and abductor pollicis longus. Note the cut proximal ends of extensor carpi ulnaris and the extensor digitorum communis.

Tendons of the extensor digitorum communis, extensor indicis, and extensor digiti minimi cross the wrist in synovial-lined tunnels, located within the extensor retinaculum (see Fig. 7–23). Distal to the extensor retinaculum, the tendons course toward the fingers in a highly variable manner (Fig. 8–45). The tendons of extensor digitorum are often interconnected by several *juncturae tendinae* (from the Latin *junctura;* joining, + *tendini;* tendon). The strips of connective tissue stabilize the angle of approach of the tendons to the base of the MCP joints. The tendons of the extensor indicis and extensor digitorum communis usually travel in a parallel fashion, blending with the connective tissue on the dorsum of the proximal phalanx (Fig. 8–46).

The anatomic organization of the extensor tendons of the fingers is very different from that of the finger flexors. The finger flexor tendons travel in a well-defined digital sheath heading toward a single discrete bony attachment. In contrast, the distal attachments of the finger extensors lack a defined digital sheath or pulley system. The extensor tendons eventually become integrated into a fibrous expansion of connective tissues, located along the entire length of the dorsum of each finger (see Fig. 8–45). The complex set of

connective tissue is called the *extensor mechanism.* Other terms are used, including the extensor expansion, extensor apparatus, and extensor assembly.[10,50] The extensor mechanism serves as a primary distal attachment for the extensor digitorum and the majority of the intrinsic muscle of the fingers. The following section describes the anatomy of the extensor mechanism. A similar but less organized extensor mechanism exists for the thumb.

### Extensor Mechanism of the Fingers

A small slip of the tendon of the extensor digitorum attaches to the base of the dorsal side of the proximal phalanx. The remaining tendon flattens into a *central band,* or slip, forming the "backbone" of the extensor mechanism. (see Figs. 8–45 and 8–47). The central band courses distally to attach to the dorsal base of the middle phalanx. Before crossing the PIP joint, two *lateral bands* diverge from the central band. The bands are located dorsal to the axis of rotation at both the PIP and DIP joints, and they fuse into a *terminal tendon* that attaches to the dorsal base of the distal phalanx. The multiple attachments of the extensor mechanism into the phalanges allow the extensor digitorum to transfer extensor force distally throughout the entire finger.

In addition to attaching into the phalanges, the extensor mechanism attaches into the palmar surface of the finger through two structures: the dorsal hood and the retinacular ligaments (see Figs. 8–45 and 8–47). The *dorsal hood* is a wide, nearly triangular sheet of thin aponeurosis located at the proximal end of the extensor mechanism. The dorsal hood contains transverse and oblique fibers. The *transverse fibers,* or "sagittal" bands, run perpendicular to the long axis of the tendon of the extensor digitorum. The transverse fibers from either side of the extensor tendon attach to the palmar plate, thereby forming a "sling" around the extreme proximal end of the proximal phalanx. The transverse fibers, therefore, transmit forces from the extensor digitorum muscle that pull the proximal phalanx into extension. In addition, the transverse fibers hold the extensor digitorum tendon over the dorsal side of the MCP joint.

The *oblique fibers* course distally and medially to fuse with the lateral and central bands. The intrinsic muscles of the hand (the lumbricals and interossei) attach into the extensor mechanism via the oblique fibers of the dorsal hood. Figure 8–47 shows this arrangement for the first dorsal interosseus and lumbrical of the index finger. The intrinsic muscles via this connection, are able to help the extensor digitorum communis extend the PIP and DIP joints.

Located at the distal end of the extensor mechanism is a pair of slender *oblique retinacular ligaments* (see Fig. 8–47). The fibers arise proximally from the fibrous digital sheath, just proximal to the PIP joint, and course obliquely and distally to insert into the lateral bands. The ligaments help coordinate movement between the PIP and DIP joints of the fingers, a point to be discussed later in this chapter. The anatomic and functional aspects of the extensor mechanism are summarized in Table 8–4.

### Action of the Extrinsic Finger Extensors

Isolated contraction of the *extensor digitorum communis* produces hyperextension of the MCP joints (Fig. 8–48). Only in the presence of activated intrinsic muscles can the extensor digitorum fully extend the PIP and DIP joints.

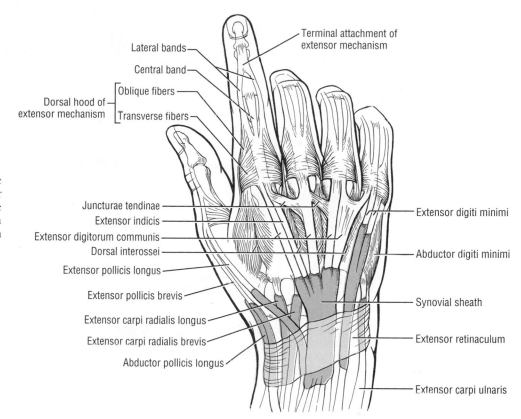

FIGURE 8-45. A dorsal view of the muscles, tendons, and extensor mechanism of the right hand. The synovial sheaths are indicated in darker red, the extensor retinaculum in lighter red.

Labels in figure:
Lateral bands
Central band
Terminal attachment of extensor mechanism
Oblique fibers
Dorsal hood of extensor mechanism
Transverse fibers
Juncturae tendinae
Extensor indicis
Extensor digitorum communis
Dorsal interossei
Extensor pollicis longus
Extensor pollicis brevis
Extensor carpi radialis longus
Extensor carpi radialis brevis
Abductor pollicis longus
Extensor digiti minimi
Abductor digiti minimi
Synovial sheath
Extensor retinaculum
Extensor carpi ulnaris

## EXTRINSIC EXTENSORS OF THE THUMB

### Anatomical Considerations

The extrinsic extensors of the thumb are the *extensor pollicis longus, extensor pollicis brevis,* and *abductor pollicis longus* (see Fig. 8-47). These radial innervated muscles have their proximal attachments on the dorsal region of the forearm. The tendons of these muscles compose the "anatomic snuffbox" located on the radial side of the wrist (Fig. 8-49). The tendons of the abductor pollicis longus and the extensor pollicis brevis travel together through a fibrous tunnel within the extensor retinaculum of the wrist (see Fig. 7-23). Distal to the extensor retinaculum, the tendon of the abductor pollicis longus inserts primarily into the radial-dorsal surface

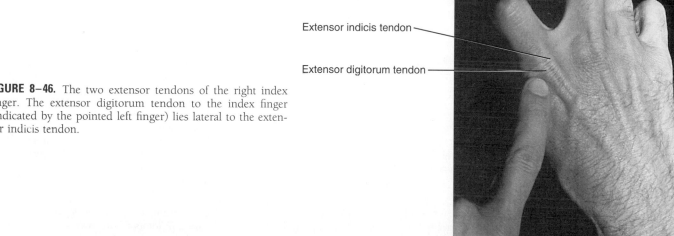

Extensor indicis tendon
Extensor digitorum tendon

FIGURE 8-46. The two extensor tendons of the right index finger. The extensor digitorum tendon to the index finger (indicated by the pointed left finger) lies lateral to the extensor indicis tendon.

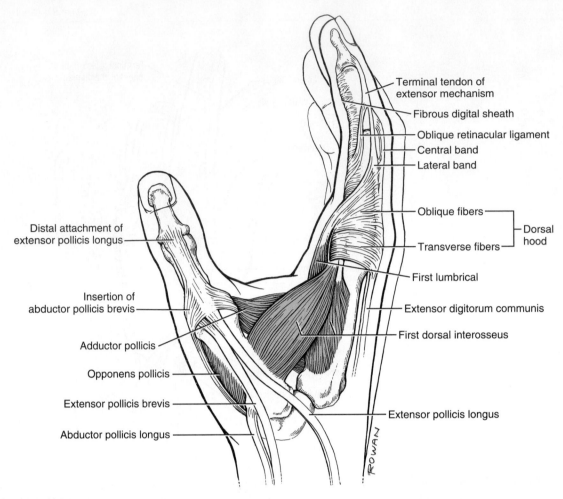

Labels on figure:
- Terminal tendon of extensor mechanism
- Fibrous digital sheath
- Oblique retinacular ligament
- Central band
- Lateral band
- Oblique fibers ⎤ Dorsal hood
- Transverse fibers ⎦
- First lumbrical
- Extensor digitorum communis
- First dorsal interosseus
- Extensor pollicis longus
- Distal attachment of extensor pollicis longus
- Insertion of abductor pollicis brevis
- Adductor pollicis
- Opponens pollicis
- Extensor pollicis brevis
- Abductor pollicis longus
- ROWAN

**FIGURE 8–47.** A radial (lateral) view of the muscles, tendons, and extensor mechanism of the right hand.

TABLE 8–4. **Anatomical and Functional Components of the Extensor Mechanism**

| Component | Pertinent Anatomy | Functional Significance |
|---|---|---|
| Central band* | Direct continuation of the extensor digitorum tendon; attaches to the dorsal side of the base of the middle phalanx. | 1) Serves as the "backbone" to the extensor mechanism.<br>2) Transmits extensor digitorum, interossei, and lumbrical extension force to the middle phalanx. |
| Lateral bands | Formed from divisions off the central band; bands fuse forming a single terminal tendon for attachment into the dorsal side of the distal phalanx. | Transmit extensor digitorum, interossei, and lumbrical extension forces to the distal phalanx. |
| Dorsal hood | *Transverse fibers*† connect the extensor tendon with either side of the palmar plate at the MCP joint. | *Transverse fibers* (1) stabilize the extensor digitorum tendon to the dorsal aspect of the MCP joint; (2) form a sling around the proximal end of the proximal phalanx. This sling is used by the extensor digitorum to extend the MCP joint. |
| | *Oblique fibers* course distally, fusing with the lateral and central bands; serve as primary or secondary attachments for lumbricals and interossei muscles. | *Oblique fibers* transfer force from lumbricals and interossei muscles into the lateral and central bands, and, in this way, the oblique fibers help extend the PIP and DIP joints. |
| Oblique retinacular ligaments | Consist of slender oblique-running fibers connecting the fibrous digital sheath to the lateral bands of the extensor mechanism. | Help coordinate movement between the PIP and DIP joints of the fingers. |

* Also called central slip.
† Also called sagittal bands.

**FIGURE 8–48.** The function of the extrinsic extensor muscles of the hand is demonstrated. Each muscle's action is determined by the orientation of the line-of-force relative to the axes of rotations at each joint (medial-lateral axes are gray; anterior-posterior axes are red). Isolated contraction of the extensor digitorum communis (EDC) hyperextends the metacarpophalangeal joints. Full extension of the interphalangeal joints requires assistance from the intrinsic muscles. The extensor pollicis longus (EPL), the extensor pollicis brevis (EPB), and the abductor pollicis longus (APL) are all primary thumb extensors. Attachments of the abductor pollicis brevis are shown blending into the distal tendon of the extensor pollicis longus.

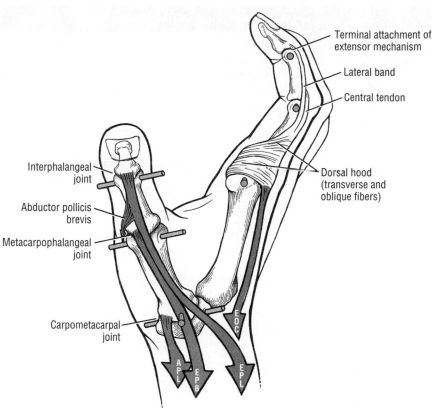

of the base of the thumb metacarpal.[54] The extensor pollicis brevis attaches distally to the dorsal base of the proximal phalanx of the thumb. The tendon of the extensor pollicis longus crosses the wrist in a separate tunnel within the extensor retinaculum in a groove just medial to the dorsal tubercle of the radius (see Fig. 7–23). The extensor pollicis longus attaches distally to the dorsal base of the distal phalanx of the thumb. Both extrinsic tendons help contribute to the extensor mechanism of the thumb.

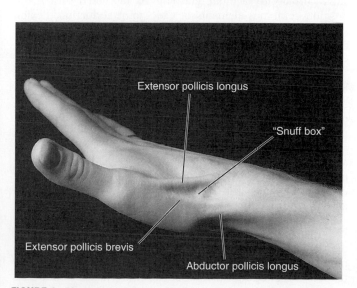

**FIGURE 8–49.** Muscles of the anatomic "snuff box" are shown.

### Functional Considerations

The multiple actions of the extensor pollicis longus, extensor pollicis brevis, and abductor pollicis longus can be understood by noting their line-of-force relative to the anterior-posterior and medial-lateral axes of rotation at the joints they cross (see Fig. 8–48). The *extensor pollicis longus* extends the IP, MCP, and CMC joints of the thumb. The muscle passes to the dorsal side of the medial-lateral axis of the CMC joint and is therefore also capable of adducting this joint. The extensor pollicis longus is unique in its ability to perform all three actions that compose the repositioning of the thumb: extension, lateral rotation, and adduction of its metacarpal.

The *extensor pollicis brevis* is an extensor of the MCP and CMC joints of the thumb; the *abductor pollicis longus* is an extensor of the CMC joint of the thumb. The muscle is also a prime abductor of the CMC joint since its line-of-force is anterior to the joint's medial-lateral axis of rotation. The dual action of the long abductor reflects its attachment on the radial-dorsal corner of the base of the thumb metacarpal. The CMC joint is reinforced by fibers of the abductor longus that attach into its capsule and adjacent trapezium. The actions of all the muscles acting on the thumb are summarized in Table 8–5.

The extensor pollicis longus and brevis, and the abductor pollicis longus, are all potent radial deviators at the wrist (see Fig. 7–21). During extension of the thumb, an ulnar deviator muscle must be activated to stabilize the wrist against unwanted radial deviation. Activation is apparent by palpating the raised tendon of the flexor carpi ulnaris, located just proximal to the pisiform, during rapid extension of the thumb.

## TABLE 8-5. Primary Actions of Muscles that Attach to the Thumb

| | | |
|---|---|---|
| CMC joint | **Flexion**<br>Adductor pollicis<br>Flexor pollicis brevis<br>Flexor pollicis longus | **Extension**<br>Extensor pollicis brevis<br>Extensor pollicis longus<br>Abductor pollicis longus |
| CMC joint | **Abduction**<br>Abductor pollicis brevis<br>Abductor pollicis longus | **Adduction**<br>Adductor pollicis<br>Extensor pollicis longus<br>First dorsal interosseus |
| CMC joint | **Opposition**<br>Opponens pollicis<br>Flexor pollicis brevis<br>Abductor pollicis brevis<br>Flexor pollicis longus<br>Abductor pollicis longus | **Reposition**<br>Extensor pollicis longus |
| MCP joint* | **Flexion**<br>Adductor pollicis<br>Flexor pollicis brevis<br>Abductor pollicis brevis<br>Flexor pollicis longus | **Extension**<br>Extensor pollicis longus<br>Extensor pollicis brevis |
| IP joint | **Flexion**<br>Flexor pollicis longus | **Extension**<br>Extensor pollicis longus<br>Abductor pollicis brevis (due to attachment into extensor mechanism) |

\* Only one degree of freedom is considered for the MCP joint.

## INTRINSIC MUSCLES OF THE HAND

The hand contains 20 intrinsic muscles. Despite their relatively small size, these muscles are essential to the fine control of the digits. Topographically, the intrinsic muscles are divided into four sets:

### 1. Muscles of the Thenar Eminence
- Abductor pollicis brevis
- Flexor pollicis brevis
- Opponens pollicis

### 2. Muscles of the Hypothenar Eminence
- Flexor digiti minimi
- Abductor digiti minimi
- Opponens digiti minimi
- Palmaris brevis

### 3. Two Heads of the Adductor Pollicis

### 4. Lumbricals and Interossei

### *Muscles of the Thenar Eminence*

#### *Anatomic Considerations*

The median nerve-innervated *abductor pollicis brevis, flexor pollicis brevis, and opponens pollicis* make up the bulk of the thenar eminence (see Fig. 8–38). The flexor pollicis brevis has two parts: a *superficial head,* which comprises most of the muscle, and a *deep head,* which comprises a small set of poorly defined fibers, often described as part of the oblique fibers of the adductor pollicis.[55] This chapter considers only the superficial head when discussing the flexor pollicis brevis. Deep to the abductor pollicis brevis is the opponens pollicis (Fig. 8–50). All three muscles have proximal attach-

ments on the transverse carpal ligament, adjacent carpal bones, and connective tissues. The short abductor and flexor have similar distal attachments to the radial side of the base of the proximal phalanx. The abductor pollicis brevis attaches to the radial side of the extensor mechanism of the thumb; the flexor pollicis brevis frequently attaches to a sesamoid bone; and the opponens pollicis attaches distally to the radial border of the thumb metacarpal.

#### *Functional Considerations*

A primary responsibility of the muscles of the thenar eminence is to position the thumb in varying amounts of opposition, usually to facilitate grasping. As discussed earlier, opposition combines elements of CMC joint abduction, flexion and medial rotation. Each muscle within the thenar eminence is a prime mover for at least one component of opposition and an assistant for several others (see Table 8–5).[28]

The action of each of the thenar muscles is based on their line-of-force relative to a particular axis of rotation (Fig. 8–51). The abductor pollicis brevis and longus abduct the metacarpal away from the plane of the palm. The flexor pollicis brevis, and to a lesser extent the medial fibers of the abductor pollicis brevis, flex the thumb at both the MCP and CMC joints. The opponens pollicis has a line-of-force to medially rotate the thumb toward the fingers. Because the opponens pollicis has its distal attachment on the metacarpal, its entire contractile force is dedicated to controlling the CMC joint.

Injury to the median nerve can disable all components of opposition. The thenar eminence becomes flat owing to muscle atrophy. The inability to oppose the thumb greatly reduces the grasping function of the entire hand. About 30%

**Palmar view**

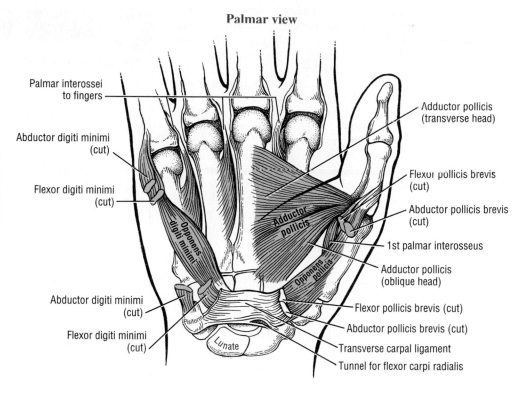

Palmar interossei to fingers

Abductor digiti minimi (cut)

Flexor digiti minimi (cut)

Abductor digiti minimi (cut)

Flexor digiti minimi (cut)

Opponens digiti minimi

Adductor pollicis

Opponens pollicis

Pisiform

Lunate

Adductor pollicis (transverse head)

Flexor pollicis brevis (cut)

Abductor pollicis brevis (cut)

1st palmar interosseus

Adductor pollicis (oblique head)

Flexor pollicis brevis (cut)

Abductor pollicis brevis (cut)

Transverse carpal ligament

Tunnel for flexor carpi radialis

**FIGURE 8–50.** A palmar view of the deep muscles of the right hand. The abductor and flexor muscles of the thenar and hypothenar eminence have been cut away to expose the underlying opponens pollicis and opponens digiti minimi.

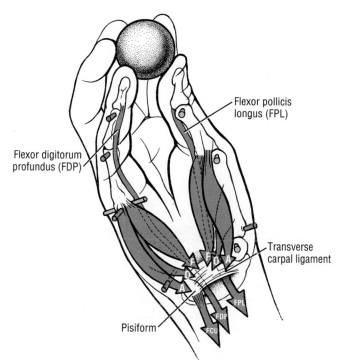

Flexor pollicis longus (FPL)

Flexor digitorum profundus (FDP)

Transverse carpal ligament

Pisiform

F O A / F O A / FPL / FDP / FCU

**FIGURE 8–51.** The action of the thenar and hypothenar muscles during opposition of the thumb and cupping of the little finger. Muscle function is based on the muscles' line-of-force relative to each joint's axes of rotation. (Medial-lateral axes are in gray; anterior-posterior axes are in red.) Other muscles shown in an active state are the flexor pollicis longus and flexor digitorum profundus of the little finger. The flexor carpi ulnaris (FCU) stabilizes the pisiform bone for the abductor digiti minimi. (F = flexor pollicis brevis and flexor digiti minimi; O = opponens pollicis and opponens digiti minimi; A = abductor pollicis brevis and abductor digiti minimi.)

of the abduction torque of the thumb is retained, however, owing to the presence of the radial-nerve innervated abductor pollicis longus.[5]

### Muscles of the Hypothenar Eminence

#### Anatomic Considerations

The muscles of the hypothenar eminence are the *flexor digiti minimi, abductor digiti minimi, opponens digiti minimi,* and *palmaris brevis* (see Fig. 8–38). The abductor digiti minimi is the most superficial and medial of these muscles, occupying the extreme ulnar border of the hand. The relatively small flexor digiti minimi is located just lateral to, and often blended with, the abductor. Deep to these muscles is the opponens digiti minimi, the largest of the hypothenar muscles. The palmaris brevis is a relatively thin and insignificant muscle about the thickness of a postage stamp. It attaches between the transverse carpal ligament and an area of skin just distal to the pisiform bone. The palmaris brevis raises the height of the hypothenar eminence to assist with the cupping of the ulnar border of the hand.

The overall anatomic plan of the hypothenar muscles is similar to that of the muscles of the thenar eminence. The flexor digiti minimi and opponens digiti minimi share proximal attachments to the transverse carpal ligament and the hook of the hamate. The abductor digiti minimi has extensive proximal attachments from the pisohamate ligament, pisiform bone, and flexor carpi ulnaris tendon. During resisted or rapid abduction of the little finger, the flexor carpi ulnaris becomes rigid to stabilize the attachment for the abductor digiti minimi. This effect can be verified by palpating the tendon of the flexor carpi ulnaris just proximal to the pisiform bone while performing this motion.

The abductor and flexor digiti minimi both have similar distal attachments to the medial border of the base of the proximal phalanx of the little finger. Some fibers from the abductor also extend to the ulnar side of the extensor mechanism. The opponens digiti minimi has its distal attachment along the ulnar border of the fifth metacarpal, proximal to the MCP joint.

### Functional Considerations

A common function of the hypothenar muscles is to cup the ulnar border of the hand and deepen the distal transverse arch (Fig. 8–51). The flexor digiti minimi flexes the fifth MCP and CMC joints. When needed, the abductor digiti minimi can spread the little finger for greater control of grasp. The opponens digiti minimi controls the rotation of the fifth metacarpal toward the middle digit. Contraction of the long finger flexors of the little finger, such as flexor digitorum profundus, also contributes to the cupping motion at the fifth CMC joint.

Injury to the ulnar nerve can cause complete paralysis of the hypothenar muscles. The hypothenar eminence becomes flat owing to muscle atrophy. Cupping of the ulnar border therefore becomes difficult or impossible.

### Two Heads of the Adductor Pollicis Muscle

The *adductor pollicis* is a two-headed muscle lying deep in the web space of the thumb, palmar to the second and third metacarpals (see Fig. 8–50). The *oblique head* has its proximal attachment on the capitate bone, the bases of the second and third metacarpals, and other adjacent connective tissues. The triangular *transverse head* has its proximal attachment on the palmar surface of the third metacarpal bone. Both heads join before attaching to the ulnar side of the base of the proximal phalanx of the thumb and often to a sesamoid bone located near the MCP joint.

Maximal force generation of the adductor pollicis exerts a vigorous flexion and adduction torque on the thumb. The force is important when firmly pinching an object between the thumb and the fingers. Figure 8–52A illustrates the large *flexion potential* of the adductor pollicis at the CMC joint. Note the very long moment arm available to the transverse head for this action. Based on leverage and tension fraction, the adductor pollicis is the most potent flexor at the CMC joint.[7] Figure 8–52B illustrates the very large moment arm available to the transverse head of the adductor pollicis for adduction at the CMC joint.[7] With the index finger well

### "Tension Fraction" of a Muscle

The adductor pollicis has a relatively large cross-sectional area and is therefore capable of generating large active forces. As a method to compare cross-sectional areas of this and other muscles, Brand and colleagues[9] have assigned each muscle below the elbow a relative *tension fraction*. This measurement is determined by dividing a muscle's physiologic cross-section by the total cross-sectional area of all muscles below the elbow (Table 8–6). This value, expressed as a percentage, provides an estimate of each muscle's relative force capability. The adductor pollicis has a tension fraction almost twice that of the average of all muscles of the thenar eminence. Data on tension fraction have been used by surgeons to help them decide on the most appropriate muscle for use in reconstructive hand surgery.

**TABLE 8–6. Tension Fractions (%) of Selected Muscles**

| Muscle | Tension Fraction |
| --- | --- |
| Supinator | 7.1 |
| Extensor carpi radialis brevis | 4.2 |
| Dorsal interosseus (index) | 3.2 |
| Abductor pollicis longus | 3.1 |
| Adductor pollicis | 3.0 |
| Pronator quadratus | 3.0 |
| Flexor digitorum profundus (index) | 2.8 |
| Flexor pollicis longus | 2.7 |
| Flexor digitorum superficialis (index) | 2.0 |
| Opponens digiti minimi | 2.0 |
| Opponens pollicis | 1.9 |
| Abductor digiti minimi | 1.4 |
| Extensor pollicis longus | 1.3 |
| Flexor pollicis brevis | 1.3 |
| Palmar interosseus (index) | 1.3 |
| Abductor pollicis brevis | 1.1 |
| Extensor digitorum communis (index) | 1.0 |
| Extensor pollicis brevis | .8 |
| Flexor digiti minimi | .4 |
| Lumbrical (index) | .2 |

Data from Brand PW, Beach RB, Thompson DE: Relative tension and potential excursion of muscles in the forearm and hand. J Hand Surg 6A:209–219, 1981.

stabilized, the first dorsal interosseus muscle can assist the adductor pollicis with this function.

### Lumbricals and Interossei Muscles

The *lumbricals* (from the Latin root *lumbricus;* an earthworm) are four very slender muscles originating from the tendons of the flexor digitorum profundus (see Fig. 8–38). Like the flexor digitorum profundus, the lumbricals have a dual source of innervation: the two lateral lumbricals are innervated by the median nerve, and the two medial lumbricals are innervated by the ulnar nerve.

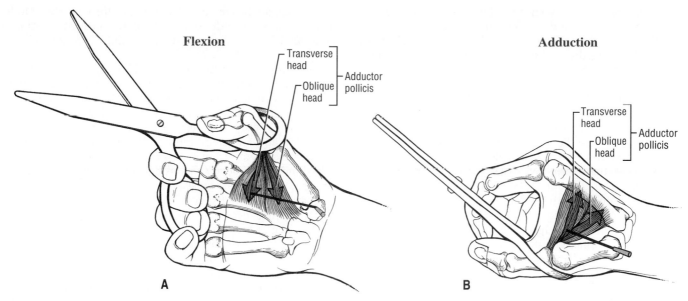

**FIGURE 8–52.** The biplanar action of the adductor pollicis muscle is illustrated using a pair of scissors for flexion *(A)* and adduction *(B)* at the carpometacarpal joint. In both *A* and *B*, the transverse head of the adductor pollicis produces a significant torque owing to its long moment arm about an anterior-posterior axis (red, *A*) and medial-lateral axis (gray, *B*). The adductor pollicis is also a potent flexor of the metacarpophalangeal joint.

All four lumbricals show marked anatomic variation in both size and attachments.[55] From their tendinous proximal attachments, the lumbricals course palmar to the deep intermetacarpal ligament, then pass around the *radial side* of the MCP joints. Distally, the lumbricals blend with the oblique fibers of the dorsal hood (see Fig. 8–47, first lumbrical). The distal attachment enables the lumbricals to exert a pull through the central and lateral bands of the extensor mechanism.

The function of the lumbricals has been a topic of study for many years (see references 2, 10, 32, 34, 43, and 52).

Muscle contraction produces extension at both the PIP and DIP joints and flexion at the MCP joints.[2] This seemingly paradoxical action is possible because the lumbricals pass *palmar* to the MCP joints and *dorsal* to the PIP and DIP joints (Fig. 8–53).

Of all the intrinsic muscles of the hand, the lumbricals have the longest fiber length, but the smallest tension fraction.[9,25] This anatomic design suggests that these muscles are capable of generating only small amounts of force over a relatively long distance.

The *interossei muscles* are named according to their loca-

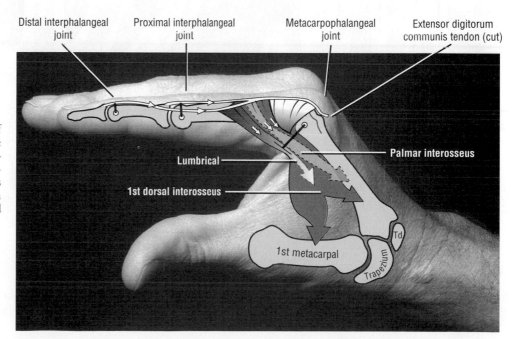

**FIGURE 8–53.** The combined action of the lumbricals and interossei are shown as flexors at the metacarpophalangeal joint and extensors at the interphalangeal joints. The lumbrical is shown with the greatest moment arm for flexion at the metacarpophalangeal joint. (Td = trapezoid bone).

tion in the regions between the shafts of the metacarpal bones (see Figs. 8–4 and 8–5).[55] In general, the interossei act at the MCP joints to spread the digits apart (abduction) or bring them together (adduction). The anatomy and precise action of each interosseus muscle is slightly different.[18,50,53]

The four *palmar interossei* are slender, single-headed muscles occupying the palmar region of the interosseous spaces.[55] The three palmar interossei to the fingers have their proximal attachments on the palmar surfaces and sides of the second, fourth, and fifth metacarpals (see Fig. 8–50). These muscles have their primary distal attachments into the oblique fibers of the dorsal hood. The palmar interossei adduct the second, fourth, and fifth MCP joints toward the midline of the hand (Fig. 8–54). The palmar interosseus muscle to the thumb occupies the first palmar interosseous space, having a primary distal attachment to the ulnar side of the proximal phalanx of the thumb, and often into a sesamoid bone at the MCP joint.[55] This muscle flexes the MCP joint of the thumb, bringing the first metacarpal toward the middle digit of the hand.

The four *dorsal interossei* fill the dorsal sides of the interosseous spaces (see Fig. 8–44). In contrast to the palmar interossei, the dorsal muscles have a bipennate shape. As a general rule, the dorsal interossei have distal attachments into the side of the base of the proximal phalanx and into the oblique fibers of the dorsal hood. The first dorsal interosseus attaches mostly into bone. The dorsal interossei abduct the MCP joints of the index, middle, and ring fingers away from an imaginary reference line through the middle digit (see Fig. 8–54). Abduction of the fifth MCP joint is performed by the abductor digiti minimi of the hypothenar group.

In addition to abducting and adducting the fingers, the interossei and abductor digiti minimi provide an important source of dynamic stability to the MCP joints. By visually superimposing the two hands shown in Figure 8–54, it is apparent that each *MCP joint* of the fingers receives a pair of abducting and adducting muscles. Each pair acts as a set of dynamic collateral ligaments, providing strength to the MCP joints and subsequently the arch system of the hand. Acting in pairs, this intrinsic musculature also controls the extent of axial rotation permitted at the MCP joints.

To varying degrees, both palmar and dorsal interossei have a line-of-force that passes palmar to the MCP joints. The interossei, via their attachments into the extensor mechanism, pass dorsal to the IP joints of the fingers (see Fig. 8–53). Like the lumbricals, therefore, contraction of the interossei causes flexion at the MCP joint and extension at the IP joints. The interossei produce greater flexion torques at the MCP joints than the lumbricals. Even though the lumbricals have the larger moment arm for this action, the 20-fold greater tension fraction of the interossei provides them with the overpowering flexion torque advantage (Table 8–6). In contrast to the lumbricals, the interossei produce relatively larger forces, but over a shorter excursion.[25] Table 8–7 summarizes some of the differences and similarities between the lumbricals and interossei.

**Palmar interossei**                              **Dorsal interossei**

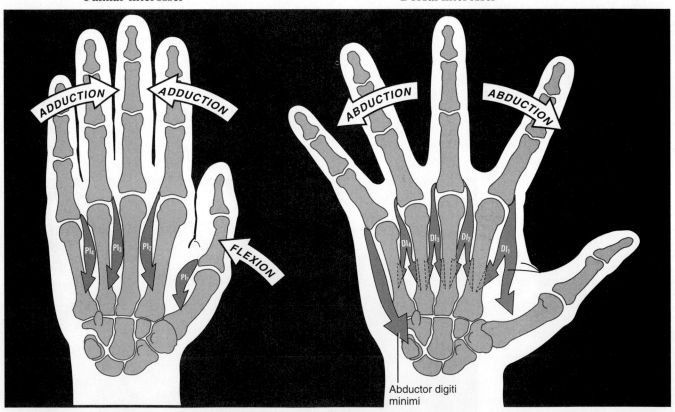

**FIGURE 8–54.** A palmar view of the frontal plane action of the palmar interossei (PI$_1$ to PI$_4$) and dorsal interossei (DI$_1$ to DI$_4$) at the metacarpophalangeal joints of the hand. The abductor digiti minimi is shown abducting the little finger.

### Muscular Biomechanics of a "Key Pinch"

Pinching an object between the thumb and the lateral side of the index finger is an important function of the hand. This action is often referred to as a key pinch. Several muscles interact to produce an effective key pinch, most notably the first dorsal interosseus and the adductor pollicis—two ulnar nerve innervated muscles.

An especially large force is demanded from the first dorsal interosseus muscle during the key pinch. This demand can be appreciated by palpating its prominent belly during the key pinch, about 2.5 cm proximal to the lateral side of the MCP joint of the index finger. For an effective pinch, the first dorsal interosseus muscle must provide a strong counteracting pinch force against the potent pinch force of the thumb (see $PF_I$ vs. $PF_T$ in Fig. 8–55). Flexion, the "strongest" of all thumb movements,[28] is driven primarily by the adductor pollicis and flexor pollicis brevis. The internal moment arm used by the first dorsal interosseus for abduction at the MCP joint of the index finger is about 1 cm. The pinch force applied by the thumb against the MCP joint of the index finger acts with an "external" moment arm of about 5 cm. This 5-fold difference in leverage across the MCP joint requires that the first dorsal interosseus must produce a force 5 times the pinching force applied by the thumb. Since many functional activities require a pinch force that exceeds 45 N (~10 lb), the first dorsal interosseus must be able to produce an abduction force of 225 N (~50 lb)! Skeletal muscle is capable of producing about 28 $N/cm^2$ (~40 lb/$in^2$); therefore, an average first dorsal interosseus muscle, with a cross-section area of about 3.8 $cm^2$, produces only about 106 N (~24 lb) of force.[15] The additional stabilizing force required to brace the index finger must be supplied by other muscles, such as the second, and perhaps the third, dorsal interosseus.

With an ulnar nerve lesion, the adductor pollicis muscle—the primary pinching muscle of the thumb—and all interossei muscles are paralyzed. The strength of a key pinch is significantly reduced following a nerve block to the ulnar nerve. The region around the dorsal web space becomes hollow owing to atrophy in the above muscles (see Fig. 8–56). A person with an ulnar nerve lesion often relies on the flexor pollicis longus (a median nerve-innervated muscle) to partially compensate for the loss of thumb pinch. This compensation is evident by the partially flexed IP joint of the thumb—known as the Froment's sign. Pinch still remains weak, however, because the dorsal interossei are not able to stabilize against the flexion force of the thumb.

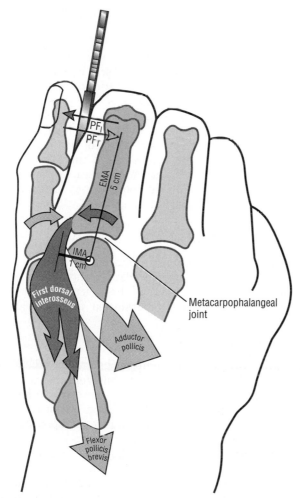

**FIGURE 8–55.** A dorsal view of the muscle mechanics of a "key pinch." Illustrated in lighter red, the adductor pollicis and flexor pollicis brevis are shown producing a pinch force through the thumb ($PF_T$). In dark red, the first dorsal interosseus is shown opposing the pinch force through the thumb by producing a pinch force though the index finger ($PF_I$). The external moment arm (EMA) at the metacarpophalangeal joint equals 5 cm; the internal moment arm (IMA) at the metacarpophalangeal joint equals 1 cm.

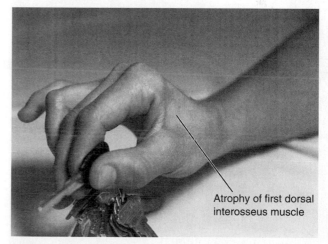

**FIGURE 8–56.** A person with an ulnar nerve lesion attempting to make a key pinch. Note the atrophy over the region of the first dorsal interosseus muscle. The flexion at the interphalangeal joint of the thumb is a way to help compensate for the paralysis of the adductor pollicis.

**TABLE 8-7.** **Anatomical and Functional Comparison Between the Lumbricals and Interossei Muscles**

|  | Lumbricals | Dorsal Interossei | Palmar Interossei |
|---|---|---|---|
| Innervation | Lateral: median nerve<br>Medial: ulnar nerve | Ulnar nerve | Ulnar nerve |
| Distal attachments | Lateral margin of the dorsal hood of the extensor mechanism | Dorsal hood of extensor mechanism and proximal phalanx | Dorsal hood of extensor mechanism |
| Contractile characteristics | Produce a relatively small force over a long excursion | Produce a relatively large force over a short excursion | Produce a relatively large force over a short excursion |
| Prime action | MCP joint flexion and IP joint extension | *Abduction;* MCP joint flexion and IP joint extension | *Adduction;* MCP joint flexion and IP joint extension |
| Comments | May have significant anatomic variation | First dorsal interosseus attaches almost exclusively to the proximal phalanx of the index finger |  |

## Interaction of the Extrinsic and Intrinsic Muscles of the Fingers

Contraction of the intrinsic muscles of the hand (lumbricals and interossei) produce MCP joint flexion with IP joint extension (see Fig. 8–53). This position is called the *intrinsic-plus position*. In contrast, contraction of the *extrinsic muscles* (extensor digitorum, flexor digitorum superficialis, and flexor digitorum profundus) produces a position of MCP joint hyperextension with IP joint flexion: the *extrinsic-plus position*. The two contrasting positions are presented in Figure 8–57. Most meaningful motions of the fingers involve a muscular interaction of both extrinsic and intrinsic muscles. As de-

scribed subsequently, the extensor mechanism provides the mechanical linkage between these sets of muscles. Interaction between the extrinsic and intrinsic muscles produces many combinations of movements at both the finger and the thumb. The following analysis addresses the muscular interaction within a typical finger during two fundamental tasks: *opening and closing of the hand*. Much of this material, especially that involving the actions of the lumbricals and interossei, remains controversial. A complicating factor is that persons often select different combinations of hand muscles to perform identical functional tasks.[26]

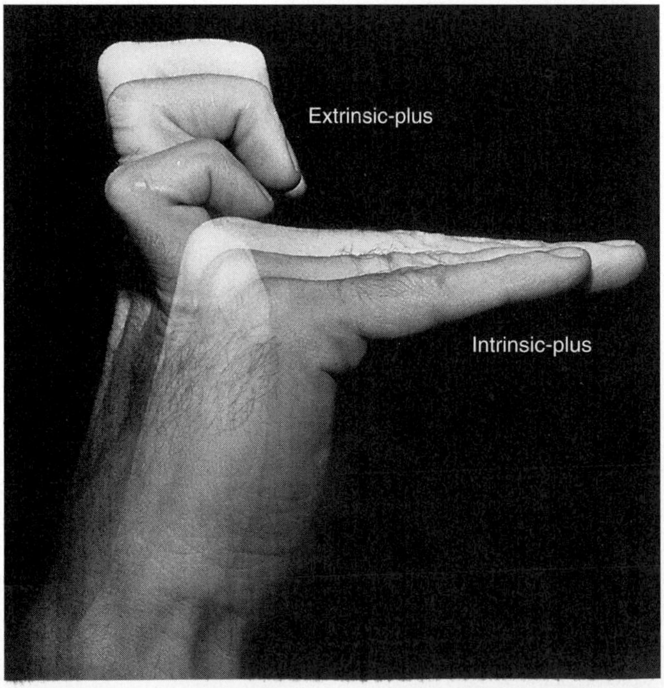

## OPENING THE HAND: FINGER EXTENSION

Opening the hand is often performed to prepare for a grasp. The action occurs through coordinated motions of extension at the MCP and the IP joints of the fingers. Extension of the thumb occurs through a coordinated action of all of its joints.

### *Primary Muscular Activity*

The greatest resistance to complete extension of the fingers is usually not from external sources, but from the passive resistance generated by the stretching of the extrinsic finger flexors, in particular the flexor digitorum profundus.[33] The passive recoil force inherent to this muscle is responsible for the partially flexed posture of a relaxed hand.

The primary extensors of the fingers are the *extensor digitorum communis* and the *intrinsic muscles,* specifically the lumbricals and interossei (Fig. 8–58).[10,34] The lumbricals show a greater and more consistent EMG level than the interossei during finger extension.[34]

Figure 8–58A shows the extensor digitorum communis exerting a force on the extensor mechanism, pulling the MCP joint toward extension. The intrinsic muscles furnish both a direct and an indirect effect on the mechanics of extension of the IP joints (Fig. 8–58B and C). The *direct effect* is provided by the proximal pull on the bands of the extensor mechanism; the *indirect effect* is provided by the production of a flexion torque at the MCP joint. The flexion torque restrains the extensor digitorum from hyperextending

**FIGURE 8-57.** The extrinsic-plus and intrinsic-plus positions of the hand.

## Opening the hand

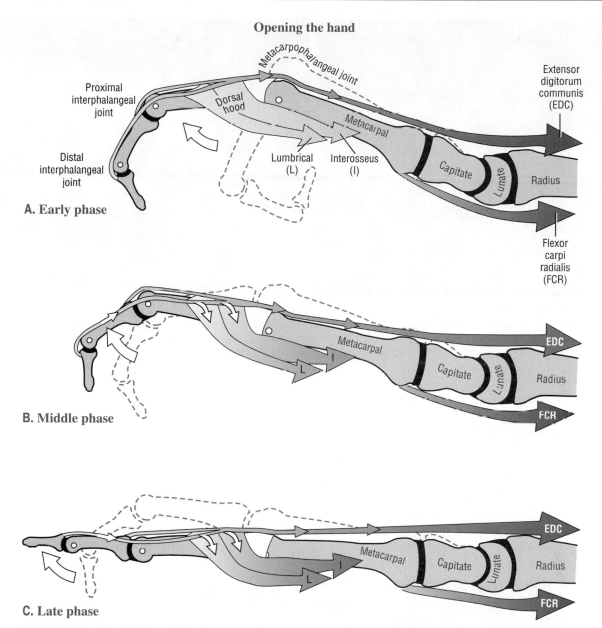

**A. Early phase**

**B. Middle phase**

**C. Late phase**

**FIGURE 8–58.** A lateral view of the intrinsic and extrinsic muscular interactions at one finger during the *opening* of the hand. The dotted outlines depict starting positions. *A*, Early phase: The extensor digitorum communis is shown extending primarily the metacarpophalangeal joint. *B*, Middle phase: The intrinsic muscles (lumbricals and interossei) assist the extensor digitorum communis with extension of the proximal and distal interphalangeal joints. The intrinsic muscles also produce a flexion torque at the metacarpophalangeal joint that prevents the extensor digitorum communis from hyperextending the metacarpophalangeal joint. *C*, Late phase: Muscle activation continues through full finger extension. Note the activation in the flexor carpi radialis to slightly flex the wrist. Observe the proximal migration of the dorsal hood between flexion and full extension. (The intensity of the red indicates the relative intensity of the muscle activity.)

the MCP joint—an action that may prematurely dissipate most of its contractile force. Only with the MCP joint blocked from hyperextending can the extensor digitorum contribute an effective IP joint extension force throughout the bands of the extensor mechanism.

The extensor digitorum and the intrinsic muscles must cooperate to perform complete finger extension. The opposing actions of these muscles at the MCP joint permit them to function synergistically at the IP joints. The importance of

this cooperative relationship is apparent by observing a person with a lesion to the ulnar nerve (Fig. 8–59A). Without active resistance from either the lumbricals or interossei in the medial two fingers, activation of the extensor digitorum communis causes the characteristic clawing of the fingers. The MCP joints hyperextend, and the IP joints remain partially flexed. This is often called the "intrinsic-minus" posture because of the lack of intrinsic-innervated muscle. (This posture is functionally similar to the "extrinsic-plus" posture

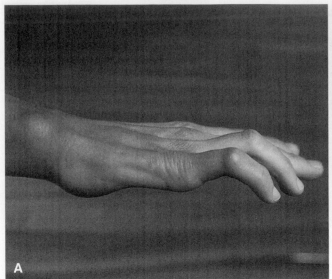
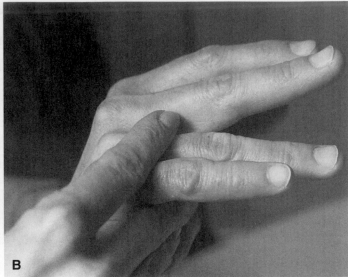

**FIGURE 8–59.** Attempts to extend the fingers with an ulnar nerve lesion and a paralysis of the most intrinsic muscles of the fingers. *A,* The medial fingers show the "claw" position with metacarpophalangeal joints hyperextended and fingers partially flexed. Note the atrophy in the hypothenar eminence and interosseous spaces. *B,* By manually holding the metacarpophalangeal joints into flexion, the extensor digitorum communis, innervated by the radial nerve, is able to fully extend the interphalangeal joints.

depicted earlier.) Without the MCP joint flexion torque normally provided by the intrinsic muscles, the extensor digitorum communis is capable of only hyperextending the MCP joints. This posture increases the passive tension in the stretched flexor digitorum profundus, thereby further limiting full IP joint extension. As shown in Figure 8–59B, by manually providing a flexion torque across the MCP joint (i.e., a force normally furnished by the intrinsic muscles), contraction of the extensor digitorum communis fully extends the IP joints. Blocking of the MCP joint from hyperextending also slackens the profundus tendon, thereby minimizing passive resistance to IP joint extension.

### Function of Wrist Flexors during Finger Extension

Activation of the wrist flexors normally accompanies finger extension. Although activity is depicted only in the flexor carpi radialis in Figure 8–58, other wrist flexors are also active. The wrist flexors offset the potent extension potential of the extensor digitorum at the wrist. The wrist actually flexes slightly throughout full finger extension, especially when performed rapidly. (Compare Figure 8–58A with Figure 8–58C.) Wrist flexion helps maintain optimal length of the extensor digitorum during active finger extension.

### Passive Forces Produced by the Oblique Retinacular Ligaments

As depicted in Figure 8–47, the oblique retinacular ligaments have proximal attachments on either side of the fibrous digital sheaths surrounding the flexor tendons, just proximal to the PIP joint. The distal ends of these ligaments attach to the lateral bands of the extensor mechanism. Each oblique ligament courses from the palmar side of the PIP joint to the dorsal side of the DIP joint. Their oblique direction helps coordinate extension between the DIP and PIP joints.[21] The extensor digitorum communis and intrinsic muscles extend the PIP joint, which stretches the oblique

retinacular ligament (Fig. 8–60, steps 1–3). The passive force in the elongated oblique ligament is transferred distally, helping to initiate extension at the DIP joint (Fig. 8–60, step 4). The oblique retinacular ligament is sometimes called the "link ligament," suggesting its probable role in synchronizing extension at both joints.

The oblique retinacular ligament may become tight owing to arthritis, trauma, or Dupuytren's contracture. Dupuytren's contracture is a condition of nodular proliferation in the palmar fascia of the hand, causing a flexed posture of the fingers, especially on the medial side of the palm. Tightness in this structure can cause flexion contracture at the PIP joint. Attempts at passively extending a PIP joint with a tight oblique retinacular ligament are often associated with a passive extension of the DIP joint.

**Active finger extension**

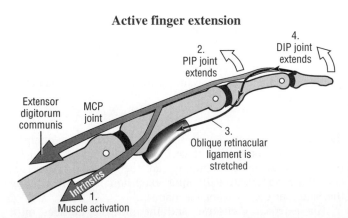

**FIGURE 8–60.** The transfer of passive force in the stretched oblique retinacular ligament during active extension of the finger. The numbered sequence (1 to 4) indicates the chronologic order of events.

# CLOSING THE HAND: FINGER FLEXION

Closing the hand requires a coordinated flexion of the MCP, PIP, and DIP joints of the fingers along with flexion and opposition of the thumb.

### *Primary Muscle Action*

The muscles needed to close the hand depend in part on the specific joints that need to be flexed and on the force requirements of the action. Flexing the fingers against a considerable resistance (i.e., making a high-powered fist) requires activation from the flexor digitorum profundus, flexor digitorum superficialis, and interossei muscles (Fig. 8–61A). Forces from the *flexor digitorum profundus* and *superficialis* combine to flex all three joints of the fingers. The flexing finger pulls the extensor mechanism distally by several millimeters.

During hand closure against a considerable resistance, the interossei muscles exhibit a very high level of EMG activity.[34] The interossei can produce relatively large flexion torques at the MCP joint. The *lumbricals*, in contrast to the interossei, show essentially no EMG activity during resisted or nonresisted closing of the hand. The lack of activation, however, does not mean that the lumbricals are incapable of producing useful forces. Recall that the lumbricals attach between the flexor profundus and the extensor mechanism. During active finger flexion, the lumbricals are stretched in a proximal direction owing to the contracting flexor profundus and, at the same time, stretched in a distal direction owing to the distal migration of the extensor mechanism (Fig. 8–61B, bidirectional arrow in lumbrical). Between full finger extension and full active flexion, a lumbrical must stretch an extraordinary distance.[43] The stretch generates a *passive flexion torque* at the MCP joint, which supplements the *active flexion torque* produced by the interossei and extrinsic musculature.

Injury to the ulnar nerve can cause paralysis of most of the intrinsic muscles, resulting in a noticeably weakened grasp. When making a fist, the sequencing of flexion across the joints is altered. Normally, at least in the radial three fingers, the PIP and DIP joints flex first, followed closely in time by flexion at the MCP joints. With paralyzed intrinsic muscles, especially if overstretched by chronic hyperextension of the MCP joints, the initiation of flexion at the MCP joints is delayed slightly. The resulting asynchronous flexion may interfere with the quality of the grasp.

**Closing the hand**

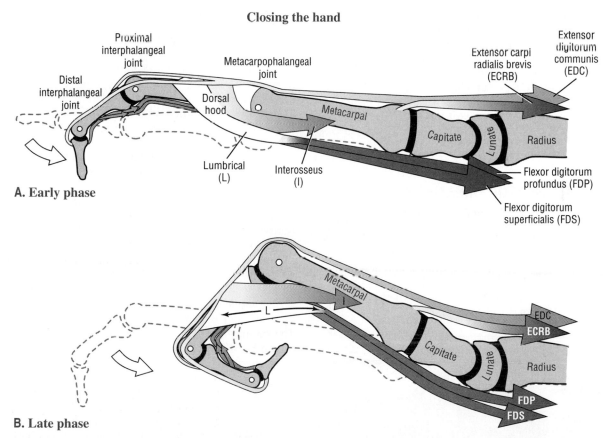

**A. Early phase**

**B. Late phase**

**FIGURE 8–61.** A side view of the intrinsic and extrinsic muscular interaction at one finger during a "high-powered" closing of the hand. The dotted outlines depict the starting positions. *A,* Early phase: The flexor digitorum profundus, flexor digitorum superficialis, and interossei muscles actively flex the joints of the finger. The lumbrical is shown as being inactive (white). *B,* Late phase: Muscle activation continues essentially unchanged through full flexion. The lumbrical remains inactive, but is stretched across both ends. The extensor carpi radialis brevis is shown extending the wrist slightly. The extensor digitorum communis helps decelerate flexion of the metacarpophalangeal joint. Note the distal migration of the dorsal hood between the early and late phases of flexion. (The intensity of the red indicates the relative intensity of the muscle activity.)

In contrast to a high-powered fist, a light, low-powered fist produces EMG activity almost exclusively from the flexor digitorum profundus. Because this muscle crosses all the joints of the fingers, its activation alone is minimally adequate to lightly close the fist. The flexor digitorum superficialis functions more as a reserve muscle, becoming active during a high-powered fist, or when isolated PIP joint flexion is required.

Extensor digitorum shows consistent EMG activity while closing the hand.[33] This activity reflects the muscle's role as an extension brake at the MCP joint. This important stabilization function allows the long finger flexors to shift their action distally to the PIP and DIP joints. Without coactivation of the extensor digitorum, the long finger flexors exhaust most of their flexion potential over the more proximal MCP joints, reducing their potential for more refined actions at the more distal joints.

### Function of Wrist Extensors During Finger Flexion

Making a strong fist requires strong synergistic activation from the wrist extensor muscles (see Fig. 8–61, extensor carpi radialis brevis). Wrist extensor activity can be verified by palpating the dorsum of the forearm while making a fist. As explained in Chapter 7, the primary function of the wrist extensors, including the extensor digitorum, is to neutralize the strong wrist flexion tendency of the activated extrinsic finger flexors (see Fig. 7–24). Wrist extension, while closing the hand, also helps to maintain an optimal length of the extrinsic finger flexors. (Compare Figure 8–61A with Figure 8–61B.) If the wrist extensors are paralyzed, attempts at making a fist result in a posture of wrist flexion and finger flexion. When combined with the increased passive tension in the overstretched extensor digitorum, the overshortened, activated finger flexors cannot produce an effective grip (see Fig. 7–26).

## HAND AS AN EFFECTOR ORGAN

The hand functions as an effector organ of the upper extremity for support, manipulation, and prehension. As a *support,* the hand acts in a nonspecific manner to brace or stabilize an object, often freeing the other hand for a more specific task. The hand may also be used as a simple platform to transfer or accept forces, such as when supporting the head when tired or when assisting in standing from a seated position.

---

**The Hand Can Be Considered to Function in the Following Ways:**

- *Support*
- *Manipulation:*
    Repetitive and blunt
    Continuous and fluid
- *Prehension* used during grip and pinch:
    Power grip
    Precision grip
    Power (key) pinch
    Precision pinch
    Hook grip

---

Perhaps the most varied function of the hand is its ability to dynamically *manipulate* objects. The number of ways the digits are used to manipulate objects is essentially infinite. In a very general sense, however, the hand manipulates objects in two fundamentally different ways: digital motions may be *repetitive and blunt,* like typing or scratching; and, in contrast, digital motions may be *continuous and fluid,* in which the rate and intensity of motion are controlled, like writing or sewing. And, of course, many if not most types of digital manipulation combine both of these elements of movement.

*Prehension* describes the ability of the fingers and thumb to grasp or to seize, often for holding, securing, and picking up objects. Over the years, several terms have evolved to describe the many forms of prehension.[31,39] Most forms of prehension can be described as a *grip* (or grasp), in which all digits are used, or as a *pinch,* in which primarily the thumb and index finger are used. Each of these forms of prehension can be further classified based on the need for *power* (loosely defined as high force without regard to the exactness of the task) or *precision* (i.e., high level of exactness with low force). Basically, most types of prehension activities fall into one of five types:

1. *Power grip* is used when stability and large forces are required from the hand, without the need for precision. The shape of the held objects tends to be spherical or cylindrical. Using a hammer is a good example of a power grip (Fig. 8–62A). This activity requires strong forces from the finger flexors, especially from the fourth and fifth digits; intrinsic muscles of the fingers, especially the interossei; and the thumb adductor and flexor musculature. Wrist extensors are needed to stabilize the partially extended wrist.

2. *Precision grip* is used when control and/or some delicate action is needed during prehension (Fig. 8–62B and C). The thumb is usually held partially abducted, and the fingers are partially flexed. Precision grip uses the thumb and one or more of the digits to improve grip security or to add variable amounts of force. The precision grip is modified to fit objects of varied sizes by altering the contour of the distal transverse arch of the hand (Fig. 8–62D to F).

3. *Power (key) pinch* is used when large forces are needed to stabilize an object between the thumb and the lateral border of the index finger (Fig. 8–62G). The power pinch is an extremely useful form of prehension, combining the force of the adductor pollicis and first dorsal interosseus with the dexterity and sensory acuity of the thumb and index finger. The biomechanics of the power key pinch are illustrated in Figure 8–55.

4. *Precision pinch* is used to provide fine control to objects held between the thumb and index finger, without the need for power. This type of pinch has many forms, such as the *tip-to-tip or pulp-to-pulp* method of holding an object (Fig. 8–62H and I). Tip-to-tip pinch is used especially for tiny objects, when skill and precision are required. Pulp-to-pulp pinch provides greater surface area for contact with larger objects, thereby increasing prehensile security.

5. *Hook grip* is a form of prehension that does not involve the thumb. A hook grip is formed by the partially flexed PIP and DIP joints of the fingers. This grip is often used in a static nature for prolonged periods of time, such as holding a luggage strap (Fig. 8–62J). The force of the

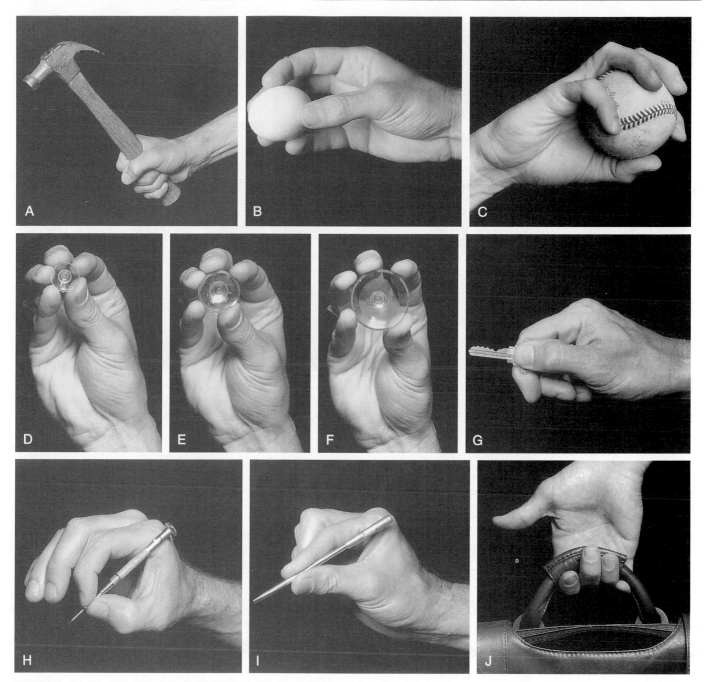

**FIGURE 8–62.** A healthy hand is shown performing common types of prehension functions. *A*, Power grip. *B*, Precision grip to hold an egg. *C*, Precision grip to throw a baseball. *D* to *F*, Modifications of the precision grip by altering the concavity of the distal transverse arch. *G*, Power key pinch. *H*, Tip-to-tip prehension pinch. *I*, Pulp-to-pulp prehension pinch. *J*, Hook grip.

hook grip is usually produced by relatively low level activity from the flexor digitorum profundus.

The categories of prehension now described do not include all of the possible ways that the hand can be used as an effector organ. These definitions can, however, establish a common reference for clinical communication. To illustrate, consider the terminology to describe methods of using three common tools. As shown in Figure 8–63A, tightening a screw involves a *precision pinch* to hold the screw and a *combined power grip* and *power pinch* to rotate the screw-

driver. The manipulation or rotation of the screwdriver in this case is performed by supination of the forearm complex. As shown in Figure 8–63B, a one-handed task of adjusting a wrench requires a *power grip* prehension of the medial fingers and a *manipulation* of the index finger and thumb. As a final example, consider the holding of a pliers (Fig. 8–63C). The thumb and index finger are in a modified *power (key) pinch*; the one upper handle of the pliers is *supported* by the palm; and the other handle is *manipulated* by action of the finger flexors.

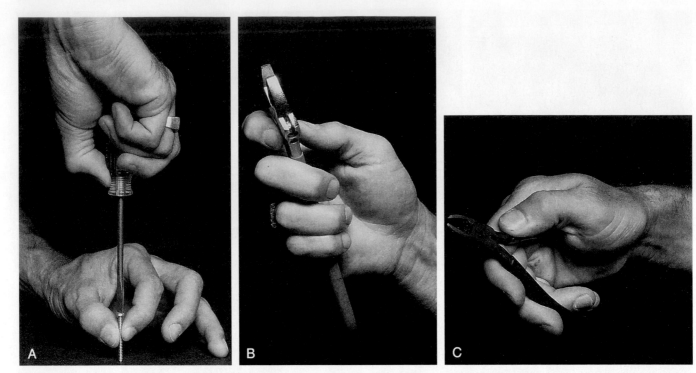

**FIGURE 8-63.** Examples of the terminology to describe the use of three common tools. *A,* Handling a screwdriver by a *precision pinch* of the right hand and a *combined power grip* and *power pinch* of the left hand. *B,* A one-handed task of adjusting a wrench requires a *power grip* by the medial fingers and a *manipulation prehension* of the index finger and thumb. *C,* Using pliers requires that the thumb and index finger produce a *power pinch.* The upper handle of the pliers *is supported* by the palm and the lower handle *is manipulated* by action of the finger flexors.

## JOINT DEFORMITIES CAUSED BY RHEUMATOID ARTHRITIS

One of the more destructive aspects of rheumatoid arthritis is chronic synovitis. Over time, synovitis tends to reduce the tensile strength of the periarticular connective tissues. Without the normal restraint provided by these tissues, forces from muscle contraction and the external environment can destroy the mechanical integrity of a joint. The joint often becomes malaligned, unstable, and frequently deformed permanently. Knowledge of the pathomechanics of common hand deformities associated with rheumatoid arthritis is a prerequisite for effective treatment.

### Zig-Zag Deformity of the Thumb

Advanced rheumatoid arthritis often results in a zig-zag deformity of the thumb. As defined in Chapter 7, zig-zag deformity describes the collapse of multiple interconnected joints in alternating directions. A common example of this deformity involves CMC joint flexion and adduction, MCP joint hyperextension, and IP joint flexion (Fig. 8–64). In this example, the collapse of the thumb starts with instability at the CMC joint.[38] Ligaments that normally reinforce the medial side of the joint, such as the anterior oblique ligament and the ulnar collateral ligaments, weaken and/or rupture owing to the disease process. Subsequently, the base of the thumb metacarpal dislocates off the lateral edge of the trapezium. Once this dislocation occurs, the adductor and short flexor muscles, which are often in spasm, hold the

thumb metacarpal rigidly against the palm. In time, rheumatoid disease may cause the muscles to become fibrotic and permanently shortened, maintaining the deformity at the CMC joint. In efforts to extend the rigid thumb out of the palm, a compensatory hyperextension deformity at the MCP joint often occurs. A weakened palmar plate offers little resistance to the forces produced by the extensor pollicis longus and brevis. Eventual bowstringing of these tendons across the MCP joint increases their leverage as extensors, thereby further contributing to the hyperextension deformity. The IP joint tends to remain flexed owing to the passive tension in the stretched flexor pollicis longus.

Clinical management of a zig-zag deformity of the thumb depends on the mechanics of the collapse and the severity of the underlying disease. Splinting and/or surgery is often indicated to reestablish proper joint alignment, especially at the CMC joint. Reconstruction of the CMC joint using the tendon of the flexor carpi radialis is often performed.[12] Because of the chronic nature of rheumatoid arthritis and the complexity of the CMC joint, artificial joint replacement is often unsuccessful.

### Destruction of the Metacarpophalangeal Joints of the Finger

Advanced rheumatoid arthritis is often associated with deformities at the MCP joint of the fingers. Two common deformities are a palmar dislocation and an ulnar drift (Fig. 8–65).

**Zig-zag deformity of the thumb**

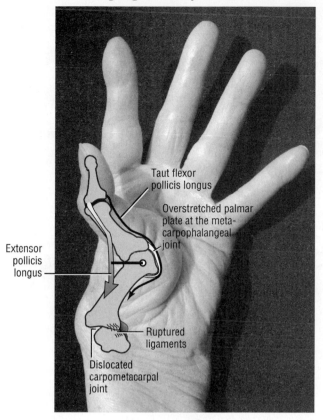

**FIGURE 8–64.** A palmar view showing the pathomechanics of a common "zig-zag" deformity of the thumb due to rheumatoid arthritis. The thumb metacarpal dislocates laterally at the carpometacarpal joint, causing hyperextension at the metacarpophalangeal joint. The interphalangeal joint remains partially flexed owing to the passive tension in the stretched and taut flexor pollicis longus. Note that the "bowstringing" of the tendon of the extensor pollicis longus across the metacarpophalangeal joint creates a large extensor moment arm, thereby magnifying the mechanics of the deformity.

## PALMAR DISLOCATION OF THE METACARPOPHALANGEAL JOINT

When the fingers flex to make a grip, the tendons of the flexor digitorum superficialis and profundus are deflected in a palmar direction, as they pass the MCP joint (Fig. 8–66A). This natural bend causes the tendons to generate a bow-stringing force in the palmar direction. The greater the degree of flexion, the greater the magnitude of the bowstringing force. The bowstringing force is transferred through the flexor pulley, the palmar plate, the collateral ligaments, and, finally, the posterior tubercle of the metacarpal head.

In the hand with severe rheumatoid arthritis, the collateral ligaments may rupture owing to the constant bowstringing force. In time, the proximal phalanx may translate in a palmar direction, resulting in a completely dislocated MCP joint (Fig. 8–66B).[49] Palmar dislocation may collapse both the longitudinal and transverse arches of the hand, causing it to appear flat.

Clinical management of palmar dislocated MCP joints depends on the severity of the rheumatoid arthritis and the amount of joint destruction. Surgery with joint replacement may or may not be indicated. Patient education on ways to "protect" the joint from further deformity is an important part of treatment. Patients are instructed in methods of performing activities that do not place excessive demands on the finger flexors. Exercises, like squeezing a rubber ball, are obviously not appropriate for a patient with markedly weakened collateral ligaments.

### ULNAR DRIFT

Ulnar drift deformity at the MCP joint consists of an excessive ulnar deviation and ulnar translation or slide of the proximal phalanx. This deformity is common in advanced rheumatoid arthritis, often seen in conjunction with a palmar dislocation of the MCP joint (see Fig. 8–65).

In all hands—healthy or otherwise—several factors favor ulnar drift of the fingers. These factors include the pull of gravity, the asymmetrical structure of the MCP joint, and the pull of the extrinsic tendons as they pass the MCP joints.[22,49,56] Possibly the most influential factor is the presence of ulnar-directed forces produced by the thumb toward the fingers. As depicted in Figure 8–67A, the contact force of the thumb causes the MCP joint of the index finger to be pushed ulnarly. This position of the joint increases the deflection or bend of the extensor digitorum communis (EDC)

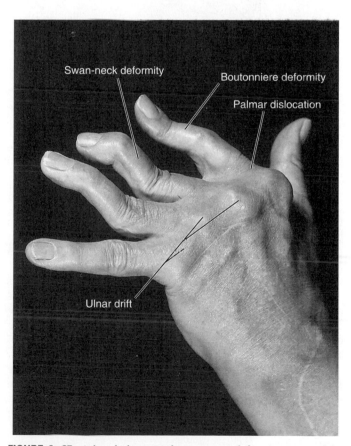

**FIGURE 8–65.** A hand showing the common deformities caused by severe rheumatoid arthritis. Particularly evident are the following: *palmar dislocation* of the metacarpophalangeal joint; *ulnar drift; swan-neck deformity;* and *boutonniere deformity.* (See text for further details) Courtesy of Teri Bielefeld, PT, CHT; Zablocki VA Hospital, Milwaukee, WI.)

**Palmar dislocation of the metacarpophalangeal (MCP) joint**

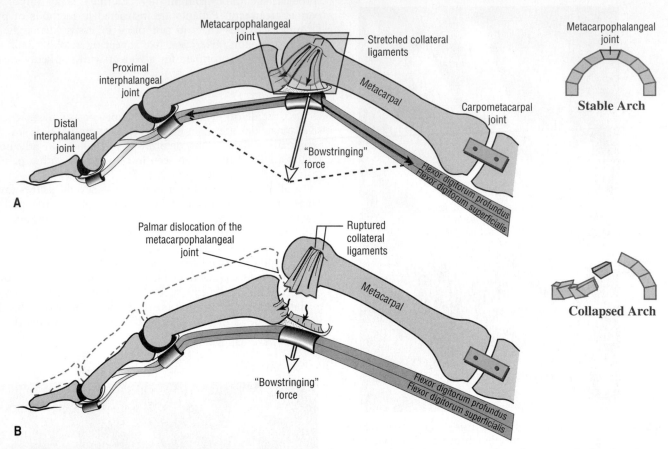

**FIGURE 8–66.** Pathomechanics of progressive palmar dislocation of the metacarpophalangeal joint of the finger. *A,* The bend in the tendons of the flexor digitorum superficialis and flexor digitorum profundus across the metacarpophalangeal joint produces a palmar-directed, bowstringing force against the palmar plate, associated pulley, and collateral ligaments. In the healthy hand, the passive tension in the stretched collateral ligaments adequately resists the palmar pull on the joint structures. *B,* In a finger with rheumatoid arthritis, the bowstringing force can rupture the weakened collateral ligaments. As a result, the proximal phalanx may eventually dislocate in a palmar direction, causing a loss in structural stability of the arch system of the hand.

tendon, as its crosses the MCP joint. Deflection causes a bowstringing force of the tendon in an ulnar direction. In the healthy hand, the transverse fibers of the dorsal hood keep the tendon centralized over the axis of rotation.

In rheumatoid arthritis, a rupture of the transverse fibers allows the tendon to slip toward the ulnar side of the joint's axis of rotation (Fig. 8–67B). In this position, forces produced by the extensor digitorum have a moment arm that can amplify the ulnar deviation posture. This situation initiates a self-perpetuating action of greater and greater ulnar deviation. The greater the ulnar deviation, the greater the moment arm available to produce ulnar deviation torque. In time, the weakened and overstretched radial collateral ligament may rupture, allowing the proximal phalanx to rotate and slide ulnarly, leading to complete joint dislocation (Fig. 8–67C).

Treatment of ulnar drift is often aimed at reducing the magnitude of the ulnar deviation forces at the MCP joint. Splinting and patient education may help decelerate the deforming cycle.[44] One surgical correction involves transferring the extensor digitorum tendon to the radial side of the MCP

joint's axis of rotation.[57] Surgical realignment of the wrist may be indicated because a deformity at the wrist can alter the angle where the extrinsic tendons approach the MCP joint.

## Zig-Zag Deformities of the Fingers

Two zig-zag patterns are often associated with advanced rheumatoid arthritis: swan-neck deformity and boutonniere deformity (see Fig. 8–65). Chronic synovitis and subsequent malalignment of the PIP joint are the primary causes of these deformities. Both deformities are often associated with ulnar drift and palmar dislocation at the MCP joints.

### SWAN-NECK DEFORMITY

*Swan-neck deformity* is characterized by hyperextension of the PIP joint with flexion at the DIP joint (see Fig. 8–65, middle finger). The position of the MCP joint is variable. The intrinsic muscles in the hand with rheumatoid arthritis often become contracted and fibrotic. With diseased and weak-

## The Development of Ulnar Drift

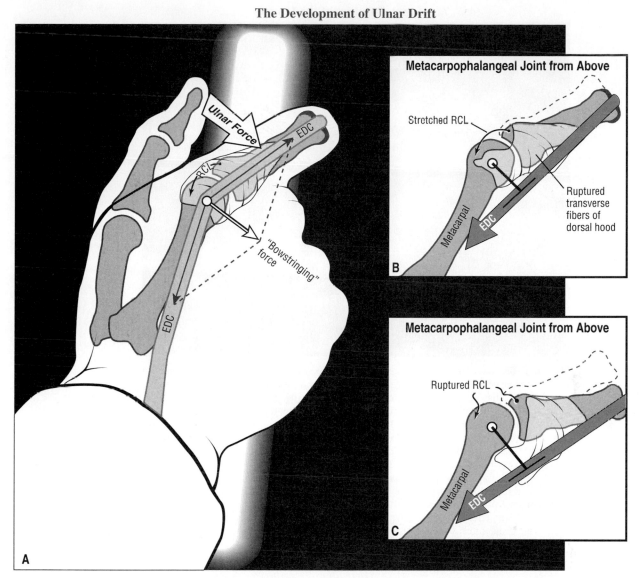

**FIGURE 8–67.** The stages of the development of ulnar drift at the metacarpophalangeal joint of the index finger. *A,* Ulnar forces from the thumb produce a natural bowstringing force on the deflected tendon of the extensor digitorum communis (EDC). *B,* In rheumatoid arthritis, rupture of the transverse fibers of the dorsal hood allows the extensor tendon to act with a moment arm that increases the ulnar deviation torque at the metacarpophalangeal joint. *C,* Over time, the radial collateral ligament (RCL) may rupture, resulting in the ulnar drift deformity.

ened palmar plates at the PIP joint, contracture of the intrinsic muscles may eventually collapse the PIP joints into hyperextension (Fig. 8–68A). The hyperextended position causes the lateral bands of the extensor mechanism to bowstring dorsally, away from the axis of rotation at the PIP joint. Bowstringing increases the moment arm for the intrinsic muscles to extend the PIP joint, thereby accentuating the hyperextension deformity. The DIP joint tends to remain flexed owing to the stretch placed on the tendon of the flexor digitorum profundus across the PIP joint.

Swan-neck deformity may also occur from trauma to the ligaments or spasticity of the intrinsic muscles. Regardless of cause, treatment often involves splinting or surgically limiting the degree of hyperextension of the PIP joint.

## BOUTONNIERE DEFORMITY

The *boutonniere deformity* is described as flexion of the PIP joint and hyperextension of the DIP joint (see Fig. 8–65, index finger). (The term boutonniere—a French word meaning buttonhole—describes the appearance of the head of the proximal phalanx, as it slips through the "buttonhole" created by the slipped lateral bands). The joints collapse in a reciprocal pattern similar to that described for swan-neck deformity. The primary cause of the boutonniere deformity is abnormal displacement of the bands of the extensor mechanism, typically the result of chronic synovitis of the PIP joint. Biomechanically, the central band ruptures and the lateral bands slip to the palmar side of the axis of rotation at the PIP joint (Fig. 8–68B). Consequently, forces transferred

## Zig-Zag Deformities of the Fingers

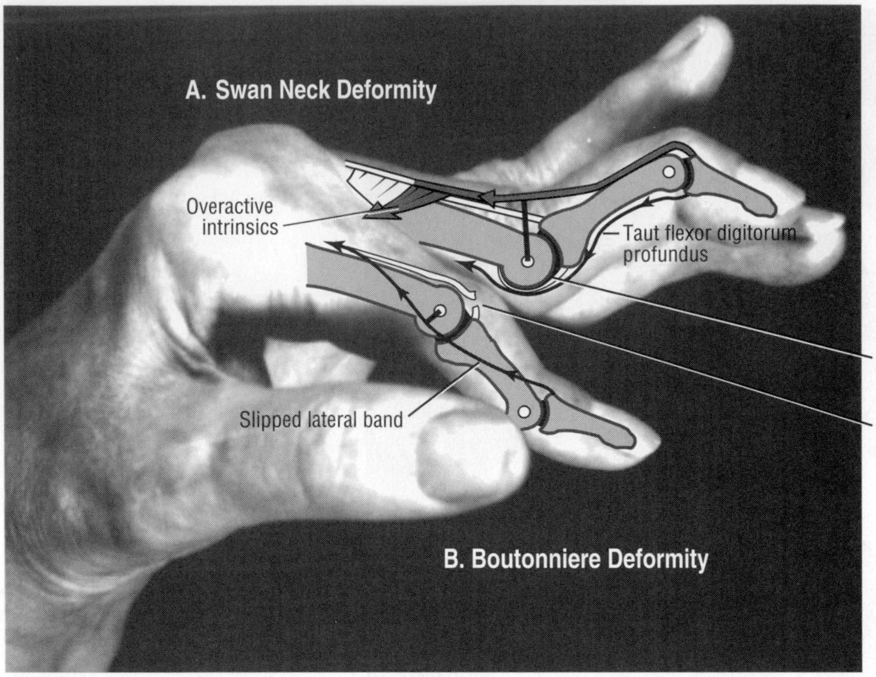

**FIGURE 8–68.** Two common zig-zag deformities of the finger with severe rheumatoid arthritis. The middle finger shows the pathomechanics of the *swan-neck deformity* (A). The overactive intrinsic muscles (red) have a chronic hyperextension effect at the proximal interphalangeal joint. Over time, the weakened palmar plates become overstretched, allowing the proximal interphalangeal joint to deform into severe hyperextension. In this position, the lateral bands produce a bowstring across the proximal interphalangeal joint, thereby accentuating the hyperextension deformity. The distal interphalangeal joint remains partially flexed owing to the increased passive tension in the stretched flexor digitorum profundus tendon.

The index finger depicts the pathomechanics of the *boutonniere deformity* (B). As a result of rheumatoid arthritis, the central band ruptures and the lateral bands slip in a *palmar* direction to the proximal interphalangeal joint; thus, the proximal interphalangeal joint loses its only means of extension. Any tension in the lateral bands now produces *flexion* at the proximal interphalangeal joint. The distal interphalangeal joint remains hyperextended owing to increased passive tension in the taut lateral bands.

across the slipped lateral bands either from active or passive sources flex the PIP joint instead of the normal extension. The DIP joint remains hyperextended owing to the increased tension in the stretched lateral bands and the shortening of the oblique retinacular ligaments. Early boutonniere deformity may be treated by splinting the PIP joint into extension. Surgery may be required to repair the central band and/or realign the lateral bands dorsal to the PIP joint. In cases of severe rheumatoid arthritis, surgery is not always beneficial if connective tissues are excessively weak.

## REFERENCES

1. An KN, Ueba Y, Chao EY, et al: Tendon excursion and moment arm of index finger muscles. J Biomech 16:419–425, 1983.
2. Backhouse KM, Catton WT: An experimental study of the functions of the lumbrical muscles in the human hand. J Anat 88:133–141, 1954.
3. Batmanabane M, Malathi S: Movements at the carpometacarpal and metacarpophalangeal joints of the hand and their effect on the dimensions of the articular ends of the metacarpal bones. Anat Rec 213:102–110, 1985.
4. Bettinger PC, Linscheid RL, Berger RA: An anatomic study of the stabilizing ligaments of the trapezium and trapeziometacarpal joint. J Hand Surg 24A:786–798, 1999.
5. Boatright JR, Kiebzak GM: The effects of low median nerve block on thumb abduction strength. J Hand Surg 22A:849–852, 1997.
6. Bowers WH, Wolf JW, Nehil JL, et al: The proximal interphalangeal joint volar plate. I. An anatomical and biomechanical study. J Hand Surg 5:79–88, 1980.
7. Brand PW: Clinical Biomechanics of the Hand. St Louis, CV Mosby, 1985.
8. Brand PW, Cranor KC, Ellis JC: Tendons and pulleys at the metacarpophalangeal joint of a finger. J Bone Joint Surg 57A: 779–784, 1975.
9. Brand PW, Beach RB, Thompson DE: Relative tension and potential excursion of muscles in the forearm and hand. J Hand Surg 6A:209–219, 1981.
10. Close JR, Kidd CC: The functions of the muscles of the thumb, the index, and long fingers. J Bone Joint Surg 51A:1601–1620, 1969.
11. Cooney WP, P Lucca MJ, Chao EYS, et al: The kinesiology of the thumb trapeziometacarpal joint. J Bone Joint Surg 63A:1371–1381, 1981.
12. Damen A, van der Lei B, Robinson PH: Bilateral osteoarthritis of the trapeziometacarpal joint treated by bilateral tendon interposition arthroplasty. J Hand Surg 22B:96–99, 1997.
13. Doyle JR, Blythe W: The finger flexor tendon sheath and pulleys: Anatomy and reconstruction. In American Academy of Orthopaedic Surgeons Symposium on Tendon Surgery in the Hand. St Louis, CV Mosby, 1975.
14. Dray GJ, Eaton RG: Dislocations and ligament injuries in the digits. In Green DP (ed): Operative Hand Surgery, 3rd ed. New York, Churchill Livingstone, 1993.

15. Dvir Z: Biomechanics of muscle. In Dvir Z (ed): Clinical Biomechanics, Philadelphia, Churchill Livingstone, 2000.

16. Eaton RG, Littler W: Ligament reconstruction for the painful thumb carpometacarpal joint. J Bone Joint Surg 55A:1655–1666, 1973.

17. El-Bacha A: The carpometacarpal joints (excluding the trapeziometacarpal). In Tubiana R (ed): The Hand, vol 1. Philadelphia, WB Saunders, 1981.

18. Eyler DL, Markee JE: The anatomy and function of the intrinsic musculature of the fingers. J Bone Joint Surg 36A:1–20, 1954.

19. Flatt AE: The Care of the Rheumatoid Hand, 3rd ed. St Louis, CV Mosby, 1974.

20. Gray DJ, Gardiner E: The innervation of the joints of the wrist and hand. Anat Rec 151:261–266, 1965.

21. Hahn P, Krimmer H, Hradetzky A, et al: Quantitative analysis of the linkage between the interphalangeal joints of the index finger. J Hand Surg 20B:696–699, 1995.

22. Hakstian RW, Tubiana R: Ulnar deviation of the fingers: The role of joint structure and function. J Bone Joint Surg 49A:299–316, 1967.

23. Imaeda T, Niebur G, Cooney WP, et al: Kinematics of the normal trapeziometacarpal joint. J Orthop Research 12:197–204, 1994.

24. Inman VT, Saunders JB: Referred pain from skeletal structures. J Nerv Ment Dis 99:660–667, 1944.

25. Jacobson MD, Raab R, Fazeli BM, et al: Architectural design of the human intrinsic hand muscles. J Hand Surg. 17A:804–809, 1992.

26. Johanson ME, Skinner SR, Lamoreux LW: Phasic relationship of the intrinsic and extrinsic thumb musculature. Clin Orthop 322:120–130, 1996.

27. Kapandji IA: The Physiology of the Joints, vol 1, 5th ed: Edinburgh, Churchill Livingstone, 1982.

28. Kaufman KR, An KN, Litchy WJ, et al: In-vivo function of the thumb muscles. Clin Biomech 14:141–151, 1999.

29. Krishnan J, Chipchase L: Passive rotation of the metacarpophalangeal joint. J Hand Surg 22B:270–273, 1997.

30. Kuczynski K: Carpometacarpal joint of the human thumb. J Anat 118:119–126, 1974.

31. Landsmeer JMF: Power grip and precision handling. Ann Rheum Dis 21:164–170, 1962.

32. Leijnse JN: Why the lumbrical muscle should not be bigger—a force model of the lumbrical in the unloaded human finger. J Biomechan 30:1107–1114, 1997.

33. Long C: Intrinsic-extrinsic muscle control of the fingers. J Bone Joint Surg 50A:973–984, 1968.

34. Long C, Brown ME: Electromyographic kinesiology of the hand: Muscles moving the long finger. J Bone Joint Surg 46A:1683–1706, 1964.

35. Marklin RW, Simoneau GG, Monroe JF: Wrist and forearm posture from typing on split and vertically inclined computer keyboards. Human Factors 41:559–569, 1999.

36. Minami A, An KN, Cooney WP, et al: Ligamentous structures of the metacarpophalangeal joint: A quantitative anatomic study. J Orthop Res 1:361–368, 1984.

37. Najima H, Oberlin C, Alnot JY, et al: Anatomical and biomechanical studies of the pathogenesis of trapeziometacarpal degenerative arthritis. J Hand Surg 22B:183–188, 1997.

38. Nalebuff EA: Diagnosis, classification, and management of rheumatoid thumb deformities. Bull Hosp Joint Dis 24:119–137, 1968.

39. Napier JR: The prehensile movements of the human hand. J Bone Joint Surg 38B:902–913, 1956.

40. Neumann DA: Observations from cineradiography analysis. Milwaukee, WI, Marquette University, 2000.

41. Pagalidis T, Kuczynski K, Lamb DW: Ligamentous stability of the base of the thumb. The Hand 13:29–35, 1981.

42. Pieron AP: The first carpometacarpal joint. In Tubiana R (ed): The Hand, vol 1. Philadelphia, WB Saunders, 1981.

43. Ranney D, Wells R: Lumbrical muscle function as revealed by a new and physiological approach. Anat Rec 222:110–114, 1988.

44. Rennie HJ: Evaluation of the effectiveness of a metacarpophalangeal ulnar deviation orthosis. J Hand Ther 9:371–377, 1996.

45. Rispler D, Greenwald D, Shumway S, et al: Efficiency of the flexor tendon pulley system in human cadaver hands. J Hand Surg 21A:444–450, 1996.

46. Seradge H, Jia YC, Owens W, et al: In vivo measurement of carpal tunnel pressure in the functioning hand. J Hand Surg 20A:855–859, 1995.

47. Shaw SJ, Morris MA: The range of motion of the metacarpophalangeal joint of the thumb and its relationship to injury. J Hand Surg 17B:164–166, 1992.

48. Shrewsbury MM, Kuczynski K: Flexor digitorum superficialis tendon in the fingers of the human hand. The Hand 6:121–133, 1974.

49. Smith RJ, Kaplan EB: Rheumatoid deformities at the metacarpophalangeal joints of the fingers. J Bone Joint Surg 49A:31–47, 1967.

50. Stack HG. Muscle function in the fingers. J Bone Joint Surg 44B:899–902, 1962.

51. Strong CL, Perry J: Function of the extensor pollicis longus and intrinsic muscle of the thumb. J Am Phys Ther 46:939–945, 1966.

52. Thomas DH, Long C, Landsmeer JMF: Biomechanical considerations of lumbricalis behavior in the human finger. J Biomechanics 1:107–115, 1968.

53. Valentin P: The interossei and the lumbricals. In Tubiana R (ed): The Hand, vol 1. Philadelphia, WB Saunders, 1981.

54. Van Oudenaarde E, Oostendorp RAB: Functional relationship between the abductor pollicis longus and the abductor pollicis brevis muscles: An EMG analysis. J Anat 186:509–515, 1995.

55. Williams PL, Bannister LH, Berry M, et al: Gray's Anatomy, 38th ed. New York, Churchill Livingstone, 1995.

56. Wise KS. The anatomy of the metacarpophalangeal joints with observations of the etiology of ulnar drift. J Bone Joint Surg 57B: 485–490, 1975.

57. Wright PE: Arthritic hand. In Crenshaw AH (ed): Campbells's Operative Orthopaedics, vol 5, 8th ed. St Louis, Mosby Year Book, 1992.

58. Zancolli EA, Ziadenberg C, Zancolli E: Biomechanics of the trapeziometacarpal joint. Clin Orthop 220:14–26, 1987.

## ADDITIONAL READING

An KN, Chao EY, Conney WP, et al: Forces in the normal and abnormal hand. J Ortho Res 3:202–211, 1985.

Buchholz B, Armstrong TJ, Goldstein SA: Anthropometric data for describing the kinematics of the human hand. Ergonomics 35:261–273, 1992.

Conney WP, Chao EY: Biomechanical analysis of static forces in the thumb during hand function. J Bone Joint Surg 59A:27–36, 1977.

Estes JP, Bochenek C, Fasler P: Osteoarthritis of the fingers. J Hand Ther 13:108–123, 2000.

Forrest WJ, Basmajian JV: Function of human thenar and hypothenar muscles: An electromyographic study of twenty-five hands. J Bone Joint Surg 47A:1585–1594, 1965.

Imaeda T, An KN, Cooney WP, et al: Anatomy of the trapeziometacarpal ligaments. J Hand Surg 18A:226–231, 1993.

Jarit P: Dominant-hand to nondominant-hand grip-strength ratios of college baseball players. J Hand Ther 4:123–126, 1991.

Johanson ME, Skinner SR, Lamoreux LW: Phasic relationships of the intrinsic and extrinsic thumb musculature. Clin Orthop 322:120–130, 1996.

Landsmeer JMF: The anatomy of the dorsal aponeurosis of the human finger and its functional significance. Anat Rec 104:31–44, 1949.

Long C, Conrad PW, Hall EW, et al: Intrinsic-extrinsic muscle control of the hand in power grip and precision handling. J Bone Joint Surg 52A:853–867, 1970.

Najima H, Oberlin C, Alnot JY, et al: Anatomical and biomechanical studies of the pathogenesis of trapeziometacarpal degenerative arthritis. J Hand Surg 22B:183–188, 1997.

Smith RJ: Balance and kinetics of the fingers under normal and pathological conditions. Clin Orthop 104 92–111, 1974.

Smutz WP, Kongsayreepong A, Hughes RE, et al: Mechanical advantage of the thumb muscles. J Biomechanics 31:565–570, 1998.

Spoor CW, Landsmeer JMF: Analysis of the zig-zag movement of the human finger under influence of the extensor digitorum tendon and the deep flexor tendon. J Biomechanics 9:561–566, 1976.

Wehbe MA, Hunter JM: Flexor tendon gliding in the hand. Part 1. In vivo excursions. J Hand Surg 10A:570–579, 1985.

# APPENDIX II

## Part A: Nerve Root Innervation of the Upper Extremity Muscles

| Muscle | $C^1$ | $C^2$ | $C^3$ | $C^4$ | $C^5$ | $C^6$ | $C^7$ | $C^8$ | $T^1$ |
|---|---|---|---|---|---|---|---|---|---|
| Serratus anterior | | | | | X | X | X | *X* | |
| Rhomboids, major and minor | | | | *X* | X | | | | |
| Subclavius | | | | | X | X | | | |
| Supraspinatus | | | | *X* | X | *X* | | | |
| Infraspinatus | | | | (x) | X | X | | | |
| Subscapularis | | | | | X | X | *X* | | |
| Latissimus dorsi | | | | | | X | X | X | |
| Teres major | | | | | *X* | X | *X* | | |
| Pectoralis major (clavicular) | | | | | X | X | X | | |
| Pectoralis major (sternocostal) | | | | | | X | X | X | X |
| Pectoralis minor | | | | | | (x) | X | X | X |
| Teres minor | | | | | X | X | | | |
| Deltoid | | | | | X | X | | | |
| Coracobrachialis | | | | | | X | X | | |
| Biceps | | | | | X | X | | | |
| Brachialis | | | | | X | X | | | |
| Triceps | | | | | | *X* | X | X | *X* |
| Anconeus | | | | | | | X | X | |
| Brachioradialis | | | | | X | X | | | |
| Extensor carpi radialis longus and brevis | | | | | *X* | X | X | *X* | |
| Supinator | | | | | *X* | X | (x) | | |
| Extensor digitorum | | | | | | X | X | X | |
| Extensor digiti minimi | | | | | | *X* | X | X | |
| Extensor carpi ulnaris | | | | | | *X* | X | X | |
| Abductor pollicis longus | | | | | | *X* | X | X | |
| Extensor pollicis brevis | | | | | | *X* | X | X | |
| Extensor pollicis longus | | | | | | *X* | X | X | |
| Extensor indicis | | | | | | *X* | X | X | |
| Pronator teres | | | | | | X | X | | |
| Flexor carpi radialis | | | | | | X | X | *X* | |
| Palmaris longus | | | | | | (x) | X | X | *X* |
| Flexor digit. superficialis | | | | | | | X | X | X |
| Flexor digit. profundus I and II | | | | | | | *X* | X | X |

| Muscle | Nerve Root | | | | | | | | |
|---|---|---|---|---|---|---|---|---|---|
| | C¹ | C² | C³ | C⁴ | C⁵ | C⁶ | C⁷ | C⁸ | T¹ |
| Flexor pollicis longus | | | | | | (x) | *X* | **X** | **X** |
| Pronator quadratus | | | | | | | *X* | **X** | **X** |
| Abductor pollicis brevis | | | | | | *X* | *X* | *X* | *X* |
| Opponens pollicis | | | | | | *X* | *X* | *X* | *X* |
| Flexor pollicis brevis | | | | | | *X* | *X* | *X* | *X* |
| Lumbricals I and II | | | | | | (x) | *X* | **X** | **X** |
| Flexor carpi ulnaris | | | | | | | *X* | **X** | *X* |
| Flexor digit. profundus III and IV | | | | | | | *X* | **X** | **X** |
| Palmaris brevis | | | | | | | (x) | **X** | **X** |
| Abductor digiti minimi | | | | | | | (x) | **X** | **X** |
| Opponens digiti minimi | | | | | | | (x) | **X** | **X** |
| Flexor digiti minimi | | | | | | | (x) | **X** | **X** |
| Palmar interossei | | | | | | | | **X** | **X** |
| Dorsal interossei | | | | | | | | **X** | **X** |
| Lumbricals III & IV | | | | | | | (x) | **X** | **X** |
| Adductor pollicis | | | | | | | | **X** | **X** |

(x), minimal literature support; *X*, moderate literature support; **X**, strong literature support.

Modified from Kendall FP, McCreary AK, Provance PG: Muscles: Testing and Function, 4th ed. Baltimore, Williams & Wilkins, 1993. Data based on a compilation from several sources in the anatomic literature.

## Part B: Key Muscles for Testing the Function of Ventral Nerve Roots (C⁵-T¹)

The table shows the key muscles typically used to test the function of individual ventral nerve roots of the brachial plexus (C⁵–T¹) in the clinic. Reduced strength in a key muscle may indicate an injury to the associated nerve root.

| Key Muscles | Ventral Nerve Roots | Sample Test Movements |
|---|---|---|
| Biceps brachii | C⁵ | Elbow flexion with forearm supinated |
| Middle deltoid | C⁵ | Shoulder abduction |
| Extensor carpi radialis longus | C⁶ | Wrist extension and radial deviation |
| Triceps brachii | C⁷ | Elbow extension |
| Extensor digitorum | C⁷ | Finger extension (metacarpophalangeal joint) |
| Flexor digitorum profundus | C⁸ | Finger flexion (distal interphalangeal joint) |
| Dorsal and palmar interossei | T¹ | Finger abduction and adduction |

## Part C: Attachments and Innervations of the Upper Extremity Muscles

### SHOULDER COMPLEX MUSCULATURE

#### Coracobrachialis
*Proximal attachment:* apex of the coracoid process by a common tendon with the short head of the biceps
*Distal attachment:* medial aspect of middle shaft of the humerus
*Innervation:* musculocutaneous nerve

#### Deltoid
*Proximal attachments*
    Anterior part: anterior surface of the lateral end of the clavicle
    Middle part: superior surface of the lateral edge of the acromion
    Posterior part: posterior border of the spine of the scapula
*Distal attachment:* deltoid tuberosity of the humerus
*Innervation:* axillary nerve

#### Infraspinatus
*Proximal attachment:* infraspinatous fossa
*Distal attachment:* middle facet of the greater tubercle of the humerus
*Innervation:* suprascapular nerve

### Latissimus Dorsi

*Proximal attachments:* posterior layer of the thoracolumbar fascia, spinous processes and supraspinous ligaments of the lower half of the thoracic vertebrae and all lumbar vertebrae, median sacral crest, posterior crest of the ilium, lower four ribs, small area near the inferior angle of the scapula, and muscular interdigitations from the obliquus external abdominis

*Distal attachment:* floor of the intertubercular groove of the humerus

*Innervation:* middle subscapular (thoracodorsal) nerve

### Levator Scapula

*Proximal attachments:* transverse processes of C1–2 and posterior tubercles of transverse processes of C3–4

*Distal attachment:* medial border of the scapula between the superior angle and root of the spine

*Innervation:* ventral rami of spinal nerves ($C^{3-4}$) and the dorsal scapular nerve

### Pectoralis Major

*Proximal attachments*

   Clavicular head: anterior margin of the medial one half of the clavicle

   Sternocostal head: lateral margin of the manubrium and body of the sternum and cartilages of the first six or seven ribs. The costal fibers blend with muscular slips from the obliquus external abdominis.

*Distal attachment:* crest of the greater tubercle of the humerus.

*Innervation*

   Clavicular head: lateral pectoral nerve

   Sternocostal head: lateral and medial pectoral nerves

### Pectoralis Minor

*Proximal attachments:* external surfaces of the third through the fifth ribs

*Distal attachment:* medial border of the coracoid process

*Innervation:* medial pectoral nerve

### Rhomboid Major and Minor

*Proximal attachments:* ligamentous nuchae and spinous processes of C7-T5

*Distal attachment:* medial border of scapula, from the root of the spine to the inferior angle

*Innervation:* dorsal scapular nerve

### Serratus Anterior

*Proximal attachments:* external surface of the lateral region of the first to ninth ribs

*Distal attachment:* entire medial border of the scapula, with a concentration of fibers near the inferior angle

*Innervation:* long thoracic nerve

### Subclavius

*Proximal attachment:* near the cartilage of the first rib

*Distal attachment:* inferior surface of the middle aspect of the clavicle

*Innervation:* branch from the upper trunk of the brachial plexus ($C^{5-6}$)

### Subscapularis

*Proximal attachment:* subscapular fossa

*Distal attachment:* lesser tubercle of the humerus

*Innervation:* upper and lower subscapular nerves

### Supraspinatus

*Proximal attachment:* supraspinatus fossa

*Distal attachment:* upper facet of the greater tubercle of the humerus

*Innervation:* suprascapular nerve

### Teres Major

*Proximal attachment:* inferior angle of the scapula

*Distal attachment:* crest of the lesser tubercle of the humerus

*Innervation:* lower subscapular nerve

### Teres Minor

*Proximal attachment:* posterior surface of the lateral border of the scapula

*Distal attachment:* lower facet of the greater tubercle of the humerus

*Innervation:* axillary nerve

### Trapezius

*Proximal attachments* (all parts): medial part of superior nuchal line and external occipital protuberance, ligamentum nuchae, spinous processes and supraspinous ligaments of the seventh cervical vertebra and all thoracic vertebrae

*Distal attachments*

   Upper part: posterior-superior edge of the lateral one third of the clavicle

   Middle part: medial margin of the acromion and upper lip of the spine of the scapula

   Lower part: Medial end of the spine of the scapula, just lateral to the root.

*Innervation:* primarily by the spinal accessory nerve (cranial nerve XI); secondary innervation directly from ventral rami of $C^{2-4}$

## ELBOW AND FOREARM MUSCULATURE

### Anconeus

*Proximal attachment:* posterior side of the lateral epicondyle of the humerus

*Distal attachments:* between the olecranon process and proximal surface of the posterior side of the ulna

*Innervation:* radial nerve

### Biceps Brachii

*Proximal attachments*

   Long head: supraglenoid tubercle of the scapula

   Short head: apex of the coracoid process of the scapula

*Distal attachments:* bicipital tuberosity of the radius; also to deep connective tissue within the forearm via the fibrous lacertus

*Innervation:* musculocutaneous nerve

### Brachialis

*Proximal attachment:* distal aspect of the anterior surface of the humerus

*Distal attachments:* coronoid process and tuberosity on the proximal ulna

*Innervation:* musculocutaneous nerve (small contribution from the radial nerve)

### Brachioradialis

*Proximal attachment:* upper two thirds of the lateral supracondylar ridge of the humerus

*Distal attachment:* near styloid process at the distal radius

*Innervation:* radial nerve

**Pronator Teres**
*Proximal attachments*
  Humeral head: medial epicondyle
  Ulnar head: medial to the tuberosity of the ulna
*Distal attachment:* lateral surface of the middle radius
*Innervation:* median nerve

**Pronator Quadratus**
*Proximal attachment:* anterior surface of the distal ulna
*Distal attachment:* anterior surface of the distal radius
*Innervation:* median nerve

**Supinator**
*Proximal attachments:* lateral epicondyle of the humerus, radial collateral and annular ligaments, and supinator crest of the ulna
*Distal attachment:* lateral surface of the proximal radius
*Innervation:* radial nerve

**Triceps Brachii**
*Proximal attachments*
  Long head: infraglenoid tubercle of the scapula
  Lateral head: posterior humerus, superior and lateral to the radial groove
  Medial head: posterior humerus, inferior and medial to the radial groove
*Distal attachment:* olecranon process of the ulna
*Innervation:* radial nerve

## WRIST MUSCULATURE

**Extensor Carpi Radialis Brevis**
*Proximal attachment:* common extensor-supinator tendon attaching to the lateral epicondyle of the humerus
*Distal attachment:* radial-posterior surface of the base of the third metacarpal
*Innervation:* radial nerve

**Extensor Carpi Radialis Longus**
*Proximal attachments:* common extensor-supinator tendon attaching to the lateral epicondyle of the humerus and the distal part of the lateral supracondylar ridge of the humerus
*Distal attachment:* radial-posterior surface of the base of the second metacarpal
*Innervation:* radial nerve

**Extensor Carpi Ulnaris**
*Proximal attachments:* common extensor-supinator tendon attaching to the lateral epicondyle of the humerus and the posterior border of the middle one third of the ulna
*Distal attachment:* posterior-ulnar surface of the base of the fifth metacarpal
*Innervation:* radial nerve

**Flexor Carpi Radialis**
*Proximal attachment:* common flexor-pronator tendon attaching to the medial epicondyle of the humerus
*Distal attachments:* palmar surface of the base of the second metacarpal and a small slip to the base of the third metacarpal
*Innervation:* median nerve

**Flexor Carpi Ulnaris**
*Proximal attachments*
  Humeral head: common flexor-pronator tendon attaching to the medial epicondyle of the humerus
  Ulnar head: posterior border of the middle one third of the ulna
*Distal attachments:* pisiform bone, pisohamate and pisometacarpal ligaments, and palmar base of the fifth metacarpal bone
*Innervation:* ulnar nerve

**Palmaris Longus**
*Proximal attachment:* common flexor-pronator tendon attaching to the medial epicondyle of the humerus
*Distal attachment:* central part of the transverse carpal ligament and palmar aponeurosis of the hand
*Innervation:* median nerve

## EXTRINSIC HAND MUSCULATURE

**Abductor Pollicis Longus**
*Proximal attachments:* posterior surface of the middle part of the radius and ulna, and adjacent interosseous membrane
*Distal attachments:* radial-dorsal surface of the base of the thumb metacarpal, including the capsule of the carpometacarpal joint of the thumb
*Innervation:* radial nerve

**Extensor Digitorum Communis**
*Proximal attachment:* common extensor-supinator tendon attaching to the lateral epicondyle of the humerus
*Distal attachments:* by four tendons, each to the base of the extensor mechanism and to the dorsal base of the proximal phalanx of the fingers
*Innervation:* radial nerve

**Extensor Digiti Minimi**
*Proximal attachment:* ulnar side of the belly of the extensor digitorum
*Distal attachments:* tendon usually divides, joining the ulnar side of the tendon of the extensor digitorum
*Innervation:* radial nerve

**Extensor Indicis**
*Proximal attachments:* posterior surface of the middle to distal part of the ulna and adjacent interosseous membrane
*Distal attachment:* tendon blends with the ulnar side of the index tendon of the extensor digitorum
*Innervation:* radial nerve

**Extensor Pollicis Brevis**
*Proximal attachments:* posterior surface of the middle to distal parts of the radius and adjacent interosseous membrane
*Distal attachment:* dorsal base of the proximal phalanx and extensor mechanism of the thumb
*Innervation:* radial nerve

**Extensor Pollicis Longus**
*Proximal attachments:* posterior surface of the middle part of the ulna and adjacent interosseous membrane

*Distal attachment:* dorsal base of the distal phalanx and extensor mechanism of the thumb
*Innervation:* radial nerve

### Flexor Digitorum Profundus
*Proximal attachments:* proximal three fourths of the anterior and medial side of the ulna and adjacent interosseous membrane
*Distal attachments:* by four tendons, each to the palmar base of the distal phalanges of the fingers
*Innervation*
　Medial half: ulnar nerve
　Lateral half: median nerve

### Flexor Digitorum Superficialis
*Proximal attachments*
　Humeroulnar head: common flexor-pronator tendon attaching to the medial epicondyle of the humerus and the medial side of the coronoid process of the ulna
　Radial head: oblique line just distal and lateral to the bicipital tuberosity
*Distal attachments:* by four tendons, each to the sides of the middle phalanges of the fingers
*Innervation:* median nerve

### Flexor Pollicis Longus
*Proximal attachments:* middle part of the anterior surface of the radius and adjacent interosseous membrane
*Distal attachment:* palmar base of the distal phalanx of the thumb
*Innervation:* median nerve

## INTRINSIC HAND MUSCULATURE

### Abductor Digiti Minimi
*Proximal attachments:* pisohamate ligament, pisiform bone, and tendon of the flexor carpi ulnaris
*Distal attachments:* ulnar side of the base of the proximal phalanx of the little finger; also attaches into the extensor mechanism of the little finger
*Innervation:* ulnar nerve

### Abductor Pollicis Brevis
*Proximal attachments:* transverse carpal ligament, palmar tubercles of the trapezium and scaphoid bones
*Distal attachments:* radial side of the base of the proximal phalanx of the thumb; also attaches into the extensor mechanism of the thumb
*Innervation:* median nerve

### Adductor Pollicis
*Proximal attachments*
　Oblique head: capitate bone, base of the second and third metacarpal, and adjacent capsular ligaments of the carpometacarpal joints
　Transverse head: palmar surface of the third metacarpal
*Distal attachments:* both heads attach on the ulnar side of the base of the proximal phalanx of the thumb and to the medial sesamoid bone at the metacarpophalangeal joint; also attaches into the extensor mechanism of the thumb
*Innervation:* ulnar nerve

### Dorsal Interossei
*Proximal attachments*
　First: adjacent sides of the first (thumb) and second metacarpal
　Second: adjacent sides of the second and third metacarpal
　Third: adjacent sides of the third and fourth metacarpal
　Fourth: adjacent sides of the fourth and fifth metacarpal
*Distal attachments*
　First: radial side of the base of the proximal phalanx of the index finger and oblique fibers of the dorsal hood
　Second: radial side of the base of the proximal phalanx of the middle finger and oblique fibers of the dorsal hood
　Third: ulnar side of the base of the proximal phalanx of the middle finger and oblique fibers of the dorsal hood
　Fourth: ulnar side of the base of the proximal phalanx of the ring finger and oblique fibers of the dorsal hood
*Innervation:* ulnar nerve

### Flexor Digiti Minimi
*Proximal attachments:* transverse carpal ligament and hook of the hamate
*Distal attachment:* ulnar side of the base of the proximal phalanx of the little finger
*Innervation:* ulnar nerve

### Flexor Pollicis Brevis
*Proximal attachments:* transverse carpal ligament and palmar tubercle of the trapezium
*Distal attachments:* radial side of the base of the proximal phalanx of the thumb; also to the lateral sesamoid bone at the metacarpophalangeal joint
*Innervation:* median nerve

### Lumbricals
*Proximal attachments*
　Medial two: adjacent sides of the flexor digitorum profundus tendons of the little, ring, and middle fingers
　Lateral two: lateral sides of the flexor digitorum profundus tendons of the middle and index fingers
*Distal attachment:* lateral margin of the extensor mechanism via the oblique fibers of the dorsal hood
*Innervation*
　Medial two: ulnar nerve
　Lateral two: median nerve

### Opponens Digiti Minimi
*Proximal attachments:* transverse carpal ligament and hook of the hamate
*Distal attachment:* ulnar surface of the shaft of the fifth metacarpal
*Innervation:* ulnar nerve

### Opponens Pollicis
*Proximal attachments:* transverse carpal ligament and palmar tubercle of the trapezium

*Distal attachment:* radial surface of the shaft of the thumb metacarpal
*Innervation:* median nerve

## Palmaris Brevis
*Proximal attachments:* transverse carpal ligament and palmar fascia just distal and lateral to the pisiform bone
*Distal attachment:* skin on the ulnar border of the hand
*Innervation:* ulnar nerve

## Palmar Interossei
*Proximal attachments*
First: ulnar side of the thumb metacarpal
Second: ulnar side of the second metacarpal
Third: radial side of the fourth metacarpal
Fourth: radial side of the fifth metacarpal
*Distal attachments*
First: ulnar side of the proximal phalanx of the thumb, blending with the adductor pollicis; also attaches to the medial sesamoid bone at the metacarpophalangeal joint
Second: ulnar side of the extensor mechanism of the index finger via oblique fibers of dorsal hood
Third: radial side of the extensor mechanism of the ring finger via oblique fibers of dorsal hood
Fourth: radial side of the extensor mechanism of the little finger via oblique fibers of dorsal hood
*Innervation:* ulnar nerve

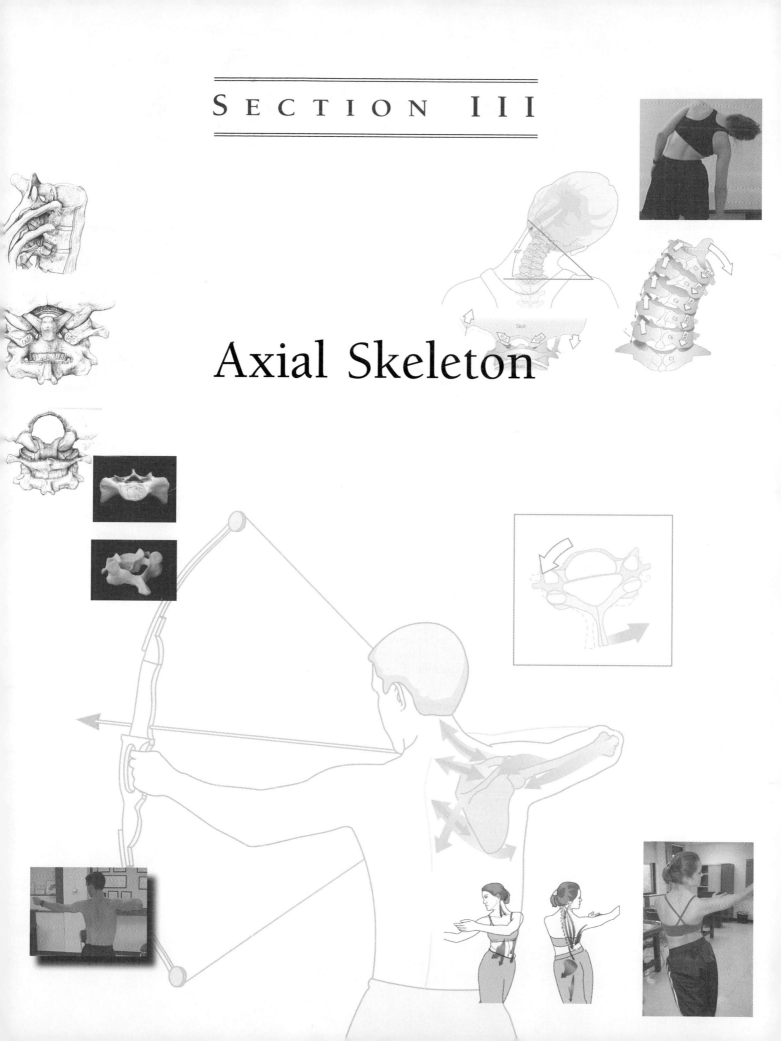

# SECTION III

# Axial Skeleton

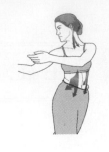

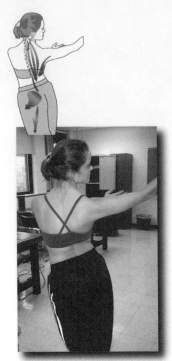

# SECTION III

# Axial Skeleton

**Section III** focuses on the kinesiology of the axial skeleton: the cranium, vertebrae, sternum, and ribs. The section is divided into three chapters, each describing a different kinesiologic aspect of the axial skeleton. Chapter 9 presents osteology and arthrology, and Chapter 10 presents muscle and joint interactions. Chapter 11 describes two special topics related to the axial skeleton: the kinesiology of mastication (chewing) and ventilation.

Section III presents several overlapping functions that involve the axial skeleton. These functions include providing (1) "core stability" plus overall mobility to the body; (2) optimal placement of the senses of vision, hearing, and smell; (3) protection to the spinal cord, brain, and internal organs; and (4) bodily activities such as the mechanics of ventilation, mastication, childbirth, coughing, and defecation. Musculoskeletal impairments within the axial skeleton can cause limitation in any of these four functions.

CHAPTER 9

# Axial Skeleton: Osteology and Arthrology

DONALD A. NEUMANN, PT, PHD

## TOPICS AT A GLANCE

## INTRODUCTION

The axial skeleton includes the cranium, vertebral column, ribs, and sternum (Fig. 9–1). This chapter presents the kinesiologic interactions between the osteology and arthrology of the axial skeleton. The focus is on the craniocervical region, vertebral column, and sacroiliac joints, and how the many articulations provide stability and movement while transferring loads through the axial skeleton. Muscles play a large role in the function of the axial skeleton, and they are the primary focus of Chapter 10.

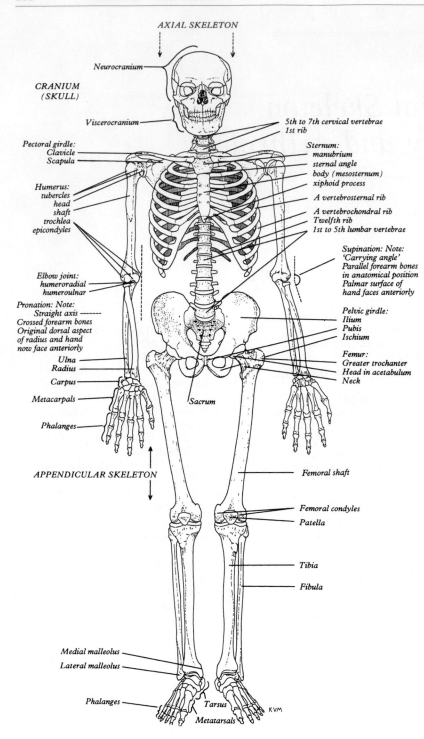

**AXIAL SKELETON**

Neurocranium

CRANIUM
(SKULL)

Viscerocranium

5th to 7th cervical vertebrae
1st rib

Pectoral girdle:
Clavicle
Scapula

Sternum:
manubrium
sternal angle
body (mesosternum)
xiphoid process

Humerus:
tubercles
head
shaft
trochlea
epicondyles

A vertebrosternal rib

A vertebrochondral rib
Twelfth rib
1st to 5th lumbar vertebrae

Elbow joint:
humeroradial
humeroulnar

Supination: Note:
'Carrying angle'
Parallel forearm bones
in anatomical position
Palmar surface of
hand faces anteriorly

Pronation: Note:
Straight axis ------
Crossed forearm bones
Original dorsal aspect
of radius and hand
now face anteriorly

Pelvic girdle:
Ilium
Pubis
Ischium

Ulna
Radius

Femur:
Greater trochanter
Head in acetabulum
Neck

Carpus

Metacarpals

Phalanges

Sacrum

APPENDICULAR SKELETON

Femoral shaft

Femoral condyles
Patella

Tibia

Fibula

Medial malleolus
Lateral malleolus

Phalanges    Tarsus
Metatarsals    KVM

**FIGURE 9-1.** Anterior view of an adult male skeleton. (From Gray's Anatomy: The Anatomical Basis of Medicine and Surgery, 38th ed. New York, Churchill Livingstone, 1995.)

Disease, trauma, and normal aging can cause a host of neuromuscular and musculoskeletal problems involving the axial skeleton. Disorders of the vertebral column are often associated with pain and impairment, primarily because of the close anatomic relationship between neural tissue (spinal cord and nerve roots) and connective tissue (vertebrae and associated ligaments, discs, and synovial joints). A "slipped disc," for example, can increase pressure on the adjacent spinal nerves or spinal cord, causing pain, muscle weakness, and reduced reflexes. To further complicate matters, certain movements and habitual postures of the vertebral column increase the likelihood of connective tissues impinging on neural tissues. An understanding of the detailed osteology and arthrology of the axial skeleton is crucial to an appreciation of the associated pathomechanics, as well as the rationale for clinical interventions.

The terminology used to describe the relative location or region within the axial skeleton can differ from that used to describe the appendicular skeleton. Table 9-1 summarizes this terminology.

## TABLE 9–1. Terminology Describing Relative Location or Region Within the Axial Skeleton

| Term | Synonym | Definition |
|------|---------|------------|
| Posterior | Dorsal | Back of the body |
| Anterior | Ventral | Front of the body |
| Medial | None | Midline of the body |
| Lateral | None | Away from the midline of the body |
| Superior | Cranial | Head or top of the body |
| Inferior | Caudal (the "tail") | Tail, or the bottom of the body |

The definitions assume a person is in the anatomic position.

# OSTEOLOGY

## Basic Components of the Axial Skeleton

### CRANIUM

The cranium is the bony encasement of the brain, which protects the brain and sensory organs (eyes, ears, nose, and vestibular system) and provides a means for ingesting food and liquid.

### Occipital and Temporal Bones

The *occipital bone* forms much of the posterior base of the skull (Figs. 9–2 and 9–3). The *external occipital protuberance* is a palpable midline point, serving as an attachment for the ligamentum nuchae and the medial part of the upper trapezius muscle. The *superior nuchal line* extends laterally from the external occipital protuberance to the base of the mastoid process of the temporal bone. This thin but distinct line marks the attachments of several extensor muscles of the

head and neck, such as the trapezius and splenius capitus muscles. The *inferior nuchal line* marks the anterior edge of the attachment of the semispinalis capitis.

---

**Relevant Osteologic Features**

*Occipital Bone*
- External occipital protuberance
- Superior nuchal line
- Inferior nuchal line
- Foramen magnum
- Occipital condyles
- Basilar part

*Temporal Bone*
- Mastoid process

---

The *foramen magnum* is a large circular hole located at the base of the occipital bone, serving as the passageway for the spinal cord. A pair of prominent *occipital condyles* project from the anterior-lateral margins of the foramen magnum, forming the convex component of the atlanto-occipital joint. The *basilar part* of the occipital bone lies just anterior to the anterior rim of the foramen magnum.

Each of the two *temporal bones* forms part of the lateral external surface of the skull, immediately surrounding and including the external auditory meatus (see Fig. 9–2). The *mastoid process*, an easily palpable structure, is just posterior to the ear. This prominent process serves as an attachment for many muscles, such as the sternocleidomastoid.

### VERTEBRAE: BUILDING BLOCKS OF THE SPINE

In addition to providing an element of stability throughout the trunk and neck, the vertebral column protects the spinal cord and exiting spinal nerves. Once outside the vertebral column, the nerve roots form a ventral ramus and a dorsal ramus of a spinal nerve (Fig. 9–4). The midthoracic vertebrae demonstrate many of the essential anatomic and functional characteristics of any given vertebra (Fig. 9–5, Table 9–2).

### RIBS

Twelve pairs of ribs enclose the thoracic cavity, forming a protective cage for the cardiopulmonary organs. The posterior end of a typical rib has a *head*, a *neck*, and an *articular tubercle* (Fig. 9–6). The head and tubercle articulate with a thoracic vertebra, forming two synovial joints: costovertebral and costotransverse, respectively (Fig. 9–5B). These joints anchor the posterior end of a rib to its respective vertebra. A *costovertebral joint* connects the head of a rib to a pair of costal facets that span two adjacent vertebrae and the intervening intervertebral disc. A *costotransverse joint* connects the articular tubercle of a rib with a costal facet on the transverse process of a corresponding vertebra.

The anterior end of a rib consists of flattened hyaline cartilage. Ribs 1 to 10 attach to the sternum, thereby completing the thoracic rib cage anteriorly (see Fig. 9–1). The

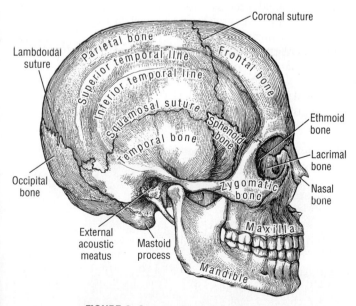

**FIGURE 9–2.** Lateral view of the skull.

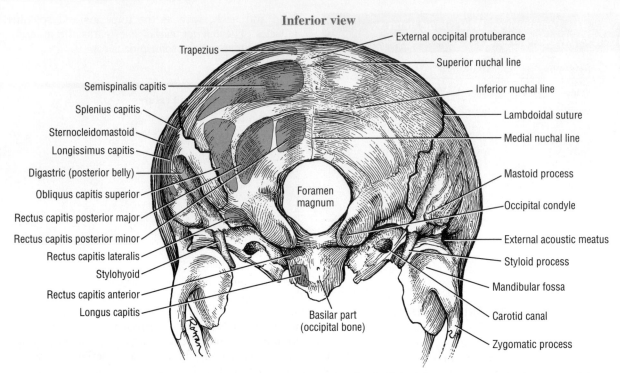

**Inferior view**

Trapezius

Semispinalis capitis

Splenius capitis

Sternocleidomastoid

Longissimus capitis

Digastric (posterior belly)

Obliquus capitis superior

Rectus capitis posterior major

Rectus capitis posterior minor

Rectus capitis lateralis

Stylohyoid

Rectus capitis anterior

Longus capitis

External occipital protuberance

Superior nuchal line

Inferior nuchal line

Lambdoidal suture

Medial nuchal line

Mastoid process

Occipital condyle

External acoustic meatus

Styloid process

Mandibular fossa

Carotid canal

Zygomatic process

Foramen magnum

Basilar part (occipital bone)

**FIGURE 9–3.** Inferior view of the occipital and temporal bones. The lambdoidal sutures separate the occipital bone medially, from the temporal bone laterally. Distal muscle attachments are indicated in gray, and proximal attachments are indicated in red.

cartilage of ribs 1 to 7 attaches directly to the lateral border of the sternum via seven sternocostal joints (Fig. 9–7). The cartilage of ribs 8 to 10 attaches to the sternum by fusing to the cartilage of the immediately superior rib. Ribs 11 and 12 do not attach to the sternum, but are anchored by lateral abdominal muscles.

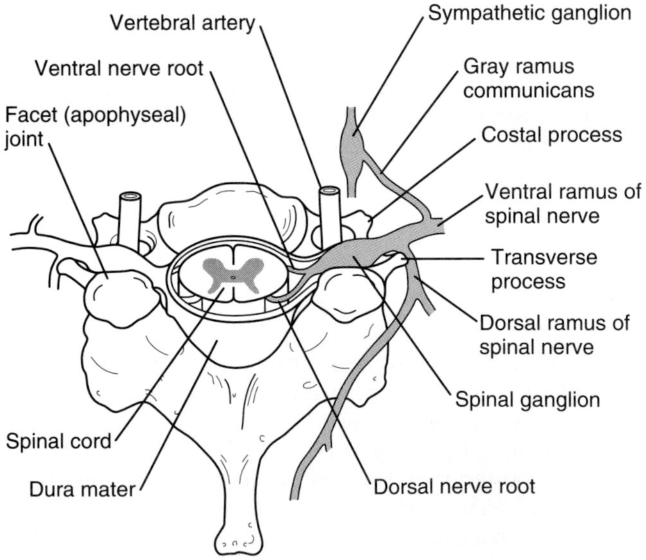

## STERNUM

The sternum is slightly convex and rough anteriorly, and slightly concave and smooth posteriorly. The bone has three parts: the manubrium (from the Latin, handle), the body, and the xiphoid process (from the Greek, sword) (see Fig. 9–7). Developmentally, the *manubrium* fuses with the body of the sternum at the *manubriosternal joint,* a fibrocartilaginous articulation that often ossifies later in life.[110] Just lateral to the *jugular notch* of the manubrium are the *clavicular facets* of the *sternoclavicular joints.* Immediately inferior to the sternoclavicular joint is a costal facet that accepts the head of the first rib at the first *sternocostal joint.*

Vertebral artery

Ventral nerve root

Facet (apophyseal) joint

Spinal cord

Dura mater

Sympathetic ganglion

Gray ramus communicans

Costal process

Ventral ramus of spinal nerve

Transverse process

Dorsal ramus of spinal nerve

Spinal ganglion

Dorsal nerve root

**FIGURE 9–4.** A cross section of a spinal cord is shown with the cervical nerve roots forming a typical spinal nerve. Note the relationship among the neural structures, bony vertebrae, dura mater, and vertebral artery. (Modified with permission from Magee DL: Orthopedic Physical Assessment, 3rd ed. Philadelphia, WB Saunders, 1997.)

---

**Osteologic Features of the Sternum**
- Manubrium
- Jugular notch
- Clavicular facets for sternoclavicular joints
- Body
- Costal facets for sternocostal joints
- Xiphoid process

**Intrasternal Joints**
- Manubriosternal joint
- Xiphisternal joint

Chapter 9   Osteology and Arthrology     **255**

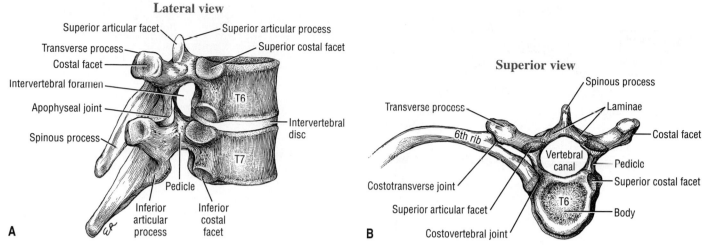

**Lateral view**

Superior articular facet — Superior articular process
Transverse process — Superior costal facet
Costal facet
Intervertebral foramen
Apophyseal joint
Spinous process
T6
T7
Intervertebral disc
Pedicle
Inferior articular process
Inferior costal facet

**A**

**Superior view**

Transverse process — Spinous process
Laminae
6th rib
Costal facet
Vertebral canal
Costotransverse joint
Pedicle
Superior costal facet
Superior articular facet
Costovertebral joint
Body
T6

**B**

**FIGURE 9–5.** The essential characteristics of a vertebra. *A,* Lateral view of the sixth and seventh vertebrae (T6 and T7). *B,* Superior view of the sixth vertebra with right rib.

**TABLE 9–2. Major Parts of a Midthoracic Vertebra**

| Part | Description | Primary Function |
|---|---|---|
| Body | Large rounded cylindrical mass of cancellous bone surrounded by a thin cortex of bone | Primary weight-bearing structure of the vertebral column |
| Intervertebral disc | Thick ring of fibrocartilage between vertebral bodies of C2 and below | Shock absorber and spacer throughout the vertebral column |
| Interbody joint | A symphysis joint formed between the superior and inferior surfaces of an intervertebral disc and adjacent vertebral bodies | Primary bond between vertebrae |
| Pedicle | Short, thick dorsal projection of bone from the mid-to-superior part of the vertebral body | Connects the vertebral body to the posterior parts of a vertebra |
| Lamina | Thin vertical plate of bone connecting the base of the spinous process to each transverse process. (The term laminae describes both right and left lamina.) | Protects the posterior aspect of the spinal cord |
| Vertebral canal | Central canal located just posterior to the vertebral body. The canal is surrounded by the pedicles and laminae. | Protects the spinal cord |
| Intervertebral foramen | Lateral opening between adjacent vertebrae | Passageway for nerve roots entering and exiting the vertebral canal |
| Transverse process | Horizontal projection of bone from the junction of a lamina and a pedicle | Attachments for muscles, ligaments, and ribs |
| Costal facet (on body) | Rounded impressions formed on the lateral sides of the thoracic vertebral bodies. Most thoracic vertebral bodies have superior and inferior facets on each side. | Attachment sites for the heads of ribs (costovertebral joints) |
| Costal facet (on transverse process) | Oval facets located at the anterior tips of each thoracic transverse process | Attachment sites for the articular tubercle of ribs (costotransverse joints) |
| Spinous process | Dorsal midline projection of bone from the laminae | Midline attachments for muscles and ligaments |
| Superior and inferior articular processes; including articular facets and apophyseal (intervertebral) joints | Paired vertical articular processes arising from the junction of a lamina and pedicle. Each process has smooth cartilage-lined articular facets. In general, superior articular facets face posteriorly; inferior articular facets face anteriorly. | Superior and inferior *articular facets* form paired *apophyseal (intervertebral)* joints. These synovial joints guide the direction and magnitude of intervertebral movement. |

**Inferior view**

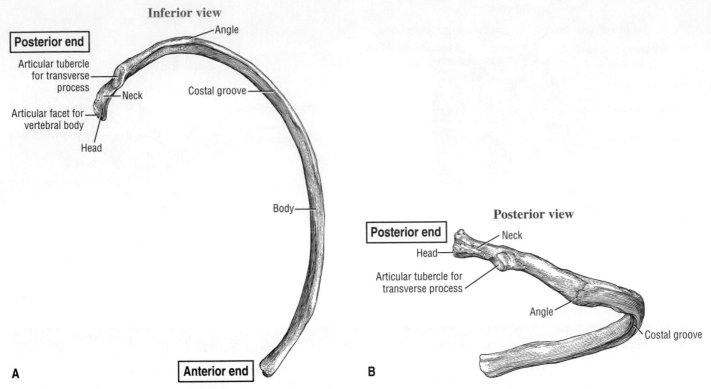

Posterior end

Articular tubercle
for transverse
process

Articular facet for
vertebral body

Head

Neck

Angle

Costal groove

Body

**A**

Anterior end

**Posterior view**

Posterior end

Head

Articular tubercle for
transverse process

Neck

Angle

Costal groove

**B**

**FIGURE 9–6.** A typical right rib. *A,* Inferior view. *B,* Posterior view.

The lateral edge of the body of the sternum is marked by a series of *costal facets* that accept the cartilages of ribs 2 to 7. The arthrology of the sternocostal joints is discussed in greater detail in Chapter 11. The *xiphoid process* is attached to the inferior end of the body of the sternum by the *xiphisternal joint.* Like the manubriosternal joint, the xiphisternal joint is connected primarily by fibrocartilage. The xiphisternal joint often ossifies by 40 years of age.[110]

## VERTEBRAL COLUMN

The word "trunk" describes the body of a person, including the sternum and ribs, but excluding the head, neck, and limbs. *Vertebral (spinal) column* describes the entire set of vertebrae, excluding the ribs, sternum, and pelvis. The terms superior and inferior are used interchangeably with the terms cranial and caudal, respectively.

The vertebral column usually consists of 33 vertebral segments, divided into five regions. Normally there are seven *cervical,* twelve *thoracic,* five *lumbar,* five *sacral,* and four *coccygeal segments.* The sacral and coccygeal vertebrae are usually fused in the adult, forming individual sacral and coccygeal bones. Individual vertebrae are abbreviated alphanumerically; for example, C2 for the second cervical, T6 for the sixth thoracic, and L1 for the first lumbar. Each region of the vertebral column (e.g., cervical and lumbar) has a distinct overall morphology that reflects its specific function. Vertebrae located at the cervicothoracic, thoracolumbar, and lumbosacral junctions often share characteristics that reflect the transition between major regions of the vertebral col-

umn. It is not uncommon, for example, for the transverse processes of C7 to have thoracic-like facets to accept a rib, or L5 may be "sacralized" (i.e., fused with the base or top of the sacrum).

### *Normal Curvatures within the Vertebral Column*

The human vertebral column consists of a series of reciprocal curvatures in the sagittal plane. While standing at rest, the curvatures define the "neutral" posture of the vertebral column (Fig. 9–8A). The cervical and lumbar regions are naturally convex anteriorly and concave posteriorly, exhibiting an alignment called *lordosis,* meaning to "bend backward." The degree of lordosis is generally less in the cervical region than in the lumbar region. The thoracic and sacrococcygeal regions, in contrast, exhibit a natural *kyphosis.* Kyphosis describes a curve that is concave anteriorly and convex posteriorly. The anterior concavity provides space for the organs within the thoracic and pelvic cavities.

The natural curvatures within the vertebral column are not fixed, but rather they are dynamic and change shape during movements and different postures. Extension of the vertebral column accentuates the cervical and lumbar lordosis, but reduces the thoracic kyphosis (Fig. 9–8B). In contrast, flexion of the vertebral column decreases, or flattens, the cervical and lumbar lordosis, but accentuates the thoracic kyphosis (Fig. 9–8C). In contrast, the sacrococcygeal curvature is fixed, being concave anteriorly, convex posteriorly. This curvature is essentially fixed by the position of the pelvis by means of the sacroiliac joints.

The embryonic vertebral column is kyphotic throughout

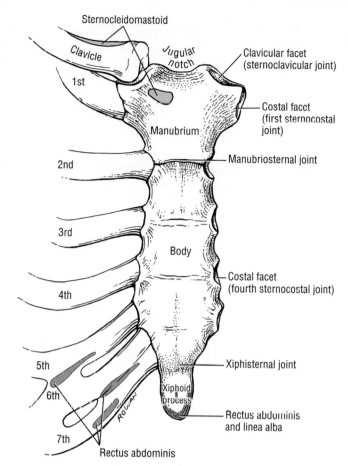

**FIGURE 9–7.** Anterior view of the sternum, part of the right clavicle, and the first seven ribs. The following articulations are seen: (1) intrasternal joints (manubriosternal and xiphisternal), (2) sternocostal joints, and (3) sternoclavicular joints. The attachment of the sternocleidomastoid muscle is indicated in red. The attachments of the rectus abdominis and linea alba are shown in gray.

its length. Lordosis in the cervical and lumbar regions occurs after birth, in association with motor maturation and upright posture. In the cervical spine, extensor muscles pull on the head and neck as the infant begins to observe the surroundings. In the lumbar spine, developing hip flexor muscles pull the convexity of the lumbar spine forward in preparation for walking. Once a child stands, the natural lordosis of the lumbar spine helps direct the body's line-of-gravity through the base of support provided by the feet.

The sagittal plane curvatures within the vertebral column provide strength and resilience to the axial skeleton. A reciprocally curved vertebral column acts like an arch. Compression forces between vertebrae are partially shared by tension in stretched connective tissues and muscles located along the convex side of each curve. As is true with long bones such as the femur, the strength and stability of the vertebral column reflect its ability to "give" slightly under a load, rather than to support large compression forces statically.

A potentially negative consequence of the natural spinal curvatures is the presence of shear forces at regions of tran-

sition between curves. Shear forces can cause premature loosening of surgical spinal fusions, especially those performed in the cervicothoracic and thoracolumbar regions.

### *Line-of-Gravity Passing through the Body*

Although highly variable, the line-of-gravity acting on a standing person with ideal posture passes through the mastoid process of the temporal bone, anterior to the second sacral vertebra, posterior to the hip, and anterior to the knee and ankle (Fig. 9–9). In the vertebral column, the line-of-gravity is on the concave side of the apex of each regions' curvature.[17] As a consequence, ideal posture allows gravity to produce a torque that helps maintain the optimal shape of each spinal curvature. The external torque due to gravity is greatest at the apex of each region: C4–5, T6, and L3.

The image depicted in Figure 9–9 is more ideal than real because each person's posture is unique and transient. Factors that alter the spatial relationship between the line-of-gravity and the spinal curvatures include fat disposition, position and magnitude of loads supported by the upper body, shapes of individual regional spinal curvatures, muscularity, connective tissue extensibility, and pregnancy. In contrast to that depicted in Figure 9–9, some describe the line-of-gravity as falling through[49] or just anterior to the lumbar vertebrae.[88] Regardless, the important point is to understand the biomechanical consequences of each possible relationship. Gravity passing posterior to the lumbar region produces a constant extension torque on the low back, facilitating natural lordosis. Alternatively, gravity passing anterior to the lumbar region produces a constant flexion torque. In either case, the external torque due to gravity, or supported external load, must be neutralized by active forces in muscles or passive forces in connective tissues. The line-of-gravity lies anterior to the lumbosacral junction and the sacroiliac joints.

Structural factors also favor the shape of the natural curves, such as wedged intervertebral discs or vertebral bodies, orientation of apophyseal joints, and tension in ligaments and muscles. The intervertebral discs in the cervical and lower lumbar regions are thicker anteriorly, for example, thereby favoring an anterior convexity in these regions.

The normal sagittal plane alignment of the vertebral column may be altered by disease, such as ankylosing spondylosis, spondylolisthesis, and muscular dystrophy, or by osteoporosis or muscle weakness associated with aging. Often, minor forms of abnormal or faulty postures occur in healthy persons (Fig. 9–10). Excessive cervical or lumbar lordosis compensates for excessive thoracic kyphosis and vice versa. The "sway back" posture shown in Figure 9–10C, for example, describes a combined exaggerated lumbar lordosis and thoracic kyphosis. The pelvis is shifted anteriorly, which forces the thighs backward. Regardless of the cause or location, abnormal curvatures alter the relationship between the line-of-gravity and each spinal region. When severe, abnormal vertebral curvatures increase stress on muscles, ligaments, bones, discs, apophyseal joints, and spinal nerve roots. Abnormal curves also change the volume of body cavities. An exaggerated thoracic kyphosis, for example, can significantly reduce the space for the lungs to expand during deep breathing (Fig. 9–11).

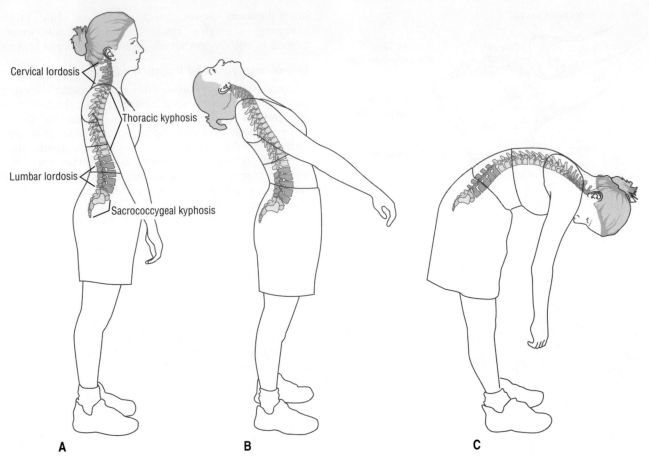

**FIGURE 9–8.** A side view shows the sagittal plane curvatures of the vertebral column. *A,* Neutral static position while one is standing. *B,* Extension of the vertebral column increases the cervical and lumbar lordosis, but reduces (straightens) the thoracic kyphosis. *C,* Flexion of the vertebral column decreases the cervical and lumbar lordosis, but increases the thoracic kyphosis.

## LIGAMENTOUS SUPPORT OF THE VERTEBRAL COLUMN

The vertebral column is supported by an extensive set of ligaments. Spinal ligaments limit motion, maintain natural spinal curvature, and indirectly protect the spinal cord. The major ligaments of the vertebral canal are depicted in Figure 9–12. The basic structure and function of each ligament are summarized in Table 9–3.

The *ligamentum flavum* originates on the anterior surface of a lamina and inserts on the posterior surface of the lamina below. The ligaments are thickest in the lumbar region. Ligamentum flavum means "the yellow ligament," reflecting its high content of yellow elastic connective tissue.[110] Passive tension in a series of stretched ligamentum flava limits flexion throughout the vertebral column, thereby protecting the intervertebral disc from excessive compression. Figure 9–13 shows the increase in tension (stress) in one ligamentum flavum. Note that between neutral extension and full flexion the ligament has elongated (strained) 35% of its original resting length.[73] Flexion beyond physiologic limits can rupture the ligament and permit compressive damage to the intervertebral disc.[2] The ligamentum flavum lies just posterior to the spinal cord. Severe hyperextension of the spine can buckle the ligamentum flavum inward and pinch the delicate spinal cord.

The *supraspinous and interspinous ligaments* extend between adjacent spinous processes. As evident by their position, they limit flexion. In the lumbar region, the supraspinous and interspinous ligaments are typically the first structures to rupture in extreme flexion.[4] The *intertransverse ligaments* extend between adjacent transverse processes, becoming taut in contralateral lateral flexion.

In the cervical region, the supraspinous ligaments thicken and extend to the cranium as the *ligamentum nuchae.* This tough membrane consists of a bilaminar strip of fibroelastic tissue that attaches between the cervical spinous processes and external occipital protuberance of the occipital bone. Because the center of mass of the head is located anterior to the cervical spine, gravity naturally flexes the craniocervical region.[21] Passive tension in a stretched ligamentum nuchae adds a small but useful element of support to the head and neck. The ligamentum nuchae also provides a midline attachment for muscles, such as the trapezius and splenius capitis and cervicis. The ligamentum nuchae accounts for the difficulty encountered when palpating the spinous process in the mid to upper cervical region (Fig. 9–14).

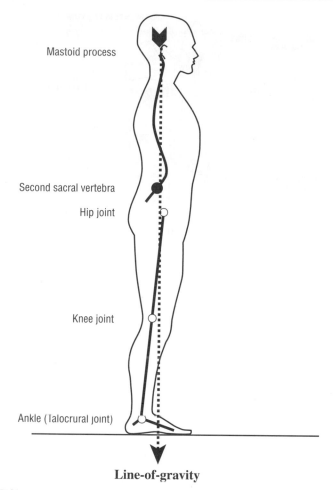

Mastoid process

Second sacral vertebra

Hip joint

Knee joint

Ankle (Talocrural joint)

**Line-of-gravity**

**FIGURE 9–9.** The line-of-gravity in a person with an ideal standing posture. (Modified from Neumann DA: Arthrokinesiologic considerations for the aged adult. In Guccione AA (ed): Geriatric Physical Therapy, 2nd ed. Chicago, Mosby-Year Book, 2000.)

The *anterior longitudinal ligament* is a long, straplike structure attaching between the basilar part of the occipital bone and the entire length of the anterior surfaces of all vertebral bodies, including the sacrum. This strong ligament is narrow at its cranial end and widens caudally. Fibers of the anterior longitudinal ligament blend with and reinforce the adjacent portion of the intervertebral disc.[110] The anterior longitudinal ligament provides stability to the vertebral column, by limiting extension or excessive lordosis in the cervical and lumbar regions.

The *posterior longitudinal ligament* is a continuous band of tissue that extends the entire length of the posterior surfaces of all vertebral bodies, between the axis (C2) and the sacrum. The posterior longitudinal ligament is located within the vertebral canal, just anterior to the spinal cord. The posterior and anterior longitudinal ligaments are named according to their relationship to the *vertebral body,* not the spinal cord. Throughout its length, the posterior longitudinal ligament blends with and reinforces the intervertebral discs.[110] Cranially, the posterior longitudinal ligament is a broad structure, narrowing as it descends toward the lumbar region. The slender lumbar portion limits its ability to restrain a posterior bulging (slipped) disc. As with the anterior longitudinal ligament, the posterior longitudinal ligament provides stability to the spine.

A *joint capsule* surrounds and reinforces each apophyseal joint (Fig. 9–15). The capsule is relatively loose, especially in the cervical region where ample range of motion is required. Although relatively loose in a neutral posture, the capsule of the apophyseal joints is under tension when stretched. In the lumbar region, the capsule is shown to accept up to 1000 N (~ 225 lb) of tension before failure.[20] This tension limits the extremes of all intervertebral motions, with the exception of extension. The capsule of the apophyseal joints is reinforced by adjacent muscles (multifidus) and connective tissue (ligamentum flava), particularly evident in the lumbar region.[96]

**FIGURE 9–10.** A diagrammatic representation of common faulty postures in the sagittal plane. (From McMorris RO: Faulty postures. Pediatr Clin North Am 8:217, 1961.)

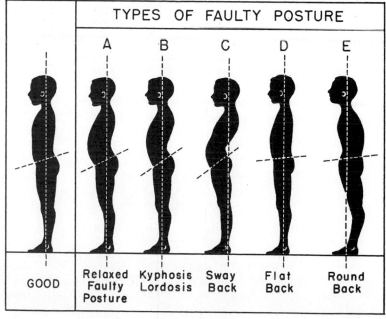

TYPES OF FAULTY POSTURE

A    B    C    D    E

GOOD    Relaxed Faulty Posture    Kyphosis Lordosis    Sway Back    Flat Back    Round Back

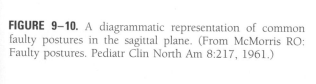

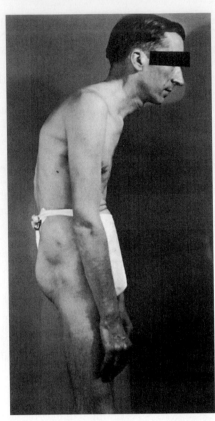

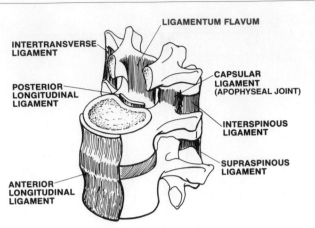

**FIGURE 9–12.** Primary ligaments that stabilize the vertebral column. (Modified from White AA, Panjabi MM: Clinical Biomechanics of the Spine, 2nd ed. Philadelphia, JB Lippincott, 1990.)

**FIGURE 9–11.** Lateral view of a person with ankylosing spondylitis. Note the severe thoracic kyphosis and flattening of the lumbar region. (From Polley HF, Hunder GG: Rheumatologic Inteviewing and Physical Examination of the Joints. Philadelphia, WB Saunders, 1978.)

**TABLE 9-3. Major Ligaments of the Vertebral Column**

| Name | Attachments | Function | Comment |
|------|-------------|----------|---------|
| Ligamentum flavum | Between the anterior surface of one lamina and the posterior surface of the lamina below | Limits flexion | Contains a high percentage of elastin Lies posterior to the spinal cord Thickest in the lumbar region |
| Supraspinous and interspinous ligaments | Between the adjacent spinous processes from C7 to the sacrum | Limits flexion | Ligamentum nuchae is the cervical and cranial extension of the supraspinous ligaments, providing a midline structure for muscle attachments, and passive support for the head. |
| Intertransverse ligaments | Between adjacent transverse processes | Limits contralateral lateral flexion | Few fibers exist in the cervical region. In the thoracic region, the ligaments are rounded and intertwined with local muscle. In the lumbar region, the ligaments are thin and membranous. |
| Anterior longitudinal ligament | Between the basilar part of the occipital bone and the entire length of the anterior surfaces of all vertebral bodies, including the sacrum | Adds stability to the vertebral column Limits extension or excessive lordosis in the cervical and lumbar regions | |

## TABLE 9-3. Major Ligaments of the Vertebral Column *Continued*

| Name | Attachments | Function | Comment |
|---|---|---|---|
| Posterior longitudinal ligament | Throughout the length of the posterior surfaces of all vertebral bodies, between the axis (C2) and the sacrum | Stabilizes the vertebral column<br>Limits flexion<br>Reinforces the posterior annulus fibrosus | Lies within the vertebral canal, just anterior to the spinal cord |
| Capsule of the apophyseal joints | Margin of each apophyseal joint | Strengthens and supports the apophyseal joint | Becomes taut at the extremes of all intervertebral motions, except for extension |

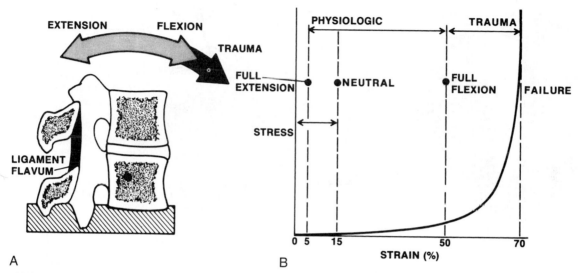

A

B

**FIGURE 9-13.** Functional biomechanics of the ligamentum flavum during extension and flexion. *A,* The ligamentum flavum is slackened in extension and stretched in flexion. Excessive flexion can cause trauma. *B,* The stress-strain relationship of the ligamentum flavum is shown between full extension to a point of failure (rupture) at extreme flexion. Note the ligament fails at a point 70% beyond its full slackened length. (Data from Nachemson A, Evans J: Some mechanical properties of the third lumbar interlaminar ligament. J Biomech 1:211–220, 1968.)

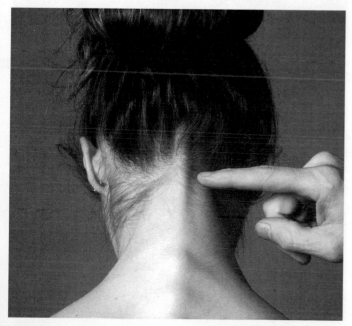

**FIGURE 9-14.** The ligamentum nuchae is shown in a thin young woman.

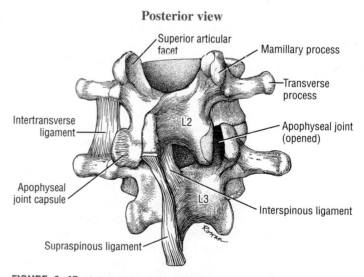

**FIGURE 9-15.** A posterior view of the second and third lumbar vertebrae. The capsule of the right apophyseal joint is removed to show the vertical alignment of the joint surfaces. The top vertebra is rotated to the right to maximally expose the articular surfaces of the right apophyseal joint.

### Intra-articular Structures Found in Apophyseal Joints

Most apophyseal joints contain *intra-articular structures* located between the internal side of the capsule and the periphery of the articular cartilage. The structures contain small fat pads mixed with thin sheets of connective tissues that extend partially into the joint. These structures—termed fibroadipose meniscoids—may help protect exposed cartilage and synovial membrane from compression forces during the extremes of movement.[66] Several different forms of intra-articular structures located within the lumbar apophyseal joints are illustrated in Figure 9–16. The meniscoids may be involved in an acute "locked back" condition. During flexion, a meniscoid may buckle on itself and become lodged under the adjacent capsule. The mensicoid may then act as a space-occupying lesion, blocking full extension.[12]

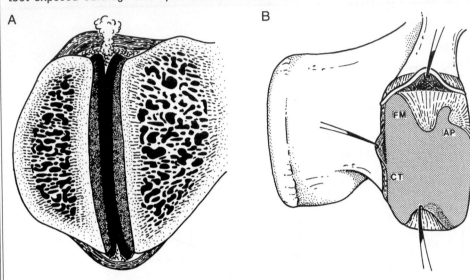

**FIGURE 9–16.** Intra-articular structures within the lumbar apophyseal joints. *A,* Frontal section shows fibroadipose meniscoids extending into the joint cavity from the capsule. *B,* Lateral view of the articular cartilage of an opened apophyseal joint shows different forms of an intra-articular structure: FM, fibroadipose meniscoid; CT, connective tissue rim; and AP, adipose tissue pad. (From Bogduk N: Clinical Anatomy of the Lumbar Spine, 3rd ed. New York, Churchill Livingstone, 1997.)

## REGIONAL OSTEOLOGIC FEATURES

The adage that "function follows structure" is very applicable in the study of the vertebral column. Although all vertebrae have a common morphologic theme, each also has a specific shape that reflects its unique function. The following section, along with Table 9–4, highlights specific osteologic features of each region of the vertebral column.

### Cervical Region

The cervical vertebrae are the smallest and most mobile of all movable vertebrae. The high degree of mobility is essential to the large range of motion required by the head. Perhaps the most unique anatomic feature of the cervical vertebrae is the presence of *transverse foramina* located within the transverse processes (Fig. 9–17). The vertebral artery ascends through these foramina, coursing toward the foramen magnum to transport blood to the brain and spinal cord. In the neck, the vertebral artery is located immediately anterior to the exiting spinal nerve roots (see Fig. 9–4).

The third through the sixth cervical vertebrae show nearly identical features and are therefore considered typical of this region. The upper two cervical vertebrae, the atlas (C1) and the axis (C2), and the seventh cervical vertebrae (C7) are atypical for reasons described in a subsequent section.

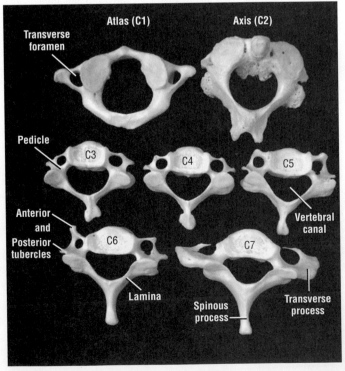

**Superior view**

**FIGURE 9–17.** A superior view of seven cervical vertebrae from the same human specimen.

## TABLE 9-4. Osteologic Features of the Vertebral Column

| | Body | Superior Articular Facets | Inferior Articular Facets | Spinous Processes | Vertebral Canal | Transverse Processes | Comments |
|---|---|---|---|---|---|---|---|
| Atlas (C1) | None | Concave, face generally superior | Flat to slightly concave, face generally inferior | None, replaced by a small posterior tubercle | Triangular, largest of cervical region | Largest of cervical region | Two large lateral masses, joined by anterior and posterior arches |
| Axis (C2) | Tall with a vertical projecting dens | Flat to slightly convex, face generally superior | Flat, face anterior and inferior | Largest of cervical region, bifid | Large and triangular | Form anterior and posterior tubercles | Contains large spinous process |
| C3-6 | Wider than deep; have uncinate processes | Flat, face posterior and superior | As above | Bifid | Large and triangular | End as anterior and posterior tubercles | Considered typical cervical vertebrae |
| C7 | Wider than deep | As above | Transition to typical thoracic vertebrae | Large and prominent, easily palpable | Triangular | Thick and prominent, may have a large anterior tubercle forming an "extra rib." | Often called "vertebral prominens" due to large spinous process |
| T2-T9 | Equal width and depth. Costal facets for attachment of the heads of ribs 2 to 9 | Flat, face mostly posterior | Flat, face mostly anterior | Long and pointed, slant inferiorly | Round, smaller than cervical | Project horizontally and slightly posterior, have costal facets for tubercles of ribs | Considered typical thoracic vertebrae |
| T1 and T10-12 | Equal width and depth. T1 has a full costal facet for rib 1 and a partial facet for rib 2. T10-12 each has a full costal facet. | As above | As above | As above | As above | T10-12 may lack costal facets. | Considered atypical thoracic vertebrae primarily by the manner of rib attachment |
| L1-5 | Wider than deep. L5 is slightly wedged (i.e., higher height anteriorly than posteriorly). | Slightly concave, face medial to posterior-medial | L1-4 slightly convex, face lateral to anterior-lateral. L5: flat, face anterior and slightly lateral | Stout and rectangular | Triangular, contains cauda equina | Slender, project laterally | Superior articular processes have mammillary bodies |
| Sacrum | Fused. Body of first sacral vertebra most evident | Flat, face posterior and slightly medial | None | None, replaced by multiple spinous tubercles | As above | None, replaced by multiple transverse tubercles | |
| Coccyx | Fusion of four rudimentary vertebrae | Rudimentary | Rudimentary | Rudimentary | Ends at the first coccyx | Rudimentary | |

### Typical Cervical Vertebrae (C3–6)

C3–6 have small rectangular-shaped *bodies*, wider from side-to-side than front-to-back (Figs. 9–17 and 9–18). The superior and inferior surfaces of the bodies are not as flat as most other vertebrae, but are curved or notched. The superior surfaces are concave side-to-side, with raised posterior-lateral hooks called *uncinate processes* (uncus means hook). The inferior surfaces, in contrast, are concave anterior-posterior, with elongated anterior and posterior margins. When articulated, small *uncovertebral joints* form between the uncinate process and adjacent part of the superior vertebra between C3 and C7. Uncovertebral joints are often called the "joints of Luschka," named after the person who first described them.[39] Small fissures extend from the uncovertebral joints into the adjacent outer rings (annuli) of the intervertebral discs. The exact function of uncovertebral joints is unclear, although they probably add stability to the cervical interbody joints.[33]

The *pedicles* of C3–6 are short and curved posterior-lateral (see Fig. 9–17). Very thin *laminae* extend posterior-medial from each pedicle (Fig. 9–20). The triangular-shaped *vertebral canal* is large in the cervical region in order to accommodate the thickening of the spinal cord associated with the formation of the cervical plexus and brachial plexus.

**Anterior view**

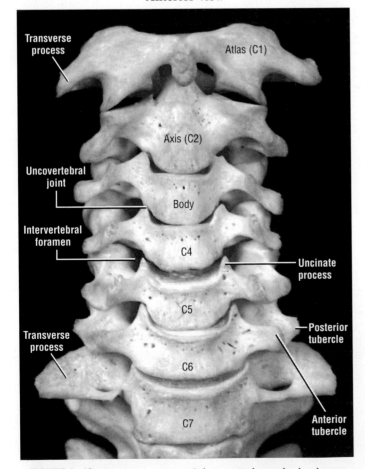

**FIGURE 9–18.** An anterior view of the cervical vertebral column.

Within the C3–6 region, consecutive superior and inferior articular processes form a continuous articular "pillar," interrupted by apophyseal joints (Fig. 9–21). The articular facets within each apophyseal joint are smooth and flat, with joint surfaces oriented midway between the vertical and horizontal planes. The *superior articular facets* face posterior and superior, whereas the *inferior articular facets* face anterior and inferior.

The *spinous processes* of C3–6 are short, with some processes being bifid (i.e., double) (see Fig. 9–17, C3). The *transverse processes* are short lateral extensions that terminate as variably shaped *anterior and posterior tubercles*. The tubercles are unique to the cervical region, serving as attachments for muscles, such as the anterior scalene, levator scapulae, and splenius cervicis.

### Atypical Cervical Vertebrae (C1–2 and C7)

#### Atlas (C1)

As indicated by its name, the primary function of the atlas is to support the head. Possessing no body, pedicle, lamina, or spinous process, the atlas is essentially two large lateral masses joined by anterior and posterior arches (Fig. 9–22). The short *anterior arch* has an *anterior tubercle* for attachment of the anterior longitudinal ligament. The much larger *posterior arch* forms nearly half the circumference of the entire atlantal ring. A small *posterior tubercle* marks the midline of the posterior arch. The lateral masses support the prominent articular processes.

The large and concave *superior articular facets* face cranially, in general, to accept the large, convex occipital condyles. The *inferior articular facets* are flat to slightly concave. These facet surfaces generally face inferiorly, with their lateral edges sloped downward, approximately 30 degrees from the horizontal plane (Fig. 9–22B). The atlas has large, palpable *transverse processes*, usually the greatest of the cervical vertebrae.

#### Axis (C2)

The axis has a large, tall *body* that serves as a base for the upwardly projecting *dens (odontoid process)* (Fig. 9–23A and B). Part of the elongated body is formed from remnants of the body of the atlas and the intervening disc. The dens provides a rigid vertical axis for rotation of the atlas and head (Fig. 9–24). Projecting laterally from the body is a pair of *superior articular processes* (Fig. 9–23A). These large flat to slightly convex processes have superior facets that are generally in a cranial position, exhibiting a 30-degree slope, which matches the slope of the inferior articular facets of the atlas. Projecting from the prominent superior articular processes of the axis are a pair of stout *pedicles* and a pair of short *transverse processes* (Fig. 9–23B). A pair of *inferior articular processes* project inferiorly from the pedicles, with articular facets facing anteriorly and inferiorly (see Fig. 9–21). The *spinous process* of the axis is bifid and very broad. This palpable spinous process serves as an attachment for many muscles, such as the semi-spinalis cervicis.

#### "Vertebral Prominens" (C7)

C7 is the most prominent of all cervical vertebrae, having many characteristics of thoracic vertebrae. C7 can have a

### Cervical Osteophytes: One Possible Consequence of Disc Disease

One important function of a healthy, well-hydrated intervertebral disc is to unload the uncovertebral joints. This unloading, or "cushioning" effect, is illustrated at the C3-C4 intervertebral junction in Figure 9–19. The effect may be reduced in the case of a degenerated or dehydrated disc. Over time, increased compression force on the uncovertebral joint may stimulate the formation of an osteophyte (bone spur), depicted at the C4-C5 intervertebral joint in Figure 9–19. Osteophytes develop in accordance with the century-old *Wolff's Law* that states "Bone is laid down in areas of high stress and reabsorbed in areas of low-stress." A large osteophyte may encroach on an exiting spinal nerve root, producing a pinched nerve syndrome with pain and weakness throughout the peripheral distribution.

**Anterior view**

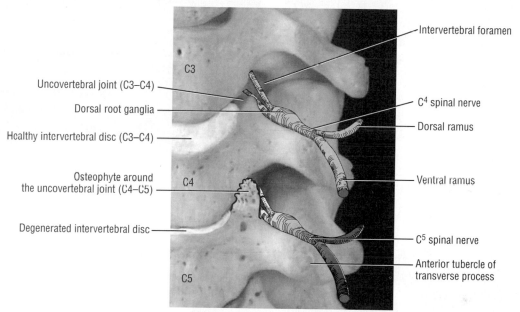

Intervertebral foramen

C3

Uncovertebral joint (C3–C4)

Dorsal root ganglia

Healthy intervertebral disc (C3–C4)

Osteophyte around the uncovertebral joint (C4–C5)

C4

Degenerated intervertebral disc

C5

$C^4$ spinal nerve

Dorsal ramus

Ventral ramus

$C^5$ spinal nerve

Anterior tubercle of transverse process

**FIGURE 9–19.** A computer-enhanced image depicts the relationship between the health of an intervertebral disc and the compression at the adjacent uncovertebral joints. The intervertebral disc between C3–C4 is shown as a healthy and fully hydrated structure. The height of the disc acts as a spacer, unloading the uncovertebral joints. In contrast, the disc between C4–C5 is shown as a degenerated, flattened structure. As a result, the adjacent C4–C5 uncovertebral joint has developed a large osteophyte owing to increased compression and resultant stress between its articular surfaces. The osteophyte is shown compressing elements of the $C^5$, which may cause radiating pain throughout the nerve's peripheral distribution.

large *transverse processes*, as illustrated in Figure 9–18. A hypertrophic anterior tubercle on the transverse process may sprout an extra cervical rib, which may impinge on the brachial plexus. This vertebra also has a large, single pointed *spinous process*, characteristic of other thoracic vertebrae (see Fig. 9–21).

### Thoracic Region

#### Typical Thoracic Vertebrae (T2–T10)

The second through the tenth thoracic vertebrae demonstrate similar features (see Fig. 9–5). *Pedicles* are directed posteriorly from the body, which reduce the size of the vertebral canal as compared with the cervical region. The large *transverse processes* project posterior-laterally, each containing a *costal facet* that articulates with the tubercle of the corresponding rib. Short, thick *laminae* form a broad base for the downward slanting *spinous processes*. The articular processes have facets that are oriented nearly vertical, with the *superior facets* facing generally posterior and the *inferior facets* facing generally anterior. The *apophyseal joints* are aligned close to the frontal plane (Fig. 9–25).

Each head of ribs 2 to 10 forms a costovertebral joint by articulating at the junction of the T1–2 through T9–10 vertebral bodies. The head of a rib articulates with a pair of costal facets that span one intervertebral junction. A thoracic (intercostal) spinal nerve root exits through a corresponding thoracic *intervertebral foramen*. The intervertebral foramen is located just anterior to the apophyseal joints.

**Posterior-lateral view**

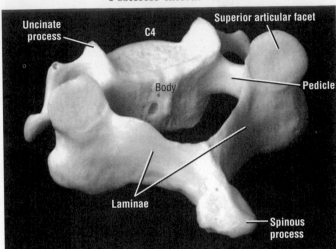

**FIGURE 9–20.** A posterior-lateral view of the fourth cervical vertebra.

**Lateral view**

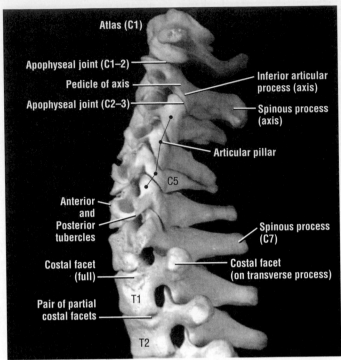

**FIGURE 9–21.** A lateral view of the cervical vertebral column.

**Superior view**

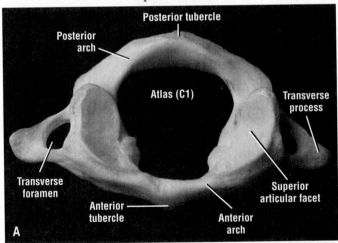

**Anterior view**

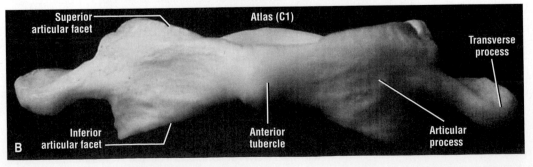

**FIGURE 9–22.** The atlas. *A,* Superior view. *B,* Anterior view.

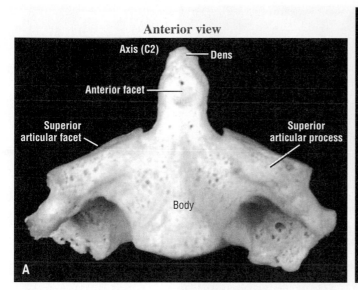

**FIGURE 9–23.** The axis. *A,* Anterior view. *B,* Superior view.

### Atypical Thoracic Vertebrae (T1 and T11–12)

The first and last two thoracic vertebrae are considered atypical mainly due to the particular manner of rib attachment. T1 has a *full costal facet* superiorly that accepts the entire head of the first rib, and a *partial facet* inferiorly that accepts part of the head of the second rib (see Fig. 9–21). The *spinous process* of T1 is especially elongated and often as prominent as the spinous process of C7. The bodies of T11 and T12 each have a single, *full costal facet* for articulation with the heads of the eleventh and twelfth ribs, respectively.

The neck of ribs 11 and 12 typically do not form articulations with corresponding transverse processes.

### Lumbar Region

Lumbar vertebrae have massive wide *bodies,* suitable for supporting the entire superimposed weight of the head, trunk, and arms (Fig. 9–26). The total mass of five lumbar vertebrae is approximately twice that of the seven cervical vertebrae (Fig. 9–27).

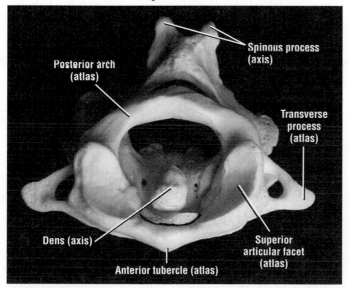

**FIGURE 9–24.** A superior view of the median atlanto-axial articulation.

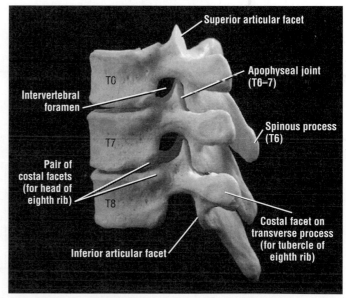

**FIGURE 9–25.** A lateral view of the sixth through eighth thoracic vertebrae.

**Superior view**

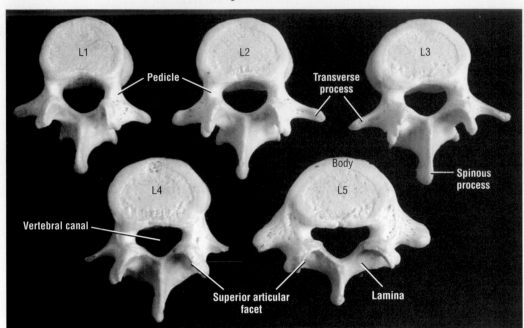

**FIGURE 9–26.** A superior view of the five lumbar vertebrae.

For the most part, the lumbar vertebrae possess similar characteristics. *Laminae and pedicles* are short and thick, forming the posterior and lateral walls of the nearly triangular-shaped vertebral canal. Thin *transverse processes* project almost laterally. *Spinous processes* are broad and rectangular, projecting horizontally from the junction of each lamina (Fig. 9–28). This shape is strikingly different from that of the pointed, sloped spinous processes of the thoracic region. Short *mammillary processes* project from the posterior surfaces of each superior articular process. These structures serve as attachment sites for the multifidi muscles.

The articular facets of the lumbar vertebrae are oriented nearly vertical. The *superior facets* are moderately concave, facing medial to posterior-medial. As depicted in Figure

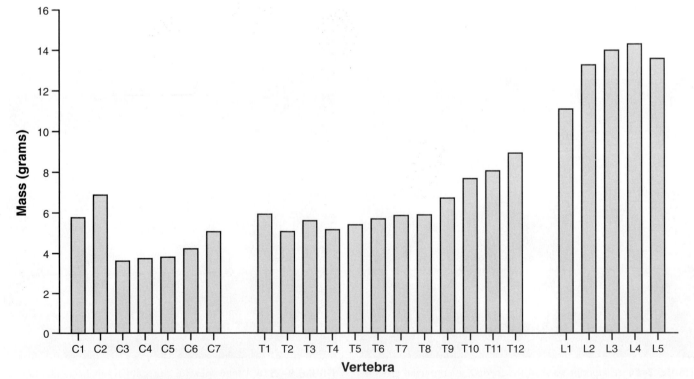

**FIGURE 9–27.** The mass, in grams, of individual vertebrae from a human adult specimen.

**Lateral view**

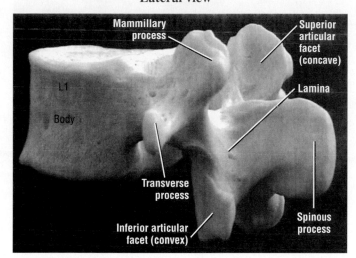

**FIGURE 9–28.** A lateral view of the first lumbar vertebra.

9–26, the superior facet surfaces in the upper lumbar region tend to be oriented close to the sagittal plane, and the superior facet surfaces in the mid-to-lower lumbar region tend to be oriented midway between the sagittal and frontal planes. The *inferior articular facets* are reciprocally matched to the shape and orientation of the superior articular facets. In general, the inferior articular facets are slightly convex, facing generally lateral to anterior-lateral (see Fig. 9–28).

The inferior facets of L5 articulate with the superior facets of the sacrum. The resulting L5-S1 apophyseal joints are typically oriented much closer to the frontal plane than are other lumbar articulations. The L5-S1 apophyseal joints provide an important source of anterior-posterior stability to the lumbosacral junction.

### Sacrum

The sacrum is a triangular bone with its base facing superiorly and apex inferiorly (Fig. 9–30). An important function of the sacrum is to transmit the weight of the vertebral column to the pelvis. In childhood, each of five separate sacral vertebrae are joined by a cartilaginous membrane. By adulthood, however, the sacrum has fused into a single bone, which still retains the typical anatomic features of a generic vertebra.

The *anterior (pelvic) surface* of the sacrum is smooth and concave, forming part of the posterior wall of the pelvic cavity (see Fig. 9–30). Four paired *ventral (pelvic) sacral foramina* transmit the ventral rami of spinal nerves that form much of the sacral plexus. The *dorsal surface* of the sacrum is convex and rough due to the attachments of muscle and ligaments (Fig. 9–31). Several *spinal and lateral tubercles* mark the remnants of fused spinous and transverse processes, respectively. Four paired *dorsal sacral foramina* transmit the dorsal rami of sacral nerves.

The superior surface of the sacrum shows a clear representation of the *body* of the first sacral vertebra (Fig. 9–32). The sharp anterior edge of the body of S1 is called the *sacral promontory*. The triangular *sacral canal* houses and protects

the cauda equina. *Pedicles* are very thick, extending laterally as the *ala* (lateral wings) of the sacrum. Stout *superior articular processes* have articular facets that face generally posterior-medial. These facets articulate with the inferior facets of L5 to form L5-S1 apophyseal joints (see Fig. 9–31). The large *auricular surface* articulates with the ilium, forming the sacroiliac joint. The sacrum narrows caudally to form its *apex,* a point of articulation with the coccyx.

### Coccyx

The coccyx is a small triangular bone consisting of four fused vertebrae (see Fig. 9–31). The base of the coccyx joins the apex of the sacrum at the *sacrococcygeal joint*. The joint has a fibrocartilaginous disc and is held together by several small ligaments. The sacrococcygeal joint usually fuses late in life. In youths, small *intercoccygeal joints* persist; however, these typically are fused in adults.[110]

## ARTHROLOGY

### Typical Intervertebral Junction

The typical intervertebral junction has three parts that are associated with movement and stability: the transverse and spinous processes, the apophyseal joints, and the interbody joint (Fig. 9–33). All three parts share common functions, although each has a predominant function (Table 9–5). The *spinous and transverse processes* function as outriggers, or levers, increasing the mechanical advantage of muscles and ligaments that move and stabilize the vertebral column.

The *apophyseal joints* are primarily responsible for guiding intervertebral motion, much like railroad tracks guide the direction of a train. The geometry, size, and spatial orientation of the articular facets within each apophyseal joint greatly influence the direction of intervertebral motion.

The *interbody joint* functions primarily for shock absorption and load distribution. In addition, the interbody joint

**TABLE 9–5. Predominant Functions of the Three Parts of a Typical Intervertebral Junction**

| Part | Function |
| --- | --- |
| Spinous process and transverse processes | Provide levers for muscles and ligaments for the purposes of causing or restricting movement, and stabilizing the vertebral column |
| Apophyseal joint | Guides intervertebral motion |
| Interbody joint | Absorbs shock and distributes load throughout the vertebral column<br>Provides intervertebral stability<br>Serves as the approximate site of the axes of rotation for movement<br>Functions as a deformable intervertebral spacer |

**SPECIAL FOCUS 9 – 3**

### Cauda Equina

The spinal cord and vertebral column have different growth rates. As a consequence, the caudal end of the adult spinal cord usually terminates adjacent to the L1-2 intervertebral foramen (Fig. 9–29). The lumbosacral nerves must travel a great distance before reaching their corresponding intervertebral foramina. As a group, the elongated nerves resemble a horse's tail, hence *cauda equina.* The cauda equina is a set of peripheral nerves that are

bathed within cerebrospinal fluid and located within the lumbosacral vertebral canal.

Severe fracture or trauma in the lumbosacral region may damage the cauda equina, but spare the spinal cord. Damage to the cauda equina may result in muscle paralysis and atrophy, altered sensation, and reduced reflexes. Spasticity with exaggerated reflexes typically occurs with damage to the spinal cord.

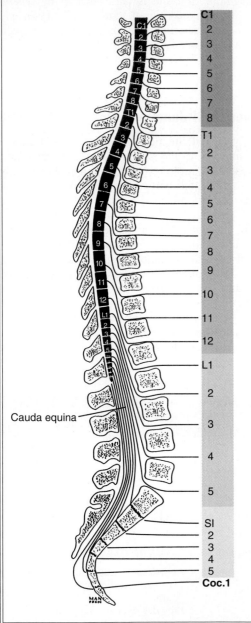

Cauda equina

**FIGURE 9–29.** Relation of the spinal cord and nerve roots to the vertebral column. The nerve roots of the spinal cord shown in black are numbered C1-S5. The intervertebral foramina through which the nerve roots pass are indicated by the numbers in the right column. In the adult, the spinal cord is shorter than the vertebral column. The spinal cord terminates adjacent to the L1-2 intervertebral foramen. (From Haymaker W, Woodhall B: Peripheral Nerve Injuries, 2nd ed. Philadelphia, WB Saunders, 1995.)

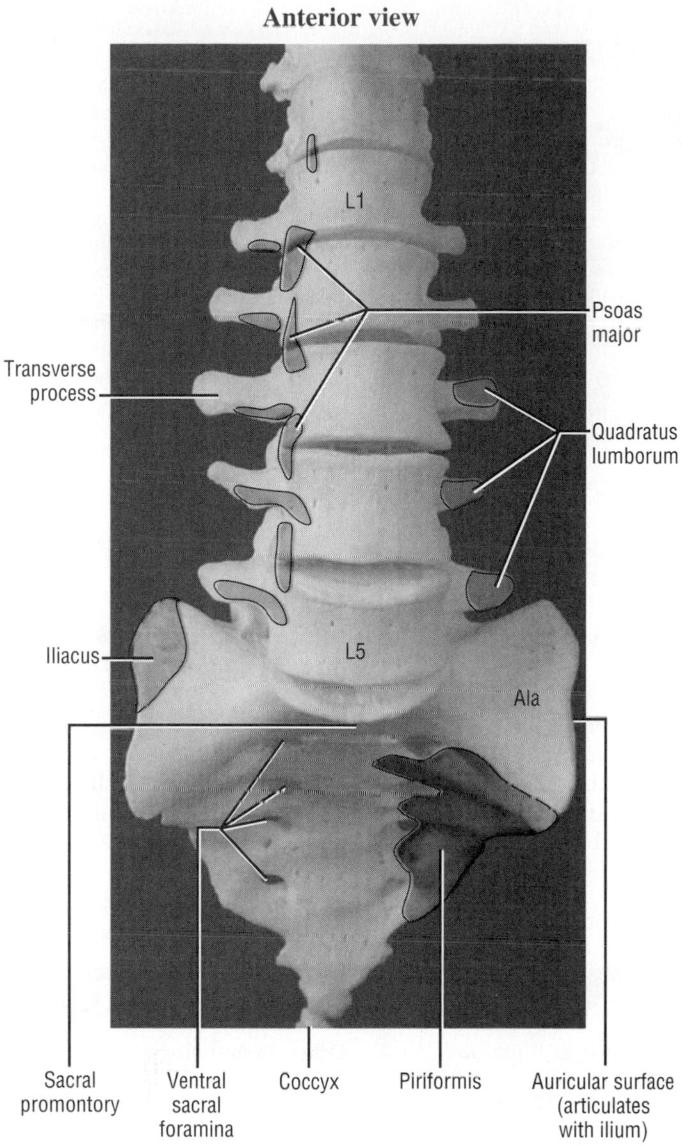

**Anterior view**

Transverse process

L1

Psoas major

Quadratus lumborum

Iliacus

L5

Ala

Sacral promontory | Ventral sacral foramina | Coccyx | Piriformis | Auricular surface (articulates with ilium)

**FIGURE 9–30.** An anterior view of the lumbosacral region. Attachments of the piriformis, iliacus, and psoas major are indicated in red. Attachments of the quadratus lumborum are indicated in gray.

**Posterior-lateral view**

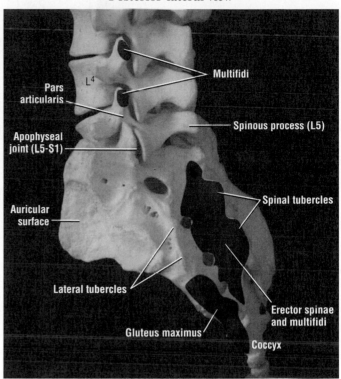

Pars articularis

L⁴

Multifidi

Spinous process (L5)

Apophyseal joint (L5-S1)

Auricular surface

Spinal tubercles

Lateral tubercles

Erector spinae and multifidi

Gluteus maximus

Coccyx

**FIGURE 9-31.** A posterior-lateral view of the lumbosacral region. Attachments of the multifidi, erector spinae, and gluteus maximus are indicated in red.

## TERMINOLOGY THAT DESCRIBES MOVEMENT

Movement within one intervertebral junction is small. When added across entire vertebral regions, however, these small movements yield considerable angular rotation. The *osteokinematics* at the vertebral column, including the head, describe

adds stability between vertebrae, serves as the approximate site of the axes of rotation, and functions as a deformable intervertebral spacer. As spacers, the intervertebral discs constitute about 25% of the total height of the vertebral column. The larger the ratio between the height of the body and the height of the disc, the greater the relative movement between consecutive bodies. The greatest space between vertebrae occurs in cervical and lumbar regions.

Interaction of all three functional parts of the vertebrae is required for normal vertebral movement. Mechanical dysfunction in any part can cause articular derangement and/or impingement of neural tissues. Understanding the spatial and physical relationships between the neurology, osteology, and arthrology of the vertebral column is an essential element in understanding the cause and treatment of spinal pain and dysfunction, regardless of etiology.

**Superior view**

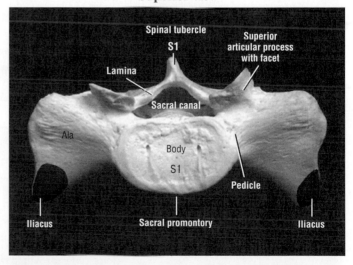

Spinal tubercle
S1

Superior articular process with facet

Lamina

Sacral canal

Ala

Body
S1

Pedicle

Iliacus | Sacral promontory | Iliacus

**FIGURE 9–32.** A superior view of the sacrum. Attachments of the iliacus muscles are indicated in red.

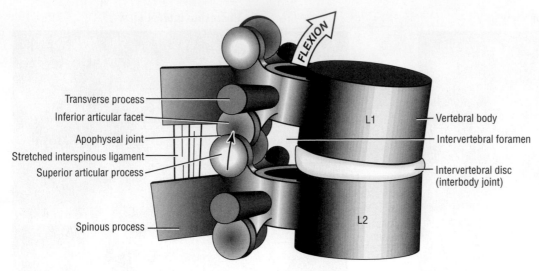

**FIGURE 9–33.** A model shows the three functional parts of a typical intervertebral junction: transverse and spinous processes, apophyseal joints, and interbody joint, including the intervertebral disc. The L1-2 junction is shown flexing and sliding between the articular facet surfaces of the apophyseal joints. The interspinous ligament is shown stretched. Note the compression of the front of the intervertebral disc.

the plane and direction of rotation for a given region. Motions are typically defined by their planes, with an associated axis of rotation located approximately through the body of the interbody joint (Table 9–6). By convention, movement throughout the vertebral column, including the head on the cervical spine, occurs in a cranial-to-caudal fashion, with the direction of movement referenced by a point on the anterior side of the more cranial (superior) vertebral segment. During

C4–5 axial rotation to the left, for example, a point on the anterior body of C4 rotates to the left, although the spinous process rotates to the right.

*Arthrokinematic terminology* describes the relative movement between articular facet surfaces within a given apophyseal joint. Most joint surfaces are flat or nearly flat, and terms such as approximation, separation, and sliding describe the arthrokinematics (Table 9–7).

### TABLE 9–6. Terminology Describing the Osteokinematics of the Axial Skeleton

| Common Terminology | Plane of Movement | Axis of Rotation | Other Terminology |
|---|---|---|---|
| Flexion and extension | Sagittal | Medial-lateral | Forward and backward bending |
| Lateral flexion to the right or left | Frontal | Anterior-posterior | Side bending to the right or left |
| Axial rotation to the right or left* | Horizontal | Vertical | Rotation, torsion |

* Axial rotation of the spine is defined by the direction of movement of a point on the *anterior side* of the vertebral body.

### TABLE 9–7. Terminology Describing the Arthrokinematics at the Apophyseal Joints

| Terminology | Definition | Functional Example |
|---|---|---|
| *Approximation* of joint surfaces | An articular facet surface tends to move closer to its partner facet. Joint approximation is usually caused by a *compression* force. | Extension or increased lordosis of the lumbar spine |
| *Separation* (gapping) between joint surfaces | An articular facet surface tends to move away from its partner facet. Joint separation is usually caused by a *distraction* force. | Therapeutic traction |
| *Sliding* (gliding) between joint surfaces | An articular facet translates in a linear or curvilinear direction within the plane of the joint. Sliding between joint surfaces is caused by a force directed tangential to the joint surfaces. Sliding between joint surfaces is resisted by a *shear* force. | Flexion-extension of the mid to lower cervical spine |

### Spinal Coupling

Movement of the vertebral column in one plane is usually associated with an automatic and, at times, nearly imperceptible movement in another plane. This kinematic phenomenon is called *spinal coupling*. Although many coupling patterns are described, the most consistent pattern involves an association between axial rotation and lateral flexion.

The mechanical reason for spinal coupling varies between regions, and it often is not clear. Explanations include muscle action, articular facet alignment, and geometry of the physiologic curve itself.[18] The latter explanation may be demonstrated by using a flexible rod as a model of the spine. Bend the rod about 30 to 40 degrees in one plane to mimic the natural lordosis or kyphosis of a particular region. While maintaining this curve, "laterally flex" the rod and note a slight automatic axial rotation. The biplanar bend placed on a flexible rod apparently creates unequal strains that are dissipated as torsion. This demonstration does not explain all coupling patterns observed clinically throughout the vertebral column, however.

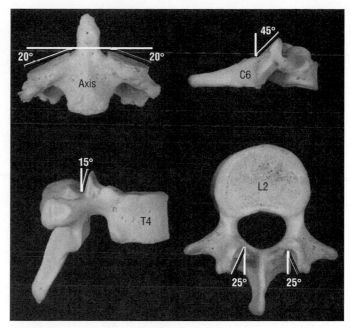

**FIGURE 9–34.** Typical spatial orientations for selected superior articular facet surfaces of cervical, thoracic, and lumbar vertebrae. The red line indicates the plane of the superior articular facet, measured against a vertical or horizontal reference line.

## STRUCTURE AND FUNCTION OF THE APOPHYSEAL AND INTERBODY JOINTS

### Apophyseal Joints

The vertebral column contains twenty-four pairs of apophyseal joints. Each apophyseal joint is formed by the articulation between opposing facet surfaces (see Fig. 9–15). Mechanically, apophyseal joints are classified as *plane joints*. Although exceptions and natural variations are common, the articular surfaces of most apophyseal joints are essentially flat. Slightly curved joint surfaces are present primarily in the upper cervical and throughout the lumbar regions.

The word *apophysis* means bony "outgrowth," illustrating the protruding nature of the articular processes. Acting as mechanical barricades, the articular processes permit certain movements and block others. The orientation of the plane of the facet surfaces within each joint influences the kinematics at different regions of the vertebral column. As a general rule, *horizontal facet surfaces favor axial rotation,* whereas *vertical facet surfaces* (in either sagittal or frontal planes) *block axial rotation*. Most apophyseal joint surfaces, however, are oriented somewhere between the horizontal and vertical. Figure 9–34 shows the typical joint orientation for articular facets in the cervical, thoracic, and lumbar regions. The plane of the facet surfaces explains, in part, why axial rotation is far greater in the cervical region than in the lumbar region. Additional factors that influence the predominant motion at each spinal region include the sizes of the intervertebral discs, shapes of the vertebrae, local muscle actions, and attachments of the ribs or ligaments.

### Interbody Joints

The interbody joint is formed by the connections between intervertebral discs, vertebral endplates, and adjacent vertebral bodies. Anatomically, this joint complex is classified as an *amphiarthrosis*.

### Structural Considerations of the Lumbar Intervertebral Disc

Most of what is known about the intervertebral disc is based on data from the lumbar region. This region-specific interest reflects the greater incidence of disc herniation (rupture). Discs in other spinal regions possess slightly different structural characteristics.[67]

#### Nucleus Pulposus and Annulus Fibrosus

The intervertebral disc consists of a central nucleus pulposus surrounded by an annulus fibrosus (Fig. 9–35). The *nucleus pulposus* is a pulplike gel located in the mid-to-posterior part of the disc. Consisting of 70 to 90% water, the nucleus functions as a modified hydraulic shock absorber that dissipates and transfers loads between consecutive vertebrae. The nucleus pulposus is thickened by relatively large branching proteoglycans. Each proteoglycan is an aggregate of many water-binding glycosaminoglycans linked to core proteins.[12] The nucleus also contains type II collagen fibers, elastic fibers, and other noncollagenous proteins. In the very young, the nucleus pulposus contains a few chondrocytes that are remnants of the primitive notochord.[110] The *annulus fibrosus* in the lumbar discs consists of 10 to 20 concentric layers, or rings, of collagen fibers. Like dough surrounding jelly in a doughnut, the collagen rings encase and physically entrap the liquid-based central nucleus. Compression force increases the hydrostatic pressure within the entrapped and water-logged nucleus pulposus. The increase

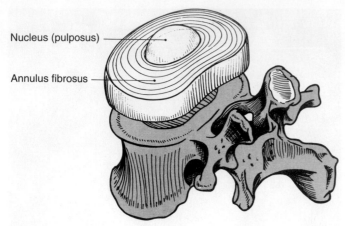

Nucleus (pulposus)

Annulus fibrosus

**FIGURE 9–35.** The intervertebral disc is shown lifted away from the underlying vertebral endplate. (Modified from Kapandji IA: The Physiology of Joints, vol. 3. New York, Churchill Livingstone, 1974.)

in pressure absorbs shock across the interbody joint. The annulus fibrosus contains material similar to that found in the nucleus pulposus, differing only in proportion. In the annulus, collagen makes up about 50 to 60% of the dry weight, as compared with only 15 to 20% in the nucleus pulposus.[12]

The intervertebral discs add considerable stability to the vertebral column, as well as being shock absorbers. The stabilizing function of the disc is due primarily to the structural configuration of the collagen fibers within the annulus fibrosus. As shown in Figure 9–36, the fibers are oriented in a precise geometric pattern. In the lumbar region, collagen rings lie about 65 degrees from the vertical, with fibers of adjacent layers traveling in opposite directions.[12,61] This structural arrangement resists distraction (vertical separation), shear (sliding), and torsion (twisting).[12] If the imbedded collagen fibers ran nearly vertical, the disc would resist distrac-

tion forces, but not sliding or torsion. In contrast, if all fibers ran parallel to the top of the vertebral body, the disc would resist shear and torsion, but not distraction forces. The 65-degree angle likely represents a geometric compromise that allows tensile resistance against the usual movements at the lumbar spine. Distraction forces are an inherent component of flexion, extension, and lateral flexion, occurring as one vertebral body tips slightly and, therefore, separates relative to its neighbor. Shear and torsion forces are produced during virtually all movements of the vertebral column. Because of the alternating pattern of layering of the annulus, only the collagen fibers oriented in the direction of the slide or twist become taut. Fibers in every other layer slacken.

### Vertebral Endplates

The *vertebral endplates* are thin caps of hyaline and fibrocartilage located on the superior and inferior surfaces of each vertebral body. The collagen fibers within the annulus fibrosus blend with the endplates of two consecutive vertebrae (Fig. 9–37). The anatomic bond between the endplates and annulus forms the primary adhesion between the vertebrae. The vertebral endplates, being semipermeable, also allow nutrients to pass from blood vessels in the vertebral body to deeper regions of the disc.

#### *Intervertebral Disc as a Hydrostatic Shock Absorber*

The vertebral column is the primary support structure for the trunk and neck. Although highly dependent on the position of the spine, approximately 80% of the load across two lumbar vertebrae is carried through the interbody joint. The remaining 20% is carried by posterior structures, such as apophyseal joints and laminae.[4]

The intervertebral discs are uniquely designed as shock absorbers, protecting the bone from the compression forces produced by body weight and muscle contraction. Compression forces push the endplates inward and toward the nucleus pulposus (Fig. 9–38). Being filled mostly with water and therefore essentially incompressible, the nucleus responds by deforming radially and outwardly against the annulus fibrosus (Fig. 9–38A). Radial deformation is resisted by the tension created within the stretched rings of collagen and elastic fibers. Internal resistance reinforces the walls of the annulus fibrosus (Fig. 9–38B). As a result, back pressure

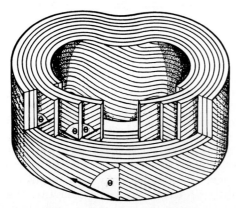

**FIGURE 9–36.** The detailed organization of the annulus fibrosus shown with the nucleus pulposus removed. Collagen fibers are arranged in multiple concentric layers, with fibers in every other layer running in identical directions. The orientation of each collagen fiber (depicted as $\theta$) is about 65 degrees from the vertical. (From Bogduk N: Clinical Anatomy of the Lumbar Spine, 3rd ed. New York, Churchill Livingstone, 1997.)

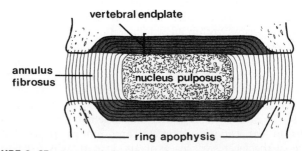

vertebral endplate

annulus fibrosus

nucleus pulposus

ring apophysis

**FIGURE 9–37.** A vertical slice through the interbody joint shows the structure of the vertebral endplates. The inner two thirds of the annulus fibrosus blends with the endplate, forming its fibrocartilaginous component. The outer one third of the annulus fibrosus blends directly with bone (i.e., ring apophysis). (From Bogduk N: Clinical Anatomy of the Lumbar Spine, 3rd ed. New York, Churchill Livingstone, 1997.)

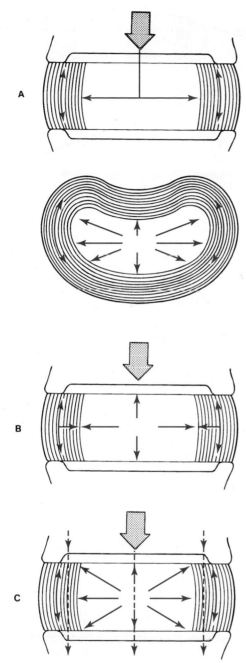

**FIGURE 9–38.** The mechanism of force transmission through an intervertebral disc. *A,* Compression force from body weight and muscle contraction (*large arrow*) raises the hydrostatic pressure in the nucleus pulposus. In turn, the increased pressure elevates the tension in the annular fibrosus (*small arrows*). *B,* The increased tension in the annulus inhibits radial expansion of the nucleus. The rising nuclear pressure is also exerted upward and downward against the endplates. *C,* The pressure within the nucleus reinforces the peripheral annulus fibrosus, converting it into a stable weight-bearing structure. The pressure is ultimately transmitted across the endplates to the next vertebra. (From Bogduk N: Clinical Anatomy of the Lumbar Spine, 3rd ed. New York, Churchill Livingstone, 1997.)

is created against the nucleus pulposus and endplates, reinforcing the entire disc and passing the load to the next vertebra (Fig. 9–38C). When compressive force is removed from the endplates, the stretched elastic and collagen fibers

return to their original preload length and prepare for another cycle of shock absorption. According to White and Panjabi,[106] two pioneers in the study of the biomechanics of the spine, the disc provides little resistance to small compressive loads, but more resistance to large ones. The disc thereby allows flexibility at low loads and provides stability at high loads.[106]

The shock absorption mechanism protects the disc in two ways (see Fig. 9–38). First, compressive forces are diverted from the nucleus, toward the annulus, and back to the nucleus and endplates. Such diversion takes time, thereby reducing the rate of loading, although not necessarily the magnitude. Second, the mechanism allows compressive forces to be shared by multiple structures, thereby limiting pressure on any single tissue.

### In Vivo Pressure Measurements from the Nucleus Pulposus

In vivo pressure measurements taken from the nucleus pulposus in the lumbar region have generally confirmed that resting in a supine position produces relatively low disc pressure.[8,9,71,72,74,108] Larger discal pressures occur from activities that combine forward bending and the need for vigorous trunk muscle contraction. These measurements have helped to increase the understanding of ways to reduce injury to the disc. Data produced by two separate studies are compared in Figure 9–39.[71,108] Both studies reinforce three points: (1) disc pressures are large when one holds a load in front of the body, especially when bending forward; (2) lifting a load with knees flexed places less pressure on the lumbar disc than does lifting a load with the knees straight, which uses more vigorous back muscle activity; and (3) sitting in a forward slouched position produces greater discal pressures than sitting erect. These points serve as the theoretical basis for many educational programs designed to prevent lumbar disc herniation.

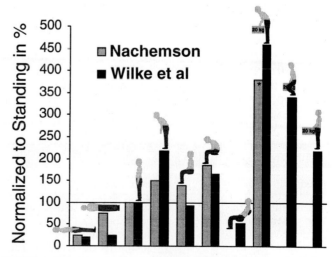

**FIGURE 9–39.** A comparison between data from two intradiscal pressure studies (see text). Each study measured in vivo pressures from a lumbar nucleus pulposus in a 70-kg subject during common postures and activities. The pressures are normalized to standing. (Modified from Wilke H-J, Neef P, Caimi M, et al: New in vivo measurements of pressures in the intervertebral disc in daily life. Spine 24:755–762, 1999.)

**Water Content within the Intervertebral Disc: Influence of Diurnal and Age-Related Changes in Overall Height**

When a healthy spine is unloaded, such as during bed rest, the pressure within the nucleus pulposus is relatively low.[71] The low pressure, combined with the hydrophilic nature of the disc, attracts water into the annulus fibrosus and nucleus pulposus. As a result, the disc swells slightly when one is sleeping. While awake and upright, however, weight bearing through the vertebral column forces water out of the disc. The cycle of swelling and contracting of the disc produces an average 1.1% daily variation in overall height.[100] One is actually taller in the morning. About 56% of the total loss in height during the day is recovered after only 2 hours of bed rest.[53]

The structure of the intervertebral disc changes with age.[99] An older disc has less proteoglycan content and, therefore, less ability to attract and retain water. The water content of the nucleus pulposus at birth is 88%, but decreases to 65 to 72% by the age of 75 years. The aged disc contains more collagen and less elastin, rendering it more fibrous and less resilient. A drier, less elastic nucleus pulposus is less able to cushion the vertebral body against excessive compression forces. As a consequence, the vertebral bodies and endplates may experience microfracture and bony reabsorption, ultimately leading to progressive and permanent age-related loss in height. The amount of loss in height is greater in persons with severe osteoporosis of the vertebral column and those with osteoporotic fractures, leading to an exaggerated kyphosis known as "widow's hump."

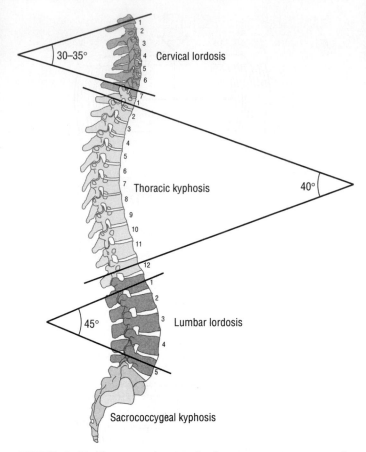

**FIGURE 9–40.** The normal sagittal plane curvatures across the regions of the vertebral column. The curvatures represent the normal resting postures of the region.

## REGIONAL KINEMATICS OF THE SPINE

This section provides both the range and predominant direction of movements at the various regions of the vertebral column. The zero or reference point used to describe the motion is the resting posture of the region while standing (Fig. 9–40).[38,52] The ranges of motion cited in this chapter

may vary from data presented in other sources. The variability reflects the differences in measurement techniques and the flexibility of the subjects. As elsewhere in the body, range of motion varies based on gender, underlying disease, activity level, and age.

The connective tissues that surround the vertebral column limit the extremes of motion (Table 9–8). By restricting motion, connective tissues—including those within muscle—help protect the delicate spinal cord and maintain optimal posture. In cases of trauma or overuse, biologic tissues

**TABLE 9–8. Connective Tissues That May Limit Motions of the Vertebral Column**

| Flexion | Extension | Axial Rotation | Lateral Flexion |
|---|---|---|---|
| Ligamentum nuchae | Cervical viscera (esophagus and trachea) | Annulus fibrosus | Intertransverse ligaments |
| Interspinous and supraspinous ligaments | Anterior annulus fibrosus | Capsule of the apophyseal joints | Contralateral annulus fibrosus |
| Ligamentum flava | Anterior longitudinal ligament | Alar ligaments | Capsule of the apophyseal joints |
| Capsule of the apophyseal joints | | | |
| Posterior annulus fibrosus | | | |
| Posterior longitudinal ligament | | | |

The list does not include limitations of motion caused by stretched muscles or by compression force created within the apophyseal and interbody joints.

### Measuring Motion of the Vertebral Column: An Overview

Motion of the vertebral column has been measured manually and radiographically and through the use of external tracking systems. Manual in vivo measurements use simple noninvasive tools, such as goniometers, inclinometers, and flexible rulers. Although these tools are simple and inexpensive, they lack high precision for measuring motion across various regions of the vertebral column. Invasive in vivo techniques are utilized to measure the rotation of pins implanted directly into the vertebral column. Although more precise, this form of measurement has its obvious practical limitations.

Perhaps the most precise in vivo kinematic measurements of the vertebral column use radiography. Planar x-rays of several individual sequences of a movement can be reconstructed with the use of a computer to measure rotation and translation of the vertebral column. Biplanar radiography has the advantage of recording movements in three dimensions. The main drawbacks of these techniques are the exposure of subjects to low doses of radiation and the time and cost of the procedure.

More complicated kinematic measurements involve computer-based external tracking systems that record and digitize movement. The relative or absolute position of targets placed on or near the trunk is recorded by specialized cameras. A more sophisticated tool has a computerized electromagnetic tracking system that can record movement in 6 degrees of freedom (three translational and three rotational). Electromagnetic fields emitted by a fixed external source are detected by remote sensors attached to the body. A computer program then calculates the near real-time position and orientation of the sensors relative to the source.

discussion begins with an overview of the functional anatomy followed by a discussion of the kinematics, organized by plane of movement.

The craniocervical region is the most mobile area within the entire vertebral column. Highly specialized joints facilitate positioning of the head, involving vision, hearing, smell, and equilibrium. As in the multiple links of the shoulder complex, the individual joints within the craniocervical region interact in a highly coordinated manner. Table 9–10 summarizes the average range of motions contributed by each region of the craniocervical region.[14,31,34,77,78,83,106]

## FUNCTIONAL ANATOMY OF THE JOINTS WITHIN THE CRANIOCERVICAL REGION

### Atlanto-occipital Joints

The atlanto-occipital joints provide independent movement of the cranium relative to the atlas. The joints are formed by the protruding convex condyles of the occipital bone fitting into the reciprocally concave superior articular facets of the atlas (Fig. 9–41). The congruent convex-concave relationship provides inherent structural stability to the articulation.

Intra-articular fat pads are commonly found between the joint capsule and the margins of the articular cartilage.[66] Anteriorly, the capsule of each atlanto-occipital joint blends with the *anterior atlanto-occipital membrane* and the anterior longitudinal ligament (Fig. 9–42). Posteriorly, the capsule is covered by a thin, broad *posterior atlanto-occipital membrane* (Fig. 9–43). As depicted on the right side of Figure 9–43,

may generate excessive tension as a means to protect an injured vertebral segment. Spasm in local muscles following acceleration-deceleration ("whiplash") injury of the neck is a common expression of this protective guarding. In cases of disease, such as severe rheumatoid arthritis, limited spinal mobility has no protective function, but is instead an intrinsic part of the pathologic process. Understanding the specific role of connective tissues in limiting motion is useful in devising therapeutic activities for persons with spinal-related pain or dysfunction.

## Craniocervical Region

The terms "craniocervical region" and "neck" are used interchangeably. Both terms refer to the combined set of three articulations: *atlanto-occipital joint, atlanto-axial joint complex,* and *intracervical apophyseal joints* (C2–7). The overall organization used to present the regional anatomy and kinematics of the craniocervical region is outlined in Table 9–9. The

**TABLE 9–9. Organization of the Joint Anatomy and Regional Kinematics at the Craniocervical Region**

| |
|---|
| **Functional Anatomy of the Joints within the Craniocervical Region** |
| Atlanto-occipital joints<br>Atlanto-axial joint complex<br>Intracervical apophyseal joints (C2-7) |
| **Sagittal Plane Kinematics at the Craniocervical Region** |
| Osteokinematics of flexion and extension<br>Arthrokinematics of flexion and extension<br>  Atlanto-occipital joint<br>  Atlanto-axial joint complex<br>  Intracervical apophyseal joints (C2-7)<br>Osteokinematics of protraction and retraction |
| **Horizontal Plane Kinematics at the Craniocervical Region** |
| Osteokinematics of axial rotation<br>Arthrokinematics of axial rotation<br>  Atlanto-axial joint complex<br>  Intracervical articulations (C2-7) |
| **Frontal Plane Kinematics at the Craniocervical Region** |
| Osteokinematics of lateral flexion<br>Arthrokinematics of lateral flexion<br>  Atlanto-occipital joint<br>  Intracervical articulations (C2-7) |

**TABLE 9–10.** Approximate Range of Motion for the Three Planes of Movement for the Joints of the Craniocervical Region

| Joint or Region | Flexion and Extension (Sagittal Plane, Degrees) | Axial Rotation (Horizontal Plane, Degrees) | Lateral Flexion (Frontal Plane, Degrees) |
|---|---|---|---|
| Atlanto-occipital joint | Flexion: 5<br>Extension: 10<br>Total: 15 | Negligible | About 5 |
| Atlanto-axial joint complex | Flexion: 5<br>Extension: 10<br>Total: 15 | 40–45 | Negligible |
| Intracervical region (C2-7) | Flexion: 35<br>Extension: 70<br>Total: 105 | 45 | 35 |
| Total across craniocervical region | Flexion: 45–50<br>Extension: 85<br>Total: 130–135 | 90 | About 40 |

The horizontal and frontal plane motions are to one side only. Data are compiled from multiple sources (see text) and subject to large intersubject variations.

the vertebral artery pierces the posterior atlanto-occipital membrane to enter the foramen magnum. This artery supplies blood to the brain. The concave-convex structure of the atlanto-occipital joints permits angular rotation in two degrees of freedom. The primary motions are flexion and extension. Lateral flexion is slight. Axial rotation is severely restricted and not considered as a degree of freedom.

### Atlanto-axial Joint Complex

The atlanto-axial joint complex consists of two joint structures: a median joint and a pair of laterally positioned apophyseal joints. The *median joint* is formed by the dens of C2 projecting through a ring created by the transverse ligament and the anterior arch of the atlas (Fig. 9–44). The joint complex has two synovial cavities. The smaller anterior cavity consists of a synovial membrane that surrounds the articulation between the anterior side of the dens and the posterior border of the anterior arch of the atlas. A small anterior facet on the anterior side of the dens marks this articulation (see Fig. 9–23A). The much larger posterior cavity has a synovial membrane that separates the posterior side of the dens and a cartilage-lined section of the *transverse*

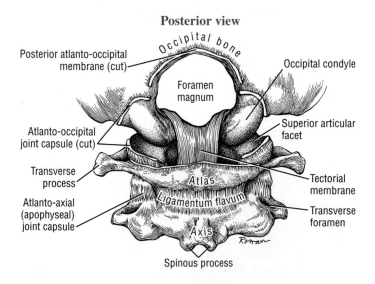

**Posterior view**

FIGURE 9–41. A posterior view of exposed atlanto-occipital joints. The cranium is rotated forward to expose the articular surfaces of the joints. Note the tectorial membrane as it crosses between the atlas and the cranium.

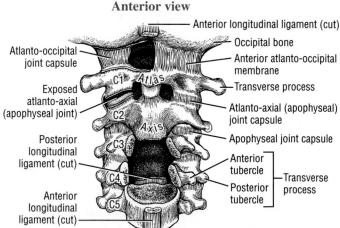

**Anterior view**

FIGURE 9–42. An anterior view illustrates the connective tissues associated with the atlanto-occipital joint and the atlanto-axial joint complex. The right side of the atlanto-occipital membrane is removed to show the capsule of the atlanto-occipital joint. The capsule of the right atlanto-axial (apophyseal) joint is also removed to expose its articular surfaces. The spinal cord and the bodies of C3 and C4 are removed to show the orientation of the posterior longitudinal ligament.

**Posterior view**

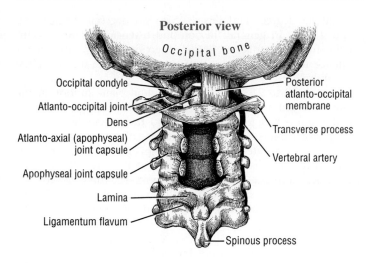

**FIGURE 9–43.** A posterior view illustrates the connective tissues associated with the atlanto-occipital joint and atlanto-axial joint complex. The left side of the posterior atlanto-occipital membrane and the underlying capsule of the atlanto-occipital joint are removed. The laminae and spinous processes of C2 and C3, the spinal cord, and the posterior longitudinal ligament and tectorial membrane are also removed to expose the posterior sides of the vertebral bodies and the dens.

*ligament of the atlas.* Because the dens acts as a vertical axis, the atlanto-axial joint is often described as a pivot joint.

The two *apophyseal joints* of the atlanto-axial joint are formed by articulation of the inferior articular facets of the atlas with the superior facets of the axis (see Fig. 9–42). The surfaces of these apophyseal joints are nearly flat and oriented close to the horizontal plane, a design that maximizes the freedom of axial rotation.

The atlanto-axial joint complex allows two degrees of freedom. About half the total horizontal plane (axial) rotation within the craniocervical region occurs at the atlanto-axial joint complex. The second degree of freedom is flexion and extension. Lateral flexion is very limited and not considered a degree of freedom.

### Tectorial Membrane and the Alar Ligaments

A review of the functional anatomy of the atlanto-axial joint complex must include a description of the tectorial membrane and the alar ligaments, connective tissues that help connect the axis with the cranium. As discussed, the transverse ligament of the atlas makes firm contact with the posterior side of the dens (see Fig. 9–44). Just posterior to the transverse ligament is a broad, firm sheet of connective tissue called the *tectorial membrane.* As a continuation of the posterior longitudinal ligament, the tectorial membrane attaches to the basilar part of the occipital bone, just anterior to the rim of the foramen magnum (see Fig. 9–41). The tectorial membrane strengthens the attachment between the cranium and the cervical column by limiting the extremes of flexion and extension.

The *alar ligaments* are tough fibrous cords that pass obliquely upward and laterally from the apex of the dens to the medial sides of the occipital condyles (Fig. 9–45). Clinically referred to as "check ligaments," the alar ligaments limit axial rotation of the head and atlas relative to the axis.[79] Evident by their position, the alar ligaments also limit lateral flexion.

### Intracervical Apophyseal Joints (C2–7)

The facet surfaces within apophyseal joints of C2–7 are orientated like shingles on a 45-degree sloped roof, approximately halfway between the frontal and horizontal planes (see Fig. 9–21, C2–3 articulation). This orientation provides great freedom of movement in all three planes, a hallmark of cervical arthrology.

## SAGITTAL PLANE KINEMATICS AT THE CRANIOCERVICAL REGION

### Osteokinematics of Flexion and Extension

Although highly variable, about 130 to 135 degrees of flexion and extension occur at the craniocervical region. The neutral resting posture of the craniocervical region is about 30 to 35 degrees of extension (see Fig. 9–40). From the extended position, the craniocervical region extends an addi-

**Superior view**

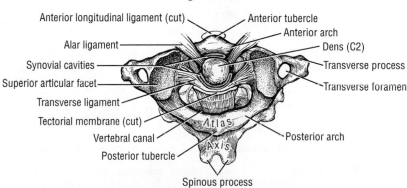

**FIGURE 9–44.** A superior view of the dens and its structural relationship to the median atlanto-axial joint. The spinal cord is removed and the tectorial membrane is cut. Synovial membranes are in red.

**Posterior view**

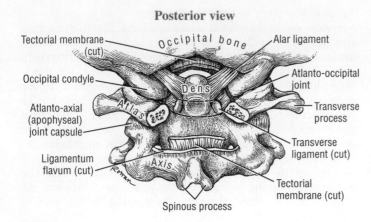

**FIGURE 9–45.** A posterior view of the atlanto-axial joint complex. The posterior arch of the atlas, tectorial membrane, and transverse ligament of the atlas are cut to expose the posterior side of the dens and the alar ligaments. The dashed lines indicate the removed segment of the transverse ligament of the atlas.

tional 85 degrees and flexes 45 to 50 degrees (Figs. 9–46 and 9–47). In general, flexion and extension occur sequentially from a cranial to caudal direction.[43] An abnormal sequence in this movement pattern may indicate intervertebral instability.

About 20 to 25% of the total sagittal plane motion at the craniocervical region occurs over the atlanto-occipital joint and atlanto-axial joint complex, and the remainder over the apophyseal joints of C2–7.[78] The axis of rotation for flexion and extension extends approximately in a medial-lateral direction through each of the three joint regions: the occipital condyles at the atlanto-occipital joint, the dens at the atlanto-axial joint complex, and the bodies of C2–C7.[23] The extremes of flexion and extension are limited primarily by tension in tissues located either posteriorly or anteriorly to the various axes of rotation (see Table 9–8). Flexion is also limited by the compression forces from the anterior margin of the annulus fibrosus, whereas extension is limited by the compression forces from the posterior margin of annulus fibrosus.

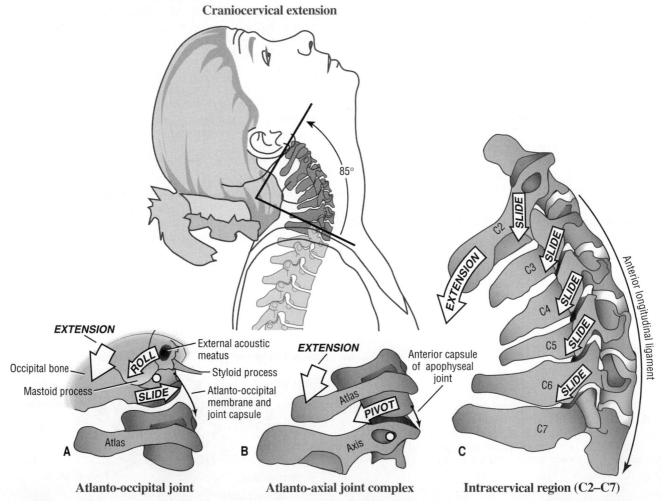

**Craniocervical extension**

**FIGURE 9–46.** Kinematics of craniocervical extension. *A,* Atlanto-occipital joint. *B,* Atlanto-axial joint complex. *C,* Intracervical region (C2-7). Elongated and taut tissues are indicated by thin black arrows.

**Craniocervical flexion**

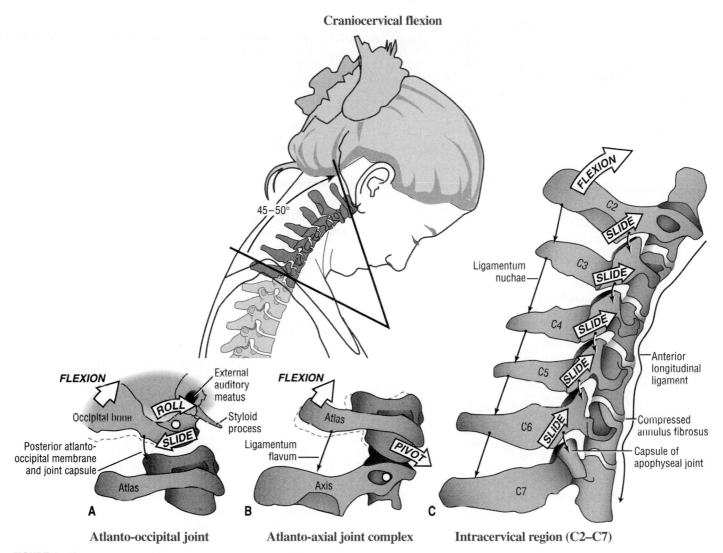

**FIGURE 9–47.** Kinematics of craniocervical flexion. *A,* Atlanto-occipital joint. *B,* Atlanto-axial joint complex. *C,* Intracervical region (C2–7). Note in *C* that flexion slackens the anterior longitudinal ligament and increases the space between the adjacent laminae and spinous processes. Elongated and taut tissues are indicated by thin black arrows; slackened tissue is indicated by a wavy black arrow.

The volume of the cervical vertebral canal is greatest in full flexion and least in full extension.[11] For this reason, a person with stenosis (narrowing) of the vertebral canal may be more prone to spinal cord injury during hyperextension activities. Repeated episodes of hyperextension-related injuries may lead to cervical myelopathy (from the Greek root *myelo,* denoting spinal cord, and *pathos,* suffering) and related neurologic deficits.

### Arthrokinematics of Flexion and Extension

#### Atlanto-occipital Joint
Like the rockers on a rocking chair, the convex occipital condyles *roll* backward in extension and forward in flexion within the concave superior articular facets of the atlas. Based on traditional convex-on-concave arthrokinematics, the condyles simultaneously *slide* slightly in the direction opposite to the roll (Fig. 9–46A and Fig. 9–47A). Tension in the tectorial membrane, articular capsules, and atlanto-occipital membranes limits the extent of the roll of the condyles.

#### Atlanto-axial Joint Complex
Although the primary motion at the atlanto-axial joint complex is axial rotation, the joint structure does allow about 15 degrees of flexion and extension. As a spacer between the cranium and axis, the ring-shaped atlas pivots forward during flexion and backward during extension (Fig. 9–46B and Fig. 9–47B). The extent of the pivot motion is limited in part by the dens that contacts the median joint of the atlanto-axial articulation.

#### Intracervical Articulations (C2–7)
Flexion and extension throughout the C2–7 occur about an arc of motion that follows the oblique plane set by the articular facets of the apophyseal joints. During *extension,* which is initiated at the lower cervical spine (C4–7), the inferior articular facets of superior vertebrae slide inferiorly and posteriorly, relative to the superior articular facets of the inferior vertebrae (Fig. 9–46C). These movements produce approximately 70 degrees of extension. Full extension is

considered the close-packed position at the cervical apophyseal joints, as well as the other regions throughout the vertebral column. This position results in maximal joint contact and load-bearing. The inferior sliding of the articular facets of superior vertebrae tends to slacken the joint capsule. The close-packed position of most synovial joints increases the tension in the surrounding capsule and associated ligaments. The apophyseal joints are one of the few exceptions to this general rule.

*Flexion* is also initiated at the lower cervical spine (C4–7).[14] The movements are the reverse of those described for extension. The inferior articular facets of the superior vertebrae slide superiorly and anteriorly, relative to the superior articular facets of the inferior vertebrae. As depicted in Figure 9–47C, the sliding between the articular facets produces approximately 35 degrees of flexion. Flexion stretches the capsule of the apophyseal joints and reduces the area for joint contact.

Overall, approximately 105 degrees of cervical flexion and extension occur as a result of the sliding between apophyseal joint surfaces. This extensive range of motion is due in part to the relatively long and unobstructed arc of motion provided by the oblique plane of the facet surfaces. On average, about 20 degrees of sagittal plane motion occur at each intervertebral junction between C2–3 and C6–7. This is a considerably greater angular motion than at the adjacent upper thoracic region. The largest angular displacement tends to occur between C5 and C6,[44] possibly accounting for the relatively high incidence of spondylosis[68] and hyperflexion-related fractures at this level (Fig. 9–48).

### Osteokinematics of Protraction and Retraction

In addition to flexion and extension in the craniocervical region, the head can also translate forward (protraction) and backward (retraction) within the sagittal plane.[78] *Protraction* of the head flexes the lower-to-mid cervical spine and extends the upper craniocervical region (Fig. 9–50A). *Retraction* of the head, in contrast, extends or straightens the lower-to-mid cervical spine and flexes the upper craniocervical region (Fig. 9–50B). In both movements, the lower-to-mid cervical spine follows the translation of the head. Although protraction and retraction of the head are physiologically normal useful motions, they may be associated with faulty posture. Prolonged periods of protraction may lead to a chronic forward head posture, causing increased strain on the craniocervical extensor muscles.

## HORIZONTAL PLANE KINEMATICS AT THE CRANIOCERVICAL REGION

### Osteokinematics of Axial Rotation

Axial rotation of the head and neck is a very important function, intimately related to vision and hearing. As shown in Figure 9–51, the craniocervical region rotates about 90 degrees to each side, for a total range of nearly 180 degrees. With an additional 150 to 160 degrees of total horizontal plane movement of the eyes, the visual field approaches 360 degrees, with little or no movement of the trunk! This wide visual field depends, of course, on factors such as range of motion and sight.

About half the axial rotation of the craniocervical region occurs at the atlanto-axial joint complex, with the remaining throughout C2–7.[106] Rotation at the atlanto-occipital joint is restricted due to the deep-seated placement of the occipital condyles within the superior articular facets of the atlas.

### Arthrokinematics of Axial Rotation

#### Atlanto-axial Joint Complex

The atlanto-axial joint complex is designed for maximal rotation within the horizontal plane. The design is most evident by the structure of the axis (C2), with its vertical dens and nearly horizontal superior articular facets (see Fig. 9–34). The ring-shaped atlas "twists" about the dens, producing about 40 to 45 degrees of axial rotation in each direction (Fig. 9–51A). The flat to slightly concave inferior articular facets of the atlas slide in a circular path across the broad "shoulders" of the superior articular facets of the axis. These surfaces have also been described as slightly convex when considering the thickness of the articular cartilage. Because of the limited axial rotation permitted at the atlanto-occipital joint, the cranium follows the rotation of the atlas, essentially degree for degree. The axis of rotation for the head and atlas is through the vertically projected dens. Horizontal plane rotation of the atlas is coupled with slight lateral flexion to the opposite side.[79]

Tension in the alar ligaments increases with rotation at the atlanto-axial joint complex, especially in the ligament located opposite to the direction of the rotation.[79] Tension in the alar ligaments and capsules of the lateral apophyseal joints, plus the many muscles about the neck, limit axial rotation.

#### Intracervical Articulations (C2–7)

Rotation throughout C2–7 is guided primarily by the spatial orientation of the facet surfaces within the apophyseal joints.

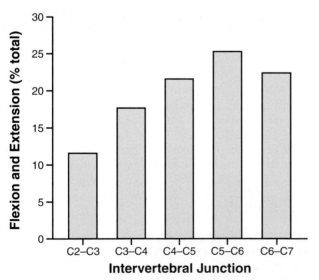

**FIGURE 9–48.** In vitro cervical flexion and extension motions averaged over ten specimens. Data are expressed as a percent of the total range of sagittal plane motion in the cervical region. (Data from Holmes A, Han ZH, Dang GT, et al: Changes in cervical canal spinal volume during in vitro flexion-extension. Spine 21:1313–1319, 1996.)

**SPECIAL FOCUS 9 – 7**

### Flexion and Extension and Its Effect on the Diameter of the Intervertebral Foramen

Flexion increases the diameter of a cervical intervertebral foramen; extension, in contrast, decreases it.[113] The mechanics of this relationship are shown for flexion at C3-4 in Figure 9–49*A* and *B*. As shown in Figure 9–49*B*, an upward and forward slide of the inferior articular facet of C3 significantly increases the diameter of the C3-4 intervertebral foramen. Flexion, therefore, allows greater room for passage of a spinal nerve. This principle has clinical relevance in cases of stenosed (narrowed) intervertebral foramen due to osteophyte formation. A large osteophyte compressing against a nerve root causes radiculopathy. Symptoms include radiating pain down the ipsilateral arm, usually the path of the cervical dermatome. Patients with this problem often describe shooting pain down the arm. This is in conjunction with craniocervical hyperextension and/or lateral flexion toward the side of the stenosis. This movement is common in men while shaving under the chin. Cervical traction performed with the neck partially flexed widens the stenosed intervertebral foramen. Therapeutic traction can decompress an irritated spinal nerve root and often reduces painful symptoms.

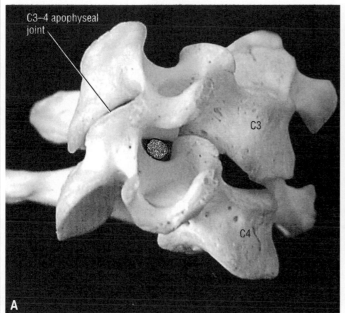

**Neutral position**

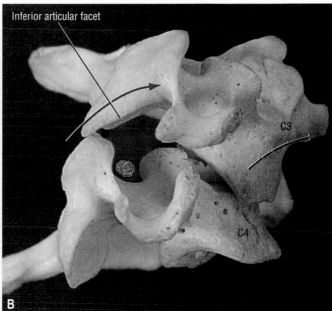

**Fully flexed**

**FIGURE 9–49.** How flexion between C3 and C4 affects the size of the intervertebral foramen is shown. *A*, In the neutral position, the facet surfaces within the apophyseal joint are in maximal contact. The size of the intervertebral foramen relative to the circumference of the exiting nerve is indicated in red. *B*, Full flexion reduces the contact area within the apophyseal joint; however, it increases the opening for passage of the nerve.

The facet surfaces are oriented about 45 degrees between the horizontal and frontal planes (see Fig. 9–34). The inferior facets slide posteriorly and somewhat inferiorly on the same side as the rotation, and anteriorly and somewhat superiorly on the side opposite the rotation (Fig. 9–51*B*). Approximately 45 degrees of axial rotation occur to each side over the C2–7 region, nearly equal to that permitted at the atlanto-axial joint complex. Rotation is greatest in the more cranial vertebral segments.

## FRONTAL PLANE KINEMATICS AT THE CRANIOCERVICAL REGION

### Osteokinematics of Lateral Flexion

Approximately 40 degrees of lateral flexion is available to each side throughout the craniocervical region (Fig. 9–52). The extremes of this movement can be demonstrated by attempting to touch the ear to the tip of the shoulder. Most of this movement occurs at the C2–7 region; however,

**Protraction**                                    **Retraction**

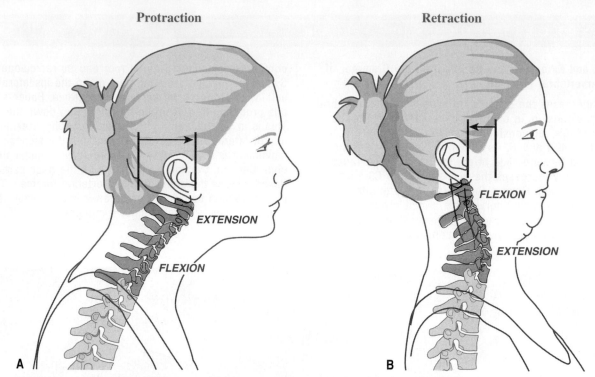

**FIGURE 9–50.** Protraction and retraction of the cranium. *A,* During protraction of the cranium, the lower-to-mid cervical spine flexes as the upper craniocervical region extends. *B,* During retraction of the cranium, in contrast, the lower-to-mid cervical spine extends as the upper craniocervical region flexes. Note the change in distance between the C1–2 spinous processes during the two movements.

about 5 degrees may occur at the atlanto-occipital joint. Lateral flexion at the atlanto-axial joint complex is negligible.

### Arthrokinematics of Lateral Flexion

#### Atlanto-occipital Joint
A small amount of side-to-side rolling of the occipital condyles occurs over the superior articular facets of the atlas. It is likely that at the extremes of lateral flexion there is a slight unilateral joint approximation on the side of the lateral flexion, and a slight joint separation on the side opposite the lateral flexion (Fig. 9–52A).

#### Intracervical Articulations (C2–7)
The arthrokinematics of lateral flexion at the C2–C7 vertebral segments are illustrated in Figure 9–52B. The inferior articular facets on the side of the lateral flexion slide inferiorly and slightly posteriorly, and the inferior articular facets on the side opposite the lateral flexion slide superiorly and slightly anteriorly.

The approximate 45-degree inclination of the articular facets of C2–7 dictates a mechanical coupling between movements in the frontal and horizontal planes. Because an upper vertebra follows the plane of the articular facet of a lower vertebra, a component of lateral flexion and axial rotation must occur simultaneously. For this reason, lateral flexion and axial rotation in the mid-and-low cervical region are mechanically coupled in an *ipsilateral fashion;* for example, lateral flexion to the right occurs with slight axial rotation to the right, and vice versa. The overall expression of the cou-

pling, however, can be altered by muscular action at the atlanto-occipital joint.

## Thoracic Region

The thorax consists of a relatively rigid rib cage, formed by the ribs, thoracic vertebrae, and sternum. The rigidity of the region provides three functions: (1) a stable base for muscles to control the craniocervical region, (2) protection for the intrathoracic organs, and (3) mechanical bellows for breathing (see Chapter 11).

### FUNCTIONAL ANATOMY OF THORACIC ARTICULAR STRUCTURES

The thoracic spine has 24 apophyseal joints, 12 on each side. Each joint consists of a pair of articular facets that are generally in the frontal plane, with a mild slope that varies between 0 and 30 degrees from the vertical (see Fig. 9–34). Although the apophyseal joints provide the primary mechanism for thoracic mobility, their potential for movement is restricted by the adjacent costovertebral and costotransverse joints. These joints mechanically tie most of the thoracic region anteriorly to the sternum. The costovertebral and costotransverse joints function during ventilation, a topic discussed in Chapter 11.

Most *costovertebral joints* connect the head of a rib with a pair of costal facets and the adjacent margin of an intervening intervertebral disc (Fig. 9–53A and B). The articular

**Craniocervical axial rotation**

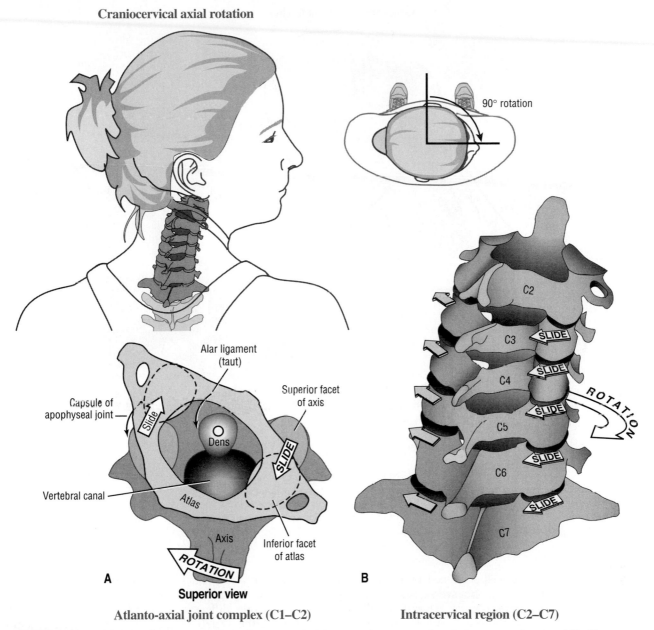

**FIGURE 9–51.** Kinematics of craniocervical axial rotation. *A,* Atlanto-axial joint complex. *B,* Intracervical region (C2–7).

surfaces of the costovertebral joints are slightly ovoid,[110] held together primarily by *capsular and radiate ligaments.*

*Costotransverse joints* connect the articular tubercle of a typical rib to the costal facet on the transverse process of a corresponding thoracic vertebra. An *articular capsule* surrounds this synovial joint (Fig. 9–53A and B). The extensive (nearly 2 cm long) *costotransverse ligament* firmly anchors the neck of a rib to the entire length of a corresponding transverse process. In addition, each costotransverse joint is stabilized by a *superior costotransverse ligament.* This strong ligament attaches between the superior margin of the neck of one rib and the inferior margin of the transverse process of the vertebra located above (Fig. 9–53A). Ribs 11 and 12 usually lack costotransverse joints.

---

**Key Anatomic Aspects of the Costovertebral and Costotransverse Joints**

*Each Costovertebral Joint*
- connects the head of a typical rib with a pair of costal facets and the adjacent margin of an intervening intervertebral disc.
- is stabilized by radiate and capsular ligaments.

*Each Costotransverse Joint*
- connects the articular tubercle of a typical rib to the costal facet on the transverse process of a corresponding thoracic vertebra.
- is stabilized by a capsular (costotransverse) ligament and the superior costotransverse ligament.

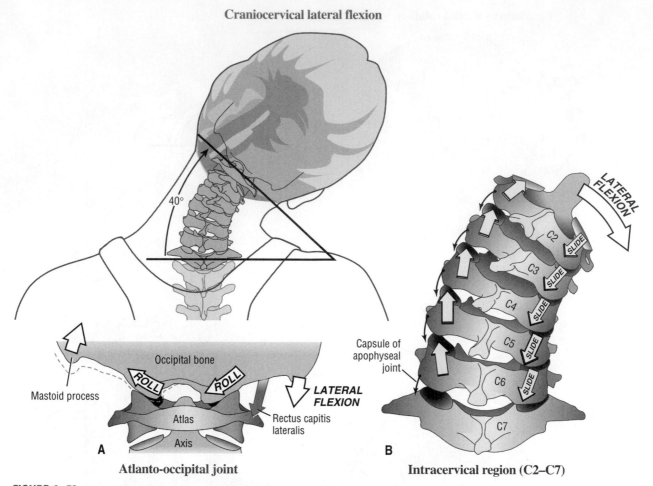

**FIGURE 9-52.** Kinematics of craniocervical lateral flexion. *A*, Atlanto-occipital joint. The primary function of the rectus capitis lateralis is to laterally flex this joint. Note the slight compression and distraction of the joint surfaces. *B*, Intracervical region (C2–7). Note the ipsilateral coupling pattern between axial rotation and lateral flexion (see text for further details). Elongated and taut tissue is indicated by thin black arrows.

The thoracic vertebrae are well stabilized by the ribs and associated costovertebral and costotransverse joints. Stability protects the spinal cord from trauma. During a fall, for example, the impact to the thoracic spine is partially absorbed and dissipated by the ribs and the associated muscles and connective tissues.

## KINEMATICS AT THE THORACIC REGION

### *Kinematics of Flexion and Extension*

Although the range of motion at each thoracic intervertebral junction is relatively small, cumulative motion is considerable over the entire thoracic spine (Table 9–11). Approximately 30 to 40 degrees of *flexion* and 20 to 25 degrees of *extension* are available throughout the thoracic region. These kinematics are shown in context with flexion and extension over the entire thoracolumbar region in Figures 9–54 and 9–55. The extremes of extension are limited owing to the potential impingement between adjacent downward-sloping spinous processes, especially of the midthoracic vertebrae. In general, the magnitude of flexion and extension increases in a cranial-to-caudal direction.

The arthrokinematics at the apophyseal joints in the thoracic spine are generally similar to those described for the C2–7. Subtle differences are related primarily to different shapes of the vertebrae and different spatial orientations of the articular facets. Flexion between T5–6, for example,

**TABLE 9-11. Approximate Range of Motion for the Three Planes of Movement for the Thoracic Region**

| Flexion and Extension (Sagittal Plane, Degrees) | Axial Rotation (Horizontal Plane, Degrees) | Lateral Flexion (Frontal Plane, Degrees) |
|---|---|---|
| Flexion: 30–40 Extension: 20–25 Total: 50–70 | 30 | 25 |

Horizontal and frontal plane motions are to one side only. Data are based on estimates by unpublished x-ray observations and goniometry.

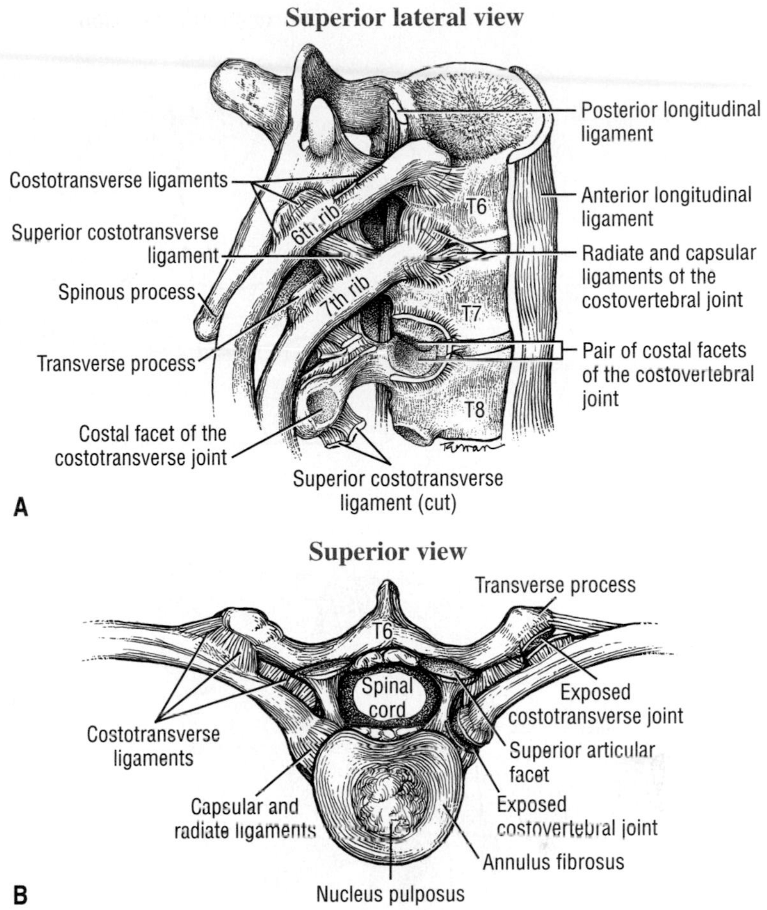

**Superior lateral view**

**Superior view**

**FIGURE 9–53.** The costotransverse and costovertebral joints of the midthoracic region. *A,* Superior-lateral view highlights the structure and connective tissues of the costotransverse and costovertebral joints associated with the sixth through the eighth thoracic vertebrae. The eighth rib is removed to expose the costal facets of the associated costovertebral and costotransverse joints. *B,* Superior view shows the capsule of the left costovertebral and costotransverse joints cut to expose joint surfaces. Note the spatial relationships between the nucleus pulposus, annulus fibrosus, and spinal cord.

occurs by a superior and slightly anterior sliding of the inferior facet surfaces of T5 on the superior facet surfaces of T6 (Fig. 9–54A). Extension occurs by a reverse process (Fig. 9–55A).

### Kinematics of Axial Rotation

Approximately 30 degrees of horizontal plane (axial) rotation occurs to each side throughout the thoracic region. This motion is depicted in conjunction with axial rotation across the entire thoracolumbar region in Figure 9–56. Rotation between T6 and T7, for instance, occurs as the near frontal plane–aligned inferior articular facets of T6 slide for a short distance against the similarly aligned superior articular facets of T7 (Fig. 9–56A). In general, the freedom of axial rotation decreases in the thoracic spine in a cranial-to-caudal direction. In the mid to lower thoracic spine, the greater vertically oriented apophyseal joints tend to block horizontal plane motion.

### Kinematics of Lateral Flexion

The predominant frontal plane orientation of the thoracic facet surfaces suggests a relative freedom of lateral flexion. This potential for movement is never fully expressed, however, because of the stabilization provided by the attachments to the ribs. Lateral flexion in the thoracic region is illustrated in context with lateral flexion over the entire thoracolumbar region in Figure 9–57. Approximately 25 degrees

of lateral flexion occurs to each side in the thoracic region. The magnitude of this intervertebral motion remains relatively constant throughout the entire thoracic region. As depicted in Figure 9–57A, lateral flexion of T6 on T7 occurs as the inferior facet surface of T6 slides superiorly on the side contralateral to the lateral flexion and inferiorly on the side ipsilateral to the lateral flexion. Note that the ribs drop slightly on the side of the lateral flexion, and rise slightly on the side opposite the lateral flexion.

As in the cervical spine, lateral flexion and axial rotation are mechanically coupled in an ipsilateral manner.[107] Coupling is most evident in the upper thoracic spine where the articular facets possess a closer orientation to those in the lower cervical region. The influence of the coupling decreases and is inconsistent in the middle and lower thoracic regions.

## STRUCTURAL DEFORMITIES OF THE THORACIC SPINE

Maintaining the spine in normal alignment throughout life requires a delicate balance between intrinsic forces, governed by muscles and osseous-ligamentous structures, and extrinsic forces governed by gravity. When the balance fails, deformity occurs. Herniated discs and nerve root impingements are relatively uncommon in the thoracic spine. This finding may be due, in part, to the relatively low intervertebral mobility and high stability provided by the rib cage. Thoracic

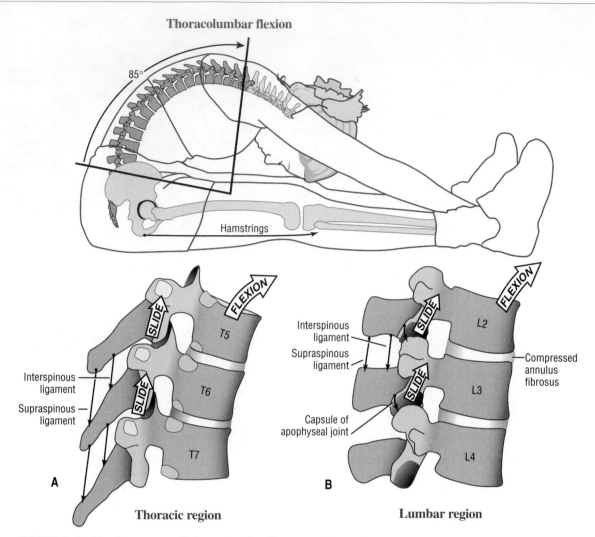

**FIGURE 9–54.** The kinematics of thoracolumbar flexion is shown through an 85-degree arc: the sum of 35 degrees of thoracic flexion and 50 degrees of lumbar flexion. *A*, Kinematics at the thoracic region. *B*, Kinematics at the lumbar region. Elongated and taut tissues are indicated by thin black arrows.

postural abnormalities, however, occur relatively frequently. The thoracic spine, constituting about half the entire length of the vertebral column, is particularly vulnerable to the effects of gravity and torsion. The two most common examples of postural abnormalities of the thoracic spine are excessive kyphosis and scoliosis. The following sections review the biomechanics of these conditions. More detailed information on the biomechanics, medical management, and physical therapy can be found in other sources (see references 25, 32, and 36).

### Excessive Kyphosis

On average, about 42 degrees of natural kyphosis is present while standing (see Fig. 9–40).[52] In some persons, however, excessive kyphosis occurs and can cause functional limitations. The acquired form of excessive kyphosis may occur as a consequence of trauma and related spinal instability, disease, or connective tissue changes that may be associated with age. In general, age-related thoracic kyphosis is usually slight and not debilitating.

The two most common conditions associated with kyphosis are Scheuermann disease and osteoporosis. *Scheuermann disease,* or "juvenile kyphosis," is a hereditary condition that starts in adolescence. Although the cause of the disease is unknown, it is characterized by wedging of the anterior side of the vertebral bodies, ultimately causing and perpetuating excessive kyphosis. Up to 10% of the adolescent population shows signs of this disorder.[111]

*Osteoporosis* of the spine is often associated with excessive thoracic kyphosis, most often observed in the elderly. Compression fractures in osteoporotic thoracic vertebrae eventually lead to reduced height in the vertebral bodies. Shortening of the midthoracic vertebrae can initiate a biomechanical cycle that accelerates the flexion deformity. Figure 9–58 demonstrates one mechanical scenario associated with the progression of a severe kyphosis.[76] In the ideal spinal posture, the line-of-force due to body weight falls slightly to the concave side of the apex of the normal cervical and thoracic curvatures (Fig. 9–58A). Gravity acts with an external moment arm that can maintain the normal thoracic and cervical

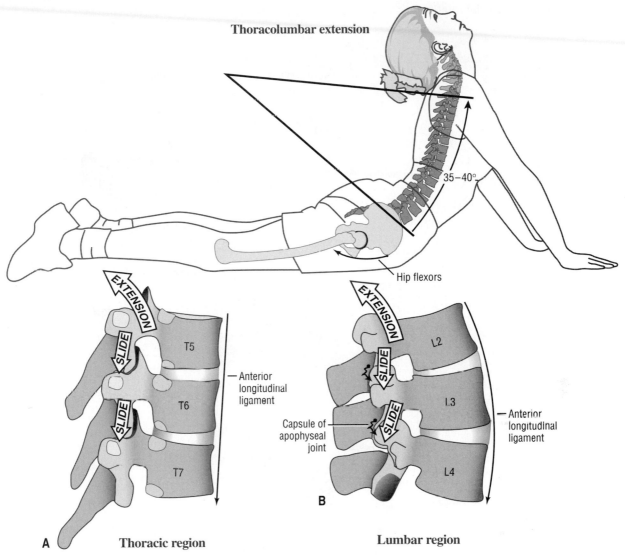

**Thoracolumbar extension**

35–40°

Hip flexors

EXTENSION

SLIDE

SLIDE

T5

T6

T7

— Anterior
longitudinal
ligament

**A**   **Thoracic region**

EXTENSION

SLIDE

SLIDE

L2

L3

L4

Capsule of
apophyseal
joint

— Anterior
longitudinal
ligament

**B**

**Lumbar region**

**FIGURE 9–55.** The kinematics of thoracolumbar extension is shown through an arc of 35 to 40 degrees: the sum of 20 to 25 degrees of thoracic extension and 15 degrees of lumbar extension. *A,* Kinematics at the thoracic region. *B,* Kinematics at the lumbar region. Elongated and taut tissue is indicated by thin black arrows; slackened tissue is indicated by a wavy black line.

curvatures. Assume that the posture shown in Figure 9–58A creates a small cervical extension torque and small thoracic flexion torque. In the thoracic spine, the natural kyphosis is limited by compression forces on the anterior side of the interbody joints. Vertebrae weakened from osteoporosis and dehydrated intervertebral discs may be unable to resist the anterior compression forces. Over time, the compression forces reduce the height of the anterior side of the interbody joint, thereby accentuating the kyphosis (Fig. 9–58B). At this point, a pathologic deforming process is initiated. The increased flexed posture shifts the line-of-force due to body-weight farther anteriorly, thus increasing the length of the external moment arm (EMA′) and magnitude of the flexed kyphotic posture. As a result, both thoracic and cervical spine regions may be subjected to a moderate flexion torque

(see Fig. 9–58B). Increased extensor muscle and ligamentous force is needed to hold the trunk, neck, and head upright. The increased force passes through the interbody joints, possibly creating small compression fractures in the vertebral bodies. At this point the vicious circle is well established.

The thoracic posture shown in Figure 9–58B may progress, in extreme cases, to that shown in Figure 9–58C. While standing, the line-of-force due to body weight has produced a small upper cervical extension torque and a large thoracic flexion torque. Note that despite the large thoracic kyphosis, the person can extend her upper craniocervical region enough to maintain a horizontal visual gaze. The main point of Figure 9–58C, however, is to appreciate the biomechanical and physiologic impact that a large external

**Thoracolumbar axial rotation**

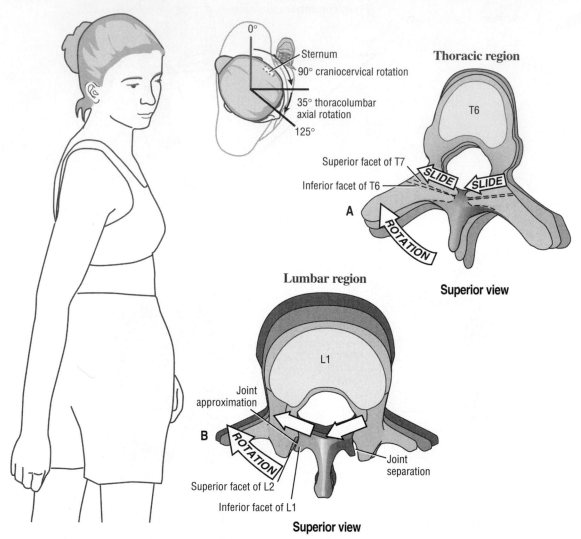

**FIGURE 9–56.** The kinematics of thoracolumbar axial rotation is depicted as the subject rotates her face 125 degrees to the right. The thoracolumbar axial rotation is shown through a 35-degree arc: the sum of 30 degrees of thoracic rotation and 5 degrees of lumbar rotation. *A,* Kinematics at the thoracic region. *B,* Kinematics at the lumbar region.

flexion torque can have in predisposing a person to an exaggerated thoracic kyphosis. Compression fractures from osteoporosis further accelerate the kyphotic process.

### Scoliosis

Scoliosis (from the Greek, meaning curvature) is a deformity of the vertebral column characterized by abnormal curvatures in all three planes, most notably in the frontal and horizontal (Fig. 9–59). The deformity most often involves the thoracic spine; however, other regions of the spine are often affected. Scoliosis is typically defined as either functional or structural. *Functional scoliosis* can be corrected by an active shift in posture, whereas *structural scoliosis* is a fixed deformity that cannot be corrected fully by an active shift in posture.

Approximately 80 to 90% of all cases of structural scoliosis are termed *idiopathic,* meaning the condition has no ap-

parent biologic or mechanical cause.[106] Idiopathic scoliosis most commonly affects adolescent girls. Most of the remaining 10 to 20% of cases are caused by neuromuscular or musculoskeletal conditions or by congenital abnormalities. In these cases, the imbalanced forces that produce the scoliosis are due most frequently to poliomyelitis, muscular dystrophy, spinal cord injury, trauma, or cerebral palsy.[25]

Typically, scoliosis is described by the location, direction, and number of fixed frontal plane curvatures (lateral bends) within the vertebral column. The most common pattern of scoliosis consists of a single lateral curve, with an apex in the T7–9 region.[19] Many other patterns involve a secondary or compensatory curve, most often in the lumbar spine. The direction of the primary lateral curve is defined by the side of the convexity of the lateral deformity. Because the thoracic vertebrae are most often involved with scoliosis, asymmetry of the rib cage is often present. The ribs on the side

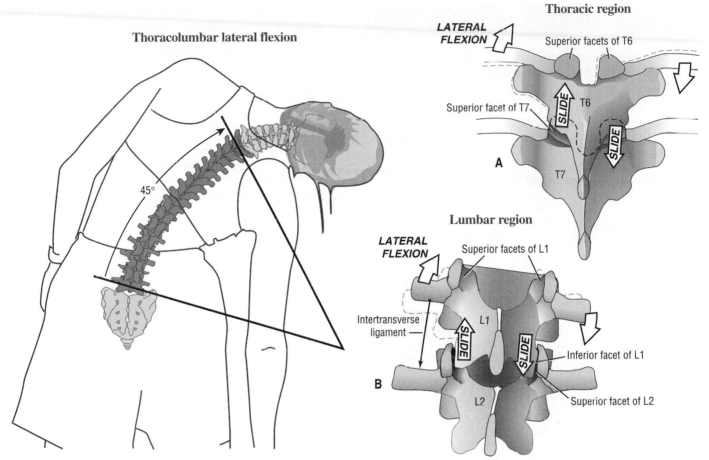

**Thoracolumbar lateral flexion**

**Thoracic region**

**Lumbar region**

**FIGURE 9–57.** The kinematics of thoracolumbar lateral flexion is shown through an approximate 45-degree arc: the sum of 25 degrees of thoracic lateral flexion and 20 degrees of lumbar lateral flexion. *A,* Kinematics at the thoracic region. *B,* Kinematics at the lumbar region. Note the slight contralateral coupling pattern between axial rotation and lateral flexion in the lumbar region. Elongated and taut tissue is indicated by a thin black arrow.

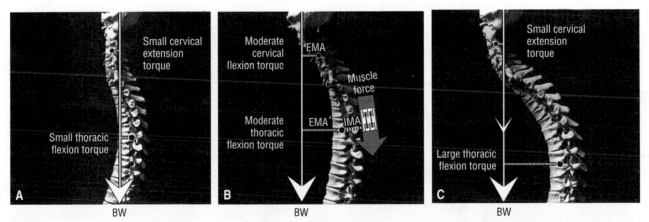

**FIGURE 9–58.** Lateral views show the biomechanical relationships between the line-of-force due to body weight (BW) and varying degrees of thoracic kyphosis. In each of the three models, the axes of rotation are depicted as the midpoint of the thoracic and cervical regions (*dark circles*). The external moment arms used by body weight are shown as dashed lines. *A,* In a person with ideal standing posture and normal thoracic kyphosis, body weight created a small cervical extension torque and a small thoracic flexion torque. *B,* In a person with moderate thoracic kyphosis, body weight created a moderate cervical and thoracic flexion torque (EMA′, external moment arm at midthoracic spine; EMA, external moment arm at midcervical spine; IMA, internal moment arm for trunk extensor muscle force). *C,* In a person with severe thoracic kyphosis, body weight caused a small cervical extension torque and a large thoracic flexion torque. All three models are based on x-rays of patients. (From Neumann DA: Arthrokinesiologic considerations for the aged adult. In Guccione AA (ed): Geriatric Physical Therapy. Chicago, Mosby-Year Book, 2000.)

**Method for Estimating Interbody Joint Compression Force Caused by Moderate Thoracic Kyphosis**

The compression force exerted on a midthoracic interbody joint while standing is equal to the sum of the forces created by body weight, any lifted load, and muscle force. The amount of intervertebral compression force required to maintain the posture depicted in Figure 9–58*B* can be estimated by assuming a condition of static equilibrium: the product of body weight (BW) force and the external moment arm (EMA′) equals the product of the muscle force times the internal moment arm (IMA). Assuming that the EMA is about twice the length of the IMA, rotary equilibrium in the sagittal plane requires a muscle force of twice BW. Assume that a 180-lb (1 pound = 4.448 Newtons) person has about 60% of BW (108 lb) located above the midthoracic region. An extensor muscle force of approximately 216 lb (2 × 108 lb) is needed to hold the flexed posture. When considering the effect of BW, a total of about 324 lb of compression force (216 lb of muscle force plus 108 lb of BW) is exerted on a midthoracic interbody joint. Applying this same biomechanical solution to the ideal posture shown in Figure 9–58*A* yields a 67% reduction in interbody joint force. This reduction is based on the ideal posture having approximately equal external and internal moment arm lengths. Although this simple mathematical model is not absolutely accurate, it emphasizes how posture can have a profound effect on the forces produced across an interbody joint.

The deformity in structural scoliosis typically has a fixed contralateral spinal coupling pattern involving lateral flexion and axial rotation. The spinous processes of the involved vertebrae are typically rotated in the horizontal plane, toward the side of the concavity of the fixed thoracic curvature. This explains why the "rib hump" is typically on the convex side of the frontal plane curvature. The ribs are forced to follow the rotation of the thoracic vertebrae. The mechanism for the fixed coupling pattern is not completely understood.

## Lumbar Region

### FUNCTIONAL ANATOMY OF THE ARTICULAR STRUCTURES WITHIN THE LUMBAR REGION (L1–S1)

#### L1–L4 Region

The facet surfaces of lumbar apophyseal joints are oriented nearly vertical, with a moderate-to-strong sagittal plane bias. The orientation of the superior articular facet of L2, for example, is about 25 degrees from the sagittal plane (see Fig. 9–34). This orientation favors sagittal plane motion at the expense of axial rotation. This trend is evident even in the mid-to-lower thoracic regions.

The facet surfaces change their orientation rather abruptly at or near the thoracolumbar junction (Fig. 9–60). The sharp frontal-to-sagittal plane transition may help to explain the relatively high incidence of traumatic paraplegia at this junction. The thorax, held relatively rigid by the rib cage, is free to flex as a unit over the upper lumbar region. A large flexion torque delivered to the thorax may concentrate an excessive hyperflexion stress at the extreme upper lumbar region. If severe enough, the stress may fracture or dislocate the bony elements and possibly injure the caudal end of the spinal cord or the cauda equina. Surgical fixation devices implanted to immobilize an unstable thoracolumbar junction are particularly susceptible to stress failure compared with other regions of the vertebral column.

#### L5–S1 Junction

As any typical intervertebral junction, the L5–S1 junction has an interbody joint anteriorly and a pair of apophyseal

of the thoracic concavity are pulled together, and the ribs on the side of the convexity are spread apart. The degree of torsion, or horizontal plane deformity, can be measured on standard x-ray by noting the rotated position of the vertebral pedicles.

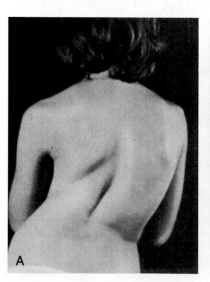

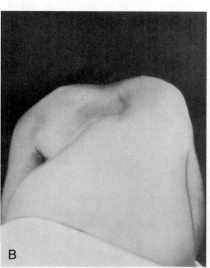

**FIGURE 9–59.** *A,* Posterior view shows excessive right thoracic and left lumbar curvatures in the frontal plane. *B,* Postural asymmetry is demonstrated in the horizontal plane. Note the abnormal rib "hump" on the right, and "hollow" on the left. (From Gartland JJ: Fundamentals of Orthopedics. Philadelphia, WB Saunders, 1979.)

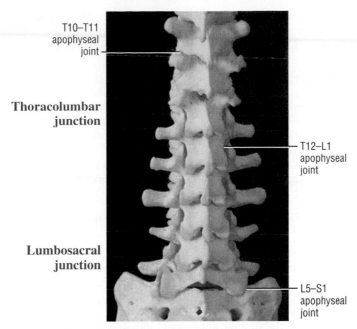

**FIGURE 9-60.** A posterior view of the thoracolumbar and lumbo-sacral junctions. Note the transition in the orientation of the facet surfaces within the apophyseal joints between the two junctions. The bony specimen demonstrates a frontal plane bias at both L4-L5 and L5-S1 apophyseal joints. This type of variation is common.

lateral aspect of the sacrum (see Fig. 9-74). As a bilateral pair, the iliolumbar ligaments provide a firm anchor between the lower lumbar vertebrae and the underlying ilium and sacrum.[112]

In addition to connective tissues, the wide, sturdy articular facets of the L5-S1 apophyseal joints provide bony stabilization to the L5-S1 junction. The near frontal plane inclination of the facet surfaces can resist part of the anterior shear at this region. This blockage creates a force within the apophyseal joint (see Fig. 9-61A, arrow labeled JF). With-

joints posteriorly. The facet surfaces of the L5-S1 apophyseal joints are usually oriented in a more frontal plane than those of other lumbar regions (Fig. 9-60).

The base (top) of the sacrum is naturally inclined anteriorly and inferiorly, forming an approximate 40-degree sacrohorizontal angle ($\alpha$) while standing (Fig. 9-61A).[52] Given this angle, the resultant force due to body weight (BW) creates an anterior shear (BW$_S$), and a compressive force (BW$_N$) acting normal (perpendicular) to the superior surface of the sacrum. The magnitude of the anterior shear is equal to the product of BW times the sine of the sacrohorizontal angle. A typical sacrohorizontal angle of 40 degrees produces an anterior shear force at the L5-S1 junction equal to 64% of superimposed BW. Increasing the degree of lumbar lordosis enlarges the sacrohorizontal angle. If the sacrohorizontal angle were increased to 55 degrees, for example, the anterior shear force would increase to 82% of superimposed BW. While standing or sitting, lumbar lordosis can be increased by this amount by anterior tilting of the pelvis (see Fig. 9-68A). (Tilting the pelvis is defined as a short-arc sagittal plane rotation of the pelvis relative to the head of the femurs. The direction of the tilt is indicated by the direction of rotation of the iliac crests of the pelvis.)

Several structures stabilize the anterior-posterior alignment of the L5-S1 junction, especially the anterior longitudinal ligament and the iliolumbar ligament. The anterior longitudinal ligament crosses anterior to the L5-S1 junction. The *iliolumbar ligament* arises from the inferior aspect of the transverse process of L5 and adjacent fibers of the quadratus lumborum muscle. The ligament attaches inferiorly to the ilium, just anterior to the sacroiliac joint, and to the upper-

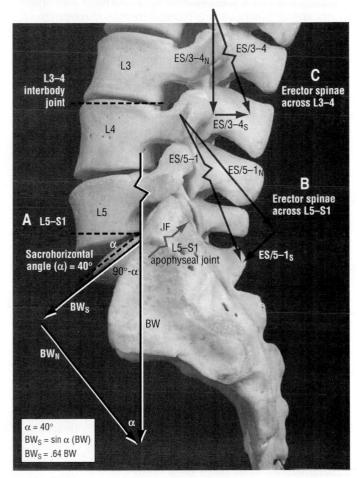

**FIGURE 9-61.** Lateral view shows the biomechanics responsible for the shear forces at the interbody joints of L5-S1 and the middle lumbar region (L3-4). The sacrohorizontal angle ($\alpha$) at L5-S1 is the angle between the horizontal plane and the superior surface of the sacrum (A). BW (body weight) is the weight of the body located above the sacrum. BW$_N$ is the normal force of body weight directed perpendicular to the superior surface of the sacrum. BW$_S$ is the shear force of body weight directed parallel to the superior surface of the sacrum. The joint force (JF) at the L5-S1 apophyseal joint is shown as a short gray arrow. The force vector of the active erector spinae is shown as it crosses L5-S1 (ES/5-1) (B). ES/5-1$_N$ is the normal force of the muscle directed perpendicular to the superior surface of the sacrum. ES/5-1$_S$ is the shear force of the muscle directed parallel to the superior surface of the sacrum. The force vector of the erector spinae is shown as it crosses L3-4 (ES/3-4) (C). ES/3-4$_N$ is the normal force of the muscle directed parallel to the superior surface of L4. ES/3-4$_S$ is the shear force of the muscle directed parallel to the superior surface of L4. See text for further details. (Created with the assistance of Guy Simoneau.)

### Anterior Spondylolisthesis at L5–S1

Anterior spondylolisthesis is a general term that describes an anterior slipping or displacement of one vertebra relative to another. This condition usually occurs at the L5–S1 junction. The term spondylolisthesis is derived from the Greek "spondylo" meaning vertebra, and "listhesis" meaning to slip. The amount of anterior slippage is often graded in severity between I and IV. Figure 9–62 shows a grade 2 spondylolisthesis. Associated with anterior spondylolisthesis is a bilateral fracture through the *pars articularis,* a section of a lumbar vertebra midway between the superior and inferior articular processes (see Fig. 9–31). Severe cases of anterior spondylolisthesis may damage the cauda equina, as this bundle of nerves passes through the L5–S1 junction.

As described for Figure 9–61*A,* increased lumbar lordosis widens the normal sacrohorizontal angle, thereby increasing the anterior shear force between L5 and S1. Exercises or other actions that create a forceful hyperextension of the lumbar spine are typically contraindicated in anterior spondylolisthesis. As shown in Figure 9–61*B,* the force vector of the erector spinae that crosses L5–S1 (ES/5-1) creates an anterior shear force (ES/5-1$_s$) parallel to the superior body of the sacrum. The direction of this shear is a function of the orientation of the adjacent erector spinae fibers and the 40-degree sacrohorizontal angle. In theory, a greater muscular force increases the anterior and inferior shear at the L5–S1 junction, especially if the muscle activation also exaggerates the regional lordosis.

The anterior-directed shear forces produced by the lumbar erector spinae occur primarily at the L5–S1 junction and not, as a rule, throughout the entire lumbar region. As indicated in Figure 9–61*C,* in normal posture, the superior surfaces of the bodies of the middle lumbar vertebrae are typically positioned in a more horizontal orientation. The erector spinae that cross these regions produce a posterior shear across the lumbar interbody joints (see Fig. 9–61*C,* ES/3–4$_S$).[63] This muscle-produced shear can offset much of the natural anterior force that occurs while lifting large loads in front of the body.

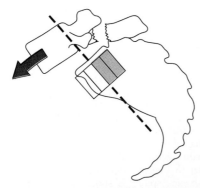

**FIGURE 9–62.** Grade 2 spondylolisthesis. (Modified from Magee DL: Orthopedic Physical Assessment, 3rd ed. Philadelphia, WB Saunders, 1997.)

out adequate stabilization, the lower end of the lumbar region can slip forward relative to the sacrum. This abnormal, potentially serious condition is known as spondylolisthesis.

## KINEMATICS AT THE LUMBAR REGION

Table 9–12 lists the average range of motion at the lumbar region. While standing, the lumbar region in the healthy adult typically exhibits about 40 to 45 degrees of lordosis.[52] Lumbar lordosis is greater in women than in men, with the greatest differences appearing after the fifth decade (Fig. 9–63).[7] Compared with standing, sitting reduces the lumbar lordosis by about 20 to 35 degrees.

### Sagittal Plane Kinematics at the Lumbar Region

Although data vary across studies and populations, about 50 degrees of flexion and 15 degrees of extension occur at the heathy lumbar spine.[80,82] This is a substantial range of motion considering it occurs across only five intervertebral junctions. This predominance of sagittal plane motion is largely due to the prevailing sagittal plane bias of the facet surfaces in the lumbar apophyseal joints. As a general principle, the amount of lumbar intervertebral flexion and extension gradually increases in a cranial-to-caudal direction. The following kinematic discussions include the lumbar kinematics and the strong kinematic relationships between the lumbar region, the trunk as a whole, and the lower extremities (Table 9–13).

#### Flexion of the Lumbar Region

Figure 9–54 shows the kinematics of flexion of the lumbar region in context with flexion of the trunk and hips. Pelvic-on-femoral (hip) flexion increases the passive tension in the stretched hamstring muscles. With the lower end of the vertebral column fixed by the sacroiliac joints, continued flexion of the middle and upper lumbar region reverses the natural lordosis in the low back.

During flexion between L2–3, for example, the inferior articular facets of L2 slide superiorly and anteriorly, relative to the superior facets of L3 (see Fig. 9–54*B*). As a consequence, muscular and gravitational forces are transferred *away* from the apophyseal joints, which generally support about 20% of the total spinal load in erect standing,[4] and toward the discs and posterior spinal ligaments. Discs are compressed while the posterior ligaments are tensed. In extreme flexion, the fully stretched articular capsule of the

| **TABLE 9–12. Approximate Range of Motion for the Three Planes of Movement for the Lumbar Region** | | |
|---|---|---|
| **Flexion and Extension (Sagittal Plane, Degrees)** | **Axial Rotation (Horizontal Plane, Degrees)** | **Lateral Flexion (Frontal Plane, Degrees)** |
| Flexion: 50 Extension: 15 Total: 65 | 5 | 20 |

Horizontal and frontal plane motions are to one side only. Data from Pearcy, et al, 1984; Pearcy and Tibrewal, 1984.

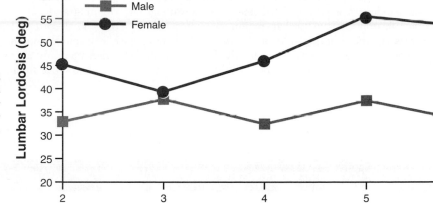

**FIGURE 9–63.** A plot shows the changes in lumbar lordosis with aging. (Data from Amonoo-Kuofi HS: Changes in the lumbo-sacral angle, sacral inclination and the curvature of the lumbar spine during aging. Acta Anat 145:373–377, 1992.)

apophyseal joints restrains additional forward migration of a superior vertebra.[96] The extreme flexed position significantly reduces the contact area within the facet surfaces of the apophyseal joints. Paradoxically, although a fully flexed lumbar spine reduces the total force on a given apophyseal joint, the pressure (force per unit area) increases on the decreased surface area under contact. High pressure may damage joints that have abnormally developed articular surfaces.

As a way of comparison, Figure 9–64 shows the relative resistance provided by local connective tissues to extreme flexion in the lumbar region.[4] Of clinical interest is the relatively large resistance provided by the stretched articular capsule that surrounds the flexed apophyseal joints. In the healthy lower back, the passive tension within the capsule of flexed apophyseal joints reduces the compression load on the intervertebral discs. A weakened or overstretched articular capsule, however, may not be able to generate sufficient tension to protect the discs from injury. The capsules of the

apophyseal joints may become overstretched from a chronic, slumped sitting posture.

### Lumbar Flexion: Its Effect on the Diameter of the Intervertebral Foramen and Migration of the Nucleus Pulposus

Relative to a neutral position, full flexion of the lumbar spine increases the diameter of the intervertebral foramina by 19% and increases the volume of the vertebral canal by 11%.[43] Therapeutically, flexion of the lumbar region is often used to temporarily reduce the pressure on a lumbar nerve root that is impinged by an obstructed foramen. In certain

| TABLE 9–13. Organization of the Discussion Sagittal Plane Kinematics at the Lumbar Region |
|---|
| **Flexion of the Lumbar Region** |
| Effect on the diameter of the intervertebral foramen and migration of the annulus pulposus |
| **Extension of the Lumbar Region** |
| Effect on the diameter of the intervertebral foramen and migration of the annulus pulposus |
| **Lumbopelvic Rhythm During Trunk Flexion and Extension** |
| **Effect of Pelvic Tilt on the Lumbar Spine** |
| Therapeutic and kinesiologic correlations between *anterior pelvic tilt* and *increased lumbar lordosis*<br>Therapeutic and kinesiologic correlations between *posterior pelvic tilt* and *decreased lumbar lordosis* |
| **Sitting Posture and Its Effect on Alignment of the Lumbar and Craniocervical Regions** |

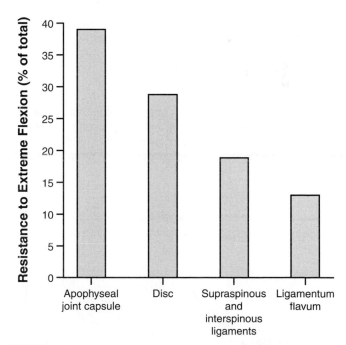

**FIGURE 9–64.** Results from cadaver experiments show the relative resistance provided by nonmuscular tissues against a flexion torque at the lumbar spine. Measurements were recorded at the extremes of lumbar flexion at the time of tissue failure. (Data from Adams MA, Hutton WC, Stott JRR: The resistance to flexion of the lumbar intervertebral joint. Spine 5:245–253, 1980.)

circumstances, however, this potential therapeutic advantage may be associated with a potential therapeutic disadvantage. For example, flexion of the lumbar region generates compression forces on the anterior side of the disc, which tend to migrate the nucleus pulposus posteriorly.[30] The magnitude of the migration is small in the healthy spine. In a person with a weakened posterior annulus, however, posterior migration of the nucleus pulposus increases pressure on the spinal cord or nerve roots. These contrasting therapeutic effects of flexion in the lumbar region are to be considered when planning an exercise program for a person with generalized low back pain.

## SPECIAL FOCUS 9–10

### Herniated Nucleus Pulposus

The formal name for a ruptured or slipped disc is *herniated nucleus pulposus.* Most herniations involve a significant posterior-lateral or posterior migration of the nucleus pulposus toward the spinal cord or spinal nerve roots (Table 9–14 and Fig. 9–65). *Nuclear protrusion,* the mildest form of herniation, may cause local back pain owing to pressure exerted against the posterior annulus and/or posterior longitudinal ligament. Herniations that result in *prolapse, extrusion, or sequestration,* however, can place pressure directly on neural elements. As a consequence, pain often radiates away from the back and toward the associated dermatomes in the lower extremities. Muscle weakness and altered deep tendon reflexes in the legs may also result from impingement on the neural tissues.

Although a herniated disc typically causes low-back pain, not everyone with low-back pain has disc involvement. Low-back pain may be caused by a number of factors besides, or in addition to, disc prolapse. Factors include muscle-ligament sprains, inflamed apophyseal or sacroiliac joints, and irritated or impinged nerve roots. Often the reason for pain is unknown, and occasionally the pain spontaneously subsides. Pain, in general, is a relatively common occurrence, even in otherwise healthy persons.

The percentage of persons with low-back pain due to a disc herniation is uncertain, but likely significant. The subject of disc herniation has generated extensive research on methods of diagnosis,[40] mechanisms of herniation,[69] associated epidemiology,[70,101] physical rehabilitation,[51] and efficacy of surgery.[85]

Two mechanisms are typically involved with disc herniation.[2,3] The first mechanism involves a very large, sudden compression force delivered over a lumbar spine that is flexed or, most likely, flexed and axially rotated (twisted).

#### TABLE 9–14. Types of Herniated Nucleus Pulposus

| Nuclear Type | Definition |
| --- | --- |
| Protrusion | Displaced nucleus pulposus remains within the annulus fibrosus, but may create a pressure bulge on the spinal cord. |
| Prolapse | Displaced nucleus pulposus reaches the posterior edge of the disc, but remains confined within the outer layers of the annulus fibrosus. |
| Extrusion | Annulus fibrosus ruptures, allowing the nucleus pulposus to completely escape from the disc into the epidural space. |
| Sequestration | Parts of the nucleus pulposus and fragments of annulus fibrosus become lodged within the epidural space. |

The types are presented in increasing magnitudes of severity.
From Magee DL: Orthopedic Physical Assessment, 3rd ed. Philadelphia, WB Saunders, 1997.

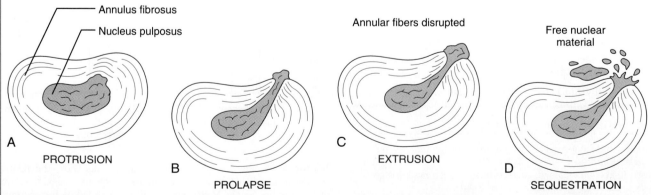

**FIGURE 9–65.** Types of disc herniations. (From Magee DL: Orthopedic Physical Assessment, 3rd ed. Philadelphia, WB Saunders, 1997.)

This mechanism of injury is often associated with a single event such as a fall or the lifting of a large load. The second mechanism involves a series of multiple, low magnitude compression forces, often imposed over a flexed lumbar spine. This mechanism of prolapse generally occurs gradually from cumulative microtrauma, such as that which may occur from many years of repetitive lifting or bending with an excessively flexed back.

A flexed and/or twisted lumbar spine renders the disc mechanically vulnerable to protrusion. A flexed spine stretches and thins the posterior side of the annulus as the nuclear gel is forced posteriorly, often under large hydrostatic pressure.[71] The amount of hydrostatic pressure increases with greater trunk muscle activation, usually in response to large external torques. With sufficiently high hydrostatic pressure, the nuclear gel creates or finds a

preexisting fissure in the posterior annulus. A partially rotated spine renders only half the posterior fibers of the annulus taut, thereby reducing the potential resistance that can be applied against approaching nuclear gel.

Despite the abundance of literature and anecdotal evidence, a single unifying cause-and-effect explanation for all forms of disc herniation is lacking. The four factors listed in the box, however, appear to be particularly important.[2] Disc prolapse can occur even in the absence of trauma or mechanical overload. A habitual, chronic sitting posture involving a rounded and flexed lumbar spine certainly may predispose a person to posterior migration of the nucleus pulposus. A chronically flexed lumbar posture may, in time, overstretch the posterior annulus to a point where it is unable to resist a potent hyperflexion-induced posterior migration of the nucleus. This explanation, however, is subject to scrutiny because the incidence of disc prolapse in the lumbar region is very low in cultures whose people habitually squat with near maximal flexed lumbar spines.[28]

The healthy lumbar disc with an intact annulus fibrosus is remarkably resistant to disc herniation, even from a large flexion force. The reason for the relatively high incidence of disc prolapse in Western cultures is still not fully understood. Several factors involving different and perhaps interrelated variables must be considered. These factors include mechanical overload, pathology, poor nutrition, age, lifestyle, earlier injury, work habits, socioeconomics, and genetics.

---

**Factors that Favor Disc Herniation in the Lumbar Spine**

1. Propensity for fissures or tears in the posterior annulus that allows a path for the flow of nuclear material
2. Sufficiently hydrated nucleus structurally capable of exerting high pressure
3. Inability of the posterior annulus to resist radial pressure from the nucleus
4. Axial loading applied over a bent (flexed) and twisted spine

---

### Extension of the Lumbar Region

Extension of the lumbar region is essentially the reverse of flexion (Fig. 9–55B), and it increases the natural lordosis. When lumbar extension is combined with full hip extension, passive tension in the stretched hip flexor muscles helps maintain lordosis by anteriorly tilting the pelvis. Extension between L2 and L3, for example, occurs as the inferior articular facets of L2 slide inferiorly and slightly posteriorly relative to the superior facets of the L3. Full extension increases both the amount of load and area of contact at the apophyseal joints.[57]

In the neutral standing posture, the healthy disc is the primary load-bearing structure in the lumbar region. As such, healthy discs reduce the load imposed on apophyseal joints and thereby protect them from excessive wear. In diseased or severely dehydrated discs, however, a greater proportion of the total load is shifted to the apophyseal joints. It is not uncommon, therefore, for a person with severe disc disease to develop osteoarthritis in the lumbar apophyseal joints.

#### Extension of the Lumbar Spine and Its Effect on the Diameter of the Intervertebral Foramen and Migration of the Nucleus Pulposus

Relative to the neutral position, full lumbar extension reduces the diameter of the intervertebral foramina by 11% and reduces the volume within the vertebral canal by 15%.[45] For this reason, clinicians often suggest that a person with nerve root impingement, from a stenosed intervertebral fora-

men, limit activities that involve hyperextension. Extension, however, tends to migrate the nucleus fibrosus anteriorly.[30] Persons with a nuclear protrusion or prolapse may find, therefore, that extension reduces the pain associated with pressure on the spinal cord or nerve roots. The normal lumbar lordotic posture may restrict the migration of the nucleus pulposus within a weakened disc from approaching the neural elements. It is uncertain whether the nucleus pulposus migrates in a similar manner in both healthy and degenerated discs.[10]

### Lumbopelvic Rhythm During Trunk Flexion and Extension

In conjunction with the hip joints, the lumbar region provides the major flexion and extension pivot point for the trunk, especially during activities such as forward bending, climbing, and lifting. The kinematic relationship between the lumbar spine and hip joints during sagittal plane movements is called *lumbopelvic rhythm*. An understanding of the normal lumbopelvic rhythm during flexion and extension of the trunk can help distinguish pathology affecting the spine and that affecting the hips.

#### Lumbopelvic Rhythm During Trunk Flexion

Consider the common action of bending forward and toward the ground while keeping the knees straight. This motion is measured as a combination of about 40 degrees of lumbar flexion and 70 degrees of hip (pelvic-on-femoral) flexion (Fig. 9–66A).[27] Although many strategies are possi-

**Three lumbopelvic rhythms used during trunk flexion**

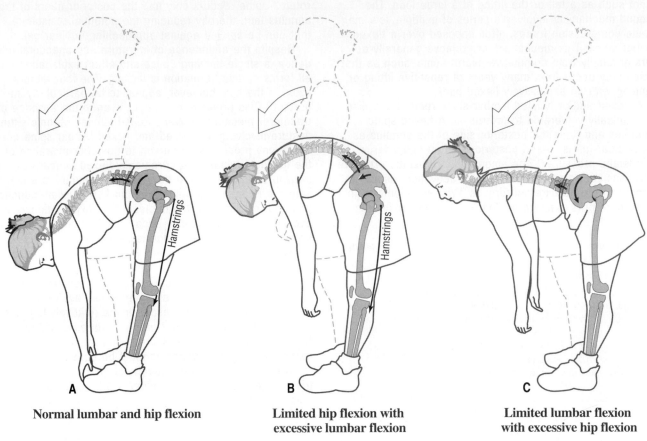

| A | B | C |
|---|---|---|
| **Normal lumbar and hip flexion** | **Limited hip flexion with excessive lumbar flexion** | **Limited lumbar flexion with excessive hip flexion** |

**FIGURE 9–66.** Three different lumbopelvic rhythms used to flex the trunk forward and toward the floor with knees held straight. *A,* Typical lumbopelvic rhythm consists of about 40 degrees of flexion of the lumbar spine and 70 degrees of flexion at the hips (pelvis on femurs). *B,* With limited flexion in the hips (for example, from tight hamstrings), greater flexion is required of the lumbar and lower thoracic spine. *C,* With limited lumbar mobility, greater flexion is required of the hip joints. Red arrows indicate limited or restricted mobility.

ble, the hips and lumbar spine typically flex simultaneously throughout the arc of trunk flexion, with motion usually initiated at the lumbar spine.[75] Figure 9–66*B* and *C* shows obvious abnormal lumbopelvic rhythms associated with marked restriction in mobility at the hip joints (*B*) or lumbar region (*C*). In both *B* and *C*, the amount of overall trunk flexion is reduced. If greater trunk flexion is required, the hip joints or lumbar region may mutually compensate for the other's limited mobility. This situation may increase the stress on the compensating region. As depicted in Figure 9–66*B*, with limited hip flexion due to restricted hamstring extensibility, for example, bending the trunk toward the floor requires greater flexion in the lumbar and lower thoracic spine. Eventually, exaggerated flexion may overstretch posterior connective tissues, such as the interspinous ligaments, posterior annular fibrosus, posterior longitudinal ligament, apophyseal joint capsule, and thoracolumbar fascia, or increase stress on the discs and apophyseal joints.

In contrast, as depicted in Figure 9–66*C*, limited mobility in the lumbar spine may require greater flexion of the hip joints. Greater forces may be required from the hip extensor muscles which, as a consequence, increase the compression

force at the hips. In persons with healthy hips, this relatively low-level increase in compression force is usually tolerated without cartilage degeneration or discomfort. In a person with a preexisting hip condition (e.g., osteoarthritis and gross joint asymmetry), however, the increased compression force may accelerate degenerative changes.

### Lumbopelvic Rhythm During Trunk Extension

The typical lumbopelvic rhythm used to extend the trunk from a forward bent position is depicted in a series of consecutive phases in Figure 9–67*A* to *C*. Extension of the trunk with knees extended is normally initiated by extension of the hips (Fig. 9–67*A*). This is followed by extension of the lumbar spine (Fig. 9–67*B* to *C*).[75] This normal lumbopelvic rhythm reduces the demands on the lumbar extensor muscles and underlying apophyseal joints and discs, thereby protecting the region against high stress. Delay in lumbar extension shifts the extensor torque demand to the powerful hip extensors (hamstrings and gluteus maximus), at the time when the external flexion torque on the lumbar region is greatest (external moment arm depicted as dark black line; see Fig. 9–67*A*). In this scenario, the demand on the lumbar extensor muscles increases only after the trunk is sufficiently

**Normal lumbopelvic rhythms used during trunk extension**

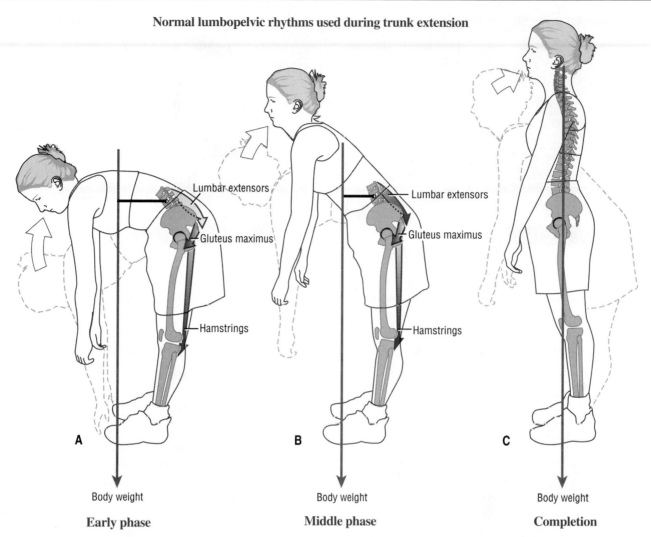

Body weight

**Early phase**                    **Middle phase**                    **Completion**

**FIGURE 9–67.** A typical lumbopelvic rhythm shown in three phases and used to extend the trunk from a forward bent position. The motion is arbitrarily divided into three chronologic phases (*A* to *C*). In each phase, the axis of rotation for the trunk extension is assumed to pierce the body of L3. *A*, In the *early phase*, trunk extension occurs to a greater extent through extension of the hips (pelvis on femurs), under strong activation of hip extensor muscles (gluteus maximus and hamstrings). *B*, In the *middle phase*, trunk extension occurs to a greater degree by extension of the lumbar spine. The middle phase requires increased activation from lumbar extensor muscles. *C*, At the *completion* of the event, muscle activity typically ceases once the line-of-force from body weight falls posterior to the hips. The external moment arm used by body weight is depicted as a solid black line. The greater intensity of red indicates relative greater intensity of muscle activation.

raised and the external moment arm, relative to body weight, is minimized (Fig. 9–67*B*). Persons with severe low-back pain may purposely delay active contraction of the lumbar extensor muscles until the trunk is nearly vertical. After standing completely upright, hip and back muscles are typically inactive, as long as the force vector due to body weight falls posterior to the hip joints (Fig. 9–67*C*).

*Effect of Pelvic Tilt on the Lumbar Spine*

Flexion and extension of the lumbar spine can occur by two fundamentally different movement strategies. The first strategy is typically used to maximally displace the upper trunk and upper extremities relative to the thighs, such as when lifting or reaching. As depicted in Figures 9–66 and 9–67, this strategy combines maximal flexion and extension of the lumbar spine with a wide arc of pelvic-on-femoral (hip) and

trunk motion. A second movement strategy involves a relatively short-arc tilt of the pelvis, with the trunk remaining nearly stationary. As depicted in Figure 9–68*A* to *D*, an anterior or a posterior pelvic tilt accentuates or reduces the lumbar lordosis. Measured while standing, an approximate one-to-one relationship exists between the change in pelvic tilt and the associated change in lumbar lordosis.[55] The change in lordosis alters the position of the nucleus pulposus within the disc and alters the diameter of the intervertebral foramina.

The axis of rotation for pelvic tilting is through both hip joints. This mechanical association strongly links the movement (pelvic-on-femoral) of the hip joints with that of the lumbar spine. This relationship is discussed further in the next section and again in Chapter 12.

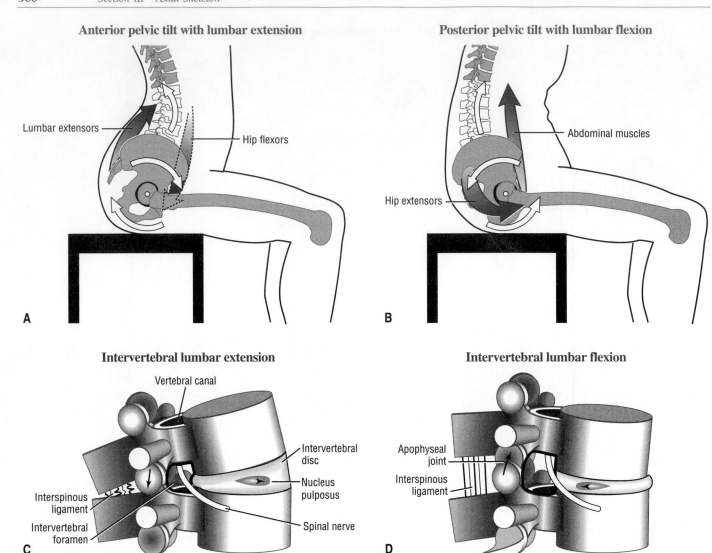

**FIGURE 9–68.** Anterior and posterior tilt of the pelvis and its effect on the kinematics of the lumbar spine. *A and C, Anterior pelvic tilt* extends the lumbar spine and increases lordosis. This action tends to shift the nucleus pulposus anteriorly and reduces the diameter of the intervertebral foramina. *B and D, Posterior pelvic tilt* flexes the lumbar spine and decreases lordosis. This action tends to shift the nucleus pulposus posteriorly and increases the diameter of the intervertebral foramina. Muscle activity is shown in red.

### Therapeutic and Kinesiologic Correlations between Anterior Pelvic Tilt and Increased Lumbar Lordosis

Active anterior tilt of the pelvis is caused by the hip flexor and back extensor muscles (Fig. 9–68A). Strengthening and increasing the control of these muscles, in theory, favors a more lordotic posture of the lumbar spine. Although this idea is intriguing, whether a person can subconsciously adopt and maintain a newly learned pelvic posture is uncertain. Nevertheless, maintaining the natural lordotic posture in the lumbar spine is a fundamental principle espoused by McKenzie[65] for persons with a herniated disc. Increased lumbar extension reduces the pressure within the disc[71] and, in some cases, reduces the contact pressure between the displaced nuclear material and the neural elements.[59] Evidence of the latter is often described clinically as "centralization" of low-back pain, meaning that discogenic pain (formerly in the lower extremities due to nerve root impingement) migrates *toward* the low back.[22] Centralization, therefore, suggests reduced disc pressure on the nerve root.

The lumbar region may demonstrate greatly exaggerated lordosis that is undesirable from a medical perspective. The pathomechanics of severe lordosis often involves a hip flexion contracture with greatly increased passive tension in the hip flexor muscles (Fig. 9–69A and B). Possible negative consequences of exaggerated lordosis include increased compression force on the apophyseal joints and increased anterior shear force at the lumbosacral junction, possibly leading to spondylolisthesis.

### Therapeutic and Kinesiologic Correlations between Posterior Pelvic Tilt and Decreased Lumbar Lordosis

Active posterior tilting of the pelvis is produced by hip extensor and abdominal muscles (see Fig. 9–68B). Strengthening and increasing the patient's conscious control over these muscles theoretically favors a reduced lumbar lordosis. This concept was the trademark of the "Williams flexion exercise," a therapeutic approach that stressed stretching the hip flexor and back extensor muscles and strengthening the

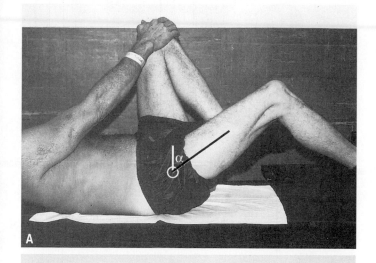

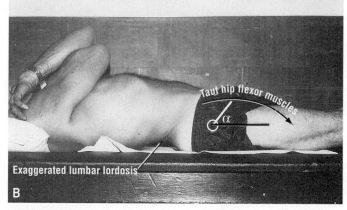

**FIGURE 9–69.** The relationship between taut hip flexor muscles, excessive anterior pelvic tilt, and exaggerated lumbar lordosis. The medial-lateral axis of rotation of the hip is shown as an open white circle. *A,* A right hip flexion contracture is shown by the angle ($\alpha$) formed between the femur (red line) and a white line representing pelvic position (i.e., a line connecting the anterior and posterior-superior iliac spines). The left normal hip is held flexed to keep the pelvis as posteriorly tilted (neutral) as possible. *B,* With both legs allowed to lie against the mat, tension created in the taut and shortened right hip flexors tilts the pelvis anteriorly, exaggerating the lumbar lordosis evident by the hollow in the low-back region. The hip flexion contracture is still present, but masked by the anteriorly tilted position of the pelvis.

abdominal and hip extensor muscles.[109] In principle, these exercises are most appropriate for persons with back pain related to excessive lumbar lordosis and significantly increased sacrohorizontal angle (see Fig. 9–61). This posture, according to Williams, was associated with degenerative disc disease, stenosis of the lumbar intervertebral foramen, osteophyte formation with nerve root irritation, and anterior spondylolisthesis of the lower lumbar region.

### Sitting Posture and Its Effect on Alignment of the Lumbar and Craniocervical Regions

For many persons, a lot of time is spent sitting, either at work, school, or home, or in a vehicle. The posture of the pelvis and lumbar spine has a large influence on the posture in other areas of the vertebral column. The topic of sitting

posture, therefore, has therapeutic implications on treatment and prevention of spinal problems. Although the posture of the pelvis can deviate in three planes about the hip joints, the following discussion highlights the effects of sagittal plane posturing of the pelvis on the lumbar and craniocervical regions.

Consider the classic contrast made between "poor" and "ideal" sitting postures (Fig. 9–70A and B). In the poor or slouched posture depicted in Figure 9–70A, the pelvis is posteriorly tilted with a slightly flexed (flattened) lumbar spine. Eventually, this posture may lead to adaptive shortening in tissues that maintain this posture (see the box). A habitually slouched sitting posture may, in time, overstretch and weaken the posterior annular fibrosus, reducing its ability to block a protruding nucleus pulposus.

---

**Tissues that, if Shortened, Predispose a Person to Slouched Sitting Posture with a Posterior Tilted Pelvis**
1. Hamstring muscles
2. Anterior longitudinal ligament
3. Anterior fibers of the annulus fibrosus

---

A slouched sitting posture typically increases the external moment arm between the line-of-force of the upper body weight and lumbar vertebrae. As a consequence, the greater flexor torque increases the compression force on the anterior margin of the lumbar discs. In vivo pressure measurements typically demonstrate larger pressures within the lumbar discs in slouched sitting compared with erect sitting.[108]

The sitting posture of the pelvis and lumbar spine strongly influences the posture of the entire axial skeleton, including the craniocervical region. Consider the contrast in sitting postures depicted in Figure 9–70. On average, the flat posture of the low back (see Fig. 9–70A) is associated with a more protracted head (i.e., a "forward head") posture.[11] Sitting with the lumbar spine flexed tips the thoracic and lower cervical regions forward into excessive flexion. In order to maintain a horizontal visual gaze—such as that typically required to view a computer monitor—the upper craniocervical region must compensate by extending slightly. Over time, this posture may result in adaptive shortening in the small posterior suboccipital muscles. As depicted in Figure 9–70B, the ideal sitting posture with natural lordosis and increased anterior pelvic tilt extends the lumbar spine. The change in posture at the base (inferior aspect) of the spine has an optimizing influence on the posture of the entire axial skeleton. The more upright and extended thoracic spine facilitates a more retracted (extended) base of the cervical spine, yielding a more desirable "chin-in" position. Because the base of the cervical spine is more extended, the upper craniocervical region tends to flex slightly to a more neutral posture.

The ideal sitting posture depicted in Figure 9–70B is difficult for many persons to maintain, especially for several hours at a time. Fatigue often develops in the lumbar extensor muscles. A prolonged, slouched sitting posture may be an occupational hazard. In addition to the possible negative effects of a chronically flexed lumbar region, the slouched sitting posture may also increase the muscular stress at the

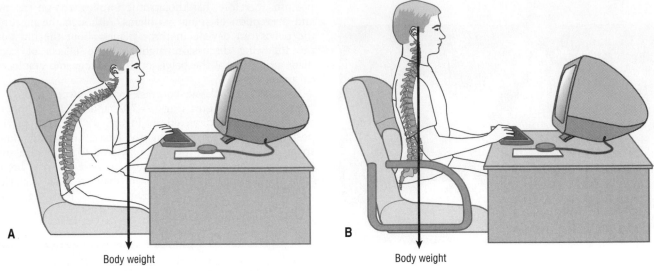

A   Body weight

B   Body weight

**FIGURE 9–70.** Sitting posture and effects on the alignment of the lumbar and craniocervical regions. *A,* With a slouched sitting posture, the lumbar spine flexes, which reduces its normal lordosis. As a consequence, the head tends to assume a "forward" posture (see text). *B,* With an ideal sitting posture aided with a cushion, the lumbar spine assumes a normal lordosis, which facilitates a more desirable "chin-in" position of the head.

base of the cervical spine. The forward-head posture increases the external flexion torque on the cervical column as a whole, requiring greater force production from the extensor muscles and local connective tissues. Sitting posture may be improved by a combination of awareness; strengthening and stretching the appropriate muscles; eyeglasses; and ergonomically designed seating, which includes adequate lumbar support.

---

**Flexion and Extension Exercises for Treatment of Low-Back Pain—Understanding the "Trade-Offs"**

As described, flexion and extension of the low back have marked and usually contrasting biomechanical consequences on intervertebral joints—from disc migration to the relative loading of the apophyseal joints (Table 9–15). Considerable controversy exists on the effectiveness of different exercise approaches for the treatment of low-back pain. An exercise approach that stresses flexion, for example, may be the most appropriate biomechanical intervention for one patient but not for another. Complicating matters is often the lack of understanding of the exact mechanical dysfunction underlying a person's low-back pain. Although the mechanics and treatment for low-back pain are sometimes obvious, the exact medical diagnosis is not in many cases.

A thorough discussion of the various physical therapy services for chronic low-back pain is not in the scope of this chapter. As a general principle, however, physical therapy is used to devise the exercises that strengthen and stabilize the low back, to educate patients on ways to reduce the load or stress on the low back during activities of daily living, and to encourage a pain-free, more normal range of movement. Regardless of the specific therapeutic approach, the therapist and physician must understand the underlying biomechanical contraindications relevant to the diagnosis. Developing this understanding requires a sound knowledge of the anatomy and kinesiology of the lumbar region and years of clinical practice.

**TABLE 9–15. Biomechanical Consequences of Lumbar Flexion and Extension**

| Movement | Biomechanical Consequences |
|---|---|
| Flexion | 1. Tends to migrate the nucleus pulposus *posteriorly,* toward neural tissue.<br>2. *Increases* the size of the opening of the intervertebral foramina.<br>3. Transfers load from the apophyseal joints to the intervertebral discs.<br>4. *Increases* tension in the posterior connective tissues (ligamentum flava, apophyseal joint capsules, interspinous and supraspinous ligaments, posterior longitudinal ligament) and posterior margin of the annulus fibrosus.<br>5. Compresses the anterior side of the annulus fibrosus. |
| Extension | 1. Tends to migrate the nucleus pulposus *anteriorly,* away from neural tissue.<br>2. *Decreases* the size of the opening of the intervertebral foramina.<br>3. Transfers load from the intervertebral disc to the apophyseal joints.<br>4. *Decreases* tension in the posterior connective tissues (see above) and posterior margin of the annulus fibrosus.<br>5. Stretches the anterior side of the annulus fibrosus. |

## *Horizontal Plane Kinematics at the Lumbar Region: Axial Rotation*

Only 5 degrees of horizontal plane rotation occurs to each side throughout the lumbar region. This motion is shown in context with the rotation of the thoracolumbar region in Figure 9–56B. Axial rotation to the right, between L1 and L2 for instance, occurs as the left inferior articular facet of L1 approximates or compresses against the left superior articular facet of L2. Simultaneously, the right inferior articular facet of L1 separates (distracts) from the right superior articular facet of L2.

The amount of actual intervertebral motion during axial rotation is very limited in the lumbar region. Only 1.1 degrees of unilateral axial rotation is measured at the L3–4 intervertebral junction.[93] The near sagittal plane orientation of the apophyseal joints physically blocks axial rotation. As indicated in Figure 9–56B, the apophyseal joints located contralateral to the side of the rotation compress, thereby blocking further movement. Axial rotation is also restricted by tension created in the stretched capsules of the apophyseal joints[35] and stretched fibers within the annulus fibrosus.[54] Axial rotation, as little as 1 to 3 degrees per intervertebral junction, has been shown to damage the articular facet surfaces and annulus fibrosus.[12]

The natural resistance to axial rotation provides vertical stability throughout the lower end of the vertebral column. The well-developed lumbar multifidi muscles and relatively rigid sacroiliac joints reinforce this stability.

## *Frontal Plane Kinematics at the Lumbar Region: Lateral Flexion*

About 15 to 20 degrees of lateral flexion occurs to each side in the lumbar region.[81] Except for differences in orientation and structure of the apophyseal joints, the arthrokinematics of lateral flexion are essentially the same in the lumbar region as in the thoracic region. Soft tissues on the side opposite the lateral flexion limit the motion (Fig. 9–57B). The nucleus pulposus migrates slightly toward the convex side of the bend.

As with the cervical and thoracic regions, lateral flexion in the lumbar region is coupled with relatively small amounts of axial rotation, and vice versa.[18,42,82] Although the precise magnitude and direction of the coupling varies between subjects and within the lumbar region, research does suggest an overall contralateral pattern. Active lateral flexion to the right, for example, is typically accompanied with slight axial rotation to the left.[93] Mechanisms to explain the coupling pattern in the lumbar spine are not clear.

## SUMMARY OF THE KINEMATICS WITHIN THE VERTEBRAL COLUMN

The following points summarize the main kinematic themes of the vertebral column:

1. The *cervical spine* permits relatively large amounts of motion in all three planes. Most notable is the high degree of axial rotation permitted at the atlanto-axial joint complex. Ample range of motion is necessary for spatial orientation of the neck and head—the site of hearing, sight, smell, and equilibrium.

2. The *thoracic spine* permits a relatively constant amount of lateral flexion. This kinematic feature reflects the general frontal plane orientation of the apophyseal joints combined with the stabilizing function of the ribs.

3. The thoracic spine supports and protects the thorax and its enclosed organs. As described in Chapter 11, an important function of the thorax is to provide a mechanical bellows for ventilation.

4. The *thoracolumbar spine,* from a cranial-to-caudal direction, permits increasing amounts of flexion and extension, at the expense of axial rotation. This feature reflects, among other things, the progressive transformation of the orientation of the apophyseal joints, from the horizontal/frontal planes in the cervical-thoracic junction to the near sagittal plane in the lumbar region. The prevailing near sagittal plane and vertical orientation of the lumbar region naturally favors flexion and extension, but restricts axial rotation.

5. The *lumbar spine,* in combination with flexion and extension of the hips, forms the primary pivot point for sagittal plane motion of the entire superimposed trunk.

## SACROILIAC JOINTS

The sacroiliac joints mark the transition between the caudal end of the axial skeleton and the lower appendicular skeleton. The analogous articulations at the cranial end of the axial skeleton are the sternoclavicular joints within the shoulder complex. Both the sternoclavicular and sacroiliac joints possess unique structural characteristics needed to satisfy equally unique functional demands. The saddle-shaped sternoclavicular joint is designed primarily for mobility. In contrast, the large, tight-fitting sacroiliac joint is designed primarily for stability, with mobility being a secondary, although nonetheless important, function.

The structural differences in the sternoclavicular and sacroiliac joints generally reflect the differences in overall functions of the upper and lower extremities. The sternoclavicular joints enjoy three degrees of freedom, a definite necessity for providing wide placement of the hands in space. The sacroiliac joints, in contrast, are stable and relatively rigid, ensuring effective load transfer among the vertebral column, lower extremities, and earth.

The exact relationship between structure and function of the sacroiliac joint is controversial.[6,37,87,97] The location of the sacroiliac joints seems to make it susceptible to abnormally large stresses due to asymmetry in leg length and abnormal posture of the lower spine or pelvis. A mechanism that describes the deterioration or malalignment of the sacroiliac joint as a common cause of low-back pain, however, is not universally agreed upon. Mixed conclusions are reached regarding the efficacy of diagnostic clinical testing and clinical intervention.[60,98,105] Adding to the clinical ambiguity of the sacroiliac joint is the lack of standard terminology to describe the related anatomy and kinesiology. As a result, the biomechanical and clinical importance of the sacroiliac joint is often either understated or exaggerated.

### Anatomic Considerations

The structural demands placed on the sacroiliac joints are considered in context with the entire *pelvic ring*. The components of the pelvic ring are the sacrum, the pair of sacroiliac

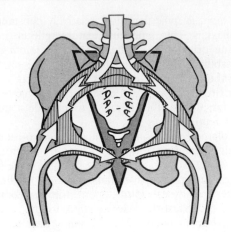

**FIGURE 9–71.** The pelvic ring. The arrows show the direction of body weight force between the trunk and the femurs (*downward and lateral arrows*), and between the femurs and the trunk (*upward and medial arrows*). The keystone of the pelvic ring is the sacrum wedged between the two ilia. (From Kapandji IA: The Physiology of Joints, vol. 3. New York, Churchill Livingstone, 1974.)

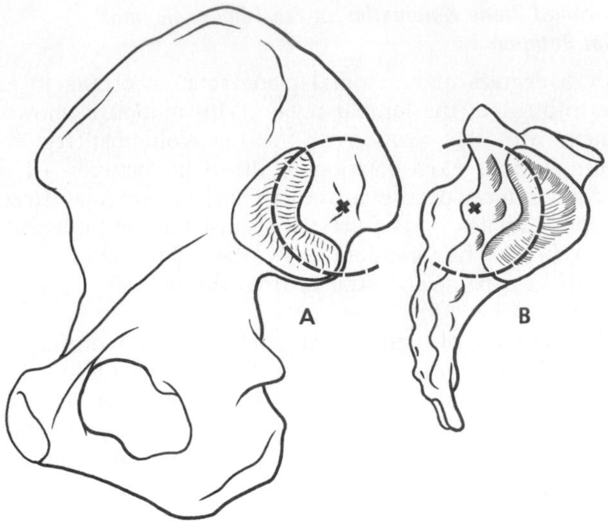

**FIGURE 9–72.** The exposed auricular surfaces of the sacroiliac joint are shown. *A,* Iliac surface. *B,* Sacral surface. (From Kapandji IA: The Physiology of Joints, vol. 3. New York, Churchill Livingstone, 1974.)

joints, the three bones of each hemipelvis (ilium, pubis, and ischium), and the pubic symphysis joint (Fig. 9–71). The pelvic ring transfers body weight bidirectionally between the trunk and femurs. The strength of the pelvic ring depends on the fit and stability of the sacrum, wedged between the two halves of the pelvis. The sacrum, anchored by the two sacroiliac joints, is the keystone of the pelvic ring.

## JOINT STRUCTURE AND LIGAMENTOUS SUPPORT

The sacroiliac joint is located just anterior to the posterior-superior iliac-spine of the ilium. Structurally, the joint consists of a relatively rigid articulation between the auricular surface (from Latin *auricle,* meaning little ear) of the sacrum and the matching auricular surface of the iliac bone. The articular surface of the joint has a semicircular, boomerang shape, with the open angle of the boomerang facing posteriorly (Fig. 9–72). Although articular cartilage covers both bony auricular surfaces of the joint, it is thicker on the side of the sacrum.[86]

In childhood, the sacroiliac joint has all the characteristics of a synovial joint, being mobile and surrounded by a pliable capsule. Between puberty and young adulthood, however, the sacroiliac joint gradually changes from a diarthrodial (synovial) joint to a modified amphiarthrodial joint.[15] Most notable is the transition from a smooth to a rough joint surface. A mature sacroiliac joint possesses numerous, reciprocally contoured elevations and depressions, deeply etched within the bone and articular cartilage (Fig. 9–73).[104] With aging, the joint capsule becomes increasingly fibrosed, less pliable, and less mobile.[87] The presence of osteophytes and defects in and around the joint are relatively common, even in the young adult. Fibrous adhesions occur in both genders—earlier in men and following menopause in women.[94] By the eighth decade, the hyaline cartilage thins and deteriorates and, in some cases, the joint may completely ossify. Anthropologists routinely use the condition of

the sacroiliac joint as a reliable method to determine the approximate age of a specimen.

The rather dramatic changes in the articular structure of the sacroiliac joints between young and old age are in some ways similar to those of joints that develop osteoarthritis.[24] For unexplained reasons, degenerative-like changes occur more frequently on the cartilage on the side of the ilium.[47] It is likely that the degenerative changes are not pathologic, in the strict sense of the word, but rather a natural response to

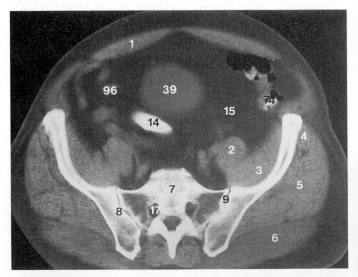

**FIGURE 9–73.** A horizontal cross-section of a computed tomography (CT) scan at the level of the sacroiliac joints. Note the irregular articular surfaces. (From Weir J, Abrahams PH: An Imaging Atlas of Human Anatomy. St. Louis, Mosby-Year Book, 1992.) KEY: #1, rectus abdominis; #2, psoas major; #3, iliacus; #4, gluteus minimus; #5, gluteus medius; #6, gluteus maximus; #7, sacrum; #8, ilium; #9, sacroiliac joint.

**Anterior view**

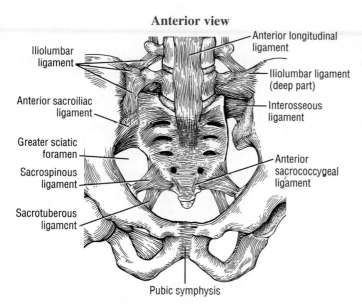

FIGURE 9–74. An anterior view of the lumbosacral region and pelvis shows the major ligaments in the region, especially those of the sacroiliac joint. On the left, part of the sacrum, the superficial parts of the iliolumbar ligament, and the anterior sacroiliac ligaments are removed to expose the auricular surface of the ilium and deeper interosseous ligament.

of the sacrum and other local ligaments. The interosseous ligament forms the most substantial bond between the sacrum and the ilium.[110]

The posterior side of the sacroiliac joint is reinforced by short and long *posterior sacroiliac ligaments* (Fig. 9–75). The extensive but relatively thin set of *short posterior sacroiliac* ligaments originates along the posterior-lateral side of the sacrum. The ligaments run superiorly and laterally to insert on the ilium, near the iliac tuberosity and the posterior-superior iliac spine. Many of these fibers blend with the deeper interosseous ligament. Fibers of the well-developed *long posterior sacroiliac ligament* originate from the regions of the third and fourth sacral segments, then course toward an attachment on the posterior-superior iliac spine of the ilium. Many fibers of the posterior sacroiliac ligament blend with the sacrotuberous ligament.

Although the sacrotuberous and sacrospinous ligaments do not actually cross the sacroiliac joint, they do assist with indirect stabilization (Fig. 9–75). The *sacrotuberous ligament* is large, arising from the posterior-superior iliac spine, lateral sacrum, and coccyx, attaching distally to the ischial tuberosity. The distal attachment blends with the tendon of the biceps femoris (lateral hamstring) muscle. The *sacrospinous ligament* is located deep to the sacrotuberous ligament, arising from the lateral margin of the caudal end of the sacrum and coccyx, attaching distally to the ischial spine.

the increased loading associated with walking and increased body-weight associated with growing. The naturally rough and irregular surfaces in the subchondral bone and articular cartilage resist movement between the sacrum and ilium.[104] The sacroiliac joint, however, is not exempt from degenerative osteoarthritis.

The sacroiliac joint is reinforced by three primary ligaments: the anterior sacroiliac, interosseous, and posterior sacroiliac.[37,110] The sacrotuberous and sacrospinous ligaments offer a secondary source of stability.

---

**Ligaments that Stabilize the Sacroiliac Joint**

*Primary*
1. Anterior sacroiliac ligament
2. Interosseous ligament
3. Short and long posterior sacroiliac ligaments

*Secondary*
4. Sacrotuberous ligament
5. Sacrospinous ligament

---

The *anterior sacroiliac ligament* is a thickening of the anterior and inferior parts of the capsule (Fig. 9–74).[46] This aspect of the joint may be strengthened by the parts of the piriformis and iliacus muscles that cross the joint.

The *interosseous ligament* is a very strong and massive set of short multiple fibers that fill most of the open space along the posterior and superior margin of the joint. This ligament is exposed on the left side in Figure 9–74, by removing part

**Posterior view**

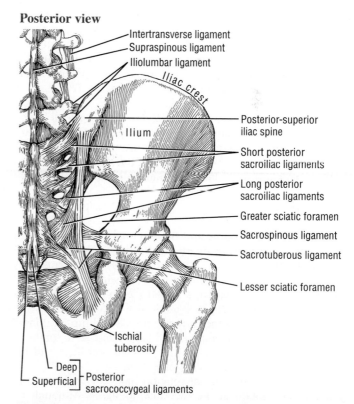

FIGURE 9–75. A posterior view of the right lumbosacral region and pelvis shows the major ligaments that reinforce the sacroiliac joint.

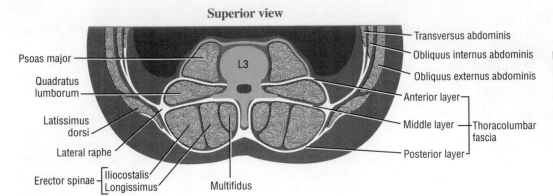

**Superior view**

Psoas major

Quadratus lumborum

Latissimus dorsi

Lateral raphe

Erector spinae ⎡ Iliocostalis
⎣ Longissimus

Multifidus

L3

Transversus abdominis

Obliquus internus abdominis

Obliquus externus abdominis

Anterior layer

Middle layer ⎤ Thoracolumbar
⎦ fascia

Posterior layer ⎦

**FIGURE 9–76.** A superior view of a horizontal cross-section through the back at the level of the third lumbar vertebra. The anterior, middle, and posterior layers of the thoracolumbar fascia are shown surrounding various muscle groups.

## THORACOLUMBAR FASCIA

The thoracolumbar fascia is believed to have an important functional role in the mechanical stability of the low back, including the sacroiliac joint.[103] This tissue is most extensive in the lumbar region, where it is organized into anterior, middle, and posterior layers. Three layers of the thoracolumbar fascia partially surround and compartmentalize the posterior muscles of the lower back (Fig. 9–76).

The *anterior and middle layers* of the thoracolumbar fascia are named according to their position relative to the quadratus lumborum muscle. Both layers are anchored medially to the transverse processes of the lumbar vertebrae, and inferiorly to the iliac crests. The *posterior layer* of the thoracolumbar fascia lies over the posterior surface of the erector spinae and, more superficially, the latissimus dorsi muscle. This layer of the thoracolumbar fascia attaches to the spinous processes of all lumbar vertebrae and the sacrum, and to the ilium near the posterior superior-iliac spines. These extensive skeletal attachments provide mechanical stability to the sacroiliac joint. Stability is enhanced by attachments made by the gluteus maximus and latissimus dorsi.

The posterior and middle layers of the thoracolumbar fascia fuse at their lateral margins, forming a *lateral raphe*. This tissue serves as an attachment for the internal obliquus abdominus and transversus abdominus muscles. The functional significance of these muscular attachments is clarified in the discussion on lifting mechanics in Chapter 10.

## Kinematics

Relatively small rotational and translational movements occur at the sacroiliac joint, primarily in the sagittal plane.[26,50,89,95] Data from the studies that measured the movements vary considerably. Typical mean values fall within the 0.2- to 2-degree range for rotation, and 1- to 2-mm range for translation.[26,50,95] Passive range of motion of 7 to 8 degrees has been measured during the extremes of bilateral hip motions.[89] Movements at the sacroiliac joint likely occur as a combination of compression force on the articular cartilage and actual slight movement between joint surfaces.

Several terms and axes of rotation have been proposed to describe the motion at the sacroiliac joints.[6,48] Although no terminology completely describes the complex multiplanar rotational and translational movements, two terms, neverthe-

less, are typically used for this purpose: nutation and counternutation. They describe movements limited to the sagittal plane, about a medial-lateral axis of rotation that traverses the interosseous ligament (Fig. 9–77). *Nutation* (meaning to nod) is defined as the relative *anterior tilt* of the base (top) of the sacrum relative to the ilium. *Counternutation* is a reverse motion defined as the relative *posterior tilt* of the base of the sacrum relative to the ilium. (Note the term *relative* used in the above definitions.) As depicted in Figure 9–77, nutation and counternutation can occur by sacral-on-iliac rotation (as previously defined), by ilium-on-sacral rotation, or by both motions performed simultaneously.

---

**Motions at the Sacroiliac Joint**

1. *Nutation* occurs by anterior sacral-on-iliac rotation, posterior ilium-on-sacral rotation, or by both motions performed simultaneously.
2. *Counternutation* occurs by posterior sacral-on-iliac rotation, anterior ilium-on-sacral rotation, or by both motions performed simultaneously.

---

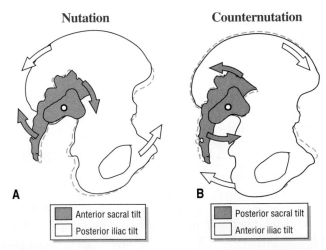

**Nutation**

**Counternutation**

A

B

| Anterior sacral tilt | Posterior sacral tilt |
| Posterior iliac tilt | Anterior iliac tilt |

**FIGURE 9–77.** The kinematics at the sacroiliac joint: *A,* Nutation. *B,* Counternutation. (See text for definitions.) Sacral rotations are indicated in gray, and iliac rotations in white. The axis of rotation for sagittal plane movement is indicated by the small circle.

## Functional Considerations

The sacroiliac joint provides two functions: (1) a stress relief within the pelvic ring and (2) a stable means for load transfer between the axial skeleton and lower limbs.

### STRESS RELIEF

The movements at the sacroiliac joint, although slight, permit an element of stress relief within the pelvic ring. This stress relief is especially important during walking and, in women, during childbirth.

While walking, the reciprocal flexion and extension pattern of the lower limbs causes each side of the pelvis to rotate slightly out of phase with the other. At normal speed of walking, the heel of the advancing lower limb strikes the ground as the toes of the opposite limb are still in contact with the ground. At this instant, tension in the hip muscles and ligaments generate oppositely directed torsions on the right and left iliac crests.[6] The torsions are most notable in the sagittal plane, as nutation and counternutation, and in the horizontal planes. Intrapelvic torsions are amplified with increased walking speed. Although slight, movements at each sacroiliac joint during walking help dissipate otherwise potentially damaging stresses that would otherwise develop throughout the pelvic ring. The pubic symphysis joint likely has a similar role in this process.

Movements at the sacroiliac joint increase during labor and delivery.[16] A significant increase in joint laxity occurs during the last trimester of pregnancy and is especially notable in women during the second pregnancy as compared with the first. Increased nutation during childbirth rotates the lower part of the sacrum posteriorly, thereby increasing the size of the pelvic outlet and favoring the passage of the infant. The articular surfaces of the sacroiliac joints are smoother in women, presenting less resistance to these slight physiologic motions.

### STABILITY DURING LOAD TRANSFER: MECHANICS OF GENERATING A NUTATION TORQUE AT THE SACROILIAC JOINT

The plane of the articular surfaces of the sacroiliac joint is nearly vertical. This orientation renders the joint vulnerable to slipping, especially when subjected to large forces. Nutation at the sacroiliac joint elevates the compression and shear (friction) forces between joint surfaces, thereby increasing stability.[104] The close-packed position of the sacroiliac joint is full nutation. Forces that create a nutation torque therefore stabilize the sacroiliac joint. Torques are created by gravity, stretched ligaments, and muscle activation.

> **Nutation Torque Increases the Stability at the Sacroiliac Joint. This Torque Is Produced by Three Forces**
> 1. Gravity
> 2. Passive tension from stretched ligaments
> 3. Muscle activation

### Stabilizing Effect of Gravity

The downward force of gravity due to body weight passes through the lumbar vertebrae, usually anterior to the midpoint of the sacroiliac joints. At the same time, gravity produces an upward hip compressive force that is transmitted from the femoral heads through the acetabula.[48] Each force acts with a moment arm that creates oppositely directed nutation torques about the sacroiliac joint (Fig. 9–78A). The

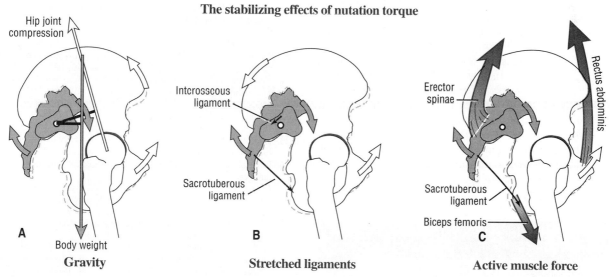

**The stabilizing effects of nutation torque**

**A**  Gravity
Hip joint compression
Body weight

**B**  Stretched ligaments
Interosseous ligament
Sacrotuberous ligament

**C**  Active muscle force
Erector spinae
Rectus abdominis
Sacrotuberous ligament
Biceps femoris

**FIGURE 9–78.** Nutation torque increases the stability at the sacroiliac joint. *A,* Two forces originating primarily by gravity—body weight and hip joint compression—generate a nutation torque at the sacroiliac joint. Each force has a moment arm (black lines) that acts from the axis of rotation (circle at joint). *B,* The nutation torque stretches the interosseous and sacrotuberous ligaments that ultimately compresses and stabilizes the sacroiliac joint. *C,* Muscle contraction (red) creates an active nutation torque across the sacroiliac joint. Note the biceps femoris transmitting tension through the sacrotuberous ligament.

torque due to body weight (shown in gray) rotates the sacrum anteriorly relative to the ilium, whereas the torque due to hip compression force (shown in white) rotates the ilium posterior relative to the sacrum. The nutation torque "locks" the joint by increasing the friction between the rough and reciprocally contoured articular surfaces.[90,104] This mechanism relies primarily on gravity and the congruity of the joint surfaces, rather than extra-articular structures such as ligaments and muscles.

### Stabilizing Effect of Ligaments and Muscles

Gravity and weight bearing through the pelvis produce the first line of stability at the sacroiliac joints. Stability is adequate for activities that involve relatively low, static loading between the pelvis and the vertebral column, such as sitting and standing. For larger and more dynamic loading, however, the sacroiliac joints are reinforced by ligaments and muscles. As described in Figure 9–78B, nutation torque stretches many of the connective tissues at the sacroiliac joint, such as the sacrotuberous and interosseous ligaments. Increased tension in these ligaments compresses the surfaces of the sacroiliac joint.

In addition to ligaments, several trunk and hip muscles reinforce and stabilize the sacroiliac joint (Table 9–16).[84] Additional stability is required during activities such as lifting, load carrying, or running. The stabilizing action of many of these muscles is based on their attachments to the thoracolumbar fascia and to the sacrospinous and sacrotuberous ligaments.[92] Contractile forces from muscles listed in Table 9–16 can stabilize the sacroiliac joint by (1) generating active compression forces against the articular surfaces, (2) increasing magnitude of nutation torque and subsequently engage an active locking mechanism, (3) pulling on connective tissues that are able to reinforce the joint,[84,102] and (4) any combination of these effects. As one example, consider the muscular interaction depicted in Figure 9–78C. Contraction of the erector spinae muscle tilts the sacrum anteriorly, whereas contraction of the rectus abdominis and biceps femoris muscles can tilt the ilium posteriorly, two elements that produce nutation torque. Through direct attachment, the biceps femoris increases tension into the sacrotuberous ligament. The muscular interaction explains, in part, why strengthening and hypertrophy of many of the muscles listed in Table 9–16 is recommended for treatment of an unstable sacroiliac joint. In addition, increased strength of the gluteus maximus, latissimus dorsi, erector spinae, internal oblique muscles and transverus abdominis increases the stability of the sacroiliac joint via their connections into the thoracolumbar fascia.

---

**TABLE 9–16. Muscles that Reinforce and Stabilize the Sacroiliac Joint**

1. Erector spinae
2. Lumbar multifidi
3. Abdominal muscle group
   a. External and internal obliques
   b. Rectus abdominis
   c. Transverus abdominis
4. Hamstrings (such as biceps femoris)

---

## REFERENCES

1. Adams MA, Hutton WC: The effect of posture on the role of the apophyseal joints in resisting intervertebral compressive forces. J Bone Joint Surg 62B:358–362, 1980.
2. Adams MA, Hutton WC: Prolapsed intervertebral disc. A hyperflexion injury. Spine 7:184–191, 1982.
3. Adams MA, Hutton WC: Gradual disc prolapse. Spine 10:524–531, 1985.
4. Adams MA, Hutton WC, Stott JRR: The resistance to flexion of the lumbar intervertebral joint. Spine 5:245–253, 1980.
5. Ahmed AM, Duncan NA, Burke DL: The effect of facet geometry on the axial torque-rotation response of lumbar motion segments. Spine 15:391–401, 1990.
6. Alderink GL: The sacroiliac joint: Review of anatomy, mechanics and function. J Orthop Sports Phys Ther 13:71–84, 1991.
7. Amonoo-Kuofi HS: Changes in the lumbosacral angle, sacral inclination and the curvature of the lumbar spine during aging. Acta Anat 145:373–377, 1992.
8. Andersson BJG, Ortengren R: Lumbar disc pressure and myoelectric back muscle activity during sitting. II. Studies on an office chair. Scand J Rehabil Med 6:115–121, 1974.
9. Andersson GBJ, Ortengren R, Nachemson A: Intradiskal pressure, intra-abdominal pressure and myoelectric back muscle activity related to posture and loading. Clin Orthop 129:156–164, 1977.
10. Beattie PF, Brooks WM, Rothstein JM, et al: Effect of lordosis on the position of the nucleus pulposis in supine subjects. A study using magnetic resonance imaging. Spine 18:2096–2102, 1994.
11. Black KM, McClure P, Polansky M: The influence of different sitting positions on cervical and lumbar posture. Spine 21:65–70, 1996.
12. Bogduk N: Clinical Anatomy of the Lumbar Spine, 3rd ed. New York, Churchill Livingstone, 1997.
13. Bogduk N, Macintosh JE, Pearcy MJ: A universal model of the lumbar back muscles in the upright position. Spine 17:897–913, 1992.
14. Bogduk N, Mercer S: Biomechanics of the cervical spine. I: Normal kinematics. Clin Biomech 15:633–648, 2000.
15. Bowen V, Cassidy D: Macroscopic and microscopic anatomy of the sacroiliac joint from embryonic life until the eighth decade. Spine 6:620–628, 1981.
16. Calguneri M, Bird HA, Wright V: Changes in joint laxity occurring during pregnancy. Ann Rheum Dis 41:126–128, 1982.
17. Calliet R: Neck and Arm Pain. Philadelphia, FA Davis, 1974.
18. Cholewicki J, Crisco JJ, Oxland TR, et al: Effects of posture and structure on three-dimensional coupled rotations in the lumbar spine. Spine 21:2421–2428, 1996.
19. Coonrad RW, Murrell GAC, Motley G, et al: A logical coronal pattern classification of 2,000 consecutive idiopathic scoliosis cases based on the scoliosis research society–defined apical vertebra. Spine 23:1380–1391, 1998.
20. Cyron BM, Hutton WC: The tensile strength of the capsular ligaments of the apophyseal joints. J Anat 132:145–150, 1981.
21. Dempster WT: Space requirements for the seated operator. WADC Technical Report 55–159. University of Michigan. Washington, DC, 1955.
22. Donelson R, Aprill C, Medcalf R, et al: A prospective study of centralization of lumbar and referred pain. Spine 22:1115–1122, 1997.
23. Dvorak J, Panjabi MM, Novotny JE, et al: In vivo flexion/extension of the normal cervical spine. Orthop Res 9:828–834, 1991.
24. Ebraheim NA, Mekhail AO, Wiley WF, et al: Radiology of the sacroiliac joint. Spine 22:869–876, 1997.
25. Edmonson AS: Scoliosis. In Crenshaw AH (ed): Campbell's Operative Orthopaedics, 8th ed, vol 5. St Louis, Mosby-Year Book, 1992.
26. Egund N, Olsson TH, Schmid H, et al: Movements in the sacroiliac joints demonstrated with roentgen stereophotogrammetry. Acta Radiol Diagn 19:833–846, 1978.
27. Esola MA, McClure PW, Fitzgerald GK, et al: Analysis of lumbar spine and hip motion during forward bending in subjects with and without a history of low back pain. Spine 21:71–78, 1996.
28. Fahrni WH, Trueman GE: Comparative radiological study of the spines of a primitive population with North Americans and North Europeans. J Bone Joint Surg 47B:552–555, 1965.
29. Farfan HF, Huberdeau RM, Dubow HI: Lumbar intervertebral disc degeneration. J Bone Joint Surg 54A:492–510, 1972.
30. Fennell AJ, Jones AP, Hukins DWL: Migration of the nucleus pulposus within the intervertebral disc during flexion and extension of the spine. Spine 21:2753–2757, 1996.

31. Fielding JW: Normal and selected abnormal motion of the cervical spine from the second cervical vertebra to the seventh cervical vertebra based on cineroentgenography. J Bone Joint Surg 46A:1779–1781, 1964.

32. Freeman B: Instrumentation and techniques for scoliosis and kyphosis. In Crenshaw AH (ed): Campbell's Operative Orthopaedics, 8th ed, vol 5. St Louis, Mosby-Year Book, 1992.

33. Goel VK, Clausen JD: Prediction of load sharing among spinal components of a C5-C6 motion segment using the finite element approach. Spine 23:684–691, 1998.

34. Goel VK, Winterbottom JM, Schulte KR, et al: Ligamentous laxity across C0-C1-C2 complex. Axial torque-rotation characteristics until failure. Spine 15:990–996, 1990.

35. Gunzburg R, Hutton W, Fraser R: Axial rotation of the lumbar spine and the effect of flexion. An in vitro and in vivo biomechanical study. Spine 16:22–28, 1991.

36. Hall CM, Brody LT: Therapeutic Exercise: Moving Towards Function. Philadelphia, Lippincott Williams & Wilkins, 1999.

37. Harrison DE, Harrison DD, Trovanovich SJ: The sacroiliac joint. A review of anatomy and biomechanics with clinical implications. J Manipulative Physiol Ther 20:607–617, 1997.

38. Harrison DD, Tadeusz JJ, Troyanovich SJ, et al: Comparisons of lordotic cervical spine curvatures to a theoretical model of the static sagittal cervical spine. Spine 21:667–675, 1996.

39. Hayashi K, Yabuki T: Origin of the uncus and of Luschka's joint in the cervical spine. J Bone Joint Surg 67A:788–791, 1985.

40. Herzog RJ: The radiologic assessment for a lumbar disc herniation. Spine 21:19S–38S, 1996.

41. Hilton RC, Ball J, Benn RT: In-vitro mobility of the lumbar spine. Ann Rheum Dis 38:378–383, 1979.

42. Hindle RJ, Pearcy MJ, Cross AT, et al: Three-dimensional kinematics of the human back. Clin Biomech 5:218–228, 1990.

43. Hino H, Abumi K, Kanayama M, et al: Dynamic motion analysis of normal and unstable cervical spines using cineradiography. Spine 24:163–168, 1999.

44. Holmes A, Han ZH, Dang GT, et al: Changes in cervical canal spinal volume during in vitro flexion-extension. Spine 21:1313–1319, 1996.

45. Inufusa A, An HS, Lim TH, et al: Anatomic changes of the spinal canal and intervertebral foramen associated with flexion-extension movement. Spine 21:2412–2420, 1996.

46. Jaovisidha S, Ryu KN, De Maeseneer M, et al: Ventral sacroiliac ligament. Anatomic and pathologic considerations. Invest Radiol 31:532–541, 1996.

47. Kampen WU, Tillmann B: Age-related changes in the articular cartilage of human sacroiliac joint. Anat Embryol 198:505–513, 1998.

48. Kapandji IA: The Physiology of Joints, vol 3. New York, Churchill Livingstone, 1974.

49. Kendall HO, Kendall FP, Boyton DA: Posture and Pain. Baltimore, Williams & Wilkins, 1952.

50. Kissling RO, Jacob HAC: The mobility of the sacroiliac joint in healthy subjects. Bull Hosp Jt Dis 54:158–164, 1996.

51. Kjellby-Wendt G, Styf J: Early active training after lumbar discectomy. A prospective, randomized, and controlled study. Spine 23:2345–2351, 1998.

52. Korovessis PG, Stamatakis MV, Baikousis AG: Reciprocal angulation of vertebral bodies in the sagittal plane in an asymptomatic Greek population. Spine 23:700–705, 1998.

53. Krag MH, Cohen MC, Haugh LD, et al: Body height change during upright and recumbent posture. Spine 15:202–207, 1990.

54. Krismer M, Haid C, Rabl W: The contribution of annulus fibers to torque resistance. Spine 21:2551–2557, 1996.

55. Levine D, Whittle MW: The effects of pelvic movement on lumbar lordosis in the standing position. J Orthop Sports Phys Ther 24:130–135, 1996.

56. Lu YM, Hutton WC, Gharpuray VM: Do bending, twisting, and diurnal fluid changes in the disc affect the propensity to prolapse? A viscoelastic finite element model. Spine 21:2570–2579, 1996.

57. Lorenz M, Patwardhan A, Vanderby R: Load-bearing characteristics of lumbar facets in normal and surgically altered spinal segments. Spine 8:122–130, 1983.

58. Magee DL: Orthopedic Physical Assessment, 3rd ed. Philadelphia, WB Saunders, 1997.

59. Magnusson ML, Aleksiev AR, Spratt KF, et al: Hyperextension and spine height changes. Spine 21:2670–2675, 1996.

60. Maigne JY, Aivaliklis A, Pfefer F: Results of sacroiliac joint double block and value of sacroiliac pain provocation tests in 54 patients with low back pain. Spine 21:1889–1892, 1996.

61. Marchand F, Ahmed AM: Investigation of the laminate structure of lumbar disc annulus fibrosus. Spine 15:402–410, 1990.

62. McClure PW, Esola M, Schreier R, et al: Kinematic analysis of lumbar and hip motion while raising from a forward, flexed position in patients with and without a history of low back pain. Spine 22:552–558, 1997.

63. McGill SM, Hughson RL, Parks K: Changes in lumbar lordosis modify the role of the extensor muscles. Clin Biomech 15:777–780, 2000.

64. McGorry RW, Hsiang SM: The effect of industrial back belts and breathing technique on trunk and pelvic coordination during a lifting task. Spine 24:1124–1130, 1999.

65. McKenzie RA: The lumbar spine: Mechanical diagnosis and therapy. Waikanae, New Zealand, Spinal Publications, 1981.

66. Mercer S, Bogduk N: Intra-articular inclusions of the cervical synovial joints. Br J Rheumatol 32:705–710, 1993.

67. Mercer S, Bogduk N: The ligaments and annulus fibrosus of human adult cervical intervertebral discs. Spine 24:619–628, 1999.

68. Milne N: The role of the zygapophyseal joint orientation and uncinate processes in controlling motion in the cervical spine. J Anat 178:189–201, 1991.

69. Moore RJ, Vernon-Roberts B, Fraser RD: The origin and fate of herniated lumbar intervertebral disc tissue. Spine 21:2149–2155, 1996.

70. Mundt DJ, Kelsey JL, Golden AL, et al: An epidemiologic study of nonoccupational lifting as a risk factor for herniated lumbar intervertebral disc. The Northeast Collaborative Group on Low Back Pain. Spine 18:595–602, 1993.

71. Nachemson A: Lumbar intradiscal pressure. Experimental studies on post-mortem material. Acta Orthop Scand Suppl 43:9–104, 1960.

72. Nachemson A: The load on lumbar discs in different positions of the body. Clin Orthop 45:107–122, 1966.

73. Nachemson A, Evans J: Some mechanical properties of the third lumbar interlaminar ligament (ligamentum flavum) J Biomech 1:211–220, 1968.

74. Nachemson A, Morris JM: In vivo measurements of intradiscal pressure. Discometry, a method for the determination of pressure in the lower lumbar discs. J Bone Joint Surg 46A:1077–1092, 1964.

75. Nelson JM, Walmsley RP, Stevenson JM: Relative lumbar and pelvic motion during loaded spinal flexion/extension. Spine 20:199–204, 1995.

76. Neumann DA: Arthrokinesiologic considerations for the aged adult. In Guccione AA (ed): Geriatric Physical Therapy. Chicago, Mosby-Year Book, 2000.

77. Ordway NR, Seymour R, Donelson RG, et al: Cervical sagittal range-of-motion analysis using three methods. Cervical range-of-motion device, 3space, and radiography. Spine 22:501–508, 1997.

78. Ordway NR, Seymour RJ, Donelson RG, et al: Cervical flexion, extension, protrusion, and retraction. A radiographic segmental analysis. Spine 24:240–247, 1999.

79. Panjabi M, Dvorak J, Crisco JJ, et al: Effects of alar ligament transection on upper cervical spine rotation. J Orthop Res 9:584–593, 1991.

80. Pearcy M, Portek I, Shepherd J: Three-dimensional X-ray analysis of normal movement in the lumbar spine. Spine 9:294–297, 1984.

81. Pearcy M, Portek I, Shepherd J: The effect of low-back pain on lumbar spinal movements measured by three-dimensional X-ray analysis. Spine 10:150–153, 1985.

82. Pearcy MJ, Tibrewal SB: Axial rotation and lateral bending in the normal lumbar spine measured by three-dimensional radiography. Spine 9:582–587, 1984.

83. Penning L: Normal movements of the cervical spine. Am J Roentgenol 130:317–326, 1978.

84. Porterfield JA, DeRosa C: Mechanical Low Back Pain: Perspectives in Functional Anatomy. Philadelphia, WB Saunders, 1998.

85. Saal JA: Natural history and nonoperative treatment of lumbar disc herniation. Spine 21:2S–9S, 1996.

86. Salsabili N, Valojerdy MR, Hogg DA: Variations in thickness of articular cartilage in the human sacroiliac joint. Clin Anat 8:388–390, 1995.

87. Sashin D: A critical analysis of the anatomy and the pathologic changes of the sacroiliac joints. J Bone Joint Surg 12:891–910, 1930.

88. Shirazi-Adl A, Parnianpour M: Effect of changes in lordosis on mechanics of the lumbar spine-lumbar curvature in lifting. J Spinal Disord 12:436–447, 1999.

89. Smidt GL, Wei SH, McQuade K, et al: Sacroiliac motion for extreme hip positions. A fresh cadaver study. Spine 22:2073–2082, 1997.

90. Snijders CJ, Vleeming A, Stoeckart R: Transfer of lumbosacral load to iliac bones and legs. Part 1: Biomechanics of self-bracing of the sacroiliac joints and its significance for treatment and exercise. Clin Biomech 8:285–294, 1993.

91. Snijders CJ, Vleeming A, Stoeckart R: Transfer of lumbosacral load to iliac bones and legs. Part II: Loading of the sacroiliac joints when lifting in a stooped posture. Clin Biomech 8:295–301, 1993.

92. Snijders CJ, Ribbers MTLM, de Bakker HV, et al: EMG recordings of abdominal and back muscles in various standing postures: Validation of a biomechanical model on sacroiliac joint stability. J Electromyogr Kinesiol 8:205–214, 1998.

93. Steffen T, Rubin RK, Baramki HG, et al: A new technique for measuring lumbar segmental motion in vivo. Spine 22:156–166, 1997.

94. Stewart TD: Pathologic changes in aging sacroiliac joints. A study of dissecting-room skeletons. Clin Orthop 183:188–196, 1984.

95. Sturesson B, Selvik G, Uden A: Movements of the sacroiliac joints. A roentgen stereophotogrammetric analysis. Spine 14:162–165, 1989.

96. Taylor JR, Twomey LT: Age changes in lumbar zygapophyseal joints. Observations on structure and function. Spine 11:739–745, 1986.

97. Tigny RL: Function and pathomechanics of the sacroiliac joint. A review. Phys Ther 65:35–44, 1985.

98. Tullberg T, Blomberg S, Branth B, et al: Manipulation does not alter the position of the sacroiliac joint. A Roentgen stereophotogrammetric analysis. Spine 23:1124–1129, 1998.

99. Twomey L, Taylor J: Flexion creep deformation and hysteresis in the lumbar vertebral column. Spine 7:116–122, 1982.

100. Tyrrell AR, Reilly T, Troup JDG: Circadian variation in stature and the effects of spinal loading. Spine 10:161–164, 1985.

101. Videman T, Battie MC, Gibbons LE, et al: Lifetime exercise and disk degeneration: An MRI study of monozygotic twins. Med Sci Sports Exerc 29:1350–1356, 1997.

102. Vleeming A, Pool-Goudzwaard AL, Hammudoghlu D, et al: The function of the long dorsal sacroiliac ligament: Its implication for understanding low back pain. Spine 21:556–562, 1996.

103. Vleeming A, Pool-Goudzwaard AL, Stoeckart R, et al: The posterior layer of the thoracolumbar fascia. Its function in load transfer from spine to legs. Spine 20:753–758, 1994.

104. Vleeming A, Stoeckart R, Volkers ACW, et al: Relation between form and function in the sacroiliac joint. Part 1: Clinical anatomical aspects. Spine 15:130–132, 1990.

105. Walker JM: The sacroiliac joint. A critical review. Phys Ther 72:903–916, 1992.

106. White AA, Panjabi MM: The clinical biomechanics of scoliosis. Clin Orthop 118:100–112, 1976.

107. White AA, Panjabi MM: Clinical Biomechanics of the Spine, 2nd ed. Philadelphia, JB Lippincott, 1990.

108. Wilke H-J, Neef P, Caimi M, et al: New in vivo measurements of pressures in the intervertebral disc in daily life. Spine 24:755–762, 1999.

109. Williams PC: Examination and conservative treatment for disk lesions of the lower spine. Clin Orthop 5:28–40, 1955.

110. Williams PL, Bannister LH, Berry M, et al: Gray's Anatomy, 38th ed. New York, Churchill Livingstone, 1995.

111. Wood GW: Other disorders of the spine. In Crenshaw AH (ed): Campbell's Operative Orthopaedics, 8th ed, vol 5. Mosby-Year Book, St Louis, 1992.

112. Yamamoto I, Panjabi MM, Oxland TR, et al: The role of the iliolumbar ligament in the lumbosacral junction. Spine 15:1138–1141, 1990.

113. Yoo JU, Zou D, Edwards WT, et al: Effect of cervical spine motion on the neuroforaminal dimensions of human cervical spine. Spine 17:1131–1136, 1992.

## ADDITIONAL READINGS

Andersson GBJ, Ortengren R, Nachemson A: Quantitative studies of the load on the back in different working postures. Scand J Rehabil Med 6:173–178, 1978.

Dunlop RB, Adams MA, Hutton WC: Disc space narrowing and the lumbar facet joints. J Bone Joint Surg 66B:706–710, 1984.

Galante JO: Tensile properties of the human lumbar annulus fibrosus. Acta Orthop Scand Suppl 100:1–91, 1967.

Lonstein JE: Congenital spine deformities. Orthop Clin North Am 30:387–405, 1999.

McGorry RW, Hsiang SM: A method for dynamic measurement of lumbar lordosis. J Spinal Disord 13:118–123, 2000.

Potvin JR, Norman RW, McGill SM: Reduction in anterior shear forces on the L4/L5 disc by the lumbar musculature. Clin Biomech 6:88–96, 1991.

Schultz A, Andersson G, Ortengren R, et al: Loads on the lumbar spine. J Bone Joint Surg 64A:713–720, 1982.

Sullivan MS, Shoaf LD, Riddle DL: The relationship of lumbar flexion to disability in patients with low back pain. Phys Ther 80:240–250, 2000.

Youdas JW, Garrett TR, Egan KS, et al: Lumbar lordosis and pelvis inclination in adults with chronic low back pain. Phys Ther 80:261–275, 2000.

# CHAPTER 10

# Axial Skeleton:
# Muscle and Joint Interactions

DONALD A. NEUMANN, PT, PHD

## TOPICS AT A GLANCE

## INTRODUCTION

Osteologic and arthrologic components of the axial skeleton are presented in Chapter 9. This chapter focuses on the muscle and joint interactions within the axial skeleton. Muscles of the axial skeleton control posture, stabilize the trunk and pelvis, produce torque about the trunk for movement, and furnish fine mobility and stability to the head and neck for optimal placement of the eyes, ears, and nose.

The anatomic structure of the muscles within the axial skeleton varies considerably in length, shape, fiber direction, cross-sectional area, and leverage across the underlying joints. Such variability reflects the diverse demands placed on the musculature, from manually lifting and transporting heavy objects, to producing subtle motions of the head for accenting a lively conversation.

In addition to the variability within muscles of the axial skeleton, they cross multiple regions of the body. The trapezius muscle, for example, attaches to the clavicle and the scapula within the appendicular skeleton, and to the vertebral column and the cranium within the axial skeleton. Protective guarding due to an inflamed upper trapezius can affect the quality of motion throughout the upper extremity and craniocervical region.

Consider the many neurologic reflexes that exist within the craniocervical region that help coordinate sight, hearing, and equilibrium. Muscular dysfunction in this region is therefore often associated with severe headache, vertigo, emotional tension, and hypersensitivity to light and sound.

The primary aim of this chapter is to elucidate the structure and function of the muscles within the axial skeleton. This information is essential to the evaluation and treatment of a wide range of musculoskeletal disorders, such as postural malalignment, muscle and soft tissue strain, and disc herniation.

## INNERVATION TO THE MUSCLES AND JOINTS WITHIN THE TRUNK AND CRANIOCERVICAL REGIONS

An understanding of the organization of the peripheral innervation of the craniocervical and trunk muscles begins with an appreciation of a typical *spinal nerve* (Fig. 10–1). Each spinal nerve is formed by the union of a ventral and a dorsal *nerve root:* the *ventral nerve root* contains primarily "outgoing" (efferent) axons that supply motor drive to muscles and other effector organs associated with the autonomic system. The *dorsal nerve root* contains primarily "incoming" (afferent) dendrites with the cell body of the neuron located in an adjacent dorsal root ganglion. Sensory neurons transmit information to the spinal cord from the muscles, joints, skin, and other organs associated with the autonomic nervous system.

Protected within the vertebral canal, the ventral and dorsal nerve roots join to form a mixed *spinal nerve.* (The adjective "mixed" indicates that the spinal nerve contains both sensory and motor fibers.) Once within the intervertebral foramen, the spinal nerve thickens owing to the merging of the motor and sensory neurons and the presence of the dorsal root ganglion.

The vertebral column contains 31 pairs of spinal nerves: 8 cervical, 12 thoracic, 5 lumbar, 5 sacral, and 1 coccygeal. The abbreviations C, T, L, and S with the appropriate superscript number designate each spinal nerve, or nerve root— for example, $C^5$ and $T^6$. The cervical region has seven vertebrae but eight cervical nerves. The suboccipital nerve ($C^1$) leaves the spinal cord between the occipital bone and posterior arch of the atlas (C1). The $C^8$ spinal nerve leaves the spinal cord between the seventh cervical vertebra (C7) and the first thoracic vertebra (T1). Spinal nerves $T^1$ and below leave the spinal cord below their respective vertebral bodies.

Once a spinal nerve exits its intervertebral foramen, it immediately divides into a *ventral and dorsal ramus* (from the Latin *ramus,* meaning "path"). The ventral ramus forms nerves that innervate the muscles, joints, and skin of the *anterior-lateral trunk and neck and all the extremities.* The dorsal ramus, in contrast, forms nerves that innervate the muscles, joints, and skin of the *posterior trunk and neck.*

### Ventral Ramus Innervation

Each ventral ramus of a spinal nerve forms a plexus or continues as a single nerve that innervates tissue in a highly segmental fashion.

### PLEXUS

A plexus is an intermingling of ventral rami that form peripheral nerves. The four major plexus, excluding the small coccygeal plexus, are formed by ventral rami: cervical ($C^{1-4}$), brachial ($C^5$-$T^1$), lumbar ($T^{12}$-$L^4$), and sacral ($L^4$-$S^4$). With the exception of the cervical plexus, most of the nerves that exit the brachial, lumbar, and sacral plexus innervate structures associated with the appendicular skeleton. Only a few nerves from the brachial, lumbar, and sacral plexus innervate structures associated with the axial skeleton (Fig. 10–2A).

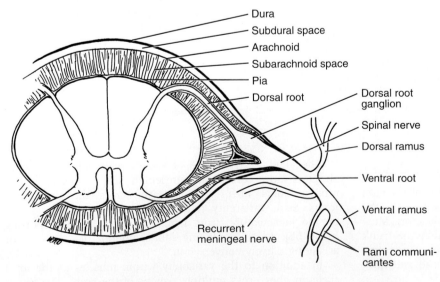

Dura
Subdural space
Arachnoid
Subarachnoid space
Pia
Dorsal root
Dorsal root ganglion
Spinal nerve
Dorsal ramus
Ventral root
Ventral ramus
Recurrent meningeal nerve
Rami communicantes

**FIGURE 10–1.** A cross-section of the spinal cord shows the dorsal (sensory) and ventral (motor) roots forming a spinal nerve. The spinal nerve divides into a relatively small dorsal ramus and a much larger ventral ramus. (Modified with permission from Jenkins DB: Hollingshead's Functional Anatomy of the Limbs and Back, 7th ed. Philadelphia, WB Saunders, 1998.)

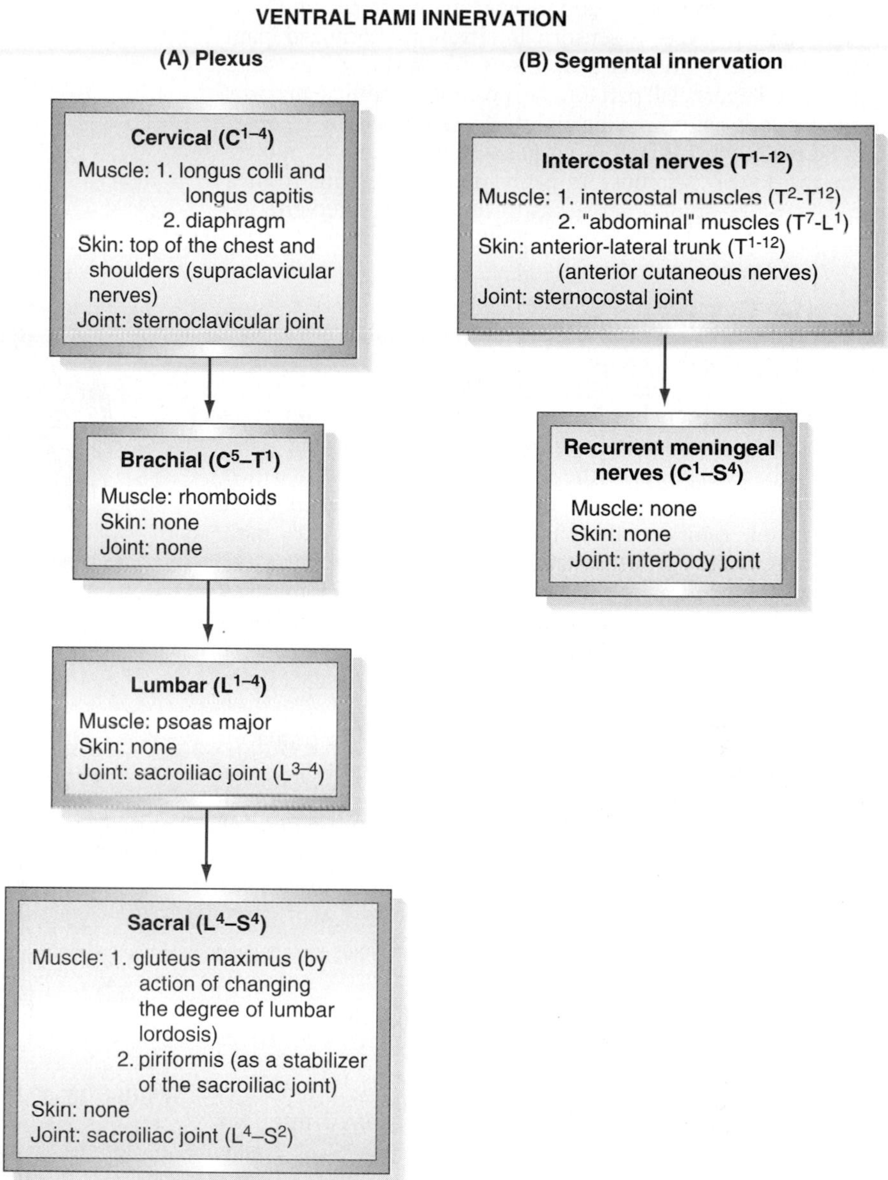

**VENTRAL RAMI INNERVATION**

**(A) Plexus**          **(B) Segmental innervation**

**Cervical (C$^{1-4}$)**

Muscle: 1. longus colli and
longus capitis
2. diaphragm
Skin: top of the chest and
shoulders (supraclavicular
nerves)
Joint: sternoclavicular joint

**Intercostal nerves (T$^{1-12}$)**

Muscle: 1. intercostal muscles (T$^2$-T$^{12}$)
2. "abdominal" muscles (T$^7$-L$^1$)
Skin: anterior-lateral trunk (T$^{1-12}$)
(anterior cutaneous nerves)
Joint: sternocostal joint

**Brachial (C$^5$–T$^1$)**

Muscle: rhomboids
Skin: none
Joint: none

**Recurrent meningeal
nerves (C$^1$–S$^4$)**

Muscle: none
Skin: none
Joint: interbody joint

**Lumbar (L$^{1-4}$)**

Muscle: psoas major
Skin: none
Joint: sacroiliac joint (L$^{3-4}$)

**Sacral (L$^4$–S$^4$)**

Muscle: 1. gluteus maximus (by
action of changing
the degree of lumbar
lordosis)
2. piriformis (as a stabilizer
of the sacroiliac joint)
Skin: none
Joint: sacroiliac joint (L$^4$–S$^2$)

**FIGURE 10–2.** Examples of tissues associated with the axial skeleton that are innervated by ventral rami of spinal nerves, via plexus *(A)* or segmental innervation *(B)*.

## SEGMENTAL INNERVATION

Ventral rami and associated branches that remain as single nerves form either intercostal or recurrent meningeal nerves. These innervate tissues throughout multiple segments or levels within the axial skeleton. This form of innervation is referred to as "segmental innervation" (Fig. 10–2B).

### Intercostal Nerves (T$^1$-T$^{12}$)

Each of the 12 ventral rami of the thoracic spinal nerves forms an intercostal nerve, innervating an intercostal dermatome and a set of intercostal muscles that share the same intercostal space. The T$^1$ ventral ramus forms the first intercostal nerve and part of the lower trunk of the brachial plexus. The ventral rami of T$^7$-T$^{12}$ also innervate the muscles of the anterior-lateral trunk (i.e., the "abdominal" muscles). The T$^{12}$ ventral ramus forms the last intercostal (sub-costal) nerve and part of the L$^1$ ventral ramus of the lumbar plexus.

### Recurrent Meningeal Nerves

Small nerves branch from the extreme proximal aspect of the ventral ramus at each spinal level. These nerves, such as the recurrent meningeal (sinuvertebral) nerve, provide mixed sensory and sympathetic nerve supply to connective tissues that surround the spinal cord or to those that reinforce each interbody joint.[10] As depicted in Figure 10–1, each recurrent meningeal nerve courses back into the intervertebral foramen, hence the name "recurrent," to supply dura mater, periosteum, blood vessels, posterior longitudinal ligament, and adjacent areas of the superficial part of the annulus fibrosus. The anterior longitudinal ligament receives sensory innervation from small branches from the ventral ramus and adjacent sympathetic connections.[10]

The nucleus pulposus and deeper parts of the annulus fibrosus do not receive sensory innervation. Localized pain from a herniated nucleus pulposis is likely due to pressure against the superficial part of the posterior annulus fibrosus or posterior longitudinal ligament. As described in Chapter 9, a herniated disc that causes pain or numbness to radiate down the lower extremity is likely due to pressure from a disc against a spinal nerve, as it exits the intervertebral foramen.

## Dorsal Ramus Innervation

### SEGMENTAL INNERVATION

A dorsal ramus branches from every spinal nerve, innervating structures in the back in a segmental fashion (Fig. 10–3). With the exception of the $C^1$ and $C^2$ dorsal rami, which are discussed separately, all dorsal rami are smaller than their ventral rami counterparts. In general, dorsal rami course a relatively short distance posteriorly, providing (1) segmental innervation to the deep layer of posterior muscles of the back, (2) dermatome sensation to the posterior back, and (3) sensation to the ligaments of the posterior aspect of each vertebrae and capsule of the apophyseal joints (Table 10–1).

The dorsal ramus of $C^1$ ("suboccipital" nerve) is primarily a motor nerve, innervating the suboccipital muscles. The dorsal ramus of $C^2$ is the largest cervical dorsal ramus. It innervates local muscles and contributes to the formation of the greater occipital nerve ($C^{2-3}$). This large nerve provides sensory innervation to the posterior scalp as far forward as the top of the head.

## TRUNK AND CRANIOCERVICAL REGIONS

### Introduction

The muscles of the axial skeleton can be organized into two categories. (1) the *trunk* and (2) the *craniocervical region*

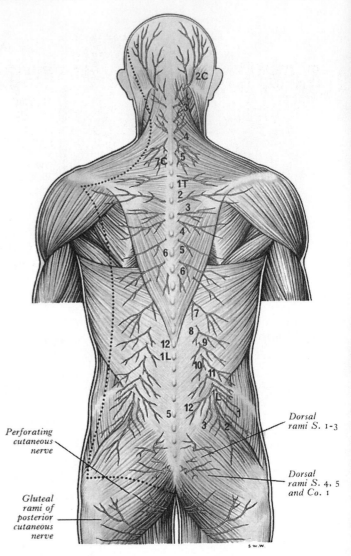

**FIGURE 10–3.** The cutaneous distribution is shown for the dorsal rami of spinal nerves. The nerves are numbered on the right side as 2C for the $C^2$ nerve, 1T for the $T^1$, and so forth. The spinous processes of various vertebral levels are numbered on the left side (7C for C7, 1L for L1, and so forth). The dotted line on the left indicates the lateral limit of skin that is innervated by the dorsal rami. (From Williams PL, Bannister LH, Berry M, et al: Gray's Anatomy, 38th ed. New York, Churchill Livingstone, 1995.)

(Table 10–2). The muscles within each category are further organized into sets, based on general location.

The material within each category is presented in two sections, the first covering anatomy and individual muscle actions, and the second covering examples of the functional interactions among the related muscles or muscle groups. Throughout this chapter, the reader is encouraged to consult Chapter 9 for a review of the pertinent osteology related to the attachments of muscles. Appendix III, Parts A to C, should be consulted for a summary of more detailed muscular anatomy and innervation to the muscles of the axial skeleton.

---

**TABLE 10–1. Examples of Tissues Innervated by Dorsal Rami of Spinal Nerves**

**$C^1$-$S^5$ Spinal Levels**

**Muscle**
1. Muscles in the deep layer of the back, such as the erector spinae and transversospinal muscles ($C^2$-$S^3$)
2. Splenius capitis ($C^{3-7}$)
3. Suboccipital muscles ($C^1$)

**Skin**
Posterior trunk ($C^2$-$S^5$)*

**Joint**
1. Capsule of apophyseal joints
2. Ligaments to the posterior aspect of a vertebrae
3. Sacroiliac joints and associated ligaments ($L^5$-$S^2$)

---

*Dorsal rami of lower sacral nerves fuse with dorsal rami of coccygeal nerves (sensory only).

| TABLE 10-2. Anatomic Organization of the Muscles of the Axial Skeleton* |
| --- |

**Muscles of the Trunk**

*Set 1: Muscles of the Posterior Trunk ("Back" Muscles)*

*Superficial layer*
    Trapezius, latissimus dorsi, rhomboids, levator scapula, and
        serratus anterior
*Intermediate layer†*
    Serratus posterior superior
    Serratus posterior inferior
*Deep layer*
    Three groups
        1. Erector spinae group (spinalis, longissimus, iliocostalis)
        2. Transversospinal group
            Semispinalis muscles
            Multifidi
            Rotatores
        3. Short segmental group
            Interspinalis muscles
            Intertransversarus muscles

*Set 2: Muscles of the Anterior-Lateral Trunk ("Abdominal" Muscles)*

    Rectus abdominis
    Obliquus internus abdominis
    Obliquus externus abdominis
    Transversus abdominis

*Set 3: Additional Muscles*

    Iliopsoas
    Quadratus lumborum

**Muscles of the Craniocervical Region**

*Set 1: Muscles of the Anterior-Lateral Craniocervical Region*

    Sternocleidomastoid
    Scalenes
        Scalenus anterior
        Scalenus medius
        Scalenus posterior
    Longus colli
    Longus capitis
    Rectus capitis anterior
    Rectus capitis lateralis

*Set 2: Muscles of the Posterior Craniocervical Region*

*Superficial group*
    Splenius cervicis
    Splenius capitis
*Deep group ("suboccipital" muscles)*
    Rectus capitis posterior major
    Rectus capitis posterior minor
    Obliquus capitis superior
    Obliquus capitis inferior

*A muscle is classified as belonging to the "trunk" or "craniocervical region" based on the location of the most of its attachments.
† These muscles are discussed in Chapter 11.

| Organization of the Presentation of the Muscles of the Trunk and Craniocervical Region |
| --- |
| *Muscles of the Trunk*<br>Section I: Anatomy and individual muscle action<br>Section II: Functional interactions among muscles<br><br>*Muscles of the Craniocervical Region*<br>Section I: Anatomy and individual muscle action<br>Section II: Functional interactions among muscles |

## Action of the Muscles of the Trunk and Craniocervical Region

### PRODUCTION OF INTERNAL TORQUE

By convention, the "strength" of a muscle action within the axial skeleton is expressed as an internal torque, defined for the sagittal, frontal, and horizontal planes. Within each plane, the maximal internal torque potential is equal to the product of (1) the muscle force generated parallel to a plane, and (2) the length of the internal moment arm available to the muscle (Fig. 10–4).

The spatial orientation of a muscle's line-of-force determines its effectiveness for producing a particular action. Consider, for example, the obliquus externus abdominis muscle producing a force across the lateral thorax, with a line-of-force oriented about 30 degrees from the vertical (Fig. 10–5). The muscle's resultant force vector can be trigonometrically partitioned into unequal vertical and horizontal force components. The vertical force component—about 86% of the muscle's maximal force—is available for producing lateral flexion or flexion torques. The horizontal force component—about 50% of the muscle's maximal force—is available for producing an axial rotation torque. (This estimation is based on cosine of 30 degrees equaling .86, and the sine of 30 equaling .5.) For a muscle to contribute *all* its force potential toward axial rotation, its overall line-of-force must be directed solely in the horizontal direction. For a muscle to contribute *all* its force potential toward either lateral flexion or flexion, its overall line-of-force must be directed vertically. The lines-of-force of muscles that control movement of the axial skeleton have a spatial orientation that varies over a wide spectrum, from nearly vertical to nearly horizontal.

More of the total muscle mass of the trunk is biased vertically than horizontally. This explains, in part, why maximal effort torques are generally greater for frontal and sagittal plane movements than for horizontal plane movements.[8,64]

### SPECIAL CONSIDERATIONS FOR THE STUDY OF MUSCLE ACTION WITHIN THE AXIAL SKELETON

To understand muscle action in the axial skeleton it is necessary to first consider the muscle during both unilateral and bilateral activations. *Bilateral activation* usually produces pure flexion or extension of the axial skeleton. Any potential for lateral flexion or axial rotation is neutralized by opposing forces in contralateral muscles. *Unilateral activation,* in contrast, tends to produce flexion or extension of the axial

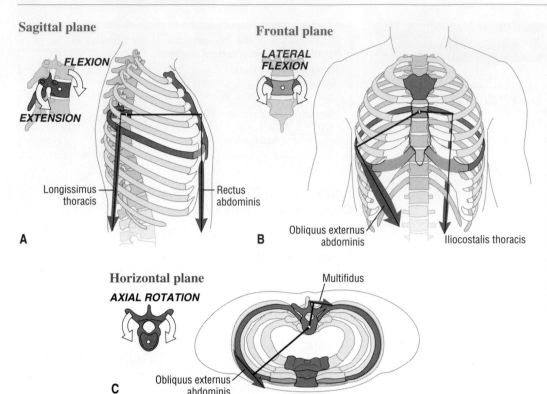

**Sagittal plane**

*FLEXION*

*EXTENSION*

Longissimus thoracis

Rectus abdominis

**A**

**Frontal plane**

*LATERAL FLEXION*

Obliquus externus abdominis

Iliocostalis thoracis

**B**

**FIGURE 10–4.** Selected muscles of the trunk are shown producing an internal torque within each of the three cardinal planes. The internal torque is equal to the product of the muscle force within a given plane and its internal moment arm, shown as dark bold lines. T6 is chosen as the representative axis of rotation (small open circle). In each case, the strength of a muscle action is determined by the distance and spatial orientation of the muscle's line-of-force relative to the axis of rotation.

**Horizontal plane**

*AXIAL ROTATION*

Multifidus

Obliquus externus abdominis

**C**

skeleton, with some combination of lateral flexion and contralateral or ipsilateral axial rotation. The term lateral flexion of the axial skeleton implies "ipsilateral" lateral flexion.

The action of a muscle within the axial skeleton depends, in part, on the relative degree of fixation, or stabilization, of the attachments of the muscle. As an example, consider the effect of a contraction of a member of the erector spinae group—a muscle that attaches to both the thorax and pel-

vis. With the pelvis stabilized, the muscle can extend the thorax; with the thorax stabilized, the muscle can rotate (tilt) the pelvis. If the thorax and pelvis are both free to move, the muscle can simultaneously extend the thorax and anteriorly tilt the pelvis. Unless otherwise stated, it is assumed that the superior (cranial) end of a muscle is less constrained and, therefore, freer to move than its inferior or caudal end.

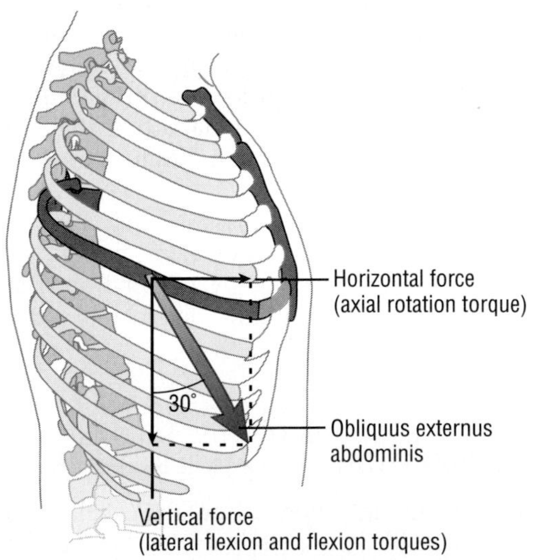

Depending on body position, gravity routinely assists or resists movements of the axial skeleton. Slowly flexing the head from the anatomic position, for example, is normally controlled by eccentric activation of the neck extensor muscles. Gravity, in this case, is the prime "flexor" of the head, whereas the extensor muscles control the speed and extent of the action. Rapidly flexing the head, however, requires a burst of concentric activation from the neck flexor muscles, because the desired speed of the motion may be greater than that produced by action of gravity alone. Unless otherwise stated, it is assumed that the action of a muscle is performed via a concentric contraction, rotating a body segment against gravity or against some other form of external resistance.

## Muscles of the Trunk—Section I: Anatomy and Individual Muscle Action

The following section describes the relationships between the anatomy and the actions of the muscles of the trunk.

Horizontal force (axial rotation torque)

30°

Obliquus externus abdominis

Vertical force (lateral flexion and flexion torques)

**FIGURE 10–5.** The line-of-force of the obliquus externus abdominis muscle is shown directed in the sagittal plane, with a spatial orientation about 30 degrees from the vertical. The resultant muscle force vector (red) is trigonometrically partitioned into a vertical force for the production of lateral flexion and flexion torques and a horizontal force for the production of axial rotation torque.

### SET 1: MUSCLES OF THE POSTERIOR TRUNK ("BACK" MUSCLES)

The muscles of the posterior trunk are organized into three layers: superficial, intermediate, and deep (see Table 10–2).

### Muscles in the Superficial and Intermediate Layers of the Back

The muscles in the superficial layer of the back are presented in the study of the shoulder (see Chapter 5). They include the trapezius, latissimus dorsi, rhomboids, levator scapula, and serratus anterior. The trapezius and latissimus dorsi are most superficial, followed by the deeper rhomboids and levator scapula. The serratus anterior muscle is located more laterally on the thorax.

In general, bilateral activation of the muscles of the superficial layer extends the adjacent region of the axial skeleton. Unilateral activation, however, laterally flexes and, in most cases, axially rotates the region.

The muscles included in the intermediate layer of the back are the serratus posterior superior and the serratus posterior inferior. They are located just deep to the rhomboids and latissimus dorsi. The serratus posterior superior and inferior are thin muscles that likely contribute little to the movement or stability of the trunk. Their function is more likely related to the mechanics of ventilation and, as such, are described in Chapter 11.

Muscles within the superficial and intermediate layers of the back are often referred to as "extrinsic muscles" because, from an embryologic perspective, they were originally associated with the front "limb buds" and only later migrated dorsally to their final position on the back. Interestingly, muscles such as the levator scapula, rhomboids, and serratus anterior, although located within the back, are actually upper limb muscles. All extrinsic muscles of the back are, therefore, innervated by ventral rami of spinal nerves (i.e., brachial plexus or intercostal nerves).

### Muscles in the Deep Layer of the Back

Muscles in the deep layer of the back are the (1) erector spinae group, (2) transversospinal group, and (3) short segmental group (Table 10–3). The anatomic organization of the erector spinae and transversospinal groups is illustrated in Figure 10–7.

In general, from superficial to deep, the fiber lengths of the muscles in the deep layer become progressively shorter. A muscle within the more superficial erector spinae group may extend virtually the entire length of the vertebral column. In contrast, muscles within the deeper short segmental group each cross only one intervertebral junction.

Although exceptions prevail, muscles in the deep layer of the back are innervated segmentally through the dorsal rami

---

### Muscles of the Superficial Layer of the Back: An Example of Muscles "Sharing" Actions Between the Axial and Appendicular Skeletons

Chapter 5 describes the actions of the muscles of the superficial layer of the back, based on their ability to rotate the appendicular skeleton (i.e., humerus, scapula, or clavicle) toward a fixed axial skeleton (i.e., head, vertebral column, or ribs). The same muscles, however, are equally capable of performing the "reverse" action (i.e., rotating segments of the axial skeleton toward the fixed appendicular skeleton). This muscular action is demonstrated by highlighting the functions of the trapezius and rhomboids while using a bow and arrow. As indicated in Figure 10–6, several muscles produce a force needed to stabilize the position of the scapula and abducted arm. Forces produced in the upper trapezius, middle trapezius, and rhomboids simultaneously rotate the cervical and upper thoracic spine to the left, indicated by the bidirectional arrows. This "contralateral" axial rotation effect is shown for C6 in the inset within Figure 10–6. As the muscle pulls the spinous process of C6 to the right, the anterior side of the vertebra is rotated to the left. The trapezius and rhomboids also stabilize the scapula against the pull of the posterior deltoid, long head of the triceps, and serratus anterior. These shared actions of the muscles of the superficial layer of the back demonstrate the inherent efficiency of the muscular system. In this example, a few muscles accomplish multiple actions that are shared across the axial and appendicular skeletons.

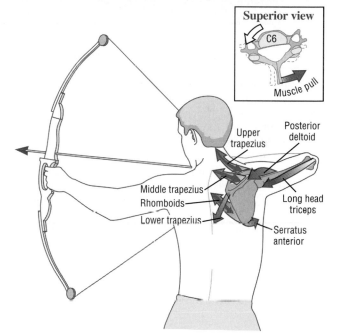

**FIGURE 10–6.** The actions of several muscles of the right shoulder and upper trunk are shown as an archer uses a bow and arrow. The upper trapezius, middle trapezius, and rhomboids demonstrate the dual action of (1) rotating the cervical and upper thoracic spine *to the left* (see inset) and (2) stabilizing the position of the right scapula relative to the thorax. The bidirectional arrows indicate the muscles simultaneously rotating the spinous process toward the scapula and stabilizing the scapula against the pull of the long head of the triceps, posterior deltoid, and serratus anterior.

### TABLE 10-3. Muscles in the Deep Layer of the Back

| Group (and Relative Depth) | Individual Muscles | General Fiber Direction | Comments |
|---|---|---|---|
| *Erector Spinae (Superficial)* | Iliocostalis lumborum<br>Iliocostalis thoracis<br>Iliocostalis cervicis | Cranial and lateral<br>Vertical<br>Cranial and medial | Most effective leverage for lateral flexion |
| | Longissimus thoracis<br>Longissimus cervicis<br>Longissimus capitis | Vertical<br>Cranial and medial<br>Cranial and lateral | Most developed of erector spinae group |
| | Spinalis thoracis<br>Spinalis cervicis<br>Spinalis capitis | Vertical<br>Vertical<br>Vertical | Poorly defined, fuses with semispinalis muscles |
| *Transversospinal (Intermediate)* | Semispinalis<br>  Semispinalis thoracis<br>  Semispinalis cervicis<br>  Semispinalis capitis | <br>Cranial and medial<br>Cranial and medial<br>Vertical | Cross six to eight intervertebral junctions |
| | Multifidi | Cranial and medial | Cross two to four intervertebral junctions |
| | Rotatores<br>  Rotator brevis<br>  Rotator longus | <br>Cranial and medial<br>Horizontal | Rotator longus crosses two intervertebral junctions; the rotator brevis crosses one intervertebral junction. The rotatores are most developed in thoracic region. |
| *Short Segmental (Deep)* | Interspinalis | Vertical | Both muscles cross one intervertebral junction. |
| | Intertransversarus | Vertical | Most developed in the cervical region. Interspinalis muscles are mixed with the interspinous ligaments. |

of spinal nerves.[84] A particularly long muscle within the erector spinae group, for instance, is innervated by multiple levels throughout the spinal cord. Embryologically, and unlike the muscles in the extremities and anterior-lateral trunk, the muscles in the deep layer of the back have retained their original location dorsal to the neuraxis. For this reason, these muscles are often called "intrinsic muscles" of the back.

As a general rule, most intrinsic muscles of the back are innervated by the dorsal rami of adjacent spinal nerves. In contrast, most extrinsic muscles of the back, such as the lastissimus dorsi and serratus posterior superior, are innervated by the ventral rami of spinal nerves, via the brachial plexus or intercostal nerves.

### Erector Spinae

The erector spinae are a large and rather poorly defined group of muscles that run on either side of the vertebral column, roughly within one hand's width from the spinous processes (Fig. 10–8). Most are located deep to the posterior layer of thoracolumbar fascia and the muscles in the intermediate and superficial layers of the back. The erector spinae consist of the spinalis, longissimus, and iliocostalis muscles. Each muscle is further subdivided topographically into three regions, producing a total of nine named muscles (see Table 10–3). Individual muscles overlap and vary greatly in size and length.

The bulk of the erector spinae muscles has a common

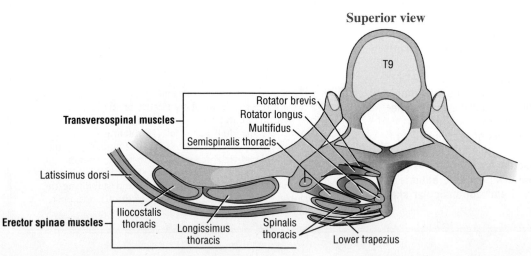

**Superior view**

**FIGURE 10–7.** Cross-sectional view through T9 highlighting the topographic organization of the erector spinae and the transversospinal group of muscles. The short segmental group of muscles is not shown.

**Posterior view**

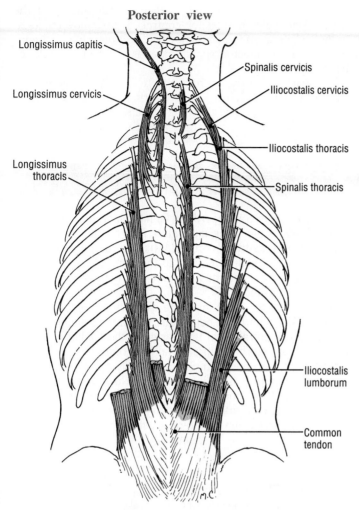

**FIGURE 10–8.** The muscles of the erector spinae group. For clarity, the left iliocostalis, left spinalis, and right longissimus muscles are cut just superior to the common tendon. (From Luttgens K, Hamilton N: Kinesiology: Scientific Basis of Human Motion, 9th ed. Madison, WI, Brown and Benchmark, 1997. The McGraw-Hill Companies.)

---

| TABLE 10–4. Attachments Made by the Common Tendon of the Erector Spinae |
|---|
| 1. Median sacral crests |
| 2. Spinous processes and supraspinous ligaments in the lower thoracic and entire lumbar region |
| 3. Iliac crests |
| 4. Sacrotuberous and sacroiliac ligaments |
| 5. Gluteus maximus |
| 6. Multifidi |

from the common tendon, attaching between the posterior end of the ribs and the transverse and articular processes of local vertebrae. In the neck, the longissimus cervicis angles slightly medially to attach to the posterior tubercles of the transverse processes of the cervical vertebrae (Fig. 10–8). The longissimus capitis, in contrast, angles slightly laterally to attach to the posterior margin of the mastoid process of the temporal bone. The more oblique angulation of the superior portion of the longissimus capitis and cervicis suggests that these muscles assist with ipsilateral axial rotation of the craniocervical region.

**Iliocostalis Muscles**

The iliocostalis muscles include the iliocostalis lumborum, iliocostalis thoracis, and iliocostalis cervicis. They occupy the most lateral column of the erector spinae group. The iliocos-

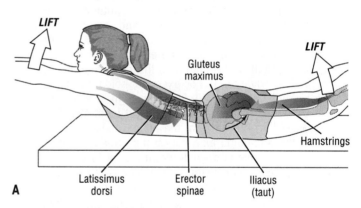

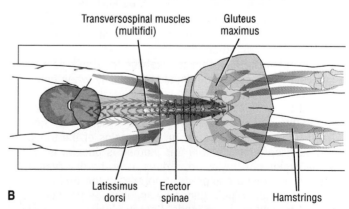

**FIGURE 10–9.** Muscle activation patterns of a healthy person while extending the trunk and head. The upper and lower extremities are also being lifted away from the supporting surface. *A,* Side view. *B,* Top view. Note in *A* that the stretched iliacus muscle contributes to the anterior tilted position of the pelvis.

---

attachment on a broad, thick tendon located superficial to the sacrum (see Fig. 10–8). This common tendon anchors the erector spinae to many locations (Table 10–4). From this common tendon arises three poorly organized vertical columns of muscle: the spinalis, longissimus, and iliocostalis.[6,49,84]

**Spinalis Muscles**

Spinalis muscles include the spinalis thoracis, spinalis cervicis, and spinalis capitis. In general, they insert superiorly on lateral aspects of the spinous processes or ligamentum nuchae in the cervical region. Spinalis muscles are usually indistinct from surrounding muscles or missing entirely. The spinalis capitis, if present, often blends with the semispinalis capitis.[84]

**Longissimus Muscles**

The longissimus muscles include the longissimus thoracis, longissimus cervicis, and longissimus capitis. As a set, they are the largest and most developed of the erector spinae group. The fibers of the longissimus muscles fan cranially

talis muscles run cranially from the common tendon. The iliocostalis lumborum and thoracis insert generally lateral to the angle of the ribs. The iliocostalis cervicis attaches to the posterior tubercles of the transverse processes of the mid cervical vertebrae, along with the longissimus cervicis.

### Summary of the Erector Spinae Group

The erector spinae muscles cross a considerable distance along the axial skeleton. This anatomic feature suggests a design more suited for control of gross movements of the entire axial skeleton than for control of finer movements at individual intervertebral junctions. As a group, bilateral contraction of the erector spinae extends the trunk, neck, or head (Fig. 10–9).

By attaching to the sacrum and to the pelvis, the erector spinae can anteriorly tilt the pelvis, thereby accentuating the lumbar lordosis. (Pelvic tilt describes a sagittal plane rotation of the pelvis about the hips. The direction of the tilt is

## SPECIAL FOCUS 10–2

### Forces Generated by the Lumbar Extensor Muscles While Carrying External Loads

Because of the ventral positioning of the eyes and arms, external loads are frequently manipulated, passed, or carried anterior to the body. The lumbar extensor muscles—such as the erector spinae—are consistently required to produce large internal forces in response to these ventrally placed external loads. The force demands on the entire set of lumbar extensor muscles are typically large due to the muscle groups' overall poor mechanical advantage (i.e., the ratio of internal-to-external moment arm; see Chapter 1). A typical erector spinae muscle in the lumbar region, for instance, may have an internal moment arm of 5 cm, whereas the external moment arm of a hand-held load could be as great as 70 cm—the horizontal distance between the lumbar vertebral body and the outstretched hand. Given a mechanical advantage of .07 (5/70), the extensor muscles must produce a force 14 times larger than the weight of the load (i.e., the reciprocal of the mechanical advantage). For example, holding a gallon of water weighing about 35.6 N (about 8 lb) at a distance 70 cm in front of the chest requires at least 498 N (about 112 lb) of force from the lumbar extensor muscles. If the additional external torque created by both outstretched arms is considered, the total force required by the lumbar extensor muscles is more than doubled! Although this muscular force is only about 25% of the total maximal force potential of the lumbar extensor muscles,[10] this example does partially explain why the lumbar spine and associated extensor muscles are inherently vulnerable to injury when one handles relatively light materials.

For persons vulnerable to disabling low-back pain, carrying loads should be limited, especially when held in front of the body. If loads must be carried, they should be as *light* as possible, and carried as *close* to the body as possible. Carrying a load directly over the head reduces the demands on all muscles of the trunk. Although carrying loads in this method is popular in some regions of the world, it does have the disadvantage of increased compression forces on the craniocervical region which, generally speaking, is not designed to support large loads. Carrying loads in a backpack is an alternative. As shown by the electromyographic (EMG) study associated with Figure 10–10,

carrying loads in a standard backpack generated, on average, about the same magnitude from the lumbar erector spinae as that produced when not carrying a load.[15] This is in sharp contrast to the large EMG response from the same muscles when carrying the same load anterior to the trunk.

Note in Figure 10–10 the large disparity in erector spinae EMG when hand-held loads are carried either ipsilateral or contralateral to the side of the lumbar extensor muscle. The contralateral load requires a large lateral flexion torque produced unilaterally by the lumbar erector spinae, as well as the other lumbar extensor muscles. This information is helpful when advising persons about safe methods of carrying hand-held loads, especially when unilateral muscle, joint, or connective tissue injury is suspected.

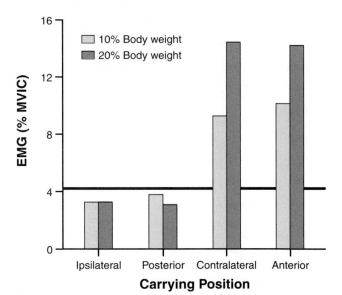

**FIGURE 10–10.** Mean electromyographic (EMG) values—expressed as a percent of maximal voluntary isometric contraction (MVIC)—from the lumbar erector spinae muscles while walking and carrying loads of two sizes and four carrying positions. The carrying position noted on the X axis is based on the position of the load relative to the erector spinae muscles. The bold horizontal line marks the EMG response while subjects walked without carrying a load. (Data from Cook TM, Neumann DA: The effects of load placement on the EMG activity of the low back muscles during load carry by men and women. Ergonomics 30: 1413–1423, 1987.)

indicated by the rotation direction of the iliac crests.) As depicted in Figure 10–9A, the anterior pelvic tilt is accentuated by the increased tension in stretched hip flexor muscles, such as the iliacus.

Contracting unilaterally, the laterally located iliocostalis muscles are the most effective lateral flexors of the erector spinae group. The cranial or cervical components of the longissimus and iliocostalis muscles assist with ipsilateral axial rotation, especially when the head and neck are fully and contralaterally rotated. The iliocostalis lumborum assists slightly with ipsilateral axial rotation.

### Transversospinal Muscles

Located immediately deep to the erector spinae muscles is the transversospinal muscle group: the semispinalis, multifidi, and rotatores (Figs. 10–11 and 10–12). Semispinalis muscles are located superficially; the multifidi, intermediately; and the rotatores, deeply.

The name transversospinal refers to the general attachments of most of the muscles, (i.e., from the transverse processes of one vertebra to the spinous processes of a more superiorly located vertebra). With a few exceptions, these attachments align most muscle fibers in a cranial and medial

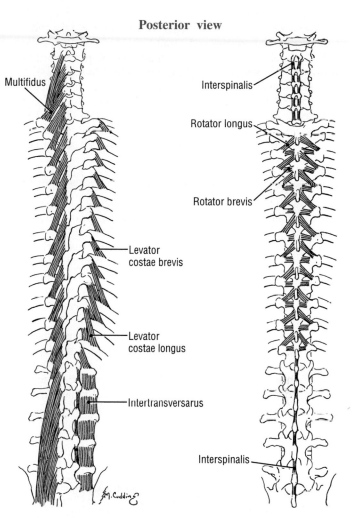

**Posterior view**

**FIGURE 10–12.** A posterior view shows the deeper muscles within the transversospinal group (multifidi and rotatores) and the muscles within the short segmental group (interspinalis and intertransversarus). The intertransversarus muscles are shown for the right side of the lumbar region only. The levator costae muscles are involved with force inspiration and are discussed in Chapter 11. (From Luttgens K, Hamilton N: Kinesiology: Scientific Basis of Human Motion, 9th ed. Madison, WI, Brown and Benchmark, 1997. The McGraw-Hill Companies.)

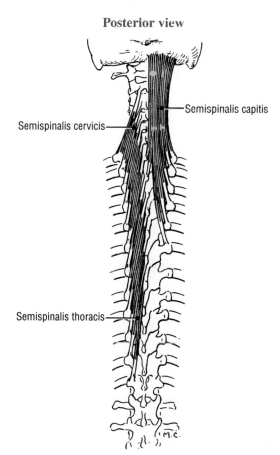

**Posterior view**

**FIGURE 10–11.** A posterior view shows the more superficial semispinalis muscles within the transversospinal group. For clarity, only the left semispinalis cervicis, left semispinalis thoracis, and right semispinalis capitis are included. (From Luttgens K, Hamilton N: Kinesiology: Scientific Basis of Human Motion, 9th ed. Madison, WI, Brown and Benchmark, 1997. The McGraw-Hill Companies.)

direction. Many of the muscles within the transversospinal group are morphologically very similar, varying primarily in length and in the number of intervertebral junctions that each muscle crosses (Table 10–5).

**TABLE 10–5. Basic Morphologic Characteristics of the Muscles within the Transversospinal Group**

| Muscle | Relative Length | Average Number of Intervertebral Junctions Crossed |
|--------|-----------------|----------------------------------------------------|
| Semispinalis | Long | 6–8 |
| Multifidi | Intermediate | 2–4 |
| Rotatores | Short | 1–2 |

### Semispinalis Muscles

The semispinalis muscles consist of the semispinalis thoracis, semispinalis cervicis, and semispinalis capitis (Fig. 10–11). In general, each muscle, or main set of fibers within each muscle, crosses six to eight intervertebral junctions. The *semispinalis thoracis* consists of many thin muscle fasciculi, interconnected by long tendons. Muscle fibers attach from transverse processes of T6-10 to spinous processes of C6-T4.

The *semispinalis cervicis,* much thicker and more developed than the semispinalis thoracis, attaches from upper thoracic transverse processes to spinous processes of C2-5. Muscle fibers that attach to the prominent spinous process of the axis (C2) are particularly well developed, serving as important stabilizers for the suboccipital muscles.

The *semispinalis capitis* lies deep to the splenius and trapezius muscles. The muscle arises primarily from upper thoracic transverse processes. The muscle thickens superiorly as it attaches to a relatively large region on the occipital bone, filling much of the area between the superior and inferior nuchal lines (see Fig. 9–3).

The semispinalis cervicis and capitis are the largest muscles that cross the posterior side of the neck. Their large size and near-vertical fiber direction provide significant extension torque to the craniocervical region. Right and left semispinalis capitis muscles are readily palpable as thick and round cords on either side of the midline of the upper neck, especially evident in infants and in thin, muscular adults (Fig. 10–13).

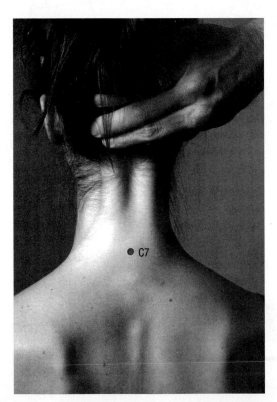

**FIGURE 10–13.** A thin, healthy 22-year-old female demonstrates the contours of the activated right and left semispinalis capitis muscles. Manual resistance is applied against an extension effort of the head. The red dot indicates the spinous process of the C7 vertebra.

---

| TABLE 10–6. Multiple Attachments of the Multifidi Throughout the Lumbosacral Region |
| --- |
| **Inferior Attachments** |
| 1. Mammillary processes of lumbar vertebrae |
| 2. Lumbosacral ligaments |
| 3. Deeper part of the common tendon of the erector spinae |
| 4. Posterior surface of the sacrum |
| 5. Posterior-superior iliac spine of pelvis |
| 6. Capsule of apophyseal joints |
| **Superior Attachments** |
| 1. Lumbar spinous processes |

### Multifidi

Multifidi lie under the semispinalis muscles. The plural "multifidi" indicates a collection of multiple fibers, rather than a set of individual muscles. All multifidi share a similar fiber direction and length, extending between the posterior sacrum and C2. In general, the multifidi originate from the transverse process of one vertebra and insert on the spinous process of a vertebra located two to four segments above (see Fig. 10–12).

Multifidi are thickest and most developed in the lumbosacral region (Table 10–6).[51] Muscle fibers within the lumbar region fill much of the concave space formed between the spinous and transverse processes. Throughout the lumbar region, the multifidi approach the spinous processes at essentially right angles to the long axis of each corresponding spinous process.[48] This angle is only apparent from a lateral view. This line-of-force maximally converts a force into a torque. The multifidi, therefore, provide an essential source of extension torque and stability to the base of the spine. Excessive force in the lumbar multifidi—due either to active contraction or protective spasm—maybe expressed clinically as an exaggerated lordosis.

### Rotatores

The rotatores are the deepest of the transversospinal group of muscles. Like the multifidi, the rotatores consist of a large set of individual muscle fibers. Although the rotatores exist throughout the entire vertebral column, they are best developed in the thoracic region (see Fig. 10–12). Each fiber attaches between the transverse process of one vertebra and the lamina and base of the spinous process of a vertebra located one or two segments above. By definition, the *rotator brevis muscle* spans one intervertebral junction, and the *rotator longus muscle* spans two intervertebral junctions.

### Summary of the Transversospinal Muscle Group

The transversospinal muscles consist of those that, on average, cross fewer intervertebral junctions than the erector spinae group. This feature suggests that, in general, the muscles are designed to produce relatively fine controlled movements across the axial skeleton, at least when compared with the erector spinae.

Contracting bilaterally, the transversospinal muscles extend the axial skeleton (Fig. 10–9B). Increased extension torque exaggerates the lumbar and cervical lordosis and decreases the thoracic kyphosis. The size and thickness of the transversospinal muscles are greatest at either end of the axial skeleton. Cranially, the semispinalis cervicis and capitis are very well-developed extensors of the craniocervical region; caudally, the lumbar multifidi are very well-developed extensors of the lumbar region.

Contracting unilaterally, the transversospinal muscles laterally flex the spine; however, their leverage for this action is limited due to their close proximity to the vertebral column. The more obliquely oriented transversospinal muscles assist with contralateral axial rotation. From a relatively fixed transverse process, contraction of a single right multifidus or rotator longus, for example, can rotate a superiorly located spinous process toward the right and, as a result, rotate the anterior side of the vertebra to the left. Compared with all the trunk muscles, however, the transversospinal muscles are secondary axial rotators. The leverage for axial rotation is relatively poor due to the muscle's proximity to the vertebral column. Compare the multifidi to the obliquus abdominis externus, for example, in Figure 10–4C. Furthermore, the prevailing line-of-force typical of transversospinal muscle fiber is directed more vertically than horizontally, thereby providing a greater force potential for extension than for axial rotation.

### Short Segmental Group of Muscles

The short segmental group of muscles consists of the *interspinalis* and the *intertransversarus muscles* (see Fig. 10–12). (The plural "interspinales and intertransversales" is often used to describe all the members within the entire set of these muscles.) They lie deep to the transversospinal group of muscles. The name "short segmental" refers to the extremely short length and highly segmented organization of the muscles. Each individual interspinalis or intertransversarus muscle crosses just one intervertebral junction. The short segmental group of muscles exists throughout the vertebral column except for the thoracic region. These muscles are most developed in the cervical region, where fine control of the head and neck is so critical.

Each pair of interspinalis muscles is located on either side of, and often blends with, the corresponding interspinous ligament. The interspinales have a relatively favorable leverage and optimal fiber direction for producing extension torque. The magnitude of this torque is relatively small, however, considering the small size of the muscles.

Each right and left pair of intertransversarus muscles is located between adjacent transverse processes. As a group, the anatomy of the intertransversales is more complex than that of the interspinales.[84] In the cervical region, for example, each intertransversarus muscle is divided into small anterior and posterior muscles, between which pass the ventral rami of spinal nerves.

As a group, unilateral contraction of the intertransversales laterally flexes the vertebral column. Although the magnitude of the lateral flexion torque is relatively small compared with other muscle groups, the torque likely provides an important source of intervertebral stability.

### Summary of the Short Segmental Group of Muscles

The interspinalis and intertransversarus muscles consist of multiple short pairs of fibers, each of which crosses only one intervertebral junction. The highly segmented nature of these muscles contributes to fine control of the axial skeleton. These muscles also provide a rich source of segmental sensory feedback, especially in the craniocervical region.[10] Feedback helps coordinate the position of the head and neck with the position of the visual and auditory systems.

## SET 2: MUSCLES OF THE ANTERIOR-LATERAL TRUNK ("ABDOMINAL" MUSCLES)

The muscles of the anterior-lateral trunk include the rectus abdominis, obliquus externus abdominis, obliquus internus abdominis, and transversus abdominis (Fig. 10–14A to D). As a group, they are often referred to as the abdominal muscles. The rectus abdominis is a long straplike muscle, located on either side of the midline of the body. The obliquus externus abdominis, obliquus internus abdominis, and transversus abdominis—the lateral abdominals—are wide and flat, layered superficial to deep, across the lateral aspect of the abdomen.

The abdominal muscles have several physiologic and kinesiologic functions (Table 10–7). This chapter emphasizes the muscles' kinesiologic functions.

### Formation of the Rectus Sheaths and Linea Alba

The obliquus externus abdominis, obliquus internus abdominis, and transversus abdominis muscles from the right and left sides of the body fuse at the midline of the abdomen through a blending of connective tissues. Each muscle contributes a thin bilaminar sheet of connective tissue that ultimately forms the *anterior and posterior rectus sheaths*. As depicted in Figure 10–15, the anterior rectus sheath is formed from connective tissues from the obliquus externus abdominis and the obliquus internus abdominis muscles. The posterior rectus sheath is formed from connective tissues from the obliquus internus abdominis and transversus abdominis. Both sheaths surround the vertically oriented rec-

| TABLE 10–7. Physiologic And Kinesiologic Functions of the Abdominal Muscles | |
| --- | --- |
| **Physiologic Functions** | **Kinesiologic Functions** |
| 1. Supports and protects the abdominal viscera<br>2. Increases intra-abdominal pressure for forced expiration of air from the lungs, vomiting, micturition, defecation, and parturition<br>3. Increases intrathoracic pressure for forced expiration of air from the lungs | 1. Moves and stabilizes the trunk<br>2. Supports the lumbar spine and sacroiliac joint during forceful conditions such as lifting heavy loads<br>3. Stabilizes the proximal bony attachments of hip and knee muscles |

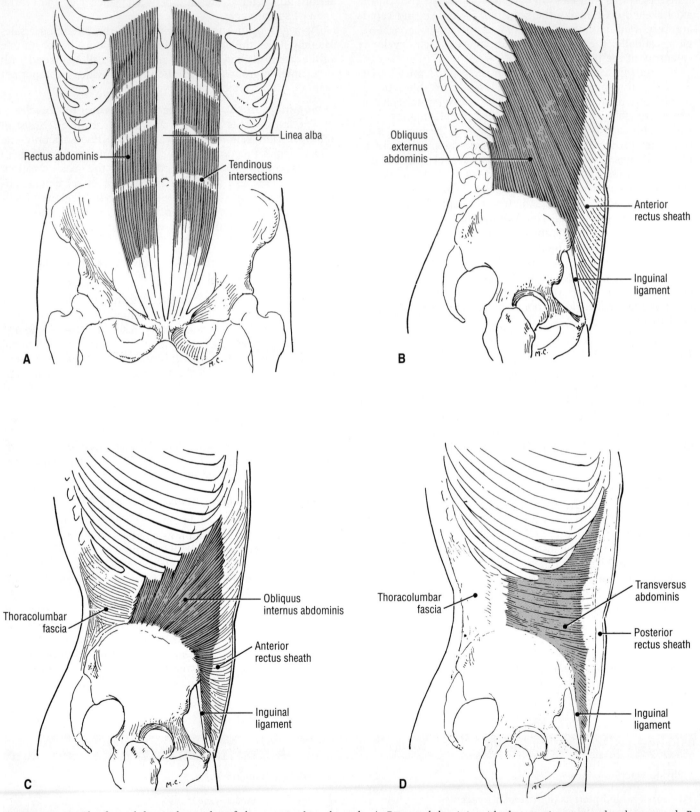

**FIGURE 10–14.** The four abdominal muscles of the anterior-lateral trunk. *A,* Rectus abdominis with the anterior rectus sheath removed. *B,* Obliquus externus abdominis. *C,* Obliquus internus abdominis, deep to the obliquus externus abdominis. *D,* Transversus abdominis, deep to other abdominal muscles. (From Luttgens K, Hamilton N: Kinesiology: Scientific Basis of Human Motion, 9th ed. Madison, WI, Brown and Benchmark, 1997. The McGraw-Hill Companies.)

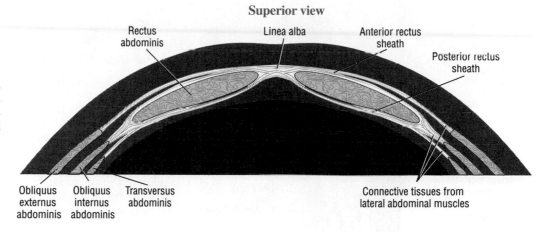

**Superior view**

**FIGURE 10–15.** Horizontal cross-sectional view of the anterior abdominal wall shown at the approximate level of the third lumbar vertebra.

tus abdominis muscle and continue medially to fuse with identical connective tissues from the other side of the abdomen.[71] (This general anatomic arrangement pertains to the abdominal wall located above the level of the iliac crests. Below this level both anterior and posterior rectus sheaths course anterior to the rectus abdominis.) The connective tissues thicken and crisscross as they traverse the midline, forming the *linea alba* (from the Latin *linea*, line, and *albus*, white). Anatomically, the linea alba is described as a "tendinous raphe," running longitudinally between the xiphoid process and pubic symphysis and pubic crest.[84]

The crisscross arrangement of the fibers within the linea alba adds considerable strength to the abdominal wall, much like the laminated structure of plywood. The linea alba also mechanically links the right and left lateral abdominal muscles, providing an effective way to transfer muscular force across the midline of the body.

### Anatomy of the Abdominal Muscles

The *rectus abdominis muscle* consists of right and left halves, separated by the linea alba. Each half of the muscle runs longitudinally, widening as it ascends within an open sleeve formed between the anterior and posterior rectus sheaths. The muscle is intersected and reinforced by three fibrous bands, known as *tendinous intersections*. These bands blend with the anterior rectus sheath. The rectus abdominis arises from the region on and surrounding the crest of the pubis, and it attaches superiorly on the xiphoid process and cartilages of the fifth through seventh ribs.

The anatomic organization of the obliquus externus abdominis, obliquus internus abdominis, and transversus abdominis muscles is different from that of the rectus abdominis. As a group, the lateral muscles originate laterally or posterior-laterally on the trunk and run in a different direction toward the midline, eventually blending with the linea alba and contralateral rectus sheaths (Table 10–8).

The *obliquus externus abdominis* is the largest and most superficial of the lateral abdominal muscles. The external oblique muscles travel in an inferior-and-medial direction, as if the hands were placed in pockets. The *obliquus internus abdominis* is located immediately deep to external oblique muscle, forming the second layer of the lateral abdominals. Most of its fibers originate on the iliac crest and adjacent thoracolumbar fascia. From this lateral attachment point, the fibers course in a cranial-and-medial direction toward the linea alba and lower ribs. As evident in Figure 10–14C, the inferior attachments of the internal oblique muscle extend to the inguinal ligament. The mean fiber direction of the internal oblique muscle is nearly perpendicular to the mean fiber direction of the overlying external oblique muscle.

| Muscle | Lateral Attachments | Midline Attachments | Actions on the Trunk |
|---|---|---|---|
| Obliquus externus abdominis | Lateral side of ribs 4–12 | Iliac crest, linea alba, and contralateral rectus sheaths | *Bilaterally:* flexion of the trunk and posterior tilt of the pelvis<br>*Unilaterally:* lateral flexion and contralateral rotation of the trunk. |
| Obliquus internus abdominis | Iliac crest, inguinal ligament, and thoracolumbar fascia | Ribs 9–12, linea alba, and contralateral rectus sheaths | *Bilaterally:* as above, plus increases tension in the thoracolumbar fascia<br>*Unilaterally:* lateral flexion and ipsilateral rotation of the trunk |
| Transversus abdominis | Iliac crest, thoracolumbar fascia, inner surface of the cartilages of ribs 6–12, and the inguinal ligament | Linea alba and contralateral rectus sheaths | *Bilaterally:* compression of the abdominal cavity, plus increases tension in the thoracolumbar fascia |

**T A B L E  10 – 8. Attachments and Individual Actions of the Lateral Abdominal Muscles**

ments to the thoracolumbar fascia. The transversus abdominis and the internal oblique muscles share many attachments, including the thoracolumbar fascia.

### Actions of the Abdominal Muscles

*Bilateral action* of the abdominal muscles reduces the distance between the xiphoid process and the pubic symphysis. Depending on which body segment is more stable, contraction of the abdominal muscles can flex the thorax and upper lumbar spine, posteriorly tilt the pelvis, or both. Figure 10–16 depicts a diagonally performed sit-up maneuver that places a relatively large demand on the oblique abdominal muscles. During a sagittal plane sit-up, the opposing axial rotation and lateral flexion tendencies of the various abdominal muscles are neutralized by opposing right and left muscles.

The axes of rotation for all motions of the vertebral column are biased posteriorly in the trunk, through the vertebral bodies. As a consequence, the abdominal muscles, most notably the rectus abdominis, possess very favorable leverage for generating trunk flexion torque (Fig. 10–17). Note in Figure 10–17 that, with the exception of the psoas major, all muscles have a moment arm to produce torques in both sagittal and frontal planes.

Contracting unilaterally, the abdominal muscles laterally flex the trunk. The external and internal obliques are particularly effective in this action owing to their relatively favorable leverage (i.e., long moment arms) (Fig. 10–17) and, as a pair, relatively large cross-sectional area. The combined cross-sectional area of the external and internal obliques at L4-L5 is almost twice that of the rectus abdominis muscle.[58]

Lateral flexion of the trunk often involves both trunk flexor and extensor muscles. For example, lateral flexion against resistance to the right demands a contraction from the right external and internal oblique, right erector spinae, and right transversospinal muscles. Coactivation amplifies the total frontal torque and simultaneously stabilizes the

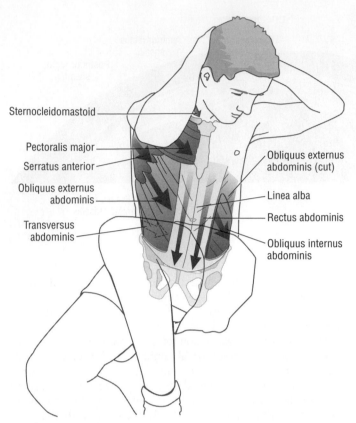

**FIGURE 10–16.** Typical muscle activation pattern is shown of a healthy person performing a diagonal sit-up maneuver that incorporates trunk flexion and axial rotation to the left.

The *transversus abdominis* is the deepest of the abdominal muscles. The muscle is also known as the "corset muscle," reflecting its primary functions of increasing intra-abdominal pressure and in stabilizing the lumbar region through attach-

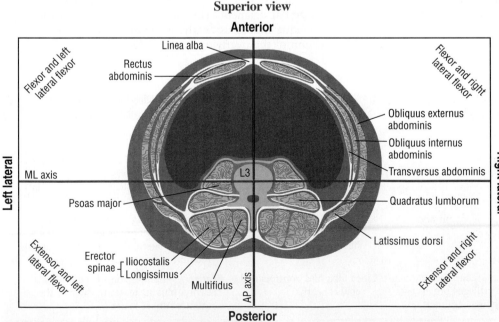

**FIGURE 10–17.** Horizontal cross-sectional view through several muscles of the trunk at the approximate level of the third lumbar vertebra. The potential of muscles to produce a torque in both sagittal and frontal planes is shown. The anterior-posterior (AP) axis of rotation (red) and medial-lateral (ML) axis of rotation (black) intersect in the center of the third lumbar vertebra. Muscles located anterior and posterior to the medial-lateral axis have the potential to flex and extend the trunk, respectively; muscles located right and left to the anterior-posterior axis have the potential to laterally flex the trunk to right and left, respectively.

trunk within the sagittal plane. Various muscle actions can be verified by studying the position of the muscles relative to the axes of rotation (see Fig. 10–17).

The internal and external oblique muscles are the most effective axial rotators of the trunk. Strong axial rotation potential is due to their relatively large combined cross-sectional area and favorable leverage (see Fig. 10–4C, extended moment arm length of the obliquus externus abdominis). During axial rotation, the external oblique muscle functions synergistically with the contralateral internal oblique muscle (see Fig. 10–16). As a pair, the external and internal oblique muscles from opposite sides of the body produce a diagonal line-of-force that crosses the midline through their mutual attachments into the linea alba. When contracting together, the two muscles reduce the distance between one shoulder and the contralateral iliac crest. By considering each muscle separately, the external oblique muscle is a contralateral rotator of the trunk, and the internal oblique muscle is an ipsilateral rotator of the trunk. Although anatomically thought of as two separate muscles, during active rotation of the trunk the external and internal oblique muscles from opposite sides function as one muscle, joined in the midline by the linea alba.

The torque demands placed on the axial rotators of the trunk vary considerably based on the nature of the given activity. Torque demands are relatively large during high

power axial rotations, such as sprinting, wrestling, and throwing a discus or javelin. The demands are very low, however, during activities that involve slow twisting of the trunk in an upright position, such as walking. Because axial rotation occurs in the horizontal plane, the muscles do not have to overcome the external torque generated by gravity.[46] Their primary resistance is that caused by the inertia of the upper body and the passive tension created by the stretching antagonist muscles.

### Trunk Flexor versus Trunk Extensor Peak Internal Torque

In the healthy adult, the magnitude of maximal effort trunk flexion torque is typically less than maximal effort trunk extension torque. Although data vary owing to gender, age, health, and angular velocity of the testing device, the flexor-to-extensor ratios determined isometrically are generally between .51 and .77.[8,65] Although the trunk flexor muscles possess greater leverage for sagittal plane torque, the trunk extensor muscles possess greater mass and, equally important, greater overall vertical orientation of muscle fibers.[24,58] The relatively greater torque potential of the back extensor muscles, at least isometrically, reflects the muscle's predominant role in counteracting gravity, either for the maintenance of upright posture or for carrying loads in front of the chest.

## SET 3: ADDITIONAL MUSCLES (ILIOPSOAS AND QUADRATUS LUMBORUM)

Although the iliopsoas and quadratus lumborum are not anatomically considered as muscles of the trunk, they are strongly associated with the movement of this region.

### Iliopsoas

The iliopsoas is a large muscle consisting of two parts: the iliacus and the psoas major (see Fig. 12–29). As are most hip flexors, the iliopsoas is innervated by the femoral nerve, a large branch from the lumbar plexus. The iliacus has a proximal attachment on the iliac fossa and lateral sacrum, just anterior and superior to the sacroiliac joint. The psoas major attaches proximally to the transverse processes of the T12 to L5, including the intervertebral discs. The two muscles fuse distal to the inguinal ligament and attach as a single tendon to the lesser trochanter of the femur.

The iliopsoas is a long muscle, exerting a potent kinetic influence across the lumbar spine, lumbosacral junction, and hip joint. Crossing anterior to the hip, it is a dominant flexor, drawing the femur toward the pelvis or the pelvis toward the femur. In the last movement, the iliopsoas can anteriorly tilt the pelvis, a motion that increases the lordosis of the lumbar region (see Fig. 9–68A).

### Function of the Psoas Major at the Lumbosacral Region

In the anatomic position, the psoas major demonstrates effective leverage for lateral flexion of the lumbar spine.[45] Little, if any, leverage exists for axial rotation. The flexor and extensor capacity of the psoas major differs throughout the lumbosacral region (Fig. 10–18). Across the L5-S1 junction, the psoas major has an approximate 2-cm moment arm for flexion.[59] The psoas major is, therefore, an effective flexor of the lower end of the lumbar spine relative to the sacrum.

Progressing superiorly toward L1, the line-of-force of the psoas major gradually shifts slightly posterior, falling either through or just posterior to the multiple medial-lateral axes

**SPECIAL   FOCUS   10 – 3**

### Role of Trunk Extensors as "Rotational Synergists" to the Oblique Abdominal Muscles

Although the external and internal obliques are considered the primary axial rotators of the trunk, they rarely act alone during this activity. Secondary axial rotators of the trunk include the ipsilateral latissimus dorsi, the more oblique components of the ipsilateral longissimus and iliocostalis muscles, and the contralateral transversospinal muscles. In addition to contributing, at least minimally, to axial rotation torque, the secondary axial rotators perform the more important function of counteracting the trunk flexion potential of the oblique abdominal muscles.[39] Axial rotation of the trunk to the left, for example, requires strong activation from both right and left transversospinal muscles in the thoracic region.[22] Bilateral activation resists the bilateral flexion tendency of the oblique abdominal muscles.

The multifidi muscles provide extension stability to the lumbar region during axial rotation.[48,83] Pathology involving the apophyseal joints or discs in the lumbar region may be associated with weakness, fatigue, or reflexive inhibition of these muscles. Without adequate activation from the multifidi during axial rotation, the partially unopposed oblique muscles would, in theory, create a subtle flexion bias to the base of the spine. Such a bias may partially explain the rounded (flexed) posture of the low back typically seen in a person with spondylosis or disc disease of the lumbar spine.

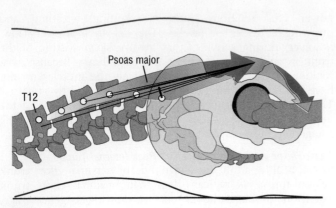

**FIGURE 10–18.** A lateral view of the psoas major highlights its multiple lines-of-force relative to the medial-lateral axis of rotation within the T12-L5 and L5-S1 intervertebral junctions. Note that the lines-of-force pass near or through the axes, with the exception of L5-S1. The flexion moment arm of the psoas major at L5-S1 is shown as the short black line.

of rotation. This reduces or eliminates its flexor and extensor capacity. Psoas major is neither a dominant flexor nor extensor of the lumbar region, but rather a dominant vertical stabilizer.[72] The term "vertical stabilizer" describes a muscular function of stabilizing a region of the axial skeleton in a near vertical position while maintaining its natural physiologic curve. Because of the lack of effective leverage in the lumbar region, the psoas major has a minimal role in directly influencing the degree of lordosis.[72] The iliopsoas, as most hip flexors, can indirectly increase the lordotic posture of the lumbar spine by tilting the pelvis anteriorly.

Through attachments on the lumbar spine, the psoas major affords excellent control of the sagittal plane positions of the trunk relative to the thighs, especially when sitting.[40]

---

**Actions of the Iliopsoas**

*Iliacus*
1. Predominant hip flexor, both femur-on-pelvis and pelvis-on-femur

*Psoas Major*
1. Lateral flexor of the lumbar region
2. Flexor of the lower lumbar spine (L5) relative to the sacrum (S1)
3. Vertical stabilizer of the lumbar spine

---

### Quadratus Lumborum

Anatomically, the quadratus lumborum is considered a muscle of the posterior abdominal wall. The muscle attaches inferiorly to the iliolumbar ligament and iliac crest, and superiorly to the 12th rib and the tips of the transverse processes of L1-4 (Fig. 10–19). The relative thickness of the muscle is evident by viewing Figure 10–17. The quadratus lumborum is innervated by the ventral rami of spinal nerves T[12]-L[3].

Contracting *bilaterally,* the quadratus lumborum is an extensor of the lumbar region. Its action is based on the line-of-force passing about 3.5 cm posterior to the medial-lateral axis of rotation at L3.[59]

Contracting *unilaterally,* the quadratus lumborum has relatively favorable leverage as a lateral flexor of the lumbar region.[59] The axial rotation potential of the quadratus lumborum, however, is minimal.

Clinically, the quadratus lumborum is often called a "hip hiker" when describing its role in walking, especially for persons with paraplegia at or below the L[1] neurologic level. By elevating (hiking) one side of the pelvis, the quadratus lumborum raises the lower limb to clear the foot from the ground during the swing phase of brace-assisted ambulation.

---

**Actions of the Quadratus Lumborum**

*Acting Bilaterally*
1. Extension of the lumbar region
2. Vertical stabilization of the lumbar spine, including the lumbosacral junction

*Acting Unilaterally*
1. Lateral flexion of the lumbar region
2. Elevation of one side of the pelvis ("hip hiking")

---

Both the psoas major and the quadratus lumborum provide substantial muscular stability to the lumbar spine. Both muscles run nearly vertical on either side of the lumbar vertebrae (see Fig. 10–17). A strong bilateral contraction of both muscles affords excellent vertical stability throughout the entire base of the spine, including the L5-S1 junction.

## Muscles of the Trunk—Section II: Functional Interactions Among Muscles

Section I describes the individual actions of the muscles of the trunk. These actions are summarized in Table 10–9. Section II highlights the functional interactions among the muscles of the trunk during two activities: (1) generating core stability to the trunk, and (2) controlling the sit-up movement. The second interaction exemplifies a classic kinesiologic relationship between the trunk and hip muscles.

**Posterior view**

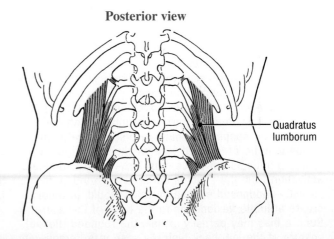

**FIGURE 10–19.** A posterior view of the quadratus lumborum muscle. (From Luttgens K, Hamilton N: Kinesiology: Scientific Basis of Human Motion, 9th ed. Madison, WI, Brown and Benchmark, 1997. The McGraw-Hill Companies.)

## TABLE 10-9. Actions of Most Muscles of the Trunk

| Muscle | Flexion | Extension | Lateral Flexion | Axial Rotation* |
|---|---|---|---|---|
| Trapezius | — | XX | XX | XX (CL) |
| Spinalis muscles (as a group) | — | XX | X | — |
| Longissimus thoracis | — | XXX | XX | — |
| Longissimus cervicis | — | XXX | XX | XX (IL) |
| Longissimus capitis | — | XXX | XX | XX (IL) |
| Iliocostalis lumborum | — | XXX | XXX | X (IL) |
| Iliocostalis thoracis | — | XXX | XXX | — |
| Iliocostalis cervicis | — | XXX | XXX | XX (IL) |
| Semispinalis thoracis | — | XXX | X | X (CL) |
| Semispinalis cervicis | — | XXX | X | X (CL) |
| Semispinalis capitis | — | XXX | X | — |
| Multifidi | — | XXX | X | XX (CL) |
| Rotatores | — | XX | X | XX (CL) |
| Interspinalis muscles | — | XX | — | — |
| Intertransversarus muscles | — | X | XX | — |
| Rectus abdominis | XXX | — | XX | — |
| Obliquus externus abdominis | XXX | — | XXX | XXX (CL) |
| Obliquus internus abdominis | XXX | — | XXX | XXX (IL) |
| Transversus abdominis† | — | — | — | — |
| Psoas major | X | X | XX | — |
| Quadratus lumborum | — | XX | XX | — |

\* CL = contralateral rotation, IL = ipsilateral rotation.

† Acts primarily to increase intra-abdominal pressure and, via attachments to the thoracolumbar fascia, to stabilize the lumbar region.

Unless otherwise stated, the actions describe movement of the muscle's superior or lateral aspect relative to its fixed inferior or medial aspect. The actions are assumed to occur from the anatomic position, against an external resistance. A muscle's relative potential to move or stabilize a region is assigned **X, minimal, XX, moderate, and XXX, maximum,** based on moment arm (leverage), cross-sectional area, and fiber direction; — indicates no effective muscular action.

---

> **Functional Interactions Among the Muscles of the Trunk**
> 1. Providing core stability to the trunk
> 2. Controlling the traditional sit-up movement

## PROVIDING CORE STABILITY TO THE TRUNK

Active muscle force provides the primary form of stability to the vertebral column. Although ligaments and other connective tissues provide a secondary source of stability, only muscles can adjust both the magnitude and timing of their forces.

Muscles of the trunk provide core stability to the trunk and, therefore, to the body as a whole. Stability allows the trunk to hold a static posture even under the influence of destabilizing external torques. The wave of muscular activation throughout the trunk muscles is experienced when attempting to stand or sit upright in an accelerating bus or train.

Core stability of the trunk establishes a base for muscles to move the limbs. During shoulder flexion, for instance, the transversus abdominis muscle is shown to become active 38.9 msec before the anterior deltoid muscle.[36] Interestingly,

for the same movement, persons with low-back pain history have a threefold delay in the onset of EMG activity in the transversus abdominis. Whether the delay in muscle activation is associated with the actual cause of the back pain is an intriguing question.

Muscular stabilizers of the trunk can be partitioned into two sets based primarily on anatomic organization: intrinsic and extrinsic. *Intrinsic muscular stabilizers* include the relatively short and segmented muscles that attach primarily within the region of the vertebral column. These muscles are involved with fine tuning of the stability within the multiple segments of the vertebral column. *Extrinsic muscular stabilizers,* in contrast, include relatively long muscles that attach, either partially or totally, to structures outside the region of the vertebral column, such as the cranium, pelvis, ribs, and lower extremities. These muscles contribute general stability to the trunk and provide a semirigid link between the vertebral column and the lower extremities.

### Intrinsic Muscular Stabilizers of the Trunk

The intrinsic muscular stabilizers of the trunk include the transversospinal and short segmental groups of muscles. Most of these muscles are organized in a relatively segmented fashion, crossing a few intervertebral junctions. The varying lines-of-force of the intrinsic muscular stabilizers

**A) Intrinsic muscular stabilizers**

**B) Spatial orientation (α) of muscle's line-of-force**

**Percent of force directed:**
*Horizontal* ($F_H$)
*Vertical* ($F_V$)

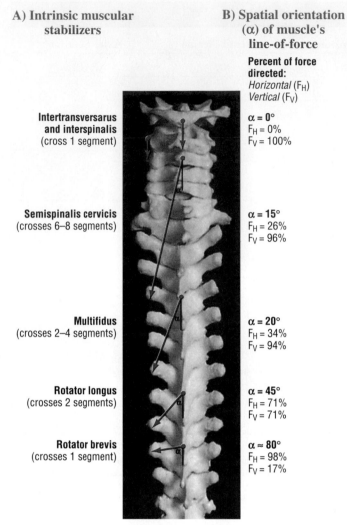

**Intertransversarus and interspinalis** (cross 1 segment)

$\alpha = 0°$
$F_H = 0\%$
$F_V = 100\%$

**Semispinalis cervicis** (crosses 6–8 segments)

$\alpha = 15°$
$F_H = 26\%$
$F_V = 96\%$

**Multifidus** (crosses 2–4 segments)

$\alpha = 20°$
$F_H = 34\%$
$F_V = 94\%$

**Rotator longus** (crosses 2 segments)

$\alpha = 45°$
$F_H = 71\%$
$F_V = 71\%$

**Rotator brevis** (crosses 1 segment)

$\alpha \approx 80°$
$F_H = 98\%$
$F_V = 17\%$

**FIGURE 10–20.** Diagrammatic representation of the spatial orientation of the lines-of-force of the intrinsic muscular stabilizers. *A,* The lines-of-force of muscles are shown within the frontal plane. The number of intervertebral junctions that each muscle crosses is noted in the parenthesis. *B,* The spatial orientation of the lines-of-force of each muscle is indicated by the angle (*α*) formed relative to the vertical position. The percentage of muscle force directed vertically is equal to the cosine of *α*; the percentage of muscle force directed horizontally is equal to the sine of *α*. Assuming adequate leverage, the vertically directed muscle forces produce extension and lateral flexion and the more horizontally directed muscle forces produce axial rotation.

out such control, the vertebral column is vulnerable to exaggerated spinal curvature and instability.

> ***Intrinsic* Muscular Stabilizers of the Trunk Include**
> 1. Transversospinal group
>    Semispinalis muscles
>    Multifidi
>    Rotatores
> 2. Short segmental group
>    Interspinalis muscles
>    Intertransversarus muscles

### *Extrinsic Muscular Stabilizers of the Trunk*

The extrinsic muscular stabilizers of the trunk include the abdominal muscles, the erector spinae, the quadratus lumborum, the psoas major, and the hip muscles that connect

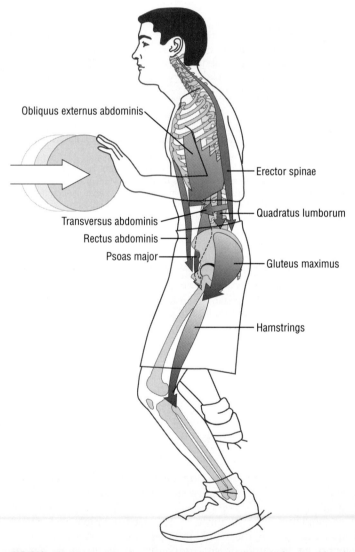

Obliquus externus abdominis
Transversus abdominis
Rectus abdominis
Psoas major
Erector spinae
Quadratus lumborum
Gluteus maximus
Hamstrings

**FIGURE 10–21.** A typical activation pattern is shown of a sample of external muscular stabilizers. The healthy person activates muscles to stabilize the body against an external force. The activation provides core stability to the trunk and the lumbosacral regions and increases the rigidity between the trunk, lower extremities, and floor.

(Fig. 10–20*A*) allow them to exert fine control of core stability in all planes. As indicated in Figure 10–20*B*, the spatial orientation of each muscle's line-of-force (*α*) produces a unique stabilization effect on the vertebral column. Vertically running interspinalis and intertransversarus muscles produce 100% of their force in the vertical direction ($F_V$). In contrast, the near horizontally oriented rotator brevis muscle produces close to 100% of its force in the horizontal direction ($F_H$). All of the remaining muscles produce forces that are directed diagonally. Muscle forces directed across the entire spectrum of the frontal plane optimize the triplanar control of core stability within the vertebral column. With-the pelvis with the lower extremities. External stabilizers provide core stability to the trunk by regulating rigidity within the trunk, and between the trunk and lower extremities. Core stability is particularly important in the lumbar and lumbosacral regions, where external forces applied against the upper body can develop substantial destabilizing leverage against the more caudal or inferior regions of the axial skeleton. Instability at the base of the spine can lead to postural malalignment throughout the entire vertebral column, as well as predispose a person to impairments related to (1) spondylolisthesis or spondylosis, (2) abnormal lordosis, and (3) damaging forces on the apophyseal, interbody, and sacroiliac joints.

---

**Primary *Extrinsic* Muscular Stabilizers of the Trunk Include**

1. Muscles of the anterior-lateral trunk
   Abdominals
      rectus abdominis
      obliquus externus abdominis
      obliquus internus abdominis
      transversus abdominis
2. Erector spinae
3. Quadratus lumborum
4. Psoas major
5. Muscles that connect the pelvis with the lower extremity—the hip muscles.

---

Figure 10–21 shows a person activating his external muscular stabilizers in response to an external force. Note the concentration of muscular activity in the lower region of the spine. (Although the intrinsic muscular stabilizers are also active for the purposes described, they are omitted from the illustration for clarity.) Activation of the psoas major, quadratus lumborum, and erector spinae muscles provides substantial vertical stability to the lumbar and lumbosacral regions, in both the frontal and sagittal planes. Co-contraction of the abdominal muscles—in particular the transversus abdominis—reinforces the stability of the lumbar region by increasing the tension within the thoracolumbar fascia, thereby creating a "corset" effect across the low back.

Activation of the abdominal muscles is essential to stabilization of the pelvis against the pull of trunk extensor muscles, especially the erector spinae, quadratus lumborum, and hip muscles (see Fig. 10–21). With the pelvis well stabilized, forces that have an impact on the trunk are effectively transferred across the sacroiliac joints, through the hips, and ultimately through the lower extremities. Strengthening exercises, designed to increase the stability of the low back and lower trunk regions, ideally include those that challenge both the trunk and the hip muscles in all planes.

## CONTROLLING THE SIT-UP MOVEMENT

The muscles of the trunk interact with each other and with the muscles of the hip joint during many activities. Consider, for instance, the combined movements of the trunk and hips while swinging a baseball bat, figure skating, or shoveling snow. To underscore this important synergistic relationship, the following discussions focus on the muscular actions of the sit-up movement.

Several strategies are used to strengthen the abdominal muscles. The common goal of the exercises is to increase the strength and control of these muscles, often as a way to improve core stability within the trunk. In a very broad sense, abdominal exercises fall into one of four categories. In column 1 of Figure 10–22, the abdominal muscles produce an isometric force to maintain a constant distance between the xiphoid process and the anterior pelvis. In columns 2 to

| #1 Isometrics | #2 Rotating the Trunk Toward the Stationary Pelvis | #3 Rotating the Trunk and Pelvis Toward the Stationary Legs | #4 Rotating the Pelvis (and/or Legs) Toward the Stationary Trunk |
|---|---|---|---|
| Examples:<br>1- Balancing the trunk upright while seated on a very large ball.<br>2- Holding a rigid trunk and low back while maintaining a "military-style" push-up.<br>3- Keeping the trunk and low back rigid while maintaining "all-fours" position, then progress to raising one arm and the contralateral leg.* | Examples:<br>1- Partial sit-ups ("crunches").*<br>2- As above, but incorporate diagonal plane movements of the trunk.<br>3- Lateral trunk curls. | Examples:<br>1- Standard full sit-up.*<br>2- As above, but incorporate diagonal plane movement of the trunk and pelvis. | Examples:<br>1- Posterior pelvic tilt while lying supine.<br>2- Antigravity or otherwise resisted hip flexion.*<br>3- Straight leg raises.*<br>4- As above, but incorporate diagonal plane movements of the legs. |
| 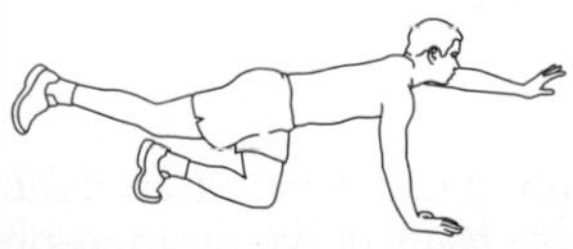 | 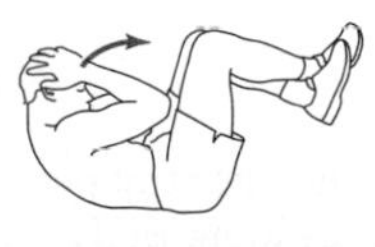 | 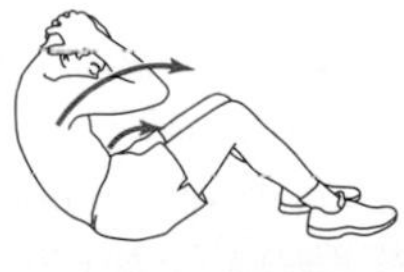 | 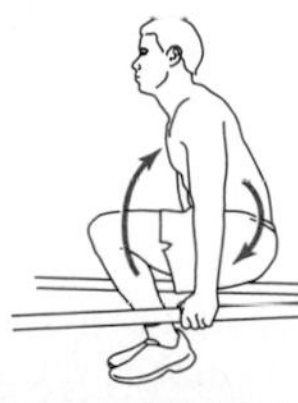 |

**FIGURE 10–22.** Categories of abdominal strengthening exercises, with selected examples. The examples marked by the asterisk are pictured below.

4, the abdominal muscles contract to reduce the distance between the xiphoid process and the anterior pelvis. Of these examples, perhaps the most well-recognized exercise is the standard sit-up, depicted in column 3.

A sit-up performed in a "hook-lying" position (i.e., hips and knees are flexed) is divided into two phases. The early trunk flexion phase terminates when both scapulae are raised off the mat (Fig. 10–23A). The later hip flexion phase involves 70 to 90 degrees of pelvic-on-femoral hip flexion

(Fig. 10–23B). As depicted in Figure 10–23A, the trunk flexion phase is driven primarily by contraction of the abdominal muscles, especially the rectus abdominis.[2] The upper and lower parts of the rectus abdominis respond with equal intensity during this motion.[47] The latissimus dorsi, passing anterior to the upper thoracic spine, may assist in flexing this region; the sternal head of the pectoralis major may assist in advancing the upper extremities and head toward the pelvis.

**A. Trunk flexion phase**

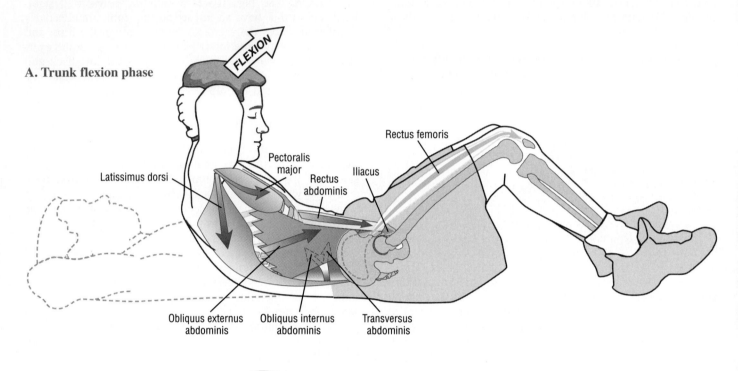

**B. Hip flexion phase**

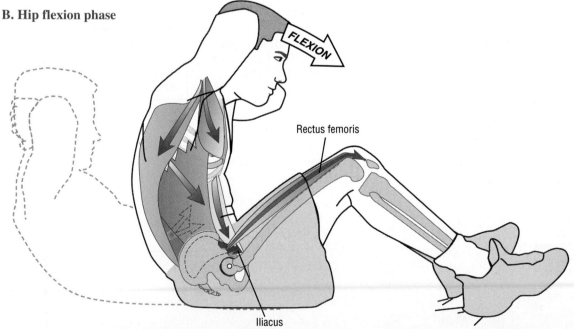

**FIGURE 10–23.** A typical activation pattern is shown of a sample of muscles, as a healthy person performs a traditional sit-up maneuver. The intensity of the red color is related to the assumed intensity of the muscle activation. *A,* The *trunk flexion phase* of the sit-up involves strong activation of the abdominal muscles, especially the rectus abdominis. *B,* The *hip flexion phase* of the sit-up involves strong activation of the abdominal and hip flexor muscles. Note in *B* the large pelvic-on-femoral kinematic contribution to the sit-up maneuver.

During the *trunk flexion phase* of the full sit-up, the thoracolumbar spine flexes, and the pelvis is tilted posteriorly, flattening the lumbar spine. The EMG level of the hip flexor muscles is relatively low, regardless of the position of the hips and knees.[2] Partially flexing the hips prior to the exercise increases the passive tension in the gluteus maximus, assisting with the posterior tilting posture of the pelvis.

During the *hip flexion phase* of the sit-up, the pelvis and trunk rotate toward the femurs. The hip flexion phase is driven by active contraction of the hip flexor muscles. Although any hip flexor muscle can assist with this action, Figure 10–23B shows the iliacus and rectus femoris as the active participants. Relative levels of EMG from the iliacus, sartorius, and rectus femoris are significantly greater when the legs are held fixed to the supporting surface.[2] The axis of rotation during the hip flexion phase of the full sit-up shifts toward the hip joints. The abdominal muscles remain isometrically active, holding the flexed thoracolumbar region against the rotating pelvis.

The full sit-up places different mechanical *workloads* on the abdominal muscles as compared with the hip flexor muscles. (Work, in this context, is the product of muscle force times the distance it contracts.) In the trunk flexion phase of the sit-up, the abdominal muscles produce work by rotating the trunk toward the pelvis; in the hip flexion phase, the hip flexor muscles produce work by contracting and rotating the pelvis and trunk toward the femurs.

Persons with moderately weakened abdominal muscles typically display a characteristic posture when attempting to perform a full sit-up. Throughout the attempt, the hip flexor muscles dominate the activity. As a result, there is minimal thoracolumbar flexion and excessive and "early" pelvic-on-femoral (hip) flexion. The dominating contraction of the hip flexor muscles exaggerates the lumbar lordosis, especially during the initiation of the maneuver.[42]

## Muscles of the Craniocervical Region—Section I: Anatomy and Individual Muscle Action

The following sections describe the anatomy and individual actions of the muscles that act exclusively within the craniocervical region. Musculature is divided into two sets: the muscles of the anterior-lateral region and the muscles of the posterior region (see Table 10–2).

Figure 10–24 depicts many of the muscles of craniocervical region as flexors or extensors, or right or left lateral flexors, depending on their attachment relative to the axes of rotation through the atlanto-occipital joints. Although Figure 10–24 describes the muscle actions at the atlanto-occipital joint only, the relative position of the muscles provides a useful guide for an understanding of the actions at other joints within the craniocervical region.

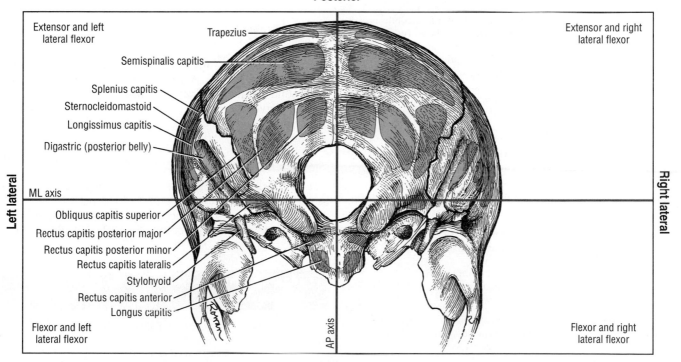

**Inferior view**

**FIGURE 10–24.** The potential action of muscles that attach to the inferior surface of the occipital and temporal bones is highlighted. The actions of the muscles across the atlanto-occipital joints are based on their location relative to the medial-lateral (ML) (black) and anterior-posterior (red) axis of rotation at the level of the occipital condyles. Note that the actions of most muscles fit into one of four quadrants.

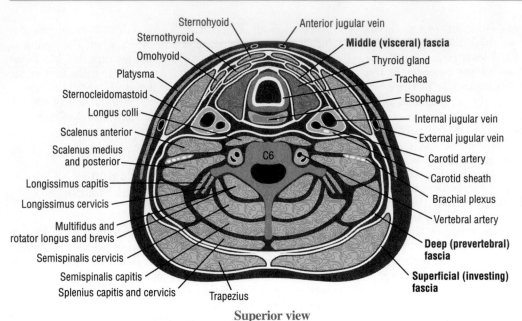

Sternohyoid
Sternothyroid
Omohyoid
Platysma
Sternocleidomastoid
Longus colli
Scalenus anterior
Scalenus medius and posterior
Longissimus capitis
Longissimus cervicis
Multifidus and rotator longus and brevis
Semispinalis cervicis
Semispinalis capitis
Splenius capitis and cervicis
Trapezius

Anterior jugular vein
**Middle (visceral) fascia**
Thyroid gland
Trachea
Esophagus
Internal jugular vein
External jugular vein
Carotid artery
Carotid sheath
Brachial plexus
Vertebral artery
**Deep (prevertebral) fascia**
**Superficial (investing) fascia**

C6

**Superior view**

**FIGURE 10–25.** A horizontal cross-sectional view through the neck at the level of the sixth cervical vertebra. Note the three components of the cervical fascia.

## CERVICAL FASCIA

Cervical fascia surrounds and compartmentalizes many structures within the neck, including muscles and neurovascular structures. The cervical fascia is subdivided into three com-ponents: superficial (investing), middle (visceral), and deep (prevertebral) (Fig. 10–25) and (Table 10–10). These components exclude the subcutaneous fascia that is imbedded within the platysma muscle. Important functions of the cervical fascia are to protect muscle, to provide structural support and protection to the cervical viscera and important neurovascular structures, and to help transfer forces between muscles.

### SET 1: MUSCLES OF THE ANTERIOR-LATERAL CRANIOCERVICAL REGION

The muscles of the anterior-lateral craniocervical region are listed in Table 10–11. With the exception of the sternocleidomastoid, which is innervated primarily by the spinal accessory nerve, the other muscles in the group are innervated by small unnamed nerves that branch from the cervical plexus.

### Sternocleidomastoid

The sternocleidomastoid is a very prominent muscle located superficially on the anterior aspect of the neck (Fig. 10–26). Inferiorly, the muscle attaches by two heads: the medial (sternal) and lateral (clavicular) (Fig. 10–27). From this at-

| TABLE **10–10.** Components of the Cervical Fascia | |
|---|---|
| **Superficial (Investing) Fascia** | Covers the entire neck region. Tissue also surrounds and interconnects the trapezius and the sternocleidomastoid muscles. Superficial fascia attaches or is continuous with many structures in the area: *Superiorly* Hyoid bone and surrounding muscular fascia Mandible Mastoid process Superior nuchal line Temporalis muscle *Inferiorly* Pectoral and deltoid fascia Acromion Clavicle Manubrium *Posteriorly* Ligamentum nuchae Spinous processes of cervical vertebrae |
| **Middle (Visceral) Fascia** | Surrounds and protects the cervical viscera: trachea, esophagus, and thyroid gland |
| **Deep (Prevertebral) Fascia** | Surrounds the large set of muscles of the craniocervical region located posterior to the cervical viscera and anterior to the trapezius. The fascia is continuous with the thoracolumbar fascia. |

| TABLE **10–11.** Muscles of the Anterior-Lateral Craniocervical Region |
|---|
| Sternocleidomastoid |
| Scalenes |
|     Scalenus anterior |
|     Scalenus medius |
|     Scalenus posterior |
| Longus colli |
| Longus capitis |
| Rectus capitis anterior |
| Rectus capitis lateralis |

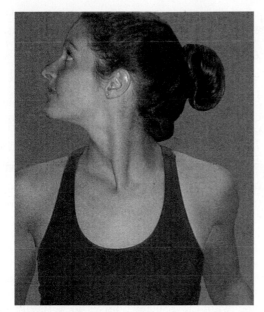

**FIGURE 10–26.** The left sternocleidomastoid muscle during active rotation of the head and neck to the right. The muscle is evident as a thick cord between the left mastoid process, just inferior to the ear, and the left sternoclavicular joint. Both sternal and clavicular heads of the muscle are visible.

tachment, the muscle ascends obliquely across the neck to attach along a thin line, extending across much of the mastoid process of the temporal bone and the lateral half of the superior nuchae line.

Acting unilaterally, the sternocleidomastoid is a lateral flexor and contralateral axial rotator of the craniocervical region. The axial rotation action is demonstrated in Figure 10–26. Bilaterally, the sagittal plane action of the sternocleidomastoid depends on the level of the craniocervical region.

From a lateral view of a person with normal posture, it can be seen that the sternocleidomastoid crosses the neck in an oblique fashion. Below approximately the C3 region, the sternocleidomastoid crosses anterior to the medial-lateral axes of rotation; above C3, however, the sternocleidomastoid crosses posterior to the medial-lateral axes of rotation. Acting together, the sternocleidomastoids have the potential to *flex* the mid to lower cervical spine and to *extend* the upper cervical spine and the atlanto-axial and atlanto-occipital joints. This muscular action varies depending on the initial posture of the craniocervical region.

**SPECIAL  FOCUS  10 – 4**

### Torticollis

Torticollis (from the Latin *tortus,* twisted; *collum,* neck) or "wryneck" describes a condition of chronic contraction of at least one of the cervical muscles, most commonly the sternocleidomastoid. The condition may be congenital or acquired. Shortening of the muscle may be due to a fibrous mass or may indicate neuromuscular disease. Often the cause of torticollis is unknown.

A person with unilateral torticollis involving a right or left sternocleidomastoid typically has an asymmetrical craniocervical posture that reflects components of the muscle's action (Fig. 10–28). Parents of a child with torticollis are often taught how to stretch the tight muscle and how to position and handle the child to promote elongation of the involved muscle. In severe cases of contracture, the muscle may be surgically released, most commonly at the sternal and clavicular heads.[85] Postsurgical treatment typically involves physical therapy to maintain the overcorrected position of the neck and reduce scar formation.

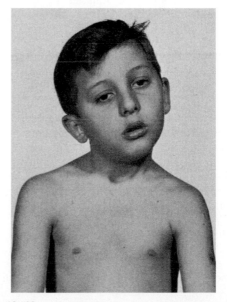

**FIGURE 10–28.** Congenital torticollis affects the right sternocleidomastoid of a 10-year-old boy. (From Tachdjian MO: Pediatric Orthopedics. Philadelphia, WB Saunders, 1972.)

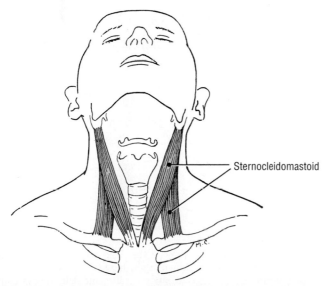
Sternocleidomastoid

**FIGURE 10–27.** An anterior view of the sternocleidomastoid muscles. (From Luttgens K, Hamilton N: Kinesiology: Scientific Basis of Human Motion, 9th ed. Madison, WI, Brown and Benchmark, 1997. The McGraw-Hill Companies.)

**Anterior view**

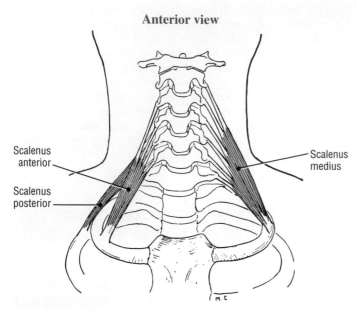

Scalenus anterior

Scalenus posterior

Scalenus medius

**FIGURE 10–29.** An anterior view of the scalene muscles. The scalenus posterior and anterior are shown on the right; the scalenus medius is shown on the left. (From Luttgens K, Hamilton N: Kinesiology: Scientific Basis of Human Motion, 9th ed. Madison, WI, Brown and Benchmark, 1997. The McGraw-Hill Companies.)

### Scalenes

As a group, the scalene muscles attach between the tubercles of the transverse processes of the middle to lower cervical vertebrae and the first two ribs (Fig. 10–29). The specific attachments of these muscles are listed in Appendix III (Part B, Set I). The brachial plexus courses between the scalene anterior and scalene medius (see Fig. 10–25). Excessive hypertrophy or spasm of these muscles or their associated fascia can compress the brachial plexus and can cause motor and sensory disturbances in the upper extremity.

The function of the scalene muscles depends on which skeletal attachments are more fixed. Assuming that the cervical spine is well stabilized, the scalene muscles raise the ribs to assist with inspiration during breathing; assuming that the scalene muscles are contracting from a fixed inferior base afforded by the first two ribs, their potential actions become evident by using a skeleton and string to mimic the line-of-force. Contracting unilaterally, the scalene muscles laterally flex the cervical spine. Axial rotation is limited in the scalenus medius and posterior due to the muscles' nearly vertical orientation. The more oblique scalenus anterior, however, has a potential for contralateral axial rotation of the cervical spine.

Contracting bilaterally, the scalenus anterior and medius have a limited moment arm to flex the cervical spine, particularly in the lower regions. The cervical attachments of all three scalene muscles split into several individual fasciculi (see Fig. 10–29). Like a system of guy wires that stabilize a large antenna, the scalene muscles provide excellent bilateral and vertical stability to the middle and lower cervical spine. Fine control of the upper craniocervical region is more likely

the responsibility of smaller more specialized muscles, such as the rectus capitis anterior and the suboccipital muscles.

### Longus Colli and Longus Capitis

The longus colli and longus capitis are located deep to the cervical viscera (trachea and esophagus), on either side of the cervical column (Fig. 10–30). These muscles function as dynamic anterior longitudinal ligaments, providing an important element of vertical stability to the region.

The *longus colli* consists of multiple fascicles that closely adhere to the anterior surfaces of the upper three thoracic and all cervical vertebrae. The muscle ascends the cervical region through multiple attachments between the vertebral bodies, anterior tubercles of transverse processes, and anterior arch of the atlas. The longus colli is the only muscle that attaches in its entirety to the anterior surface of the vertebral column. Compared with the scalene and sternocleidomastoid muscles, the longus colli is a relatively thin muscle (see Fig. 10–25). The more anterior fibers of the longus colli flex the cervical region. The more lateral fibers act in conjunction with the scalene muscles to vertically stabilize the region.

The *longus capitis* arises from the anterior tubercles of the transverse processes of the mid to lower cervical vertebrae and inserts into the basilar part of the occipital bone (see Fig. 10–24). The primary action of the longus capitis is to flex and stabilize the upper craniocervical region. Lateral flexion is a secondary action.

### Rectus Capitis Anterior and Rectus Capitis Lateralis

The rectus capitis anterior and rectus capitis lateralis are two short muscles that arise on the elongated transverse processes of the atlas (C1) and insert on the inferior surface of occipital bone (see Fig. 10–30). The rectus capitis lateralis

**Anterior view**

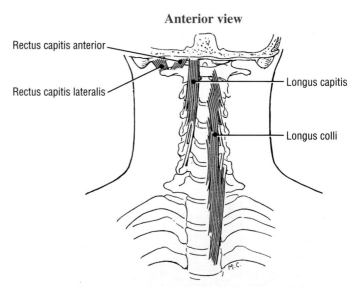

Rectus capitis anterior

Rectus capitis lateralis

Longus capitis

Longus colli

**FIGURE 10–30.** An anterior view of the deep muscles in the neck. The following muscles are shown: right longus capitis, right rectus capitis anterior, right rectus capitis lateralis, and left longus colli. (From Luttgens K, Hamilton N: Kinesiology: Scientific Basis of Human Motion, 9th ed. Madison, WI, Brown and Benchmark, 1997. The McGraw-Hill Companies.)

### SPECIAL FOCUS 10–5

#### Vulnerability of the Longus Colli and Longus Capitis to Acceleration Injury

The cervical spine is vulnerable to acceleration (whiplash) injury, especially as a result of an automobile accident. Vulnerability is due, in part, to the large mass moment of inertia of the relatively heavy head. An impact that creates a large angular velocity of the head generates a proportionally large angular momentum throughout the entire craniocervical region. If directed in the sagittal plane, the momentum of the flexing or extending head can damage tissues that are excessively strained or compressed. Momentum directed in the frontal plane can create lateral flexion whiplash, which also damages tissue.

Whiplash associated with cervical hyperextension generally creates greater strain on muscles and soft tissues than does whiplash associated with cervical flexion.[68] The greater range of hyperextension can severely strain the flexor muscles and cervical viscera, and it can excessively compress the apophyseal joints and posterior aspects of the cervical spine (Fig. 10–31*A*). The maximum extent of flexion is partially blocked by the chin striking the chest (Fig. 10–31*B*).

Research on replicas of the human head, neck, and torso has shown that the longus colli and longus capitis are particularly vulnerable to strain injury from hyperextension-associated whiplash. Whiplash from excessive hyperextension produced a 56% strain (elongation) in the longus colli, and whiplash from excessive lateral flexion produced a 57% strain in the longus capitis.[18] Both these levels of strain can cause tissue damage.

Clinically, a person with a hyperextension injury often shows marked tenderness and protective spasm in the region of the longus colli. Tenderness may also be associated with excessive strain in other flexor muscles, such as the sternocleidomastoid and scalenus anterior, and the cervical viscera. Spasm in the longus colli tends to produce a straight cervical spine, lacking the normal lordosis. Persons with a strained and painful longus colli often have difficulty shrugging their shoulders. Without the adequate stabilization provided by the longus colli and other flexors, the upper trapezius muscle loses stable cranial attachment and, therefore, becomes an ineffective elevator of the shoulder girdle.[68] This clinical scenario is an excellent example of the interdependence of muscle function, in which one muscle's action depends on the stabilization force of another.

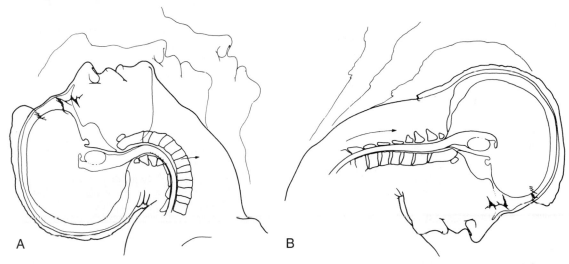

A                                    B

**FIGURE 10–31.** During acceleration (whiplash) injuries, cervical extension (*A*) typically exceeds cervical flexion (*B*). As a result, the anterior structures of the cervical region are more vulnerable to strain injury. (From Porterfield JA, DeRosa C: Mechanical Neck Pain: Perspectives in Functional Anatomy. Philadelphia, WB Saunders, 1995.)

attaches laterally to the occipital condyle; the rectus capitis anterior, the smaller of the recti, attaches immediately anterior to the occipital condyle (see Fig. 10–24).

The actions of the rectus capitis anterior and lateralis muscles are limited to the atlanto-occipital joint, where each muscle controls one of the joint's two degrees of freedom (see Chapter 9). The rectus capitis anterior is primarily a flexor, and the rectus capitis lateralis is primarily a lateral flexor.

### SET 2: MUSCLES OF THE POSTERIOR CRANIOCERVICAL REGION

The muscles of the posterior craniocervical region are listed in Table 10–12. They are innervated by dorsi rami of cervical spinal nerves.

#### Splenius Cervicis and Capitis

The splenius cervicis and capitis muscles are a long and thin pair of muscles, named by their resemblance to a bandage

**TABLE 10–12. Muscles of the Posterior Craniocervical Region**

Splenius muscles
    Splenius cervicis
    Splenius capitis
Suboccipital muscles
    Rectus capitis posterior major
    Rectus capitis posterior minor
    Obliquus capitis superior
    Obliquus capitis inferior

(from the Greek *splenion,* bandage) (Fig. 10–32). As a pair, the splenius muscles arise from the inferior half of the ligamentum nuchae and spinous processes of C7-T6, just deep to the trapezius muscle. The *splenius capitis* attaches cranially just deep to the sternocleidomastoid, along a thin line that extends across the mastoid process and the lateral one third of the superior nuchae line (see Fig. 10–24). The *splenius cervicis* attaches to the posterior tubercles of the transverse processes of C1-3. Much of this cervical attachment is shared by the levator scapula muscle.

Contracting unilaterally, the splenius muscles perform lateral flexion and ipsilateral axial rotation of the head and cervical spine. Contracting bilaterally, the splenius muscles extend the upper craniocervical region.

### Suboccipital Muscles

The suboccipital muscles consist of four paired muscles located very deep in the neck, immediately superficial to the

atlanto-occipital and atlanto-axial joints (Fig. 10–33). These relatively short, thick muscles attach between the atlas, axis, and occipital bone. Their specific muscular attachments are listed in Appendix III (Part B, Set II). The suboccipital muscles are not easily palpable. They lie deep to the upper trapezius, splenius group, and semispinalis capitis muscles (see Fig. 10–24).

The primary function of the suboccipital muscles is to provide fine control of movement at the atlanto-occipital and atlanto-axial joints. In conjunction with the rectus capitis anterior and lateralis, these specialized joints increase the number of movements possible within the upper craniocervical region to orient the eyes, ears, and nose. As indicated in Figure 10–34, no two muscles have identical actions at both joints.

## Muscles of the Craniocervical Region— Section II: Functional Interactions Among Muscles that Cross the Craniocervical Region

Nearly 30 muscles cross the craniocervical region. They include the muscles that act exclusively within the craniocervical region (Table 10–13), plus those classified as muscles of the posterior trunk that cross the craniocervical region (e.g., trapezius and longissimus capitis).

This section highlights the functional interactions among the muscles that cross the craniocervical regions during two activities: (1) stabilizing the craniocervical region and (2) producing the movements of the head and neck that optimize the function of visual, auditory, and olfactory systems. Although other functional interactions exist for these muscles, the two activities provide a format for describing key kinesiologic principles involved in this important region of the body.

**Functional Interactions Among Muscles that Cross the Craniocervical Region**
1. Stabilization of the head and neck
2. Production of the movements of the head and neck that optimize vision and hearing

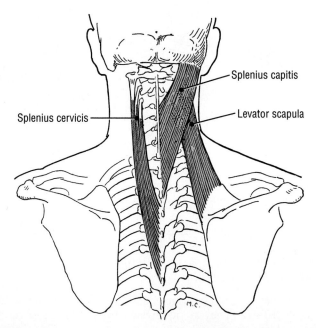

**FIGURE 10–32.** A posterior view of the left splenius cervicis, right splenius capitis, and right levator scapula. Although not visible, the levator scapula has similar cervical attachments as the splenius cervicis. (From Luttgens K, Hamilton N: Kinesiology: Scientific Basis of Human Motion, 9th ed. Madison, WI, Brown and Benchmark, 1997. The McGraw-Hill Companies.)

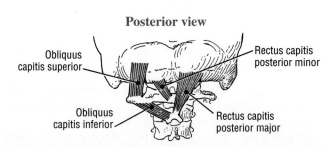

**FIGURE 10–33.** A posterior view of the suboccipital muscles. The left obliquus capitis superior, left obliquus capitis inferior, left rectus capitis posterior minor, and right rectus capitis posterior major are shown. (From Luttgens K, Hamilton N: Kinesiology: Scientific Basis of Human Motion, 9th ed. Madison, WI, Brown and Benchmark, 1997. The McGraw-Hill Companies.)

**SPECIAL FOCUS 10-6**

**Specialized Muscles that Control the Atlanto-Axial and Atlanto-Occipital Joints: An Example of Fine-Tuning of the Cervical Coupling Pattern**

The specialized muscles that control the atlanto-axial and atlanto-occipital joints exert fine control over the movement of the upper craniocervical region. One benefit of this fine level of control is related to the coupling pattern of the cervical region. As described in Chapter 9, an ipsilateral coupling pattern exists in the C2-C7 region between the motions of axial rotation and lateral flexion. Axial rotation, due primarily to the orientation of the apophyseal joints, is associated with slight ipsilateral lateral flexion and vice versa. The expression of this coupling pattern can be obscured, however, by the specialized muscles that control the atlanto-occipital and atlanto-axial joints. Consider, for example, the coupling

between right axial rotation and right lateral flexion (see Fig. 9–52*B*). In order to maintain a level horizontal visual gaze throughout axial rotation, the left rectus capitis lateralis, for instance, produces a slight left lateral flexion torque to the head via the atlanto-occipital joints. This muscular action offsets the tendency for the head to bend to the right with the rest of the cervical region during the right axial rotation. Similarly, right lateral flexion of the C2-7 region, which also results in right axial rotation of this cervical region, may be accompanied by a slight, offsetting left axial rotation torque to the head by the left obliquus capitis inferior muscle. In both examples, movement of the head and eyes can be more precisely maintained within the horizontal plane, thereby facilitating the visual tracking of a moving object while rotating the head.

## STABILIZING THE CRANIOCERVICAL REGION

The muscles that cross the craniocervical region compose much of the bulk of the neck, especially in the regions lateral and posterior to the cervical vertebrae (see Fig. 10–25). When strongly activated, this mass of muscle can protect the cervical viscera, intervertebral discs, apophyseal joints, and neural tissues. Resistive exercises are often performed by athletes involved in contact sports as a means to hypertrophy this musculature. Hypertrophy alone, however, may not necessarily prevent neck injury. Data on the biomechanics of whiplash injury, for example, suggest that the time required to react to an impending injury and generate a substantial stabilizing force may exceed the time of the

## TABLE 10-13. Actions of Muscles Located Exclusively within the Craniocervical Region

| Muscle | Flexion | Extension | Lateral Flexion | Axial Rotation* |
|---|---|---|---|---|
| Sternocleidomastoid | XXX | X* | XXX | XXX (CL) |
| Scalenus anterior | XX | — | XXX | X (CL) |
| Scalenus medius | X | — | XXX | — |
| Scalenus posterior | — | — | XX | — |
| Longus colli | XX | — | XX | — |
| Longus capitis | XX | — | XX | — |
| Rectus capitis anterior | XX (AOJ only) | — | X (AOJ only) | — |
| Rectus capitis lateralis | — | — | XX (AOJ only) | — |
| Splenius capitis | — | XXX | XX | XXX (IL) |
| Splenius cervicis | — | XXX | XX | XXX (IL) |
| Rectus capitis posterior major | — | XXX (AOJ and AAJ) | XX (AOJ only) | XX (IL) (AAJ only) |
| Rectus capitis posterior minor | — | XX (AOJ only) | X (AOJ only) | — |
| Obliquus capitis inferior | — | XX (AAJ only) | — | XXX (IL) (AAJ only) |
| Obliquus capitis superior | — | XXX (AOJ only) | XXX (AOJ only) | — |

* Upper parts of sternocleidomastoid extend the upper cervical region, atlanto-axial joint, and atlanto-occipital joint.
   A muscle's relative potential to move or stabilize a region is scored **X, minimal, XX, moderate,** and **XXX, maximum;** — indicates no effective muscular action. AOJ, atlanto-occipital joint; AAJ, atlanto-axial joint; CL, contralateral rotation; IL, ipsilateral rotation.

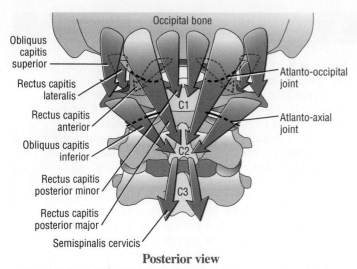

Posterior view

*Occipital bone*

Obliquus capitis superior

Rectus capitis lateralis

Rectus capitis anterior

Obliquus capitis inferior

Rectus capitis posterior minor

Rectus capitis posterior major

Semispinalis cervicis

Atlanto-occipital joint

Atlanto-axial joint

C1

C2

C3

**Posterior view**

| MUSCLES | ATLANTO-OCCIPITAL JOINT | | | ATLANTO-AXIAL JOINT | | |
|---|---|---|---|---|---|---|
| | FLEXION | EXTENSION | LATERAL FLEXION | FLEXION | EXTENSION | AXIAL ROTATION* |
| Rectus capitis anterior | XX | – | X | – | – | – |
| Rectus capitis lateralis | – | – | XX | – | – | – |
| Rectus capitis posterior major | – | XXX | XX | – | XXX | XX(IL) |
| Rectus capitis posterior minor | – | XX | X | – | – | – |
| Obliquus capitis inferior | – | – | – | – | XX | XXX(IL) |
| Obliquus capitis superior | – | XXX | XXX | – | – | – |

*CL = contralateral rotation, IL = ipsilateral rotation

**FIGURE 10–34.** A posterior view depicts the lines-of-force of muscles that exert exclusive control of the atlanto-occipital and atlanto-axial joints. The joints each allow two primary degrees of freedom. Note that the attachment of the semispinalis cervicis muscle provides a stable base for the rectus capitis posterior major and the obliquus capitis inferior, two of the larger and more dominant suboccipital muscles. The chart summarizes the actions of the muscles at the atlanto-occipital and atlanto-axial joints. A muscle's relative potential to perform a movement is assigned one of three scores: **X, minimal; XX, moderate; and XXX, maximum.** The dash indicates no effective torque production.

whiplash event.[18] For this reason, athletes need to anticipate a potentially harmful situation and contract the neck musculature *before* impact. The timing of muscle contraction appears as important in protecting the neck as does the magnitude of muscle force.

In addition to protecting the neck, forces produced by muscles provide the primary source of vertical stability to the craniocervical region. The "critical load" of the cervical spine (i.e., maximum compressive load that the neck, unsupported by muscle, can sustain before buckling) is between 10.5 and 40 N (between ~2.4 and 9 lb). This is less than the actual weight of the head![66,67] A coordinated interaction of muscles generates forces that are, on average, directed *through* the axis of rotation at each intervertebral junction. By passing through these multiple axes, the forces compress the intervertebral segments together, thereby stabilizing them without buckling.

The muscular interaction associated with the stabilization of the craniocervical region likely involves the more precise control afforded by relatively short, segmented muscles such as the multifidi, rotatores, and interspinalis muscles. The stability in the region is augmented by other longer muscles, including the scalenes, sternocleidomastoid, levator scapula, semispinalis capitis and cervicis, and trapezius. As a group, they form an extensive guy wire system that ensures vertical stability, most notably in frontal and sagittal planes. Figure 10–35A highlights a sample of muscles that act as guy wires to maintain ideal anterior-posterior alignment throughout the craniocervical region. Ideally, the co-contraction of flexor and extensor muscles counterbalance each other and, as a consequence, vertically stabilize the region. Note that the muscles depicted in Figure 10–35A are anchored inferiorly to several different structures: the sternum, clavicle, ribs, scapula, and vertebral column. These bony structures must be stabilized by other muscles, such as the lower trapezius and subclavius muscles for securing the scapula and clavicle, respectively.

## PRODUCING EXTENSIVE AND WELL-COORDINATED MOVEMENTS OF THE HEAD AND NECK: OPTIMIZING THE PLACEMENT OF THE EYES, EARS, AND NOSE

The craniocervical region allows the greatest triplanar mobility of any region of the axial skeleton. Ample movement is essential to optimal spatial orientation of the eyes, ears, and nose. Although all planes of motion are important in this regard, the following section highlights movement within the horizontal plane.

Figure 10–36 illustrates a total body movement that exhibits a sample of the muscular interactions used to maximize the extent of axial rotation of the craniocervical region. Note that full axial rotation of the craniocervical region provides the eyes with at least 180 degrees of visual scanning. As depicted, rotation to the right is driven by simultaneous activation of the left sternocleidomastoid and scalenus anterior (Fig. 10–36A); right splenius capitis and cervicis; right upper erector spinae, such as the longissimus capitis; and left transversospinal muscles, such as the multifidi (Fig. 10–36B). Activation of these muscles provides the required rotational power to the head and neck, as well as simultaneously stabilizing the craniocervical region in both the frontal and sagittal planes. For example, the extension potential provided by the splenius capitis and cervicis and the upper erector spinae is offset by the flexion potential of the sternocleidomastoid and scalenus anterior. Furthermore, the left lateral flexion potential of the left sternocleidomastoid is offset by the right lateral flexion potential of the right splenius capitus and cervicis.

Full axial rotation of the craniocervical region requires muscular interactions that extend into the trunk and lower extremities. Consider, for example, the activation of the right and left oblique abdominal muscles (see Fig. 10–36A). They

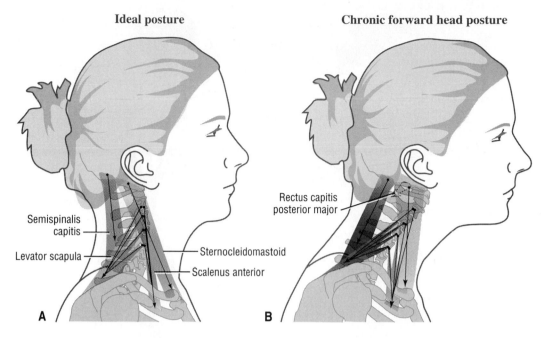

**FIGURE 10–35.** *A,* Four muscles acting as guy wires to maintain an ideal posture within the craniocervical region. *B,* Mechanics associated with a chronic forward head posture as discussed in Special Focus 10–7. The protracted position of the craniocervical region places greater stress on the levator scapula and semispinalis capitis muscles. The rectus capitis posterior major—one of the suboccipital muscles—is shown actively extending the upper craniocervical region. The highly active and stressed muscles are depicted in brighter red.

provide much of the torque needed to rotate the base of the craniocervical region. As shown in Figure 10–36*B*, the erector spinae and transversospinal muscles throughout the entire posterior trunk are active to offset the potent trunk flexion tendency of the oblique abdominal muscles.

The latissimus dorsi is an ipsilateral rotator of the trunk when the glenohumeral joint is well stabilized by other muscles. Selected left hip muscles actively rotate the pelvis and attached lumbosacral region to the right, relative to the fixed left femur.

---

### SPECIAL FOCUS 10–7

**Muscular Imbalance Associated with Chronic Forward Head Posture**

The ideal posture shown in Figure 10–35*A* depicts an optimally balanced craniocervical guy wire system. Excessive muscular tension in any of the muscles, however, can disrupt the vertical stability of the region. One such disruption is a chronic forward head posture, involving excessive protraction of the craniocervical region (Fig. 10–35*B*). Habitual forward head posture can occur for two different reasons. First, a hyperextension (whiplash) to the neck can injure anterior muscles, such as the sternocleidomastoid, longus colli, and scalenus anterior. As a result, chronic spasm in the strained muscles translates the head forward, resulting in excessive flexion, especially at the cervicothoracic junction. A clinical sign often associated with forward head posturing is a realignment of sternocleidomastoid muscle within the sagittal plane. The cranial end of the muscle, normally aligned posterior to the sternoclavicular joint, shifts anteriorly to a position directly above the sternoclavicular joint (compare Fig. 10–35*A* with *B*).

A second cause of a chronic forward head posture may be related to a progressive shortening of several anterior neck muscles. One such scenario involves pur-posely protracting the craniocervical region to improve visual contact with objects manipulated in front of the body. This activity is typical when viewing a computer screen. This position, if held for an extended period, may alter the functional resting length of the muscles, eventually transforming the forward posture into a "natural" posture.

Regardless of the factors that predispose a person to a chronic forward head posture, the posture itself stresses extensor muscles, such as the levator scapula and semispinalis capitis (see Fig. 10–35*B*). The suboccipital muscle, such as the rectus capitis posterior major, may be fatigued as a result of its prolonged extension activity required to "level" the head and eyes. Over time, increased muscular stress throughout the entire craniocervical region can lead to localized and painful muscle spasms, or "trigger points," common in the levator scapula and suboccipital muscles. This condition is often associated with headaches and radiating pain into the scalp. The key to most treatment for chronic forward head posture is to restore optimal craniocervical posture, accomplished through improved postural awareness, ergonomic workplace design, and therapeutic exercise.

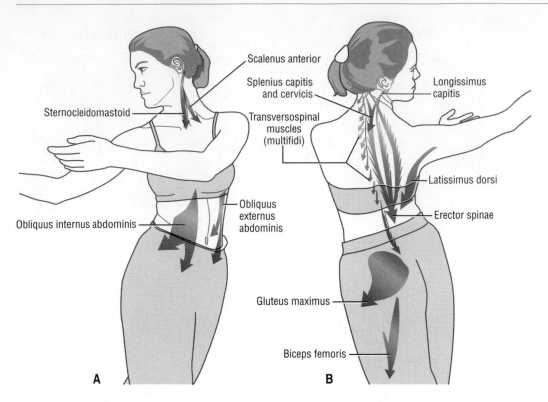

Sternocleidomastoid

Scalenus anterior

Splenius capitis and cervicis

Transversospinal muscles (multifidi)

Obliquus internus abdominis

Obliquus externus abdominis

Longissimus capitis

Latissimus dorsi

Erector spinae

Gluteus maximus

Biceps femoris

A

B

**FIGURE 10–36.** A typical activation pattern of selected muscles of the craniocervical region, trunk, and hip is shown, as a healthy person rotates the entire body to the right within the horizontal plane. *A,* Anterior view. *B,* Posterior view.

## SELECTED BIOMECHANICAL ISSUES OF LIFTING: A FOCUS ON REDUCING BACK INJURY

Lifting heavy objects places considerable demands on many muscles throughout the body (Fig. 10–37). Lifting can generate large compression, tension, and shear forces throughout the body, most notably at the base of the spine. At some critical level, forces that have an impact on the low-back region may exceed the structural tolerance of the local muscles, ligaments, and apophyseal and interbody joints. Lifting is a leading risk factor associated with low-back pain in the United States and is especially related to occupation.[25,41,43,53] Disability associated with low-back pain is a significant problem, both in terms of cost and suffering. An estimated 30% of the workforce in the United States regularly handles materials in a potentially harmful manner, including lifting.[63]

This topic of the biomechanics of lifting describes (1) why the low-back region is vulnerable to lifting-related injury and (2) how the forces in the low-back region can be minimized in order to reduce the chance of injury.

### Muscular Mechanics of Extension of the Low Back While Lifting

The amount of force produced by the extensor muscles of the posterior trunk is strongly correlated with the amount of force placed on the connective tissues (tendons, ligaments, fascia, discs) within the low back. The following sections, therefore, focus on the role of the muscles during lifting, and how forces produced by muscles can be modified to reduce the stress on the structures in the low-back region.

## ESTIMATING THE MAGNITUDE OF FORCE IMPOSED ON THE LOW BACK WHILE LIFTING

Considerable research has been undertaken to quantify the relative forces and torques imposed on the various structures in the low back while lifting.[1,3,31,56,70] This research helps clinicians and members of governmental agencies develop safety guidelines and limits for lifting, especially in the workplace.[12,13,23,29,35,37,44] Of particular interest during lifting are the variables of peak force, or torque, produced by muscles; tension developed within stretched ligaments; and compression and shear forces developed against the intervertebral discs and apophyseal joints. Measurement of these variables is typically not made directly, but rather through relatively sophisticated equipment that permits indirect estimates or model-based estimates of a desired variable. Such equipment is usually not available in most clinical settings. A more simple but less accurate method of estimating forces imposed on the low back uses calculations based on the assumption of static equilibrium (see Chapter 4).

The following section presents the steps used in making these calculations in order to estimate the compression force on the L2 vertebra while lifting a load in the sagittal plane. Although this hypothetic example provides a limited amount of information on a rather complex biomechanical event, it does yield valuable insight into the mathematical relationship between the force produced by the muscle and the compression force imposed on a representative structure within the low back.

Figure 10–38 shows the data required to make a general estimate of the compression force against the L2 vertebra while lifting. The subject is depicted midway through a vertical lift of a moderately heavy load, weighing 25% of his

calculating the external torque imposed by the external forces. Note that two external torques are described: one due to the external load (EL) and one due to the subject's body weight (BW) located above L2. The extensor muscle force (MF) is defined as the MF generated on the posterior (extensor) side of the axis of rotation. As shown in Step 1, the back extensor muscles produce an internal torque of 125.6 Nm to support the combined external torque of the load and body weight.

**Static Equilibrium Method for Estimating the Compression Force on the L2 Vertebra Requires Three Steps**

*Step 1* Formulate a static equilibrium equation in which the sum of the internal and external torques in the sagittal plane is equal to zero. This step allows the determination of the *internal torque* produced by the back extensor muscles.

*Step 2* Determine the *extensor muscle force* required to generate the internal extensor torque.

*Step 3* Determine the *compression (reaction) force* (RF) on the superior surface of L2 as the sum of the vectors produced by (1) the back extensor muscle force, (2) external load, and (3) body weight. L2 must produce an upward reaction force (labeled RF) that opposes EL, BW, and MF.

*Step 2* estimates the amount of extensor muscle force needed to sustain the internal torque. By assuming that the back extensor muscles have an average internal moment arm of 5 cm, the extensor muscles must produce at least 2512 N (565.1 lb) of force to lift the load.

*Step 3* estimates the total compression reaction force imposed on the L2 vertebra while lifting. (The term reaction implies that the L2 vertebra must "push" back against the other downward acting forces.) A rough estimate of this force can be made by assuming static equilibrium ($\Sigma$ forces = 0). It is assumed that the muscle, body weight, and external load forces are parallel to each other and are directed perpendicular to the superior surface of L2. (This assumption creates a small error in the estimation of the compression force. A more valid approach requires the use of trigonometry to determine the components of body weight and external load that truly act perpendicular to L2.) The compression reaction force (see Fig. 10–38, RF vector) is equal in magnitude but opposite in direction to the sum of MF, BW, and EL.

The solution to this hypothetic example suggests that a compression force of 3232 N (over 725 lb) is exerted on L2 while lifting an external load weighing 200 N (about 45 lb). To put this magnitude of force into clinical perspective, consider the following two points. First, the National Institute of Occupational Safety and Health (NIOSH) has set guidelines to protect workers from excessive loads on the lumbar region caused by lifting and handling materials. NIOSH has recommended an upper safe limit of 3400 N (764 lb) of compression force on L5-S1.[63,81] Second, the maximal load-carrying capacity of the lumbar spine is estimated to be 6400 N (1439 lb),[38] almost twice the maximal safe force recommended by NIOSH. The limit of 6400 N of force applies to a 40-year-old man. This is a maximal limit

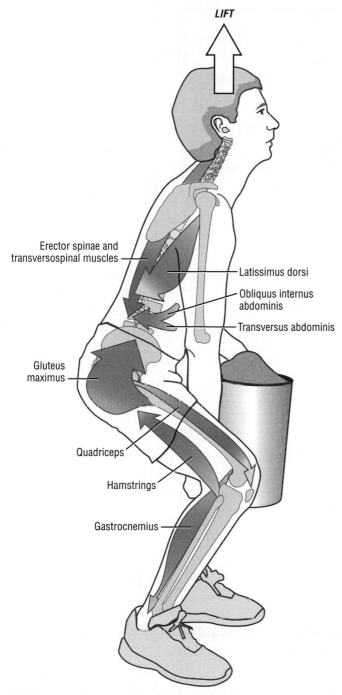

**FIGURE 10–37.** The typical activation pattern of selected muscles is shown as a healthy person lifts a load.

body weight. The axis of rotation for the sagittal plane motion is oriented in the medial-lateral direction in the region of L2 (see Fig. 10–38, open circle). Estimating the compression force is a three-step process.

*Step 1* establishes an equation that demonstrates static rotary equilibrium about the axis of rotation. The equation specifies that the sum of the internal and external torques within the sagittal plane is equal to zero. This assumption allows the internal (muscular) torque to be estimated by

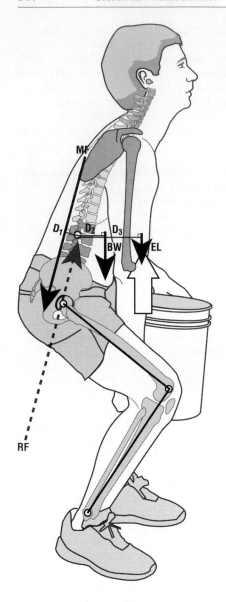

**Data**

- Internal moment arm ($D_1$) = **5 cm.**
- Total body weight = **800 N** (~180 lbs).
- Partial body weight (BW) above L2= 65% of total body weight, or ~ **520 N.**
- External moment arm from BW ($D_2$) = **13 cm.**
- External load (EL) = 25% of total body weight = **200 N** (~45 lbs).
- External moment arm from EL ($D_3$) = 29 cm.

**Step 1 — Establish Sagittal Plane Equilibrium**

Internal Torque = External Torque (BW x $D_2$ + EL x $D_3$)

Internal Torque = (520 N x .13 m) + (200 N x .29m)

**Internal Torque = 125.6 Nm**

**Step 2 — Estimate the Extensor Muscle Force (MF)**

Internal Torque (MF x $D_1$) = External Torque (BW x $D_2$ + EL x $D_3$)

$$MF = \frac{(520\ N \times .13\ m) + (200\ N \times .29\ m)}{.05\ m}$$

**MF = 2512 N (~565.1 lbs)**

**Step 3 — Estimate the Compression Reaction Force (RF) on L2**

Σ Forces = 0

-MF + -EL + -BW + RF = 0

RF = 2512 N + 520 N + 200 N

**CF ≈ 3232 N (726.6 lbs)**

**FIGURE 10–38.** The steps used to estimate the compression reaction force (RF) on the L2 vertebra while lifting a load are shown. The biomechanics are limited to the sagittal plane, about an axis of rotation at L2 (open circle). The calculations are shown in three steps: (1) establish sagittal plane equilibrium, (2) estimate the extensor muscle force, and (3) estimate the compression reaction force acting on L2. The mathematical solutions assume a condition of static equilibrium. (All abbreviations are defined in the boxes.)

that decreases by 1000 N each subsequent decade. These force values are general estimates that do not apply equally to all persons in all lifting situations.

The static model very likely underestimates the actual compressive force on the L2 vertebra for the following two reasons. First, the model accounts for muscle force produced by the back extensors only. Other muscles, especially those with near-vertical fiber orientation such as the rectus abdominis and the psoas major, certainly add to the muscular-based compression on the lumbar spine. Second, the model contains an assumption of a condition of static equilibrium, thereby ignoring the additional forces needed to accelerate the body and load upward. A rapid lift requires greater muscle force and imposes greater compression and shear on the joints and connective tissues in the low back. For this reason, it is usually recommended that a person lift loads slowly and smoothly, a condition not always practical in occupational settings.

## WAYS TO REDUCE THE FORCE DEMANDS ON THE BACK MUSCLES WHILE LIFTING

An essential point to recognize, from the calculations performed in Step 3 of Figure 10–38, is that the MF vector is by far the most influential variable for determining the magnitude of the compression force. Proportional reductions in muscle force have the greatest effect on reducing the overall compression force on the structures in the low back.

The primary factor responsible for the large force required by the low-back muscles while lifting is the disparity in the length of the internal and external moment arms. The internal moment arm ($D_1$) depicted in Figure 10–38 is assumed to be 5 cm. The extensor muscles are therefore at a sizable mechanical disadvantage and must produce a force many times larger than the weight of the load being lifted. As previously demonstrated, lifting an external load weighing 25% of one's body weight produces a compression force on L2 of four times body weight!

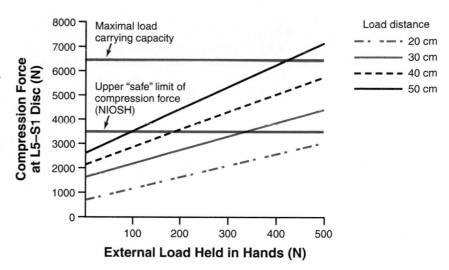

**FIGURE 10-39.** Graph shows the predicted compression force at the L5-S1 disc as a function of load size and the distance the loads are held in front of the body (1 lb = 4.448 N.). The two red horizontal lines indicate (1) the maximal load-carrying capacity of the lumbar region before structural failure, and (2) the upper safe limits of compression force on the lumbar spine as determined by the National Institute of Occupational Safety and Health. (Plot modified from Chaffin DB, Andersson GBJ: Occupational Biomechanics, 2nd ed. New York, John Wiley and Sons, 1991.

Therapeutic and educational efforts directed toward reduction of the likelihood of back injury are often directed toward reduction of the muscle force demands by four methods. *First,* reduce the rate of lifting. As previously stated, reducing the lifting velocity proportionately decreases the amount of back extensor muscle force.

*Second,* reduce the weight of the external load. This point is obvious, but not always possible.

*Third,* reduce the length of the external moment arm of the external load. This is likely the most effective and practical method of decreasing compression forces on the low back. As demonstrated in Figure 10-38, a load should be lifted from between the legs, thereby minimizing the distance between the load and the lumbar region. As estimated, lifting a heavy load using ideal technique produced a compression force on the lumbar region that remained close to the upper limits of safety proposed by NIOSH. Lifting the same load with a longer external moment arm creates very large and potentially dangerous compression forces on the low back. Figure 10-39 shows a plot of predicted compression forces on the L5-S1 disc as a function of both load size and distance between the load and the front of the chest.[12] Although an extreme example, the plot predicts that holding an external load that weighs 200 N (45 lb) 50 cm in front of the body creates about 4500 N of compression force, greatly exceeding the upper safe limit of 3400 N. In everyday life, lifting an object from between the legs is not always practical. Consider the act of sliding an obese patient toward the head of a hospital bed. Inability to reduce the distance between the patient's center of mass (located anterior to S2) and the lifter can dramatically compromise the safety of the lifter.

*Fourth,* increase the internal moment arm available to the low-back extensor muscles. A larger internal moment arm for extension allows a given extension torque to be generated with less muscle force. As stated, less muscle force typically equates to less force on the vertebral elements. Increased lumbar lordosis does indeed raise the internal moment arm available to the lumbar erector spinae muscles.[77] Lifting with an accentuated lumbar lordosis, however, is not always practical or even desirable. Lifting a very heavy load

off the floor, for example, tends to flex the lumbar spine, thereby decreasing the lordosis. Even if lifting while maintaining an exaggerated lumbar lordosis, the associated increased compression force on the apophyseal joints may not be well tolerated.

> **Four Ways to Reduce the Amount of Force Required of the Back Extensor Muscles While Lifting**
> 1. Reduce the speed of lifting
> 2. Reduce the magnitude of the external load
> 3. Reduce the length of the external moment arm
> 4. Increase the length of the internal moment arm

## ROLE OF INCREASING INTRA-ABDOMINAL PRESSURE WHILE LIFTING

In 1957, Bartelink[7] introduced the notion that the Valsalva maneuver (named after the Italian anatomist, 1666–1723), typically used while lifting loads, may help unload and thereby protect the lumbar spine. The Valsalva maneuver describes the action of voluntarily increasing intra-abdominal pressure by vigorous contraction of the abdominal muscles against a closed glottis. The Valsalva maneuver creates a rigid, vertical column of high pressure within the abdomen that pushes upward against the diaphragm and downward against the pelvic floor. Acting as an inflated "intra-abdominal balloon," Bartelink proposed that activating this mechanism while lifting may partially reduce the demands on the lumbar extensor muscles and, therefore, lower the compression force on the lumbar spine.

Although the notion of increasing intra-abdominal pressure as a way to reduce compression forces on the spine is intriguing, studies have refuted the biomechanical validity of the concept.[5,34,57,61] Contraction of the abdominal muscles produces forces that *increase* the vertical compression on the lumbar spine. Because the abdominal muscles flex the lumbar spine, their strong activation requires increased counterbalancing torques from the extensor muscles, thereby adding to the overall myogenic compression on the lumbar spine. Most persons, however, likely do benefit from the Valsalva maneuver while lifting. In a healthy person, increased compression on the lumbar spine, especially when produced through co-contraction of the surrounding muscles, provides an effective source of vertical stability to the region. Muscles such as the transversus abdominis and obliquus internus abdominis are very active while lifting,[16,17] providing an additional corset effect across the posterior lumbar region. Strong contraction of these muscles also resists unwanted torsions created by the asymmetrical lifting of an external load.

In summary, the Valsalva maneuver, typically performed while lifting, is likely a beneficial action that provides an important element of stability to the lumbar spine. The increased stability is the result of the increased myogenic lumbar compression and direct splinting action on the low back. The increased intra-abdominal pressure while lifting is more a consequence of strong contraction of the abdominal muscles and not a method, in itself, to unload the lumbar spine.

## ADDITIONAL SOURCES OF EXTENSION TORQUE USED FOR LIFTING

The maximal force-generating capacity of the low-back extensor muscles in a typical young adult in estimated to be approximately 4000 N (900 lb).[10] By assuming an average internal moment arm of 5 cm, this muscle group is expected to produce about 200 Nm of trunk extension torque. Although this estimation varies for any given person, it serves as a useful reference for the following discussion. Given a hypothetic maximal voluntary trunk extensor torque of about 200 Nm, how is the fact explained that lifting typically requires extensor torques that greatly exceed 200 Nm? For instance, the person depicted lifting the load in Figure 10–38 would have exceeded his theoretical 200 Nm threshold if the external load were increased to about 80% of his body weight. Although this is a considerable weight, it is not unusual for a person to successfully lift much greater loads, such as those regularly encountered by heavy labor workers and by competitive "power lifters." In attempts to explain this apparent dilemma, two secondary sources of extension torque are proposed: (1) passive tension generated from stretching the posterior ligamentous system, and (2) muscular-generated tension transferred through the thoracolumbar fascia.

### *Passive Tension Generation from Stretching the Posterior Ligamentous System*

When stretched, healthy ligaments and fascia exhibit some degree of natural elasticity. This quality allows connective tissue to temporarily store a small part of the force that initially causes the elongation. Bending forward in preparation for lifting progressively elongates several connective tissues in the lumbar region and, presumably, the passive tension developed in these tissues can assist with an extension torque.[21] These connective tissues, collectively known as the *posterior ligamentous system*, include the posterior longitudinal ligament, ligamentum flavum, apophyseal joint capsule, interspinous ligament, and the posterior layer of the thoracolumbar fascia.[30]

In theory, about 72 Nm of total passive extensor torque is produced by maximally stretching the posterior ligamentous system (Table 10–14).[10] Adding this passive torque to the hypothetic 200 Nm of active torque yields a total of 272 Nm of extension torque available for lifting. A fully engaged (stretched) posterior ligamentous system can, therefore, generate about 25% of the total extension torque for lifting. Note, however, that this 25% passive torque reserve is only available after the lumbar spine is maximally flexed, which

---

**TABLE 10-14. Maximal Passive Extensor Torque Produced by Stretched Lumbar Ligaments**

| Ligament | Average Maximum Tension (N)[1] | Extensor Moment Arm (m)[2] | Maximal Passive Extension Torque (Nm)[3] |
|---|---|---|---|
| Posterior longitudinal ligament | 90 | .02 | 1.8 |
| Ligamentum flava | 244 | .03 | 7.3 |
| Capsule of apophyseal joints | 680 | .04 | 27.2 |
| Interspinous ligament | 107 | .05 | 5.4 |
| Posterior layer of thoracolumbar fascia, including supraspinous ligaments and the aponeurosis covering the erector spinae muscles | 500 | .06 | 30 |
| Total | | | 71.7 |

[1]*Average maximum tension* is the tension within each stretched tissue at the point of rupture.
[2]*Extensor moment arm* is the perpendicular distance between the attachment sites of the ligaments and the medial-lateral axis of rotation within a representative lumbar vertebra.
[3]*Maximal passive extensor torque* is estimated by the product of [1] and [2] above.
Data from Bogduk N, Twomey L: Clinical Anatomy of the Lumbar Spine, 2nd ed. New York, Churchill Livingstone, 1991.

in reality is rare while lifting. Even some competitive power lifters, who appear to lift with a fully rounded low back, avoid the extremes of flexion.[14] It is generally believed that maximum flexion of the lumbar spine should be avoided while lifting.[54,55] The lumbar region should be held in a near neutral lordotic position—"neither hyperlordotic or hypolordotic."[55] The neutral position of the lumbar spine apparently aligns the local extensor muscles to more effectively resist anterior shear produced at the lumbar spine while lifting.[54] Although the neutral position of the lumbar spine may reduce the chance of injury to the low back, it engages only a small portion of the total passive torque reserve available to assist with extension. Most of the extension torque must be generated by active muscle contraction.[69] Muscle tissue can be significantly strengthened through resistive exercise in order to meet the large demands imposed by lifting.

### SPECIAL FOCUS 10-8

#### Period of "Electrical Silence" of the Erector Spinae Muscles

As described, flexing the lumbar spine engages the posterior ligamentous system to produce a passive extension torque, thereby potentially relieving some of the force demands placed on the extensor muscles. The full expression of this unloading phenomenon can be demonstrated by placing surface EMG electrodes over the lumbar erector spinae muscle group. The subject then slowly bends the trunk forward while keeping the hips and knees as extended as possible. Throughout this motion a variable amount of EMG activity from the erector spinae is observed, reflecting this muscle's eccentric activity while lowering the trunk. Once in full lumbar flexion, however, the EMG signal from the erector spinae group typically ceases.[26] The weight of the flexed trunk is supported totally by the passive torque generated by the fully stretched posterior ligamentous system, as well as the stretched connective tissues within the electrically silent erector spinae. From the flexed position, the subject actively and swiftly returns the trunk to an erect position. As the lumbar spine progressively extends, the passive torque reserve of the posterior ligamentous system progressively falls. The extension torque is then generated actively by contracting the erector spinae muscles, as evident by the large increase in the EMG signal.

### *Muscular-Generated Tension Transferred Through the Thoracolumbar Fascia*

The thoracolumbar fascia is thickest and most extensively developed in the lumbar region (see Fig. 9–76). Much of the tissue attaches to the lumbar spine, sacrum, and pelvis in a position well posterior to the axis of rotation at the lumbar region. Theoretically, therefore, passive tension within stretched thoracolumbar fascia can produce an exten-

sion torque in the lumbar region and, as such, may augment the torque created by the low-back musculature.

In order for the thoracolumbar fascia to generate useful tension, it must be stretched and rendered taut. This can occur in two ways. First, the fascia is stretched simply by bending forward and flexing the lumbar spine in preparation for lifting. Second, the fascia is stretched by active contraction of muscles that attach into the thoracolumbar fascia, such as the obliquus internus abdominis, transversus abdominis, latissimus dorsi, and gluteus maximus. These muscles are active during lifting.

Vigorous contraction of the abdominal muscles naturally occurs as a person lifts. This phenomenon is associated with an increase in intra-abdominal pressure. In theory, a contraction force generated by the obliquus internus abdominis and transversus abdominis can be transferred posteriorly to the thoracolumbar fascia to generate an extension torque in the lumbar region. The prevailing horizontal fiber direction of most of the thoracolumbar fascia limits the amount of extension torque that can be produced.[9] The force generated by the abdominal muscles may indirectly produce 6 Nm of extensor torque across the lumbar spine[50] compared with the approximately 200 Nm of active torque generated by the low-back extensor muscles. Although the actual extension torque may be small, the tension transferred through the thoracolumbar fascia may provide important static bracing to the lumbar region, much like a corset.

The latissimus dorsi and gluteus maximus may also indirectly contribute to lumbar extension torque via attachments to the thoracolumbar fascia. The two muscles attach extensively into the thoracolumbar fascia. Both are active during lifting, but for different reasons (Fig. 10–40). The gluteus maximus stabilizes and controls the hips. The latissimus dorsi helps transfer the external load being lifted from the arms to the trunk. In addition to attaching into the thoracolumbar fascia, the latissimus dorsi attaches into the posterior aspect of the pelvis, sacrum, and spine. Based on these attachments and its relative moment arm for producing lumbar extension (see Fig. 10–17), the latissimus dorsi has all the attributes of an extensor of the low back. The oblique fiber direction of the muscle as it ascends the trunk can also provide torsional stability to the axial skeleton, especially when bilaterally active. This stability may be especially useful when handling large loads in an asymmetrical fashion.

## A Closer Look at Lifting Technique

Extensive research has been conducted in the attempt to define the safest technique for lifting, especially with regard to the posture of the lumbar spine.[19,20,28,33,60,75,78] No technique is considered the safest for all persons across the wide spectrum of lifting situations.

### TWO CONTRASTING LIFTING TECHNIQUES: THE STOOP VERSUS THE SQUAT LIFT

The stoop lift and the squat lift represent the biomechanical extremes of a broad continuum of possible lifting strategies (Fig. 10–41). The *stoop lift* is performed primarily by extending the hips and lumbar region, while the knees remain

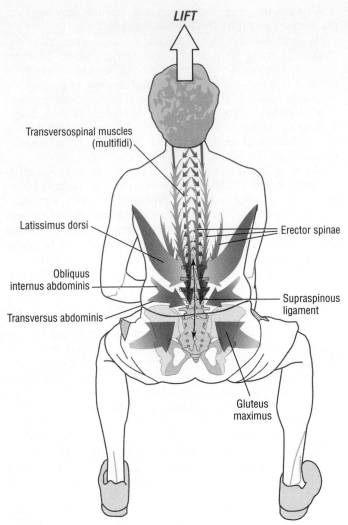

**FIGURE 10–40.** A posterior view of a typical activation pattern of selected muscles as a healthy person lifts a load by the hands. The supraspinous ligament is shown elongated and subjected to increased tension.

slightly flexed. This lifting strategy is associated with greater flexion of the low back, especially at the initiation of the lift. Furthermore, the stoop lift creates long external moment arms between the trunk and the low back, and between the load and the low back. The greater external torque requires greater extension torque from the trunk extensor muscles. In combination with a maximally flexed lumbar spine, the stoop lift can create large and possibly damaging compression and shear forces on the discs.

The *squat lift,* in contrast, typically begins with maximally flexed knees. The knees are extended during the lift, powered by the quadriceps muscles (Fig. 10–41*B*). Depending on the physical characteristics of the load and the initial depth of the squat, the lumbar region may remain nearly hyperextended, neutral (normal lordosis), or flexed throughout the lift. Perhaps the greatest advantage of the squat lift is that it typically allows the load to be raised more naturally from between the knees. The squat lift can, in theory, reduce the moment arm of the load and trunk and, as a

consequence, diminish the extensor torque demands on the muscles of the back.

The squat lift is most often advocated as the safer of the two techniques in terms of preventing back injuries. No overwhelming scientific evidence, however, supports this strongly held clinical belief.[79] As with many espoused clinical principles, the advantage of one particular concept or technique is often at least partially offset by a disadvantage. This holds true for the apparent advantage of the squat lift over the stoop lift. Although the squat lift may reduce the demands on the extensor muscles in the low back, it usually creates greater demands on the knees.[32,74] The extreme degree of initial knee flexion associated with the full squat places high force demands on the quadriceps muscle to extend the knees. The forces impose very large pressures across the tibiofemoral and patellofemoral joints. Healthy persons may tolerate high pressures at these joints without negative consequences; however, someone with painful or arthritic knees may not. The adage that lifting with the legs "spares the back and spoils the knees" does, therefore, have some validity.

Another factor to consider when evaluating the benefits of the squat lift over the stoop lift is the total work required to lift the load. The mechanical work performed while lifting is equal to the product of the weight of the body and external load multiplied by the vertical displacement of the body and load. The stoop lift is 23% to 34% more metabolically "efficient" than the squat lift—in terms of work performed per level of oxygen consumption.[82] The squat lift requires greater work because a greater proportion of the total body mass must be moved through space.

## Summary: Factors that Contribute to Safe Lifting

Rather than a squat lift or stoop lift, people usually choose an individualized (freestyle) technique. A freestyle technique

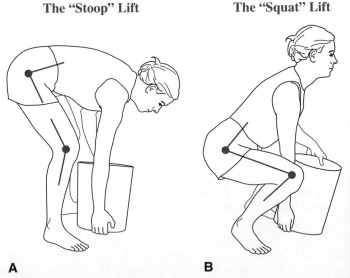

**FIGURE 10–41.** Two contrasting styles of lifting. *A,* The initiation of the stoop lift. *B,* The initiation of the squat lift. The axes of rotation are shown at the hip and knee joints.

## TABLE 10–15. Factors Considered to Contribute to Safe Lifting Techniques

| Consideration | Rationale | Comment |
|---|---|---|
| Maintain the external load as close to the body as possible. | Minimizes the external moment arm of the load, thereby reduces torque and force demands on back muscle. | Holding the load between the knees while lifting is ideal but not always possible. |
| Lift with the lumbar spine held as close to a neutral lordotic posture as possible. Avoid the *extremes* of flexion and extension. Exact position of the spine can vary based on comfort and practicality. | Concentrating on holding the lumbar spine in a neutral lordotic position may help prevent the spine from extremes of flexion and extension. Vigorous contraction of the back extensor muscles, with the lumbar spine maximally *flexed,* may produce damaging forces on the intervertebral discs. In contrast, vigorous contraction of the back extensor muscles with the lumbar spine maximally *extended* may damage the apophyseal joints. | Lifting with minimal-to-moderate flexion or extension in the lumbar spine may be acceptable for some persons, depending on the health and experience of the lifter and the situation. Minimal-to-moderate flexion or extension both have a biomechanical advantage:<br>  *Minimal-to-moderate flexion* increases the passive tension generated by the posterior ligamentous system, possibly reducing the force demands on extensor muscles.<br>  *Minimal-to-moderate extension* places the apophyseal joints nearer to their close-packed position, thereby providing greater stability to the region. |
| When lifting, fully utilize the hip and knee extensor muscles to minimize the force demands on the low-back muscles. | Very large forces produced by low-back extensor muscles can injure the muscles themselves, intervertebral discs, vertebral endplates, or apophyseal joints. | Persons with hip or knee arthritis may be unable to effectively use the muscles in the legs to assist the back muscles.<br>The squat lift may encourage the use of the leg muscles but also increases the overall work demands on the body. |
| Minimize the vertical and horizontal distance that a load must be lifted. | Minimizing the distance that the load is moved reduces the total work of the lift, thereby reducing fatigue; minimizing the distance that the load is moved reduces the extremes of movement in the low back and lower extremities. | Using handles or an adjustable-height platform may be helpful. |
| Avoid twisting when lifting. | Torsional forces applied to vertebrae can predispose the person to intervertebral disc injury. | Properly designed work environment can reduce the need for twisting while lifting. |
| Lift as slowly and smoothly as conditions allow. | A slow and smooth lift reduces the large peak force generated in muscles and connective tissues. | |
| Lift with a moderately wide and slightly staggered base of support provided by the legs. | A relatively wide base of support affords greater overall stability of the body, thereby reducing the chance of a fall or slip. | |
| When possible, use the assistance of a mechanical device or additional people while lifting. | Using assistance while lifting can reduce the demand on the back of the primary lifter. | Using a mechanical hoist (Hoyer lift) or a "two-man" transfer may be prudent in many settings. |

allows the lifter to combine some of the benefits of the squat lift with the more metabolically efficient stoop lift. Workers have reported a higher, self-perceived, maximal safe limit when allowed to lift in a freestyle technique rather than in a set technique.[76] Although not ideal for everyone and every lifting task, the technique depicted in Figure 10–38 illustrates two safety features: (1) the lumbar spine is held in a near-neutral lordotic position, and (2) the load is lifted from between the legs. These and additional considerations for safe lifting techniques are also listed in Table 10–15.

Those persons with a history of or propensity for low-back injury should heed the following three common sense considerations: (1) know your physical limits, (2) think the lift through before the event, and (3) within practical and health limits, stay in optimal physical and cardiovascular condition.

## REFERENCES

1. Adams MA, Dolan P: A technique for quantifying the bending moment acting on the lumbar spine in vivo. J Biomech 24:117–126, 1991.

2. Andersson EA, Nilsson J, Ma Z, et al: Abdominal and hip flexor muscle activation during various training exercises. Eur J Appl Physiol 75:115–123, 1997.

3. Andersson GBJ, Ortengren R, Nachemson A: Quantitative studies of back loads in lifting. Spine 1:178–185, 1976.

4. Andersson GBJ, Ortengren R, Nachemson A: Quantitative studies of the load on the back in different working postures. Scand J Rehabil Med 6:173–181, 1978.

5. Aspden RM: Intra-abdominal pressure and its role in spinal mechanics. J Biomech 2:168–174, 1987.

6. Aspden RM: Review of the functional anatomy of the spinal ligaments and the lumbar erector spinae muscles. Clin Anat 5:372–387, 1992.

7. Bartelink DL: The role of abdominal pressure in relieving the pressure on the lumbar intervertebral discs. Bone Joint Surg 39B:718–725, 1957.

8. Beimborn DS, Morrissey MC: A review of the literature related to trunk muscle performance. Spine 13:655–660, 1988.

9. Bogduk N, Macintosh JE: The applied anatomy of the thoracolumbar fascia. Spine 9:164–170, 1984.

10. Bogduk N, Twomey L: Clinical Anatomy of the Lumbar Spine, 2nd ed. New York, Churchill Livingstone, 1991.

11. Burgess-Limerick R, Abernethy B: Toward a quantitative definition of manual lifting postures. Hum Factors 39:141–148, 1997.

12. Chaffin DB, Andersson GBJ: Occupational Biomechanics, 2nd ed. New York, John Wiley and Sons, 1991.

13. Chaffin DB, Page GB: Postural effects on biomechanical and psychophysical weight-lifting limits. Ergonomics 37:663–676, 1994.

14. Cholewicki J, McGill SM: Lumbar posterior ligament involvement during extremely heavy lifts estimated from fluoroscopic measurements. J Biomech 25:17–28, 1992.

15. Cook TM, Neumann DA: The effects of load placement on the EMG activity of the low back muscles during load carrying by men and women. Ergonomics 30:1413–1423, 1987.

16. Cresswell AG, Grundstrom H, Thorstensson A: Observations on intra-abdominal pressure and patterns of abdominal intra-musuclar activity in man. Acta Physiol Scand 144:409–418, 1992.

17. de Looze MP, Groen H, Horemans H, et al: Abdominal muscles contribute in a minor way to peak spinal compression in lifting. J Biomech 32:655–662, 1999.

18. Deng YC, Goldsmith W: Response of a human head/neck/upper-torso replica to dynamic loading. Part I: Physical model. J Biomech 20:471–486, 1987.

19. Delitto RS, Rose SJ, Apts DW: Electromyographic analysis of two techniques for squat lifting. Phys Ther 67:1329–1334, 1987.

20. Dolan P, Earley M, Adams MA: Bending and compressive stresses acting on the lumbar spine during lifting activities. J Biomech 27:1237–1248, 1994.

21. Dolan P, Mannion AF, Adams MA: Passive tissues help the back muscles to generate extensor moments during lifting. J Biomech 27:1077–1085, 1994.

22. Donisch EW, Basmajian JV: Electromyography of deep back muscles in man. Am J Anat 133:25–36, 1972.

23. Drury CG, Deeb JM, Hartman B, et al: Symmetric and asymmetric manual materials handling. Part 2: Biomechanics. Ergonomics 32:565–583, 1989.

24. Dumas GA, Poulin MJ, Roy B, et al: Orientation and moment arms of some trunk muscles. Spine 16:293–303, 1991.

25. Ferguson SA, Marras WS: A literature review of low back disorder surveillance measures and risk factors. Clin Biomech 12:211–226, 1997.

26. Floyd WF, Silver PHS: The function of the erectores spinae muscles in certain movements and postures in man. J Physiol 129:184–203, 1955.

27. Freivalds A, Chaffin DB, Garg A, et al: A dynamic biomechanical evaluation of lifting maximum acceptable loads. J Biomech 17:251–262, 1984.

28. Garg A, Moore JS: Prevention strategies and the low back in industry. Occup Med 7:629–640, 1992.

29. Genaidy AM, Waly SM, Khalil TM, et al: Spinal compression tolerance limits for the design of manual material handling operations in the workplace. Ergonomics 36:415–434, 1993.

30. Gracovetsky S, Farfan HF, Lamy C: The mechanism of the lumbar spine. Spine 6:249–262, 1981.

31. Granata KP, Marras WS: An EMG-assisted model of loads on the lumbar spine during asymmetric trunk extensions. J Biomech 26:1429–1438, 1993.

32. Hagen KB, Hallen JH, Ringdahl-Harms K: Physiological and subjective responses to maximal repetitive lifting employing stoop and squat technique. Eur J Appl Physiol 67:291–297, 1993.

33. Hart DL, Stobbe TJ, Jaraiedi M: Effect of lumbar posture on lifting. Spine 12:138–145, 1987.

34. Hemborg B, Moritz U, Lowing H: Intra-abdominal pressure and trunk muscle activity during lifting. Part IV: The causal factors of intra-abdominal pressure rise. Scand J Rehabil Med 17:25–38, 1985.

35. Hidalgo J, Genaidy A, Karwowski W, et al: A comprehensive lifting model: Beyond the NIOSH lifting equation. Ergonomics 40:916–927, 1997.

36. Hodges PW, Richardson CA: Inefficient muscular stabilization of the lumbar spine associated with low back pain: A motor control evaluation of transversus abdominis. Spine 21:2640–2650, 1996.

37. Hsiang SM, McGorry RW: Three different lifting strategies for controlling the motion patterns of the external load. Ergonomics 40:928–939, 1997.

38. Jager M, Luttmann A: The load on the lumbar spine during asymmetrical bimanual material handling. Ergonomics 35:783–805, 1992.

39. Juker D, McGill S, Kropf P, et al: Quantitative intramuscular myoelectric activity of lumbar portions of psoas and the abdominal wall during a wide variety of tasks. Med Sci Sports Exerc 30:301–310, 1998.

40. Keagy RD, Brumlik J, Bergan JJ: Direct electromyography of the psoas major muscle in man. J Bone Joint Surg 48A:1377–1382, 1966.

41. Kelsey JL, Githens PB, White AA, et al: An epidemiologic study of lifting and twisting on the job and risk for acute prolapsed lumbar intervertebral disc. J Orthop Res 2:61–66, 1984.

42. Kendall FP, McCreary AK, Provance PG: Muscles: Testing and Function, 4th ed. Baltimore, Williams & Wilkins, 1993.

43. Keyserling WM: Workplace risk factors and occupational musculoskeletal disorders. Part 1: A review of biomechanical and psychophysical research on risk factors associated with low back pain. Am Ind Hyg Assoc J 61:39–50, 2000.

44. Kingma I, van Dieen JH, de Looze M, et al: Asymmetric low back loading in asymmetric lifting movements is not prevented by pelvic twist. J Biomech 31:527–534, 1998.

45. Kumar S: Moment arms of spinal musculature determined from CT scans. Clin Biomech 3:137–144, 1988.

46. Kumar S, Narayan Y, Zedka M: An electromyographic study of unresisted trunk rotation with normal velocity among healthy subjects. Spine 21:1500–1512, 1996.

47. Lehman GJ, McGill SM: Quantification of the differences in electromyographic activity magnitude between the upper and lower portions of the rectus abdominis muscles during selected trunk exercises. Phys Ther 81:1096–1101, 2001.

48. Macintosh JE, Bogduk N: The biomechanics of the lumbar multifidus. Clin Biomech 1:205–213, 1986.

49. Macintosh JE, Bogduk N: The attachments of the lumbar erector spinae. Spine 16:783–792, 1991.

50. Macintosh JE, Bogduk N, Gracovetsky S: The biomechanics of the thoracolumbar fascia. Clin Biomech 2:78–83, 1987.

51. Macintosh JE, Valenica F, Bogduk N, et al: The morphology of the human lumbar multifidus. Clin Biomech 1:196–204, 1986.

52. Madsen OR: Trunk extensor and flexor strength measured by the Cybex 6000 dynamometer. Spine 21:2770–2776, 1996.

53. Marras WS, Lavender SA, Leurgans SE, et al: Biomechanical risk factors for occupationally related low back disorders. Ergonomics 38:377–410, 1995.

54. McGill SM: Biomechanics of the thoracolumbar spine. In Dvir Z (ed): Clinical Biomechanics. Philadelphia, Churchill Livingstone, 2000.

55. McGill SM, Hughson RL, Parks K: Changes in lumbar lordosis modify the role of the extensor muscles. Clin Biomech 15:777–780, 2000.

56. McGill SM, Norman RW: Dynamically and statically determined low back moments during lifting. J Biomech 18:877–885, 1985.

57. McGill SM, Norman RW: Reassessment of the role of intra-abdominal pressure in spinal compression. Ergonomics 30:1565–1588, 1987.

58. McGill SM, Patt N, Norman RW: Measurement of the trunk musculature of active males using CT scan radiography: Implications for force and moment generating capacity about the L4/L5 joint. J Biomech 21:329–341, 1988.

59. McGill SM, Santaguida L, Stevens J: Measurement of the trunk musculature from T5 to L5 using MRI scans of 15 young males corrected for muscle fibre orientation. Clin Biomech 8:171–178, 1993.

60. McGorry RW, Hsiang SM: The effect of industrial back belts and

breathing technique on trunk and pelvic coordination during a lifting task. Spine 24:1124–1130, 1999.

61. Nachemson AL, Andersson GBJ, Schultz AB: Valsalva maneuver biomechanics: Effects on lumbar trunk loads of elevated intraabdominal pressures. Spine 11:476–479, 1986.

62. National Institute for Occupational Safety and Health (NIOSH): The National Occupational Exposure Survey (Publication No. 89–103). Cincinnati, OH, NIOSH, 1989.

63. National Institute for Occupational Safety and Health (NIOSH): Work Practices Guide for Manual Lifting (Report No. 81–122). Cincinnati, OH, NIOSH, 1992.

64. Newton M, Thow M, Somerville D, et al: Trunk strength testing with iso-machines. Part 2: Experimental evaluation of the Cybex II back testing system in normal subjects and patients with chronic low back pain. Spine 18:812–824, 1993.

65. Nordin M, Kahanovitz N, Verderame R, et al: Normal trunk muscle strength and endurance in women and the effect of exercises and electrical stimulation. Part 1: Normal endurance and trunk muscle strength in 100 women. Spine 12:105–111, 1987.

66. Panjabi MM, Cholewicki J, Nibu K, et al: Critical load of the human cervical spine: An in vitro experimental study. Clin Biomech 13:11–17, 1998.

67. Patwardhan AG, Havey RM, Ghanayem AJ, et al: Load-carrying capacity of the human cervical spine in compression is increased under a follower load. Spine 25:1548–1554, 2000.

68. Porterfield JA, DeRosa C: Mechanical Neck Pain: Perspectives in Functional Anatomy. Philadelphia, WB Saunders, 1995.

69. Potvin JR, McGill SM, Norman RW: Trunk muscle and lumbar ligament contributions to dynamic lifts with varying degrees of trunk flexion. Spine 16:1099–1107, 1991.

70. Potvin JR, Norman RW, McGill SM: Reduction in anterior shear forces on the L4/L5 disc by the lumbar musculature. Clin Biomech 6:88–96, 1991.

71. Rizk NN: A new description of the anterior abdominal wall in man and mammals. J Anat 131:373–385, 1980.

72. Santaguida PL, McGill SM: The psoas major muscle: A three-dimensional geometric study. J Biomech 28:339–345, 1995.

73. Schipplein OD, Reinsel TE, Andersson GBJ, et al: The influence of initial horizontal weight placement on the loads at the lumbar spine while lifting. Spine 20:1895–1898, 1995.

74. Schipplein OD, Trafimow JH, Andersson GBJ, et al: Relationship between moments at the L5/S1 level, hip and knee joint when lifting. J Biomech 23:907–912, 1990.

75. Shirazi-Adl A, Parnianpour M: Effect of changes in lordosis on mechanics of the lumbar spine-lumbar curvature in lifting. J Spinal Dis 5:436–447, 1999.

76. Stevenson J, Bryant T, Greenhorn D, et al: The effect of lifting protocol on comparisons with isoinertial lifting performance. Ergonomics 33:1455–1469, 1990.

77. Tveit P, Daggfeldt K, Hetland S, et al: Erector spinae lever arm length variations with changes in spinal curvature. Spine 19:199–204, 1994.

78. Vakos JP, Nitz AJ, Threlkeld AJ, et al: Electromyographic activity of selected trunk and hip muscles during a squat lift. Spine 19:687–695, 1994.

79. van Dieen JH, Hoozemans MJM, Toussaint HM: Stoop or squat: A review of biomechanical studies on lifting technique. Clin Biomech 14:685–696, 1999.

80. Vitti M, Fujiwara M, Basmajian JV, et al: The integrated roles of longus colli and sternocleidomastoid muscles: An electromyographic study. Anat Rec 177:471–484, 1973.

81. Waters TR, Putz-Anderson V, Garg A, et al: Revised NIOSH equation for the design and evaluation of manual lifting tasks. Ergonomics 36:749–776, 1993.

82. Welbergen E, Kemper HCG, Knibbe JJ, et al: Efficiency and effectiveness of stoop and squat lifting at different frequencies. Ergonomics 34:613–624, 1991.

83. Wilke H-J, Wolf S, Claes LE, et al: Stability increase of the lumbar spine with different muscle groups. Spine 20:192–198, 1995.

84. Williams PL, Bannister LH, Berry M, et al: Gray's Anatomy, 38th ed. New York, Churchill Livingstone, 1995.

85. Wolfort FG, Kanter MA, Miller LB: Torticollis. Plast Reconstr Surg 84:682–692, 1989.

## ADDITIONAL READINGS

Adams MA, McNally DS, Chinn H, et al: Posture and the compressive strength of the lumbar spine. Clin Biomech 9:5–14, 1994.

Chaffin DB, Park KS: A longitudinal study of low back pain as associated with occupational weight lifting factors. Am Ind Hyg Assoc J 34:513–525, 1973.

Ekholm J, Arborelius UP, Nemeth G: The load on the lumbosacral joint and trunk muscle activity during lifting. Ergonomics 25:145–161, 1982.

Halpern AA, Bleck EE: Sit up exercises: An electromyographic study. Clin Orthop 145:172–178, 1979.

Keshner EA, Campbell D, Katz RT, et al: Neck muscle activation patterns in humans during isometric head stabilization. Exp Brain Res 75:335–344, 1989.

Moroney SP, Schultz AB, Miller JAA: Analysis and measurement of neck loads. J Orthop Res 6:713–720, 1988.

# CHAPTER 11

# Kinesiology of Mastication and Ventilation

DONALD A. NEUMANN, PT, PHD

## TOPICS AT A GLANCE

## PART 1: MASTICATION

Mastication is the process of chewing, tearing, and grinding food with the teeth. This process involves an interaction of the muscles of mastication, the teeth, and the pair of temporomandibular joints (TMJs). The joints form the pivot point between the lower jaw (mandible) and the base of the cranium. The TMJs are one of the most continuously used pairs of joints in the body, not only during mastication, but also during swallowing and speaking. The first part of this chapter focuses on the kinesiologic role of the TMJ during mastication.

## OSTEOLOGY AND TEETH

### Regional Surface Anatomy

Figure 11–1 highlights the surface anatomy associated with the TMJ. The *mandibular condyle* fits within the mandibular fossa of the temporal bone. The condyle can be palpated just

anterior to the *external auditory meatus* (i.e., the opening into the ear). The cranial attachment of the temporalis muscle is within a broad, slightly concave region of the skull known as the *temporal fossa*. The temporal, parietal, frontal, sphenoid, and zygomatic bones all contribute to the temporal fossa.

Additional surface anatomy associated with the TMJ is the *mastoid process* of the temporal bone, the *angle of the mandible,* and the *zygomatic arch*. The zygomatic arch is formed by the union of the zygomatic process of the temporal bone and the temporal process of the zygomatic bone.

### Individual Bones

The mandible, maxillae, temporal, zygomatic, sphenoid, and hyoid bones are all related to the structure or function of the TMJ.

#### MANDIBLE

The mandible is the largest of the facial bones (see Fig. 11–1). It is a very mobile bone, suspended from the cranium by

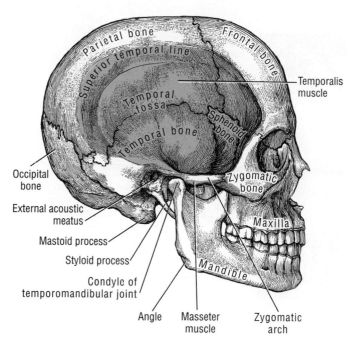

**FIGURE 11–1.** Lateral view of the skull with emphasis on bony landmarks associated with the temporomandibular joint. The proximal attachments of the temporalis and masseter muscles are indicated in red.

muscles, ligaments, and capsule of the TMJ. Muscles of mastication attach either directly or indirectly to the mandible. Muscle contraction brings the teeth embedded within the mandible against the teeth embedded within the fixed maxillae.

---

| **Relevant Osteologic Features of the Mandible** |
| --- |
| • Body |
| • Ramus |
| • Angle |
| • Coronoid process |
| • Condyle |
| • Neck |
| • Mandibular notch |
| • Pterygoid fossa |

---

The two main parts of the mandible are the body and the two rami (Fig. 11–2). The *body*, the horizontal portion of the bone, accepts the lower 16 adult teeth (see Fig. 11–3). The *rami* of the mandible project vertically from the posterior aspect of the body (see Fig. 11–2). Each ramus has an external and internal surface, four borders, and two processes at its superior aspect—the coronoid process and the condylar process. Extending between the coronoid and condylar process is the *mandibular notch*. The posterior and inferior borders of the ramus join at the readily palpable *angle of the mandible*. The masseter and medial pterygoid muscles—two powerful muscles of mastication—share similar attachments in the region of the angle of the mandible.

The *coronoid process* is a triangular projection of thin bone that extends upward from the anterior border of the ramus. This process is the primary inferior attachment of the tem-

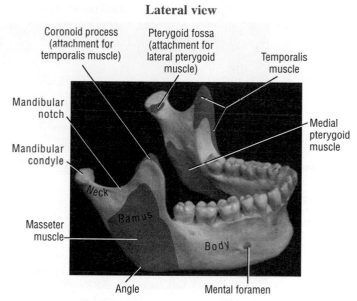

**Lateral view**

**FIGURE 11–2.** Lateral view of the mandible. Muscle attachments are shown.

poralis muscle. The *condyle* of the mandible extends upward from the posterior border of the ramus. The condyle forms the convex bony component of the TMJ. The *mandibular neck* is a slightly constricted region located immediately below the condyle. The lateral pterygoid muscle attaches to the anterior-medial surface of the mandibular neck, within a small depression called the *pterygoid fossa* (Figs. 11–2 and 11–4).

## MAXILLAE

The right and left maxillae fuse to form a single maxilla, or upper jaw. The maxilla is fixed within the skull through

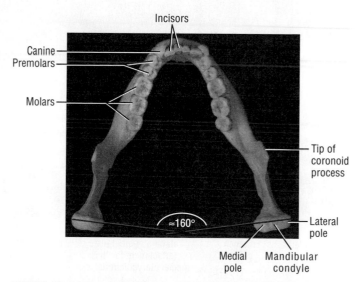

**FIGURE 11–3.** The mandible as viewed from above. The names of the permanent teeth are indicated. The long (side-to-side) axis through each mandibular condyle intersects at an approximate 160-degree angle.

**Internal (medial) view**

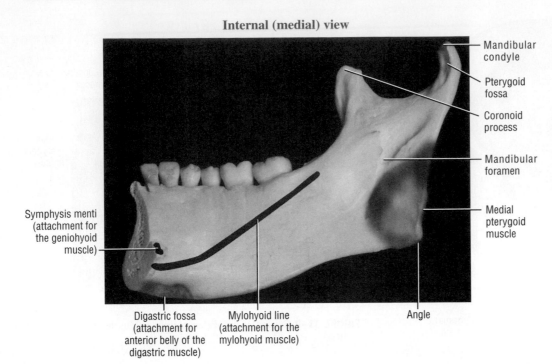

**FIGURE 11–4.** Internal view of the right side of the mandible. The bone is bisected in the midsagittal plane. The attachments of the mylohyoid and geniohyoid muscles are indicated in red; the attachment of the anterior belly of the digastric and medial pterygoid muscles are indicated in gray. Note the one missing wisdom tooth (third molar).

rigid articulations to adjacent bones (see Fig. 11–1). The maxillae extend superiorly forming the floor of the nasal cavity and the orbit of the eyes. The lower horizontal portions of the maxillae accept the upper teeth.

## TEMPORAL BONE

Two temporal bones exist—one on each side of the cranium. The *mandibular fossa* forms the bony concavity of the TMJ (Fig. 11–5). The fossa is bound anteriorly by the *artic-*

**Inferior view**

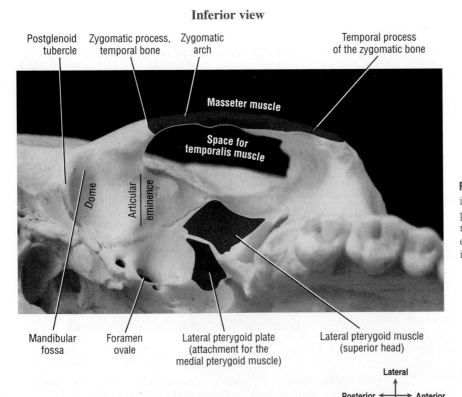

**FIGURE 11–5.** Inferior view of the skull highlighting the right mandibular fossa, lateral pterygoid plate, and zygomatic arch. The proximal attachments of the masseter, medial pterygoid, and lateral pterygoid (superior head) muscles are shown in red.

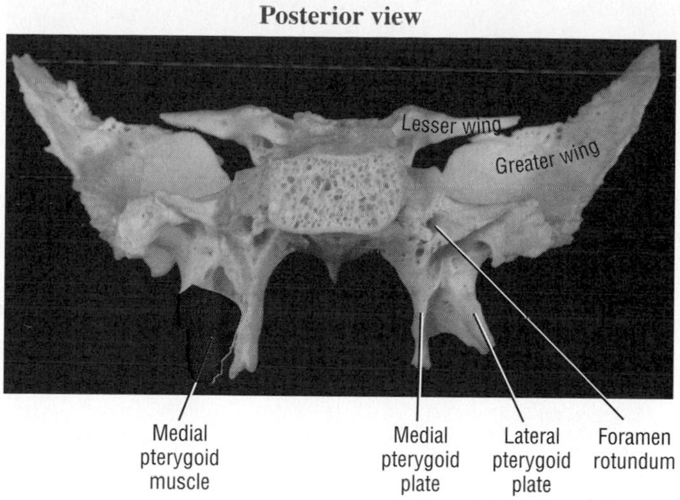

**Posterior view**

![Posterior view of sphenoid bone]

FIGURE 11–6. Posterior view of a sphenoid bone removed from the cranium. The proximal attachment of the medial pterygoid muscle is indicated in red.

*ular eminence,* and posteriorly by the *postglenoid tubercle* and the tympanic part of the temporal bone. On full opening of the mouth, the condyles of the mandible slide anteriorly and inferiorly across the pair of sloped articular eminences.

---

**Relevant Osteologic Features of the Temporal Bone**
- Mandibular fossa
- Articular eminence
- Postglenoid tubercle
- Styloid process
- Zygomatic process

---

The *styloid process* is a long slender extension of bone that protrudes from the inferior aspect of the temporal bone (see Fig. 11–1). The pointed process serves as an attachment for the stylomandibular ligament (to be discussed further) and three small muscles (styloglossus, stylohyoid, and stylopharyngeus). The *zygomatic process* of the temporal bone forms the posterior half of the zygomatic arch (see Fig. 11–5).

## ZYGOMATIC BONE

The right and left zygomatic bones constitute the major part of the cheeks and the lateral orbits of the eyes (see Fig. 11–1). The *temporal process* of a zygomatic bone contributes the anterior half of the zygomatic arch (see Fig. 11–5). A large part of the masseter muscle attaches to the zygomatic bone and the adjacent zygomatic arch.

## SPHENOID BONE

Although the sphenoid bone does not contribute to the structure of the TMJ, it does provide proximal attachments for the medial and lateral pterygoid muscles. When articulated within the cranium, the sphenoid bone lies transversely

across the base of the skull. The relevant osteologic features of the sphenoid bone are its *greater wing, medial pterygoid plate,* and *lateral pterygoid plate* (Fig. 11–6). By removing a section of the zygomatic arch, the lateral surfaces of the greater wing and lateral pterygoid plate are revealed (Fig. 11–7).

---

**Relevant Osteologic Features of the Sphenoid Bone**
- Greater wing
- Medial pterygoid plate
- Lateral pterygoid plate

---

## HYOID BONE

The hyoid is a **U**-shaped bone located at the base of the throat, just anterior to the body of the third cervical vertebra. The *body of the hyoid* is convex anteriorly. The bilateral *greater horns* form its slightly curved sides. The hyoid is suspended primarily by its bilateral stylohyoid ligaments. Several muscles involved with moving of the tongue, swallowing, and speaking attach to the hyoid bone (see Fig. 11–20).

## Teeth

The maxillae and mandible each contain 16 permanent teeth (see Fig. 11–3, for names of lower teeth). The structure of each tooth reflects its function in mastication (Table 11–1).

Each tooth has two basic parts: crown and root (Fig. 11–8). Normally the *crown* is covered with enamel and is located above the gingiva (gum). The *root* of each tooth is embedded in alveolar bone. The *peridontal ligaments* help attach the roots of the teeth within their sockets.

*Cusps* are conical elevations that arise on the surface of a tooth. *Maximal intercuspation* describes the position of the mandible when the cusps of the opposing teeth are in maximal contact. The term is frequently used interchangeably with *centric relation,* especially in describing the relative position of the articular surfaces within the TMJ. The relaxed *postural position* of the mandible allows a slight "freeway

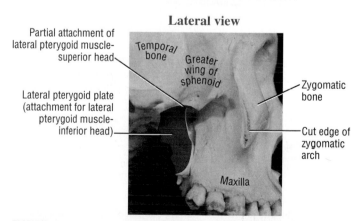

FIGURE 11–7. Lateral view of the right side of the cranium with a section of the zygomatic arch removed. The greater wing and lateral side of the lateral pterygoid plate are visible. Note the attachments in red of the two heads of the lateral pterygoid muscle.

**TABLE 11–1. Permanent Teeth**

| Names | Functions | Numbers | Structural Characteristics |
|---|---|---|---|
| Incisors | Cut food | Maxillary, 4<br>Mandibular, 4 | Sharp edges |
| Canines | Tear food | Maxillary, 2<br>Mandibular, 2 | Longest permanent teeth; crown has a single cusp. |
| Premolars | Crush food into smaller particles | Maxillary, 4<br>Mandibular, 4 | Crown has two cusps (bicuspid); lower second premolars may have three cusps. |
| Molars | Grind food into small particles for swallowing | Maxillary, 6<br>Mandibular, 6 | Crown has four or five cusps. |

space" (interocclusal clearance) between the upper and lower teeth. Normally, the teeth make contact (occlude) only during chewing and swallowing.

## ARTHROLOGY

The TMJ is formed by the condyle of the mandible that fits loosely within the mandibular fossa of the temporal bone (see Fig. 11–1). It is a synovial joint that permits a wide range of rotation as well as translation. An *articular disc* cushions the potentially large and repetitive muscle forces inherent to mastication. The disc separates the joint into two synovial joint cavities (Fig. 11–9). The *inferior joint cavity* is between the inferior aspect of the disc and the mandibular condyle. The larger *superior joint cavity* is between the superior surface of the disc and the bone formed by the mandibular fossa and the articular eminence.

Although both right and left TMJs function together, each retains its ability to function relatively independently. Mastication is typically performed asymmetrically, with one side of the mandible exerting a greater biting force than the other. The dominant side is often referred to as the "working" side, whereas the nondominant side is referred to as the "balancing" side.[20] Different demands are placed on the muscles and joints of the working and balancing sides.

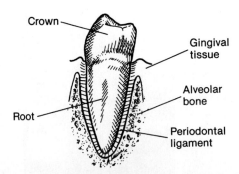

**FIGURE 11–8.** The tooth and its periodontal supportive structures. The width of the periodontal ligaments is greatly exaggerated for illustrative purposes. (From Okeson JP: Management of Temporomandibular Disorders and Occlusion, 4th ed. Chicago, Mosby, 1998.)

## Osseous Structure

### MANDIBULAR CONDYLE

The mandibular condyle is flattened from front to back, with its medial-lateral length twice as long as its anterior-posterior length (see Fig. 11–3).[46] The condyle is generally convex, possessing short projections of bone known as *medial* and *lateral poles*. The medial pole is more prominent than the lateral. When opening and closing the mouth, the outside edge of the lateral pole can be palpated as a point under the skin just anterior to the external auditory meatus.

The articular surface of the mandibular condyle is lined with a thin but dense layer of *fibrous connective tissue*. This tissue absorbs loads associated with mastication better than hyaline cartilage, and it has a superior reparative process.[56] Both of these functions are important when considering the extraordinary demands placed on the joint surfaces.[48]

### MANDIBULAR FOSSA

The mandibular fossa of the temporal bone is divided into two surfaces: articular and nonarticular. The *articular surface* of the fossa is formed by the articular eminence, occupying the sloped anterior wall of the fossa (see Figs. 11–5 and 11–9). This thick and smooth loadbearing surface is lined with a dense layer of fibrocartilage. Full opening of the mouth requires that each condyle slides forward across the articular eminence. The slope of the articular eminence varies considerably among persons but typically is oriented about 70 degrees from the horizontal plane.[29] The slope affects the path taken by the condyles during the opening and closing of the mouth.

The *nonarticular surface* of the fossa consists of a very thin layer of bone and fibrocartilage that occupies much of the superior (dome) and posterior walls of the fossa (see Fig. 11–5). The thin region is not an adequate loadbearing surface. A large force applied to the chin can fracture this region of the fossa, possibly even sending bone fragments into the cranium.

## Articular Disc

The articular disc within the TMJ consists primarily of dense fibrous connective tissue that, with the exception of its periphery, lacks a blood supply (see Fig. 11–9). The tissue is

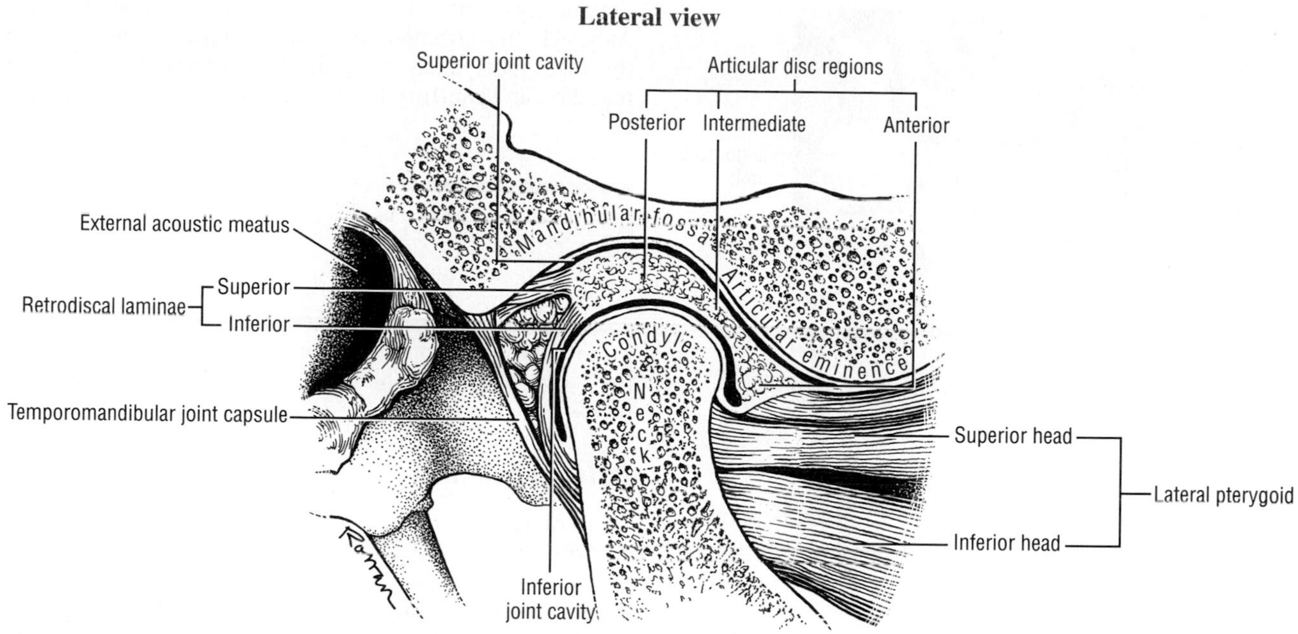

**Lateral view**

**FIGURE 11–9.** A lateral view of a sagittal plane cross-section through a normal right temporomandibular joint. The mandible is in a position of maximal intercuspation, with the disc in its ideal position relative to the condyle and the temporal bone.

flexible but firm owing to its high collagen content. The entire periphery of the disc attaches to the surrounding capsule of the joint.

The disc is divided into three regions: posterior, intermediate, and anterior (see Fig. 11–9). The shape of each region allows the disc to accommodate the contour of the condyle and the fossa. The *posterior region* of the disc is convex superiorly and concave inferiorly. The concavity accepts most of the condyle much like a ball-and-socket joint. The extreme posterior region attaches to a loosely organized *retrodiscal laminae,* containing collagen and elastin fibers. Connections made by the laminae anchor the disc posteriorly to bone (see the box). A meshwork of fat, blood vessels, and sensory nerves fills the space between the superior and inferior laminae.

---

**The *Posterior* Region of the Articular Disc Attaches to the**

1. Collagen-rich *inferior retrodiscal lamina* which, in turn, attaches to the periphery of the superior neck of the mandible along with the capsule of the TMJ.
2. Elastin-rich *superior retrodiscal lamina* which, in turn, attaches to the tympanic plate of the temporal bone just posterior to the fossa.

---

The *intermediate region* of the disc is concave inferiorly and generally flat superiorly. The *anterior region* is nearly flat inferiorly and slightly concave superiorly to accommodate the maximal convexity of the articular eminence. The anterior region of the disc attaches to several tissues (see the box).

The thickness of the disc varies between its anterior and posterior regions. The thinnest intermediate region is only 1 mm thick.[25] The anterior and posterior regions, however, are about two to three times thicker. The disc is constricted at

its intermediate region.[47] The constriction, flanked by the adjacent thicker anterior and posterior regions, forms a dimple on the disc's inferior surface. In maximal intercuspation, the dimpled region of the intermediate region of the disc fits between the anterior-superior edge of the condyle and the articular eminence of the fossa.[33] The disc position protects the condyle as it slides forward across the articular eminence during the later phase of opening the mouth widely.

---

**The *Anterior* Region of the Articular Disc Attaches to the**

1. Periphery of the superior neck of the mandible along with the anterior capsule of the TMJ.
2. Tendon of the superior head of the lateral pterygoid muscle.
3. Temporal bone just anterior to the articular eminence.

---

The articular disc maximizes the congruency within the TMJ to reduce contact pressure. The disc adds stability to the joint and helps guide the condyle of the mandible during movement. In the healthy TMJ, the disc slides with the translating condyle. Movement is governed by intra-articular pressure, by muscle forces, and by collateral ligaments that attach the condyle to the periphery of the disc.

## Capsular and Ligamentous Structures

### FIBROUS CAPSULE

The TMJ and disc are surrounded by a loose *fibrous capsule.* The internal surfaces of the capsule are lined with a synovial membrane. Superiorly, the capsule attaches to the rim of the mandibular fossa, as far anterior as the articular eminence. Inferiorly, the capsule forms *collateral ligaments* that attach to the periphery of the articular disc. Anteriorly, the capsule,

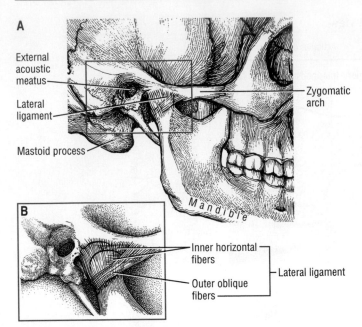

**A**

External
acoustic
meatus

Lateral
ligament

Mastoid process

Zygomatic
arch

*Mandible*

**B**

Inner horizontal
fibers

Outer oblique
fibers

Lateral ligament

**FIGURE 11–10.** *A,* The lateral ligament of the temporomandibular joint. *B,* The lateral ligament's main fibers: oblique and horizontal.

and part of the anterior edge of disc, attaches to the tendon of the superior head of the lateral pterygoid muscle (see Fig. 11–9).

The capsule supports the joint, produces synovial fluid, and contains sensory nerve endings. Medially and laterally the capsule is firm, providing stability to the joint during lateral movements such as those produced during chewing. Anteriorly and posteriorly, however, the capsule is lax, allowing the condyle and disc to translate forward when the mouth is opened.

### LATERAL LIGAMENT

The primary ligament reinforcing the TMJ is the *lateral (temporomandibular) ligament* (Fig. 11–10A). The lateral ligament is typically described as a combination of horizontal and oblique fibers (Fig. 11–10B).[59] The more superficial *oblique fibers* course in an anterior-superior direction, from the posterior neck of the mandible to the lateral margins of the articular eminence and zygomatic arch. The deeper, *horizontal fibers* share similar temporal attachments. They course horizontally and posteriorly to attach into the lateral pole of the mandibular condyle.

The primary function of the lateral ligament is to stabilize the lateral side of the capsule. Tears or excessive elongation of the lateral ligament may cause the disc to be moved medially by an unopposed pull of the superior head of the lateral pterygoid muscle. As described in Arthrokinematics, the oblique fibers have a special function in guiding the movement of the condyle during opening of the mouth.[47]

### ACCESSORY LIGAMENTS

The *stylomandibular and sphenomandibular ligaments* are the accessory ligaments of the TMJ. Both are located medial to the joint capsule (Fig. 11–11). The ligaments help suspend the mandible from the cranium. The base of the sphenoman-

dibular ligament attaches to the medial side of the disc. Although this ligament may have some stabilizing effect on the disc, most likely both the stylomandibular and sphenomandibular ligaments have a very limited role in TMJ function.

---

**Supporting Connective Tissues within the TMJ**

- Articular disc
- Fibrous capsule
- Collateral ligaments
- Lateral TMJ ligament
- Sphenomandibular ligament
- Stylomandibular ligament

---

## Osteokinematics

The osteokinematics descriptors of mandibular motion are protrusion and retrusion, lateral excursion, and depression and elevation (Figs. 11–12 to 11–14). All of these movements are used during mastication. For a more detailed analysis of mandibular movements, the reader is encouraged to consult the classic work by Posselt,[51] thoroughly summarized by Okeson.[47]

### PROTRUSION AND RETRUSION

*Protrusion* of the mandible occurs as it translates *anteriorly* without significant rotation (Fig. 11–12A). Protrusion is an important component of the mouth's opening maximally. *Retrusion* of the mandible occurs in the reverse direction (Fig. 11–12B). Retrusion provides an important component of closing the widely opened and protruded mouth.

### LATERAL EXCURSION

*Lateral excursion* of the mandible occurs primarily as a side-to-side translation (Fig. 11–13A). The direction (right or left) of active lateral excursion can be described as either contralateral or ipsilateral to the side of the primary muscle action. In the adult, an average of 11 mm of maximal unilateral excursion is considered normal.[60] Lateral excursion of the mandible is usually combined with other relatively slight

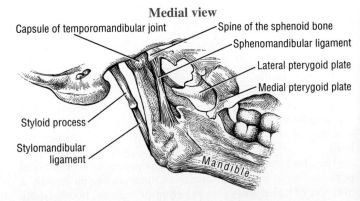

**Medial view**

Capsule of temporomandibular joint

Spine of the sphenoid bone

Sphenomandibular ligament

Lateral pterygoid plate

Medial pterygoid plate

Styloid process

Stylomandibular
ligament

*Mandible*

**FIGURE 11–11.** A medial view of the temporomandibular joint capsule shows the stylomandibular and sphenomandibular ligaments.

**Protrusion**

**Retrusion**

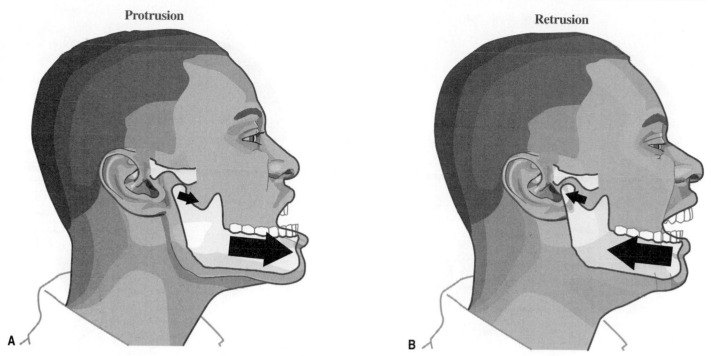

**FIGURE 11–12.** Protrusion (*A*) and retrusion (*B*) of the mandible.

translations and rotations. Normally, the specific path of movement is guided by the contact made between the opposed teeth and the shape of the mandibular fossa.

## DEPRESSION AND ELEVATION

*Depression* of the mandible *opens* the mouth, a fundamental component of eating (Fig. 11–14A). Maximal opening of the mouth typically occurs during actions such as yawning and singing. In the adult, the mouth can be opened an average of 50 mm as measured between the incisal edges of the upper and lower front teeth.[60] The interincisal opening is typically large enough to fit three adult "knuckles" (proximal interphalangeal joints). Typical mastication, however, requires an average maximal opening of 18 mm or about 36% of maximum. Being unable to fit two knuckles between the

**Lateral excursion**

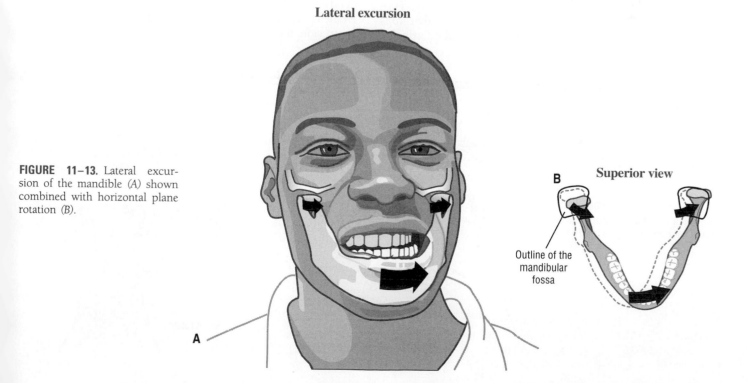

**FIGURE 11–13.** Lateral excursion of the mandible (*A*) shown combined with horizontal plane rotation (*B*).

**B**   **Superior view**

Outline of the mandibular fossa

**Depression**

**Elevation**

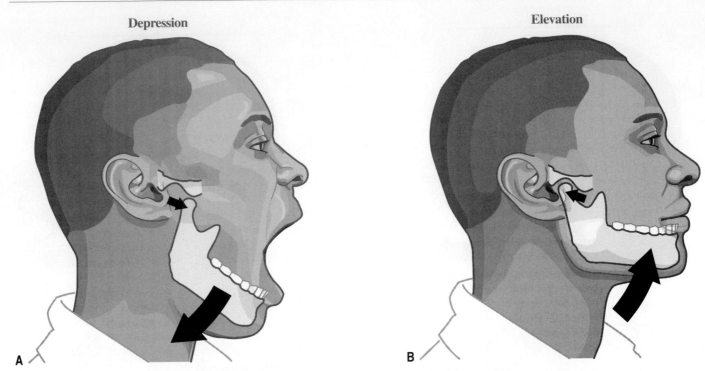

**FIGURE 11–14.** Depression (A) and elevation (B) of the mandible.

edges of the upper and lower incisors is considered abnormal. *Elevation* of the mandible *closes* the mouth—an action used to grind food during mastication (Fig. 11–14B).

## Arthrokinematics

Movement of the mandible typically involves bilateral action of the TMJs. Abnormal function in one joint interferes with the function of the other. The following principles are helpful in an understanding of the arthrokinematics at the TMJ: (1) during *rotational movement*, the mandibular condyle rolls relative to the inferior surface of the disc, *and* (2) during

*translational movement*, the mandibular condyle *and* disc slide essentially together. This is referred to as *condyle-disc complex translation*. The disc is stretched in the direction of the translating condyle.

## PROTRUSION AND RETRUSION

During protrusion and retrusion, the mandibular condyle and disc complex translates anteriorly and posteriorly, respectively, relative to the fossa (Fig. 11–12A and B). The condyle and disc follow the downward slope of the articular eminence. The mandible slides slightly downward during protrusion and slightly upward during retrusion. The path of

**Opening the mouth**

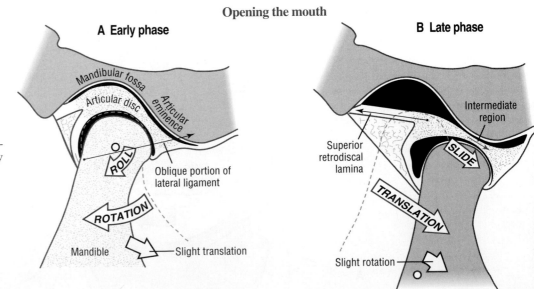

**FIGURE  11–15.** Arthrokinematics of opening the mouth: early phase (A) and late phase (B).

SPECIAL FOCUS 11-1

### Internal Derangement of the Disc-Condyle Complex

Mechanical problems within the TMJ can cause impairments in mastication. A common cause of impairment is *internal derangement* of the *disc-condyle complex*.[47] The condition is defined as an abnormal position of the disc relative to the condyle and fossa. The derangement can be caused by abnormal disc shape, overstretched collateral ligaments, chronic inflammation, loss of elasticity within the superior retrodiscal lamina, or abnormal forces from the lateral pterygoid muscle.[34]

---

**Internal Derangement of the Disc-Condyle Complex**
- *Disc displacement*
  Pain, clicking sounds, and limited range in opening the mouth
- *Chronic disc dislocation*
  Pain, very limited range in opening the mouth, inflammation possibly leading to osteoarthritis

---

Regardless of the cause of the derangement, the disc and condyle translate out of phase with each other. This condition is referred to as *disc displacement*. Even at rest, the intermediate region of the disc is displaced *anterior* and *medial* to the anterior margin of the condyle. Attempts at fully opening the mouth may abruptly relocate the disc to its ideal position. The abrupt movement may create a single or a reciprocal clicking sound, depending on the degree of the disc displacement.[47,52]

A displaced disc can deteriorate to *chronic dislocation*. The disc remains abnormally anterior and medial to the condyle both at rest ("closed-lock position") and throughout the entire opening and closing cycle. A TMJ with a chronically dislocated disc typically does not emit clicking sounds because the disc usually does not relocate or "reduce" to its ideal position during movement. The abnormal position of the disc blocks forward translation of the condyle. Mouth opening is limited, often associated with a deviation of the mandible toward the affected side. A joint with chronic disc dislocation or malalignment often becomes inflamed and painful. In severe cases, the joint tissues may degenerate and eventually become arthritic (Fig. 11-16). As in other synovial joints, an arthritic TMJ may demonstrate crepitus during movement and, in extreme cases, may ankylose or fuse.

The clinical course of a patient with internal derangement of the disc-condyle complex is highly variable. Often the patient offers an extended history of nonpainful movements that emit clicking sounds. The condition may gradually or suddenly worsen, with recurring periods of increased pain, cessation of clicking, and episodes of locking or severely limited motion.[26] The condition is often exacerbated by a forced yawn, a minor trauma to the jaw, or a dental procedure that requires prolonged opening of the mouth.

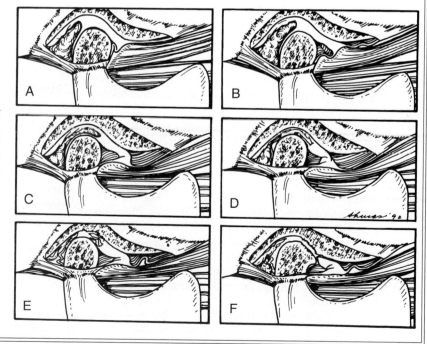

**FIGURE 11-16.** Stages of internal derangement of the temporomandibular joint. Normal joint (*A*), displacement of the disc (*B*), dislocation of the disc (*C*), impingement of the retrodiscal tissues (*D*), retrodiscitis and tissue breakdown (*E*), and osteoarthritis (*F*). (Modified from Farrar WB, McCarty WL: A Clinical Outline of Temporomandibular Joint Diagnosis and Treatment, 7th ed. Montgomery, AL, Normandic Publications, 1983.)

movement varies depending on the degree of opening of the mouth.

## LATERAL EXCURSION

Lateral excursion involves primarily a side-to-side translation of the condyle and disc within the fossa. Slight multiplanar rotations are typically combined with lateral excursion.[47] Figure 11–13B shows an example of lateral excursion combined with slight horizontal plane rotation. The left condyle forms a pivot point within the fossa as the right condyle rotates slightly anteriorly and medially. Slight rotations also occur in sagittal and frontal planes, owing primarily to the effect of the condyle and disc sliding across the sloped articular eminence.

## DEPRESSION AND ELEVATION

Opening and closing of the mouth occur by depression and elevation of the mandible, respectively. During these movements, each TMJ experiences a combination of rotation and translation between the mandibular condyle, articular disc, and fossa. Because rotation and translation occur simultaneously, the axis of rotation is constantly moving. In the ideal case, the movements within both joints result in a maximal range of mouth opening with a minimal stress placed on the articular surfaces.

The arthrokinematics of opening the mouth are depicted for an early and a late phase in Figure 11–15. The *early phase,* constituting the first 35 to 50% of the range of motion, involves primarily *rotation* of the mandible relative to the cranium.[57, 67] As depicted in Figure 11–15A, the condyle rolls posteriorly within the concave inferior surface of the disc. The direction of the roll is in relation to the rotation of a point on the ramus of the mandible. The rolling motion swings the body of the mandible inferiorly and posteriorly. The axis of rotation is not fixed but migrates within the vicinity of the condyles.[20, 50]

The rolling motion of the condyle stretches the oblique portion of the lateral ligament. The increased tension in the ligament helps to initiate the late phase of the mouth's opening.[49, 59]

The *late phase* of opening the mouth comprises the final 50 to 65% of the total range of motion. This phase is marked by a gradual transition from primary rotation to primary translation. The transition can be readily appreciated by palpating the condyle of the mandible during the full opening of the mouth. During the translation, the condyle *and* disc slide together in a forward and inferior direction against the slope of the articular eminence (Fig. 11–15B). At the end of opening, the axis of rotation shifts inferiorly. The exact point of the axis is difficult to define because it depends on the person's unique rotation-to-translation ratio.[30] At the later phase of opening, the axis is usually below the neck of the mandible.[20]

Full opening of the mouth maximally stretches and pulls the disc anteriorly. The extent of the forward translation (protrusion) is limited, in part, by tension in the stretched, elastic superior retrodiscal lamina. The intermediate region of the disc translates forward while remaining between the superior aspect of the condyle and the articular eminence. This placement of the disc maximizes joint congruency and reduces large variation in intra-articular stress.

The arthrokinematics of *closing the mouth* occur in the reverse order of that described for opening. When the mouth is fully opened and prepared to close, tension in the superior retrodiscal lamina starts to retract the disc, initiating the early phase of closing. The later phase is dominated by rotation of the condyle within the concavity of the disc, terminated when contact is made between the upper and lower teeth.

## MUSCLE AND JOINT INTERACTION

### Innervation to the Muscles and Joints

The muscles of mastication and their innervation are listed in Table 11–2. Based primarily on size, the muscles of mastication are divided into two groups: primary and secondary. The primary muscles are the masseter, temporalis, medial pterygoid, and lateral pterygoid. The secondary muscles are much smaller. The primary muscles of mastication are innervated by the mandibular nerve, a division of the trigeminal nerve (cranial nerve V). This nerve exits the skull via the foramen ovale (see Fig. 11–5).

### TABLE 11–2. Primary and Secondary Muscles of Mastication and Their Innervation

| Primary Muscles | Innervation |
| --- | --- |
| Masseter | Branch of the mandibular nerve, a division of cranial nerve V |
| Temporalis | Branch of the mandibular nerve, a division of cranial nerve V |
| Medial Pterygoid | Branch of the mandibular nerve, a division of cranial nerve V |
| Lateral Pterygoid | Branch of the mandibular nerve, a division of cranial nerve V |

| Secondary Muscles | Innervation |
| --- | --- |
| *Suprahyoid Group* | |
| Digastric (posterior belly) | Facial nerve (cranial nerve VII) |
| Digastric (anterior belly) | Inferior alveolar nerve (branch of the mandibular nerve, a division of cranial nerve V) |
| Geniohyoid | $C^1$ via the hypoglossal nerve (cranial nerve XII) |
| Mylohyoid | Inferior alveolar nerve (branch of the mandibular nerve, a division of cranial nerve V) |
| Stylohyoid | Facial nerve (cranial nerve VII) |
| *Infrahyoid Group* | |
| Omohyoid | Ventral rami of $C^{1-3}$ |
| Sternohyoid | Ventral rami of $C^{1-3}$ |
| Sternothyroid | Ventral rami of $C^{1-3}$ |
| Thyrohyoid | Ventral rami of $C^1$ (via cranial nerve XII) |

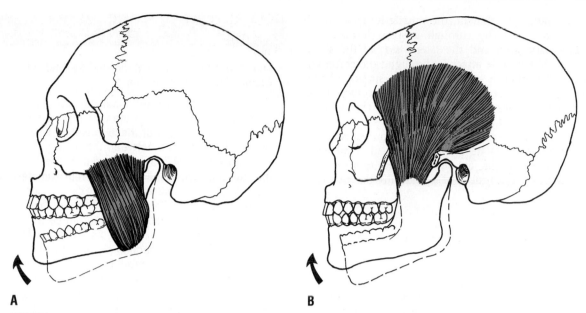

**A**    **B**

**FIGURE 11–17.** The masseter (*A*) and temporalis (*B*) muscles. (Modified from Okeson JP: Management of Temporomandibular Disorders and Occlusion, 4th ed. Chicago, Mosby, 1998.)

The synovial membrane and the central part of the articular disc within the TMJ lack sensory innervation. The periphery of the disc, capsule, lateral ligament, and retrodiscal tissues, however, possess pain fibers and mechanoreceptors.[64,66] Mechanoreceptors and sensory nerves, from oral mucosa, periodontal ligaments, and muscles, provide the nervous system with a rich source of proprioception. This source of information helps to protect the tissues through neuromuscular reflex actions and allows coordination between the muscles and joint. The sensory innervation to the TMJ is carried through two branches of the mandibular nerve: auriculotemporal and masseteric.

## Muscular Anatomy and Function

### PRIMARY MUSCLES OF MASTICATION

The primary muscles of mastication are the masseter, temporalis, medial pterygoid, and lateral pterygoid. Refer to Appendix III, Part D, for a summary of muscle attachments.

### *Masseter*

The masseter is a thick, powerful muscle, easily palpable just above the angle of the mandible (Fig. 11–17A). It originates from the zygomatic arch and zygomatic bone (see Figs. 11–1 and 11–5) and inserts inferiorly on the external surface of the ramus of the mandible (see Fig. 11–2).

The masseter has two sets of fibers: superficial and deep. The larger, more superficial fibers travel inferiorly and posteriorly, attaching near the angle of the mandible. The deeper fibers travel more vertically, attaching to the upper regions of the ramus of the mandible.

Bilateral contraction of the masseters elevates the mandible to bring the teeth into contact during mastication. The line-of-force of the superficial fibers is nearly perpendicular to the biting surface of the molars. The primary function of the masseter, therefore, is to develop large forces between the molars for effective grinding and crushing of food. Bilateral action of the masseters also protrudes the mandible

slightly. Unilateral contraction of the masseter, however, causes slight *ipsilateral excursion* of the mandible. Such an action may occur during a lateral grinding motion while chewing (Fig. 11–18). The multiple actions of the masseter are useful for effective mastication.

### *Temporalis*

The temporalis is a flat, fan-shaped muscle that fills much of the concavity of the temporal fossa of the skull (Fig. 11–

**Active lateral excursion**

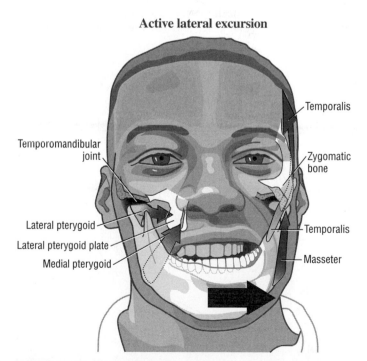

**FIGURE 11–18.** Frontal plane view shows the muscular interaction during *left active lateral excursion* of the mandible. This action may occur during a side-to-side grinding motion while chewing. The muscles producing the movement are indicated in red.

17*B*). From its cranial attachment, the muscle forms a broad tendon that narrows distally through a space formed between the zygomatic arch and the lateral side of the skull (see Fig. 11–5). The muscle attaches distally to the coronoid process and to the anterior edge and medial surface of the ramus of the mandible (see Fig. 11–2). Bilateral contractions of the temporalis muscles *elevate the mandible.* The oblique posterior fibers *elevate and retrude the mandible.*

Similar to the masseter, the temporalis courses slightly medially as its approaches its distal attachment. Unilateral contraction of the temporalis, as when chewing in a side-to-side manner, causes slight *ipsilateral excursion of the mandible* (Fig. 11–18).

### Medial Pterygoid

The medial pterygoid and masseter have a very similar line-of-force and size (compare Fig. 11–17*A* with Fig. 11–19*A*). The medial pterygoid arises from the medial surface of the lateral pterygoid plate of the sphenoid bone (see Figs. 11–5 and 11–6). From this attachment, it courses parallel to the superficial fibers of the masseter to attach on the internal surface of the ramus near the angle of the mandible (see Figs. 11–2 and 11–4). Acting bilaterally, contraction of the medial pterygoid muscles *elevates* and, to a limited extent, *protrudes* the mandible. Because of the oblique line-of-force of the muscle relative to the frontal plane, a unilateral contraction produces a very effective *contralateral excursion* of the mandible (see Fig. 11–18).

### Lateral Pterygoid

The lateral pterygoid has a superior and an inferior head (Fig. 11–19*B*). The *superior head* arises from the greater wing of the sphenoid bone. The considerably larger *inferior head* arises from the lateral surface of the lateral pterygoid plate. As a whole, the muscle traverses nearly horizontally to insert into (1) the neck of the mandible at the pterygoid fossa, (2) the articular disc, and (3) the capsule of the TMJ

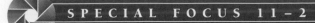

**Functional Interactions Between the Masseter and Medial Pterygoid Muscles**

The medial pterygoid and masseter muscles form a sling around the angle of the mandible. Simultaneous bilateral contractions of these muscles exert a very powerful biting force between the molars. These forces average 419 N (94.2 lb) in the adult.[34] The bite force measured between the molars is approximately double the bite force measured between the incisors.

Acting on opposite sides of the mandible, the masseter and medial pterygoid also coproduce a laterally directed force on the mandible. As shown in Figure 11–18, simultaneous contraction of the right medial pterygoid and left masseter produces left lateral deviation. Contraction of these muscles in this synergistic fashion can produce a potent shear force between the molars and food on both sides of the mouth. The combined muscular action is very effective at grinding and crushing food prior to swallowing.

(Fig. 11–9).[1,5,65] The precise distal attachments are still a subject of debate.[27] About 65% of the fibers of the superior head attach into the pterygoid fossa (see Fig. 11–2); the remaining attach into the medial wall of the capsule, and a relatively small portion into the medial side of the articular disc. Activation of the superior head exerts an anterior-medial force on the capsule and disc. This muscular action may be involved in the pathomechanics of excessive anterior-

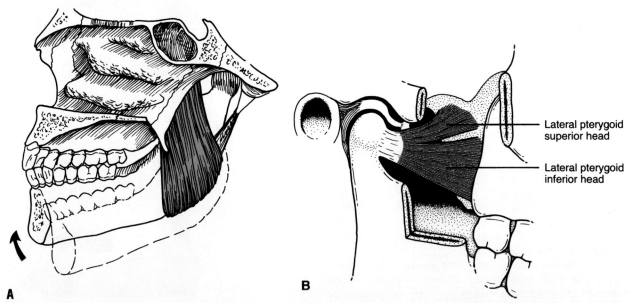

Lateral pterygoid superior head

Lateral pterygoid inferior head

**A**                                                    **B**

**FIGURE 11–19.** *A,* The medial view of the right medial pterygoid. *B,* The lateral view of the two heads of the lateral pterygoid. (*A* with permission from Okeson JP: Management of Temporomandibular Disorders and Occlusion, 4th ed. Chicago, Mosby, 1998. *B* modified from Kaplan AS and Assael LA: Temporomandibular Disorders: Diagnosis and Treatment. Philadelphia, WB Saunders, 1991.)

the right lateral and medial pterygoid and by the left masseter and temporalis.

Bilateral contraction of the lateral pterygoids produces strong *protrusion* of the mandible.[34] As described in Muscular Control of Opening and Closing of the Mouth, the two heads of the lateral pterygoid muscles have antagonistic roles during opening and closing of the mouth. Most data suggest that the *inferior head* is the primary depressor of the mandible, especially during resisted opening of the mouth.[31,37,42] The *superior head* helps control the position of the disc and joint during elevation of the mandible.[31,37] This function is especially important during resisted, unilateral closure of the jaw, such as when biting down on a hard object between the molars.

## SECONDARY MUSCLES OF MASTICATION

The suprahyoid and infrahyoid muscles are considered secondary muscles of mastication (see Table 11-2). Forces produced by these muscles are transferred either directly or indirectly to the mandible (Fig. 11-20). The *suprahyoid muscles* attach between the base of the cranium, the hyoid, and the mandible; the *infrahyoid muscles* attach superiorly to the hyoid and inferiorly to the thyroid cartilage, sternum, and scapula. The mandibular attachments of three of the suprahyoid muscles—anterior belly of the digastric, geniohyoid, and mylohyoid—are shown in Figure 11-4. Appendix III, Parts E and F, includes the attachments and innervations of the suprahyoid and infrahyoid muscles.

With the hyoid bone stabilized by activation of the infrahyoid muscles, the suprahyoid muscles assist with depression of the mandible.[6] The suprahyoid and infrahyoid muscles are also involved in speech, tongue movement, and swallowing, and in controlling of boluses of food prior to swallowing.

## SUMMARY OF INDIVIDUAL MUSCLE ACTION

Table 11-3 provides a summary of the individual actions of the muscles of mastication.

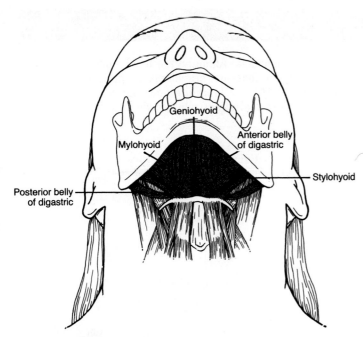

**FIGURE 11-20.** The suprahyoid (red) and infrahyoid muscles are shown, attaching to the hyoid bone. The sternothyroid and thyrohyoid muscles are deep to the sternohyoid and are not visible. (Modified with permission from Kaplan AS and Assael LA: Temporomandibular Disorders: Diagnosis and Treatment. Philadelphia, WB Saunders, 1991.)

medial disc displacement.[34] The entire inferior head attaches within the pterygoid fossa.

Unilateral contraction of both heads of the lateral pterygoid produces effective *contralateral excursion* of the mandible (see Fig. 11-18). Unilateral muscle contraction rotates the ipsilateral condyle anterior-medially within the horizontal plane. Usually a given right or left lateral pterygoid muscle contracts synergistically with other muscles during mastication. For example, as depicted in Figure 11-18, a chewing motion that involves left lateral excursion is controlled by

## TABLE 11-3. Actions of the Muscles of Mastication on the Mandible

| Muscle | Elevation (closing of the mouth) | Depression (opening of the mouth) | Lateral Excursion* | Protrusion | Retrusion |
|---|---|---|---|---|---|
| Masseter | XXX | — | X (IL) | X | — |
| Medial pterygoid | XXX | — | XXX (CL) | X | — |
| Lateral pterygoid (superior head) | † | — | XXX (CL) | XXX | — |
| Lateral pterygoid (inferior head) | — | XXX | XXX (CL) | XXX | — |
| Temporalis | XXX | — | X (IL) | — | XXX (posterior fibers) |
| Suprahyoid muscle group | — | XXX | — | — | X‡ |

\* CL = contralateral excursion, IL = ipsilateral excursion
† Stabilizes or adjusts the position of the disc.
‡ By direct action of the geniohyoid, mylohyoid, and digastric (anterior belly) only.
A muscle's relative potential to move the mandible is assigned one of three scores: **X = minimal, XX = moderate,** and **XXX = maximum.** A dash indicates no effective muscular action.

### SPECIAL FOCUS 11-3

**Passive Muscular Tension and its Possible Influence on the Posture of the Mandible**

Based on muscular anatomy, it is logical to assume that the posture of the head can influence the resting posture of the mandible.[8,22,39] Consider, for example, the chronic forward head posture described previously in Chapters 9 and 10. The person depicted in Figure 11–21 shows a variant of this posture. Observe that the protracted (forward) head is combined with a flexed upper thoracic and lower cervical spine and with an extended upper cervical and craniocervical region. This posture stretches infrahyoid muscles, such as the sternohyoid and omohyoid, which can create an inferior and posterior traction on the hyoid. The traction is transferred to the mandible through suprahyoid muscles such as the anterior belly of the digastric. As a result, the mandible is pulled in a direction of retrusion and depression. Because of the attachment of the omohyoid to the scapula, poor posture of the shoulder girdle could indirectly place additional tension against the mandible.

Altering the resting posture of the mandible changes the position of its condyle within the fossa. A posteriorly displaced condyle could, in theory, compress the delicate retrodiscal tissues, creating inflammation and muscle spasm. Spasm in the lateral pterygoid muscle may be a natural protective mechanism to *protrude* the mandible away from the compressed retrodiscal tissues. Chronic spasm within this muscle may, however, abnormally position the disc anterior and medial to the condyle. As described in Special Focus 11–1, this situation may predispose a person to a condition of derangement of the disc-condyle complex. Although the data suggest an association between abnormal craniocervical posture and disorders of the TMJ, the literature does not unequivocally support a cause-and-effect relationship between these variables.[69]

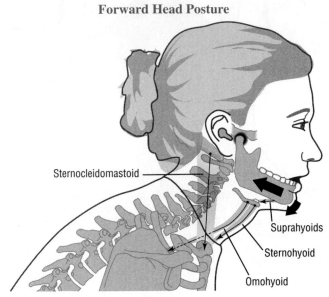

**Forward Head Posture**

**FIGURE 11–21.** A forward head posture shows one mechanism by which passive tension in selected suprahyoid and infrahyoid muscles alters the resting posture of the mandible. The mandible is pulled inferiorly and posteriorly, changing the position of the condyle within the temporomandibular joint.

## MUSCULAR CONTROL OF OPENING AND CLOSING OF THE MOUTH

### Opening of the Mouth

Opening of the mouth is performed primarily through contraction of the *inferior head of the lateral pterygoid* and *the suprahyoid group of muscles*. This action is depicted in Figure 11–22A as the mouth opens in preparation to bite on a grape. The inferior head of the lateral pterygoid is primarily responsible for the forward translation (protrusion) of the mandibular condyle.[34] This muscle is also involved in a force-couple with the contracting suprahyoid muscles. The force-couple rotates the mandible about its axis of rotation, shown as a white circle below the neck of the mandible. Although mandibular rotation is minimal during the later phase of opening the mouth, it does facilitate the extremes of this action. Gravity also assists with opening of the mouth.

As described previously, the disc and condyle slide forward as a unit during the late phase of opening of the mouth. The disc is stretched and pulled anteriorly by (1) collateral ligaments attaching the disc to the translating condyle, and (2) increased intra-articular pressure created by activation of the inferior head of the lateral pterygoid. Although the superior head of the lateral pterygoid attaches directly to the disc, it is relatively inactive while the mouth is opening.

### Closing of the Mouth

Closing of the mouth against resistance is performed primarily by contraction of the *masseter, medial pterygoid,* and the *temporalis muscles* (Fig. 11–22B). They all have a very favorable moment arm (leverage) for this action. The more oblique posterior fibers of the temporalis muscles also *retrude* the mandible. This action translates the mandible in a posterior-superior direction, helping to reseat the condyle deep within the fossa.

The *superior head of the lateral pterygoid* is active eccentrically while closing the mouth. The activation tends to be greatest on the "working" side of the mandible (i.e., that side most involved with chewing).[47] Eccentric activation exerts a forward tension on the disc and neck of the mandible. The tension stabilizes and optimally positions the disc between the condyle and articular eminence. The muscle activation also helps balance the retrusion force generated by the posterior fibers of the temporalis.

**Opening the mouth**

**Closing the mouth**

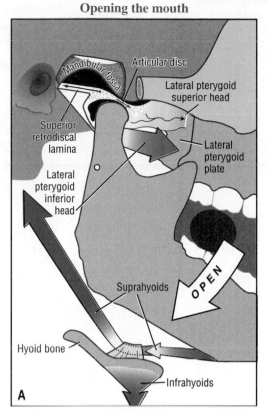

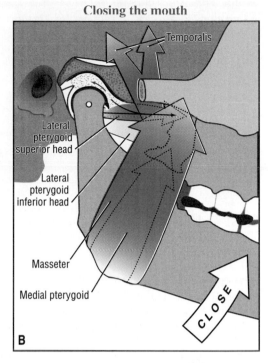

**FIGURE 11–22.** The muscle and joint interaction while opening (*A*) and closing (*B*) the mouth. The relative degree of muscle activation is indicated by the different intensity of red. In *B* the superior head of the lateral pterygoid muscle is shown eccentrically active. (These locations of the axes of rotation in *A* and *B* are estimates only.)

**The Special Role of the Superior Head of the Lateral Pterygoid in Adjusting Disc Position**

The specific position of the disc relative to the condyle while biting depends on the type of resistance created by the objects being chewed. While closing of the mouth against a relatively low bite resistance, such as on a soft grape as depicted in Figure 11–22*B*, the thin intermediate region of the disc is typically in its ideal position between the condyle and articular eminence. During the application of a large, asymmetrical bite force, however, the position of the disc may need to be adjusted. Unilaterally biting on a hard piece of candy between the molars, for example, momentarily reduces the intra-articular pressure within the ipsilateral TMJ. Until the candy is crushed, it acts as a spacer between the upper and lower jaw, which reduces joint contact. During this event, a forceful *concentric contraction* of the superior head of the lateral pterygoid muscle can protrude the disc forward, thereby sliding its thicker, posterior region between the condyle and articular eminence. The thicker surface increases the congruency within the joint, helping to stabilize it against the uneven forces applied to the mandible as a whole. Fibers of the lateral pterygoid that attach to the neck of the mandible can brace, if necessary, the condyle against the articular eminence.

## TEMPOROMANDIBULAR DISORDERS

*Temporomandibular disorder (TMD)* is a broad and often vague term that defines a number of clinical problems that involve the masticatory system.[33,40] TMDs are typically associated with a primary dysfunction involving either the muscles or the joint structure.[43,61] Muscular dysfunctions typically respond more favorably to conservative treatment.[53] In addition to pain in the muscles and joint during movement, the signs and symptoms include joint sounds, reduced molar bite forces, limited ranges in opening of the mouth, tension headaches, joint locking, referred pain to the face and scalp, and nocturnal bruxism (i.e., excessive grinding of the teeth while sleeping).

No single mechanical or physiologic explanation can account for the myriad of symptoms associated with TMD.[62] The pathomechanics involved with a particular disorder may stem from an isolated traumatic event, such as a fall, blow to the face, or severe cervical hyperextension/hyperflexion (whiplash). Often, however, the exact pathomechanics are unknown. Little scientific evidence supports a direct cause-and-effect relationship between poor occlusion of the teeth and TMD.[9,38]

The treatment for TMD is mixed and depends primarily on the nature of the underlying problem.[17,23,28,38] Dentists, physical therapists, and counselors occasionally collaborate in the treatment of TMD. Surgical intervention is rare and usually performed only when the pain is so great or motion so limited that the quality of life is significantly reduced. The more common conservative, nonsurgical treatments for TMD are listed in the box on the following page.

## PART 2: VENTILATION

*Ventilation* is the mechanical process by which air is inhaled and exhaled through the lungs and airways. This rhythmic process persists 12 to 20 times per minute at rest and is essential to the maintenance of life. This chapter now focuses on the kinesiology of ventilation.

Ventilation allows for the exchange of oxygen and carbon dioxide between the alveoli of the lungs and the blood. This exchange is essential to oxidative metabolism within muscle fibers. The process converts chemical energy stored in ATP into the mechanical energy needed to move and stabilize the joints of the body.

The relative intensity of ventilation can be described as "quiet" or "forced." In the healthy population, *quiet ventilation* occurs during relatively sedentary activities that have low metabolic demands. In contrast, *forced ventilation* occurs during strenuous activities that require rapid and voluminous exchange of air, such as exercising, or in the presence of some respiratory diseases. A wide and continuous range of ventilation intensity exists between quiet and forced ventilation.

Figure 11–23 shows the lung volumes and capacities in

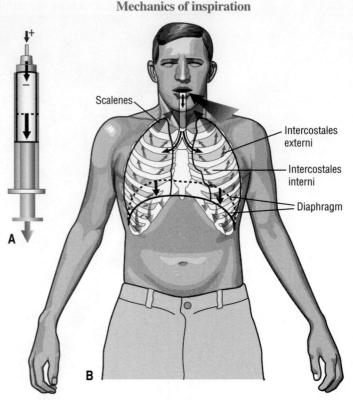

**Mechanics of inspiration**

Scalenes

Intercostales externi

Intercostales interni

Diaphragm

**FIGURE 11–24.** The muscular mechanics of inspiration. *A,* This analogy shows Boyle's law. Increasing the volume within a piston reduces the air pressure within the chamber of the piston. The negative air pressure creates suction that draws the outside, higher pressure air into the piston through an aperture at the top of the piston. *B,* A healthy adult shows how contraction of the primary muscles (diaphragm, scalenes, intercostales) of inspiration increases intrathoracic volume, which in turn expands the lungs and reduces alveolar pressure. The negative alveolar pressure draws atmospheric air into the lungs. The descent of the diaphragm is indicated by the pair of thick, black, vertical arrows.

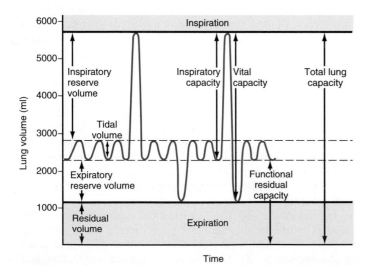

**FIGURE 11–23.** The lung volumes and capacities in the normal adult are shown. Lung capacity is the sum of two or more volumes. (With permission from Guyton AC and Hall JE: Textbook of Medical Physiology, 10th ed. Philadelphia, WB Saunders, 2000.)

the normal adult. As depicted, the *total lung capacity* is about 5½ liters of air. *Tidal volume* is defined as the volume of air moved in and out of the lungs during each ventilation cycle. At rest, tidal volume is about ½ liter, increasing to about 60% of *vital capacity* during exercise.

Ventilation is driven by a combination of active and passive forces that alters the volume within the expandable thorax. In accordance with *Boyle's law,* the *volume* occupied by a gas, such as air, is inversely proportional to the *pressure* exerted by the gas. Increasing the volume within the chamber of a piston, for example, lowers the pressure of the contained air (Fig. 11–24A). Because air flows spontaneously from high to low pressure, the relatively high air pressure outside the piston forces air into an opening at the top of the piston. In other words, the negative pressure in the piston sucks air into the piston.

Boyle's law states that the *volume* and *pressure* exerted by a gas are inversely proportional.

Much of the physics of human ventilation is based on the inverse relationship between volume and pressure of a gas. During *inspiration,* the intrathoracic volume is increased by contraction of the muscles that attach to the ribs and sternum (Fig. 11–24*B*). As the thorax expands, the pressure within the interpleural space, which is already negative, is further reduced, creating a suction that expands the lungs. The resulting expansion of the lungs reduces alveolar pressure below atmospheric pressure, ultimately drawing air from the atmosphere to the lungs.

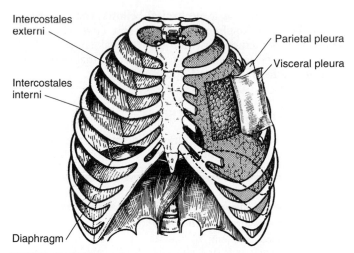

**FIGURE 11–25.** The bony housing of the thorax is shown along with the enclosed lungs, parietal and visceral pleural, and intercostal and diaphragmatic muscles. (Modified with permission from McNaught AB and Callander R: Illustrated Physiology. New York, Churchill Livingstone, 1975.)

**Factors that Can Oppose Expansion of the Thorax**

The work performed by the muscles of inspiration must overcome the natural elastic recoil of the lung tissue and the joints that compose the thorax. Additional work is performed to overcome the resistance of the inspired air as it passes through the extensive airways. The amount of air that reaches the alveoli depends on the reduced alveolar pressure, which is determined in part by the net effect of muscle contraction and the mechanical properties that oppose thoracic expansion.

Several factors can oppose expansion of the thorax. Advanced age, for example, is associated with *increased stiffness* of the joints and connective tissues that make up the thorax.[18] The lung parenchyma, however, loses elastic recoil and becomes *more compliant* with aging. Compliance, in this context, is a measure of the distensibility of the lungs produced for a given drop in transpulmonary pressure or the slope of the volume-pressure curve. When combined, the total system (thorax and lungs) shows a net decrease in compliance with aging.[68] A greater reduction in pressure is required to inspire a given volume of air. In effect, muscles have to work harder during inspiration. This partially explains why aging is typically associated with a slight decrease in tidal volume and slight increase in respiratory frequency.

Diseases or abnormal postures can also oppose thoracic expansion. Rheumatoid arthritis, for example, can increase the stiffness of the cartilage of the sternocostal joints, thereby resisting an increase in intrathoracic volume. Severe scoliosis or kyphosis may physically limit the expansion of the thorax.

*Expiration* is the process of expiring (exhaling) air from the lungs into the environment. In accord with the analogy to the piston previously described, *decreasing* the volume within the chamber of a piston *increases* the pressure on the contained air, forcing it outward. Expiration in the human occurs by a similar process. Reducing the intrathoracic volume increases the alveolar pressure, thereby driving air from the alveoli to the atmosphere.

*Quiet expiration* is primarily a passive process that does not depend on muscle activation. When the muscles of inspiration relax after contraction, the intrathoracic volume is naturally decreased by the elastic recoil of lungs, thorax, and connective tissues of stretched inspiratory muscles. *Forced expiration,* such as that required to cough or blow out a candle, requires the active force produced by expiratory muscles, such as the abdominals.

## ARTHROLOGY

### Thorax

The rib cage, or thorax, is a closed system that functions as the mechanical bellows of ventilation (Fig. 11–25). The internal aspect of the thorax is sealed from the outside by several structures (Table 11–4). Although this chapter fo-

**TABLE 11–4. Tissues that Seal the Thorax**

| |
| --- |
| **Posterior-laterally** |
| thoracic vertebrae |
| ribs |
| intercostal muscles and membrane |
| **Anteriorly** |
| costal cartilages |
| sternum |
| intercostal muscles and membranes |
| **Superiorly** |
| upper ribs and clavicles |
| cervical fascia that surrounds the esophagus and trachea |
| cervical muscles |
| **Inferiorly** |
| diaphragm muscle |

cuses on the thorax as a mechanical bellows, the thorax also (1) protects cardiopulmonary organs and large vessels; (2) serves as a structural base for the cervical spine; and (3) provides a site for attachment of muscles that move and stabilize the head, neck, and upper extremities.

## Articulations within the Thorax

The thorax changes shape during ventilation by movement at five articulations: manubriosternal, sternocostal, interchondral, costotransverse, and costovertebral joints.

---

**Articulations within the Thorax**
- Manubriosternal joint
- Sternocostal joints (including the costochondral and chondrosternal junctions)
- Interchondral joints
- Costotransverse joints
- Costovertebral joints

---

### MANUBRIOSTERNAL JOINT

The manubrium fuses with the body of the sternum at the *manubriosternal joint* (Fig. 11–26). This fibrocartilaginous articulation is an amphiarthrosis, similar to the structure of the pubic symphysis. A partial disc fills the cavity of the manubriosternal joint, completely ossifying late in life. Before ossification, the joint may contribute modestly to expansion of the thorax.

### STERNOCOSTAL JOINTS

Bilaterally, the anterior cartilaginous ends of the first seven ribs articulate with the lateral sides of the sternum. In a broad sense, these articulations may be called *sternocostal joints* (see Fig. 11–26). Because of the intervening cartilage between the bone of the ribs and the sternum, however, each sternocostal joint is structurally divided into a costochondral and chondrosternal junction.

The *costochondral junctions* represent the transition between the bone and cartilage of the anterior ends of each rib. No capsule or ligament reinforces these junctions. The periosteum of the ribs gradually transforms into the perichondrium of the cartilage. Costochondral junctions permit very little movement.

The *chondrosternal junctions* are formed between the medial ends of the cartilage of the ribs and the small concave costal facets on the sternum. The first chondrosternal junction is a synarthrosis, providing a relatively stiff connection with the sternum.[64] The second through the seventh joints, however, are synovial in nature, permitting slight gliding motions. Fibrocartilaginous discs are sometimes present, especially in the lower joints where cavities are frequently absent. Each synovial joint is surrounded by a capsule that is strengthened by *radiate ligaments*. An *intra-articular ligament* is frequently encountered in the second chondrosternal junction.[64]

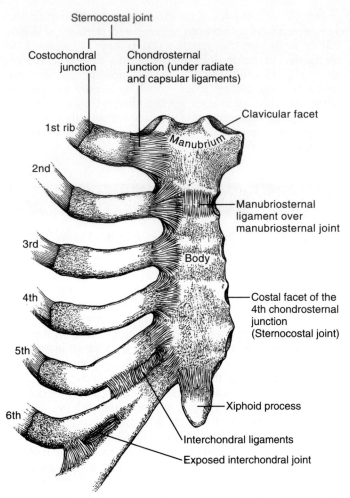

**FIGURE 11–26.** Anterior view of part of the thoracic wall highlights the manubriosternal joint, sternocostal joints with costochondral and chondrosternal junctions, and interchondral joints. The ribs are removed on the left side to expose the costal facets.

### INTERCHONDRAL JOINTS

The opposed borders of the cartilages of ribs 6 to 10 form small, synovial-lined *interchondral joints,* strengthened by *interchondral ligaments* (see Fig. 11–26). Ribs 11 and 12 do not attach anteriorly to the sternum.

### COSTOTRANSVERSE AND COSTOVERTEBRAL JOINTS

The posterior end of the ribs attaches to the vertebral column via the costotransverse and costovertebral joints. The *costovertebral joints* connect the heads of each of the twelve ribs to the corresponding sides of the bodies of the thoracic vertebrae. The *costotransverse joints* connect the articular tubercles of ribs 1 to 10 to the transverse processes of the corresponding thoracic vertebrae. Ribs 11 and 12 usually lack costotransverse joints. The anatomy and ligament structures of these joints are described and illustrated in Chapter 9 (see Fig. 9–53).

# Changes in Intrathoracic Volume During Ventilation

## VERTICAL CHANGES

During inspiration, the vertical diameter of the thorax is increased primarily by contraction and subsequent lowering of the dome of the diaphragm muscle (see Fig. 11–24B). During quiet expiration, the diaphragm relaxes, allowing the dome to recoil upward to its resting position.

## ANTERIOR-POSTERIOR AND MEDIAL-LATERAL CHANGES

Elevation and depression of the ribs and sternum produce changes in the anterior-posterior and medial-lateral diameters of the thorax. To varying degrees, all five articulations within the thorax contribute to these changes in diameter.

During *inspiration,* the shaft of the ribs elevates in a path generally perpendicular to the axis of rotation that courses between the costotransverse and costovertebral joints (Fig. 11–27). The downward sloped shaft of the ribs rotates upward and outward, increasing the intrathoracic volume in both anterior-posterior and medial-lateral diameters. Only a slight rotation at the posterior joints produces a relatively large displacement of the shaft of the ribs. This mechanism is somewhat similar to the rotation of a bucket handle.

The specific path of movement of a given rib depends partially on its unique shape, and on the spatial orientation of the axis of rotation that runs through the costotransverse and costovertebral joints. In the *upper six ribs,* the axis makes an approximate 25- to 35-degree angle with the frontal plane; in the *lower six ribs,* the axis makes an approximate 35- to 45-degree angle with the frontal plane. The anatomic specimen used to illustrate Figure 11–27A shows an approximate 35-degree angle. This slight difference in angulation causes the upper ribs to elevate slightly more in the anterior direction, thereby facilitating the forward and upward movement of the sternum.

The elevating ribs and sternum create slight bending and twisting movements within the pliable cartilages associated with the joints of the thorax. As depicted in Figure 11–27B, torsion created in the twisted cartilage within a sternocostal joint stores a component of the energy used to elevate the ribs. The energy is partially recaptured during expiration, as the rib cage recoils to its relatively constricted state.

Because of the contrast in length of the first seven ribs and the differences in stiffness between the first and the remainder of the sternocostal joints, elevation of the ribs places dissimilar stresses on the lateral edge of the sternum. Part of the stress may be dissipated by slight movement at the manubriosternal joint.

During *expiration,* the muscles of inspiration relax, allowing the ribs and the sternum to return to their preinspiration position. The lowering of the body of the ribs combined with the inferior and posterior movements of the sternum decreases the anterior-posterior and medial-lateral diameters of the thorax.

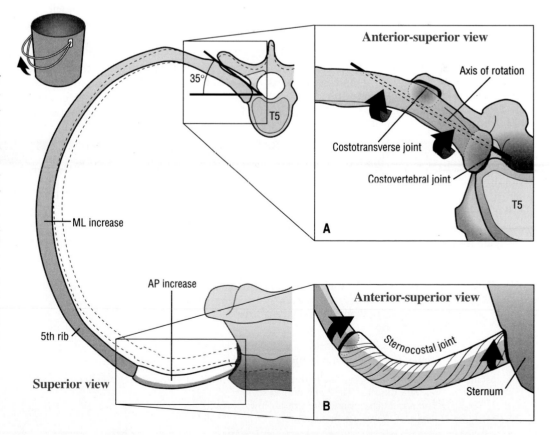

**FIGURE 11–27.** A top view of the 5th rib shows the "bucket-handle" mechanism of elevation of the ribs during inspiration. The ghosted outline of the rib indicates its position prior to inspiration. Elevation of the rib increases both the anterior-posterior (AP) and medial-lateral (ML) diameters of the thorax. The rib connects to the vertebral column via costotransverse and costovertebral joints (*A*) and to the sternum via the sternocostal joint (*B*). During elevation, the neck of the rib moves about an axis of rotation that courses between each costotransverse and costovertebral joint. The elevating rib creates a torsion in the cartilage associated with the sternocostal joint.

# MUSCULAR ACTIONS DURING VENTILATION

An extraordinarily large number of muscles and joints interact during ventilation. The actions of many different muscles can produce similar effects on changing intrathoracic volume. The redundancy provides for a very adaptable and responsive system, a necessity considering the complexity and simultaneous demands placed on the muscles that attach to the thorax. With the exception of the diaphragm, the muscles of ventilation may be concurrently used for other functions, such as control of movements of the trunk, neck, and upper extremities.

A great deal is still to be learned about the function of the muscles of ventilation. Much of what is known is assumed through indirect analysis of muscle activation. The indirect analysis includes measurement of fiber type and cross-sectional data,[44] ventilatory pressures,[7] human and animal EMG,[16,55] optical[45] and ultrasonic imaging,[4] and determining the effects of nerve stimulation.[3] Clinical observations of the effects of muscle paralysis following spinal cord injury have helped in the understanding of the normal function of the muscles.[45]

Any muscle that attaches to the thorax can potentially assist with the mechanics of ventilation. A muscle that increases intrathoracic volume is considered a *muscle of inspiration*. A muscle that decreases intrathoracic volume is considered a *muscle of expiration*. The detailed anatomy and innervation of the muscles of ventilation are found throughout Appendix III, Part G in particular.

## Muscles of Quiet Inspiration

The muscles of quiet inspiration are the diaphragm, scalenes, and intercostales. These muscles are considered primary because they are active during all work intensities. Active contraction of the diaphragm muscle is dedicated totally toward the mechanics of inspiration. The intercostales and scalene muscles, however, also stabilize and rotate parts of the axial skeleton. The mode of action and innervation of the primary muscles of inspiration are summarized in Table 11–5.

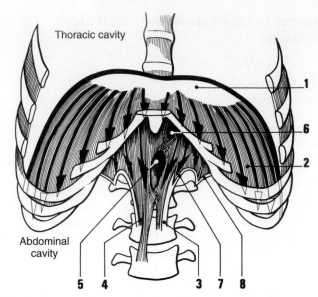

**FIGURE 11–28.** The action of the diaphragm during the initiation of inspiration. *Key:* 1, central tendon; 2, muscle fibers (costal part); 3, left crus; 4, right crus; 5, opening for the aorta; 6, opening for the esophagus; 7, part of the psoas muscle; and 8, part of the quadratus lumborum muscle. (Modified from Kapandji IA: The Physiology of Joints, vol. 3. New York, Churchill Livingstone, 1974).

## DIAPHRAGM

The *diaphragm* is a dome-shaped, thin, musculotendinous sheet of tissue that separates the thoracic cavity from the abdominal cavity (Fig. 11–28). Its convex upper surface is the floor of the thoracic cavity, and its concave lower surface is the roof of the abdominal cavity.

The diaphragm has three parts based on bony attachments: the *costal part* arises from the upper margins of the lower six ribs; the relatively small and variable *sternal part* arises from the posterior side of the xiphoid process; and the thicker *crural part* is anchored to the bodies of the upper three lumbar vertebrae through two distinct tendinous at-

| TABLE 11–5. Primary Muscles of Inspiration | | | |
|---|---|---|---|
| **Muscle** | **Mode of Action** | **Innervation** | **Location of Illustrations** |
| Diaphragm | 1. The diaphragm increases the vertical diameter of the thorax by lowering and flattening its dome.<br>2. The increasing intra-abdominal pressure caused by the lowering of the diaphragm expands the lower ribs laterally.<br>3. Once stabilized by increased intra-abdominal pressure, continued contraction of the costal fibers of diaphragm elevates the middle and lower ribs. | Phrenic nerve (ventral ramus $C^{3-5}$) | Chapter 11 |
| Scalenes | The scalene anterior, medius, and posterior elevate the upper ribs and the sternum. | Ventral rami of spinal nerves ($C^{3-7}$) | Chapter 10 |
| Intercostales | The intercostales, especially the parasternal interni, elevate the ribs. The intercostales stabilize the intercostal spaces and prevent an inward collapse of the upper thoracic wall. | Intercostal nerves (ventral rami $T^{2-12}$) | Chapter 11 |

**SPECIAL   FOCUS   11–6**

### The Variable Positions of the Diaphragm

Because of the position of the liver within the abdomen, the right side of the diaphragm lies slightly higher than the left. In quiet inspiration, the dome of the diaphragm drops about 1.5 cm. During forced inspiration, the diaphragm flattens and may drop 6 to 10 cm.[64] At maximum inspiration, the right sides descend to the level of the body of T11; the left side descends to the level of the body of T12.

In the upright position, gravity lowers the position of the abdominal contents. For this reason, the dome of the diaphragm rests lower while standing or sitting compared with being supine. Persons with dyspnea, or "shortness of breath" associated with respiratory disease, often feel that they can breathe more easily while sitting. The diaphragm can contract a greater distance before encountering resistance from the abdominal contents in the sitting position.

tachments known as the *right and left crus.* Two aponeurotic arches attach the diaphragm to the external surfaces of the quadratus lumborum and psoas major muscles. The crural part of the diaphragm contains the longest and most vertically oriented fibers.

The three sets of peripheral attachments of the diaphragm converge to form a *central tendon* at the upper dome of the muscle. Each half of the diaphragm receives its innervation via the phrenic nerve, with nerve roots originating from ventral roots $C^{3-5}$, but primarily $C^4$.

The diaphragm is the most important and efficient muscle of inspiration, performing 70 to 80% of the work of inspiration.[36] This function is due in part to the muscle's ability to increase intrathoracic volume in three diameters; vertical, medial-lateral, and anterior-posterior.

With the lower ribs stabilized, the initial contraction of the diaphragm lowers and flattens its dome. This piston action *increases* the vertical diameter of the thorax as it simultaneously *decreases* the vertical diameter of the abdomen. The descent of the diaphragm is resisted by an increase in intra-abdominal pressure; by compressed abdominal contents; and by passive tension in stretched abdominal muscles, such as the transversus abdominis. The increased intra-abdominal pressure causes the lower ribs to expand laterally. The natural resistance provided by the abdomen stabilizes the dome of the diaphragm, allowing continued contraction of the costal part of the muscle to elevate the ribs. The elevation can be visualized by reversing the direction of the arrowheads in Figure 11–28. The action of the diaphragm on the ribs expands the middle and lower thorax in both *anterior-posterior and medial-lateral diameters.*

## SCALENE MUSCLES

The *scalenus anterior, medius, and posterior muscles* attach between the cervical spine and the upper two ribs (see Chapter 10). By assuming that the cervical spine is well stabilized, bilateral contraction of the muscles increases intrathoracic volume by elevating the upper ribs and attached sternum. The scalene muscles are active along with the diaphragm during every inspiration cycle.[12]

## INTERCOSTALES MUSCLES

### Anatomy of the Intercostales Muscles

The *intercostales* are a thin, three-layer set of muscles that occupy the intercostal spaces. Each set of intercostal muscles within a given intercostal space is innervated by an adjacent intercostal nerve.

The *intercostales externi* are most superficial, analogous in depth and fiber direction to the obliquus abdominis externus muscles (see Chapter 10). There are eleven per side, and each intercostalis externi arises from the lower border of a rib and inserts on the upper border of the rib below (see Fig. 11–25, see right side). Fibers travel obliquely between ribs in an inferior and medial direction. The intercostales externi are most developed laterally. Near the sternum, the intercostales externi are very thin and terminate as the *anterior intercostal membrane.*

The *intercostales interni* are deep to the externi and are analogous in depth and fiber direction to the obliquus abdominis internus. There are also eleven per side, and each intercostalis interni occupies one intercostal space, in a manner similar to the intercostalis externi. A major difference, however, is that the fibers of the intercostales interni travel perpendicular to the fibers of the intercostales externi (Fig. 11–25, see right side). The intercostales interni are most developed in the parasternal region; posteriorly, they terminate as the *posterior intercostal membrane.*

The *intercostales intimi muscles* are the deepest and least developed of the intercostales. They run parallel and deep to the intercostales interni. Fibers of the intercostales intimi near the angle of the ribs, often called the subcostales, may cross one or two intercostal spaces. The intercostales intimi are most developed in the lower thorax.

### Function of the Intercostales Muscles

By spanning each intercostal space, an intercostalis muscle has the potential to alter the volume within the thorax by elevating a lower rib, depressing an upper rib, or performing both actions. The specific strategy used by the different intercostales muscles during the different phases of ventilation is an uncertain and a controversial topic.[24] The conventional teaching is that the intercostales *externi* are more associated with *inspiration,* and the *interni* are more associated with *expiration.*[63,64] Although this association has been shown in EMG studies, simple functional distinction is not clear.[12,35,55] For instance, both the intercostales externi *and* interni have been shown to be active during inspiration.[16] Research also suggests that the parasternal intercostales interni are consistently more active during inspiration than the more lateral set of intercostales muscles.[24] The lateral set of intercostales (interni and externi) show considerable activation during axial rotation of the trunk. In a similar manner as the "oblique abdominals" (see Chapter 10), the more lateral intercostales externi are most active during contralateral trunk rotation, and the more lateral intercostales interni are most active during ipsilateral trunk rotation.[55]

In summary, the human body apparently has several strategies available for activating the intercostales. Both sets of muscles may elevate or depress the ribs, depending on the workload placed on the ventilatory system and the torque demands placed on the trunk as a whole, and which of the two adjacent ribs is freest to move.[14]

One function of the intercostales that is clear is their ability to *stabilize the intercostal spaces.* During inspiration, the intercostales muscles contract to stiffen the rib cage.[4] With the assistance of the scalene muscles, the splinting action prevents the thoracic wall from being partially sucked inward by the reduced intrathoracic pressure caused by contraction of the diaphragm.[13]

## Muscles of Forced Inspiration

Forced inspiration requires additional muscles to assist the primary muscles of inspiration. As a group, the additional muscles are referred to as *muscles of forced inspiration,* or *accessory muscles of inspiration.* Table 11–6 shows a sample of the mode of action of several muscles of forced inspiration. Each muscle has a line-of-action that can directly or indirectly increase intrathoracic volume. The muscles listed in Table 11–6 are illustrated elsewhere in this textbook. The serratus posterior superior and serratus posterior inferior, however, are illustrated in Figure 11–29; the levator costae muscles are illustrated in Figure 10–12.

The muscles of forced inspiration are typically used in healthy persons to increase both the rate and volume of inspired air. These muscles may also compensate for the dysfunction of one or more of the primary muscles of inspiration, such as the diaphragm. This compensation is frequently employed in persons with severe chronic obstructive pulmonary disease.

### Chronic Obstructive Pulmonary Disease: Altered Muscle Mechanics

*Chronic obstructive pulmonary disease (COPD)* is a disorder that typically incorporates three components: (1) chronic bronchitis, (2) emphysema, and (3) asthma. Symptoms include chronic inflammation and narrowing of the bronchioles, chronic cough, and mucus-filled airways, with overdistension and destruction of the alveolar walls. A significant complication of COPD is elastic recoil loss within the lungs and collapsed bronchioles. As a result, air remains trapped in the lungs at the end of quiet or forced expiration. This

### SPECIAL FOCUS 11–7

#### "Paradoxical Breathing" Following Cervical Spinal Cord Injury

In the healthy person, ventilation typically involves a characteristic pattern of movement between the thorax and abdomen. During inspiration, the thorax expands outwardly owing to the elevation of the ribs and sternum. The abdomen may protrude slightly because of the anterior displacement of the abdominal viscera, compressed by the descending diaphragm.

A complete cervical spinal cord injury below the C4 vertebra does not paralyze the diaphragm because its innervation is primarily from the C[4] nerve root. The intercostales and abdominal muscles, however, are typically totally paralyzed. The patient with this level of spinal cord injury often displays a "paradoxical breathing" pattern.[45] The pathomechanics of this breathing pattern provide insight into the normal interaction of the diaphragm, intercostales, and abdominal muscles during inspiration.

Without the splinting action of the intercostales across the intercostal spaces, the lowering of the dome of the diaphragm creates an internal suction within the chest that constricts the upper thorax, especially in its anterior-posterior diameter. The term paradoxical breathing describes the constriction, rather than the normal expansion, of the rib cage during inspiration.[45] The constriction of the thorax can reduce the vital capacity of a person with an acute cervical spinal cord injury. In the healthy adult, vital capacity is about 4000 mL. About 3000 mL of this capacity is accounted for by contraction and full descent of the diaphragm. The vital capacity of a person immediately following a C4 spinal cord injury may fall as low as 300 mL.[64] Although the diaphragm may be operating at near normal capacity, the constricting, rather than the normally expanding, thorax limits the inhalation of 2700 mL of air. Several weeks following a spinal injury, however, the atonic (flaccid) intercostales typically become hypertonic. The increased muscle tone can act as a splint to the thoracic wall, as evident by the fact that vital capacity in an average size adult with a C4 or below injury often returns to near 3000 mL.

In addition to the constriction of the upper thorax during inspiration, a person with an acute cervical injury often displays marked forward protrusion of the abdomen during inspiration. The atonic and paralyzed abdominal muscles offer little resistance to the forward migration of the abdominal contents. Without this resistance, the contracting diaphragm has little leverage to expand the middle and lower ribs. These pathomechanics also contribute to the loss of vital capacity following a cervical injury.

While seated, the person with an acute cervical spinal cord injury may benefit from an elastic abdominal binder. In the seated position, the dome of the diaphragm rests lower than in the supine position. An abdominal binder can offer beneficial resistance to the descent of the diaphragm until the anticipated return of firmness in the muscles that support the anterior abdominal wall.[21]

## TABLE 11-6. Muscles of Forced Inspiration

| Muscle | Mode of Action | Innervation | Location of Illustrations |
|---|---|---|---|
| Serratus posterior superior | Increases intrathoracic volume by elevating the upper ribs | Intercostal nerves (ventral rami $T^{2-5}$) | Chapter 11 |
| Serratus posterior inferior | Stabilizes the lower ribs for contraction of the diaphragm | Intercostal nerves (ventral rami $T^{9-12}$) | Chapter 11 |
| Levator costae (longus and brevis) | Increases intrathoracic volume by elevating the upper ribs | Branches of dorsi rami of adjacent thoracic spinal nerves | Chapter 10 |
| Sternocleidomastoid | Increases intrathoracic volume by elevating the sternum and upper ribs | Primary source: spinal accessory nerve (cranial nerve XI) | Chapter 10 |
| Latissimus dorsi | Increases intrathoracic volume by elevating ribs; this function requires the arms to be fixed. | Thoracodorsal nerve ($C^{6-8}$) | Chapter 5 |
| Iliocostalis thoracis and cervicis (erector spinae) | Increases intrathoracic volume by extending the trunk; stabilizes the neck for contraction of the sternocleidomastoid and scalenes. | Adjacent dorsal rami of spinal nerves | Chapter 10 |
| Pectoralis minor | Increases intrathoracic volume by elevating the upper ribs; requires activation from muscles such as trapezius and levator scapulae to stabilize the scapula. | Medial pectoral nerve ($C^{7-8}$) | Chapter 5 |
| Pectoralis major (sternal head) | Increases intrathoracic volume by elevating the middle ribs and sternum; this function requires the arms to be fixed.<br>Greater flexion or abduction of the shoulders increases the vertical line-of-force of the muscle fibers relative to its thoracic attachments: this strategy increases the effectiveness of this muscle in expanding intrathoracic volume. | Lateral and medial pectoral nerves ($C^{5}$-$T^{1}$) | Chapter 5 |
| Serratus anterior | Increases intrathoracic volume by elevating the ribs. | Long thoracic nerve ($C^{5-7}$) | Chapter 5 |
| Quadratus lumborum | Stabilizes the lower ribs for contraction of the diaphragm during early forced inspiration. | Ventral rami of $T^{12}$-$L^{3}$ | Chapter 10 |

complication is called *hyperinflation of the lungs.*[10,54] In advanced cases, the thorax remains in a chronic state of near full inflation, regardless of the actual phase of ventilation. The thorax of a person with COPD, therefore, typically develops a barrel-shaped appearance.

The excessive air in the lungs at the end of expiration alters the geometry of the muscles of inspiration, especially the diaphragm. Throughout the ventilation cycle, the diaphragm flattens and remains abnormally low in the thorax. The change in position and shape of the diaphragm alters its *resting length* and *line-of-force.*[41] These two factors reduce the effectiveness of the diaphragm during inspiration. Operating at a shortened length on its length-tension curve compromises force production. Furthermore, functioning in a lowered position redirects the line-of-force of the costal fibers of the diaphragm more horizontally. This robs the muscle's effectiveness at elevating the ribs. At a low enough position,

the line-of-force of the muscle can paradoxically draw the lower ribs *inward,* thereby inhibiting inspiration.

Because of the compromised function of the diaphragm, persons with advanced COPD often depend on muscles of forced inspiration in addition to other primary muscles of inspiration. Even at rest, ventilation appears labored. Muscles such as the scalenes, sternocleidomastoid, erector spinae, and pectoralis major can be observed contracting. Often, a person with COPD may stand or walk with the body partially bent over while placing one or both arms on a stable object, such as the back of a chair, grocery cart, or walker.[2] This strategy stabilizes the distal attachments of arm muscles, such as the sternal head of the pectoralis major and latissimus dorsi. As a consequence, these muscles can assist with inspiration by elevating the sternum and ribs. Although this method increases the number of muscles available to assist with inspiration, it also increases the workload of standing

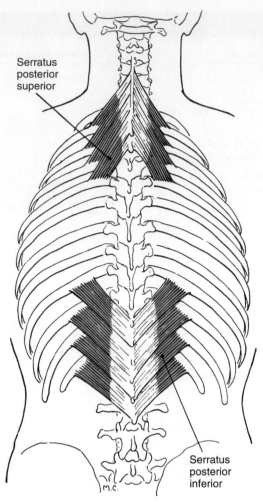

Serratus
posterior
superior

Serratus
posterior
inferior

**FIGURE 11–29.** A posterior view shows the serratus posterior superior and serratus posterior inferior muscles. These are considered as the intermediate muscles of the back, located deep to the rhomboids and the latissimus dorsi. (Modified with permission from Luttgens K and Hamilton N: Kinesiology: Scientific Basis of Human Motion, 9th ed. New York, McGraw-Hill, 1997. With permission of the McGraw-Hill Companies.)

and walking, often starting a vicious circle of increased fatigue and dyspnea.

## Muscles of Forced Expiration

Quiet expiration is normally a passive process, driven primarily by the elastic recoil of the thorax, lungs, and relaxing diaphragm. In the healthy lungs, the increased alveolar pressure associated with the passive process is sufficient to exhale the approximately 500 mL of air normally associated with quiet expiration.

During forced expiration, active muscle contraction is required to rapidly reduce intrathoracic volume. *Muscles of forced expiration* include the four abdominal muscles, transversus thoracis, and intercostales. The modes of action of the muscles of forced expiration are summarized in Table 11–7.

### ABDOMINAL MUSCLES

The abdominal muscles include the rectus abdominis, obliquus externus abdominis, obliquus internus abdominis, and

transversus abdominis (see Chapter 10). Contraction of these muscles has a direct and indirect effect on forced expiration (Fig. 11–30). By acting directly, contraction of the abdominal muscles flexes the thorax and depresses the ribs and sternum. These actions can rapidly and forcefully reduce intrathoracic volume, such as when coughing, sneezing, or vigorously exhaling to the limits of the expiratory reserve volume (see Fig. 11–23). When acting indirectly, contraction of the abdominal muscles—especially the transversus abdominis—increases the intra-abdominal pressure and compresses the abdominal viscera. The increased pressure can forcefully push the relaxed diaphragm upward, well into the thoracic cavity. In this manner, active contraction of the abdominal muscles takes advantage of the parachute-shaped diaphragm to help expel air from the thorax. As described in Chapter 10, the increased intra-abdominal pressure is also used during activities involving the Valsalva maneuver, including defecation, childbirth, and lifting of heavy loads.

Although the abdominal muscles are described here as muscles of forced expiration, their contraction also enhances inspiration. As the diaphragm is forced upward at maximal expiration, it is stretched to an optimal point on its length-tension curve. As a consequence, the muscle is more pre-

**Mechanics of forced expiration**

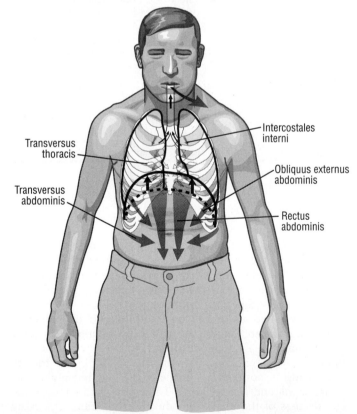

Transversus
thoracis

Transversus
abdominis

Intercostales
interni

Obliquus externus
abdominis

Rectus
abdominis

**FIGURE 11–30.** Muscle activation during forced expiration. Contraction of abdominal muscles, transversus thoracis, and intercostales interni are shown increasing both intrathoracic and intra-abdominal pressures. The passive recoil of the diaphragm is indicated by the pair of thick, black, vertical arrows. The intercostales externi may be active in varying degrees; however, that is not shown.

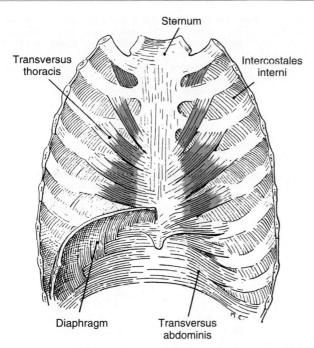

Sternum

Transversus
thoracis

Intercostales
interni

Diaphragm

Transversus
abdominis

**FIGURE 11–31.** An internal view of the anterior thoracic wall shows the transversus thoracis (red), intercostales interni, diaphragm, and transversus abdominis. (Modified with permission from Luttgens K and Hamilton N: Kinesiology: Scientific Basis of Human Motion, 9th ed. New York, McGraw-Hill, 1997. With permission of the McGraw-Hill Companies.)

**SPECIAL FOCUS 11 – 8**

**Important Physiologic Functions of the Abdominal Muscles**

Forceful expiration is driven primarily by the abdominal muscles. These muscles are included in several physiologic functions, including singing, laughing, coughing, and adequately responding to a "gag" reflex when choking. The latter two functions are particularly vital to health and safety. Coughing or vigorously "clearing the throat" is a natural way to remove secretions from the bronchial tree, thereby reducing the likelihood of lung infection. A strong contraction of the abdominal muscles is also used to dislodge objects lodged in the trachea.

Persons with weakened or completely paralyzed abdominal muscles must learn alternative methods of coughing or have others "manually" assist with this function. Consider, for example, a person with a complete spinal cord lesion at the T4 level. Because of the innervation of the abdominal muscles (ventral rami of $T^7$-$L^1$), that person would likely have completely paralyzed abdominal muscles. Persons with paralyzed or very weakened abdominal muscles must exercise extra caution to prevent choking.

pared to initiate a more forceful contraction at the next inspiration cycle.

## TRANSVERSUS THORACIS AND INTERCOSTALES

The transversus thoracis muscle, also known as the triangularis sterni or sternocostalis, is a muscle of forced expiration.

The muscle is located on the internal side of the thorax, fanning in an oblique and inferior direction between the upper five ribs and the sternum (Fig. 11–31). The muscle's neural activation is coupled with that of the abdominal muscles during forced expiration.[15]

The intercostales, especially the interni fibers, depress the ribs during forced expiration.[12]

**TABLE 11–7. Muscles of Forced Expiration**

| Muscle | Mode of Action | Innervation | Location of Illustrations |
|---|---|---|---|
| Abdominal muscles<br>rectus abdominis<br>obliquus externus abdominis<br>obliquus internus abdominis<br>transversus abdominis | 1. Decreases intrathoracic volume by flexing the trunk and depressing the ribs.<br>2. Compresses the abdominal wall and contents, which increases intra-abdominal pressure; as a result, the relaxed diaphragm is pushed upward, decreasing intrathoracic volume. | Intercostal nerves; ventral rami $T^7$-$L^1$. | Chapter 10 |
| Transversus thoracis | Decreases intrathoracic volume by depressing the ribs. | Intercostal nerves (adjacent ventral rami) | Chapter 11 |
| Intercostales | The intercostales, especially the interni fibers, decrease intrathoracic volume by depressing the ribs. | Intercostal nerves; ventral rami $T^2$-$T^{12}$ | Chapter 11 |

## REFERENCES

1. Abe S, Ouchi Y, Ide Y, et al: Perspectives on the role of the lateral pterygoid muscle and the sphenomandibular ligament in temporomandibular joint function. J Craniomand Pract 15:203–207, 1997.
2. Berman JE: Personal communication, Marquette University, Milwaukee, 2001.
3. Budzinska K, Supinski G, DiMarco AF: Inspiratory action of separate external and parasternal intercostal muscle contraction. J Appl Physiol 67:1395–1400, 1989.
4. Cala SI, Kenyon CM, Lee A, et al: Respiratory ultrasonography of human parasternal intercostal muscles in vivo. Ultrasound Med Biol 24: 313–326, 1998.
5. Carpentier P, Yung JP, Marguelles-Bonnet R, et al: Insertions of the lateral pterygoid muscles. J Oral Maxillofac Surg 46:477–482, 1988.
6. Castro HA, Resende LA, Berzin F, et al: Electromyographic analysis of superior belly of the omohyoid muscle and anterior belly of the digastric muscle in mandibular movements. Electromyogr Clin Neurophysiol 38:443–447, 1998.
7. Clanton TL, Diaz PT: Clinical assessment of the respiratory muscles. Phys Ther 75:983–995, 1995.
8. Darnell MW: A proposed chronology of events for forward head posture. J Craniomand Pract 1:50–54, 1983.
9. De Boever JA, Carlsson GE, Klineberg IJ: Need for occlusal therapy and prosthodontic treatment in the management of temporomandibular disorders. Part I. Occlusal interferences and occlusal adjustment. J Oral Rehabil 27:367–379, 2000.
10. Decramer M: Hyperinflation and respiratory muscle interaction. Eur Respir J 10:934–941, 1997.
11. De Troyer A, Estenne M: Coordination between rib cage muscles and diaphragm during quiet breathing in humans. J Appl Physiol 57:899–906, 1984.
12. De Troyer A, Estenne M: Functional anatomy of the respiratory muscles. Clin Chest Med 9:175–193, 1988.
13. De Troyer A, Heilporn A: Respiratory mechanics in quadriplegia. The respiratory function of the intercostal muscles. Am Rev Respir Dis 122: 591–600, 1980.
14. De Troyer A, Kelly S, Zin WA: Mechanical action of the intercostal muscles on the ribs. Science 220:87–88, 1983.
15. De Troyer A, Ninane V, Gilmartin JJ, et al: Triangularis sterni muscle use in supine humans. J Appl Physiol 62:919–925, 1987.
16. DiMarco AF, Romaniuk JR, Supinski GS: Action of the intercostal muscles on the rib cage. Respir Physiol 82:295–306, 1990.
17. Dunn J: Physical therapy. In Kaplan AS, Assael LA (eds): Temporomandibular Disorders, Treatment and Disorders. Philadelphia, WB Saunders, 1991.
18. Estenne M, Yernault JC, De Troyer A: Rib cage and diaphragm-abdomen compliance in humans: Effects of age and posture. J Appl Physiol 59:1842–1848, 1985.
19. Ferrario VF, Sforza C: Biomechanical model of the human mandible in unilateral clench: Distribution of temporomandibular joint reaction forces between working and balancing sides. J Prosthet Dent 72:169–176, 1994.
20. Ferrario VF, Sforza C, Miani A, et al: Open-close movements in the human temporomandibular joint: Does a pure rotation around the intercondylar hinge axis exist? J Oral Rehabil 23:401–408, 1996.
21. Goldman JM, Rose LS, Williams SJ, et al: Effect of abdominal binders on breathing in tetraplegic patients. Thorax 41:940–945, 1986.
22. Goldstein DF, Kraus SL, Williams WB, et al: Influence of cervical posture on mandibular movement. J Prosthet Dent 52:421–426, 1984.
23. Hall CM, Brody LT: Therapeutic Exercise: Moving Towards Function. Philadelphia, Lippincott Williams & Wilkins, 1999.
24. Han JN, Gayan-Ramirez G, Dekhuijzen R, et al: Respiratory function of the rib cage muscles. Eur Respir J 6:722–728, 1993.
25. Hansson T, Oberg T, Carlsson GE, et al: Thickness of the soft tissue layers and the articular disk in the temporomandibular joint. Acta Odontol Scand 35:77–83, 1977.
26. Helms CA, Katzberg RW, Dolwick MF: Internal Derangements of the Temporomandibular Joint. Radiology Research and Education Foundation, San Francisco, 1983.
27. Heylings DJ, Nielsen IL, McNeill C: Lateral pterygoid muscle and the temporomandibular disc. J Orofac Pain 9:9–15, 1995.
28. Iglarsh ZA, Snyder-Mackler L: Temporomandibular joint and the cervical spine. In Richardson JV, Iglarsh ZA (eds): Clinical Orthopaedic Physical Therapy. Philadelphia, WB Saunders, 1994.
29. Isberg A, Westesson PL: Steepness of articular eminence and movement of the condyle and disk in asymptomatic temporomandibular joints. Oral Surg Oral Med Oral Pathol Oral Radiol Endod 86:152–157, 1998.
30. Jinbao W, Xiaoming X, Jingen S: Analysis of opening-closing movement of the temporomandibular joint. Acta Anat 133:213–216, 1988.
31. Juniper RP: Temporomandibular joint dysfunction: A theory based upon the electromyographic studies of the lateral pterygoid muscle. Br J Oral Maxillofac Surg 22:1–8, 1984.
32. Kapandji IA: The Physiology of the Joints, vol 3, 5th ed. Edinburgh, Churchill Livingstone, 1982.
33. Katzberg RW, Westesson PL: Diagnosis of the temporomandibular joint. Philadelphia, WB Saunders, 1993.
34. Lafreniere CM, Lamontagne M, El-Sawy R: The role of the lateral pterygoid muscles in TMJ disorders during static conditions. J Craniomand Pract 15:38–52, 1997.
35. Le Bars P, Duron B: Are the external and internal intercostal muscles synergists or antagonists in the cat? Neurosci Lett 51:383–386, 1984.
36. Loring SH, De Troyer A: Actions of the respiratory muscles. In Roussos C, Macklem PT (eds): The Thorax. New York, Marcel Dekker, 1985.
37. Mahan PE, Wilkinson TM, Gibbs CH, et al: Superior and inferior bellies of the lateral pterygoid muscle EMG activity at basic jaw positions. J Prosthet Dent 50:710–718, 1983.
38. Major PW, Nebbe B: Use and effectiveness of splint appliance therapy: Review of literature. J Craniomand Pract 15:159–166, 1997.
39. Mannheimer JS, Dunn J: Cervical spine. In Kaplan AS, Assael LA (eds): Temporomandibular Disorders, Treatment and Disorders. Philadelphia, WB Saunders, 1991.
40. Marbach JJ, Ballard GT, Frankel MR, et al: Patterns of TMJ surgery: Evidence of sex differences. J Am Dent Assoc 128:609–614, 1997.
41. Marchand E, Decramer M: Chronic obstructive pulmonary disease. Clin Chest Med 21:679–692, 2000.
42. McNamara JA: The independent functions of the two heads of lateral pterygoid muscle. Am J Anat 138:197–206, 1973.
43. Miller A: TMD epidemiology. In McNeill C (ed): Current Controversies in Temporomandibular Disorders. Quintessence Publishing Co., Chicago, IL, 1992.
44. Mizuno M: Human respiratory muscles: Fibre morphology and capillary supply. Eur Resp J 4:587–601, 1991.
45. Morgan MDL, Gourlay AR, Silver JR, et al: Contribution of the rib cage to breathing in tetraplegia. Thorax 40:613–617, 1985.
46. Oberg T, Carlsson GE, Fajers CM: The temporomandibular joint. A morphologic study on human autopsy material. Acta Odontol Scand 29: 349–384, 1971.
47. Okeson JP: Management of Temporomandibular Disorders and Occlusion. Mosby, St. Louis, 1998.
48. Osborn JW: The disc of the human temporomandibular joint: Design, function, and failure. J Oral Rehabil 12:279–293, 1985.
49. Osborn JW: The temporomandibular ligament and the articular eminence as constraints during jaw opening. J Oral Rehabil 16:323–333, 1989.
50. Piehslinger E, Celar AG, Celar RM, et al: Computerized axiography: Principles and methods. J Craniomand Pract 9:344–355, 1991.
51. Posselt U: Movement areas of the mandible. J Prosthet Dent 7:375–385, 1957.
52. Prinz JF: Physical mechanisms involved in the genesis of temporomandibular joint sounds. J Oral Rehabil 25:706–714, 1998.
53. Rauhala K, Oikarinen KS, Raustia AM: Role of temporomandibular disorders (TMD) in facial pain: Occlusion, muscle and TMJ pain. J Craniomand Pract 17:254–261, 1999.
54. Reid WD, Dechman G: Considerations when testing and training the respiratory muscles. Phys Ther 75:971–982, 1995.
55. Rimmer KP, Ford GT, Whitelaw WA: Interaction between postural and respiratory control of human intercostal muscles. J Appl Physiol 79: 1556–1561, 1995.
56. Robinson PD: Articular cartilage of the temporomandibular joint: Can it regenerate? Ann R Coll Surg Engl 75:231–236, 1993.
57. Rocabado M: Arthrokinematics of the temporomandibular joint. Dent Clin North Am 27:573–594, 1983.
58. Sari S, Sonmez H, Oray GO, et al: Temporomandibular joint dysfunction and occlusion in the mixed and permanent dentition. J Clin Pediatr Dent 24:59–62, 1999.
59. Sato H, Strom D, Carlsson GE: Controversies on anatomy and function of the ligaments associated with the temporomandibular joint: A literature survey. Orofac Pain 9:308–316, 1995.

60. Sinn DP, de Assis EA, Throckmorton GS: Mandibular excursions and maximum bite forces in patients with temporomandibular joint disorders. J Oral Maxillofac Surg 54:671–679, 1996.

61. Stohler CS: Muscle-related temporomandibular disorders. J Orofac Pain 13:273–284, 1999.

62. Suvinen TI, Reade PC, Sunden B, et al: Temporomandibular disorders. Part 1: A comparison of symptom profiles in Australian and Finnish patients. J Orofac Pain 11:58–66, 1997.

63. Whitelaw WA, Ford GT, Rimmer KP, et al: Intercostal muscles are used during rotation of the thorax in humans. J Appl Physiol 72:1940–1944, 1992.

64. Williams PL, Bannister LH, Berry M, et al: Gray's Anatomy, 38th ed. New York, Churchill Livingstone, 1995.

65. Wilkinson TM: The relationship between the disk and the lateral pterygoid muscle in the human temporomandibular joint. J Prosthet Dent 60:715–724, 1988.

66. Wink CS, Onge MS, Zimmy ML: Neural elements in the human temporomandibular articular disc. J Oral Maxillofac Surg 50:334–337, 1992.

67. Yustin DC, Rieger MR, McGuckin RS, et al: Determination of the existence of hinge movements of the temporomandibular joint during normal opening by Cine-MRI and computer digital addition. J Prosthodont 2:190–195, 1993.

68. Zaugg M, Lucchinetti E: Geriatric anesthesia: Respiratory function in the elderly. Anesth Clin North Am 18:47–58, 2000.

69. Zonnenberg AJ, Van Maanen CJ, Oostendorp RA, et al: Body posture photographs as a diagnostic aid for musculoskeletal disorders related to temporomandibular disorders (TMD). J Craniomand Pract 14:225–232, 1996.

## ADDITIONAL READINGS

Campbell EJM: The role of the scalene and sternomastoid muscles in breathing in a normal subject: An electromyographic study. J Anat 89: 378–386, 1955.

Di Fabio RP: Physical therapy for patients with TMD: A descriptive study of treatment, disability, and health status. J Orofacial Pain 12:124–134, 1998.

Goldman MD, Loh L, Sears TA: The respiratory activity of human levator costae muscles and its modification by posture. J Physiol 362:189–204, 1985.

Goodheart G: Applied kinesiology in dysfunction of the temporomandibular joint. Dent Clin North Am 27:613–630, 1983.

Krumpe PE, Knudson RJ, Parsons G, et al: The aging respiratory system. Clin Geriatric Med 1:143–175, 1985.

Lipton JA, Ship JA, Larach-Robinson D: Estimated prevalence and distribution of reported orofacial pain in the United States. J Am Dent Assoc 124:115–121, 1993.

McKay GS, Yemm R, Cadden SW: The structure and function of the temporomandibular joint. Br Dent J 173:127–132, 1992.

Passero PL, Wyman BS, Bell JW, et al: Temporomandibular joint dysfunction syndrome. Phys Ther 65:1203–1207, 1985.

Widmark G: On surgical intervention in the temporomandibular joint. Swed Dent J 123S:1–87, 1997.

## Part A: Muscles of the Trunk

### SET 1: MUSCLES OF THE POSTERIOR TRUNK

See Appendix II for attachments and innervations of the muscles in the superficial layer of the posterior trunk (trapezius, latissimus dorsi, serratus anterior, and so forth).

#### Erector Spinae Group

Iliocostalis, Longissimus, and Spinalis Muscles

**Iliocostalis Lumborum**
*Inferior attachments:* common tendon*
*Superior attachments:* inferior surface of the angle of ribs 6 to 12

**Iliocostalis Thoracis**
*Inferior attachments:* upper surface of the angle of ribs 6 to 12
*Superior attachments:* angle of ribs 1 to 6

**Iliocostalis Cervicis**
*Inferior attachments:* angle of ribs 3 to 7
*Superior attachments:* posterior tubercles of the transverse processes of C4–6

**Longissimus Thoracis**
*Inferior attachments:* common tendon
*Superior attachments:* transverse processes of T1–12 and areas between the tubercle and angle of ribs 3 to 12

**Longissimus Cervicis**
*Inferior attachments:* transverse processes of T1–4
*Superior attachments:* posterior tubercles of the transverse processes of C2–6

**Longissimus Capitis**
*Inferior attachments:* transverse processes of T1–5 and articular processes of C4–7
*Superior attachments:* posterior margin of the mastoid process of the temporal bone

**Spinalis Thoracis**
*Inferior attachments:* common tendon
*Superior attachments:* spinous processes of T1–6

**Spinalis Cervicis**
*Inferior attachments:* ligamentum nuchae and spinous processes of C7–T1
*Superior attachments:* spinous process of C2

**Spinalis Capitis**
Blends with semispinalis capitis

*Innervation to the erector spinae:* dorsal rami of adjacent spinal nerves ($C^3$–$L^5$)

#### Transversospinal Group

Multifidi, Rotatores, and Semispinalis Muscles

**Multifidi**
*Inferior attachments (lumbar):* mammillary processes of lumbar vertebrae, lumbosacral ligaments, deep part of the common tendon of the erector spinae, posterior surface of the sacrum, posterior-superior iliac spine of the pelvis, and the capsule of the lumbar and lumbosacral apophyseal joints
*Inferior attachments (thoracic):* transverse processes of T1–12
*Inferior attachments (cervical):* articular processes of C3–7
*Superior attachments:* spinous processes of vertebrae located 2–4 intervertebral segments superior
*Innervation:* dorsal rami of adjacent spinal nerves ($C^4$–$S^3$)

**Rotatores: Longus and Brevis**
*Inferior attachments:* transverse processes of all vertebrae
*Superior attachments:* spinous processes of vertebrae located 1 to 2 intervertebral segments superior
*Note:* the rotator longus crosses two intervertebral junctions; the more horizontal rotator brevis crosses only one intervertebral junction.
*Innervation:* dorsal rami of adjacent spinal nerves ($C^4$–$L^4$)

**Semispinalis Thoracis**
*Inferior attachments:* transverse processes of T6–10
*Superior attachments:* spinous processes of C6–T4

**Semispinalis Cervicis**
*Inferior attachments:* transverse processes of T1–6
*Superior attachments:* spinous processes of C2–5, primarily C2

**Semispinalis Capitis**
*Inferior attachments:* transverse processes of C7–T7 and articular processes of C4–6
*Superior attachments:* between the superior and inferior nuchal lines of the occipital bone

---

*This broad tendon connects the inferior end of most of the erector spinae to the base of the axial skeleton. The specific attachments of the central tendon include median sacral crests, spinous processes and supraspinous ligaments in the lower thoracic and entire lumbar region, iliac crests, sacrotuberous and sacroiliac ligaments, gluteus maximus, and multifidi muscles.

*Innervation to the semispinalis muscles:* dorsal rami of adjacent spinal nerves ($C^1$–$T^6$)

### Short Segmental Group

Interspinalis and Intertransversarus Muscles

#### Interspinalis Muscles

These paired muscles attach regularly between adjacent spinous processes within the cervical vertebrae, except C1 and C2, and the lumbar vertebrae. In the thoracic spine, the interspinalis muscles exist only at the extreme upper and lower regions.

*Innervation:* dorsal rami of adjacent spinal nerves ($C^3$–$L^5$)

#### Intertransversarus Muscles

These paired right and left muscles attach between adjacent transverse processes of all cervical, lower thoracic, and lumbar vertebrae. In the cervical region, the intertransversarus muscles are subdivided into small anterior and posterior muscles, indicating their position relative to the anterior and posterior tubercles of the transverse processes, respectively. In the lumbar region, the intertransversarus muscles are subdivided into small lateral and medial muscles, indicating their relative position between the transverse processes.

*Innervation:* the anterior, posterior, and lateral intertransversarus muscles are innervated by ventral rami of adjacent spinal nerves ($C^3$–$L^5$); the medial intertransversarus muscles, within the lumbar region, are innervated by the dorsal rami of adjacent spinal nerves ($L^1$–$L^5$).

## SET 2: MUSCLES OF THE ANTERIOR-LATERAL TRUNK: "ABDOMINAL" MUSCLES

#### Obliquus Externus Abdominis

*Lateral attachments:* lateral side of ribs 4 to 12

*Medial attachments:* anterior half of the outer lip of the iliac crest, linea alba, and contralateral rectus sheaths

*Innervation:* intercostal nerves ($T^8$–$T^{12}$), iliohypogastric ($L^1$), and ilioinguinal ($L^1$) nerves

#### Obliquus Internus Abdominis

*Lateral attachments:* anterior two thirds of the middle lip of the iliac crest, inguinal ligament, and thoracolumbar fascia

*Medial attachments:* ribs 9 to 12, linea alba, and contralateral rectus sheaths

*Innervation:* intercostal ($T^8$–$T^{12}$), iliohypogastric ($L^1$), and ilioinguinal ($L^1$) nerves

#### Rectus Abdominis

*Superior attachments:* xiphoid process and cartilages of ribs 5 to 7

*Inferior attachments:* crest of pubis and adjacent ligaments supporting the pubic symphysis joint

*Innervation:* intercostal nerves ($T^7$–$T^{12}$)

#### Transversus Abdominis

*Lateral attachments:* anterior two thirds of the inner lip of the iliac crest, thoracolumbar fascia, inner surface of the cartilages of ribs 6 to 12, and inguinal ligament

*Medial attachments:* linea alba and contralateral rectus sheaths

*Innervation:* intercostal ($T^7$–$T^{12}$), iliohypogastric ($L^1$), and ilioinguinal ($L^1$) nerves

## Part B: Muscles of the Craniocervical Region

### SET 1: MUSCLES OF THE ANTERIOR-LATERAL CRANIOCERVICAL REGION

#### Longus Capitis

*Inferior attachments:* anterior tubercles of transverse processes of C3–6

*Superior attachment:* inferior surface of the basilar part of the occipital bone, immediately anterior to the attachment of the rectus capitis anterior

*Innervation:* ventral rami of spinal nerves ($C^1$–$C^3$)

#### Longus Colli
##### Superior Oblique Portion

*Inferior attachments:* anterior tubercles of transverse processes of C3–5

*Superior attachment:* tubercle on anterior arch of C1

##### Vertical Portion

*Inferior attachments:* anterior surface of the bodies of C5–T3

*Superior attachments:* anterior surface of the bodies of C2–4

##### Inferior Oblique Portion

*Inferior attachments:* anterior surface of the bodies of T1–3

*Superior attachments:* anterior tubercles of transverse processes of C5–6

*Innervation:* ventral rami of spinal nerves ($C^2$–$C^8$)

#### Rectus Capitis Anterior

*Inferior attachment:* anterior surface of the transverse process of C1

*Superior attachment:* inferior surface of the basilar part of the occipital bone immediately anterior to the occipital condyle

*Innervation:* ventral rami of spinal nerves ($C^1$–$C^2$)

#### Rectus Capitis Lateralis

*Inferior attachment:* superior surface of the transverse process of C1

*Superior attachment:* inferior surface of the occipital bone immediately lateral to the middle section of the occipital condyle

*Innervation:* ventral rami of spinal nerves ($C^1$–$C^2$)

### Scalenes

#### Scalenus Anterior

*Superior attachments:* anterior tubercles of the transverse processes of C3–6

*Inferior attachment:* inner border of first rib

#### Scalenus Medius

*Superior attachments:* posterior tubercles of the transverse processes of C2–7

*Inferior attachment:* upper border of the first rib, posterior to the attachment of the scalenus anterior

#### Scalenus Posterior

*Superior attachments:* posterior tubercles of the transverse processes of C5–7

*Inferior attachment:* external surface of the second rib

*Innervation to the scalene muscles:* ventral rami of spinal nerves ($C^3$–$C^7$)

## Sternocleidomastoid

*Inferior attachments:* sternal head, anterior surface of the upper aspect of the manubrium of the sternum; clavicular head; posterior-superior surface of the medial one third of the clavicle

*Superior attachments:* lateral surface of the mastoid process of the temporal bone and lateral one half of the superior nuchal line of the occipital bone

*Innervation:* spinal accessory nerve (cranial nerve XI). A secondary source of innervation is through the ventral rami of the mid and upper cervical plexus, which may carry sensory (proprioceptive) information.

## SET 2: MUSCLES OF THE POSTERIOR CRANIOCERVICAL REGION

### Splenius Capitis

*Inferior attachments:* inferior half of the ligamentum nuchae and spinous process of C7–T4

*Superior attachments:* mastoid process of the temporal bone and the lateral one third of the superior nuchal line of the occipital bone. These attachments are immediately medial to the attachments of the sternocleidomastoid.

*Innervation:* dorsal rami of spinal nerves ($C^2$–$C^8$)

### Splenius Cervicis

*Inferior attachments:* spinous process of T3–6

*Superior attachments:* posterior tubercles of the transverse processes of C1–3

*Innervation:* dorsal rami of spinal nerves ($C^2$–$C^8$)

#### Suboccipital Muscles

### Obliquus Capitis Inferior

*Inferior attachment:* apex of the spinous process of C2

*Superior attachment:* inferior margin of the transverse process of C1

### Obliquus Capitis Superior

*Inferior attachment:* superior margin of the transverse process of C1

*Superior attachments:* between the lateral end of the inferior and superior nuchal lines; lateral to the attachment of the semispinalis capitis

### Rectus Capitis Posterior Major

*Inferior attachment:* spinous process of C2

*Superior attachment:* immediately medial to the lateral end of the inferior nuchal line

### Rectus Capitis Posterior Minor

*Inferior attachment:* tubercle on the posterior arch of C1

*Superior attachment:* immediately anterior to the medial end of the inferior nuchal line, just posterior to the foramen magnum

*Innervation to suboccipital muscles:* suboccipital nerve (dorsal ramus $C^1$)

## Part C: Miscellaneous: Quadratus Lumborum

### Quadratus Lumborum

*Inferior attachment:* iliolumbar ligament and crest of the ilium

*Superior attachments:* rib 12 and tips of the transverse processes of the L1–4

*Innervation:* $T^{12}$–$L^3$ (ventral rami)

## Part D: Muscles of Mastication

### Masseter: Combined Superficial and Deep Fibers

*Proximal attachments:* lateral-inferior surfaces of the zygomatic bone and inferior surfaces of the zygomatic arch

*Distal attachment:* external surface of the mandible, between the angle and just below the coronoid process

*Innervation:* branch of the mandibular nerve, a division of cranial nerve V

### Temporalis

*Proximal attachments:* temporal fossa and deep surfaces of temporal fascia

*Distal attachments:* apex and medial surfaces of the coronoid process of the mandible and the entire anterior edge of the ramus of the mandible

*Innervation:* branch of the mandibular nerve, a division of cranial nerve V

### Medial Pterygoid

*Proximal attachment:* medial surface of the lateral pterygoid plate

*Distal attachment:* internal surface of the mandible between the angle and mandibular foramen

*Innervation:* branch of the mandibular nerve, a division of cranial nerve V

### Lateral Pterygoid

**Superior Head**

*Proximal attachment:* greater wing of the sphenoid bone

**Inferior Head**

*Proximal attachment:* lateral surface of the lateral pterygoid plate

*Distal attachments:* pterygoid fossa on the mandible and the articular disc and capsule of the temporomandibular joint

*Innervation:* branch of the mandibular nerve, a division of cranial nerve V

## Part E: Suprahyoid Muscles

### Digastric: Posterior Belly

*Proximal attachment:* mastoid notch of the temporal bone

*Distal attachment:* facial sling attached to the lateral aspect of the hyoid bone

*Innervation:* facial nerve (cranial nerve VII)

### Digastric: Anterior Belly

*Proximal attachment:* fascial sling attached to the lateral aspect of the hyoid bone

*Distal attachment:* base of the mandible near its midline (digastric fossa)

*Innervation:* inferior alveolar nerve (branch of the mandibular nerve, a division of cranial nerve V)

### Geniohyoid

*Proximal attachment:* small region at the midline of the anterior aspect of the mandible's internal surface (symphysis menti)

*Distal attachment:* body of the hyoid bone

*Innervation:* C$^1$ via the hypoglossal nerve (cranial nerve XII)

### Mylohyoid
*Proximal attachment:* the internal surface of the mandible, bilaterally on the mylohyoid line
*Distal attachment:* body of the hyoid bone
*Innervation:* inferior alveolar nerve (branch of the mandibular nerve, a division of cranial nerve V)

### Stylohyoid
*Proximal attachment:* base of the styloid process of the temporal bone
*Distal attachment:* anterior edge of the greater horn of the hyoid bone
*Innervation:* facial nerve (cranial nerve VII)

## Part F: Infrahyoid Muscles

### Omohyoid
*Inferior attachment:* upper border of the scapula near the scapular notch
*Superior attachment:* body of the hyoid bone
*Innervation:* ventral rami of C$^{1-3}$

### Sternohyoid
*Inferior attachments:* posterior surface of the medial end of the clavicle, superior-posterior part of the manubrium sternum, and posterior sternoclavicular ligament
*Superior attachment:* body of the hyoid bone
*Innervation:* ventral rami of C$^{1-3}$

### Sternothyroid
*Inferior attachments:* posterior part of the manubrium of the sternum and the cartilage of the first rib
*Superior attachment:* thyroid cartilage
*Innervation:* ventral rami of C$^{1-3}$

### Thyrohyoid
*Inferior attachment:* thyroid cartilage
*Superior attachment:* junction of the body and greater horn of the hyoid bone
*Innervation:* ventral rami of C$^1$ via cranial nerve VII

## Part G: Muscles Related Primarily to Ventilation

### Diaphragm
*Inferior attachments*
*Costal part:* inner surfaces of the cartilages and adjacent bony regions of ribs 6–12
*Sternal part:* posterior side of the xiphoid process
*Crural (lumbar) part:* (1) two aponeurotic arches covering the external surfaces of the quadratus lumborum and psoas major muscles; (2) right and left crus, originating from the bodies of L1–3 and their intervertebral discs

*Superior attachment*
Central tendon near the center of the dome of the muscle

*Innervation:* phrenic nerve (C$^{3-5}$)

### Intercostales Externi
*Attachments*
Eleven per side, each muscle arises from the lower border of a rib and inserts on the upper border of the rib below. Fibers are the most superficial of the intercostales muscles, running in an inferior and medial direction. Fibers are most developed laterally.

### Intercostales Interni
*Attachments*
Eleven per side, each muscle arises from the lower border of a rib and inserts on the upper border of the rib below. Fibers run in a plane immediately deep to the intercostales externi. Fibers of the intercostales interni run in an inferior and slightly lateral direction, nearly perpendicular to the direction of the intercostales externi. Fibers of the intercostales interni are most developed adjacent to the sternum, parasternally.

### Intercostales Intimi
*Attachments*
Each muscle arises from the lower border of a rib near its angle and inserts on the upper border of the second or third rib below. Fibers run parallel and deep to the intercostales interni. Fibers of the intercostales intimi located near the angle of the ribs, often called *subcostales,* may cross two intercostal spaces. The intercostales intimi are most developed in the lower thorax.

*Innervation to the intercostales:* intercostal nerves (ventral rami T$^{2-12}$)

### Levatores Costarum
*Superior attachments:* ends of the transverse processes of C7–T11
*Inferior attachments:* external surfaces of ribs, between the tubercle and angle. Each of the twelve muscles attach to the rib immediately inferior to its vertebral attachment.

*Innervation:* Branches of dorsi rami of adjacent thoracic spinal nerves

### Serratus Posterior Inferior
*Superior attachments:* posterior surfaces of ribs 9–12, near their angles
*Inferior attachments:* spinous processes and supraspinous ligaments of T11–L3
*Innervation:* intercostal nerves (ventral rami T$^{9-12}$)

### Serratus Posterior Superior
*Superior attachments:* spinous processes of C6–T3, including supraspinous ligaments and ligamentum nuchae
*Inferior attachments:* posterior surfaces of ribs 2–5, near their angles
*Innervation:* intercostal nerves (ventral rami T$^{2-5}$)

### Transversus Thoracis
*Inferior attachments:* inner surfaces of the lower third of the body of the sternum and adjacent surfaces of the xiphoid process
*Superior attachments:* internal surfaces of the cartilages of ribs 2 to 6
*Innervation:* intercostal nerves (adjacent ventral rami)

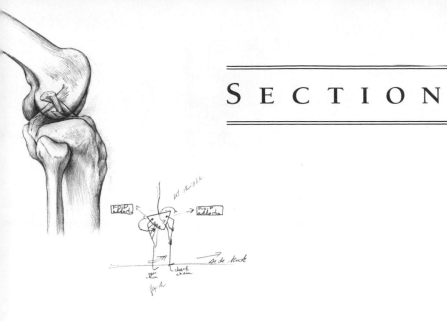

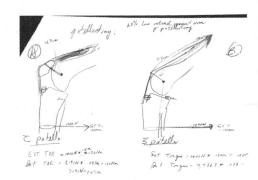

# SECTION IV

# Lower Extremity

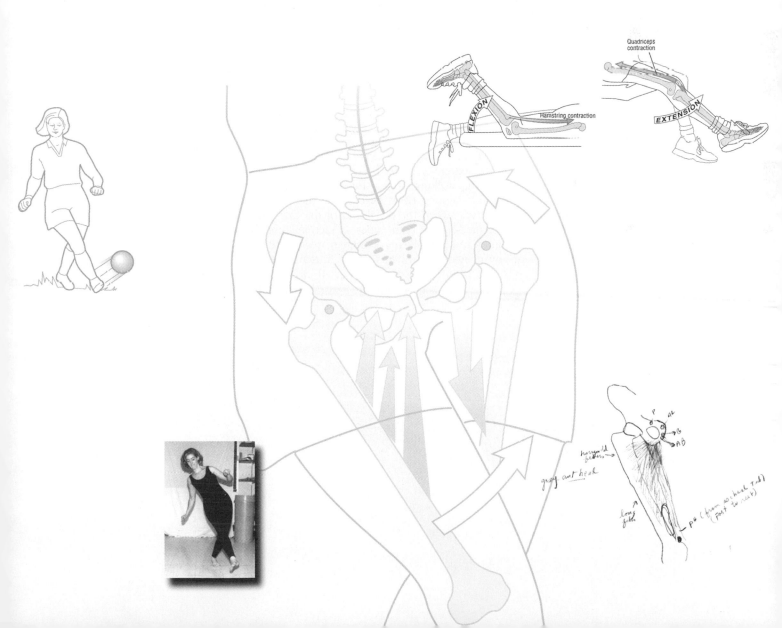

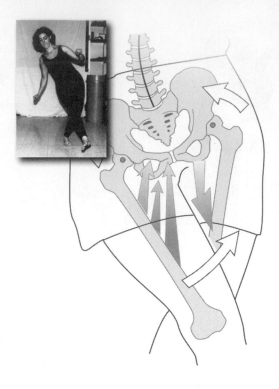

# Lower Extremity

**Section IV** is divided into four chapters. Chapters 12 to 14 describe the kinesiology of the major articular region within the lower extremity; Chapter 15 describes the kinesiology of walking, an ultimate functional expression of the kinesiology of the lower extremity. For either limb, about 60% of the walking cycle is involved in the "stance phase" in which the distal end of the extremity is fixed to the ground. During the "swing phase"—the remaining 40% of the walking cycle—the distal end of the extremity is unconstrained and free to move. Chapters 12 to 14 describe the function of the muscles and joints from two perspectives: when the distal end of the extremity is fixed, and when it is free. An understanding of both types of actions greatly increases the ability to appreciate the beauty and complexity of human movement, as well as to diagnose, treat, and prevent any related impairments of the musculoskeletal system.

# Hip

## DONALD A. NEUMANN, PT, PhD

### TOPICS AT A GLANCE

## INTRODUCTION

The hip is the articulation between the large spherical head of the femur and the deep socket provided by the acetabulum of the pelvis. This major joint provides simultaneous movement between the lower extremity and the pelvis. Because of its location within the body, a pathologic or traumatized hip typically causes a wide range of functional limitations, including difficulty in walking, dressing, driving a car, lifting and carrying loads, and climbing stairs.

The hip has many anatomic features that are well suited for stability during standing, walking, and running. The femoral head is stabilized by a deep socket that is surrounded by an extensive set of capsular ligaments. Many large forceful muscles provide the necessary torques needed to propel the body upward and forward. Weakness in these muscles has profound impact on the mobility of the body as a whole.

Hip disease and injury are relatively common, particularly in the very young and in the elderly. The abnormally formed hip in an infant is prone to dislocation. The hip in the aged is vulnerable to degenerative joint disease. Increased osteoporosis coupled with increased risk of falling predispose the elderly to a higher incidence of hip fracture.

This chapter describes the structure of the hip, its associated capsule and ligaments, and the actions of the surrounding musculature. This information is the basis for treatment and diagnosis of musculoskeletal problems in this region of the body.

## OSTEOLOGY

### Innominate

Each *innominate* (from the Latin *innominatum,* meaning nameless) is the union of three bones: the *ilium, pubis,* and *ischium* (Figs. 12–1 and 12–2). The right and left innominates connect with each other anteriorly at the pubic symphysis and posteriorly at the sacrum. The innominate bones and the sacrum form the bony *pelvis* (from the Latin, meaning *basin* or *bowl*). While a person stands, the pelvis is normally oriented so that when viewed laterally, a vertical line passes between the anterior-superior iliac spine and the pubic tubercle (see Fig. 12–1).

The external surface of the innominate has three conspicuous features. The large fan-shaped *wing* (or *ala*) of the ilium forms the superior half of the innominate. Just below the wing is the deep, cup-shaped *acetabulum.* Just inferior and slightly medial to the acetabulum is the large *obturator foramen.* This foramen is covered by an *obturator membrane* (see Fig. 12–2).

---

**Osteologic Features of the Ilium**

*External Surface*
- Posterior, anterior, and inferior gluteal lines
- Anterior-superior iliac spine
- Anterior-inferior iliac spine
- Iliac crest
- Posterior-superior iliac spine
- Posterior-inferior iliac spine
- Greater sciatic notch
- Greater sciatic foramen
- Sacrotuberous and sacrospinous ligaments

*Internal Surface*
- Iliac fossa
- Auricular surface
- Iliac tuberosity

---

### ILIUM

The external surface of the ilium is marked by rather faint *posterior, anterior,* and *inferior gluteal lines* (see Fig. 12–1). These lines help to identify attachment sites of the gluteal muscles to the pelvis. At the most anterior extent of the ilium is the easily palpable *anterior-superior iliac spine* (see Figs. 12–1 and 12–2). Below this spine is the *anterior-inferior iliac spine.* The prominent *iliac crest,* the most supe-

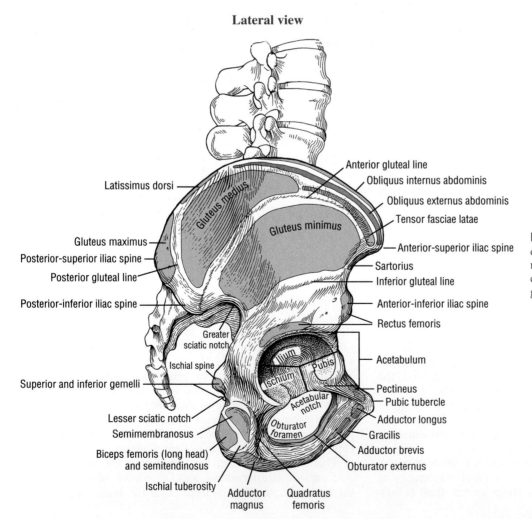

**Lateral view**

Latissimus dorsi
Gluteus medius
Gluteus minimus
Gluteus maximus
Posterior-superior iliac spine
Posterior gluteal line
Posterior-inferior iliac spine
Greater sciatic notch
Ischial spine
Superior and inferior gemelli
Lesser sciatic notch
Semimembranosus
Biceps femoris (long head) and semitendinosus
Ischial tuberosity
Adductor magnus
Quadratus femoris
Ilium
Ischium
Pubis
Acetabular notch
Obturator foramen

Anterior gluteal line
Obliquus internus abdominis
Obliquus externus abdominis
Tensor fasciae latae
Anterior-superior iliac spine
Sartorius
Inferior gluteal line
Anterior-inferior iliac spine
Rectus femoris
Acetabulum
Pectineus
Pubic tubercle
Adductor longus
Gracilis
Adductor brevis
Obturator externus

**FIGURE 12–1.** A view from the side of the right innominate bone. Proximal attachments of muscle are indicated in red, distal attachments in gray.

**Anterior view**

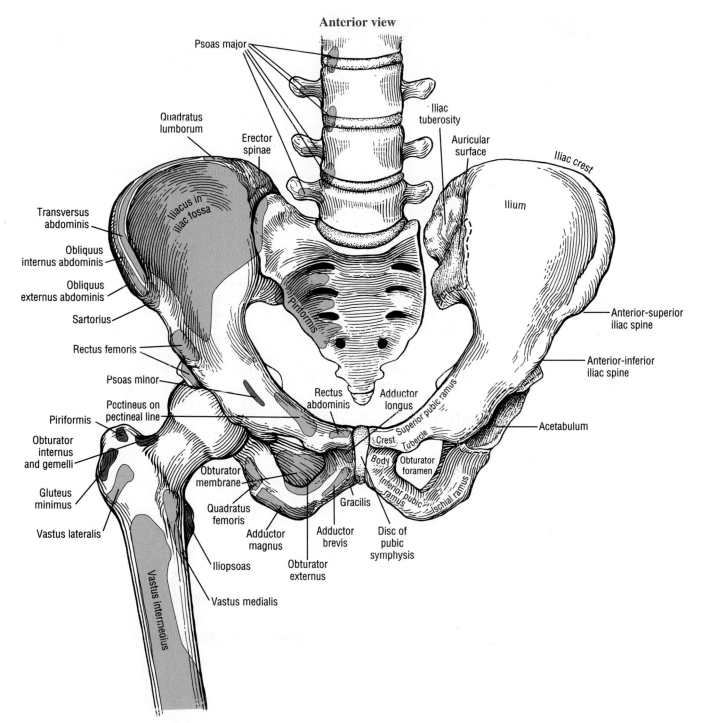

**FIGURE 12–2.** The anterior aspect of the pelvis, sacrum, and right proximal femur. Proximal attachments are indicated in red, distal attachments in gray. A section of the left side of the sacrum is removed to expose the auricular surface of the sacroiliac joint. The pelvic attachments of the capsule around the sacroiliac joint are indicated by dashed lines.

rior rim of the ilium, continues posteriorly and ends at the *posterior-superior iliac spine* (Fig. 12–3). The soft tissue superficial to the posterior-superior iliac spine is often marked by a dimple in the skin. The less prominent *posterior-inferior iliac spine* marks the superior rim of the *greater sciatic notch*. The opening of this notch is bridged by the *sacrotuberous* and *sacrospinous ligaments* to form the *greater sciatic foramen*.

The internal aspect of the ilium has two surfaces (see Fig. 12–2). Anteriorly, the smooth concave *iliac fossa* is filled by the iliacus muscle. Posteriorly, the *auricular surface* articulates with the sacrum at the sacroiliac joint, shown on the right side in Figure 12–2. Just posterior to the auricular surface is the large, rough *iliac tuberosity* formed by attachments of sacroiliac ligaments.

**Osteologic Features of the Pubis**
- Superior pubic ramus
- Body
- Pectineal line
- Pubic tubercle
- Pubic symphysis joint and disc
- Inferior pubic ramus

## PUBIS

The *superior pubic ramus* extends anteriorly from the anterior wall of the acetabulum to the large flattened *body* of the pubis (see Fig. 12–2). On the upper surface of the superior ramus is the *pectineal line,* marking the attachment of the pectineus muscle. The *pubic tubercle* projects anteriorly from the superior pubic ramus, serving as an attachment for the inguinal ligament.

**Posterior view**

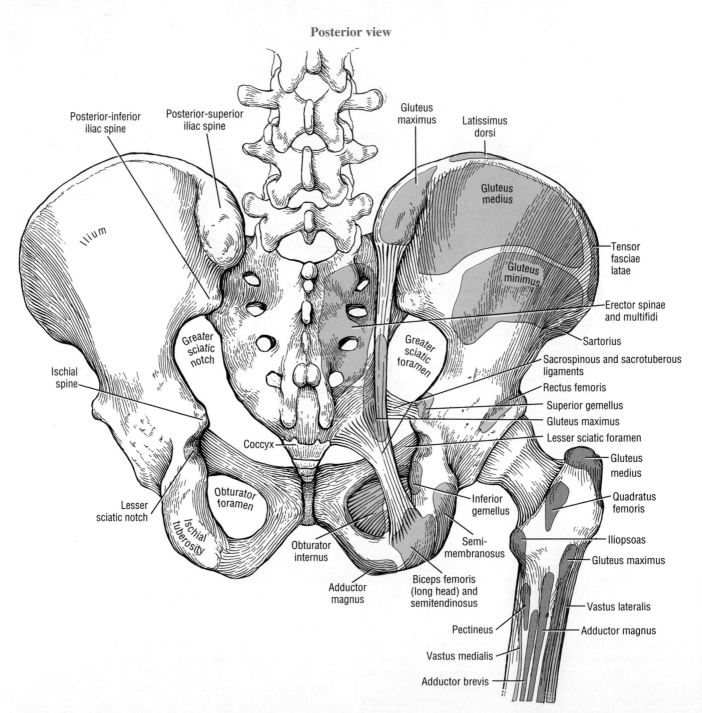

**FIGURE 12–3.** The posterior aspect of the pelvis, sacrum, and right proximal femur. Proximal attachments of muscles are indicated in red, distal attachments in gray.

The two pubic bones articulate in the midline by way of the fibrocartilaginous *pubic symphysis joint.* This joint—typically classified as an amphiarthrosis—is lined with hyaline cartilage and held together by a fibrocartilaginous, interpubic disc and supportive ligaments. Up to 2 mm of translation and 3 degrees of rotation occur at the pubic symphysis joint.[83,85] Structurally, the pubic symphysis completes the anterior pelvic ring. As described in Chapter 9, other components that form the pelvic ring are the sacrum, the pair of sacroiliac joints, and the innominate. The pubic symphysis provides stress relief throughout the pelvic ring during walking and, in women, during childbirth. The *inferior pubic ramus* extends from the body of the pubis posteriorly to the junction of the ischium (see Fig. 12–2).

## ISCHIUM

The sharp *ischial spine* projects from the posterior side of the ischium, just inferior to the greater sciatic notch (see Fig. 12–3). The *lesser sciatic notch* is located just inferior to the spine. The sacrotuberous and sacrospinous ligaments convert the lesser sciatic notch into a *lesser sciatic foramen.*

---

**Osteologic Features of the Ischium**
- Ischial spine
- Lesser sciatic notch
- Lesser sciatic foramen
- Ischial tuberosity
- Ischial ramus

---

Projecting posteriorly and inferiorly from the acetabulum is the large, stout *ischial tuberosity* (see Fig. 12–3). This palpable structure serves as the proximal attachment for many muscles of the lower extremity, most notably the hamstrings. The *ischial ramus* extends anteriorly from the ischial tuberosity, ending at the junction with the inferior pubic ramus (see Fig. 12–2).

## ACETABULUM

Located just above the obturator foramen is the large cup-shaped acetabulum (see Fig. 12–1). The acetabulum forms the socket of the hip. All three bones of the pelvis form part of the acetabulum: the ilium and ischium contributing 80% and the pubis the remaining 20%. The specific features of the acetabulum are discussed in the section, Arthrology.

---

**Osteologic Features of the Femur**
- Femoral head
- Femoral neck
- Intertrochanteric line
- Greater trochanter
- Trochanteric fossa
- Intertrochanteric crest
- Quadrate tubercle
- Lesser trochanter
- Linea aspera
- Pectineal (spiral) line
- Gluteal tuberosity
- Lateral and medial supracondylar lines
- Adductor tubercle

---

## Femur

The femur is the longest and strongest bone of the human body (Fig. 12–4). Its shape and robust stature reflect the powerful action of muscles and contribute to the long stride length during walking. At its proximal end, the femoral *head,* projects medially for an articulation with the acetabulum. The femoral *neck* connects the femoral head to the shaft. The neck serves to displace the proximal shaft of the femur laterally away from the joint, thereby reducing the likelihood of bony impingement against the pelvis. Distal to the neck, the femoral shaft courses slightly medial, thereby placing the knees and feet closer to the midline of the body.

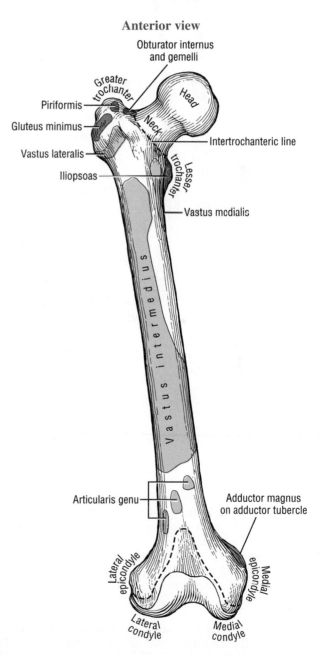

**Anterior view**

Obturator internus and gemelli · Greater trochanter · Head · Piriformis · Neck · Gluteus minimus · Vastus lateralis · Intertrochanteric line · Iliopsoas · Lesser trochanter · Vastus medialis · Vastus intermedius · Articularis genu · Adductor magnus on adductor tubercle · Lateral epicondyle · Medial epicondyle · Lateral condyle · Medial condyle

**FIGURE 12–4.** The anterior aspect of the right femur. Proximal attachments of muscles are indicated in red, distal attachments in gray. The femoral attachments of the hip joint capsule and the knee joint capsule are indicated by dashed lines.

**Medial view**

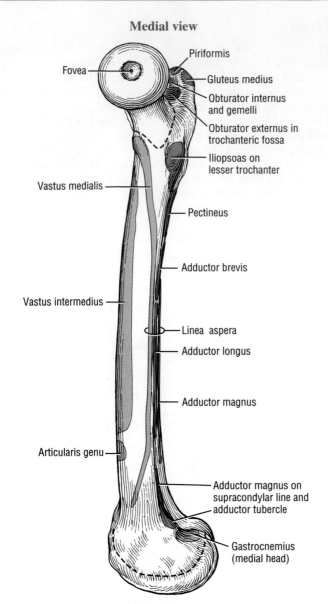

**FIGURE 12–5.** The medial aspect of the right femur. Proximal attachments of muscles are indicated in red, distal attachments in gray. The femoral attachments of the hip joint capsule and the knee joint capsule are indicated by dashed lines.

The shaft of the femur displays a slight anterior convexity (Fig. 12–5). As a long, eccentrically loaded column, the femur bows slightly when subjected to body weight. As a consequence, stress along the bone is dissipated through compression along its posterior shaft and through tension along its anterior shaft. This bowing allows the femur to bear a greater load than if the femur were perfectly straight.

Anteriorly, the *intertrochanteric line* marks the distal attachment of the capsular ligaments (see Fig. 12–4). The *greater trochanter* extends laterally and posteriorly from the junction of the femoral neck and shaft (Fig. 12–6). This prominent and easily palpable structure serves as the distal

attachment for many muscles. On the medial surface of the greater trochanter is a small pit called the *trochanteric fossa* (Figs. 12–5 and 12–7). This fossa accepts the distal attachment of the obturator externus muscle.

Posteriorly, the femoral neck joins the femoral shaft at the raised *intertrochanteric crest* (see Fig. 12–6). The *quadrate tubercle*, the distal attachment of the quadratus femoris muscle, is a slightly raised area on the crest just inferior to the trochanteric fossa. The *lesser trochanter* projects sharply from the inferior end of the crest in a posterior-medial direction. The lesser trochanter serves as the major distal attachment for the iliopsoas muscle, an important hip flexor.

The middle third of the posterior side of the femoral shaft is clearly marked by a vertical ridge called the *linea aspera* (from the Latin *linea*, line + *aspera*, rough). This raised line serves as an attachment site for the vasti muscles of the quadriceps group, many of the adductor muscles, and the intermuscular fascia of the thigh. Proximally, the linea aspera splits into the *pectineal (spiral) line* medially and the *gluteal tuberosity* laterally (see Fig. 12–6). At the distal end of the femur, the linea aspera divides into the *lateral* and *medial supracondylar lines*. The *adductor tubercle* is located at the extreme distal end of the medial supracondylar line.

## "ANGLE OF INCLINATION"

The *angle of inclination* of the femur describes the angle within the frontal plane between the femoral neck and the medial side of the femoral shaft (Fig. 12–8). At birth, this angle measures about 140 to 150 degrees. Because of the loading across the femoral neck during walking, this angle usually reduces to its normal adulthood value of about 125 degrees.[62] As depicted in Figure 12–8, this angle provides optimal alignment of the joint surfaces.

A change in the angle of inclination can occur owing to acquired or congenital factors. In general, *coxa vara* (Latin *coxa*, hip, + *vara*, to bend inward) describes an angle of inclination markedly less than 125 degrees. *Coxa valga* (Latin *valga*, to bend outward) describes an angle of inclination markedly greater than 125 degrees (Fig. 12–8*B* and *C*). These abnormal angles alter the alignment between the femoral head and the acetabulum, thereby altering hip biomechanics. In a severe case, malalignment may lead to abnormal joint wear or hip dislocation.

## "TORSION ANGLE"

The *torsion angle* of the femur describes the relative rotation (twist) that exists between the shaft and neck of the femur. Normally, as viewed from above, the femoral neck projects on average 10 to 15 degrees anterior to a medial-lateral axis through the femoral condyles. This degree of torsion is called *normal anteversion* (Fig. 12–9*A*). In conjunction with the normal angle of inclination, a 15-degree angle of anteversion affords optimal alignment and joint congruence (see alignment of red dots in Figs. 12–8*A* and 12–9*A*).

A torsion angle that is markedly different from 15 degrees

**Posterior view**

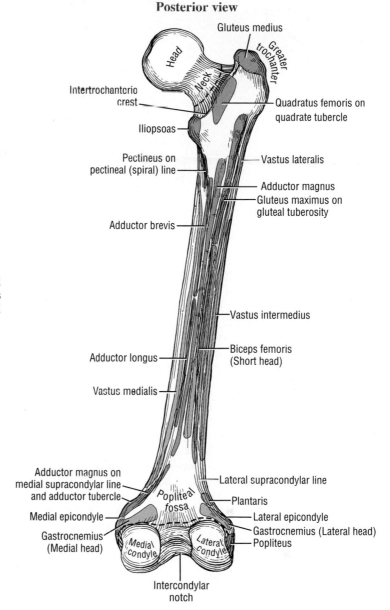

FIGURE 12–6. The posterior aspect of the right femur. Proximal attachments of muscles are indicated in red, distal attachments in gray. The femoral attachments of the hip joint capsule and the knee joint capsule are indicated by dashed lines.

is considered abnormal. A torsion angle significantly greater than 15 degrees is called *excessive anteversion* (Fig. 12–9B). In contrast, a torsion angle significantly less than 15 degrees (i.e., approaching 0 degrees) is in *retroversion* (Fig. 12–9C).

Typically, an infant is born with about 30 degrees of femoral anteversion.[18] With bone growth and increased muscle activity, this angle usually decreases to 15 degrees by 6 years of age.[71,87] Excessive anteversion is often associated with congenital dislocation, marked joint incongruence, and increased wear on articular cartilage. Excessive anteversion in children may also be associated with an abnormal gait pattern called "in-toeing."[70] "In-toeing" is a walking pattern with exaggerated posturing of hip internal rotation. This gait pattern apparently is a compensatory mechanism used to guide the excessively anteverted femoral head more directly into

**Superior view**

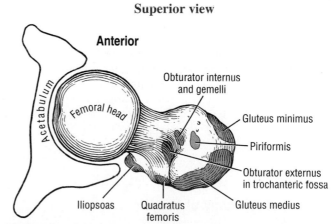

FIGURE 12–7. The superior aspect of the right femur. Distal attachments of muscles are shown in gray.

**Angle of inclination**

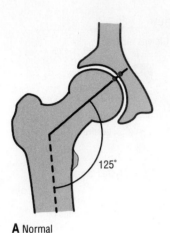
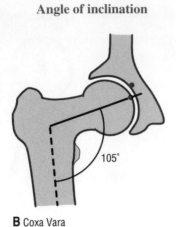
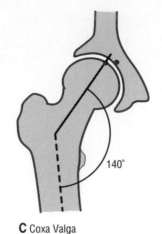

125°

**A** Normal

105°

**B** Coxa Vara

140°

**C** Coxa Valga

**FIGURE 12–8.** The proximal femur is shown: *A,* normal angle of inclination; *B,* coxa vara; and *C,* coxa valga. The pair of red dots in each figure indicates the different alignments of the hip joint surfaces. Optimal alignment is shown in *A.*

the acetabulum (Fig. 12–10*A* and *B*). Over time, children may develop contracture of the internal rotator muscles and various ligaments, thereby reducing external rotation range of motion.[23] Approximately 50% of the children with "in-toeing" eventually walk normally.[18] The gait pattern improves primarily because of structural compensation in other parts of the lower extremity, most commonly the tibia.

### INTERNAL STRUCTURE OF THE PROXIMAL FEMUR

#### *Compact and Cancellous Bone*

Walking produces tension, compression, bending, shear, and torsion on the proximal femur (see Chapter 1). Each type of force produces a different kind of stress on the proximal femur. (Stress is a *resistance* produced by tissue in response to an external load.) In order to tolerate repetitive stresses throughout a lifetime, the proximal femur must resist and absorb mechanical energy. These two functions are accomplished by two strikingly different compositions of bone. *Compact bone* is very dense and unyielding, with an ability to withstand large external loads. This type of bone is particularly thick in the cortex, the outer shell, of the lower femoral neck and entire shaft (Fig. 12–12). These regions are subjected to large shear and torsion forces. *Cancellous bone*, in contrast, consists of a three-dimensional lattice of branching trabeculae. The relative "spongy" consistency of cancellous bone absorbs external forces. Cancellous bone tends to concentrate along lines of stress, forming *trabecular networks*.[74] A *medial trabecular* and an *arcuate trabecular network* are visible within the femur shown in Figure 12–12.[65] The overall pattern of the trabecular network changes when the proximal femur is subjected to abnormal forces over an extended time.

### ARTHROLOGY

#### Functional Anatomy of the Hip Joint

The hip is the classic ball-in-socket joint of the body. Extensive ligaments and large muscles maintain the femoral head

securely in the acetabulum. Thick layers of articular cartilage, muscle, and cancellous bone in the proximal femur help dampen the large forces that routinely cross the hip. Failure of any of these protective mechanisms due to disease or injury often leads to deterioration of the joint structure.

### FEMORAL HEAD

The femoral head is located just inferior to the middle third of the inguinal ligament. On average, the centers of the two adult femoral heads are 17.5 cm (6.9 in) apart from each other.[53] The head of the femur forms about two thirds of a nearly perfect sphere (Fig. 12–13).[26] Located slightly posterior to the center of the head is a prominent pit, or *fovea* (see Fig. 12–5). The entire surface of the femoral head is covered by articular cartilage, except for the region of the fovea. The cartilage tends to be thickest in a broad region above and anterior to the fovea (Fig. 12–14).[42]

---

**Osteologic Features of the Femoral Head and Acetabulum**

*Femoral Head*
- Fovea and ligamentum teres

*Acetabulum*
- Acetabular notch
- Transverse acetabular ligament
- Acetabular labrum
- Lunate surface
- Acetabular fossa

---

The *ligamentum teres* (ligament to the head of the femur) runs between the transverse acetabular ligament and the fovea of the femoral head (see Fig. 12–13). The ligamentum teres is a tubular sheath of synovial-lined connective tissue, which adds little stability to the joint. Within the teres ligament is a small branch of the obturator artery. This small and inconstant vessel provides only minimal blood to the femoral head, the major supply provided by arteries that course through the joint capsule.

## ACETABULUM

The acetabulum is a deep, hemispheric cup-like socket that accepts the femoral head. The bony rim of the acetabulum is

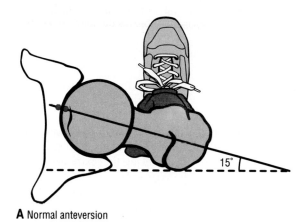

**A** Normal anteversion

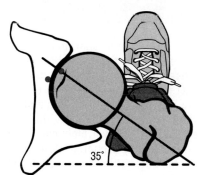

**B** Excessive anteversion

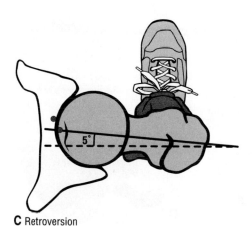

**C** Retroversion

**FIGURE 12–9.** The angle of torsion is shown between the neck and shaft of the femur: *A*, normal anteversion; *B*, excessive anteversion; and *C*, retroversion. The pair of red dots in each figure indicates the different alignments of the hip joint surfaces. Optimal alignment is shown in *A*.

incomplete near its inferior pole, creating the *acetabular notch* (see Fig. 12–1). The *transverse acetabular ligament* spans the acetabular notch.

The *acetabular labrum* is a ring of fibrocartilage that surrounds the circumference of the acetabulum (see Fig. 12–13). The labrum is triangular in cross-section, with its base attaching along the rim of the acetabulum. Adjacent to the acetabular notch, the labrum blends with the transverse acetabular ligament. The labrum deepens the concavity of the socket and securely grips the periphery of the femoral head. The acetabular labrum, therefore, adds significantly to the stability of the articulation. Traumatic dislocation of the hip usually tears the labrum.

The femoral head contacts the acetabulum only along its horseshoe-shaped *lunate surface* (see Fig. 12–13). This surface is covered with articular cartilage, thickest along the superior-anterior region of its dome (see Fig. 12–14).[42] The regions of thickest cartilage correspond to roughly the regions of highest joint pressures when walking.[13] During walking, hip forces fluctuate between 13% of body-weight during mid swing phase to over 300% body-weight during stance phase (Fig. 12–15).[13] During stance phase, the lunate surface flattens slightly as the acetabular notch widens, thereby increasing contact area and reducing peak pressure.[47] Forces on the acetabulum during walking are also transferred to the sacroiliac joint and pubic symphysis joint.[13] Hypomobility at these joints may increase stress at the hip, possibly causing excessive wear.

The *acetabular fossa* is a depression located deep within the floor of the acetabulum. Because the fossa does not normally make contact with the femoral head, it is devoid of cartilage. Instead, the fossa contains the teres ligament, fat, synovial membrane, and blood vessels.

## ACETABULAR ALIGNMENT

In the anatomic position, the acetabulum projects laterally from the pelvis with a varying amount of inferior and anterior tilt. Acetabular dysplasia describes a congenital or an acquired condition in which the acetabulum is abnormally shaped and poorly aligned. A malaligned acetabulum does not adequately cover the femoral head, often causing chronic dislocation and osteoarthritis.[50] Two angles describe the extent to which the shape of the acetabulum naturally covers the femoral head: the center-edge angle and the acetabular anteversion angle.

### Center-Edge Angle

The *center-edge angle* (also called the angle of Wiberg) describes the extent to which the acetabulum covers the femoral head within the frontal plane (Fig. 12–16A). The center-edge angle is highly variable but, on average, measures about 35 to 40 degrees in the x-rays of adults.[1] The normal center-edge angle provides a protective shelf over the femoral head. A more vertical alignment (i.e., a smaller angle) offers less containment of the femoral head and is associated with an increased risk of dislocation.[1]

### Acetabular Anteversion Angle

The *acetabular anteversion angle* describes the extent to which the acetabulum surrounds the femoral head within

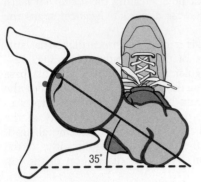
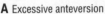
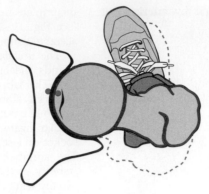

35°

**A** Excessive anteversion

**B** Excessive anteversion with "in-toeing"

**FIGURE 12–10.** Two situations show the same individual with excessive anteversion of the proximal femur. *A,* Offset red dots indicate malalignment of the hip while standing in the anatomic position. *B,* As evident by the alignment of the red dots, standing with the hip internally rotated ("in-toeing") improves the joint congruity.

the horizontal plane.[1] A normal acetabular anteversion angle of about 20 degrees exposes part of the anterior side of the femoral head (Fig. 12–16*B*). The thick anterior capsular ligament of the hip and the iliopsoas tendon cover this side of the hip. Persons with excessive anteversion of both the femur and the acetabulum are susceptible to anterior joint dislocation, especially at the extremes of external rotation.

### SPECIAL FOCUS 12–1

**Natural Anteversion of the Femur: A Reflection of the General Prenatal Development of the Lower Limb**

During prenatal development, the upper and lower extremities both undergo significant axial rotation (Fig. 12–11). By about 54 days after conception, the lower limbs have rotated *internally* (medially) about 90 degrees. This rotation turns the knee cap region to its final anterior position. In essence, the lower limbs have become permanently "pronated." This helps to explain why the "extensor" muscles—such as the quadriceps and tibialis anterior—face anteriorly, and the "flexor" muscles—such as the hamstrings and gastrocnemius—face posteriorly after birth.

The final torsion angle between the shaft and the neck of the femur reflects the degree of this medial rotation.

The functional consequence of the medial rotation of the lower limbs is that the plantar surfaces of the feet assume a plantigrade and pronated position suitable for walking. This pronated position is evident by the medial position of the great toe on the lower limb, similar to the thumb when the forearm is fully pronated. Other anatomic features, such as the oblique nature of the lower extremity dermatomes and the twisted ligaments of the hip (see Figs. 12–17 and 12–18), reflect the developmental medial rotation of the lower extremity.

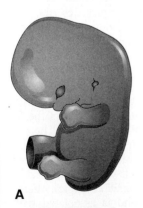
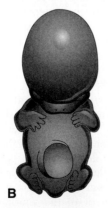
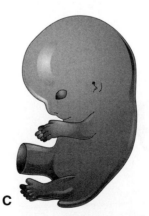
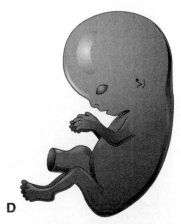

**A**      **B**      **C**      **D**

**FIGURE 12–11.** The morphologic rotation of the limb buds during prenatal development. *A,* At about 48 days, the limbs extend ventrally and the hands and feet face each other. *B,* At about 51 days, the elbows flex and the hands are curved over the thorax. *C,* About 54 days, the soles of the feet face each other. *D,* By about 54 days, the entire lower limb buds have "internally rotated" almost 90 degrees. By this phase of development, the elbows face caudally and the knees cranially. (From Moore KL: The Developing Human, 6th ed. Philadelphia, WB Saunders, 1998.)

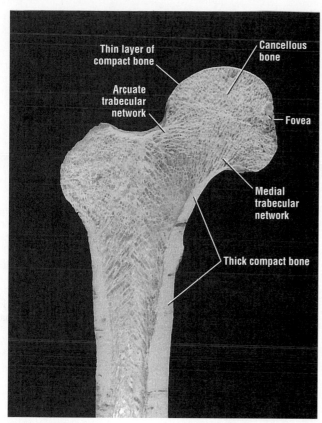

**FIGURE 12–12.** A frontal plane cross-section showing the internal architecture of the proximal femur. Note the thicker areas of compact bone around the shaft, and the cancellous bone occupying most of the medullary (internal) region. Two trabecular networks within the cancellous bone are also indicated. (From Neumann DA: An Arthritis Home Study Course: The Synovial Joint: Anatomy, Function, and Dysfunction. The Orthopedic Section of the American Physical Therapy Association, 1998.)

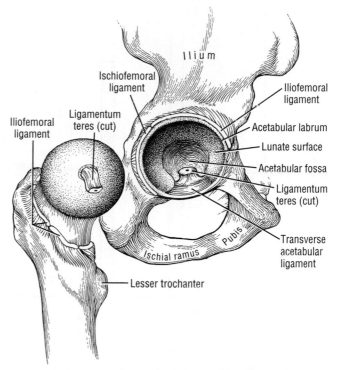

**FIGURE 12–13.** The right hip joint is opened to expose its internal components.

## CAPSULE AND LIGAMENTS OF THE HIP

A *synovial membrane* lines the internal surface of the hip capsule. The external surface of the capsule is reinforced by the iliofemoral, pubofemoral, and ischiofemoral ligaments (Figs. 12–17 and 12–18). Passive tension in these ligaments and in surrounding muscles limits the extremes of all move-

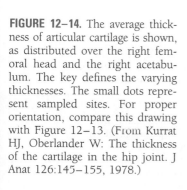

**FIGURE 12–14.** The average thickness of articular cartilage is shown, as distributed over the right femoral head and the right acetabulum. The key defines the varying thicknesses. The small dots represent sampled sites. For proper orientation, compare this drawing with Figure 12–13. (From Kurrat HJ, Oberlander W: The thickness of the cartilage in the hip joint. J Anat 126:145–155, 1978.)

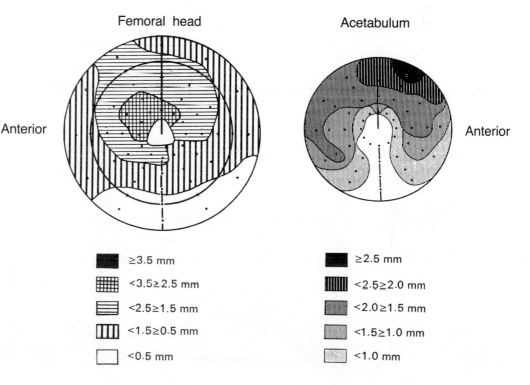

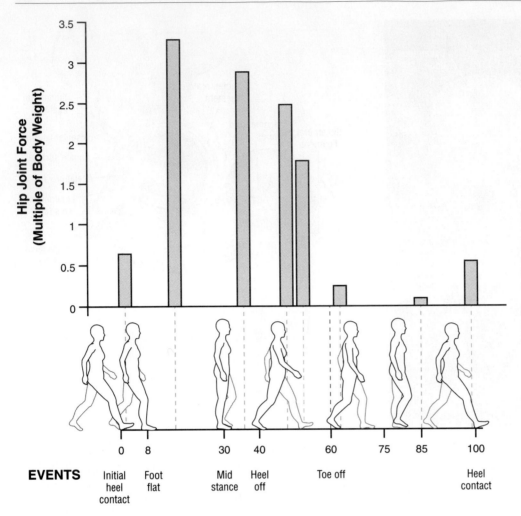

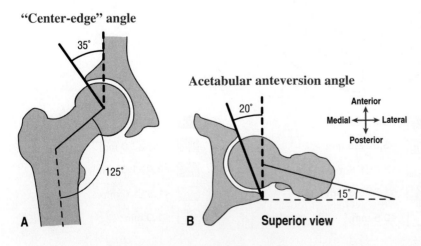

**Percent of Gait Cycle**

**FIGURE 12–15.** Graph shows a computer model's estimate of the hip joint force during various times in the gait cycle. Stance phase is between 0% and 60% of the gait cycle, and the swing phase is between 60% and 100% of the gait cycle. (Data from Dalstra M, Huiskes R: Load transfer across the pelvic bone. J Biomechan 28:715–724, 1995.)

ments of the hip (Table 12–1).[21] All three ligaments are at least partially taut in full hip extension.

The *iliofemoral ligament* (or **Y**-ligament) is a very thick and strong sheet of connective tissue, resembling an inverted **Y**. Proximally, the iliofemoral ligament attaches near the anterior-inferior iliac spine and along the adjacent margin of the acetabulum. Fibers form distinct medial and lateral fasciculi, each attaching to either end of the intertrochanteric line of the femur. The motion of full hip extension stretches the iliofemoral ligament and anterior capsule.[85] Full external rotation elongates the lateral fasciculus of the iliofemoral ligament.[21]

**FIGURE 12–16.** Two angles describe the extent to which the shape of the acetabulum naturally covers the femoral head. *A,* The *center-edge angle* indicates the relative coverage provided by the acetabulum over the femoral head within the frontal plane. This angle is formed by the intersection of a vertical reference line (stippled) and a line that connects the upper edge of the acetabulum to the center of the femoral head. The normal 125-degree angle of inclination of the proximal femur is also indicated. *B,* The *acetabular anteversion angle* describes the extent to which the acetabulum surrounds the femoral head within the horizontal plane. Measured from above, this angle is normally about 20 degrees. As shown, the angle is formed by the intersection of an anterior-posterior reference line (stippled) and a line across the rim of the acetabulum. The 15 degrees of normal anteversion of the proximal femur is also indicated.

### "Developmental Dysplasia of the Hip": A Case of Acetabular Malalignment

Developmental dysplasia of the hip (DDH) is a childhood condition usually involving abnormal formation (i.e., dysplasia) of the hip.[3] The cause of DDH is not completely clear, but abnormal physical stress on the hip—in utero or in early childhood—may interfere with joint formation and alignment.

DDH is often associated with a shallow and abnormally aligned acetabulum (i.e., a small center-edge angle). The femoral head, therefore, is allowed to "drift," usually superiorly and posteriorly from the acetabulum. The loss of a stable fulcrum for hip motion can change the moment arms and operational lengths of hip muscles, thereby causing functional weakness of the joint.

A child born with cerebral palsy has a particularly high likelihood of DDH. Hip dysplasia is often the result of muscle "imbalance," retained primitive reflexes, and absence of weight-bearing stimulation to the bones. Hip deformities, such as coxa valga and excessive femoral or acetabular anteversion, are often associated with DDH.[75]

Treatment of DDH depends on the age of the child and the underlying etiology. In the newborn, splinting or casting the hip in abduction is often performed in an attempt to "seat" the femoral head directly into the acetabulum. Over time, this position may stimulate the formation of a more normal joint shape. In the older child, surgery is often indicated. Osteotomy with realignment of the pelvis and/or the proximal femur is performed to improve stability and increase surface area for weight bearing.[14,30,64]

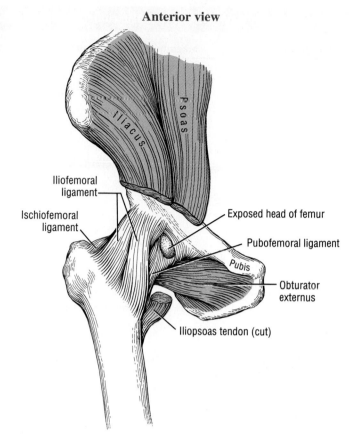

**FIGURE 12–17.** The anterior capsule and ligaments of the right hip. The iliopsoas is cut to expose the anterior side of the joint. Note that part of the femoral head protrudes just medial to the iliofemoral ligament. This region is normally covered by a bursa.

The iliofemoral ligament is one of the thickest and thus one of the strongest ligaments of the body. When a person stands with the hip fully extended, the anterior surface of the femoral head rests against the iliofemoral ligament. Passive tension in this ligament forms an important stabilizing force that resists further extension of the pelvis on the femur. Persons with paraplegia often use the passive tension of an elongated (or taut) iliofemoral ligament to assist with standing (Fig. 12–19).

Although thinner and more circular than the fibers of the iliofemoral ligament, the pubofemoral and ischiofemoral ligaments blend with and strengthen the inferior and posterior aspects of the capsule. The *pubofemoral ligament* attaches along the anterior and inferior rim of the acetabulum and adjacent parts of the superior pubic ramus and obturator membrane (see Fig. 12–17). The fibers blend with the medial fasciculus of the iliofemoral ligament, becoming taut in hip abduction and extreme extension.

The *ischiofemoral ligament* attaches from the posterior and inferior aspects of the acetabulum, primarily from the adjacent ischium (see Fig. 12–18). Fibers from this ligament join circular fibers located deeper within the capsule. Other

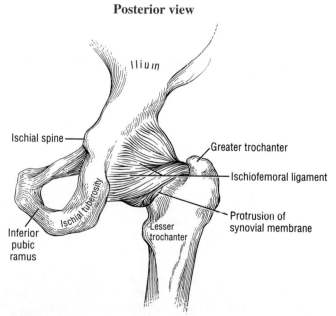

**FIGURE 12–18.** The posterior capsule and ligaments of the right hip.

**TABLE 12–1. Ligamentous and Muscular Tissues that Limit the Extremes of Hip Motion**

| Hip Motion | Magnitude of Hip Motion | Examples of Tissue that may Limit the Extremes of Motion |
| --- | --- | --- |
| Flexion | 80° (with knee extended) | Hamstrings and gracilis muscles |
| | 120° (with knee fully flexed) | Inferior fibers of ischiofemoral ligament<br>Inferior capsule |
| Extension | 20° of extension (with knee extended)* | Predominantly iliofemoral ligament and anterior capsule; some components of the pubofemoral and ischiofemoral ligaments |
| | 0° (with knee fully flexed) | Rectus femoris muscle |
| Abduction | 40° | Pubofemoral ligament, inferior capsule, adductor and hamstring muscles |
| Adduction | 25° | Superior fibers of ischiofemoral ligament, iliotibial band, and abductor muscles such as the tensor fasciae latae |
| Internal Rotation | 35° | Ischiofemoral ligament, external rotator muscles (e.g., piriformis) |
| External Rotation | 45° | Lateral fasciculus of iliofemoral ligament, iliotibial band, and internal rotator muscles (e.g., gluteus minimus, tensor fasciae latae) |

* Implies 20 degrees of extension *beyond* the neutral zero degree position.

more superficial fibers spiral superiorly and laterally across the posterior neck of the femur to attach near the apex of the greater trochanter (see Fig. 12–17). These superficial fibers become taut in full internal rotation and extension; superior fibers of the ischiofemoral ligament become taut in full adduction; and inferior fibers and a portion of the nearby inferior capsule become taut in flexion.

In addition to the three primary ligaments, the capsule consists of dense longitudinal and circular fibers. These fibers are covered by more superficial ligaments. *Longitudinal fibers* are most extensive within the anterior capsule, deep to and partially imbedded within the iliofemoral ligament. *Circular fibers*—known as the *zona orbicularis* of the capsule—are located more extensively on the inner layer of the capsule, forming a ring around the base of the femoral neck.[85]

### Close-packed Position of the Hip

Full extension (i.e., about 20 degrees beyond the neutral position) of the hip twists or "spirals" much of the capsular ligaments to their most taut position. Adding slight internal rotation and abduction to full extension elongates some component of *all* the capsular ligaments (Fig. 12–20). This fact is useful when attempting to provide a maximum stretch to the hip's capsular ligaments.

Because the position of full extension, slight internal rotation, and abduction of the hip elongates most of the capsular ligaments, it is considered the *close-packed position* at the hip. The increased passive tension generated by the stretched capsular ligaments lends stability to the joint and reduces passive accessory movement or "joint play." Interestingly, the hip is unique in that its close-packed position is not associated with its position of maximal joint congruency.[85] The joint surfaces fit most congruently in 90 degrees of flexion with moderate abduction and external rotation. In this position, much of the capsule and associated ligaments have "unraveled" to a more slackened state, adding only little passive tension to the joint.

## Osteokinematics

This section describes the range of motion allowed at the hip, including the factors that permit and restrict this motion. Reduced hip motion may be an early indicator of hip disease or trauma. It is often associated with pain, muscle

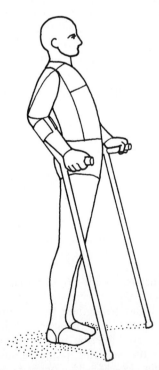

**FIGURE 12–19.** A person with paraplegia is shown standing with the aid of braces at the knees and ankles. Leaning of the pelvis and trunk posteriorly, relative to the hip joints, stretches the iliofemoral ligaments. This stretch provides a passive flexor torque at the hip, which helps to stabilize the pelvis and trunk while standing. (From Somers MF: Spinal Cord Injury: Functional Rehabilitation. Norwalk, Appleton & Lange, 1992.)

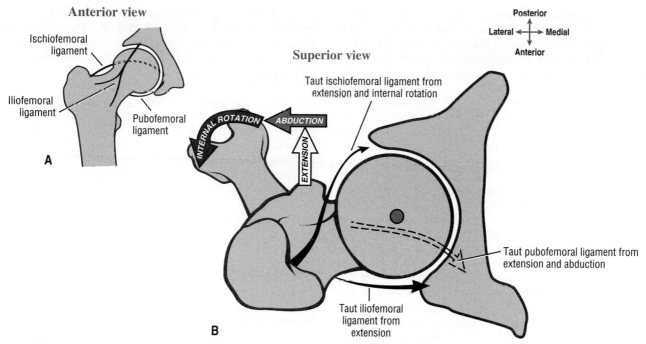

**Anterior view**

Ischiofemoral ligament

Iliofemoral ligament

Pubofemoral ligament

**A**

**Superior view**

Posterior

Lateral ←→ Medial

Anterior

Taut ischiofemoral ligament from extension and internal rotation

INTERNAL ROTATION

ABDUCTION

EXTENSION

Taut pubofemoral ligament from extension and abduction

Taut iliofemoral ligament from extension

**B**

**FIGURE 12–20.** *A,* The hip is shown in a neutral position, with all three capsular ligaments identified. *B,* Superior view of the hip in its close-packed position, i.e., fully extended with slight abduction and internal rotation. This position elongates at least some component of all three capsular ligaments.

weakness, or trauma to bone and joint. Limited hip motion can impose significant functional limitations when walking or tying shoelaces.

Two terms describe the range of motion of the hip. *Femoral-on-pelvic hip osteokinematics* describes the rotation of the femur about a relatively fixed pelvis. *Pelvic-on-femoral hip osteokinematics,* in contrast, describes the rotation of the pelvis, and often the superimposed trunk, over relatively fixed femurs. Regardless of whether the femur or the pelvis is considered the moving segment, the osteokinematics are de-

---

**SPECIAL FOCUS 12–3**

**Intracapsular Pressure Within the Hip**

The intracapsular pressure in the healthy hip is normally less than atmospheric pressure. This relatively low pressure creates a partial suction that resists distraction of the articular surfaces, providing an additional element of stability to the hip.

Wingstrand and colleagues[86] studied the effect of joint position and capsular swelling on the intracapsular pressure within cadaveric hips. Except in the extremes of motion, pressures remained relatively low throughout most of flexion and extension. When fluid was injected into the joint to simulate capsular swelling, pressures rose dramatically throughout a greater portion of the range of motion (Fig. 12–21). Regardless of the amount of injected fluid, however, pressures always remained lowest in the mid range of motion. These data help to explain why persons with capsulitis and swelling within the hip tend to feel most comfortable holding the hip in partial flexion. Reduced intracapsular pressure decreases distension of the inflamed capsule. Unfortunately, over time, the flexed position may lead to contracture caused by the adaptive shortening of the hip flexor muscles and capsular ligaments.

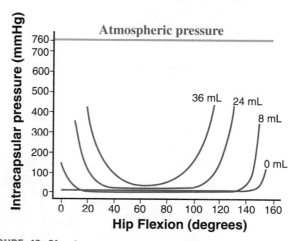

**Atmospheric pressure**

Intracapsular pressure (mmHg)

760
700
600
500
400
300
200
100
0

36 mL    24 mL    8 mL

0 mL

0   20   40   60   80   100   120   140   160

**Hip Flexion (degrees)**

**FIGURE 12–21.** The intracapsular pressure in the hip joint of cadavers as a function of hip flexion angle. The four curved lines indicate the pressure-angle relationships after the injection of different volumes of fluid into the capsule. (Data from Wingstrand H, Wingstrand A, Krantz P: Intracapsular and atmospheric pressure in the dynamics and stability of the hip. Acta Orthop Scand 61:231–235, 1990.)

scribed from the anatomic position. The names of the movements are as follows: *flexion and extension* in the sagittal plane, *abduction and adduction* in the frontal plane, and *internal and external rotation* in the horizontal plane. The term horizontal is used with the assumption that a subject is standing in the anatomic position.

Reporting the range of motion at the hip uses the anatomic position as the 0-degree or neutral reference point. In the sagittal plane, for example, femoral-on-pelvic flexion is described by the rotation of the femur anterior to the 0-degree position. Extension, the reverse movement, is described as the rotation of the femur posterior to the 0-degree position. The term hyperextension is not used to describe normal range of motion at the hip.

As depicted in Figure 12–22, each plane of motion is associated with a unique axis of rotation. The axis of rotation for internal and external rotation is often referred to as the "longitudinal" axis of rotation. The longitudinal axis of rotation is also referred to as a *vertical* axis. The latter description, however, assumes the subject is standing with the hip in the anatomic position. This axis extends as a line between the center of the femoral head and the center of the knee joint. Because of the angle of inclination of the proximal femur and the anterior bowing of the femoral shaft,

most of the longitudinal axis of rotation lies *outside* the femur itself (see Fig. 12–22*A* and *B*). The extramedullary location of the axis has implications in the understanding of some of the actions of muscles, a point discussed later in this chapter.

Unless otherwise specified, the following discussions on osteokinematics include average *passive* ranges of motion at the hip. The connective tissues and muscles that limit motion are also described (see Table 12–1). The muscles used to produce and control the hip motion are discussed later in this chapter. Although femoral-on-pelvic and pelvic-on-femoral movements often occur simultaneously, they are presented here separately.

## FEMORAL-ON-PELVIC OSTEOKINEMATICS

### Rotation of the Femur in the Sagittal Plane

On average, with the knee fully flexed, the hip *flexes* to 120 degrees (Fig. 12–23*A*).[72] Tasks such as squatting and tying a shoelace typically require near full hip flexion.[35] With the knee extended, hip flexion is limited to about 80 degrees because of the passive tension within the stretched hamstring and gracilis muscles.[10] Full hip flexion slackens most ligaments, but stretches the inferior capsule.

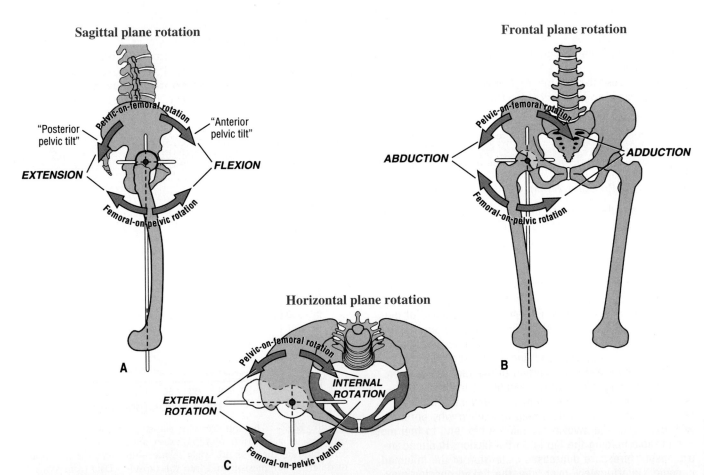

**FIGURE 12–22.** The osteokinematics of the right hip joint. Femoral-on-pelvic and pelvic-on-femoral rotations occur in three planes, depicted as red arrows. The axis of rotation for each plane of movement is shown as a red dot, located at the center of the femoral head. *A,* Side view shows *sagittal plane rotations* about a medial-lateral axis of rotation. *B,* Front view shows *frontal plane rotations* about an anterior-posterior axis of rotation. *C,* Top view shows *horizontal plane rotations* about a longitudinal, or vertical, axis of rotation.

**Femoral-On-Pelvic Hip Rotation**

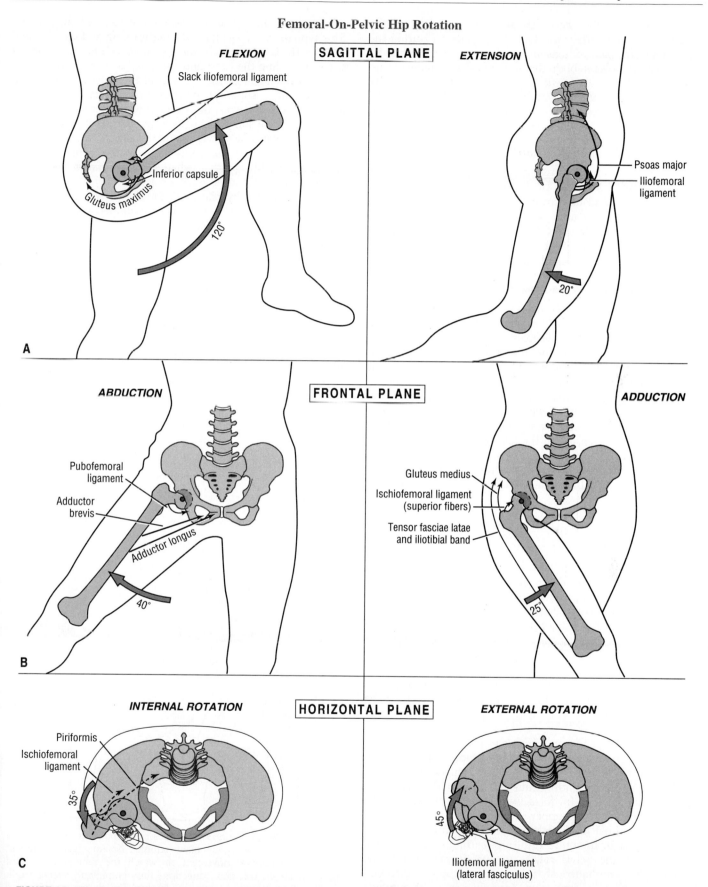

**FIGURE 12-23.** The approximate maximal range of passive femoral-on-pelvic (hip) motion is depicted in the sagittal plane (*A*), frontal plane (*B*), and horizontal plane (*C*). Ligaments and muscles, elongated and pulled taut, are indicated by straight black (or dashed) arrows. Slackened tissue is indicated by a wavy black arrow.

The hip normally *extends* about 20 degrees beyond the neutral position.[72] When the knee is fully flexed during the hip extension, passive tension in the stretched rectus femoris, which crosses both the hip and knee, reduces hip extension to about the neutral position. Full hip extension increases the passive tension in most capsular connective tissues, especially the iliofemoral ligament, and the hip flexor muscles.

### Rotation of the Femur in the Frontal Plane

On average, the hip *abducts* 40 degrees (Fig. 12–23B).[72] This motion is limited primarily by the pubofemoral ligament and by the adductor and hamstring muscles. The hip *adducts* 25 degrees beyond the neutral position.[7] In addition to interference with the contralateral limb, passive tension in stretched hip abductor muscles, iliotibial band, and superior fibers of the ischiofemoral ligament all limit full adduction.

### Rotation of the Femur in the Horizontal Plane

Like most movements, internal and external rotation of the hip shows large intersubject variability. On average, the hip *internally rotates* about 35 degrees from the neutral position (Fig. 12–23C).[72,77] With the hip fully extended, maximal internal rotation elongates external rotator muscles, such as the piriformis, and parts of the ischiofemoral ligament. In healthy young adults, the amount of internal rotation remains essentially unchanged with the hip flexed or extended.[72]

The extended hip *externally rotates* on average about 45 degrees. Excessive tension in the tensor fasciae latae, iliotibial band, and lateral fasciculus of the iliofemoral ligament may limit full external rotation. The position of hip flexion decreases active external rotation motion to 30 to 35 degrees.

## PELVIC-ON-FEMORAL OSTEOKINEMATICS

### Lumbopelvic Rhythm

The lower, caudal end of the axial skeleton is firmly attached to the pelvis by way of the sacroiliac joints. As a consequence, rotation of the pelvis over the femoral heads typically changes the configuration of the lumbar spine. This important kinematic relationship is known as lumbopelvic rhythm, introduced in Chapter 9. This concept is revisited in this chapter with a focus on the kinesiology at the hip.

Figure 12–24 shows two contrasting types of lumbopelvic rhythms frequently used during pelvic-on-femoral hip flexion. Although the kinematics depicted are limited to the sagittal plane, the concepts apply to pelvic rotations in all planes.

Figure 12–24 shows an example of an *ipsi-directional lumbopelvic rhythm,* where the pelvis and lumbar spine rotate in the *same* direction. This movement maximizes the angular displacement of the entire trunk relative to the lower extremities, and it is useful for activities such as extending the reaching capacity of the upper extremities. The kinematics of the ipsi-directional lumbopelvic rhythm are discussed in detail in Chapter 9. In contrast, during *contra-directional lumbopelvic rhythm,* the pelvis rotates in one direction while the lumbar spine simultaneously rotates in the opposite direction (Fig. 12–24B). The important consequence of this movement is that the supralumbar trunk (i.e., that part of the body located *above* the first lumbar vertebra) can remain essentially stationary as the pelvis rotates over the femurs. This type of rhythm is used during walking and dancing and other activities in which the position of the supralumbar trunk, including the head and eyes, needs to be held fixed in space, independent of the rotation of the pelvis. In this manner, the lumbar spine functions as a mechanical "de-coupler," allowing the pelvis and the supralumbar trunk to move independently. A person with a fused lumbar spine, therefore, is unable to rotate the pelvis about the hips without a similar rotation of parts of the supralumbar trunk. This abnormal situation is readily apparent when the individual walks.

Figure 12–25 shows pelvic-on-femoral osteokinematics at the hip, organized by plane of motion. These kinematics are all based on the *contra-directional* lumbopelvic rhythm. The range of motions depicted in each figure have been estimated using photographs of healthy young adults. In most cases, the amount of pelvic-on-femoral rotation is restricted by the natural limitations of movement at the lumbar spine.

### Pelvic-on-Femoral Rotation in the Sagittal Plane: The Anterior and Posterior Pelvic Tilt

Hip flexion can occur through a limited arc via an *anterior tilt* (Fig. 12–25A) of the pelvis over stationary femoral heads. As defined in Chapter 9, pelvic "tilt" is a sagittal plane rotation of the pelvis relative to the femur. The direction of the tilt—either anterior or posterior—is based on the direction of rotation of a point on the iliac crest. The associated increased lumbar lordosis offsets most of the un-

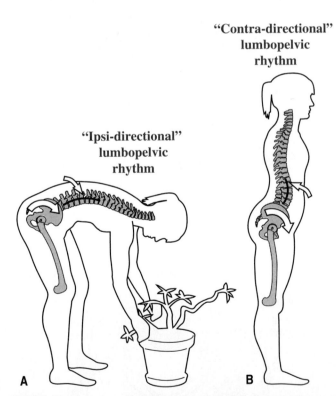

**FIGURE 12–24.** Two contrasting types of lumbopelvic rhythms used to rotate the pelvis over fixed femurs. *A,* An "ipsi-directional" rhythm describes a movement in which the lumbar spine and pelvis rotate in the same direction, thus amplifying overall trunk motion. *B,* A "contra-directional" rhythm describes a movement in which the lumbar spine and pelvis rotate in opposite directions. See text for further explanation.

**Pelvic-On-Femoral Hip Rotation**
**(With Supralumbar Trunk Stationary)**

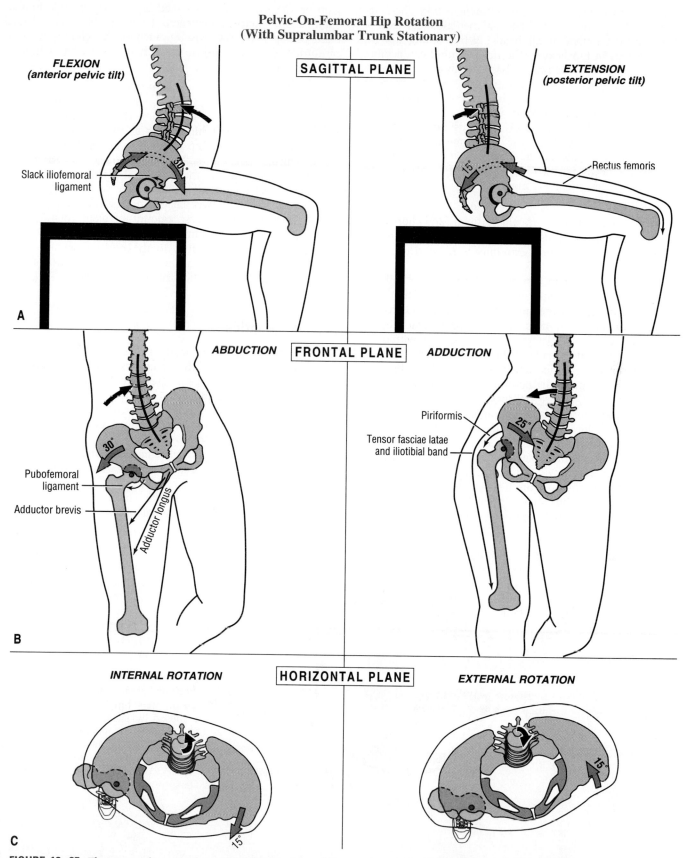

**FIGURE 12–25.** The maximal range of passive pelvic-on-femoral hip motion in the sagittal plane (*A*), frontal plane (*B*), and horizontal plane (*C*). The motion assumes that the supralumbar trunk remains essentially stationary during the hip motion. Ligaments and muscles elongated and pulled taut are indicated by straight black arrows; tissues slackened are indicated by wavy black arrows.

desired forward motion of the supralumbar trunk. The anterior tilt of the pelvis occurs about a medial-lateral axis of rotation through both femoral heads. While sitting upright with 90 degrees of hip flexion, the normal adult can achieve about 30 degrees of additional pelvic-on-femoral hip flexion before being restricted by a completely extended lumbar spine. Full anterior tilt of the pelvis slackens the iliofemoral ligament and elongates the inferior capsule.

As depicted in Figure 12–25A, the hips can be *extended* about 10 to 20 degrees from the 90-degree sitting posture via a *posterior tilt* of the pelvis. The lumbar spine flexes or flattens as the pelvis is tilted. The iliofemoral ligament and iliopsoas muscle are slightly elongated.

### Pelvic-on-Femoral Rotation in the Frontal Plane

Pelvic-on-femoral rotations in the frontal and horizontal planes are best described assuming a person is standing on one limb. The weight-bearing extremity is referred to as the *support hip.*

*Abduction* of the support hip occurs by raising or "hiking" the iliac crest on the side of the nonsupport hip (Fig. 12–25B). Assuming that the supralumbar trunk remains stationary, the lumbar spine must bend in the direction opposite the rotating pelvis. A lateral convexity occurs within the lumbar region toward the side of the abducting hip.

Pelvic-on-femoral hip abduction is restricted to about 30 degrees, primarily due to the natural limits of lateral bending in the lumbar spine. Severe tightness in the adductor muscles and/or restriction in the pubofemoral ligament limits pelvic-on-femoral hip abduction. In the event of marked adductor contracture, the iliac crest on the side of the nonsupport hip remains *lower* than the iliac crest of the support hip, markedly interfering with walking.

*Hip adduction* of the support hip occurs by a *lowering* of the iliac crest on the side of the nonsupport hip. This motion causes a slight lateral concavity within the lumbar region on the side of the adducted hip. A hypomobile lumbar spine and/or marked decreased length within the iliotibial band or hip abductor muscles, such as the gluteus medius, piriformis, or tensor fasciae latae, may restrict the extremes of this motion.

### Pelvic-on-Femoral Rotation in the Horizontal Plane

Pelvic-on-femoral rotation occurs in the horizontal plane about a longitudinal axis of rotation (Fig. 12–25C). *Internal rotation* of the support hip occurs as the iliac crest on the side of the nonsupport hip rotates *forward* in the horizontal plane. During *external rotation,* in contrast, this same iliac crest rotates *backward* in the horizontal plane. If the pelvis is rotating beneath a relatively stationary trunk, the lumbar spine must rotate or twist in the opposite direction as the rotating pelvis. The modest amount of axial rotation normally permitted in the lumbar spine limits the full rotation potential of the support hip. In the healthy person, therefore, the ligaments and capsule at the hip are not significantly stretched during horizontal plane pelvic-on-femoral rotation.

## Arthrokinematics

During hip motion, the nearly spherical femoral head remains snugly seated within the confines of the acetabulum. The steep walls of the acetabulum, in conjunction with the tightly fitting acetabular labrum, limit significant translation between the joint surfaces. Hip arthrokinematics are based on the traditional convex-on-concave or concave-on-convex principles (see Chapter 1).

Figure 12–26 shows a highly mechanically based illustration of a hip opened to enable visualization of the paths of articular motion. *Abduction and adduction* occur across the longitudinal diameter of the joint surfaces (red). With the hip extended, *internal and external rotation* occur across the

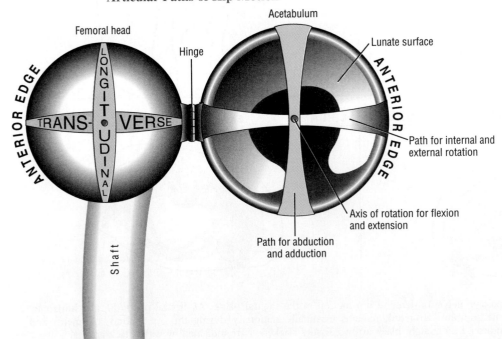

**Articular Paths of Hip Motion**

**FIGURE 12–26.** A "mechanical" drawing of the right hip. The joint surfaces are exposed by swinging the femur open like a door on a hinge. The articular paths of hip frontal and horizontal plane motion occur along the longitudinal (red) and transverse (gray) diameters, respectively.

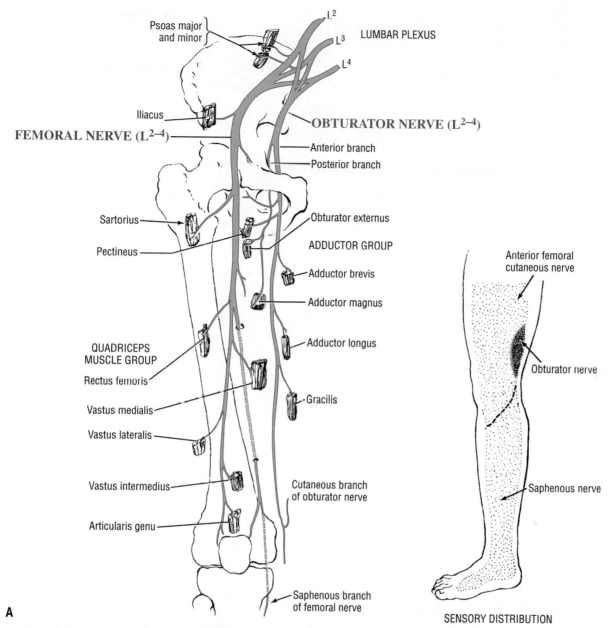

**A**

**FIGURE 12–27.** The path and general proximal-to-distal order of muscle innervation for the femoral nerve and obturator nerve (A) and the sciatic nerve (B). The locations of certain muscles relative to the joint are altered slightly for clarity. The roots for each nerve are shown in parenthesis. (Modified from deGroot J: Correlative Neuroanatomy, 21st ed. Norwalk, Appleton & Lange, 1991.)

*Illustration continued on following page*

transverse diameter of the joint surfaces (gray). *Flexion and extension* occur as a spin between the femoral head and the lunate surfaces of the acetabulum. The axis of rotation for this spin passes through the femoral head.

## MUSCLE AND JOINT INTERACTION

### Innervation to the Muscles and Joint

#### INNERVATION TO MUSCLES

The lumbar plexus and the sacral plexus arise from nerve roots of T[12] through S[4]. Nerves from the lumbar plexus innervate the muscles of the anterior and medial thigh, in-

cluding the quadriceps femoris. Nerves from the sacral plexus innervate the muscles of the posterior and lateral hip, posterior thigh, and entire lower leg.

#### Lumbar Plexus

The lumbar plexus is formed from the ventral rami of T[12]–L[4]. This plexus gives rise to the femoral and obturator nerves (Fig. 12–27A). The *femoral nerve,* the largest branch of the lumbar plexus, is formed by L[2]–L[4] nerve roots. *Motor branches* innervate most hip flexors and all knee extensors. Within the pelvis, proximal to the inguinal ligament, the femoral nerve innervates the psoas major, psoas minor, and iliacus. Distal to the inguinal ligament, the femoral nerve innervates the sartorius, part of the pectineus, and the quad-

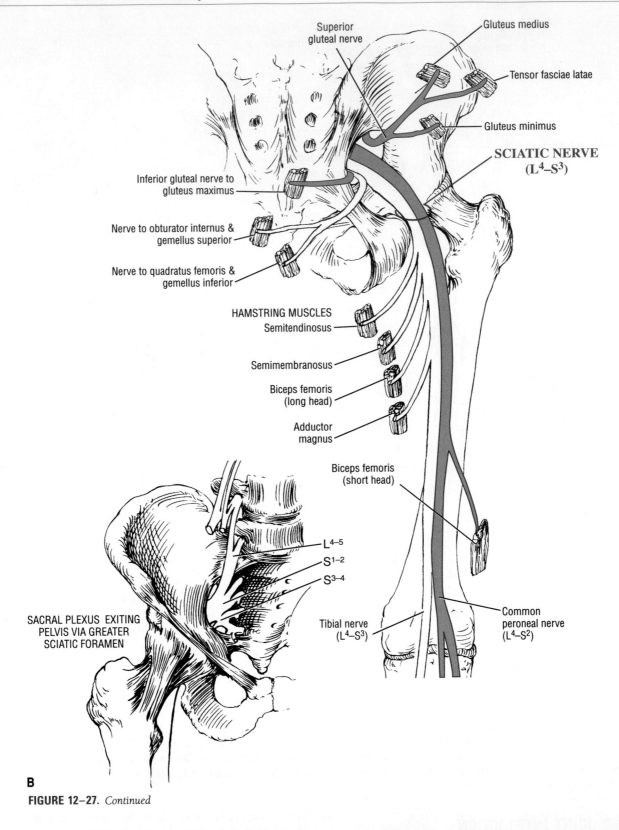

Superior gluteal nerve

Gluteus medius

Tensor fasciae latae

Gluteus minimus

**SCIATIC NERVE**
**(L⁴–S³)**

Inferior gluteal nerve to gluteus maximus

Nerve to obturator internus & gemellus superior

Nerve to quadratus femoris & gemellus inferior

HAMSTRING MUSCLES
Semitendinosus

Semimembranosus

Biceps femoris (long head)

Adductor magnus

Biceps femoris (short head)

L⁴⁻⁵
S¹⁻²
S³⁻⁴

SACRAL PLEXUS EXITING PELVIS VIA GREATER SCIATIC FORAMEN

Tibial nerve (L⁴–S³)

Common peroneal nerve (L⁴–S²)

**B**

**FIGURE 12–27.** *Continued*

riceps muscle group. The femoral nerve has an extensive *sensory distribution* covering much of the skin of the anterior-medial aspect of the thigh. The sensory branches of the femoral nerve innervate the skin of the anterior-medial aspect of the lower leg, via the saphenous cutaneous nerve.

**Primary Sources of Muscular Innervation from the Lumbar Plexus**

- Femoral nerve (L²–L⁴)
- Obturator nerve (L²–L⁴)

Like the femoral nerve, the *obturator nerve* is formed from the ventral rami of L²–L⁴ nerve roots. *Motor branches* innervate the hip adductor muscles. The obturator nerve divides into anterior and posterior branches as it passes through the obturator foramen. The posterior branch innervates the obturator externus and anterior head of the adductor magnus. The anterior branch innervates part of the pectineus, the adductor brevis, the adductor longus, and the gracilis. The obturator nerve has a *sensory distribution* to the skin of the medial thigh.

### Sacral Plexus

The sacral plexus, located on the posterior wall of the pelvis, is formed from the ventral rami of (L⁴–S⁴).[85] Most nerves from the sacral plexus exit the pelvis via the greater sciatic foramen to innervate the posterior hip muscles (Fig. 12–27B).

---

**Primary Sources of Lower Limb Muscular Innervation from the Sacral Plexus**

- Nerve to the piriformis (S¹⁻²)
- Nerve to the obturator internus and gemellus superior (L⁵–S²)
- Nerve to the quadratus femoris and gemellus inferior (L⁴–S¹)
- Superior gluteal nerve (L⁴–S¹)
- Inferior gluteal nerve (L⁵–S²)
- Sciatic nerve (L⁴–S³) with tibial and common peroneal portions

---

Three small nerves innervate five of the six "short external rotators" of the hip. The nerves are named simply by the muscles that they innervate. The *nerve to the piriformis* (S¹⁻²) innervates the piriformis within the pelvis. External to the pelvis, the *nerve to the obturator internus and gemellus superior* (L⁵–S²) and the *nerve to the quadratus femoris and gemellus inferior* (L⁴–S¹) travel to and innervate their respective muscles.

The *superior and inferior gluteal nerves* are named according to their position as they exit the greater sciatic notch. The *superior gluteal nerve* (L⁴–S¹) innervates the gluteus medius, gluteus minimus, and tensor fasciae latae. The *inferior gluteal nerve* (L⁵–S²) is the sole innervation to the gluteus maximus.

The *sciatic nerve* (L⁴–S³), the widest and longest nerve in the body, exits the pelvis through the greater sciatic foramen, usually inferior to the piriformis. The sciatic nerve actually consists of two nerves: the tibial and the common peroneal, both enveloped in one connective tissue sheath. In the posterior thigh, the *tibial portion* of the sciatic nerve innervates all the biarticular muscles within the hamstring group and the posterior (extensor) head of the adductor magnus. The *common peroneal portion* of the sciatic nerve innervates the short head of the biceps femoris.

The sciatic nerve branches into separate tibial and common peroneal components usually just proximal to the knee. It is not uncommon, however, that the division occurs more proximally near the pelvis. A division proximal to the greater sciatic foramen usually results in the common peroneal nerve piercing the piriformis as the nerve exits the pelvis.[85]

The motor nerve roots that supply the muscles of the lower extremity are listed in Appendix IVA. Appendix IVB shows key muscles typically used to test the functional status of the L²–S³ ventral nerve roots.

## SENSORY INNERVATION TO THE HIP

As a general rule, the hip capsule receives sensory innervation by the same nerve roots that supply the overlying muscle. The femoral nerve sends nerve filaments into the anterior aspect of the hip capsule. Nerve branches enter the posterior joint capsule from all roots of the sacral plexus.[32,85] The obturator nerve sends filaments into the medial aspect of the hip and of the knee joint. This explains why inflammation of the hip may be perceived as pain in the medial knee region.

## Muscular Function at the Hip

Throughout this chapter, the line-of-force of several muscles is illustrated relative to the axes of rotation at the hip. Figure 12–28, for example, shows a sagittal plane representation of the significant flexor and extensor muscles of the

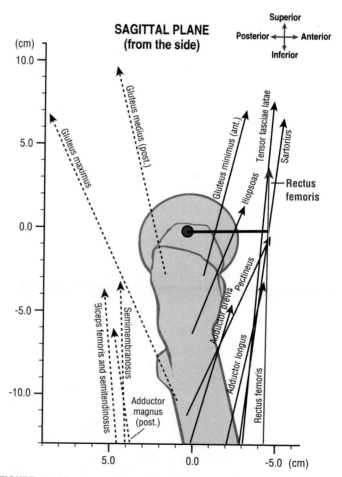

**FIGURE 12–28.** A view from the side that depicts the sagittal plane line-of-force of several muscles that cross the hip. The axis of rotation (red) is directed in the medial-lateral direction through the femoral head. The flexors are indicated by solid lines and the extensors by dashed lines. The internal moment arm, used by the rectus femoris, is represented by the thick black line. (For clarity, the gracilis is not shown.)

hip.[16,17] Although Figure 12–28 provides useful insight into the potential function of several muscles of the hip, two limitations are considered. First, the line-of-force of each muscle does *not* represent a force vector, only the overall direction of the muscle's force. The figure does not provide the information needed to compare the "strength"—or torque—potential of each muscle. This comparison requires additional data, especially the muscle's cross-sectional area. Second, the lines-of-force and subsequent lengths of the moment arms depicted in Figure 12–28 apply only to the anatomic position. Once the hip moves out of this position, the potential action and torque potential of each muscle change. This partially explains why the maximal-effort, internal torque of a muscle group varies throughout the range of motion.

Throughout this chapter, a muscle's action is considered either primary or secondary (Table 12–2). The designation of muscle action is based on data such as moment arm, muscle size, and, when available, reports from EMG-based and anatomic studies. Unless otherwise specified, muscle actions are based on a concentric contraction, originating from the anatomic position. A muscle with a relatively insignificant action, or an action that is more substantial outside the anatomic position, is not included in Table 12–2. Consult Appendix IVC for a listing of detailed attachments of muscles of the hip.

## HIP FLEXOR MUSCLES

The primary hip flexors are the iliopsoas, sartorius, tensor fasciae latae, rectus femoris, pectineus, and adductor longus (Fig. 12–29).[17] Figure 12–28 shows the excellent flexion leverage of many of these muscles. Secondary hip flexors are the adductor brevis, gracilis, and anterior fibers of the gluteus minimus.

### Anatomy and Individual Action

The *iliopsoas* is large and long, spanning between the last thoracic vertebra and the proximal femur (see Fig. 12–29). Anatomically, the iliopsoas consists of two muscles: the iliacus and the psoas major. The *iliacus* attaches on the iliac fossa and extreme lateral edge of sacrum, just over the sacroiliac joint. The *psoas major* attaches along the transverse processes of the last thoracic and all lumbar vertebrae, including the intervertebral discs. The fibers of the iliacus and the psoas major fuse just anterior to the femoral head (see Fig. 12–29, right side). A tendon forms that anchors the muscle to the femur, near and on the lesser trochanter. In route to its distal insertion, the broad tendon of the iliopsoas is deflected posteriorly about 35 to 45 degrees, immediately after it crosses the rim of the pubis. With the hip in full extension, this deflection raises the tendon's angle-of-insertion to the femur, thereby increasing the muscle's leverage for hip flexion.

The iliopsoas is a potent hip flexor, from both a femoral-on-pelvic and pelvic-on-femoral perspective. From the anatomic position, the iliopsoas is not an effective rotator. In the hip abducted position, the iliopsoas can assist in external rotation.[99]

The iliopsoas muscle produces forces that cross the lumbar and lumbosacral regions as well as the hip.[2,37,76] The iliacus, by anterior tilting of the pelvis, can accentuate the lumbar lordosis if the pelvis is not well stabilized by a muscle such as the rectus abdominis. The psoas major provides excellent vertical stability to the lumbar spine (see Chapter 10).

The *psoas minor* lies anterior to the muscle belly of the psoas major. This slender muscle attaches proximally between the twelfth thoracic and first lumbar vertebra, and distally to the pelvis near the pectineal line. Unlike the psoas major, the psoas minor has little, if any, functional significance in hip motion. The psoas minor is absent in about 40% of people.[85]

The *sartorius,* the longest muscle in the body, originates at the anterior-superior iliac spine (see Fig. 12–29). This thin, fusiform muscle courses inferiorly and medially across the thigh to attach distally on the medial surface of the proximal tibia (see Fig. 13–7). The name sartorius is based on the Latin root *sartor,* referring to a tailor's position of crossed-legged sitting. This name describes the muscle's combined action of hip flexion, external rotation, and abduction.

## TABLE 12–2. Muscles of the Hip Organized According to Their Action*

| Flexors | Adductors | Internal Rotators | Extensors | Abductors | External Rotators |
|---|---|---|---|---|---|
| **Primary** | **Primary** | **Secondary** | **Primary** | **Primary** | **Primary** |
| Iliopsoas | Adductor longus | Gluteus minimus | Gluteus maximus | Gluteus medius | Gluteus maximus |
| Tensor fasciae latae | Adductor brevis | (anterior fibers) | Biceps femoris | Gluteus minimus | Piriformis |
| Sartorius | Pectineus | Gluteus medius | (long head) | Tensor fasciae latae | Obturator internus |
| Rectus femoris | Gracilis | (anterior fibers) | Semitendinosus | **Secondary** | Gemellus superior |
| Adductor longus | Adductor magnus | Tensor fasciae latae | Semimembranosus | Piriformis | Gemellus inferior |
| Pectineus | (both heads) | Adductor longus | Adductor magnus | Sartorius | Quadratus femoris |
| **Secondary** | **Secondary** | Adductor brevis | (posterior head) | | Sartorius |
| Adductor brevis | Biceps femoris | Pectineus | **Secondary** | | **Secondary** |
| Gracilis | (long head) | Semitendinosus | Gluteus medius | | Gluteus medius |
| Gluteus minimus | Quadratus femoris | Semimembranosus | (posterior fibers) | | (posterior fibers) |
| (anterior fibers) | Gluteus maximus | | | | Gluteus minimus |
| | (lower fibers) | | | | (posterior fibers) |
| | | | | | Obturator externus |
| | | | | | Biceps femoris |
| | | | | | (long head) |

*Each action assumes a muscle contraction originating from the anatomic position. Many of these muscles will have different actions if they contract from a position other than the anatomic position.

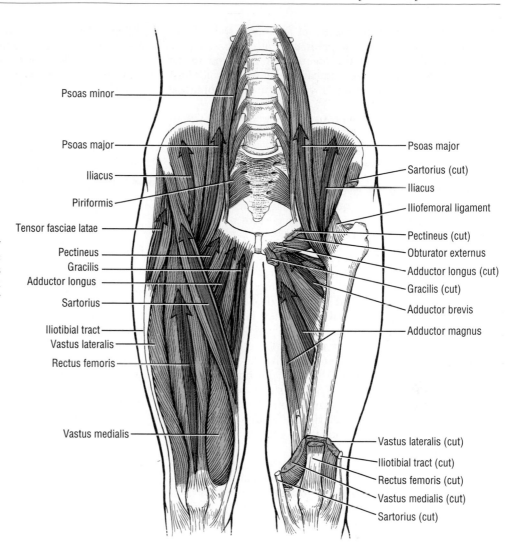

**FIGURE 12–29.** Muscles of the anterior hip region. The right side shows the primary flexors and adductor muscles of the hip. Many muscles on the left side are cut to expose the adductor brevis and adductor magnus.

The *tensor fasciae latae* attaches to the ilium just lateral to the sartorius (see Fig. 12–29). This relatively short muscle attaches distally to the proximal part of the iliotibial band or tract.[85] The band extends distal to the knee to the lateral tubercle of the tibia.

The iliotibial tract is a component of a more extensive connective tissue known as the *fascia lata of the thigh.*[36] Laterally, the fascia lata is thickened by attachments from the tensor fasciae latae and the gluteus maximus. At multiple locations, the fascia lata turns inward between muscles, forming distinct fascial sheets known as intermuscular septa. These septa partition each of the main muscle groups of the thigh according to innervation. The septa, along with most attachments of the adductor muscles, are anchored to the femur along the linea aspera.

From the anatomic position, the tensor fasciae latae is a primary flexor and abductor of the hip. The muscle is also a secondary internal rotator of the hip.[66] As indicated by its name, the tensor fasciae latae increases tension throughout the fascia lata. Tension passed inferiorly through the iliotibial tract may help stabilize the lateral aspect of the extended knee. Repetitive tension within the iliotibial band may cause inflammation at its insertion site near the lateral tubercle of the tibia. Stretching an excessively tight iliotibial band with

the knee extended often incorporates various combinations of hip adduction and extension.

The proximal part of the *rectus femoris* emerges between an inverted **V**, formed by the sartorius and tensor fasciae latae (see Fig. 12–29). This large bipennate-shaped muscle has its proximal attachment at the anterior-inferior iliac spine and along the superior rim of the acetabulum and into the joint capsule. Along with the other members of the quadriceps, the rectus femoris attaches to the tibia via the ligamentum patellae. The rectus femoris is responsible for about one third of the total isometric, flexor torque at the hip.[48] In addition, the rectus femoris is a primary knee extensor. The combined two-joint actions of this important muscle are considered in Chapter 13. The anatomy and function of the pectineus and adductor longus are described in the section on the adductors of the hip.

### Overall Function of the Hip Flexors

#### Pelvic-on-Femoral Hip Flexion: Anterior Pelvic Tilt

The anterior pelvic tilt is performed by a force-couple between the hip flexors and low-back extensor muscles (Fig. 12–30). With fixed femurs, contraction of the hip flexors rotates the pelvis about the medial-lateral axis through both hips. Although Figure 12–30 illustrates the iliopsoas and rectus femoris, *any muscle capable of femoral-on-pelvic flexion is equally capable of tilting the pelvis anteriorly.* Clinically, the most important aspect of the anterior tilt is related to the increase in lordosis at the lumbar spine. Greater lordosis increases the compressive loads on the lumbar apophyseal joints.

A lumbopelvic posture with normal lumbar lordosis optimizes the alignment of the entire spine (see Chapter 9). Some persons have difficulty maintaining lumbar lordosis while standing. Increased stiffness in connective tissue around the lumbar spine and/or increased passive resistance from hamstring muscles favors a relatively flat (i.e., slightly flexed) lumbar spine. The quantitative relationship between the degree of hamstring tightness and posture of the pelvis and lumbar spine remains controversial.[44]

### Femoral-on-Pelvic Hip Flexion

Femoral-on-pelvic hip flexion is performed through a synergy between the hip flexors and abdominal muscles. This cooperation is most apparent during activities that require large amounts of hip flexor force. Consider, for example, the straight-leg-raise exercise often used to strengthen the abdominal muscles. This action requires that the rectus abdominis generate a potent *posterior* pelvic tilt in order to neutralize the strong *anterior* pelvic tilt potential of the hip flexor muscles (Fig. 12–31A). Without sufficient stabilization from the rectus abdominis, contraction of the hip flexor muscles is inefficiently spent tilting the pelvis anteriorly (Fig. 12–31B). The excessive anterior tilt of the pelvis accentuates the lumbar lordosis.

The pathomechanics depicted in Figure 12–31B are most severe in situations in which the abdominal muscles are weak, but the hip flexors remain relatively strong. With the exception of poliomyelitis or muscular dystrophy, this pattern of weakness is relatively rare. More commonly, the abdominal muscles are only moderately weak, secondary to disuse atrophy or abdominal surgery. In this case, persons may develop low-back pain due to the increased compression force on the apophyseal joints of the chronically, fully extended lumbar vertebrae.

## HIP ADDUCTOR MUSCLES

The primary adductors of the hip are the pectineus, adductor longus, gracilis, adductor brevis, and adductor magnus (see Fig. 12–29). Secondary adductors are the biceps femoris (long head), the gluteus maximus, especially the inferior fibers, and the quadratus femoris. The line-of-force of these muscles is shown in Figure 12–33.

### Functional Anatomy

The adductor muscle group occupies the medial quadrant of the thigh. Topographically, the adductor muscles are organized into three layers (Fig. 12–34). The pectineus, adductor longus, and gracilis occupy the *superficial layer.* Proximally, these muscles attach along the superior and inferior pubic ramus and adjacent body of the pubis. Distally, the pectineus and the adductor longus attach to the posterior surface of the femur—near and along varying regions of the linea aspera. The long and slender gracilis attaches distally to the medial side of the proximal tibia (see Fig. 13–7).

The *middle layer* of the adductor group is occupied by the triangular-shaped *adductor brevis.* The adductor brevis attaches to the pelvis on the inferior pubic ramus, and to the femur along the proximal one third of the linea aspera.

The *deep layer* of the adductor group is occupied by the massive, triangular-shaped *adductor magnus* (see Fig. 12–29, left side, and Fig. 12–40, right side). This large muscle attaches primarily from the entire ischial ramus and part of the ischial tuberosity. From its proximal attachment, the adductor magnus forms anterior and posterior heads.

The *anterior head of the adductor magnus* has two sets of fibers: horizontal and oblique. The relatively small set of horizontally directed fibers crosses from the inferior pubic ramus to the extreme proximal end of the linea aspera, often called the adductor minimus. The larger obliquely directed fibers run from the ischial ramus to nearly the entire length of the linea aspera, as far distally as the medial supracondylar line. Both parts of the anterior head are innervated by the obturator nerve, which is typical of the adductor muscles.

The *posterior head of the adductor magnus* consists of a thick mass of the fibers arising from the region of the pelvis adjacent to the ischial tuberosity. From this posterior attachment, the fibers run vertically and attach as a tendon on the adductor tubercle on the medial side of the distal femur. The posterior head of the adductor magnus is innervated by the tibial branch of the sciatic nerve, as are the hamstring muscles. Because of a similar location, innervation, and action as the hamstring muscles, the posterior head is often referred to as the extensor head of the adductor magnus.

### Overall Function of the Hip Adductors

The line-of-force of the adductors approaches the hip from many different orientations. Functionally, therefore, the adductor muscles produce torques in all planes at the hip.[17,61] The following section considers the primary actions of the

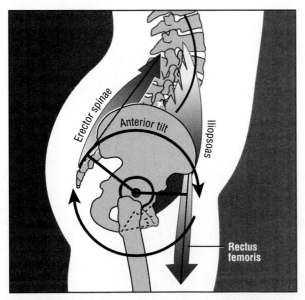

**FIGURE 12–30.** The force-couple is shown between two representative hip flexor muscles and the erector spinae to anteriorly tilt the pelvis. The moment arms for the erector spinae and rectus femoris are indicated by the dark black lines. Note the increased lordosis at the lumbar spine.

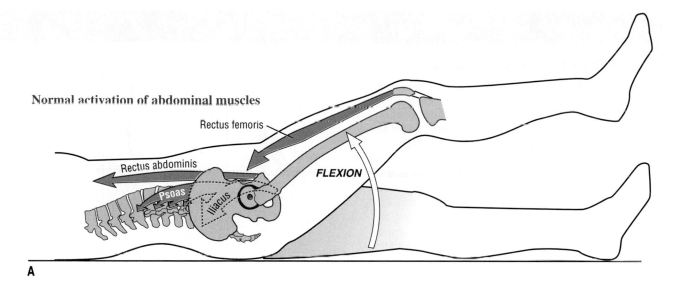

### Normal activation of abdominal muscles

Rectus femoris

Rectus abdominis

Psoas

Iliacus

**FLEXION**

**A**

### Reduced activation of abdominal muscles

Rectus abdominis

**ANTERIOR TILT**

Rectus femoris

Psoas

Iliacus

**FLEXION EFFORT**

**B**

**FIGURE 12–31.** The stabilizing role of the abdominal muscles is shown during a unilateral straight-leg raise. *A,* With normal activation of the rectus abdominis, the pelvis is stabilized and prevented from anterior tilting by the pull of the hip flexor muscles. *B,* With reduced activation of the rectus abdominis, contraction of the hip flexor muscles causes a marked anterior tilt of the pelvis. Note the increase in lumbar lordosis that accompanies the anterior tilt of the pelvis. The reduced activation in the abdominal muscle is indicated by the lighter red.

adductors in the frontal and sagittal planes. The secondary action of these muscles as internal rotators is discussed later in this chapter.

### *Frontal Plane Function of the Adductors*

The most obvious function of the adductor muscles is production of adduction torque. The torque controls the kinematics of both femoral-on-pelvic as well as pelvic-on-femoral hip adduction. Figure 12–35 shows an example of the adductor muscles contracting bilaterally to control both forms of motion. On the right side, several adductors are shown accelerating the femur toward the ball. Adding to the forcefulness of this action is the downward rotation or lowering of the right iliac crest—a motion controlled through pelvic-on-femoral hip adduction at the left hip. Although only the adductor magnus is shown on the left side, other adductor muscles assist in this action.

### *Sagittal Plane Function of the Adductors*

Regardless of hip position, the posterior fibers of the adductor magnus are powerful extensors of the hip, similar to the hamstring muscles. In general, the remaining adductor muscles, however, are flexors *or* extensors, depending on hip position.[17,69] Consider, for example, the adductor longus as a representative adductor muscle during a fast sprint (Fig. 12–36A). From a position of at least about 50 to 60 degrees of hip flexion, the line-of-force of the adductor longus is *posterior* to the medial-lateral axis of the joint. At this position, the adductor longus has an extensor moment arm and is capable of generating an extension torque—similar to the posterior head of the adductor magnus. From a hip position *less than* 60 degrees of hip flexion, however, the line-of-force of the adductor longus shifts *anteriorly* to the medial-lateral axis of rotation (Fig. 12–36B). The adductor longus now has a flexor moment arm and generates a flexor torque similar to the rectus femoris, for example.

The adductors provide a useful source of flexor and extensor torque at the hip. The bidirectional torques are useful during high power, cyclic motions such as sprinting, cycling, running up a steep hill, and descending and rising from a deep squat. When the hip is near full flexion, the adductors

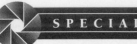

## SPECIAL FOCUS 12-4

**Effect of Hip Flexor Contracture on Standing**

Hips that remain flexed for a prolonged time often develop flexion contracture. This situation is often associated with spasticity of the hip flexors, weakness of the hip extensors, arthritis or dysplasia of the hip, or confinement to a wheelchair. In time, adaptive shortening in the flexor muscles and capsular ligaments limits full extension of the hip.

One consequence of a hip flexion contracture is a disruption in the normal biomechanics of standing. Normally, standing requires very little muscular energy. While standing, the hip is stabilized through an interaction of two opposing torques: body weight and passive tension from taut anterior capsular ligaments of the hip. As shown in Figure 12-32A, standing with the hips near full extension directs the force of body weight slightly posterior to the medial-lateral axis of rotation at the hip. The force of body weight, therefore, is converted to a small, but nevertheless useful, hip extensor torque. The hip is prevented from further extension by passive flexor torque created by the stretched capsular ligaments. The static equilibrium formed between the forces of gravity and stretched connective tissues minimizes the need for metabolically "expensive" muscle activation.

With a hip flexion contracture, the hip remains partially flexed while the person attempts to stand. This posture redirects the force of body weight anterior to the hip, creating a flexion torque (Fig. 12-32B). Whereas gravity normally extends the hip while standing, *gravity now acts as a hip flexor.* In order to prevent flexing into a full squat, active extensor torques are required from muscles such as the gluteus maximus. In turn, the metabolic cost of standing increases and, over time, increases the desire to sit. Often, prolonged sitting perpetuates the circumstances that initiated the flexion contracture.

Standing with a hip flexion contracture interferes with the joint's ability to optimally dissipate compression loads. Normally, standing with hips near full extension places the highest regions of joint pressure over the regions of thickest articular cartilage. Standing, or walking, with a partially flexed hip, however, causes the higher regions of joint pressure to pass through the thinner regions of cartilage. This arrangement cannot optimally dissipate compression loads, which cross the joint (see Fig. 12-32A and B, compare red dots at joint interface). As a result, the articular cartilage is not able to protect the underlying bone from large forces that are usually produced by activated muscles.

Clinically, persons with painful arthritis or bursitis of the hip are susceptible to flexion contracture. It is important to reduce the inflammation through medicine and physical therapy so that activities that favor the extended position can be tolerated. Hip extension exercises can strengthen the extensor muscles, while stretching the hip flexors and anterior capsular structures.

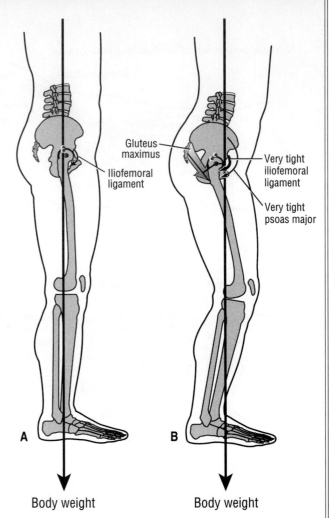

**FIGURE 12-32.** The effect of a hip flexion contracture on the biomechanics of standing. *A*, When standing with hips fully extended, the force of body weight falls slightly posterior to the axis of rotation at the hip. Body weight, therefore, causes an extension torque at the hip. The anterior capsule and ligaments at the hip are pulled taut, which prevents further hip extension. *B*, An attempt to stand upright with a hip flexion contracture redirects the force of body weight anterior to the hip joints, causing a hip flexor torque. The gluteus maximus (red) is active to prevent the hip joints from further flexion. The very tight iliofemoral ligament and psoas major muscle are indicated by the black arrows. In *A* and *B*, the red circle at the center of the femoral head represents the axis of rotation. The pair of red dots denote the relative overlap of articular cartilage. (See text for further description.) (From Neumann DA: An Arthritis Home Study Course: The Synovial Joint: Anatomy, Function, and Dysfunction. The Orthopedic Section of the American Physical Therapy Association, 1998.)

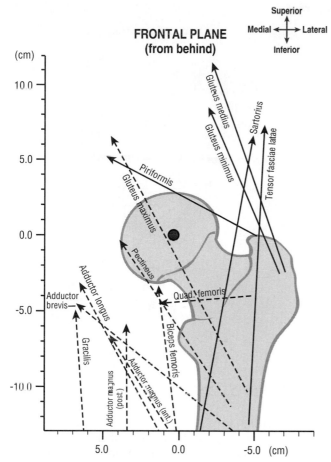

**FRONTAL PLANE**
**(from behind)**

Superior
Medial ←→ Lateral
Inferior

**FIGURE 12–33.** A posterior view depicts the frontal plane line-of-force of several muscles that cross the right hip. The axis of rotation (red) is directed in the anterior-posterior direction through the femoral head. The abductors are indicated by solid lines and the adductors by dashed lines.

are mechanically prepared to augment the extensors. In contrast, when the hip is near full extension, they are mechanically prepared to augment the flexors. This utilitarian function of the adductors may partially explain their relatively high susceptibility to strain injury while running.

## HIP INTERNAL ROTATOR MUSCLES

From the anatomic position, there are no primary internal rotators of the hip because no muscle is optimally positioned in the horizontal plane to produce internal rotation torque. Many secondary internal rotators exist, including the anterior fibers of the gluteus minimus and the gluteus medius, tensor fasciae latae, adductor longus, adductor brevis, and pectineus (Fig. 12–37). The tensor fascia latae and the medial hamstrings (i.e., semitendinosus and semimembranosus)[45] also function as secondary internal rotators of the hip.

With the hip flexed toward 90 degrees, the internal rotation torque potential of the internal rotator muscles dramatically increases. This becomes clear with the help of a skeleton model and piece of string to mimic the line-of-force of muscles, such as the gluteus minimus and anterior fibers of the gluteus medius. Flexing the hip close to 90 degrees orients the line-of-force of these muscles nearly perpendicu-

lar to the longitudinal axis of rotation. The internal rotation moment arm of the anterior part of the gluteus medius, for example, increases 8 fold between 0 and 90 degrees of flexion.[15] Interestingly, even several external rotator muscles, such as the piriformis, switch leverage to become internal rotators at 90 degrees of flexion. These changes in leverage explain why internal rotation torque in healthy persons is about 50% greater with the hip flexed rather than extended.[45] This phenomena may partially explain the excessively internally rotated gait pattern typically observed in a person with cerebral palsy. With poor control of hip extensor muscles, the resulting flexed posture of the hip enhances the torque potential of the internal rotator muscles. This gait pattern may be better controlled by enhanced activation of the gluteus maximus, a potent extensor and external rotator.[15] The anatomy of each of the internal rotators is described under other sections (see Figs. 12–29 and 12–44).

### Overall Function of the Hip Internal Rotators

*Biomechanics of the Adductor Muscles as Internal Rotators of the Hip*

Many of the adductor muscles are capable of producing at least modest internal rotation torque at the hip when the body is in the anatomic position.[17,84,85] This action, however, may be difficult to reconcile considering that most adductors attach to the posterior side of the femur along the linea aspera. A shortening of these muscles appears to rotate the femur externally instead of internally. What must be considered, however, is the effect that the natural bowing of the femoral shaft has on the line-of-force of the muscles. Bowing places much of the linea aspera *anterior* to the longitudinal axis of rotation at the hip (Fig. 12–38A). As depicted in Figure 12–38B, the horizontal force component of an adductor muscle, such as the adductor longus, lies *anterior* to the axis of rotation. Force from this muscle, therefore, acts with a moment arm necessary to produce internal rotation, although torque is minimal.

*Functional Potential of the Internal Rotator Muscles While Walking*

From a pelvic-on-femoral perspective, the internal rotators perform a subtle but nevertheless important function during gait. During the stance phase, the internal rotators move the pelvis in the horizontal plane over a relatively fixed femur (Fig. 12–39).[33,66] The pelvic rotation about the right hip is evident by the forward rotation of the *left* iliac crest. The right internal rotator muscles, therefore, can provide some of the drive to the contralateral (left) swinging limb. During relatively fast walking speed, a greater demand is placed on the internal rotator muscles to increase the stride length of the contralateral lower limb.

## HIP EXTENSOR MUSCLES

### Anatomy and Individual Action

The primary hip extensors are the gluteus maximus, the hamstrings (i.e., the long head of the biceps femoris, the semitendinosus, and the semimembranosus), and the posterior head of the adductor magnus (Fig. 12–40).[17,25] The posterior fibers of the gluteus medius are secondary extensors. As described earlier, the adductor muscles can extend the hip provided that it is flexed beyond about 50 degrees.[17]

## Adductor Muscle Group

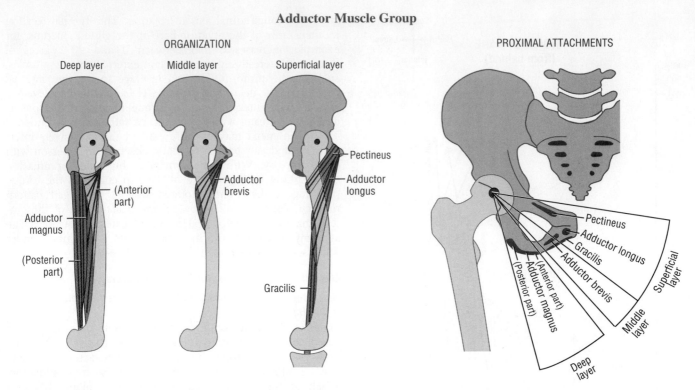

**FIGURE 12–34.** The anatomic organization and proximal attachments of the adductor muscle group.

The *gluteus maximus* has numerous proximal attachments from the posterior side of the ilium, sacrum, coccyx, sacro-tuberous and posterior sacroiliac ligaments, and adjacent fascia. The muscle attaches into the iliotibial band of the fascia lata, along with the tensor fasciae latae, and the gluteal tuberosity on the femur. The gluteus maximus is a primary extensor and external rotator of the hip.

The *hamstring muscles* have their proximal attachment on the posterior side of the ischial tuberosity, and attach distally to the tibia and fibula. Based on these attachments, the hamstrings extend the hip *and* flex the knee. The anatomy and function of the posterior head of the *adductor magnus* is described under the section on adductors of the hip.

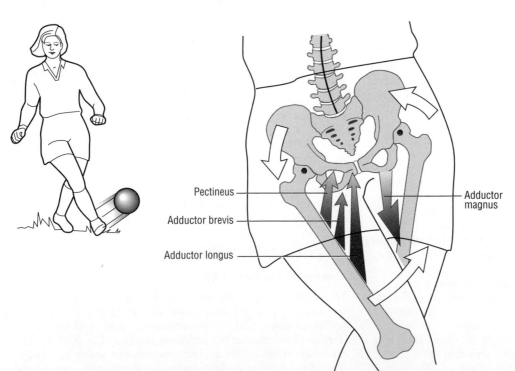

**FIGURE 12–35.** The bilateral cooperative action of the adductor muscles while kicking a soccer ball. The left adductor magnus is shown actively producing *pelvic-on-femoral adduction.* Several right adductor muscles are shown actively producing *femoral-on-pelvic adduction torque,* needed to accelerate the ball.

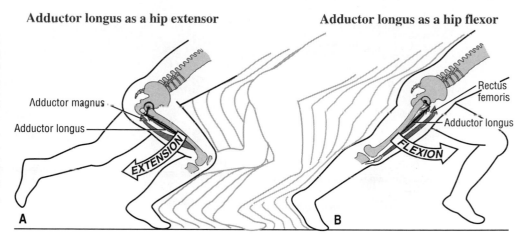

**Adductor longus as a hip extensor**                    **Adductor longus as a hip flexor**

**FIGURE 12–36.** The dual sagittal plane action of the adductor longus muscle is demonstrated while sprinting. *A*, With the hip flexed, the adductor longus is in position to extend the hip, along with the adductor magnus. *B*, With hip extended, the adductor longus is in position to flex the hip, along with the rectus femoris. These contrasting actions are based on the change in line-of-action of the adductor longus, relative to the medial-lateral axis of rotation at the hip.

Figure 12–28 depicts the line-of-force of the primary hip extensors. In the extended position, the posterior head of the adductor magnus has the greatest moment arm for extension, followed closely by the biceps femoris and the semitendinosus. The semimembranosus and the gluteus maximus have the greatest cross-sectional areas of all the extensors.[69]

From a position of 75 degrees of flexion, the hamstrings and adductor magnus produce about equal magnitudes of extension torque, or about 90% of the total extensor torque potential at the hip.[69] Most of the remaining torque is generated by the gluteus maximus.

### Overall Function of the Hip Extensors

*Pelvic-on-Femoral Hip Extension*

The following sections describe two different situations in which the hip extensor muscles control pelvic-on-femoral extension.

**Hip Extensors Performing a Posterior Pelvic Tilt.** With the supralumbar trunk held relatively stationary, the hip extensor and abdominal muscles act as a force-couple to

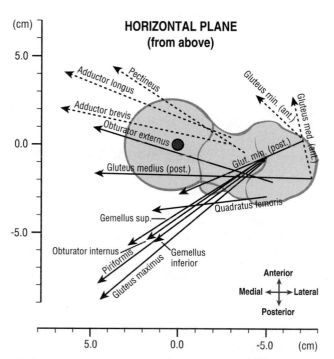

**FIGURE 12–37.** A superior view depicts the horizontal plane line-of-force of several muscles that cross the hip. The longitudinal axis of rotation is in the superior-inferior direction through the femoral head. For clarity, the tensor fasciae latae, sartorius, and hamstring muscles are not shown. The external rotators are indicated by solid lines and the internal rotators by dashed lines.

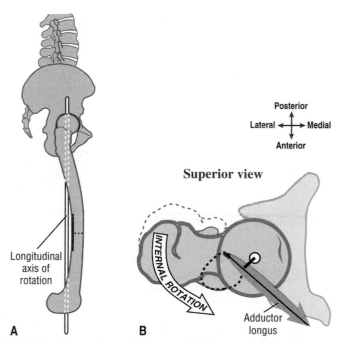

**FIGURE 12–38.** The function of the adductor muscles as internal rotators of the hip: *A*, Because of the anterior bowing of the femoral shaft, a large segment of the linea aspera (red) runs anterior to the longitudinal axis of rotation. *B*, A superior view of the right hip shows the horizontal line-of-force of the adductor longus. The muscle causes an internal rotation torque by producing a force that passes anterior to the axis of rotation (white dot at femoral head). The moment arm used by the adductor longus is indicated by the thick dark line. The dashed circle represents the outline of the midshaft of the femur at the region of the distal attachment of the adductor longus.

**Superior view**

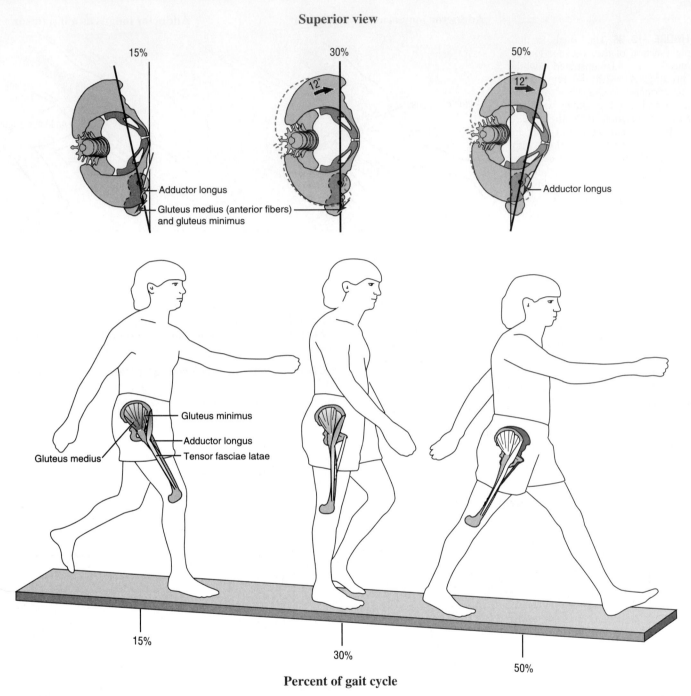

**Percent of gait cycle**

**FIGURE 12–39.** The activation pattern of several muscles of the right hip is depicted during various parts of the gait cycle. The hip internal rotators (tensor fasciae latae, gluteus minimus, anterior parts of the gluteus medius, and adductor longus) are shown rotating the pelvis in the horizontal plane over a relatively fixed right femur. (Compare the bottom and top views.) The tensor fasciae latae and the gluteal muscles function as hip abductors by controlling the frontal plane stability of the pelvis. (The images were prepared from photographs of a subject walking at a relatively fast speed of about 1.9 m/s. This relatively fast walking speed has exaggerated the normal amount of horizontal plane rotation used during walking.)

posteriorly tilt the pelvis (Fig. 12–41). The posterior tilt extends the hips and reduces the lumbar lordosis.

The muscular mechanics involved with posterior tilting of the pelvis are similar to those described for the anterior tilting of the pelvis (compare Figs. 12–30 and 12–41). In both tilting actions, a force-couple exists between the hip and trunk muscles. As a consequence, the pelvis rotates through a relatively short arc, using the femoral heads as a pivot point.

**Hip Extensors Controlling a Forward Lean of the Body.** Leaning forward while standing is a very common activity. Consider, for example, the forward lean used to wash the face over a sink. The muscular support of this near static posture at the hips is primarily the responsibility of the hamstring muscles. Consider the two phases of a forward lean shown in Fig. 12–42. During a slight forward lean (Fig. 12–42A), body weight force is displaced just anterior to the medial-lateral axis of rotation at the hip. This

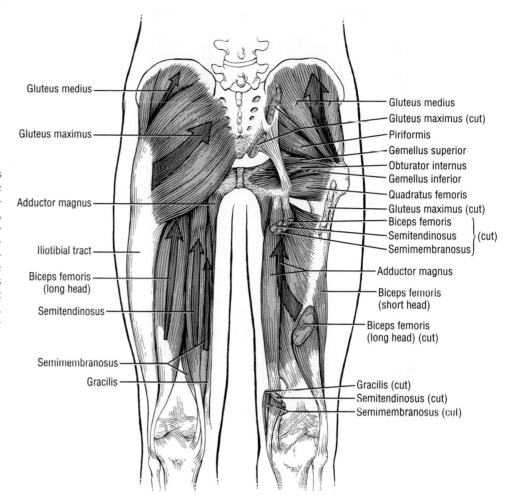

**FIGURE 12–40.** The posterior muscles of the hip. The left side highlights the gluteus maximus and hamstring muscles (long head of the biceps femoris, semitendinosus, and semimembranosus). The right side shows the hamstring muscles cut to expose the adductor magnus and short head of the biceps femoris. The right side shows the gluteus medius and five of the six short external rotators, i.e., piriformis, gemellus superior and inferior, obturator internus, and quadratus femoris.

slightly flexed posture of the hips is restrained by minimal activation from the gluteus maximus and hamstring muscles. During a more significant forward lean, however, body weight force is displaced farther in front of the medial-lateral axis of rotation at the hips (Fig. 12–42B). Supporting this markedly flexed posture requires greater muscle activation from the hamstring muscles. The gluteus maximus, however, remains relatively inactive in this position—a point verifiable by palpation and inferred from EMG data.[20] This apparent increased responsibility of the hamstrings, in contrast to the gluteus maximus, can be explained biomechanically and physiologically. A significant forward lean *increases* the hip extension moment arm of the hamstring muscles, while it decreases the hip extensor moment arm of the gluteus maximus.[69] (Compare the 15-degree and 30-degree points in the graph in Fig. 12–42.) Leaning forward mechanically optimizes the extensor torque potential of hamstrings. A significant forward lean elongates the hamstring muscles across both the hip and knee joints. Elongation significantly increases the passive force in these muscles which, in turn, helps support the partially flexed position of the hips. For these reasons, the hamstrings appear uniquely equipped to support the hip posture associated with forward lean. Apparently, the nervous system recruits the large gluteus maximus for activities that require more substantial hip extension torque, such as those needed for climbing a steep flight of stairs.

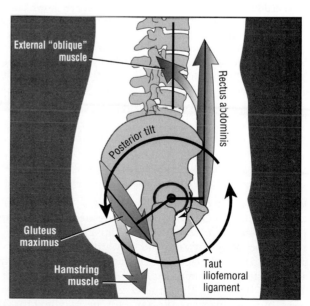

**FIGURE 12–41.** The force-couple between representative hip extensors (gluteus maximus and hamstrings) and abdominal muscles (rectus abdominis and obliquus externus abdominis) that posteriorly tilt the pelvis. The moment arms for each muscle group are indicated by the dark black line. Note the decreased lordosis at the lumbar spine. The extension at the hip stretches the iliofemoral ligament.

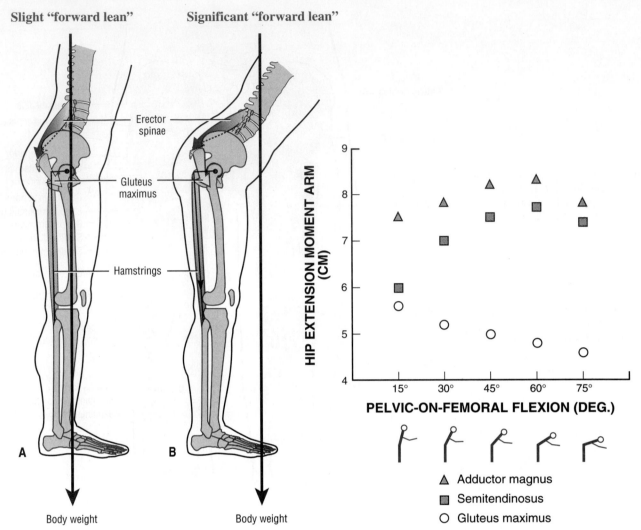

**FIGURE 12–42.** The hip extensor muscles are shown controlling a forward lean of the pelvis over the thighs. *A,* Slight forward lean of the upper body displaces the body-weight force slightly anterior to the medial-lateral axis of rotation at the hip. *B,* A more significant forward lean displaces the body-weight force even farther anteriorly. The greater flexion of the hips rotates the ischial tuberosities posteriorly, thereby increasing the hip extension moment arm of the hamstrings. The taut line (with arrow head within the stretched hamstring muscles) indicates the increased passive tension. In both *A* and *B,* the relative demands placed on the muscles are shown by relative shades of red. At right is a graph showing the length of hip extension moment arms of selected hip extensors as a function of forward lean. (Data from Pohtilla JF: Kinesiology of hip extension at selected angles of pelvifemoral extension. Arch Phys Med Rehabil 50:241–250, 1969.)

*Femoral-on-Pelvic Hip Extension*

As a group, the hip extensor muscles are frequently required to produce large femoral-on-pelvic hip extensor torque to accelerate the body forward and upward. Consider, for example, the demands placed on the right hip extensors while climbing a steep mountain (Fig. 12–43). The flexed position of the right hip while the climber is carrying a heavy pack imposes a large external (flexion) torque at the hip. The flexed position, however, favors greater extensor torque generation from the hip extensor muscles.[69] Furthermore, with the hip markedly flexed, many of the adductor muscles can produce an extensor torque, thereby assisting the primary hip extensors.

## HIP ABDUCTOR MUSCLES

### *Anatomy and Individual Action*

The primary hip abductor muscles are the gluteus medius, gluteus minimus, and tensor fasciae latae.[9,17] The piriformis and sartorius are considered secondary hip abductors (see Figs. 12–29, 12–40, and 12–44).

The *gluteus medius* attaches on the external surface of the ilium above the anterior gluteal line. The muscle attaches distally on the lateral aspect of the greater trochanter. The distal attachment provides the gluteus medius with the greatest abductor moment arm of all the abductor muscles (see Fig. 12–33). The gluteus medius is also the largest of the

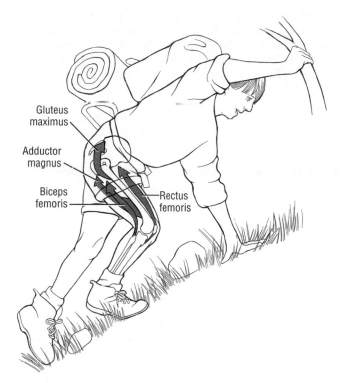

**FIGURE 12-43.** Relatively high demands are placed on hip extensor muscles while climbing a mountain and supporting an external load.

hip abductor muscles, occupying about 60% of the total abductor cross-sectional area.[9]

Based on anatomic and EMG-based studies, the gluteus medius is classified into three independent anatomic and functional sets of fibers: anterior, middle, and posterior.[9,80] Although all fibers contribute to abduction, from the anatomic position the anterior fibers internally rotate the hip and the posterior fibers extend and externally rotate it. These actions change considerably when motion is performed out of the anatomic position.[16]

The *gluteus minimus* lies deep and slightly anterior to the gluteus medius. This muscle attaches proximally on the ilium—between the anterior and inferior gluteal lines—and distally on the anterior aspect of the greater trochanter. The gluteus minimus is smaller than the gluteus medius, occupying about 20% of the total abductor cross-sectional area.[9]

The actions of the gluteus minimus are similar to those of the gluteus medius,[9] especially in regard to abduction.[41] One notable exception, however, is the flexion potential of the anterior fibers of the gluteus minimus (see Fig. 12–28).

The *tensor fasciae latae* is the smallest of the three primary hip abductors, occupying about 11% of the total abductor cross-sectional area.[9] The anatomy of the tensor fasciae latae is discussed elsewhere in this text.

### Hip Abductor Mechanism

*Control of Frontal Plane Stability of the Pelvis during Walking*

The abduction torque produced by the hip abductor muscles is essential to the control of frontal plane, pelvic-on-femoral

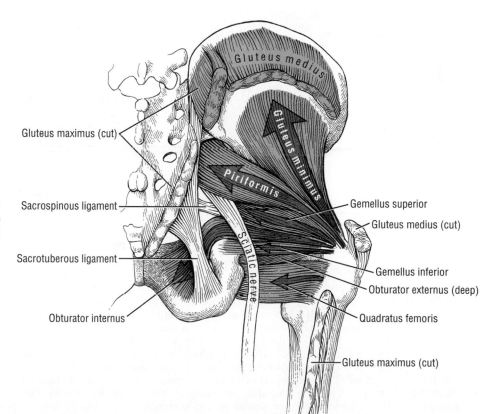

**FIGURE 12-44.** Deep muscles of the posterior and lateral hip region. The gluteus medius and the gluteus maximus are cut to expose deeper muscles.

kinematics during walking. During most of the stance phase, the hip abductors stabilize the pelvis over the relatively fixed femur (see Fig. 12–39).[31,51] During the stance phase, therefore, the hip abductors have a role in controlling the pelvis in the frontal plane and, as discussed earlier, in the horizontal plane.

The abduction torque produced by the hip abductor muscles is particularly important during the single-limb support phase of gait. During this time, the opposite leg is off the ground and swinging forward. Without adequate abduction torque on the stance limb, the pelvis and trunk may drop uncontrollably toward the side of the swinging limb. The activation of the hip abductor muscle is verified by palpating the gluteus medius just superior to the greater trochanter. The right muscle, for example, becomes firm as the left leg lifts off the ground. The bursa located at the point of distal attachment of the hip abductor muscles may become inflamed. Trochanteric bursitis can be very painful, especially during activation of the abductor muscles during single-limb support.

The frontal plane stabilizing function of hip abductor muscles is an extremely important component of walking. The force produced by the abductors during stance accounts for most of the compressive forces generated at the hip.

### Role of the Hip Abductors in the Production of Hip Force

Figure 12–45 shows the major factors involved with frontal plane stability of the right hip during single-limb support

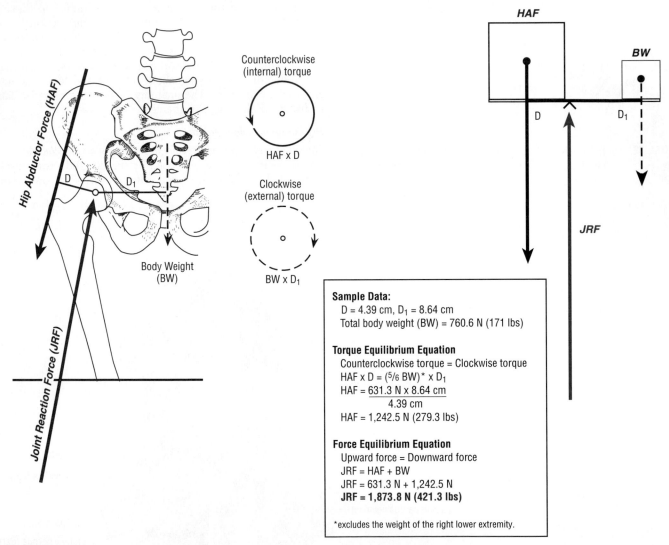

**Sample Data:**
D = 4.39 cm, $D_1$ = 8.64 cm
Total body weight (BW) = 760.6 N (171 lbs)

**Torque Equilibrium Equation**
Counterclockwise torque = Clockwise torque
HAF $\times$ D = ($5/6$ BW)* $\times D_1$
HAF = $\dfrac{631.3 \text{ N} \times 8.64 \text{ cm}}{4.39 \text{ cm}}$
HAF = 1,242.5 N (279.3 lbs)

**Force Equilibrium Equation**
Upward force = Downward force
JRF = HAF + BW
JRF = 631.3 N + 1,242.5 N
**JRF = 1,873.8 N (421.3 lbs)**

*excludes the weight of the right lower extremity.

**FIGURE 12–45.** A frontal plane diagram shows the function of the right hip abductor muscles during single-limb support on the right hip. On the left, the pelvis-and-trunk are in static equilibrium about the right hip. The sum of the torques in the frontal plane equal zero. The *counterclockwise torque* (solid circle) is the product of the hip abductor force (HAF) times moment arm (D); the *clockwise torque* (dashed circle) is the product of body weight (BW) times moment arm ($D_1$). Static stability occurs when HAF $\times$ D = BW $\times D_1$. The see-saw model (right) simplifies the major kinetic events during single-limb support. A joint reaction force (JRF) is directed through the fulcrum of the see-saw (hip joint). The sample data in the box are used in the torque and force equilibrium equations. These equations determine the magnitude of the hip abductor force and joint reaction force needed during single-limb support. (See text.) Note that for simplicity, the calculations assume static equilibrium and that all force vectors are acting in a vertical direction. (From Neumann DA: Biomechanical analysis of selected principles of hip joint protection. Arthritis Care Res 2:146–155, 1989. Reprinted with permission from *Arthritis Care and Research.* © American College of Rheumatology.)

in walking. The hip abductor and body weight forces act as two opposing forces that balance the pelvis over the stance femoral head. The pelvis is comparable to a see-saw, with its fulcrum represented by the femoral head. When the see-saw is balanced, the counterclockwise (internal) torque produced by the hip abductor force (HAF) equals the clockwise (external) torque caused by body weight (BW). Balance of opposing torques is called static rotary equilibrium (see Chapter 4).

During single-limb support, the hip abductor muscles—in particular the gluteus medius—produce most of the forces at the hip.[13] This important point is demonstrated by the model in Figure 12–45. Note that the internal moment arm (D) used by the hip abductor muscles is about half the length of the external moment arm (D₁) used by body weight.[53,63] Given this length disparity, the hip abductor muscles must produce a force *twice* that of body weight in order to achieve stability during single-limb support. On every step, therefore, the pelvis is forced against the femoral head by the combined force created by the hip abductor muscles and the pull of body weight. To achieve static linear equilibrium, the downward force is counteracted by a joint reaction force of equal magnitude, but oriented in nearly the opposite direction (see Fig. 12–45, JRF).[60] Inman calculated that the joint reaction force is directed 10 to 15 degrees from vertical, an angle that is strongly influenced by the orientation of the hip abductor muscle force vector.[31]

The sample data supplied in Figure 12–45 allow the magnitude of the hip abductor force and joint reaction force to be estimated. The torque and force equilibrium equations assume that the sum of frontal plane torques about the right hip and vertical forces are both equal to zero. As shown, a hip joint reaction force of 1873.8 N (421.3 lb) occurs when a 760.6 N (171 lb)–person is in single stance over the right limb during gait. About 66% of the joint reaction force comes from the hip abductor muscles. These calculations demonstrate that a joint reaction force of about 2.4 times body weight is generated through the hip during single-limb support. While the person is walking, this force is greater due to accelerations of the pelvis over the femoral head. Research using strain gauges implanted into a hip prosthesis show that joint compression forces reach 2.5 to 3 times body weight in walking. These forces increase to 5.5 times body weight in running.[4,74] Even ordinary daily functional activities can generate very high joint forces. Hodge and colleagues[29] reported pressures (forces per unit area) of 18 MPa (1 MPa equals 145 lb/in²) on the acetabulum while the healthy adult is rising from a chair. To appreciate the magnitude of this pressure, consider that the air pressure within a car tire is about 29 lb/in² (0.2 MPa). During sit-to-stand, therefore, pressures on the acetabulum reach 90 times the pressure in a full tire.[19] Joint forces have important physiologic functions, such as stabilizing the femoral head within the acetabulum, assisting in the nutrition of the articular cartilage, and providing the stimulus for normal development and shape of joint structure in childhood. The articular cartilage and trabecular bone must, however, protect the joint by dispersing these large forces. A hip with arthritis may no longer be able to provide this protection.

**SPECIAL FOCUS 12–5**

### Hip Abductor Muscle Weakness

Several medical conditions are associated with weakness of the hip abductor muscles. These conditions include muscular dystrophy, Guillain-Barré syndrome, and poliomyelitis. The abductors may also be weakened owing to hip arthritis, hip instability, or hip surgery. The classic indicator of hip abductor weakness is the positive *Trendelenburg sign*.[27] The patient is asked to stand in single-limb support over the weak hip. A positive sign occurs if the pelvis drops to the side of the unsupported limb; in other words, the weak hip "falls" into pelvic-on-femoral adduction (see Fig. 12–25*B*). The clinician needs to be cautious in interpreting and documenting the results of this test. The patient with a weak right hip abductor, for example, may drop the pelvis to the left. Weakness is often masked, however, by a compensatory lean of the *trunk* to the right. Leaning the trunk *to the side of the weakness* reduces the external torque demand on the abductor muscles by reducing the length of the external moment arm (see Fig. 12–45, D₁). When seen in gait, this compensatory lean to the side of weakness is referred to as a "gluteus medius limp" or "compensated Trendelenburg gait." Using a cane in the hand opposite the weakened hip abductors corrects this abnormal gait pattern.[6]

## HIP EXTERNAL ROTATOR MUSCLES

The primary external rotator muscles of the hip are five of the six "short external rotators," the gluteus maximus, and the sartorius. In the anatomic position, muscles considered as secondary external rotators are the posterior fibers of the gluteus medius and the gluteus minimus, the long head of the biceps femoris, and the obturator externus. The last muscle is a secondary rotator because in the anatomic position its line-of-force lies only a few millimeters posterior to the longitudinal axis of rotation (see Fig. 12–37).

### *Functional Anatomy of the "Short External Rotators"*

The six "short external rotators" of the hip are the piriformis, obturator internus, gemellus superior, gemellus inferior, quadratus femoris, and obturator externus (see Figs. 12–17, 12–40, and 12–44). The line-of-force of these muscles is oriented primarily in the horizontal plane. This orientation is optimal for the production of external rotation torque. In a manner similar to the infraspinatus and teres minor at the shoulder, the short external rotators also provide stability to the posterior side of the joint.

The *piriformis* attaches proximally on the anterior surface of the sacrum, among the exiting ventral rami of sacral spinal nerves (see Fig. 12–29). Exiting the pelvis through the greater sciatic foramen, the piriformis attaches on the superior aspect of the greater trochanter (see Fig. 12–44).

In addition to the action of external rotation, the piriformis also has a secondary action as a hip abductor. Both actions are apparent by the muscle's line-of-force rela-

**Standing at rest**                    **Active pelvic-on-femoral external rotation**

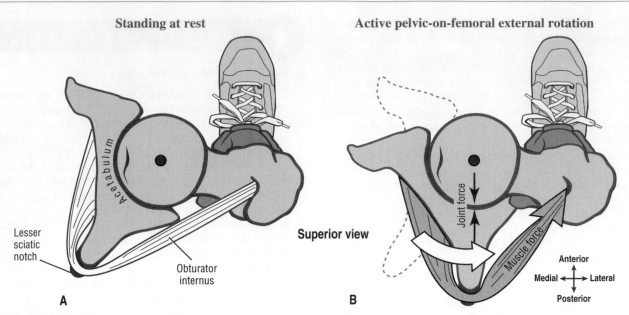

**FIGURE 12–46.** Superior view depicts the orientation and action of the obturator internus muscle. *A,* While standing at rest, the obturator internus muscle makes a 130-degree deflection as it courses through the pulley formed by the lesser sciatic notch. *B,* With the femur fixed during standing, contraction of this muscle causes pelvic-on-femoral external rotation. Note that the compression force generated into the joint is the result of the muscle contraction.

tive to the axis of rotation at the hip (see Figs. 12–33 and 12–37).

The sciatic nerve usually exits the pelvis below the piriformis. As described earlier in this chapter, the sciatic nerve may pass *through* the belly of the piriformis. A shortened piriformis may, for example, compress and irritate the sciatic nerve. This condition, known as "piriformis syndrome,"[85] is often treated by stretching the muscle through a combination of adduction and internal rotation, from a position near full hip extension.

The *obturator internus* muscle arises from the internal side of the obturator membrane and from the adjacent ilium (see Fig. 12–44). From this origin, the fibers converge to a tendon and exit the pelvis through the lesser sciatic foramen. The fixed pulley provided by the lesser sciatic notch deflects the tendon about 130 degrees on its approach to the trochanteric fossa of the femur (Fig. 12–46A). Contraction of this muscle with the femur held fixed, causes the pelvis to rotate on the femur (Fig. 12–46B). Force produced by the obturator internus compresses the joint surface. This compression force may help stabilize the joint during active pelvic rotation.

The *gemellus superior and gemellus inferior* muscles are located on either side of the central tendon of the obturator internus (see Fig. 12–44). The gemelli (from the Latin root *geminus,* meaning twins) are two small muscles with proximal attachments on either side of the lesser sciatic notch. Each muscle blends in with the central tendon of the obturator internus for a common attachment to the femur. Immediately below the gemellus inferior is the *quadratus femoris* muscle. This flat muscle arises from the external side of the ischial tuberosity and inserts on the posterior side of the proximal femur.

The *obturator externus* muscle arises from the external side of the obturator membrane and adjacent ilium (see Fig. 12–

17). The belly of this muscle is visible from the anterior side after removal of the adductor longus and pectineus muscles (Fig. 12–29). The muscle attaches posteriorly on the femur at the introchanteric fossa (see Figs. 12–5 and 12–7).

### Overall Function of the External Rotators

As described for the internal rotators of the hip, the functional potential of the external rotators is most evident during pelvic-on-femoral rotation. Consider, for example, the right external rotator muscles contracting to rotate the pelvis over the femur (Fig. 12–47). With the right lower extremity firmly in contact with the ground, concentric contraction of the right external rotators accelerates the anterior side of the pelvis and attached trunk *away* from the fixed femur. This horizontal plane action of planting a foot and cutting to the opposite side is a natural way to abruptly change direction while running. If needed, eccentric activation of the internal rotators may decelerate this action. Extremely rapid coactivation of the adductor muscles to help decelerate external rotation of the pelvis may cause "strain" injury to these muscles. The mechanism of injury may further explain the relatively high incidence of adductor muscle "pulls" during many sporting activities, which involve rapid rotation of the pelvis-and-trunk while running.

## MAXIMAL TORQUE PRODUCED BY THE HIP MUSCLES

Several studies have measured the maximal-effort torque production of hip muscles.[34,45] Table 12–3 summarizes the average maximal (isokinetic) torques produced by healthy men and women of different age groups.[8] These normative data are useful when assessing progress and setting goals for persons involved in strength training programs of the hip muscles.

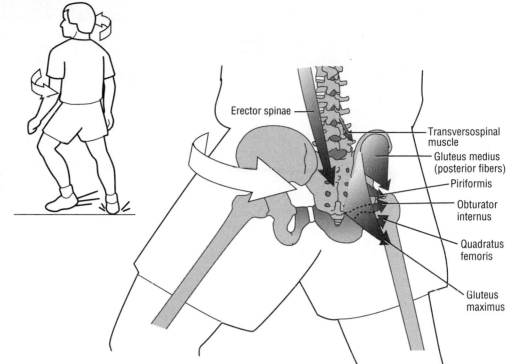

**FIGURE 12–47.** Action of the external rotator muscles during pelvic-on-femoral external rotation of the right hip. Back extensor muscles are also shown rotating the trunk.

Labels on figure: Erector spinae · Transversospinal muscle · Gluteus medius (posterior fibers) · Piriformis · Obturator internus · Quadratus femoris · Gluteus maximus

### Maximal Torque Versus Hip Joint Angle Relationship

In contrast to the isokinetic data presented in Table 12–3, maximal-effort torque produced by hip muscles is often measured isometrically, across several different joint angles. The unique shape of a muscle group's torque-joint angle curve can identify the points in the range of motion where functional demands are greatest on the muscle. Consider, for example, the isometric torque-angle curve of the hip abductor muscles in healthy young adults (Fig. 12–48).[53] The hip abductor muscles produce their greatest torque at full *adduction* (i.e., near the position associated with single-limb support). In contrast, abductor torque potential is least at the fully shortened muscle length that corresponds to 40 degrees of abduction. Ironically, the near maximally abducted hip is the position suggested for manually testing the strength of the hip abductors.[39]

## Examples of Hip Disease

### RATIONALE FOR SELECTED THERAPEUTIC AND SURGICAL INTERVENTION

Two of the most common causes of hip impairment occur from fracture of the proximal femur and osteoarthritis. This

| TABLE 12–3. Average Maximal-Effort Torque (N · m) for the Six Major Muscle Groups at the Hip* | | | | |
|---|---|---|---|---|
| Muscle Group | Younger Men ($\overline{X}$ = 28 yrs) | Older Men ($\overline{X}$ = 54 yrs) | Younger Women ($\overline{X}$ = 27 yrs) | Older Women ($\overline{X}$ = 53 yrs) |
| Extensors | 177 (42) | 157 (22) | 110 (37) | 101 (27) |
| Flexors | 152 (50) | 113 (21) | 91 (24) | 67 (21) |
| Adductors | 121 (26) | 99 (18) | 82 (26) | 63 (17) |
| Abductors | 103 (26) | 75 (18) | 66 (19) | 48 (14) |
| Internal rotators | 72 (17) | 61 (21) | 47 (13) | 34 (9) |
| External rotators | 65 (24) | 50 (15) | 43 (13) | 32 (11) |

*Standard deviations in parenthesis. Torques were measured isokinetically at 30°/sec and then averaged over the full range of motion. The torques are presented in order from greatest to least values. Data are based on 72 healthy subjects between 20 and 81 years of age. (Modified from Cahalan TD, Johnson ME, Liu S, et al: Quantitative measurements of hip strength in different age groups. Clin Orthop 246: 136–145, 1989.)
Conversion: 1.36 N · m = 1 ft-lb

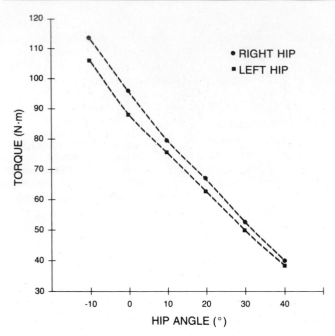

**FIGURE 12–48.** This plot shows the effect of frontal plane range of hip motion on the maximal effort, isometric hip abductor torque in 30 healthy persons. The −10-degree hip angle represents a fully adducted position where the muscles are at a relatively long length. (Data from Neumann DA, Soderberg GL, Cook TM: Comparison of maximal isometric hip abductor muscle torques between hip sides. Phys Ther 68:496–502, 1988.)

section describes each of these conditions, followed by a discussion on clinical biomechanics associated with selected therapeutic and surgical interventions.

### Fracture of the Hip

Fracture of the hip (i.e., proximal femur) is a major health and economic problem in the United States.[11] About 20% of persons with hip fractures die within a year owing to factors directly related to these fractures.[43] Nearly 80% of persons over 65 years of age who sustain hip fractures are female.[38]

The risk of hip fracture doubles each decade after the age of 50 years.[22] Two primary factors most often associated with the higher incidence of hip fracture in the elderly are age-related osteoporosis and the higher incidence of falling. Additional factors proposed by Cummings and Nevitt[12] are included in Table 12–4.

### Hip Osteoarthritis

Hip osteoarthritis is a disease manifested primarily by the deterioration of the joint's articular cartilage. Without an adequate mechanism to dissipate loads, the joint surfaces may rapidly degenerate and change shape.

Clinical signs of hip osteoarthritis are listed in the box. Hip osteoarthritis is often referred to as degenerative arthritis of the hip. The term "arthrosis" is often used to describe a condition in which a joint is degenerated but not inflamed.

---

| **Sustaining a Fracture of the Hip Following a Fall** |
| :---: |
| Loss of Balance |
| ↓ |
| **Failure of Protective Reflexes** |
| (e.g., slowed reaction time, sedation, dementia, muscle weakness) |
| ↓ |
| **Fall** |
| ↓ |
| **Potential Energy Dissipated Primarily over Hip Region** |
| ↓ |
| **Failure of Local Shock Absorption** |
| (e.g., reduced fat around hip, weakness/atrophy of hip muscles, hard impact surface) |
| ↓ |
| **Diminished Strength of Bone** |
| (e.g., osteoporosis, thinned bone cortex, loss of major trabeculae) |
| ↓ |
| **Fractured Hip** |

From Cummings SR, Nevitt MC: A hypothesis: The causes of hip fractures. J Gerontol Med Sci 44: M107–M111, 1989.

---

### Clinical Signs of Hip Osteoarthritis Include

- Pain
- Synovitis
- Loss of joint space
- Muscle atrophy
- Hypertrophic bone formation
- Reduced range of motion
- Abnormal gait

---

 **SPECIAL FOCUS 12–6**

### What Causes Primary Osteoarthritis of the Hip?

The exact cause of primary hip osteoarthritis remains unclear. Although the frequency of osteoarthritis—at any joint—increases with age, the disease is not triggered solely *by* the aging process.[46] If this were true, then *all* elderly persons would develop this disease. The causes of osteoarthritis are complicated and not exclusively based on a simple wear-and-tear phenomenon. Although physical stress may increase the rate and amount of wear at a joint,[68] this does not always lead to osteoarthritis. Other mechanisms related to osteoarthritis are metabolism of the ground matrix of the cartilage, genetics, immune system factors, neuromuscular dysfunctions,[78] and biochemical factors.[46]

Hip osteoarthritis may be classified as either a primary or secondary disease. *Primary* or idiopathic *hip osteoarthritis* refers to an arthritic condition without a known cause. *Secondary hip osteoarthritis,* in contrast, refers to an arthritic condition resulting from a known mechanical disruption of the joint. This may occur from trauma, structural failure such as slipped capital femoral epiphysis, anatomic asymmetry such as excessive acetabular anteversion, leg length discrepancy, avascular necrosis of the femoral head (i.e., Legg-Calvé-Perthes disease), or congenital dislocation. Persons who perform heavy physical work are more likely to require hospitalization because of osteoarthritis of the hip.[82]

### Therapeutic Intervention for a Painful or Structurally Unstable Hip

#### Using a Cane and Proper Methods for Carrying External Loads

Physical rehabilitation of a painful or structurally unstable hip often includes instructions in assisted gait[40] and func-tional activities, exercise,[24,81] modalities for relieving pain, and aerobic conditioning. In addition, clinicians frequently give advice on how to protect the hip from large forces while a person is walking.[54] One method of protecting the hip is to use a cane in the hand opposite to the affected hip. Use of the cane reduces joint forces that are caused by the activation of the hip abductor muscles.[59,60] Figure 12–49 shows that applying a cane force in the left hand results in a joint reaction force at the right hip of 1195.4 N (268.8 lb). This correlates with a 36% reduction in joint reaction force compared with that produced when not using a cane (see Fig. 12–45, for comparison).

Methods of carrying external loads influence the demands placed on the hip abductor muscles and therefore on the underlying hip joint.[52,56,57] Persons with painful, unstable, or surgically replaced hips are to be cautioned about the consequences of carrying a hand-held load *opposite,* or contralateral, to the affected hip.[4,49,58] As shown in Figure 12–50, the contralateral load has a very large external moment arm ($D_2$), creating a substantial clockwise torque about the right hip. For frontal plane stability, the right hip abductors must

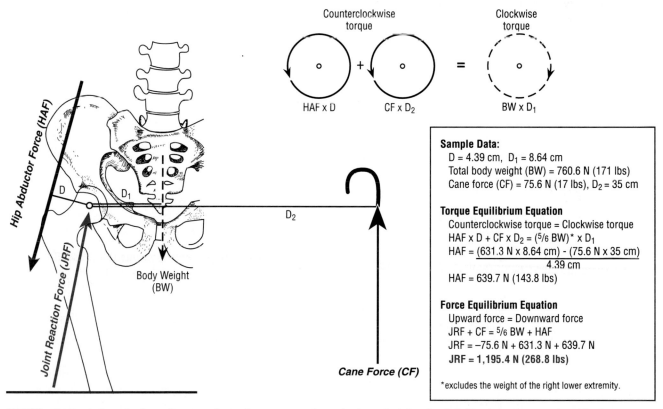

**FIGURE 12–49.** A frontal plane diagram shows how a cane force (CF) applied by the left hand produces a frontal plane torque about the right hip in single-limb support. This cane-produced torque can minimize the torque demands on the right hip abductor muscles. Note that the *clockwise torque* (dashed circle) due to body weight (BW × $D_1$) is balanced by the *counterclockwise torques* (solid circles) due to the hip abductor force (HAF × D) and the cane force (CF × $D_2$). The data shown in the box are used in the torque and force equilibrium equations to solve for hip abductor force and joint reaction force (JRF). The moment arm used by cane force is represented by $D_2$. (See Fig. 12–45 for additional abbreviations and background.) For simplicity, the calculations in the inset assume static equilibrium and that all force vectors are acting in a vertical direction. (From Neumann DA: Hip abductor muscle activity in persons with a hip prosthesis while carrying loads in one hand. Phys Ther 76:1320–1330, 1996. With permission of the APTA.)

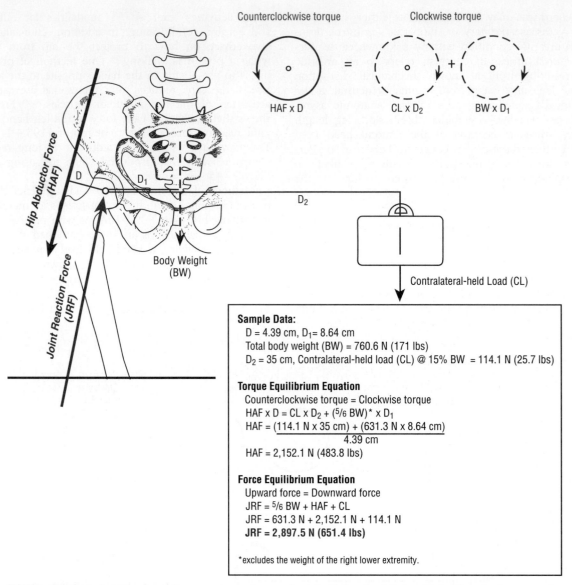

Counterclockwise torque    Clockwise torque

HAF x D    =    CL x $D_2$    +    BW x $D_1$

Hip Abductor Force (HAF)

Joint Reaction Force (JRF)

Body Weight (BW)

$D_2$

Contralateral-held Load (CL)

**Sample Data:**
D = 4.39 cm, $D_1$= 8.64 cm
Total body weight (BW) = 760.6 N (171 lbs)
$D_2$ = 35 cm, Contralateral-held load (CL) @ 15% BW  = 114.1 N (25.7 lbs)

**Torque Equilibrium Equation**
Counterclockwise torque = Clockwise torque
HAF x D = CL x $D_2$ + ($^5/_6$ BW)* x $D_1$
HAF = $\dfrac{(114.1 \text{ N x } 35 \text{ cm}) + (631.3 \text{ N x } 8.64 \text{ cm})}{4.39 \text{ cm}}$
HAF = 2,152.1 N (483.8 lbs)

**Force Equilibrium Equation**
Upward force = Downward force
JRF = $^5/_6$ BW + HAF + CL
JRF = 631.3 N + 2,152.1 N + 114.1 N
**JRF = 2,897.5 N (651.4 lbs)**

*excludes the weight of the right lower extremity.

**FIGURE 12–50.** A frontal plane diagram shows how a load held in the left hand significantly increases the amount of right hip abductor force (HAF) during single-limb support. Two clockwise torques (dashed circles) are produced about the right hip due to body weight (BW × $D_1$) and the contralaterally held load (CL × $D_2$). For equilibrium about the right hip, the clockwise torques must be balanced by a counterclockwise torque (solid circle) produced by the hip abductor force (HAF × D). The data shown in the box are used in the torque and force equilibrium equations to solve for hip abductor force and joint reaction force (JRF). $D_2$ is equal to the moment arm used by the contralateral-held load (CL). Refer to Figure 12–45 for background and other abbreviations. For simplicity, the calculations assume static equilibrium and that all force vectors are acting in vertical directions. (From Neumann DA: Hip abductor muscle activity in persons with a hip prosthesis while carrying loads in one hand. Phys Ther 76:1320–1330, 1996. With permission of the APTA.)

create a counterclockwise torque large enough to balance the clockwise torques because of the load (CL × $D_2$) *and* body weight (BW × $D_1$). As a result of the relatively small moment arm available to the hip abductor muscles (D), the amount of hip abductor force during single-limb support is very large. As shown by the calculations in Figure 12–50, a contralaterally held load of only 15% of body weight (i.e., 114.1 N or 25.7 lb) results in a joint reaction force of

2897.5 N (651.4 lb). A healthy hip can usually tolerate this amount of force without difficulty. Caution must be exercised, however, if structural stability of the hip is compromised.

The previous discussion focuses on methods that reduce the force demands on the hip abductor muscles as a means to reduce the force on a painful or an unstable hip. Although these methods may have their desired effect, the

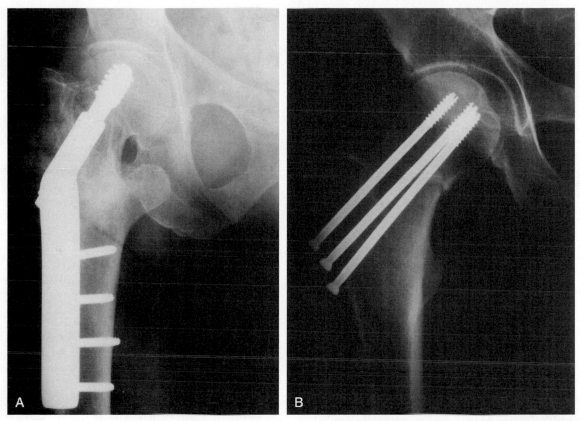

**FIGURE 12–51.** X-rays show two common forms of internal fixation for treatment of a fracture of the proximal femur. *A,* A compression screw is used to repair an intertrochanteric fracture. The screw is designed like a piston, compressing slightly when under the load of body weight. The compression increases bone-to-bone contact across the fracture site. *B,* Three pins are used to stabilize a fracture through the femoral neck. (Courtesy of Michael Anderson, M.D., Blount Orthopedic Clinic, Milwaukee, WI.)

reduced functional demand placed on the hip may also perpetuate prolonged weakness in the hip abductor muscles which, in turn, causes deviations in gait.[67] Clinicians must meet the dual challenge of protecting a vulnerable hip from excessive and potentially damaging abductor forces, while simultaneously increasing the functional strength and endurance of the abductors. This requires knowledge of the normal and abnormal frontal plane mechanics of the hip, the pathology specific to the patient's condition, and the symptoms that suggest the hip is being subjected to potentially damaging forces. The signs and symptoms include excessive pain, marked gait deviation, generalized hip instability, and abnormal positioning of the lower limb.

### Surgical Intervention Following Fracture or Osteoarthritis

Surgery is often indicated to repair a fractured hip. The type of surgical repair depends on the location and severity of the fracture.[73] Figure 12–51 shows two common types of *internal fixation* used for a fractured proximal femur. The amount of weight placed on the hip after surgery is usually limited until the fracture site shows ample evidence of healing.

A *total hip arthroplasty* is often indicated when a person with hip disease, most often osteoarthritis, has constant pain that significantly limits function and quality of life. This operation replaces the diseased joint with biologically inert materials (Fig. 12–52). A prosthetic hip is secured by cement or through biologic fixation, provided by bone growth into the surface of the implanted components. Although the total hip arthroplasty is typically a successful procedure, premature loosening of the femoral and/or acetabular component can be a postoperative problem.[78] Large torsional loads between the prosthetic implant and the bony interface may contribute to the loss of fixation.[5] Until sufficient long-term data emerge from clinical trials, debate regarding the most durable materials and effective methods of fixation continue.

### Biomechanical Consequences of Coxa Vara and Coxa Valga

The average angle of inclination of the femoral neck is 125 degrees. The angle may be changed as a result of a surgical repair of a fractured hip or an angle of inclination designed into a prosthesis. Additionally, an operation known as a *coxa vara (or valga) osteotomy* intentionally alters a preexisting angle of inclination. This operation involves cutting a wedge of bone from the proximal femur, thereby changing the orientation of the femoral head to the acetabulum.[64] A goal of this operation is often to improve the congruency of the weight-bearing surfaces of the hip (Fig. 12–53).

Regardless of the type and rationale of the hip surgery, changing the angle of inclination of the proximal femur alters the stability, stress, and function of the muscles. These alterations can have positive and negative biomechanical effects. Figure 12–54A shows two positive biomechanical effects of coxa vara. The varus position increases the moment arm of the hip abductor force (compare the dashed lines indicated by $D_1$ and D). The greater leverage increases the abduction torque produced per unit of hip abductor muscle force. This situation is useful for persons with hip abductor weakness. Reducing the force demands on the hip abductors while walking also helps to protect an arthritic or a prosthetic hip from excessive wear. A varus osteotomy is performed to improve the stability of the joint by aligning the femoral head more directly into the acetabulum.

A potentially negative effect of coxa vara is an increased bending moment generated across the femoral neck (Fig. 12–54B). The bending moment arm (dashed line indicated by I′) increases as the angle of inclination approaches 90 degrees. Increasing the bending moment raises the tension across the superior aspect of the femoral neck. This situation may cause a fracture of the femoral neck or a structural failure of the prosthesis. Marked coxa vara increases the

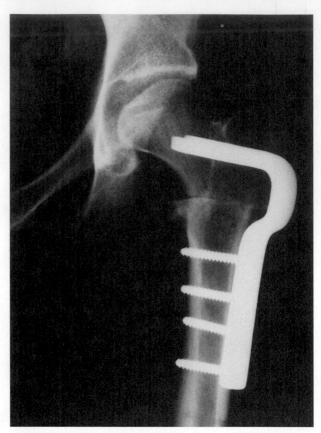

**FIGURE 12–53.** A varus osteotomy was performed on a hip with avascular necrosis of the femoral head. The removed wedge of bone is apparent at the extreme proximal femoral shaft. The increased varus position in this particular patient improved the congruency of the weight-bearing surface of the hip. The osteotomy site was stabilized with a blade plate. (Courtesy of Michael Anderson, M.D., Blount Orthopedic Clinic, Milwaukee, WI.)

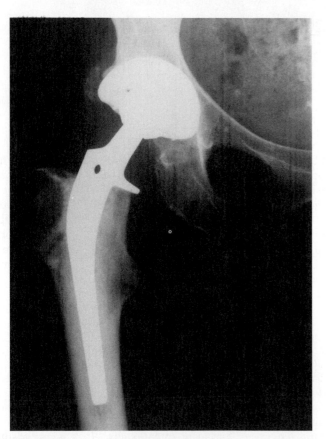

**FIGURE 12–52.** An x-ray shows a total hip arthroplasty. The femoral component is made of a high-strength steel alloy that is cemented into the medullary canal. The socket is porous coated, allowing the pelvic bone to grow into the device and provide biologic fixation. (Courtesy of Michael Anderson, M.D., Blount Orthopedic Clinic, Milwaukee, WI.)

vertical shear between the femoral head and the adjacent epiphysis. In children, this situation may lead to a condition known as a slipped capital femoral epiphysis. Coxa vara may decrease the functional length of the hip abductor muscles, thereby reducing the force generating capability of these muscles and increasing the likelihood of a "gluteus medius limp." The loss in muscle force may offset the increased abductor torque potential gained by the increased hip abductor moment arm.

Coxa valga may result from a surgical intervention or from pathology such as hip dysplasia. A potentially positive effect of the valgus position is a decreased bending moment arm across the femoral neck (see Fig. 12–54C, compare I″ with I′). This situation decreased the vertical shear across the femoral neck. The valgus position, however, may increase the functional length of the hip abductor muscles, thus their force generating capability may increase. In contrast, a potentially negative effect of coxa valga is the decreased moment arm available to the hip abductor force (see Fig. 12–54D, compare D″ with D). In extreme coxa valga, the femoral head is positioned more lateral to the acetabulum, possibly favoring dislocation.

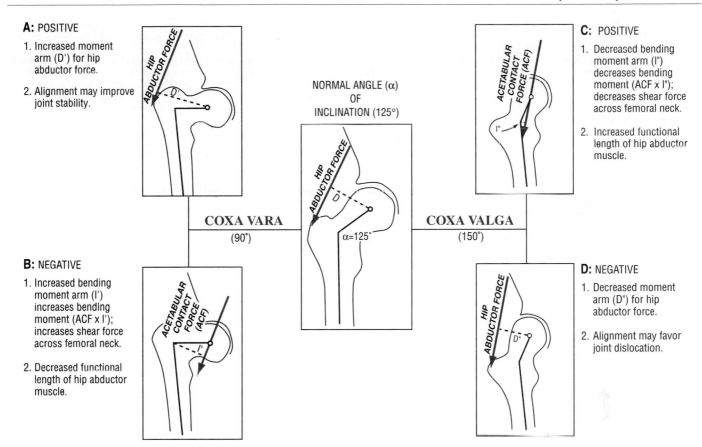

**A:** POSITIVE

1. Increased moment arm (D') for hip abductor force.

2. Alignment may improve joint stability.

**B:** NEGATIVE

1. Increased bending moment arm (I') increases bending moment (ACF x I'); increases shear force across femoral neck.

2. Decreased functional length of hip abductor muscle.

NORMAL ANGLE (α) OF INCLINATION (125°)

COXA VARA (90°)

COXA VALGA (150°)

**C:** POSITIVE

1. Decreased bending moment arm (I") decreases bending moment (ACF x I"); decreases shear force across femoral neck.

2. Increased functional length of hip abductor muscle.

**D:** NEGATIVE

1. Decreased moment arm (D") for hip abductor force.

2. Alignment may favor joint dislocation.

**FIGURE 12–54.** The negative and positive biomechanical effects of coxa vara and coxa valga are contrasted. As a reference, a hip with a normal angle of inclination (α = 125 degrees) is shown in the center of the display. D is the internal moment arm used by hip abductor force; I is the bending moment arm across the femoral neck.

## REFERENCES

1. Anda S, Svenningsen S, Dale LG, et al: The acetabular sector angle of the adult hip determined by computed tomography. Acta Radiol Diagn 27:443–447, 1986.
2. Andersson E, Oddsson L, Grundstrom H, et al: The role of the psoas and iliacus muscles for stability and movement of the lumbar spine, pelvis and hip. Scand J Med Sci Sports 5:10–16, 1995.
3. Beaty JH: Congenital anomalies of hip and pelvis. In Crenshaw AH (ed): Campbells' Operative Orthopaedics, 3rd vol, 8th ed. St. Louis, Mosby-Year Book, 1992.
4. Bergmann G, Graichen F, Rohlmann A. Hip joint loading during walking and running, measured in two patients. J Biomechan 26:969–990, 1993.
5. Bergmann G, Graichen F, Rohlmann A, et al: Hip joint forces during load carrying. Clin Orthop 335:190–201, 1997.
6. Blount WP: Don't throw away the cane. J Bone Joint Surg 38A:695–708, 1956.
7. Boone DC, Azen SP: Normal range of motion of joints in male subjects. J Bone Joint Surg 61A:756–759, 1979.
8. Cahalan TD, Johnson ME, Liu S, et al: Quantitative measurements of hip strength in different age groups. Clin Orthop 246:136–145, 1989.
9. Clark JM, Haynor DR: Anatomy of the abductor muscles of the hip as studied by computed tomography. J Bone Joint Surg 69A:1021–1031, 1987.
10. Cornbleet SL, Woolsey NB: Assessment of hamstring muscle length in school-aged children using the sit-and-reach test and the inclinometer measure of hip joint angle. Phys Ther 76:850–855, 1996.
11. Craik RL: Disability following hip fracture. Phys Ther 74:387–398, 1994.
12. Cummings SR, Nevitt MC: A hypothesis: The causes of hip fractures. J Gerontol Med Sci 44:M107–M111, 1989.
13. Dalstra M, Huiskes R: Load transfer across the pelvic bone. J Biomechan 28:715–724, 1995.
14. Delp SL, Bleck EE, Zajac FE, et al: Biomechanical analysis of the Chiari pelvic osteotomy—preserving hip abductor strength. Clin Orthop 254:189–198, 1990.
15. Delp SL, Hess WE, Hungerford DS, et al: Variation of rotation moment arms with hip flexion. Biomechanics 32:493–501, 1999.
16. Dostal WF, Andrews JG: A three-dimensional biomechanical model of hip musculature. J Biomech 14:803–812, 1981.
17. Dostal WF, Soderberg GL, Andrews JG: Actions of hip muscles. Phys Ther 66:351–359, 1986.
18. Fabry G, MacEwen GD, Shands AR: Torsion of the femur: A follow-up study in normal and abnormal conditions. J Bone Joint Surg 55A:1726–1738, 1973.
19. Fagerson TL: Personal communication, 1999.
20. Fischer FJ, Houtz SJ: Evaluation of the function of the gluteus maximus muscle. Am J Phys Med 47:182–191, 1968.
21. Fuss FK, Bacher A: New aspects of the morphology and function of the human hip joint ligaments. Am J Anat 192:1–13, 1991.
22. Gallagher JC, Melton LJ, Riggs BL, et al: Epidemiology of fractures of the proximal femur in Rochester, Minnesota. Clin Orthop 150:163–171, 1980.
23. Gelberman RH, Cohen MS, Desai SS, et al: Femoral anteversion: A clinical assessment of idiopathic in toeing gait in children. J Bone Joint Surg 69B:75–79, 1987.
24. Givens-Heiss DL, Krebs DE, Riley PO, et al: In vivo acetabular contact pressures during rehabilitation. Part II: Postacute phase. Phys Ther 72:700–705, 1992.
25. Green DL, Morris JM: Role of adductor longus and adductor magnus in postural movements and in ambulation. Am J Phys Med 49:223–240, 1970.
26. Hammond BT, Charnley J: The sphericity of the femoral head. Med Biol Engng 5:445–453, 1967.
27. Hardcastle P, Nade S: The significance of the Trendelenburg test. J Bone Joint Surg 67B:741–746, 1985.

28. Harris WH: The first 32 years of total hip arthroplasty. Clin Orthop 274:6–11, 1992.
29. Hodge WA, Carlson KL, Fijan RE: Contact pressures from an instrumented hip endoprosthesis. J Bone Joint Surg 71A:1378–1386, 1989.
30. Hsin J, Saluja R, Eilert RE, et al: Evaluation of the biomechanics of the hip following a triple osteotomy of the innominate bone. J Bone Joint Surg 78A:855–862, 1996.
31. Inman VT: Functional aspects of the abductor muscles of the hip. J Bone Joint Surg 29A:607–619, 1947.
32. Inman VT, Saunders JB: Referred pain from skeletal structures. J Nerv Ment Dis 99:660–667, 1944.
33. Inman VT, Ralston HJ, Todd F: Human Walking. Baltimore, Williams & Wilkins, 1981.
34. Jensen RH, Smidt GL, Johnston RD: A technique for obtaining measurements of force generated by hip muscles. Arch Phys Med 52:207–215, 1971.
35. Johnston RC, Smidt GL: Hip motion measurements for selected activities of daily living. Clin Orthop 72:205–215, 1970.
36. Kaplan EB: The iliotibial tract: Clinical and morphological significance. J Bone Joint Surg 40A:817–832, 1958.
37. Keagy RD, Brumlik J, Bergan JJ: Direct electromyography of the psoas major muscle in man. J Bone Joint Surg 48A:1377–1382, 1966.
38. Kelsey J: The epidemiology of diseases of the hip: A review of the literature. Int J Epidemiol 6:269–282, 1977.
39. Kendall FP, McCreary AK, Provance PG: Muscles: Testing and Function, 4th ed. Baltimore, Williams & Wilkins, 1993.
40. Krebs DE, Elbaum L, Riley PO, et al: Exercise and gait effects on in vivo hip contact pressures. Phys Ther 71:301–309, 1991.
41. Kumagai MK, Shiba N, Higuchi F, et al: Functional evaluation of hip abductor muscles with use of magnetic resonance imaging. J Orthop Res 15:888–893, 1997.
42. Kurrat HJ, Oberlander W: The thickness of the cartilage in the human joint. J Anat 126:145–155, 1978.
43. Lewinnek GE, Kelsey J, White AA, et al: The significance and a comparative analysis of the epidemiology of hip fractures. Clin Orthop 152:35–43, 1980.
44. Li Y, McClure PW, Pratt N: The effect of hamstring muscle stretching on standing posture and on lumbar and hip motions during forward bending. Phys Ther 76:836–849, 1996.
45. Lindsay DM, Maitland ME, Lowe RC, et al: Comparison of isokinetic internal and external hip rotation torques using different testing positions. J Orthop Phys Ther 16:43–50, 1992.
46. Lohmander LS: Articular cartilage and osteoarthrosis. The role of molecular markers to monitor breakdown, repair, and disease. J Anat 184:477–492, 1994.
47. Lohe F, Eckstein F, Sauer T, et al: Structure, strain and function of the transverse acetabular ligament. Acta Anat 157:315–323, 1996.
48. Markhede G, Stener B: Function after removal of various hip and thigh muscles for extirpation of tumors. Acta Orthop Scand 52:373–395, 1981.
49. McGibbon CA, Krebs DE, Mann RW: In vivo hip pressures during cane and load-carrying gait. Arthritis Care Res 10:300–307, 1997.
50. Michaeli DA, Murphy SB, Hipp JA: Comparison of predicted and measured contact pressures in normal and dysplastic hips. Med Eng Phys 19:180–186, 1997.
51. Merchant AC: Hip abductor muscle force. J Bone Joint Surg 47A:462–476, 1965.
52. Neumann DA, Cook TM: Effect of load and carry position on the electromyographic activity of the gluteus medius muscle during walking. Phys Ther 65:305–311, 1985.
53. Neumann DA, Soderberg GL, Cook TM: Comparison of maximal isometric hip abductor muscle torques between hip sides. Phys Ther 68:496–502, 1988.
54. Neumann DA: Biomechanical analysis of selected principles of hip joint protection. Arthritis Care Res 2:146–155, 1989.
55. Neumann DA, Soderberg GL, Cook TM: Electromyographic analysis of hip abductor musculature in healthy right-handed persons. Phys Ther 69:431–440, 1989.
56. Neumann DA, Cook TM, Sholty RL, Sobush DC: An electromyographic analysis of hip abductor muscle activity when subjects are carrying loads in one or both hands. Phys Ther 72:207–217, 1992.
57. Neumann DA, Hase A: An electromyographic analysis of hip abductors during load carriage: Implications for hip joint protection. J Orthop Sports Phys Ther 19:296–304, 1994.
58. Neumann DA: Hip abductor muscle activity in persons with a hip prosthesis while carrying loads in one hand. Phys Ther 76:1320–1330, 1996.
59. Neumann DA: Hip abductor muscle activity as subjects with hip prosthesis walk with different methods of using a cane. Phys Ther 78:490–501, 1998.
60. Neumann DA: An electromyographic study of the hip abductor muscles as subjects with a hip prosthesis walked with different methods of using a cane and carrying a load. Phys Ther 79:1163–1173, 1999.
61. Nemeth G, Ohlsen H: Moment arms of the hip abductor and adductor muscles measured in vivo by computed tomography. Clin Biomechan 4:133–136, 1989.
62. Ogus O: Measurement and relationship of the inclination angle, Alsberg angle and the angle between the anatomical and mechanical axes of the femur in males. Surg Radiol Anat 18:29–31, 1996.
63. Olson VL, Smidt GL, Johnston RC: The maximum torque generated by the eccentric, isometric, and concentric contractions of the abductor muscles. Phys Ther 52:149–157, 1972.
64. Osborne GV, Fahrni WH: Oblique displacement osteotomy for osteoarthritis of the hip joint. J Bone Joint Surg 32B:148–160, 1950.
65. Pauwels F: Biomechanics of the Normal and Diseased Hip. Berlin, Springer-Verlag, 1976.
66. Pare EB, Stern JT, Schwartz JM: Functional differentiation within the tensor fasciae latae. J Bone Joint Surg 63A:1457–1471, 1981.
67. Perron M, Malouin F, Moffet H, et al: Three-dimensional gait analysis in women with a total hip arthroplasty. Clin Biomech 15:504–515, 2000.
68. Peyron JG: Osteoarthritis: The epidemiologic viewpoint. Clin Orthop 213:13–19, 1986.
69. Pohtilla JF: Kinesiology of hip extension at selected angles of pelvifemoral extension. Arch Phys Med Rehabil 50:241–250, 1969.
70. Reikeras O, Bjerkreim I: Idiopathic increased anteversion of the femoral neck. Acta Orthop Scand 53:839–845, 1982.
71. Reikeras O, Bjerkreim I, Kolbenstvedt A: Anteversion of the acetabulum and femoral neck in normals and patients with osteoarthritis of the hip. Acta Orthop Scand 54:18–23, 1983.
72. Roach KE, Miles TP: Normal hip and knee active range of motion: The relationship to age. Phys Ther 71:656–665, 1991.
73. Russell TA: Fractures of Hip and Pelvis. In Crenshaw AH (ed): Campbells' Operative Orthopaedics, 2nd vol, 8th ed. St. Louis, Mosby Year Book, 1992.
74. Rydell N: Biomechanics of the hip joint. Clin Orthop 92:6–15, 1973.
75. Sage FP: Cerebral palsy. In Crenshaw AH (ed): Campbells' Operative Orthopaedics, 2nd vol, 8th ed. St. Louis, Mosby Year Book, 1992.
76. Santaguida PL, McGill SM: The psoas major muscle: A three-dimensional geometric study. J Biomech 28:339–345, 1995.
77. Simoneau GG, Hoenig K, Lepley J, et al: Influence of hip position and gender on active hip internal and external rotation. J Orthop Sports Phys Ther 28:158–164, 1998.
78. Sims K: The development of hip osteoarthritis: Implications for conservative management. Man Ther 4:127–135, 1999.
79. Skyrme AD, Cahill DJ, Marsh HP, et al: Psoas major and its controversial rotational action. Clin Anat 12:264–265, 1999.
80. Soderberg GL, Dostal WF: Electromyographic study of three parts of the gluteus medius muscle during functional activities. Phys Ther 58:691–696, 1978.
81. Strickland EM, Fares M, Krebs DE, et al: In vivo acetabular contact pressures during rehabilitation. Part I: Acute phase. Phys Ther 72:691–699, 1992.
82. Vingard E, Alfredsson L, Goldie I, et al: Occupation and osteoarthritis of the hip and knee: A register-based cohort study. Int J Epidemiol 20:1025–1031, 1991.
83. Walheim GG, Selvik G: Mobility of the symphysis pubis. Clin Orthop 191:129–135, 1984.
84. Williams M, Wesley W: Hip rotator action of the adductor longus muscle. Phys Ther Rev 31:90–92, 1952.
85. Williams PL, Bannister LH, Berry M, et al: Gray's Anatomy, 38th ed, New York, Churchill Livingstone, 1995.
86. Wingstrand H, Wingstrand A, Krantz P: Intracapsular and atmospheric pressure in the dynamics and stability of the hip. Acta Orthop Scand 61:231–235, 1990.
87. Yoshioka Y, Cooke TO: Femoral anteversion: assessment based on function axes. J Orthop Res 5:86–91, 1987.

## ADDITIONAL READING

Baker AS, Bitounis VC: Abductor function after total hip replacement. J Bone Joint Surg 71B:47–50, 1989.

Basmajian JV, Greenlaw RK: Electromyography of the iliacus and psoas with inserted fine wire electrodes. Anat Rec 160:310–311, 1968.

Bergstrom G, Bjelle A, Sorenssen L, et al: Prevalence of rheumatoid arthritis, osteoarthritis, chondrocalcinosis and gouty arthritis at age 79. J Rheumatol 13:150–157, 1986.

Borja F, Latta LL, Stinchfield FE, et al: Abductor muscle performance in total hip arthroplasty with and without trochanteric osteotomy. Clin Orthop 197:181–190, 1985.

Evans BG, Salvati EA, Huo MH, Huk OL: The rationale for cemented total hip arthroplasty. Clin Orthop 24:599–610, 1993.

Free SA, Delp SL: Trochanteric transfer in total hip replacement: Effects on the moment arms and force-generating capacities of the hip abductors. J Orthop Res 14:245–250, 1996.

Greenwald AS, Haynes DW: Weight-bearing areas in the human hip joint. J Bone Joint Surg 54B:157–163, 1972.

Mann RA, Moran GT, Dougherty SE: Comparative electromyography of the lower extremity in jogging, running, and sprinting. Am J Sports Med 6:501–510, 1986.

McKibbin B: The action of the iliopsoas muscle in the newborn. J Bone Joint Surg 50B:161–165, 1968.

Murray MP, Seireg AH, Scholz RC: A survey of the time, magnitude, and orientation of forces applied to walking sticks by disabled men. Am J Phys Med 48:1–13, 1969.

Neumann DA: Arthrokinesiologic considerations in the aged adult. In Guccione AA (ed): Geriatric Physical Therapy, 2nd ed. St. Louis, Mosby Year Book, 2000.

Spoor CW, van Leeuven JL, de Windt FHJ: A model study of muscle forces and joint-force direction in normal and dysplastic neonatal hips. J Biomech 22:873–884, 1989.

Staheli LT, Corbett M, Wyss C, et al: Lower-extremity rotational problems in children. J Bone Joint Surg 67A:39–47, 1985.

Van den Bogert AJ, Read L, Nigg BM: An analysis of hip joint loading during walking, running, and skiing. Med Sci Sports Exerc 31:131–142, 1999.

Vas MD, Kramer JF, Rorabeck CH, et al: Isometric hip abductor strength following hip replacement and its relationship to functional assessment. J Orthop Sports Phys Ther 18:526–531, 1993.

Vasvada AN, Delp SL, Mahoney WJ, et al: Compensating for changes in muscle length in total hip arthroplasty—effects on the moment generating capacity of the muscles. Clin Orthop 302:121–133, 1994.

Vrhas MS, Brand RA, Brown TD: Contribution of passive tissues to the intersegmental moments at the hip. J Biomech 23:357–362, 1990.

Waters RL, Perry J, McDaniels JM, et al: The relative strength of the hamstrings muscles during hip extension. J Bone Joint Surg 56A:1592–1597, 1974.

Woolson ST, Mohoney WJ, Schurman DJ: Time-related improvement in the range of motion of the hip after total hip replacement. J Bone Joint Surg 67A:1251–1254, 1985.

# *Knee*

## DONALD A. NEUMANN, PT, PhD

## TOPICS AT A GLANCE

## INTRODUCTION

The knee consists of the lateral and medial tibiofemoral joints and the patellofemoral joint (Fig. 13–1). Motion at the knee occurs in two planes, allowing flexion and extension in the sagittal plane, and internal and external rotation in the horizontal plane. Functionally, however, these movements rarely occur independent of movement at other joints of the lower limb. Consider, for example, the interaction among the hip, knee, and ankle during running or climbing or standing from a seated position. The strong functional association within the joints of the lower limb is reflected by the fact that most muscles that cross the knee also cross either the hip or ankle.

The knee has important biomechanical functions, many of which are expressed during walking and running. During the swing phase of walking, the knee flexes to shorten the functional length of the lower limb; otherwise, the foot would not easily clear the ground. During the stance phase, the knee remains slightly flexed, allowing shock absorption, conservation of energy, and transmission of forces through the lower limb. Running requires that the knee moves through a large range of motion, especially in the sagittal plane. Rapidly changing directions while running (i.e., cutting) requires additional freedom of movement in the horizontal plane.

Stability of the knee is based primarily on its soft tissue constraints rather than on its bony configuration. The massive femoral condyles articulate with the nearly flat surfaces of the tibia, held in place by an extensive ligamentous capsule and large muscles. With the foot firmly in contact with the ground, these soft tissues are often subjected to large

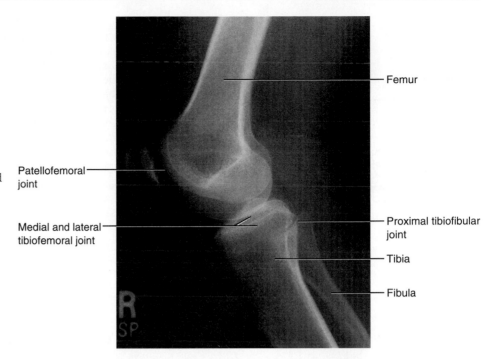

**FIGURE 13-1.** X-ray shows the bones and associated articulations of the knee.

Femur

Patellofemoral joint

Medial and lateral tibiofemoral joint

Proximal tibiofibular joint

Tibia

Fibula

---

forces, from both muscles and external sources. Injury to ligaments and to cartilage are two common consequences of the large functional demands placed on the knee. Knowledge of the anatomy and kinesiology of the knee is an essential prerequisite to the understanding of the mechanism of injury and the most effective therapeutic intervention.

## OSTEOLOGY

### Distal Femur

At the distal end of the femur are the large *lateral and medial condyles* (from the Greek *kondylos,* knuckle) (Figs. 13–2 to 13–4). *Lateral and medial epicondyles* project from each condyle, providing elevated attachment sites for the collateral ligaments. A large *intercondylar notch* separates the lateral and medial condyles, forming a passageway for the cruciate ligaments (Fig. 13–4). Interestingly, a narrower than average notch may increase the likelihood of injury to the anterior cruciate ligament.[106]

Articular cartilage covers much of the surface of the femoral condyle. The articular surface for the tibia follows a curve that is a flat-to-convex path from front to back (Fig. 13–5). The most distal end of each femoral condyle is nearly flat, thereby increasing the area for weight bearing.

*Lateral and medial grooves* are etched faintly in the cartilage of the femoral condyles (see Fig. 13–4). When the knee is fully extended, the anterior edge of the tibia is aligned with these grooves. The position of the grooves highlights the asymmetry in the shape of the medial and lateral articular surfaces of the femur. The medial surface curves slightly laterally from back to front, and extends farther anteriorly than the lateral articular surface. As explained later in this chapter, the asymmetry in shape of the condyles affects the sagittal plane kinematics.

| **Osteologic Features of the Distal Femur** |
| --- |
| • Lateral and medial condyles |
| • Lateral and medial epicondyles |
| • Intercondylar notch |
| • Lateral and medial grooves (etched in the cartilage of the femoral condyles) |
| • Intercondylar or trochlear groove |
| • Lateral and medial facets for the patella |

The femoral condyles fuse anteriorly to form the *intercondylar* (or *trochlear*) *groove* (see Fig. 13–4). This pulley-shaped structure articulates with the posterior side of the patella, forming the patellofemoral joint. The intercondylar groove is concave from side to side and slightly convex from front to back. The sloping sides of the groove form *lateral and medial facets.* The more pronounced lateral facet extends more proximally and projects farther anteriorly than the medial facet. The shape of the lateral facet helps to stabilize the patella within the groove during knee movement.

### Proximal Tibia and Fibula

The fibula is essentially a non-weight-bearing bone. Although it has no direct function at the knee, the slender bone splints the lateral side of the tibia and helps maintain its alignment.

The *head of the fibula* serves as an attachment for the biceps femoris and the lateral collateral ligament. The fibula is attached to the lateral side of the tibia by proximal and distal tibiofibular joints (see Fig. 13–2). The structure and function of these joints are discussed in Chapter 14.

## Anterior view

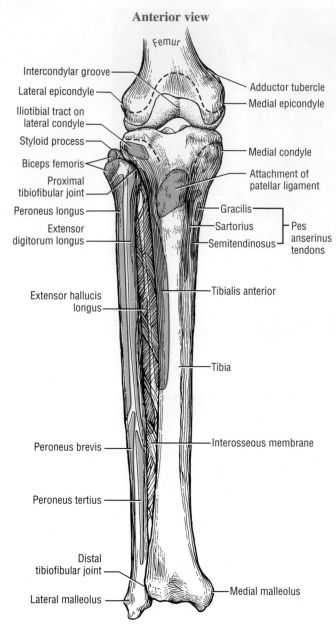

**FIGURE 13–2.** Anterior view of the right distal femur, the tibia, and the fibula. Proximal attachments of muscles are shown in red, distal attachments in gray. The dashed lines show the attachments of the capsule of the knee joint.

---

The primary function of the tibia is to transfer weight across the knee to the ankle. Its proximal end flares into *medial and lateral condyles,* which form articular surfaces with the distal femur (see Fig. 13–2). The superior surfaces of the condyles form a flat, broad region, often referred to as the tibial plateau. The plateau supports two smooth articular surfaces that accept the large femoral condyles, forming the tibiofemoral joints of the knee (see Fig. 13–4). The larger, medial articular surface is flat to slightly concave, whereas the lateral articular surface is flat to slightly convex. The articular surfaces are separated down the midline by an *in-*

## Posterior view

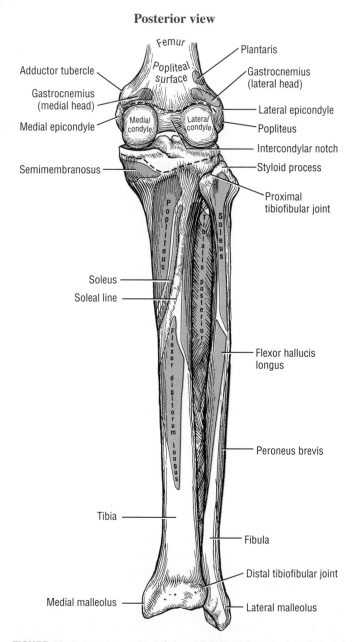

**FIGURE 13–3.** Posterior view of the right distal femur, the tibia, and the fibula. Proximal attachments of muscles are shown in red, distal attachments in gray. The dashed lines show the attachment of the joint capsule of the knee.

---

**Osteologic Features of the Proximal Tibia and Fibula**

*Proximal Fibula*
- Head

*Proximal Tibia*
- Medial and lateral condyles
- Intercondylar eminence
- Anterior intercondylar fossa
- Posterior intercondylar fossa
- Tibial tuberosity
- Soleal (popliteal) line

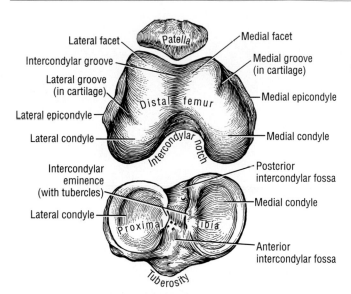

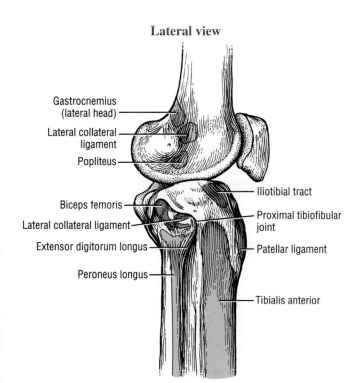

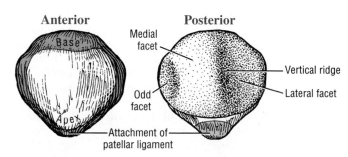

ity serves as the distal attachment for the quadriceps femoris muscle. On the posterior side of the proximal tibia is a roughened *soleal (popliteal) line,* coursing diagonally in a distal-to-medial direction (see Fig. 13–3).

## Patella

The patella (from the Latin, "small plate") is a nearly triangular-shaped bone embedded within the quadriceps tendon. It is the largest sesamoid bone in the body. The patella has a curved *base* superiorly and a pointed *apex* inferiorly (Figs. 13–6 and 13–7). In a relaxed standing position, the apex of the patella lies just proximal to the knee joint line. The subcutaneous *anterior surface* of the patella is convex in all directions. The base of the patella is rough due to the attachment of the quadriceps tendon. The patellar ligament attaches between the apex of the patella and the tibial tuberosity.

> **Osteologic Features of the Patella**
> - Base
> - Apex
> - Anterior surface
> - Posterior articular surface
> - Vertical ridge
> - Lateral, medial, and "odd" facets

The *posterior articular surface* of the patella is covered with articular cartilage up to 4 to 5 mm thick.[32] This surface contacts the intercondylar groove of the femur, forming the patellofemoral joint. The thick cartilage helps to disperse the large compression forces that cross the joint. A rounded *vertical ridge* runs longitudinally from top to bottom across the posterior surface of the patella. On either side of this ridge are lateral and medial facets. The larger and slightly concave *lateral facet* matches the general contour of the lateral facet of the intercondylar groove of the femur (see Fig. 13–4). The *medial facet* shows significant anatomic variation. A third *"odd"* facet exists along the extreme medial border of the medial facet.

**FIGURE 13–4.** Osteology of the right patella, articular surface of the distal femur and of the proximal tibia.

*tercondylar eminence* formed by medial and lateral tubercles. A shallow anterior and a posterior *intercondylar fossa* flank either side of the eminence. The cruciate ligaments and menisci attach along the intercondylar regions.

The prominent *tibial tuberosity* is located on the anterior surface of the proximal shaft of the tibia. The tibial tuberos-

**FIGURE 13–5.** Lateral view of the right knee. Proximal attachments of muscles and ligaments are shown in red, distal attachments in gray. Note the curved shape of the articular surface of the femoral condyles.

**FIGURE 13–6.** Anterior and posterior surfaces of the right patella. The attachment of the tendon of the quadriceps muscles is in gray; the proximal attachment of the patellar ligament is in red. Note the smooth articular cartilage covering the posterior articular surface of the patella.

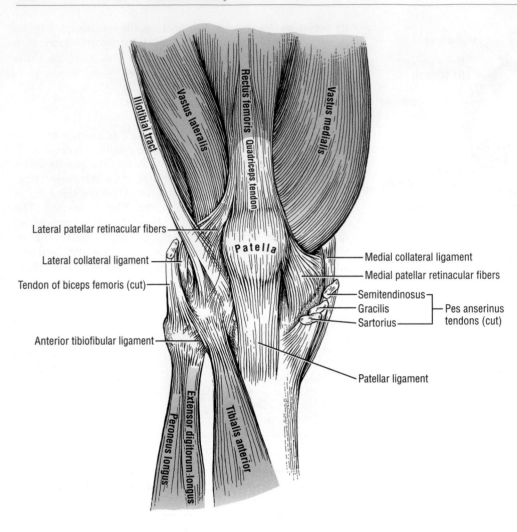

Lateral patellar retinacular fibers

Lateral collateral ligament

Tendon of biceps femoris (cut)

Anterior tibiofibular ligament

Iliotibial tract

Vastus lateralis

Rectus femoris

Quadriceps tendon

Vastus medialis

Patella

Medial collateral ligament

Medial patellar retinacular fibers

Semitendinosus

Gracilis

Sartorius

Pes anserinus tendons (cut)

Patellar ligament

Extensor digitorum longus

Peroneus longus

Tibialis anterior

**FIGURE 13–7.** Anterior view of the right knee, highlighting many muscles and connective tissues. The pes anserinus tendons are cut to expose the medial patellar retinaculum.

## ARTHROLOGY

### General Anatomic and Alignment Considerations

#### NORMAL ALIGNMENT OF THE KNEE

The shaft of the femur angles slightly medially as it descends toward the knee. This oblique orientation is due to the natural 125-degree angle of inclination of the proximal femur (Fig. 13–8A). Because the articular surface of the proximal tibia is oriented nearly horizontal, the knee forms an angle on its lateral side of about 170 to 175 degrees. This normal alignment of the knee within the frontal plane is referred to as *genu valgum*.

Variation in normal frontal plane alignment at the knee is not uncommon. A lateral angle less than 170 degrees is called *excessive genu valgum,* or "knock-knee" (Fig. 13–8B). In contrast, a lateral angle that exceeds about 180 degrees is called *genu varum,* or "bow-leg" (Fig. 13–8C).

The longitudinal or vertical axis of rotation at the hip is defined in Chapter 12 as a line connecting the femoral head with the center of the knee joint. As depicted in Figure 13–

8A, this longitudinal axis can be extended inferiorly through the knee to the ankle and foot. The axis mechanically links the horizontal plane movements of the major joints of the entire lower limb. Horizontal plane rotations that occur in the hip, for example, affect the posture of the joints as far distal as those in the foot. This topic is developed further in Chapter 14.

### Capsule and Related Structures

The fibrous capsule of the knee encloses the medial and lateral tibiofemoral joints and the patellofemoral joint. The proximal and distal attachments of the capsule to bone are indicated by the dotted lines in Figures 13–2 and 13–3. The capsule of the knee receives significant reinforcement from muscles, ligaments, and fascia. Five reinforced regions of the capsule are described next and summarized in Table 13–1.

The *anterior capsule* of the knee attaches to the margins of the patella and the patellar ligament, being reinforced by the quadriceps muscle and *patellar retinacular fibers*. The retinacular fibers are extensions of the connective tissue covering the vastus lateralis, vastus medialis, and iliotibial tract (see Fig. 13–7). This extensive set of netlike fibers connects the femur, tibia, patella, patellar ligament, collateral ligaments, and menisci.

The *lateral capsule* of the knee is reinforced by the lateral (fibular) collateral ligament, lateral patellar retinacular fibers,

### Normal genu valgum

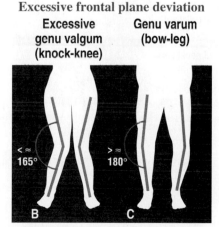

**FIGURE 13–8.** Frontal plane deviations of the knee. *A,* Normal genu valgum. The normal 125-degree angle of inclination of the proximal femur and the longitudinal axis of rotation throughout the entire lower extremity are also shown. *B* and *C* illustrate excessive frontal plane deviations.

and iliotibial tract (Fig. 13–9). Muscular stability is provided by the biceps femoris, the tendon of the popliteus, and the lateral head of the gastrocnemius.

The *posterior capsule* is reinforced by the oblique popliteal ligament and the arcuate popliteal ligament (Fig. 13–10). The *oblique popliteal ligament* spans between the semimembranosus tendon—from which much of the ligament originates—and the lateral femoral condyle. This ligament is pulled taut in full knee extension, when the tibia is rotated externally relative to the femur. The *arcuate popliteal ligament* originates from the fibular head, then divides into two limbs. The larger and more prominent limb arches across the tendon of the popliteus muscle to attach to the posterior intercondylar area of the tibia. An inconsistent and smaller limb attaches to the posterior side of the lateral femoral condyle, and often to a sesamoid bone (or *flabella,* meaning "bean") imbedded within the lateral head of the gastrocnemius. The posterior capsule is further reinforced by the popliteus, gastrocnemius, and hamstring muscles, especially by the fibrous extensions of the semimembranosus tendon. Unlike the elbow, the knee has no bony block against hyperextension. The muscles and posterior capsule limit hyperextension.

The *posterior-lateral capsule* of the knee is reinforced by the arcuate popliteal ligament, lateral collateral ligament, and popliteus muscle and tendon. This set of tissues is often referred to as the arcuate complex.

The *medial capsule* of the knee is very extensive, covering the entire posterior-medial to anterior-medial region of the knee.[109] The capsule is reinforced by the medial collateral ligament and medial patellar retinacular fibers, and by the expansions from the tendon of the semimembranosus (Fig. 13–11). The medial capsule is further reinforced by the flat tendons of the sartorius, gracilis, and semitendinosus—collectively referred to as the pes anserinus (from the Latin, "goose's foot") tendons. The medial capsule and associated structures provide stabilization to the knee.

### SYNOVIAL MEMBRANE AND ASSOCIATED STRUCTURES

#### *Bursae, Fat Pads, and Plicae*

The internal surface of the capsule of the knee is lined with a synovial membrane. The anatomic organization of this membrane is the most complex and extensive in the body.[120] The complexity is due in part to the convoluted embryonic development of the knee.[71]

The knee has as many as 14 bursae, which form at intertissue junctions that encounter high friction during movement.[120] These intertissue junctions involve tendon, ligament, skin, bone, capsule, and muscle (Table 13–2). Although some bursae are simply extensions of the synovial membrane, others are formed external to the capsule. Activities that involve excessive and repetitive forces at these intertissue junctions frequently lead to bursitis, an inflammation of the bursa.

Fat pads are often associated with bursae around the knee. Fat and synovial fluid reduce friction between moving parts. At the knee, the most extensive fat pads are associated with the suprapatellar and deep infrapatellar bursae.

**TABLE 13-1. Ligaments, Fascia, and Muscles That Reinforce the Capsule of the Knee**

| Region of the Capsule | Connective Tissue Reinforcement | Muscular-Tendinous Reinforcement |
|---|---|---|
| Anterior | Patellar ligament<br>Patellar retinacular fibers | Quadriceps |
| Lateral | Lateral collateral ligament<br>Lateral patellar retinacular fibers<br>Iliotibial tract | Biceps femoris<br>Tendon of the popliteus<br>Lateral head of the gastrocnemius |
| Posterior | Oblique popliteal ligament<br>Arcuate popliteal ligament | Popliteus<br>Gastrocnemius<br>Hamstrings |
| Posterior-lateral | Arcuate popliteal ligament<br>Lateral collateral ligament | Tendon of the popliteus |
| Medial | Medial collateral ligament<br>Medial patellar retinacular fibers | Expansions from the tendon of the semimembranosus<br>Tendons of the sartorius, gracilis, and semitendinosus |

## Tibiofemoral Joint

### ARTICULAR STRUCTURE

#### Bony Fit

The medial and lateral tibiofemoral joint consists of the articulations between the large, convex femoral condyles and the nearly flat and smaller tibial condyles. The large surface area of the femoral condyles permits extensive knee motion in the sagittal plane for activities such as running, squatting, and climbing. Joint stability is provided not by a tight congruous bony fit, but by forces and physical containment provided by muscles, ligaments, capsule, menisci, and body weight.

#### Menisci

##### Anatomic Considerations

The medial and lateral menisci are crescent-shaped, fibrocartilaginous discs located within the knee joint (Fig. 13–12A and B). The menisci transform nearly flat articular surfaces of the tibia into shallow seats for the femoral condyles.

The menisci are anchored to the intercondylar region of the tibia by their *anterior and posterior horns*. The external edge of each meniscus is attached to the tibia and the adjacent capsule by *coronary* (or *meniscotibial*) *ligaments* (see Fig. 13–12A). The coronary ligaments are relatively loose, thereby allowing the menisci, especially the lateral, to pivot freely during movement. A slender *transverse ligament* connects the two menisci anteriorly.

Several muscles have secondary attachments into the menisci. The quadriceps and semimembranosus attach to both menisci.[67] The popliteus attaches to the lateral meniscus. Through these attachments, the muscles help stabilize the position of the menisci during active knee movement.

Blood supply to the menisci is greatest near the peripheral (external) border. Blood comes from capillaries located within the adjacent synovial membrane and capsule.[18] The internal border of the menisci, in contrast, is essentially avascular. The menisci are essentially aneural, except near their horns.

The two menisci have different shapes and methods of

attaching to the tibia. The medial meniscus has an oval or C shape, with its external border attaching to the deep surface of the medial collateral ligament and adjacent capsule; the lateral meniscus has a circular or O shape, with its external

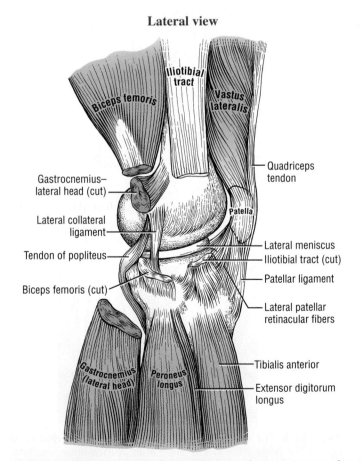

**Lateral view**

**FIGURE 13–9.** Lateral view of the right knee shows many muscles and connective tissues. The iliotibial tract, lateral head of the gastrocnemius, and biceps femoris are cut to better expose the lateral collateral ligament, popliteus tendon, and lateral meniscus.

**Posterior view**

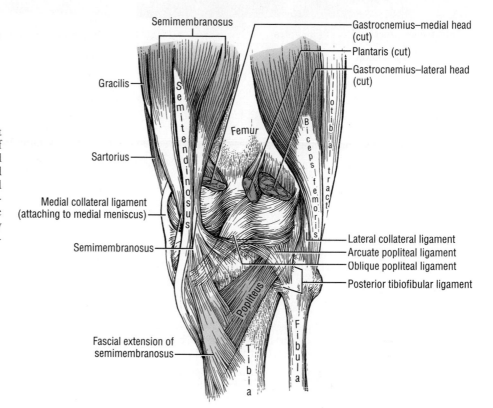

FIGURE 13–10. Posterior view of the right knee that emphasizes the major parts of the posterior capsule: the oblique popliteal and arcuate popliteal ligaments. The lateral and medial heads of the gastrocnemius and plantaris muscles are cut to expose the posterior capsule. Observe the popliteus muscle deep in the popliteal fossa, lying partially covered by the fascial extension of the semi-membranosus.

**Medial view**

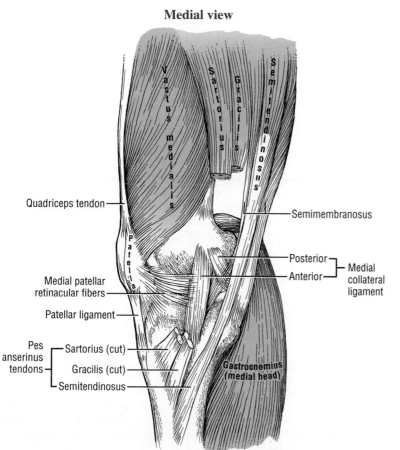

FIGURE 13–11. Medial view of the right knee shows many muscles and connective tissues. The tendons of the sartorius and gracilis are cut to better expose the anterior and posterior parts of the medial collateral ligament.

## TABLE 13-2. Examples of Bursae at Various Intertissue Junctions

| Intertissue Junction | Examples |
| --- | --- |
| Ligament and tendon | Bursa between the lateral collateral ligament and tendon of the biceps femoris |
| | Bursa between the medial collateral ligament and tendons of the pes anserinus (i.e., gracilis, semitendinosus, and sartorius) |
| Muscle and capsule | Unnamed bursa between the medial head of the gastrocnemius and the medial side of the capsule |
| Bone and skin | *Subcutaneous prepatellar bursa* between the inferior border of the patella and the skin |
| Tendon and bone | *Semimembranosus bursa* between the tendon of the semimembranosus and medial condyle of the tibia |
| Bone and muscle | *Suprapatellar bursa* between the femur and the quadriceps femoris (largest of the knee) |
| Bone and ligament | *Deep infrapatellar bursa* between the tibia and patellar ligament |

## SPECIAL FOCUS 13-1

### Development and Function of Plicae

During embryonic development, the knee experiences significant physical transformation. Mesenchymal tissues thicken and then reabsorb, forming primitive compartments, ligaments, and menisci. Incomplete resorption of mesenchymal tissue during development forms tissues known as *plicae*.[23] Plicae, or synovial pleats, appear as folds in the synovial membranes. Plicae may be very small and unrecognizable, or so large that they nearly separate the knee into medial and lateral compartments. Plicae reinforce the synovial membrane of the knee.

Three plicae in the knee are the (1) superior or suprapatellar plica, (2) inferior plica (first called ligamentum mucosum by Vesalius in 1515),[23] and (3) medial plica. The most prominent medial plica is known by about 20 names, including alar ligament, synovialis patellaris, and intraarticular medial band. Plicae exist in approximately 25 to 50% of knees.

Plicae that are unusually large, or are thickened owing to irritation or trauma, cause knee pain. The medial plica is most commonly involved with a painful plica syndrome. Treatment includes rest, anti-inflammatory medication, isometric exercise, and arthroscopy resection.

---

border attaching only to the lateral capsule (Fig. 13–13). The tendon of the popliteus passes between the lateral collateral ligament and the external border of the lateral meniscus.

### Ligaments Associated with the Menisci
- Coronary (meniscotibial) ligaments
- Transverse ligament
- Posterior meniscofemoral ligament

The lateral meniscus also attaches to the femur via the *posterior meniscofemoral ligament* (see Figs. 13–12A and 13–13). The ligament arises from the posterior horn of the lateral meniscus and attaches to the femur along with the posterior cruciate ligament. This and other meniscofemoral ligaments are sometimes the only bony attachment made by the posterior horn of the lateral meniscus.[120]

### Functional Considerations
The primary function of the menisci is to reduce the compressive stress at the tibiofemoral joint. Other functions include stabilizing the joint during motion, lubricating the articular cartilage, reducing the friction, and guiding the knee's arthrokinematics. The following section

describes the role of the menisci in transferring loads across the knee.

**Menisci as Shock Absorbers.** While walking, compression forces at the knee joint routinely reach approximately 2 to 3 times body weight. Forces as high as nine times body weight may occur during maximal-effort isokinetic knee extension.[88] By nearly tripling the area of joint contact, the menisci significantly reduce pressure (i.e., force per unit area) on the articular cartilage.[103] A complete lateral meniscectomy increases the peak contact pressures by 230%,[91] which likely increases the risk of developing stress-related arthritis. Surgically repairing a meniscus instead of removing it is clearly the treatment of choice.[102]

The menisci support about half the total load across the knee.[68] At every step, the menisci deform peripherally as they are compressed.[108] This mechanism allows part of the compression force at the knee to be absorbed as a circumferential tension throughout each meniscus. A torn meniscus therefore loses its capacity to absorb loads.

## Osteokinematics at the Tibiofemoral Joint

The tibiofemoral joint possesses two degrees of freedom: flexion and extension in the sagittal plane and, provided the knee is slightly flexed, internal and external rotation in the horizontal plane. These motions are shown for both *tibial-on-*

**Superior view**

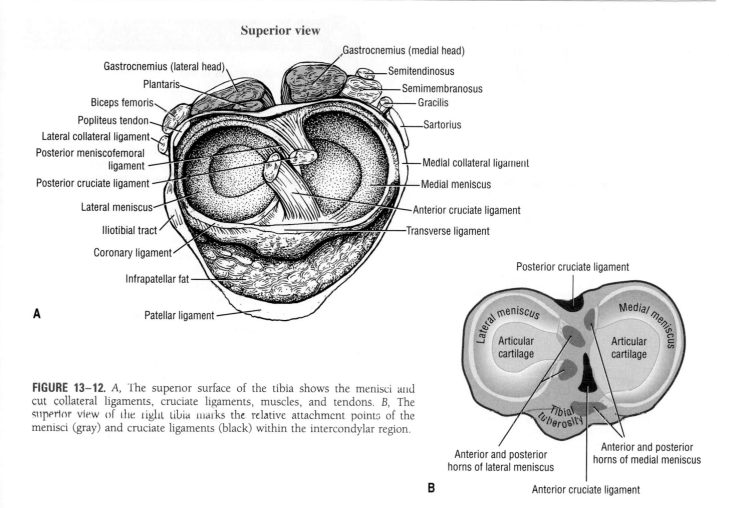

**FIGURE 13–12.** *A,* The superior surface of the tibia shows the menisci and cut collateral ligaments, cruciate ligaments, muscles, and tendons. *B,* The superior view of the right tibia marks the relative attachment points of the menisci (gray) and cruciate ligaments (black) within the intercondylar region.

*femoral* and *femoral-on-tibial* situations in Figures 13–14 and 13–15. Frontal plane motion at the knee occurs passively only, limited to about 6 to 7 degrees.[81]

## FLEXION AND EXTENSION

Flexion and extension at the knee occur about a medial-lateral axis of rotation. Range of motion varies with age and gender, but in general the healthy knee rotates from 130 to 140 degrees of flexion to about 5 to 10 degrees of hyperextension.[7,101]

The medial-lateral axis of rotation for flexion and extension is not fixed, but migrates within the femoral condyles. The curved path of the axis is known as an "evolute," or instant center of rotation (Fig. 13–16).[111] The path of the axis is influenced by the eccentric curvature of the femoral condyles.[30,50,110]

The migrating axis of rotation has biomechanical and clinical implications. First, the migrating axis alters the length of the internal moment arm of the flexor and extensor muscles. This fact explains, in part, why maximal-effort internal torque varies across the range of motion. Second, many external devices that attach to the knee, such as a goniometer or a hinged knee orthosis, rotate about a fixed axis of rotation. During knee motion, therefore, the external devices may rotate in a dissimilar plane as the leg. As a consequence, a hinged orthosis, for example, may act as a piston relative to the leg, causing rubbing against and abrasion to the skin.

## INTERNAL AND EXTERNAL ROTATION

Internal and external rotation of the knee occurs in a horizontal plane about a vertical or longitudinal axis of rotation. This motion is also called "axial" rotation. In general, horizontal plane rotation increases with greater knee flexion. A knee flexed to 90 degrees permits about 40 to 50 degrees of total rotation.[86,89] External rotation range of motion generally exceeds internal rotation by a ratio of 2:1.[86] In full extension, however, horizontal plane rotation is essentially absent. Rotation is blocked by passive tension in the stretched ligaments and by increased bony congruity within the joint.

As depicted in Figure 13–15, horizontal plane rotation at the knee occurs by either tibial-on-femoral or femoral-on-tibial rotation. Both forms of rotation provide a functional and very important element of mobility to movement of the lower extremity as a whole. Consider, for

**Posterior view**

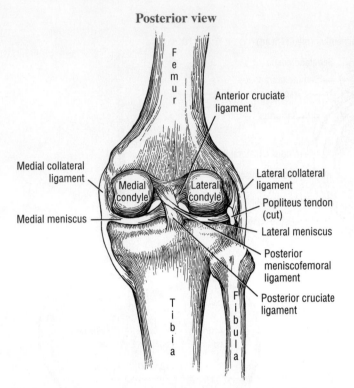

**FIGURE 13–13.** Posterior view of the deep structures of the right knee after all muscles and the posterior capsule are removed. Observe the menisci, collateral ligaments, and cruciate ligaments. Note the popliteus tendon that courses between the lateral meniscus and lateral collateral ligament.

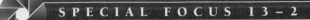

### SPECIAL FOCUS 13-2

**Common Mechanism of Injury of the Menisci of the Knee**

Tears of the meniscus often occur by forceful, horizontal plane rotation of the femoral condyles over a partially flexed and weight-bearing knee. The torsion within the compressed knee can pinch and dislodge the meniscus. A dislodged or folded flap of meniscus can block knee movement, causing the "locked-knee" syndrome.

The medial meniscus is injured more frequently than the lateral meniscus. The mechanism of injury often involves an external force applied to the lateral aspect of the knee. This force—often described as a "valgus force"—causes an excessive valgus position of the knee and subsequently strains the medial collateral ligament. The medial meniscus may tear as it is stretched between the compressed joint surfaces and its connection to the taut medial collateral ligament.

example, a sharp 90-degree "cutting" maneuver used to change directions while running. The trunk and pelvis rotate over the femur, as the femur rotates over the tibia. Chapter 14 describes how the tibia rotates over the relatively fixed foot.

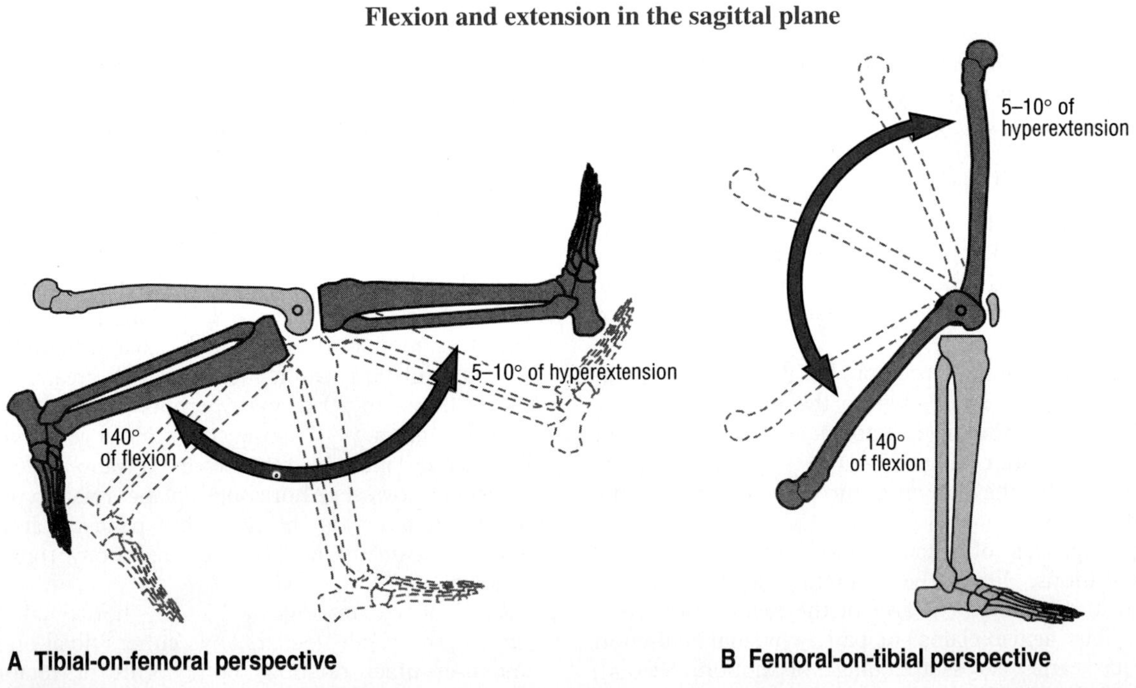

**Flexion and extension in the sagittal plane**

**A  Tibial-on-femoral perspective**

**B  Femoral-on-tibial perspective**

**FIGURE 13–14.** Sagittal plane motion at the knee. *A,* Tibial-on-femoral perspective. *B,* Femoral-on-tibial perspective.

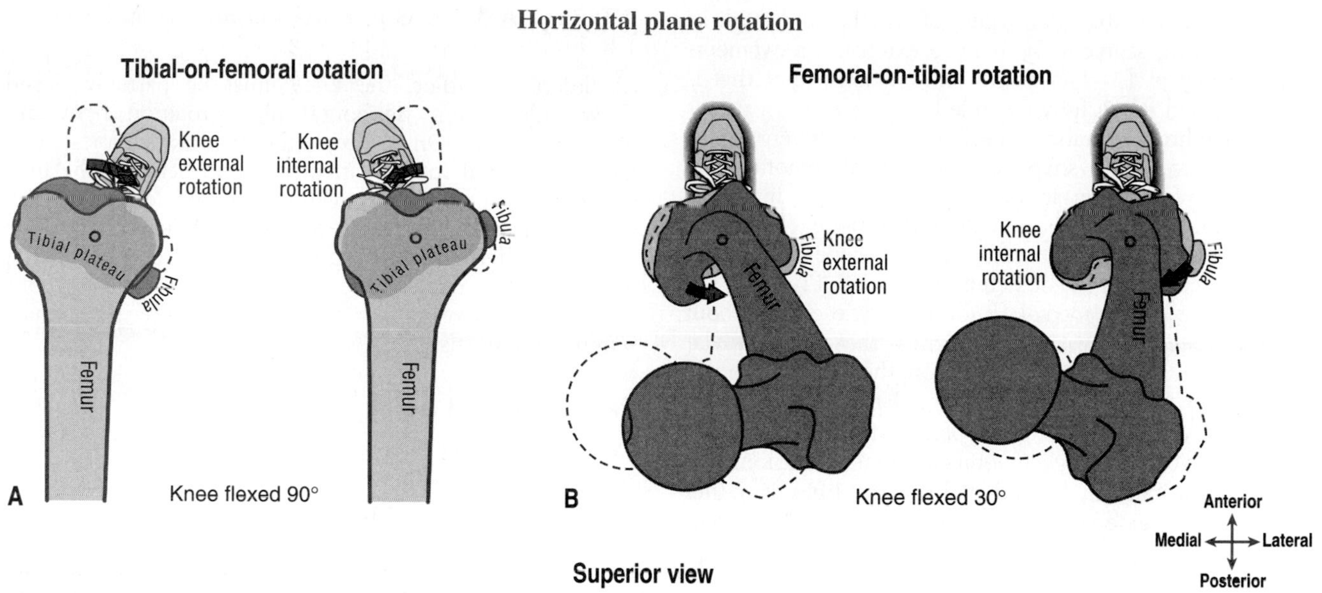

**Horizontal plane rotation**

**Tibial-on-femoral rotation**

Knee external rotation

Knee internal rotation

Tibial plateau

Fibula

Femur

**A**      Knee flexed 90°

**Femoral-on-tibial rotation**

Knee external rotation

Knee internal rotation

Fibula

Femur

**B**      Knee flexed 30°

Anterior
Medial ←→ Lateral
Posterior

**Superior view**

**FIGURE 13–15.** Horizontal plane (axial) rotation at the knee. *A,* Tibial-on-femoral rotation. *B,* Femoral-on-tibial rotation.

## Arthrokinematics at the Tibiofemoral Joint

### ACTIVE EXTENSION OF THE KNEE

Figure 13–17 depicts the arthrokinematics of the last 90 degrees of active knee extension. During *tibial-on-femoral extension,* the articular surface of the tibia rolls and slides anteriorly on the femoral condyles (Fig. 13–17A). The menisci are shown pulled anteriorly by the contracting quadriceps muscle.

During *femoral-on-tibial extension,* as in standing up from a deep squat position, the femoral condyles simultaneously roll anteriorly and slide posteriorly on the articular surface of the tibia (Fig. 13–17B). These "off-setting" arthrokinematics may help limit the magnitude of anterior translation of the femur on the tibia. The quadriceps direct the roll of the femoral condyles. The quadriceps also stabilize the menisci against the posterior shear caused by the sliding femur.

### *"Screw-Home" Rotation of the Knee*

Locking the knee in full extension requires about 10 degrees of external rotation.[59] The rotary locking action is called *"screw-home" rotation,* based on the observable twisting of the knee during the last 30 degrees of extension. External rotation is different from the axial rotation illustrated in Figure 13–15. Screw-home rotation has been kinematically described as a "conjunct rotation."[120] This type of rotation is mechanically linked to the flexion and extension kinematics and cannot be performed independently.

To observe the screw-home rotation at the knee, have a partner sit with the knee flexed to about 90 degrees. Draw a line on the skin between the tibial tuberosity and the apex of the patella. After completing full tibial-on-femoral extension, redraw this line between the same landmarks and note the change in position of the externally rotated tibia. A

similar but less obvious locking mechanism also takes place during femoral-on-tibial extension (compare Fig. 13–17A with B). Rising up from a squat position, for example, the knee locks into extension as the femur internally rotates

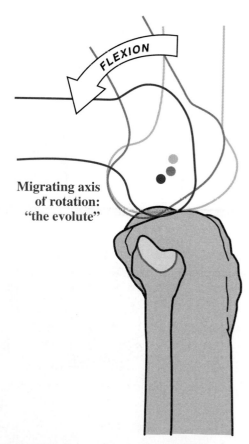

FLEXION

**Migrating axis of rotation: "the evolute"**

**FIGURE 13–16.** The flexing knee generates a migrating medial-lateral axis of rotation. This migration is described as "the evolute."

relative to the fixed tibia. Regardless of whether the thigh or leg is the moving segment, both knee extension movements depicted in Figure 13–17A and B show a knee joint that is externally rotated when fully extended.

The screw-home rotation mechanics are driven by at least three factors: the shape of the medial femoral condyle, the passive tension in the anterior cruciate ligament, and the lateral pull of the quadriceps muscle (Fig. 13–18).[33,99] The most important factor is the shape of the medial femoral condyle. As depicted in Figure 13–18B, the articular surface of the medial femoral condyle curves about 30 degrees laterally, as it approaches the intercondylar groove. Because the articular surface on the medial condyle extends farther anteriorly than on the lateral condyle, the tibia "follows" this laterally curved path during full tibial-on-femoral extension. During femoral-on-tibial extension, the femur follows a medially curved path on the tibia. In either case, the result is external rotation of the knee at full extension.

## ACTIVE FLEXION OF THE KNEE

The arthrokinematics of active knee flexion occur by a reverse fashion depicted in Figure 13–17A and B. To unlock a knee that is fully extended, the joint must first internally rotate. This action is driven primarily by the popliteus muscle. The muscle can rotate the femur externally to initiate femoral-on-tibial flexion, or rotate the tibia internally to initiate tibial-on-femoral flexion.

## INTERNAL AND EXTERNAL (AXIAL) ROTATION OF THE KNEE

As described earlier, the knee must be partially flexed to allow independent horizontal plane rotation between the tibia and femur. Once flexed, the arthrokinematics of internal and external rotation involve a spin between the menisci and the articular surfaces of the tibia and femur. Horizontal plane rotation of the femur over the tibia causes the menisci to deform slightly, as they are compressed between the spinning femoral condyles. The menisci are stabilized by connections from active musculature such as the popliteus and semimembranosus.

## Patellofemoral Joint

The patellofemoral joint is the interface between the articular side of the patella and the intercondylar groove on the femur. The quadriceps muscle, the articular joint surfaces, and the retinacular fibers stabilize the joint (see Fig. 13–7). As the knee flexes and extends, the articular surface of the patella slides over the intercondylar groove of the femur. During tibial-on-femoral flexion, the patella slides against the femur; during femoral-on-tibial flexion, the femur slides against the patella.

### PATELLOFEMORAL JOINT KINEMATICS

#### *Path and Area of Patellar Contact on the Femur*

Studies on cadavers have provided detailed descriptions of the regions of joint contact and pressure in the patellofemo-

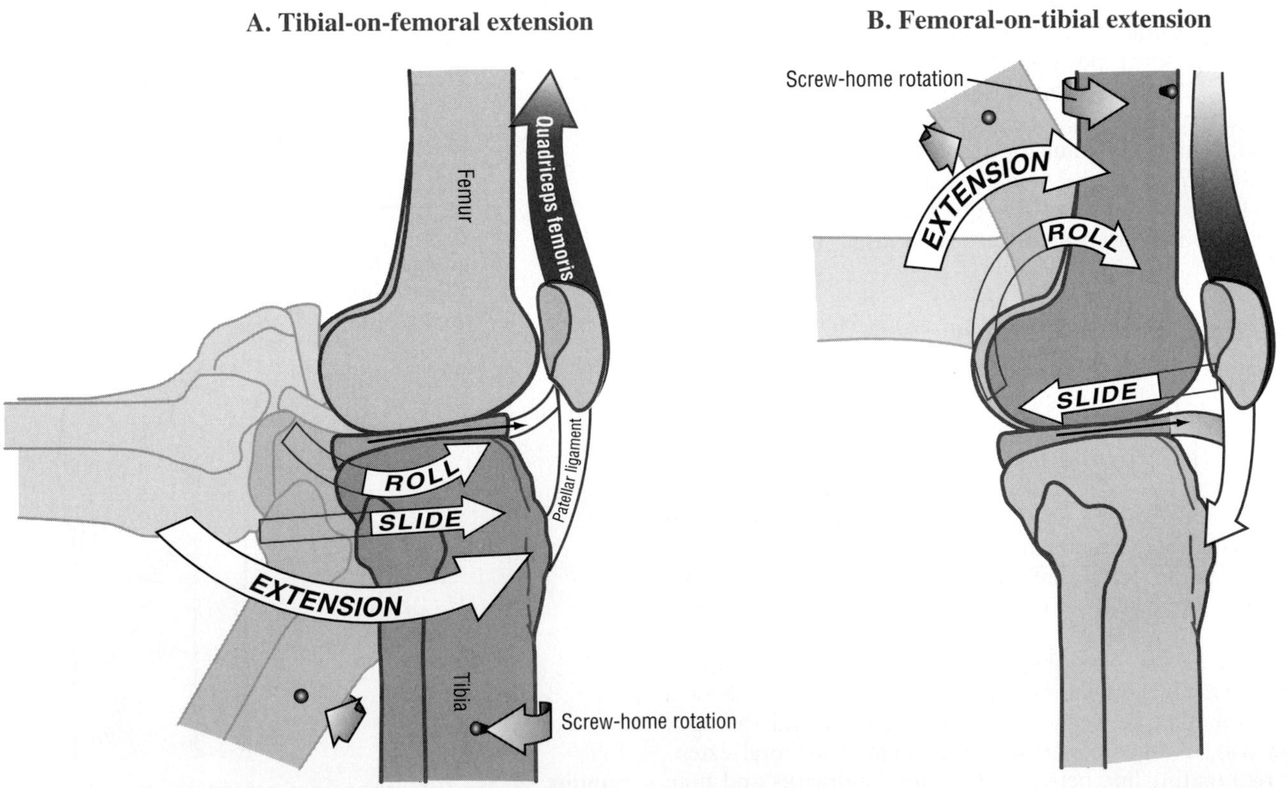

**FIGURE 13–17.** The active arthrokinematics of knee extension. *A*, Tibial-on-femoral perspective. *B*, Femoral-on-tibial perspective. In both *A* and *B*, the meniscus is pulled toward the contracting quadriceps.

## A. Factors guiding "screw-home" rotation

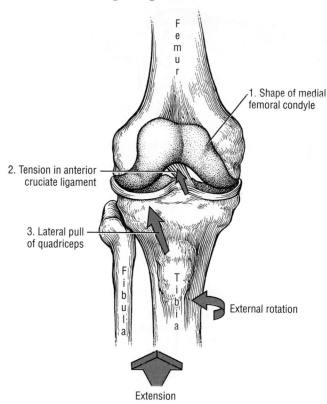

1. Shape of medial femoral condyle

2. Tension in anterior cruciate ligament

3. Lateral pull of quadriceps

External rotation

Extension

## B. Path of the tibia on the femoral condyles

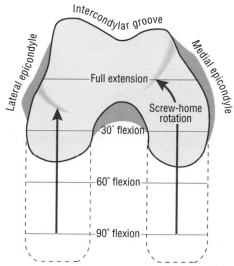

Intercondylar groove

Lateral epicondyle

Medial epicondyle

Full extension

Screw-home rotation

30° flexion

60° flexion

90° flexion

**FIGURE 13–18.** The "screw-home" locking mechanism of the knee. *A,* During terminal tibial-on-femoral extension, three factors contribute to the locking mechanism of the knee. Each factor contributes bias to external rotation of the tibia, relative to the femur. *B,* The two red arrows depict the path of the tibia across the femoral condyles during the last 90 degrees of extension. Note that the curved medial femoral condyle helps to direct the tibia to its externally rotated and locked position.

ral joint.[37,56,82] Data from these studies and cineradiographic observations were used to construct the model illustrated in Figure 13–19. At 135 degrees of flexion, the patella contacts the femur near its superior pole (Fig. 13–19A). At this flexed position, the patella rests below the intercondylar groove, bridging the intercondylar notch of the femur (Fig. 13–19D). At this position, the lateral edge of the lateral facet and the "odd" facet of the patella share articular contact with the femur (Fig. 13–19E). As the knee extends toward 90 degrees of flexion, the contact region on the patella starts to migrate inferiorly (Fig. 13–19B). Between 90 and 60 degrees of flexion, the patellofemoral joint occupies its greatest contact area with the femur (Fig. 13–19D, E).[82] At its maximum, this contact area is only about 30% of the total surface area of the patella. Joint pressure (i.e., compression force per unit area), therefore, can rise to significant levels within the patellofemoral joint.

As the knee extends through the last 20 degrees of flexion, the primary contact point on the patella migrates to the inferior pole (Fig. 13–19C). In full extension the patella rests completely above the intercondylar groove, against the suprapatellar fat pad. In this position with quadriceps relaxed, the patella can be moved freely within the intercondylar groove. Flexing the knee to about 20 or 30 degrees, however, reduces this mobility. The patella becomes seated in the intercondylar groove and stabilized by tension in the stretched quadriceps and local connective tissues.

## Collateral Ligaments

### ANATOMIC CONSIDERATIONS

The *medial collateral ligament* (MCL) is a flat, broad structure that spans the medial side of the joint (see Fig. 13–11). Several structures blend with and reinforce the MCL, most notably the medial patellar retinacular fibers and medial capsule.

The MCL consists of anterior and posterior parts. The larger *anterior part* consists of a relatively well-defined set of superficial fibers about 10 cm long. Distally these fibers blend with medial patellar retinacular fibers before attaching to the medial-proximal aspect of the tibia. The fibers' attachments are just posterior to the attachments of the pes anserinus group. From proximal to distal, the anterior part of the MCL runs in a slightly oblique posterior-to-anterior direction.

The *posterior part* of the MCL consists of a short set of fibers, deep to the anterior fibers. These fibers have extensive distal attachments to the posterior-medial joint capsule, medial meniscus, and thick tendon of the semimembranosus muscle.

The *lateral (fibular) collateral ligament* consists of a round, strong cord that runs nearly vertical between the lateral epicondyle of the femur to the head of the fibula (see Fig. 13–9). Distally, the lateral collateral ligament blends with the tendon of the biceps femoris muscle. Unlike its medial counterpart, the MCL, the lateral collateral ligament does not attach to the adjacent meniscus (see Fig. 13–13).

### FUNCTIONAL CONSIDERATIONS

The primary function of the collateral ligaments is to limit excessive motion in the frontal plane. With the knee ex-

**A. Knee flexed 135°**     **B. Knee flexed 90°**     **C. Knee flexed 20°**

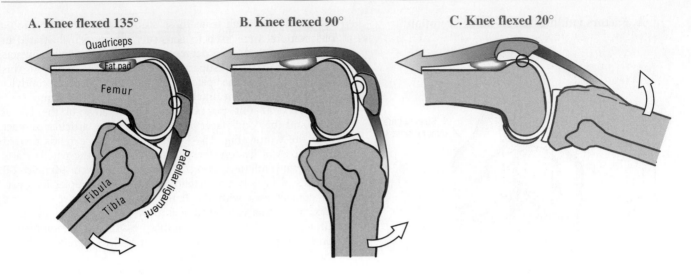

**D. Path of sliding patella on the femur**     **E. Posterior articular surface of patella**

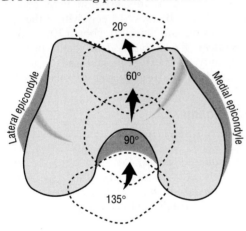

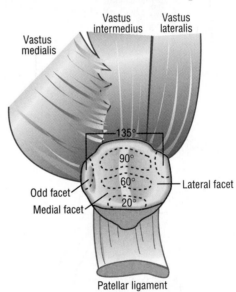

**FIGURE 13–19.** The kinematics at the patellofemoral joint during active tibial-on-femoral extension. The circle depicted in *A–C* indicates the point of maximal contact between the patella and the femur. As the knee is extended, the contact point on the patella migrates from its superior pole to its inferior pole. Note the suprapatellar fat pad deep to the quadriceps. *D* and *E* show the path and contact areas of the patella on the intercondylar groove of the femur. The values 135, 90, 60, and 20 degrees indicate flexed positions of the knee.

tended, the anterior part of the MCL provides the primary resistance against a valgus, or an abduction, stress. The lateral collateral ligament, in comparison, provides the primary resistance against a varus, or an adduction, stress.[104] Many other tissues provide varying amounts of restraint to valgus and varus forces applied to the knee (Table 13–3).[104,118]

A secondary function of the collateral ligaments is to limit the extremes of knee extension. This function is shared, however, by the posterior capsule, oblique popliteal ligament, knee flexor muscles, and anterior cruciate ligament. Figure 13–20*A* and *B* demonstrates the increase in passive tension in both MCL and posterior capsule, as the knee assumes the locked position of full femoral-on-tibial ex-

sion. In flexion, the capsule and ligaments are relatively slack (see Fig. 13–20*A*). Full extension—which includes the screw-home rotation—elongates the collateral ligaments roughly 20% beyond their length at full flexion.[118] Although a valuable stabilizer, a taut MCL is especially vulnerable to injury from a valgus (i.e., an abduction) stress delivered over a planted foot. This mechanism of injury is part of the classic "clip" in football.

The collateral ligaments also provide limited resistance to the extremes of internal and external rotation while the knee is partially flexed.[118] Table 13–4 provides a summary of the functions and common mechanisms of injury for the major ligaments of the knee, including the posterior capsule.

**TABLE 13-3.** **Tissues That Provide Primary and Secondary Restraint to the Knee***

|  | Valgus Force | Varus Force |
| --- | --- | --- |
| Primary restraint | Medial collateral ligament, especially the anterior fibers | Lateral collateral ligament |
| Secondary restraint | Medial capsule<br>Posterior-medial capsule (includes semimembranosus tendon)<br>Anterior and posterior cruciate ligaments<br>Bony contact laterally<br>Compression of the lateral meniscus<br>Medial retinacular fibers<br>Pes anserinus (i.e., tendons of the sartorius, gracilis, and semitendinosus)<br>Gastrocnemius (medial head) | Arcuate complex (includes lateral collateral ligament, posterior-lateral capsule, popliteus tendon, and arcuate popliteal ligament)<br>Iliotibial tract<br>Biceps femoris tendon<br>Bony contact medially<br>Compression of the medial meniscus<br>Anterior and posterior cruciate ligaments<br>Gastrocnemius (lateral head) |

*Assume a fully extended knee.

## Anterior and Posterior Cruciate Ligaments

### GENERAL CONSIDERATIONS

Cruciate, meaning cross-shaped, describes the spatial relation of the ligaments as they cross within the intercondylar notch of the femur (Fig. 13–21A and B). The cruciate ligaments are intracapsular structures that are covered by an extensive synovial lining. Since most of the surface of the ligaments lies between the synovial membrane and the capsule, the cruciates are considered "extrasynovial." The ligaments are supplied with blood from small vessels in the synovial membrane and nearby soft tissue.

The cruciate ligaments are named according to their attachment to the tibia (see Fig. 13–12A and B). Both ligaments are thick and strong, reflecting their important role in providing stability to the knee. Acting together, the anterior and posterior cruciate ligaments resist the extremes of all knee motions (see Table 13–4). The cruciate ligaments, however, provide most of the resistance to *anterior-posterior shear forces* between the tibia and femur. These forces arise primarily from the sagittal plane progression intrinsic to walking, squatting, running, and jumping.[17] The ligaments help to guide the arthrokinematics at the knee.

Injury to the cruciate ligaments can lead to marked instability of the knee. Because the cruciates do not spontaneously heal on their own, surgical reconstruction often requires autograft (patellar tendon or hamstring/adductor tendon), and less frequently, an allograft (artificial ligament). Although these reconstructions are reasonably successful at restoring basic stability, the natural kinematics at the repaired knee are never completely normal. A retrospective review of the literature suggests that the likelihood of gonarthrosis (or arthrosis) of the knee increases significantly following injury to the anterior cruciate ligament.[35]

**A. Ligaments slack in flexion**

**B. Ligaments pulled taut in extension**

**FIGURE 13–20.** Medial view of the knee shows the elongation of the medial collateral ligament and the posterior capsule and oblique popliteal ligament during active femoral-on-tibial extension. *A*, In knee flexion, the medial collateral ligament, oblique popliteal ligament, and posterior capsule are relatively slackened. *B*, The structures are pulled taut as the knee actively extends by contraction of the quadriceps. Note the "screw-home" rotation of the knee during end-range extension.

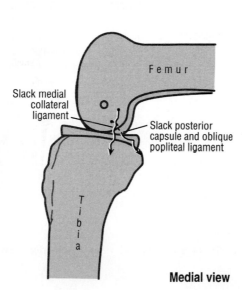
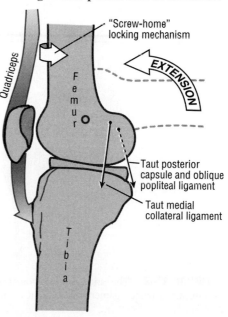

**Medial view**

**TABLE 13–4. Function of Ligaments at the Knee and Common Mechanisms of Injury**

| Structure | Function(s) | Common Mechanisms of Injury |
|---|---|---|
| Medial collateral ligament | 1. Resists valgus (abduction)<br>2. Resists excessive knee extension<br>3. Resists axial rotation | 1. Valgus force with foot planted (e.g., "clip" in football)<br>2. Severe hyperextension of the knee |
| Lateral collateral ligament | 1. Resists varus (adduction)<br>2. Resists knee extension<br>3. Resists axial rotation | 1. Varus force with foot planted<br>2. Severe hyperextension of the knee |
| Posterior capsule | 1. Resists full knee extension<br>2. Oblique popliteal ligament resists external rotation<br>3. Posterior-lateral capsule resists varus | 1. Hyperextension or combined hyperextension with external rotation of the knee |
| Anterior cruciate ligament | 1. Most fibers resist excessive anterior translation of the tibia or excessive posterior translation of the femur<br>2. Most fibers limit full knee extension<br>3. Resists extremes of varus, valgus, and axial rotation | 1. Hyperextension of the knee<br>2. Large valgus force with foot planted<br>3. Either of the above combined with large internal axial rotation torque (e.g., the femur forcefully externally rotates over a fixed tibia) |
| Posterior cruciate ligament | 1. Most fibers resist excessive posterior translation of the tibia or excessive anterior translation of the femur<br>2. Most fibers become taut at full flexion<br>3. Some fibers become taut at maximal hyperextension and the extremes of varus, valgus, and axial rotation | 1. Hyperflexion of the knee<br>2. "Dashboard" injuries with excessive posterior translation of the tibia relative to the femur<br>3. Severe hyperextension of the knee with a gapping of the posterior side of the joint<br>4. Large valgus or varus force with foot planted<br>5. Any of the above combined with large axial rotation torque |

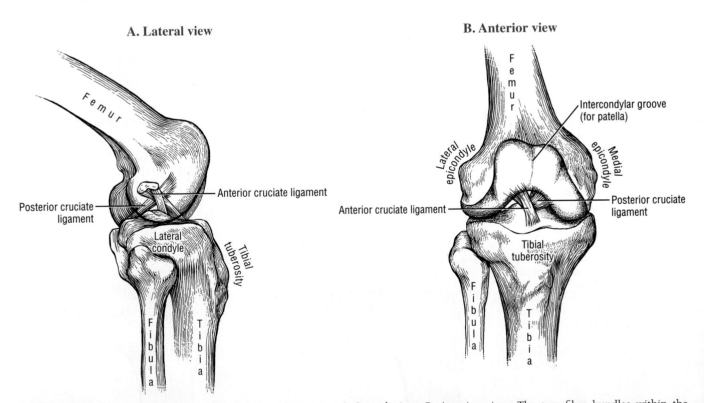

**FIGURE 13–21.** The anterior and posterior cruciate ligaments. *A,* Lateral view. *B,* Anterior view. The two fiber bundles within the anterior cruciate ligament are evident in *A.*

# ANTERIOR CRUCIATE LIGAMENT

## *Functional Anatomy*

The anterior cruciate ligament (ACL) attaches along an approximate 30-mm impression on the anterior intercondylar area of the tibial plateau.[36] From this attachment, the ligament runs obliquely in a posterior, slightly superior, and lateral direction to attach on the medial side of the lateral femoral condyle (see Fig. 13–21A and B). The collagen fibers within the ACL twist upon one another, thereby forming spiraling fascicles, or bundles. The bundles are often referred to as posterior-lateral and anterior-medial, named according to their relative attachment on the tibia.[36] The posterior-lateral bundle is the main component of the ACL.

The length and orientation of the twisting ACL change as the knee joint rotates. Although some fibers of the ACL remain taut throughout the full range of motion, most fibers, especially within the posterior-lateral bundle, become more taut as the knee approaches full extension (Fig. 13–22A).[49] Along with the posterior capsule, collateral ligaments, and hamstring muscles, the ACL produces useful tension that helps stabilize the extended or near-extended knee.

## *Mechanism of Injury to the Anterior Cruciate Ligament*

The ACL is the most frequently injured ligament of the knee, occurring often during sports activities such as football, downhill skiing, basketball, and soccer. An ACL injury may occur in conjunction with injury to other structures, such as the medial collateral ligament and medial meniscus. One of the most common and relatively simple manual exams for ACL integrity is called the *"anterior drawer"* test. The basic component of this test involves pulling the leg forward with the knee flexed to about 90 degrees (see Fig. 13–22A and B). In the normal knee, the ACL provides about 85% of the total passive resistance to the anterior translation of the tibia.[11] An anterior laxity of 8 mm (1/3 in) greater than the contralateral knee is indicative of an ACL tear. With the knee flexed and "unlocked," secondary restraint structures such as the posterior capsule, collateral ligaments, and flexor muscles offer less resistance to an anteriorly translating tibia. Spasm in the hamstring muscles may limit anterior translation of the tibia, thereby masking a torn ACL.

The oblique manner in which the ACL courses through the knee allows at least a part of this structure to resist the extremes of all movements. Although the spatial orientation of the ACL provides a wide range of stability, it also predisposes the person to ligament injury. As listed in Table 13–4, the ACL is pulled taut as a result of many tibial-on-femoral or femoral-on-tibial movements. One finding common to many ACL injuries is a high-velocity stretch while the ligament is under tension. This may occur, for example, when the foot is firmly planted and the femur is vigorously externally rotated and/or translated posteriorly. As noted by observing a skeletal model or Figure 13–21, this movement in conjunction with a valgus force can elongate and potentially tear the ACL.

Another common mechanism for injuring the ACL involves excessive hyperextension of the knee while the foot is planted on the ground. Very large forces produced by the quadriceps muscle during this event may add to the severity of the injury. Marked hyperextension frequently involves trauma to the collateral ligaments and the posterior capsule.

# POSTERIOR CRUCIATE LIGAMENT

## *Functional Anatomy*

The posterior cruciate ligament (PCL) provides another important source of resistance to the anterior-posterior shear forces at the knee. Slightly thicker than the ACL, the PCL attaches from the posterior intercondylar area of the tibia to the lateral side of the medial femoral condyle (see Figs. 13–12A and B, 13–13, and 13–21A and B). The course of this ligament is more vertical and slightly less oblique than that of the ACL.

The specific anatomy of the PCL is variable. It has two bundles: a larger *anterior set* (anterior-lateral), forming the bulk of the ligament, and a smaller *posterior set* (posterior-medial).[15,42,84]

Two accessory components of the PCL are often present. In about 70% of knees, either an anterior meniscofemoral ligament or a posterior meniscofemoral ligament is present.[45] These ligaments have a mass of only 20% of the PCL and, therefore, play a minor role in stability. Figures 13–12A and 13–13 show a segment of the more common posterior meniscofemoral ligament, originating from the lateral meniscus and blending into the posterior fibers of the PCL.

Like the ACL, some fibers within the PCL remain taut throughout the entire range of motion. The majority of the ligament (i.e., the larger anterior fibers), however, becomes taut at the extremes of flexion.[36] As depicted in Figure 13–22C, the PCL is pulled taut by the hamstring muscle contraction and subsequent posterior slide of the tibia. Adding a forceful quadriceps contraction to an existing hamstring contraction reduces the tension and stretch on the PCL.[48]

One of the most common exams of the integrity of the PCL is the *"posterior drawer"* test. This test involves pushing the leg posteriorly with the knee flexed to 90 degrees (Fig. 13–22D). Normally, the PCL provides about 95% of the total passive resistance to the posterior translation of the tibia.[11] Often, following a PCL injury, the tibia sags posteriorly against the femur. This observation, in conjunction with a positive posterior drawer sign, suggests a ruptured PCL.

Another important function of the PCL is to limit the extent of anterior translation of the femur over the fixed tibia. Activities, such as rapidly descending into a squat and landing from a jump with knee partially flexed, create a large anterior shear force on the femur against the tibia. The femur is held from sliding off the anterior edge of the tibia by forces in the PCL, joint capsule, and muscle. The popliteus muscle, by crossing the posterior side of the knee, may share a portion of the force naturally placed on the PCL.[42]

## *Mechanism of Injury to the Posterior Cruciate Ligament*

Injury to the PCL accounts for only 5% to 20% of all such injuries to the knee.[14] Half of PCL injuries occur with injuries to other knee structures, most often the ACL and posterior-lateral capsule. Three mechanisms are proposed for rup-

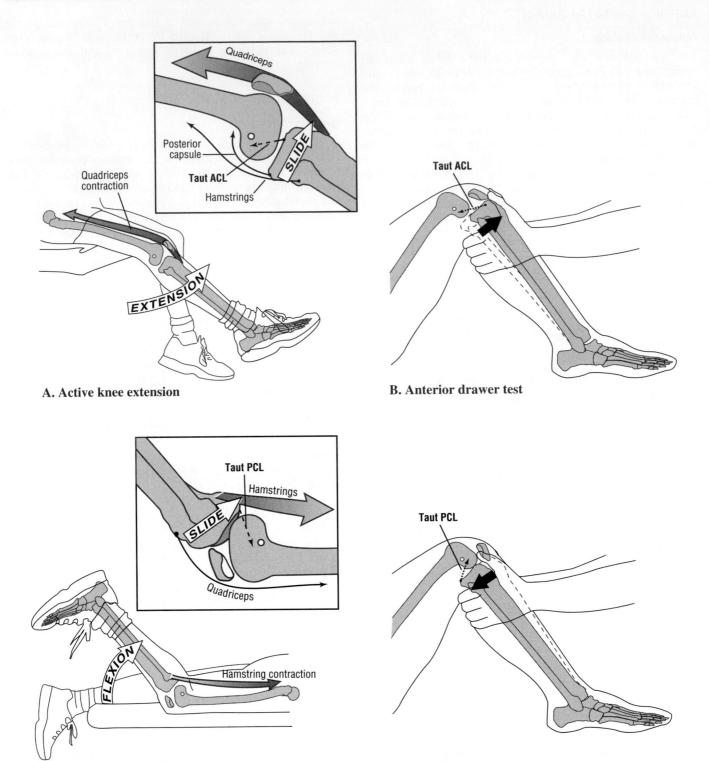

**A. Active knee extension**

**B. Anterior drawer test**

**C. Active knee flexion**

**D. Posterior drawer test**

**FIGURE 13–22.** The interaction between muscle contraction and tension changes in the cruciate ligaments is shown. *A,* Contraction of the quadriceps muscle extends the knee and slides the tibia anterior relative to the femur. Knee extension also elongates most of the anterior cruciate ligament (ACL), posterior capsule, hamstring muscles, and collateral ligaments (not shown). Note that the quadriceps and ACL have an antagonistic relationship throughout most of the terminal range of extension. *B,* The anterior drawer test evaluates the integrity of the ACL. *C,* Contraction of the hamstring muscles flexes the knee and slides the tibia posterior relative to the femur. Knee flexion elongates the quadriceps muscle and most of the fibers within the posterior cruciate ligament (PCL). *D,* The posterior drawer test checks the integrity of the PCL. Tissues pulled taut are indicated by thin black arrows.

### Altered Muscle Activation Pattern Following Anterior Cruciate Ligament Injury

Contraction of the quadriceps muscle causes an anterior translation of the tibia relative to the femur. This translation can increase the tension in most fibers of the ACL.[105] Contraction of the hamstring muscles, in contrast, causes a posterior translation of the tibia that slackens most fibers of the ACL.[79] Following an ACL injury, the hamstrings often experience spasm. The resulting flexed knee may be a mechanism that is employed to limit the stretch on a reconstructed or damaged ACL.[1] Stimulation from stretch receptors in an injured but intact ACL may trigger spasm in the hamstring muscles. This, in turn, may reflexively inhibit the quadriceps muscle.[69] This muscular-based "flexion bias" of the knee places the tibia relatively posterior to the femoral condyles, thereby unloading most fibers of the ACL.

Following an ACL injury or reconstruction, a pattern of muscle activation while walking may develop that favors greater activation of the hamstrings and inhibition of the quadriceps.[119] In theory, increased activation of the hamstrings in an ACL-deficient knee may partially compensate for an excessive anterior displacement of the tibia relative to the femur.[77]

ture of the PCL (see box).[60] Falling over a hyperflexed knee is the most common mechanism of injury. The most common high-energy injury to the PCL is the "dashboard" injury, in which a passenger's knee strikes an automobile's dashboard, driving the tibia posteriorly relative to the femur. Severe hyperextension with an associated gapping of the posterior side of the joint can cause combined injury to the ACL, PCL, and posterior capsule. Additional mechanisms of injury to the PCL are included in Table 13–4.

> **Three Common Mechanisms of Injury to the PCL**
> 1. Hyperflexion
> 2. Pretibial trauma ("dashboard" injury)
> 3. Hyperextension

## MUSCLE AND JOINT INTERACTION

### Innervation to the Muscles and Joints

INNERVATION TO MUSCLES

The quadriceps femoris is innervated by the *femoral nerve* (see Fig. 12–27A). Like the triceps at the elbow, the knee's sole extensor group is innervated by just one peripheral nerve. A complete femoral nerve lesion, therefore, can cause total paralysis of the knee extensors. The flexors and rotators

### Considerations Regarding Resistive Exercises During Postsurgical Rehabilitation of the Anterior Cruciate Ligament

Volumes of material have been written on the ACL, especially related to the topics of biomechanics[66,73,92] surgical reconstruction and healing[22,29,43,121,122] long-term results following surgical repair,[80] and postsurgical[2,4,5,24,114,116] and nonsurgical rehabilitation.[28] Much of the debate and controversy associated with this literature about the ACL is beyond the scope of this text. One topic, however, that is highlighted here is the issue of strengthening the quadriceps as a part of ACL rehabilitation.

Some persons following ACL reconstructive surgery limit quadriceps activity while walking. Persistent weakness of the muscle may ensue, despite improvement in many functional measures.[64] Reduced functional strength in the quadriceps may cause a loss of active terminal extension, poor gait, and excessive wear on the knee's articular cartilage. Strengthening and general activation of the quadriceps are therefore important goals in any ACL repair rehabilitation program.

Depending on the patient's age, time since surgery, and injury severity, it may be prudent to limit the amount of tension placed on a healing ACL graft. Certain methods for strengthening the quadriceps are contraindicated or at least questionable, especially during the early course of

rehabilitation. Many reports have warned against resisted (tibial-on-femoral) knee extension at angles that are less than 70 degrees of full extension.[12,25,61,88,126] As the knee approaches full extension, the active quadriceps produces an anterior shear on the tibia, which can strain the ACL (see Fig. 13–22A and B). The larger the force in the quadriceps, the greater the anterior shear and subsequent load placed on the ACL.[47] As a response to these reports, clinicians routinely advocate exercises that concentrate on loading the quadriceps muscle during the last 45 degrees of *femoral-on-tibial extension*.[12,46] These exercises are often referred to as "closed kinetic chain" exercises. Exercises such as "mini squats," squats against elastic resistance, single-leg half squats, and leg presses produce equal,[4] or less, strain on the ACL than tibial-on-femoral resistance exercises, such as lifting ankle weights.[46,113,125] Femoral-on-tibial extension may demand a coactivation of the knee extensor and flexor muscles, thereby increasing stability of the knee and limiting anterior-posterior shear forces. This method of exercise may limit tension placed on the ACL and, at the same time, provide adequate resistance against the quadriceps. At some point in the rehabilitation process, however, tension in the ACL may actually facilitate healing and can be considered therapeutic.[115]

of the knee are innervated by several nerves from both the lumbar and sacral plexus, but primarily by the *tibial portion of the sciatic nerve* (see Fig. 12–27B). Table 13–5 summarizes the motor innervation to the knee.

The motor nerve roots that supply all the muscles of the lower extremity are listed in Appendix IVA. Appendix IVB shows key muscles typically used to test the functional status of the $L^2$–$S^3$ ventral nerve roots.

## SENSORY INNERVATION TO THE JOINT

Sensory innervation to the knee is supplied primarily from the $L^3$ through $L^5$ nerve roots, carried by anterior and posterior sets of nerves.[58,65] The *posterior set* is derived from the posterior tibial and obturator nerves. The posterior tibial nerve (a branch from the tibial portion of the sciatic) is the largest afferent supply to the knee joint. It supplies sensation to the posterior capsule and associated ligaments, and most of the internal structures of the knee as far anterior as the infrapatellar fat pad. The afferent fibers within the obturator nerve are the reason why inflammation of the hip joint is often perceived as "referred pain" in the medial knee region.

The *anterior set* of sensory nerves to the knee consists primarily of sensory branches from the femoral nerve. Articular branches of the femoral nerve supply most of the anterior-medial and anterior-lateral capsule and the associated ligaments. The anterior set also contains sensory branches from the common peroneal nerve and the saphenous nerve ($L^{3-4}$).

## Muscular Function at the Knee

### EXTENSOR AND FLEXOR-ROTATOR MUSCLES

Muscles of the knee are described here as two groups: the knee extensors (i.e., quadriceps) and the knee flexor-rotators. The anatomy of many of these muscles is presented in Chapter 12. Consult Appendix IV, Part C, for a summary of the attachments and nerve supply to the muscles of the knee.

### *Quadriceps: Knee Extensor Mechanism*

#### *Functional Considerations*

By isometric, eccentric, and concentric activations, the quadriceps femoris muscle is able to perform multiple functions at the knee. Through *isometric activation*, the quadriceps stabilizes and helps to protect the knee; through *eccentric activation,* the quadriceps controls the rate of descent of the body's center of mass, such as in sitting or stooping. Eccentric activation provides shock absorption to the knee. At the heel contact phase of walking, the knee flexes slightly in response to the posteriorly located ground reaction force. Eccentrically active quadriceps controls flexion. Acting as a spring, the muscle helps dampen the impact of loading on the joint. This protection is especially useful during high impact loading, such as landing from a jump, running, or descending from a high step. A person whose knee is braced or fused in full extension lacks this natural shock absorption mechanism.

In the previous examples, eccentric activation of the

---

**TABLE 13–5. Actions and Innervation of Muscles That Cross the Knee***

| Muscle | Action | Innervation | Plexus |
|---|---|---|---|
| Sartorius | Hip flexion, external rotation, and abduction<br>**Knee flexion and internal rotation** | Femoral nerve | Lumbar |
| Gracilis | Hip flexion and adduction<br>**Knee flexion and internal rotation** | Obturator nerve | Lumbar |
| Quadriceps femoris<br>  Rectus femoris<br>  Vastus group | **Knee extension and hip flexion**<br>**Knee extension** | Femoral nerve | Lumbar |
| Popliteus | **Knee flexion and internal rotation** | Tibial nerve | Sacral |
| Semimembranosus | Hip extension<br>**Knee flexion and internal rotation** | Sciatic nerve (tibial portion) | Sacral |
| Semitendinosus | Hip extension<br>**Knee flexion and internal rotation** | Sciatic nerve (tibial portion) | Sacral |
| Biceps femoris<br>  (short head) | **Knee flexion and external rotation** | Sciatic nerve (common peroneal portion) | Sacral |
| Biceps femoris<br>  (long head) | Hip extension<br>**Knee flexion and external rotation** | Sciatic nerve (tibial portion) | Sacral |
| Gastrocnemius | **Knee flexion**<br>Ankle plantar flexion | Tibial nerve | Sacral |
| Plantaris | **Knee flexion**<br>Ankle plantar flexion | Tibial nerve | Sacral |

\* The actions involving the knee are shown in **bold**. Muscles are listed in descending order of nerve root innervation.

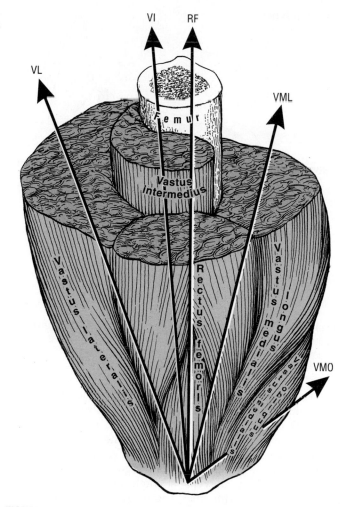

**FIGURE 13–23.** A cross-section through the right quadriceps muscle. The arrows depict the approximate line-of-force of each of part of the quadriceps: vastus lateralis (VL), vastus intermedius (VI), rectus femoris (RF), vastus medialis longus (VML), and vastus medialis obliquus (VMO).

quadriceps is employed to decelerate knee flexion. *Concentric contraction* of this muscle, in contrast, accelerates the tibia or femur into knee extension. This action is often used to raise the body's center of mass, such as running uphill, jumping, or standing from a seated position.

## Anatomic Considerations

The *quadriceps femoris* is a large and powerful extensor muscle, consisting of the rectus femoris, vastus lateralis, vastus medialis, and deeper vastus intermedius (Figs. 13–7 and 13–23). The large vastus group produces about 80% of the total extension torque at the knee, and the rectus femoris produces about 20% (Fig. 13–24).[54] Contraction of the vasti extends the knee only. Contraction of the rectus femoris, however, causes hip flexion and knee extension.

All heads of the quadriceps unite to form a strong tendon that attaches to the base of the patella. The quadriceps tendon continues distally as the patellar ligament, joining the apex of the patella to the tibial tuberosity. The vastus lateralis and vastus medialis attach into the capsule and menisci via patellar retinacular fibers (see Fig. 13–7). The quadriceps muscle and tendon, patella, and patellar ligament are often described as the knee extensor mechanism.

The *rectus femoris* attaches to the pelvis near the anterior-inferior iliac spine. The vastus muscles, however, attach to an extensive part of the femur, particularly the anterior-lateral shaft and the linea aspera (see Figs. 12–4 to 12–6). Although the *vastus lateralis* is the largest of the quadriceps muscles, the vastus medialis extends farther distally toward the knee.

The *vastus medialis* consists of fibers that form two distinct fiber directions. The more distal oblique fibers (the vastus medialis "obliquus") approach the patella at 50 to 55 degrees, medial to the quadriceps tendon; the remaining more longitudinal fibers (the vastus medialis "longus") approach the patella at 15 to 18 degrees, medial to the quadriceps tendon (see Fig. 13–23).[74] These two sets of fibers are a subset of one anatomically distinct muscle: the vastus medialis.[35] The two sets of fibers, however, have different lines-of-force on the patella. Although the oblique fibers account for only 30% of the cross-sectional area of the entire vastus medialis muscle,[97] the oblique pull on the patella has important implications for the stabilization and orientation of the patella as it tracks or slides through the intercondylar groove of the femur.

The deepest quadriceps muscle, the *vastus intermedius*, is located under the rectus femoris. Deep to the vastus intermedius is the *articularis genu*. This muscle contains a few slips of muscle fibers that attach proximally to the anterior side of the distal femur, and distally into the anterior capsule. This muscle pulls the capsule and synovial membrane

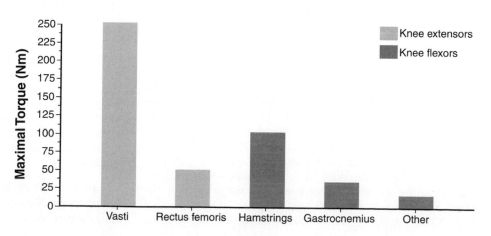

**FIGURE 13–24.** The maximal knee torque produced by muscles that cross the knee is displayed. Note the relatively large torque potential of the vastus group. (Data from Hoy MG, Zajac FE, Gordon ME: Musculoskeletal model of the human lower extremity. J Biomechan 23:157–169, 1990.)

**A. Crane**                                          **B. Human Knee**

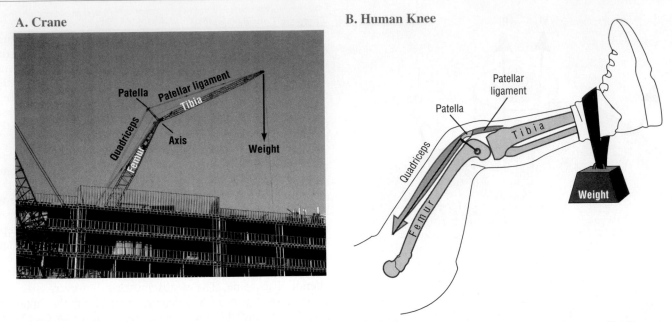

**FIGURE 13–25.** An analogy is made between a crane (*A*) and the human knee (*B*). In the crane, the moment arm is the distance between the axis and the tip of the piece of metal that functions like a patella.

proximally during active knee extension.[120] The articularis genu is analogous to the articularis cubiti at the elbow.

**Patella: Augmentation of Knee Extension Leverage.** Functionally, the patella displaces the tendon of the quadriceps anteriorly, thereby increasing the internal moment arm of the knee extensor mechanism. In this way, the patella augments the torque potential of the quadriceps. Figure 13–25 shows an analogy between a mechanical crane and the human knee. Both use a "spacer" to increase the distance between the axis of rotation and the internal "lifting" force. The larger the internal moment arm, the greater the internal torque produced per level of force generated by the quadriceps of the human knee (or transferred by the cable in the crane).

*Quadriceps Action at the Knee: Understanding the Biomechanical Interactions Between External and Internal Torques*

In many upright activities, the external (flexor) torque at the knee is the product of the external load being moved multiplied by its external moment arm. The internal (extensor) torque, in contrast, is the product of quadriceps force multiplied by its internal moment arm. An understanding of how these opposing torques are produced and how they interact is an important consideration in knee rehabilitation.

**External Torque Demands Against the Quadriceps: Contrasting "Tibial-on-Femoral" with "Femoral-on-Tibial" Methods of Knee Extension.** Strengthening exercises for the quadriceps muscle typically are reliant on resistive, external torques generated by gravity acting on the body. The magnitude of external torques varies depending on how the knee is being extended. During tibial-on-femoral knee extension, the external moment arm of the weight of the lower leg increases from 90 to 0 degrees of knee flexion (Fig. 13–27 *A* to *C*). In contrast, during femoral-on-tibial

knee extension, the external moment arm of the upper body weight decreases from 90 to 0 degrees of knee flexion (Fig. 13–27 *D* to *F*). Figure 13–27 shows the relationships between the relative external torque for the two methods of extending the knee over a selected range of motion.

Information from the graph in Figure 13–27 is useful when designing quadriceps strengthening exercises, especially for persons with knee pathology. By necessity, exercises that significantly challenge the quadriceps also stress the knee joint and its associated connective tissues. Clinically, this stress is considered either therapeutic or damaging, depending on the type and severity of the pathology or injury. A person with marked patellofemoral joint pain or painful arthritis, for example, is typically advised to avoid large forces created by the quadriceps.[112] Muscle forces are typically large when responding to large external torques. As depicted by the red shading in the graph in Figure 13–27, external torques are relatively large from 90 to 45 degrees of flexion via femoral-on-tibial extension, and from 45 to 0 degrees of flexion via tibial-on-femoral extension. Reducing relatively large external torques can be accomplished by modifying the manner of applying resistance against the knee extensor muscles. An external load, for example, can be applied at the ankle during tibial-on-femoral knee extension between 90 and 45 degrees of flexion. This exercise can be followed by an exercise that involves rising from a partial squat position, a motion that incorporates femoral-on-tibial extension between 45 and 0 degrees of flexion. Combining both exercises in the manner described provides moderate to minimal external torques against the quadriceps, throughout a continuous range of motion.

**Internal Torque-Joint Angle Relationship of the Quadriceps Muscle.** Maximal knee extension torque typically occurs between 45 and 60 degrees of flexion (Fig.

13–28).[54,98,110] As depicted by the dashed red line in Figure 13–28A, the maximal-effort knee extension torque remains at least 90% of maximum between 80 and 30 degrees of flexion. This 50-degree, high-torque potential of the quadriceps is used during many activities that incorporate femoral-on-tibial kinematics, such as ascending a high step[72] or holding a partial squat position while participating in sports, such as basketball and football. Note the rapid decline in internal torque potential as the knee angle approaches full extension. Interestingly, the *external torque* applied against the knee during femoral-on-tibial extension also declines rapidly during the same range of motion (see Fig. 13–27, graph). There appears to be a biomechanical match in the internal torque potential of the quadriceps and the external torques applied against the quadriceps during the last 45 to 60 degrees of femoral-on-tibial knee extension. This match accounts, in part, for the popularity of "closed-kinetic chain" exercises that focus on applying resistance to the quadriceps while the person is standing upright and moving through the last 45 to 60 degrees of femoral-on-tibial knee extension.

The variables of internal moment arm and muscle length strongly influence the shape of the knee extension torque-angle curve (Fig. 13–28B). Moment arm influences torque, and muscle length influences muscle force potential (see Chapter 3). It is not possible to determine with certainty which variable—leverage or muscle length—has the greater influence on the maximal torque production of the quadriceps. Knee extensor torque potential (see Fig. 13–28A) and internal moment arm length of the quadriceps (see Fig. 13–28B) both peak at about 45 degrees of flexion.

**Loss of Full Knee Extension.** The inability to extend the knee fully is a relatively common clinical phenomenon. Factors that often prevent full knee extension can be broadly classified into three categories: (1) reduced force production from the quadriceps, (2) excessive resistance from the connective tissues, and (3) faulty arthrokinematics. Table 13–6 presents clinical examples for each of these categories.

### Patellofemoral Joint Kinetics

Patellofemoral joint compression forces may reach 3.3 times body weight while climbing stairs and may rise to 7.8 times body weight in performing deep knee bends.[100] Such large joint forces reflect the magnitude of the forces produced within the quadriceps muscle. An additional factor is the angle of the knee joint at the time of muscle activation. To

---

**SPECIAL FOCUS 13–5**

#### Consequences of a Patellectomy

According to one study, an approximate 20% loss of internal moment arm occurs following a patellectomy.[63] Averaged over full range of motion, the internal moment arm of a patellectomized knee was reduced from 4.7 cm to 3.8 cm. These data suggest that, in theory, a knee without a patella needs to generate 25% more force to produce an equivalent pre-patellectomized extensor torque. The increased muscle force is needed to compensate for the proportional loss in leverage. As a consequence, the greater muscle force increases the compression force on the tibiofemoral joint, creating additional wear on the articular cartilage (Fig. 13–26).

**A. With patella**    **B. Without patella**

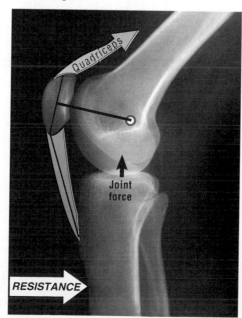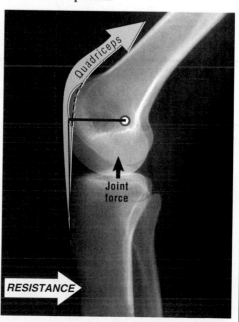

**FIGURE 13–26.** The quadriceps is shown contracting with a patella (A) and without a patella (B). In each case, the quadriceps maintains equilibrium at the knee by responding to two equal magnitudes of external resistance. The moment arm (black line) is reduced in B owing to the patellectomy. As a consequence, the quadriceps must produce a greater force to extend the knee. This greater joint force is transferred across the tibiofemoral joint.

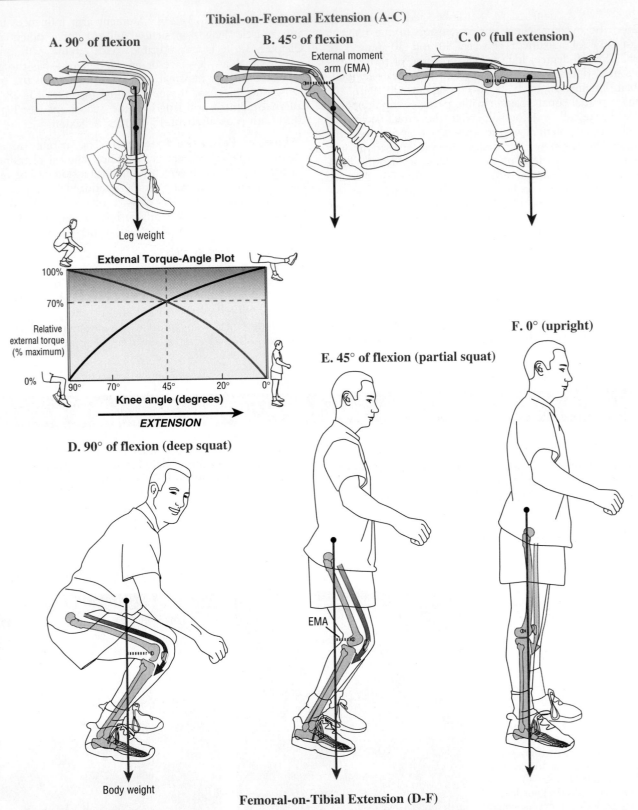

**Tibial-on-Femoral Extension (A-C)**

**A. 90° of flexion**

**B. 45° of flexion**

External moment arm (EMA)

**C. 0° (full extension)**

Leg weight

**External Torque-Angle Plot**

100%

70%

Relative external torque (% maximum)

0%

90°    70°    45°    20°    0°

**Knee angle (degrees)**

**EXTENSION**

**D. 90° of flexion (deep squat)**

**E. 45° of flexion (partial squat)**

**F. 0° (upright)**

EMA

Body weight

**Femoral-on-Tibial Extension (D-F)**

**FIGURE 13–27.** The external (flexion) torques are shown imposed on the knee between flexion (90 degrees) and full extension (0 degrees). Tibial-on-femoral extension is shown in *A–C,* and femoral-on-tibial extension is shown in *D–F.* The external torques are equal to the product of body or leg weight times the external moment arm (EMA). The graph shows the relationship between the external torque—normalized to a maximum (100%) torque for each method of extending the knee—for selected knee joint angles. (Tibial-on-femoral extension shown in black; femoral-on-tibial extension shown in gray.) External torques above 70% for each method of extension are shaded in light red. The increasing red color of the quadriceps muscle denotes the increasing demand on the muscle and underlying joint, in response to the increasing external torque.

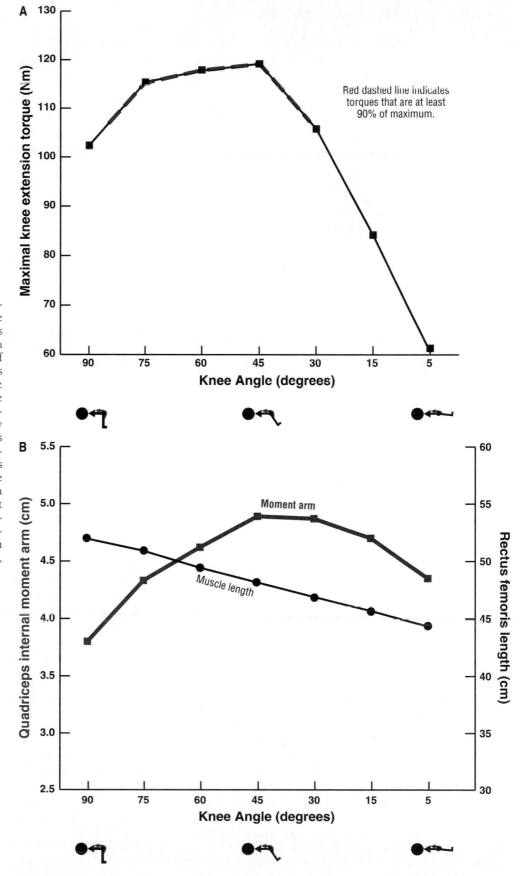

**FIGURE 13–28.** Biomechanical variables related to maximal-effort knee extension torque. *A*, The plot depicts knee extension torque between 90 degrees and near 0 degrees of knee flexion. Knee extensor torques are produced isometrically, with the hip extended. *B*, The plot shows the relationship between the internal moment arm of the quadriceps (left y axis, in red) and rectus femoris length (right y axis, in black) between 90 degrees and near 0 degrees of knee flexion. Data on muscle length were estimated using a human skeleton. Data on torque and moment arm are based on a healthy male population. (Data from Smidt GL: Biomechanical analysis of knee flexion and extension. J Biomechan 6:79–92, 1973.)

### TABLE 13-6. Selected Factors that Contribute to the Inability to Completely Extend the Knee

| Factor | Clinical Examples |
|---|---|
| Reduced force production from the quadriceps | Disuse atrophy of quadriceps following trauma and/or prolonged immobilization<br>Lacerated femoral nerve<br>Herniated disc compressing $L^3$ or $L^4$ nerve roots<br>Severe pain<br>Excessive swelling in the knee |
| Excessive resistance from connective tissues | Excessive tightness in hamstring or other knee flexor muscles<br>Excessive stiffness in the anterior cruciate ligament, posterior capsule, or collateral ligaments<br>Scarring of the skin in the popliteal fossa |
| Faulty arthrokinematics | Lack of "screw-home" rotation mechanics<br>Lack of anterior slide of the tibia*<br>Meniscal block or other derangement<br>Lack of superior slide of the patella* |

\* Assume tibial-on-femoral knee extension.

illustrate these factors, consider the force on the patellofemoral joint while in a partial squat position (Fig. 13–29A). The force within the extensor mechanism is transmitted proximally and distally through the quadriceps tendon (QT) and patellar ligament (PL), much like a cable crossing a fixed pulley. The resultant, or combined effect, of these forces is directed toward the intercondylar groove of the femur as a joint force (JF). Increasing knee flexion by descending into a deeper squat significantly raises the force demands throughout the extensor mechanism, ultimately on the patellofemoral joint (Fig. 13–29B). The increased knee flexion associated with the deeper squat also reduces the angle formed by the intersection of force vectors QT and PL. As shown by the vector addition, reducing the angle of these force *increases* the magnitude of the JF directed between the patella and the femur.

---

**Two Interrelated Factors That Increase the Compression Force in the Patellofemoral Joint**

1. Increased force demands on the quadriceps muscle
2. Increased knee flexion

---

While performing a squat maneuver, the pressure (force/area) within the patellofemoral joint is greatest at 60 to 90 degrees of knee flexion. The contact area within the patellofemoral joint is also greatest at 60 to 90 degrees of knee flexion (Fig. 13–19E).[10,56,82] Without this large area to dis-

perse the forces, the pressure at the patellofemoral joint can rise to an intolerable level. Having the contact area within the joint greatest at the positions that receive the largest compression forces protects the joint against degeneration. This mechanism allows a healthy patellofemoral joint to tolerate large compression forces over a lifetime, often with little or no appreciable wear or discomfort.

**Tracking Within the Patellofemoral Joint.** During active knee extension, several structures guide, or "track," the patella through the intercondylar groove of the femur (see the next box). Acting alone, each structure exerts a medial or lateral pull on the patella as it slides in the groove (Fig. 13–31). When these forces balance each other, they cooperate to track the patella through the groove with as little stress to the articular surfaces as possible.[44] If the forces do not balance one another, the patella may not track optimally and may even dislocate. Increased stress due to abnormal tracking may lead to arthritis, chondromalacia, recurrent patellar dislocation, or patellofemoral joint pain syndrome.

---

### SPECIAL FOCUS 13-6

**Quadriceps Weakness: Pathomechanics of "Extensor Lag"**

Persons with moderate weakness in the quadriceps often show considerable difficulty completing the full range of tibial-on-femoral extension of the knee, commonly displayed while sitting. This difficulty persists even when the external load is limited to just the weight of the lower leg. Although the knee can be fully extended passively, efforts at active extension typically fail to produce the last 15 to 20 degrees of extension. Clinically, this characteristic demonstration of quadriceps weakness is often referred to as an "extensor lag."

Extensor lag at the knee is often a persistent and perplexing problem during rehabilitation of the post-surgical knee. The mechanics that create this condition during the seated position are as follows: As the knee approaches terminal extension, the maximal internal torque potential of the quadriceps is least while the opposing external (flexor) torque is greatest. This natural disparity is hardly evident in persons with normal quadriceps strength. With moderate muscle weakness, however, the disparity often results in extensor lag.

Swelling or effusion of the knee increases the likelihood of an extensor lag. Swelling increases intraarticular pressure, which can physically impede full knee extension.[123] Increased intraarticular pressure can reflexively inhibit the neural activation of the quadriceps muscle.[19,83] Methods that reduce swelling of the knee, therefore, have an important role in a therapeutic exercise program of the knee.

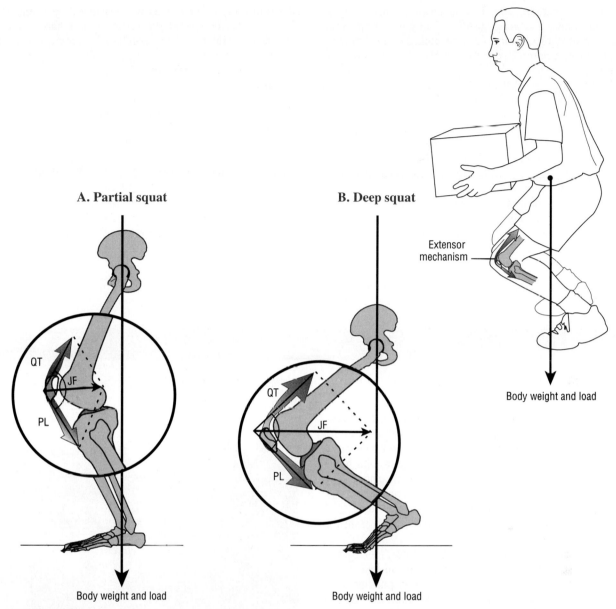

**A. Partial squat**

**B. Deep squat**

Extensor
mechanism

Body weight and load

Body weight and load

Body weight and load

**FIGURE 13–29.** The relationship between the depth of a squat position and the compression force within the patellofemoral joint is shown. *A,* Maintaining a partial squat requires that the quadriceps transmit a force through the quadriceps tendon (QT) and the patellar ligament (PL). The vector addition of QT and PL provides an estimation of the patellofemoral joint force (JF). *B,* A deeper squat requires greater force from the quadriceps owing to the greater external (flexion) torque on the knee. Furthermore, the greater knee flexion (*B*) decreases the angle between QT and PL and, consequently, produces a greater joint force between the patella and femur.

---

**Structures that Guide the Patella through the Intercondylar Groove of the Femur**

- Quadriceps muscle
- Quadriceps tendon
- Patellar ligament
- Iliotibial tract
- Patellar retinacular fibers
- Shape of the articular surfaces

The overall line-of-force of the quadriceps tends to pull the patella superiorly and laterally relative to its ligament. The degree of lateral pull exerted by the quadriceps is often referred to as the *Q-angle* (Fig. 13–32).[52] This angle is formed between (1) a line representing the resultant pull of the quadriceps, made by connecting a point near the anterior-superior iliac spine to the midpoint of the patella, and (2) a line connecting the tibial tuberosity with the midpoint of the patella. Different Q-angles exist between the genders:

15.8 degrees in women, and 11.2 degrees in men.[53] A Q-angle greater than 15 degrees is often thought to contribute to patellofemoral joint pain, chondromalacia, and patellar dislocation. Little scientific evidence, however, supports this assumption.[78]

The lateral bias in pull of the quadriceps produces a natural bowstringing force against the patella (see Fig. 13–31). An important function of the oblique fibers of the vastus medialis is to counteract the tendency of the quadriceps muscle as a whole to dislocate the patella laterally.[74] The medial patellofemoral (retinacular) fibers[21] and the normally raised lateral facet within the intercondylar groove of the femur resist the laterally encroaching patella.

A combination of several structural and functional factors can lead to excessive lateral tracking of the patella (Table 13–7). Abnormal tracking is often associated with an abnor-

mal tilting of the patella as it rides in the groove. A shallow intercondylar groove of the femur is a reliable predictor of excessive lateral tilt of the patella in women, especially near full knee extension.[96] Over time, an abnormal tilt can lead to increased stress on the articular cartilage and recurrent lateral dislocation.[38]

Increased Q-angle due to bony malalignment is a possible factor contributing to excessive lateral tracking of the patella.[78] The greater the Q-angle, the greater the lateral bowstringing effect on the patella. Factors that increase the Q-angle also tend to increase genu valgum. These factors include an overstretched medial collateral ligament, internal rotation/adduction hip posturing, excessive foot pronation, and gender. Data collected at a large sports medicine clinic showed that recurrent dislocation of the patella accounted for 58.4% of all dislocations in women, compared with only 14% in men.[20]

### SPECIAL FOCUS 13–7

#### Two Common Painful Conditions Involving the Patellofemoral Joint

*Patellofemoral joint pain syndrome* is a common condition in persons involved in sports, ranking first in track and second in American football and soccer.[20] Joint pain also occurs in persons not involved in sports. Those who have no history of trauma can also experience joint pain. Cases may be mild, involving only a generalized aching about the anterior knee, or they may be severe and involve recurrent dislocation or subluxation of the patella from the intercondylar groove.

Over time, some of those with patellofemoral joint pain syndrome develop degenerative changes in the joint surfaces, a condition known as chondromalacia patellae. *Chondromalacia patellae* (from the Greek *chondros,* cartilage, + *malakia,* softness) is a general term that describes excessive cartilage degeneration on the posterior side of the patella.[90,109] Those with this condition often experience retropatellar pain and crepitus, especially while squatting or climbing steep stairs or after sitting for a prolonged period. The cartilage becomes soft, pitted, and fragmented. Depending on the amount of cartilage wear and associated inflammation, chondromalacia can be very painful.

The exact causes of chondromalacia are unknown. The condition occurs frequently in the young and old and in the active and sedentary, and it does not always develop into a more generalized osteoarthritis of the knee. In some cases, however, chondromalacia may be associated with osteoarthritis of the entire knee. Figure 13–30 shows an extreme case of osteoarthritis of a cadaveric knee with degeneration throughout its entirety. Based on the biomechanics described, persons with chondromalacia, active arthritis, or generalized patellofemoral joint pain are often

advised against performing squatting activities, especially while carrying loads.

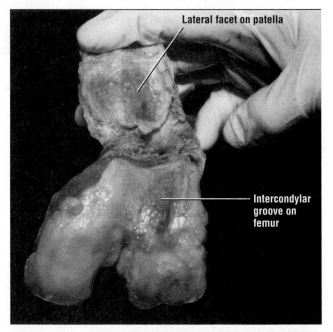

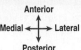

**FIGURE 13–30.** The distal surface of the left femur and the patella is shown in the knee of a cadaver. This specimen is from an individual who had chondromalacia patellae and generalized osteoarthritis of the knee. Note the irregular surfaces and marked degeneration on the cartilage of the femur and patella.

## Major Guiding Forces Acting on the Patella

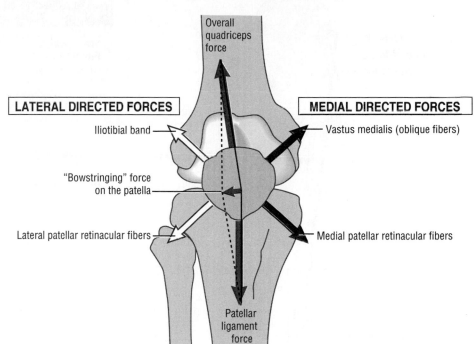

**FIGURE 13–31.** The major guiding forces acting on the patella are shown as it moves through the intercondylar groove of the femur. Each structure has a natural tendency to pull the patella laterally or medially. In most cases, the opposing forces counteract one another so that the patella moves optimally during flexion and extension.

(See Table 13–8 for a partial summary of these data.) The greater Q-angle reported in women may partially account for this large disparity.

### Knee Flexor-Rotator Muscles

With the exception of the gastrocnemius, all muscles that cross posterior to the knee have the ability to flex and to internally or externally rotate the knee. The so-called flexor-rotator group of the knee includes the hamstrings, sartorius, gracilis, and popliteus. Unlike the knee extensor group, which are all innervated by the femoral nerve, the flexor-rotator muscles have three sources of innervation: femoral, obturator, and sciatic.

#### Functional Anatomy

The *hamstring muscles* (i.e., semimembranosus, semitendinosus, and long head of the biceps femoris) have their proximal attachment on the ischial tuberosity. The short head of the biceps has its proximal attachment on the lateral lip of the linea aspera of the femur. Distally, the three hamstrings cross the knee joint and attach to the tibia and fibula (see Figs. 13–9 to 13–11).

The *semimembranosus* attaches distally to the posterior side of the medial condyle of the tibia. Additional distal attachments of this muscle include the medial collateral ligament, both menisci, oblique popliteal ligament, and popliteus muscle. For most of its course, the sinewy *semitendinosus* tendon lies immediately posterior to the semimembranosus muscle. Just proximal to the knee, however, the tendon of the semitendinosus courses anteriorly toward the distal attachment on the anterior-medial aspect of tibia. Both heads of the *biceps femoris* attach on the head of the fibula, beside the fibular collateral ligament.

All hamstring muscles, except the short head of the biceps femoris, cross the hip and knee. As described in Chapter 12, the three biarticular hamstrings are very effective hip extensors, especially in the control of the position of the pelvis and trunk over the femur.

In addition to flexing the knee, the medial hamstrings (i.e., semimembranosus and semitendinosus) internally rotate the knee. The biceps femoris externally rotates the knee. Horizontal rotation occurs when the knee is flexed. This horizontal plane action of the hamstrings can be appreciated by palpating the tendons of semitendinosus and biceps femoris behind the knee as the leg is internally and externally rotated repeatedly. This is performed while the subject is sitting with the knee flexed 70 to 90 degrees. As the knee is gradually extended, the pivot point for the rotating lower leg shifts from the knee to the hip. At full extension, rotation at the knee ceases because the knee becomes mechanically locked and most ligaments are pulled taut. Furthermore, the moment arm of the hamstrings for internal and external rotation of the knee is reduced significantly at full extension.

The *sartorius* and *gracilis* have their proximal attachments on different parts of the pelvis (see Chapter 12). At the hip, both muscles are hip flexors, but they have opposite actions in the frontal and horizontal planes. Distally, the tendons of the sartorius and gracilis travel side by side across the medial side of the knee to attach to the proximal shaft of the tibia, near the semitendinosus (see Fig. 13–11). The three juxtaposed tendons of the sartorius, gracilis, and semitendinosus attach to the tibia using a common, broad sheet of connective tissue known as the *pes anserinus*. As a group, the "pes muscles" are effective internal rotators of the knee. Connective tissues hold the tendons of the pes group just

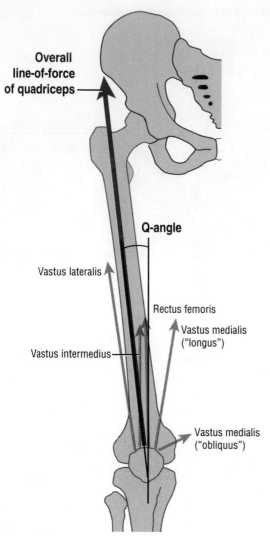

Overall
line-of-force
of quadriceps

Q-angle

Vastus lateralis

Rectus femoris

Vastus medialis
("longus")

Vastus intermedius

Vastus medialis
("obliquus")

**FIGURE 13–32.** The overall line-of-force of the quadriceps is shown as well as the separate line-of-force of the muscles within the quadriceps. The vastus medialis is divided into its two predominant fiber groups: the obliquus and the longus. The net lateral pull exerted on the patella by the quadriceps is indicated by the Q-angle. (See text for further details.)

## TABLE 13–7. Possible Causes and Examples of Excessive Lateral Tracking of the Patella

| Structural or Functional Abnormality | Specific Examples |
|---|---|
| Excessive tightness in lateral soft tissues | Tight iliotibial tract and/or lateral patellar retinacular fibers |
| Excessive laxity in medial soft tissues | Laxity of medial collateral ligament and/or medial patellar retinacular fibers |
| Bony dysplasia | Hypoplastic lateral facet on the intercondylar groove of the femur (i.e., a shallow intercondylar groove) Small or dysplastic patella |
| Abnormal patellar position | Patella alta (high-riding patella) |
| Knee malalignment | Increased Q-angle Increased genu valgum Excessive anteversion of the hip Excessive external tibial torsion |
| Muscle weakness | Weakness and atrophy of the oblique fibers of the vastus medialis |

*posterior* to the medial-lateral axis of rotation. Although these muscle do not attach to the femur, their indirect attachment via connective tissues allows them to flex and internally rotate the knee.

The pes anserinus group adds significant dynamic stability to the medial side of the knee. Along with the medial collateral ligament, active tension in the pes muscles resists knee external rotation and valgus stress at the knee. Surgical repositioning of the pes tendons is recommended to reinforce the medial side of the knee in persons with chronic laxity in the medial collateral ligament.[109]

The *popliteus* is a triangular muscle located deep to the gastrocnemius within the popliteal fossa (see Fig. 13–10).

## TABLE 13–8. Frequency of Joint Dislocation by Gender*†

| Dislocation | % of Dislocation by Gender | | % of Total Injuries by Gender | |
|---|---|---|---|---|
| | *Men* | *Women* | *Men* | *Women* |
| Shoulder (recurrent) | 38.1 | 1.9 | 1.9 | 0.1 |
| Shoulder (acute) | 22.1 | 3.8 | 1.1 | 0.3 |
| Patella (recurrent) | 14.0 | **58.4** | 0.7 | 4.6 |
| Patella (acute) | 11.0 | 34.0 | 0.5 | 2.7 |
| Finger | 5.1 | — | 0.3 | — |
| Elbow | 5.1 | 1.9 | 0.3 | 0.1 |

\* Data collected on athletic injuries over a 7-year period at University of Rochester, Section of Sports Medicine. Note in **bold** the high percentage of recurrent patellar dislocation for women.

† The dislocation is expressed as a percentage of the total injuries by gender.

Data from DeHaven KE, Lintner DM: Athletic injuries: Comparison by age, sport, and gender. Am J Sports Med 14:218–224, 1986.

By a strong intracapsular tendon, the popliteus attaches proximally to the lateral condyle of the femur, between the lateral collateral ligament and the lateral meniscus (see Fig. 13–9). The popliteus is the only muscle of the knee that attaches within the capsule. After exiting the posterior capsule, the popliteus has an extensive attachment to the posterior side of the tibia. Fibers from the popliteus attach to the lateral meniscus and blend with the arcuate popliteal ligament.

The anatomy and action of the gastrocnemius and plantaris are considered in Chapter 14.

### Group Action of Flexor-Rotator Muscles

The flexor-rotator muscles of the knee best perform their actions during walking and running. Examples of these actions are considered separately for tibial-on-femoral and femoral-on-tibial movements of the knee.

**Control of Tibial-on-Femoral Osteokinematics.** An important action of the flexor-rotator muscles is to accelerate or decelerate the tibia during walking or running. Typically, these muscles produce relatively low-to-moderate forces but at relatively high shortening or lengthening velocities. One of the more important functions of the hamstring muscles, for example, is to decelerate the advancing tibia at the late swing phase of walking. Through eccentric action, the muscle helps dampen the impact of full knee extension. Consider also sprinting or rapidly walking uphill. These same muscles rapidly contract to accelerate knee flexion in order to shorten the functional length of the lower limb during the swing phase.

**Control of Femoral-on-Tibial Osteokinematics.** The muscular demand needed to control femoral-on-tibial motions is generally larger and more complex than that needed to control most ordinary tibial-on-femoral knee motions. A muscle like the sartorius, for example, may have to simultaneously control up to five degrees of freedom (i.e., two at the knee and three at the hip). To illustrate, consider the action of several knee flexor-rotator muscles while running to catch a ball (Fig. 13–33A). While the right foot is firmly fixed to the ground, the right femur, pelvis, trunk, neck, head, and eyes all rotate to the left. Note the diagonal flow of contracting muscles between the right fibula and left side of the neck. The muscle action epitomizes intermuscular synergy. In this case, the short head of the biceps femoris anchors the diagonal kinetic chain to the fibula. The fibula, in turn, is anchored to the tibia via the interosseous membrane and other muscles.

Stability and control at the knee require interaction of forces produced by muscles and ligaments.[9] Interaction is especially important for control of movements in the horizontal and frontal planes. To illustrate, refer to Figure 13–33B. With the right foot planted, the short head of the biceps femoris accelerates the femur internally. By way of eccentric activation, the pes anserinus muscles help decelerate the internal rotation of the femur and pelvis over the tibia. The pes anserinus group of muscles functions as a dynamic medial collateral ligament by resisting the external rotation and valgus torques produced at the knee. Muscle action may help compensate for a weak or lax medial collateral ligament.

### Maximal Torque Production of the Knee Flexor-Rotator Muscles

Maximal effort knee flexion torque is generally greatest near full extension, then declines steadily as the knee is progressively flexed (Fig. 13–34A).[110] Although the hamstrings have

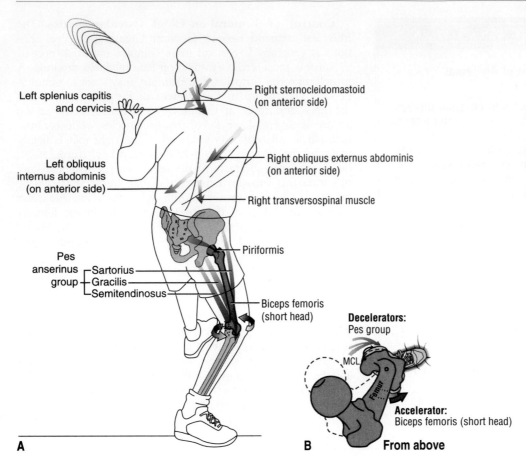

Left splenius capitis
and cervicis

Left obliquus
internus abdominis
(on anterior side)

Pes
anserinus
group

Sartorius
Gracilis
Semitendinosus

Right sternocleidomastoid
(on anterior side)

Right obliquus externus abdominis
(on anterior side)

Right transversospinal muscle

Piriformis

Biceps femoris
(short head)

Decelerators:
Pes group

MCL

Femur

Accelerator:
Biceps femoris (short head)

From above

A

B

**FIGURE 13–33.** *A,* Several muscles are shown controlling the rotation of the head, neck, trunk, pelvis, and femur toward the approaching ball. Since the right foot is fixed to the ground, the right knee functions as an important pivot point. *B,* Control of the movement of the right knee within the horizontal plane is illustrated from above. The short head of the biceps femoris contracts to accelerate the femur internally (i.e., the knee joint moves into external rotation). Active force from the pes anserinus muscles in conjunction with a passive force from the stretched medial collateral ligament (MCL) helps to decelerate, or limit, the external rotation at the knee.

their greatest internal moment arm at about 45 degrees of knee flexion (Fig. 13–34*B*), the muscles produce their greatest knee flexor torque when fully elongated. Flexing the hip to elongate the hamstrings promotes even greater knee flexion torque.[6] Length-tension relationship appears to be a very influential factor in determining the flexion torque potential of the hamstrings.

Few data are available on the maximal torque potential of the internal and external rotator muscles of the knee. With the hip and knee each flexed to 90 degrees, the internal and external rotators at the knee produce peak torques of about 30 Nm.[107] With hips and knees flexed to only about 20 degrees, the peak internal rotation torque exceeds external rotation torque by about 40%.

### Maximal Torque Production at the Knee: Effects of Type and Speed of Muscle Activation

Clinically, internal torque at the knee is typically measured using isokinetic dynamometry (see Chapter 4). In this type of measurement, the joint is typically rotating so that both the length and moment arm of the muscles are constantly changing across a range of motion. Isokinetic dynamometry allows internal torques to be measured during concentric, isometric, and eccentric muscle activations. In general, internal torques produced through eccentric or isometric activations are greater than those produced through concentric contraction. Based on the force-velocity curve of muscle (see Chapter 2), concentrically produced muscle torques decline

as the contraction speed increases.[6,8,40,52] Figure 13–35 shows a plot of the peak torque produced by the knee extensors and flexors during nonisometric (isokinetic) activations.[52] The decline in peak torque occurs during concentric contractions for both knee extensors and knee flexors. In contrast, the peak torques remain essentially constant during increasing eccentric activated velocities.

### Synergy Among Monoarticular and Biarticular Muscles of the Hip and Knee

#### Typical Movement Combinations: Hip-and-Knee Extension or Hip-and-Knee Flexion

Many movements performed by the lower extremities involve the cyclic actions of hip-and-knee extension or hip-and-knee flexion. These patterns of movement are fundamental components of walking, running, jumping, and climbing. Hip-and-knee extension propels the body forward or upward, whereas hip-and-knee flexion advances or swings the lower limb. These movements are controlled, in part, through a synergy among monoarticular and polyarticular muscles, many of which cross the hip and knee.

Figure 13–36 shows an interaction of muscles during the hip-and-knee extension phase of running. The vastius and gluteus maximus—two monoarticular muscles—are shown contracting synergistically with the biarticular semitendinosus and rectus femoris. The vastus group of the quadriceps and the semitendinosus are both electrically active, yet their net torque at the knee favors extension. The active shortening of

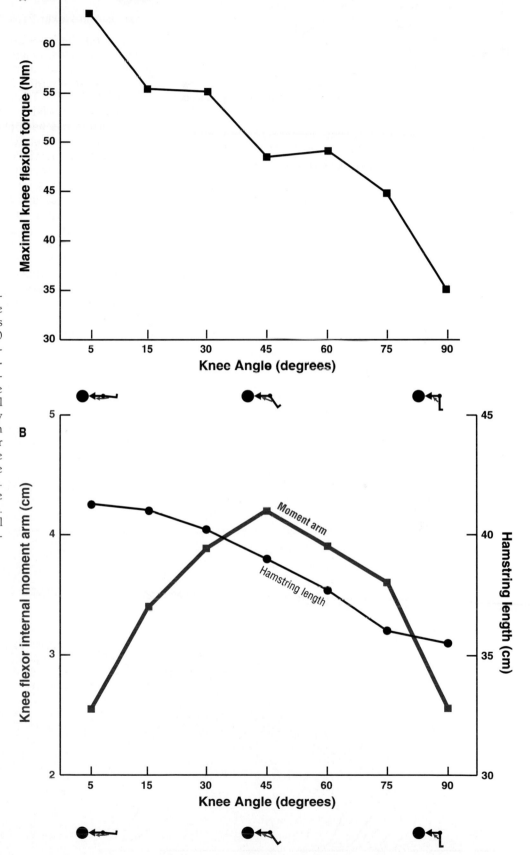

**FIGURE 13–34.** Biomechanical variables related to maximal-effort knee flexion torque. *A,* The plot depicts knee flexion torque between near 0 degrees and 90 degrees of knee flexion. Knee flexor torques are produced isometrically, with the hip extended. *B,* This plot shows the relationships between the internal moment arm of the hamstrings (left y axis, in red) and hamstring length (right y axis, in black) between near 0 degrees and 90 degrees of knee flexion. Data on muscle length were estimated using a human skeleton. Data on torque and moment arm are based on a healthy male population. (Data from Smidt GL: Biomechanical analysis of knee flexion and extension. J Biomechan 6:79–92, 1973.)

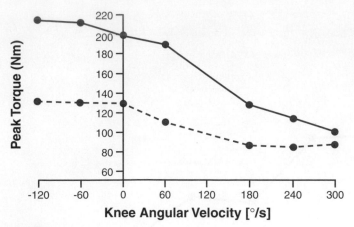

**Peak Torque (Nm)** vs **Knee Angular Velocity [°/s]**

**FIGURE 13–35.** Peak torque generated by the knee extensor muscles (top, solid line) and knee flexor muscles (bottom, dashed line). Positive velocities denote concentric (muscle shortening) activity and negative velocities denote eccentric (muscle lengthening) activity. Data are from 64 untrained, healthy males. (From Horstmann T, Maschmann J, Mayer F, et al: The influence of age on isokinetic torque of the upper and lower leg musculature in sedentary men. Int J Sports Med 20:362–367, 1999. Georg Thieme Verlag.)

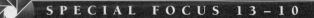

SPECIAL FOCUS 13–10

**Extensor-to-Flexor Peak Torque Ratios**

In general, the knee extensor muscles produce a torque about two-thirds greater than the knee flexor muscles.[13] A major factor accounting for this difference is the relatively large torque produced by the vastus muscles (see Fig. 13–24).[54] The patella significantly increases the moment arm available to the quadriceps.

Research has been performed to define a normative extensor-to-flexor peak torque ratio at the knee to help clinicians set appropriate goals for isokinetic strength training.[13,51] Unfortunately, the torque ratios have been found to vary considerably, therefore limiting clinical usefulness. Grace and colleagues[39] reported an extensor-to-flexor torque ratio of 1.67:1 (i.e., extensors produced 67% greater peak torque than flexors) in 172 high school–age males. In another study, the peak knee extensor-to-flexor torque ratios were measured at three different isokinetic test speeds in 100 healthy subjects.[124] Results were 1.39:1 at 60 degrees/sec, 1.27:1 at 180 degrees/sec, and 1.19:1 at 300 degrees/sec. The difference in peak torques between the extensor and flexor muscles decreased as the speed of contraction increased.

the overpowering vastus not only extends the knee, but lengthens or stretches the active semitendinosus. Because the semitendinosus is lengthened across the knee as it simultaneously produces hip extension, little overall change occurs in the muscle's length. The semitendinosus, therefore, extends the hip but actually contracts or shortens a relatively short distance.

The action of the semitendinosus muscle favors relatively high force output per level of neural drive or effort. The physiologic basis for this phenomenon rests on the force-velocity and length-tension relationships of muscle. Consider primarily the effect of muscle velocity on muscle force production. Muscle force per level of effort increases sharply as the contraction velocity is reduced (see Chapter 3). As an

example, a muscle contracting at 6.3% of its maximum shortening velocity produces a force of about 75% of its maximum. Slowing the contraction velocity to only 2.2% of maximal (i.e., very near isometric) raises force output to 90% of maximum.[75] In the movement of hip-and-knee extension, the vastus muscles, by extending the knee, indirectly augment hip extension force by reducing the contraction velocity of the semitendinosus.

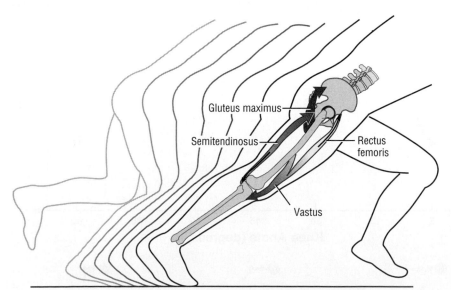

**FIGURE 13–36.** The action of several monoarticular and biarticular muscles are depicted during the hip-and-knee extension phase of running. Observe that the vasti extend the knee, which then stretches the distal end of the semitendinosus. The gluteus maximus extends the hip, which then stretches the proximal end of the rectus femoris. The stretched biarticular muscles are depicted by thin black arrows. The stretch placed on the active biarticular muscles reduces the rate and amount of their overall contraction. (See text for further details.)

**TABLE 13–9. Examples of Muscle Synergies at the Hip and Knee**

| | Monoarticular Muscles | Action | Biarticular Transducers | Action Augmented |
|---|---|---|---|---|
| Active hip *and* knee *extension* | Vasti | Knee *extension* | Two-joint hamstrings | Hip *extension* |
| | Gluteus maximus | Hip *extension* | Rectus femoris | Knee *extension* |
| Active hip *and* knee *flexion* | Iliopsoas | Hip *flexion* | Two-joint hamstrings | Knee *flexion* |
| | Biceps femoris (short head), popliteus | Knee *flexion* | Rectus femoris | Hip *flexion* |

After Leiber RL: Skeletal Muscle Structure and Function. Baltimore, Williams & Wilkins, 1992.

Consider next the effect of muscle length on the passive force produced by a muscle. Based on a muscle's passive length-tension relationship, the internal resistance or force within a muscle, such as the semitendinosus, increases as it is stretched. The semitendinosus—as well as all biarticular hamstrings—functions as a "transducer" by transferring force from the contracting vastus muscles to the extending hip.

During active hip-and-knee extension, the gluteus maximus and rectus femoris have a relationship similar to that

### A. Hip flexion and knee extension

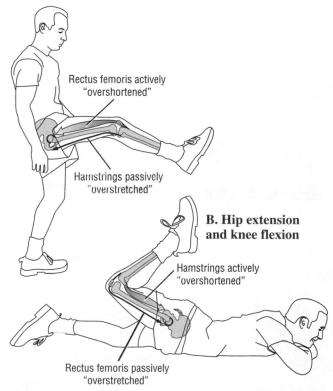

Rectus femoris actively "overshortened"

Hamstrings passively "overstretched"

### B. Hip extension and knee flexion

Hamstrings actively "overshortened"

Rectus femoris passively "overstretched"

**FIGURE 13–37.** The motions of (*A*) hip flexion and knee extension and (*B*) hip extension and knee flexion. For both movements, the near-maximal contraction of the biarticular muscles (red) causes a near-maximal stretch in the biarticular antagonist muscles (thin black arrows).

between the vasti and semitendinosus. In essence, the powerful monoarticular gluteus maximus augments knee extension force by extending the hip. This, in turn, stretches the activated rectus femoris. In this example, the rectus femoris is the biarticular transducer, transferring force from the gluteus maximus to knee extension. A summary of these and other muscular interactions used during hip-and-knee flexion are listed in Table 13–9.

The interdependence between the hip and knee extensor muscles allows for the most efficient force development. This interdependence is considered when evaluating functional activities that require combined hip-and-knee extension, such as standing from a chair. Weakness of the vasti could cause difficulty in extending the hip, whereas weakness of the gluteus maximus could cause difficulty in extending the knee.

#### Atypical Movement Combinations: Hip Flexion-and-Knee Extension or Hip Extension-and-Knee Flexion

Consider movement patterns of the hip and knee that are out of phase with the more typical movement patterns described here. Hip flexion can occur with knee extension (Fig. 13–37A), or hip extension can occur with knee flexion (Fig. 13–37B). The physiologic consequences of these movements are very different from those described in Figure 13–36. In Figure 13–37A, the biarticular rectus femoris must shorten a great distance, and with relatively higher velocity, in order to flex the hip and extend the knee. Even with maximal effort, active knee extension is usually limited during this action. Based on the length-tension and force-velocity relationships of muscle, the rectus femoris is not able to develop maximal knee extensor force. The hamstrings are overstretched across both the hip and knee, thereby passively resisting knee extension.

The situation described in Figure 13–37A applies to the movement described in Figure 13–37B. The biarticular hamstrings must contract to a very short length—a movement that is often accompanied by cramping. Furthermore, the biarticular rectus femoris is overstretched across both the hip and knee, thereby passively resisting knee flexion. For both reasons, knee flexion force and range of motion are usually limited by the out-of-phase movement.

The atypical movements depicted in Figure 13–37A and B may have a useful purpose. Consider the movement of kicking a football. Elastic energy is stored in the stretched rectus femoris by the preparatory movement of combined

## Reaction Forces through the Normal Knee

### A. Standing          B. Walking

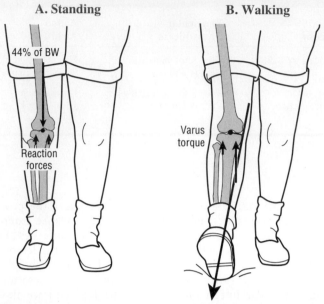

**FIGURE 13–38.** *A,* While standing, a force equal to about 44% of body weight (BW) passes close to the center of each knee joint. The lateral and medial articular surfaces of the tibia respond with forces equal to about 22% of body weight. *B,* While walking, a force equal to about three times body weight passes medial to the knee joint, creating a varus torque at every step. The direction of this force causes the medial articular surface of the tibia to respond with a greater reaction force than the lateral articular surface. (Force vectors are not drawn to scale.)

hip extension and knee flexion. The action of kicking the ball involves a rapid and full contraction of the rectus femoris to simultaneously flex the hip and extend the knee. The goal of this action is to dissipate all force in the rectus femoris as quickly as possible. In contrast, activities such as walking or jogging use biarticular muscles so that forces are developed more slowly and in a repetitive or cyclic fashion. The rectus femoris and semitendinosus, for instance, tend to remain at a relatively fixed length throughout much of the activation cycle. In this way, muscles avoid repetitive cycles of storing and immediately releasing relatively large amounts of energy. More moderate levels of active and passive forces are cooperatively shared between muscles, thereby optimizing the metabolic efficiency of the movement.

## Abnormal Alignment of the Knee

### FRONTAL PLANE

In the frontal plane, the knee is normally aligned in about 5 to 10 degrees of valgus. Deviation from this alignment is referred to as excessive genu valgum or genu varum.

### *Genu Varum with Unicompartmental Osteoarthritis of the Knee*

In the normally aligned knee, joint reaction forces during standing pass almost equally through the lateral and medial knee compartments (Fig. 13–38*A*). Assuming that 44% of

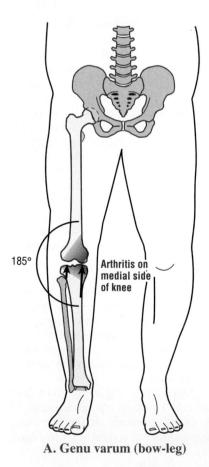

**A. Genu varum (bow-leg)**

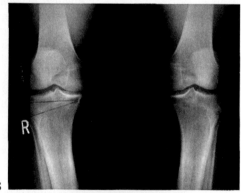

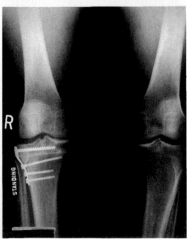

**FIGURE 13–39.** Bilateral genu varum with osteoarthritis in the medial compartment of the right knee. *A,* The varus deformity of the right knee is shown with associated increased joint reaction force on the medial compartment. The area in red indicates arthritic changes. *B,* An anterior x-ray view with subject (a 43-year-old man) standing, showing bilateral genu varum and medial joint osteoarthritis. Both knees have a loss of medial joint space and hypertrophic bone around the medial compartment. To correct the deformity on the right (R) knee, a wedge of bone will be surgically removed by a procedure known as a high tibial osteotomy. *C,* The x-ray shows the right knee after the removal of the wedge of bone. Note the change in joint alignment compared with the same knee in *B.* (Courtesy of Joseph Davies, M.D., Milwaukee Orthopedic Group, Sinai Samaritan Medical Center, Milwaukee.)

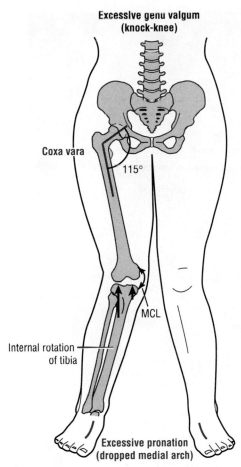

**Excessive genu valgum (knock-knee)**

Coxa vara

115°

Internal rotation of tibia

MCL

Excessive pronation (dropped medial arch)

**FIGURE 13–40.** Excessive genu valgum of the right knee. In this example, the valgus deformity is the result of abnormal alignment at both proximal and distal ends of the lower limb (red). Coxa vara and/or excessive pronation of the foot can increase the valgus stress at the knee. Over time, greater valgus stress at the knee can increase the strain in the medial collateral ligament (MCL), and can increase the compression force on the lateral compartment of the knee. Note that the excessive pronation of the foot, from a dropped medial arch, causes the tibia to rotate internally while standing.

body weight is located above the knees, each compartment theoretically receives joint reaction forces equal to about 22% of body weight. (See the two small arrows in Fig. 13–38A.) While walking, however, total knee reaction forces increase to about three times body weight. The increase is due to the combined effect of muscle activation and reaction forces produced by the ground at heel contact. Because the heel normally strikes the ground just lateral to its midline, the resulting ground reaction force passes just medial to the knee (Fig. 13–38B). A net varus torque, therefore, is created with every step. For this reason, joint reaction forces while walking are typically greater on the medial compartment.

Most persons tolerate the asymmetrical dynamic loading of the knee with little or no difficulty. In some persons, however, the medial compartment experiences excessive wear, ultimately leading to unicompartmental osteoarthritis.[76] Thinning of the articular cartilage on the medial side can tilt

the knee into genu varum, or bow-legged deformity (Fig. 13–39A). A vicious circle may erupt: the varus deformity increases medial compartment loading, resulting in greater loss of medial joint space, causing greater varus deformity, and so on. Figure 13–39B is an anterior view of an x-ray showing bilateral genu varum. Both knees illustrate signs of medial joint osteoarthritis (i e , loss of medial joint space and hypertrophic reactive bone around the medial compartment). Management of genu varum often involves surgery, such as a high tibial (wedge) osteotomy. The goal of this surgery is to correct the varus deformity and reduce the stress over the medial compartment (Fig. 13–39C).[117] In addition to surgery, foot orthoses are worn to reduce stress on knees with medial joint arthritis. Laterally wedged insoles decrease the varus torque on the knee, and thereby decrease the load on the medial compartment.[16]

### Excessive Genu Valgum

Several biomechanical factors can lead to excessive genu valgum, or "knock-knee" (Fig. 13–40). Genu valgum is often the result of abnormal alignment at either end of the lower extremity. As indicated in Figure 13–40, coxa vara (i.e., a femoral neck-shaft angle less than 125 degrees) or excessively pronated feet may increase the valgus stress on the knee. Over time, this stress may strain and subsequently weaken the medial collateral ligament. Standing with a valgus deformity of approximately 10 degrees greater than normal directs most of the joint force to the lateral compartment.[62] Knee replacement surgery may be indicated to correct a valgus deformity, especially if it is painful or causes loss of function or lessens quality of life. Figure 13–41 shows severe bilateral osteoarthritis of the knee, with severe genu valgum on the right and genu varum on the left. This "wind-swept" deformity was corrected surgically with bilateral knee replacements (Fig. 13–41C).

## SAGITTAL PLANE

### Genu Recurvatum

Full extension with slight external rotation is the knee's close-packed, stable position. While standing in this locked position, the knee is typically hyperextended about 5 to 10 degrees owing in part to the posterior slope of the tibial plateau. Hyperextension directs the line-of-gravity from body weight slightly anterior to the medial-lateral axis of rotation at the knee. Gravity, therefore, produces a slight knee extension torque that can naturally assist with locking of the knee, allowing the quadriceps to relax while standing. Normally, this gravity-assisted extension torque is adequately resisted by passive tension in the stretched posterior capsule and stretched flexor muscles of the knee.

Hyperextension beyond 10 degrees is called *genu recurvatum* (from the Latin *genu,* knee; + *recurvare,* to bend backward). The primary cause of genu recurvatum is a chronic, overpowering knee extensor torque that eventually overstretches the posterior structures in the knee. The overpowering knee extension torque may stem from poor postural control or from neuromuscular disease that causes spasticity of the quadriceps muscles and/or paralysis of the knee flexors.

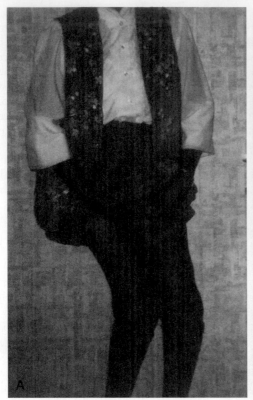

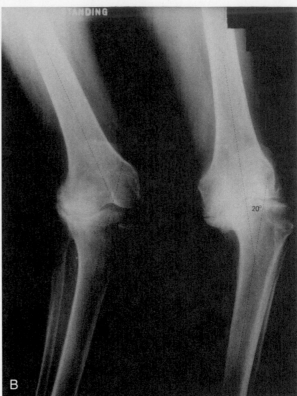

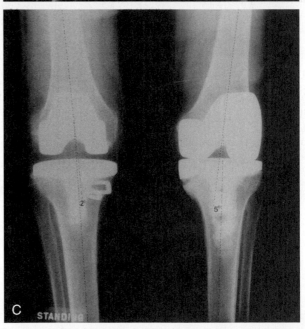

**FIGURE 13–41.** Bilateral frontal plane malalignment in the knees of an 83-year-old female. *A,* The classic "wind-swept" deformity, with excessive genu valgum on right and genu varum on the left. *B* and *C* are the x-rays of the patient in *A,* before and after knee replacement. Note in *B,* the hypertrophic bone formation in areas of increased stress. With excessive genu valgum, the stress is greater on the lateral compartment; with genu varum, the stress is greater on the medial compartment. (Courtesy of Joseph Davies, M.D., Milwaukee Orthopedic Group, Sinai Samaritan Medical Center, Milwaukee.)

## SPECIAL FOCUS 13–11

**Case Report: Pathomechanics and Treatment of Severe Genu Recurvatum**

Figure 13–42*A* shows a case of severe genu recurvatum of the left knee, caused by a flaccid muscle paralysis from polio, contracted 30 years earlier. The deformity has progressed slowly over the last 20 years as the individual

continued to walk without a knee brace. She has partial paralysis of the left quadriceps and hip flexors, but complete paralysis of the left knee flexors. Her completely paralyzed left ankle joint was surgically fused in about 25 degrees of plantar flexion.

**A. Uncorrected**

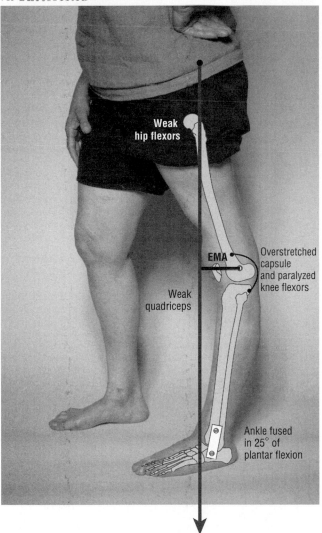

Weak
hip flexors

EMA

Overstretched
capsule
and paralyzed
knee flexors

Weak
quadriceps

Ankle fused
in 25° of
plantar flexion

Body weight

**B. Corrected**

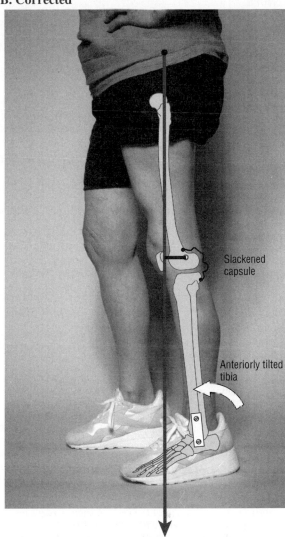

Slackened
capsule

Anteriorly tilted
tibia

Body weight

**FIGURE 13–42.** Subject showing marked genu recurvatum of the left knee secondary to polio. In addition to sporadic muscle weakness throughout the left lower extremity, the left ankle was surgically fused in 25 degrees of plantar flexion. *A,* When standing barefoot, the subject's body weight acts with an abnormally large external moment arm (EMA) at the knee. The resulting large extensor torque amplifies the magnitude of the knee hyperextension deformity. *B,* Subject is able to reduce the severity of the recurvatum deformity by wearing a tennis shoe with a built-up heel. The shoe tilted her tibia and knee forward, thereby reducing the length of the deforming external moment arm at the knee.

Several interrelated factors are responsible for the development of the deformity depicted in Figure 13–42A. Because of the fixed plantar flexion position of the ankle, the tibia must be tilted posteriorly so that the bottom of the foot makes full contact with the ground. Over the years, this tilted position of the tibia hyperextended the knee and overstretched the posterior structures of the knee. Of particular importance is the fact that total paralysis of the knee's flexor muscles provided no direct muscular resistance against the knee's hyperextension deformity. Furthermore, the greater the hyperextension deformity, the longer the external moment arm available to body weight to perpetuate the deformity. Without bracing of the knee, the hyperextension deformity produced a vicious circle, allowing continuous stretching of the posterior structures of the knee and continuous progression of the deformity.

The knee functions as the middle link of the lower limb. Consequently, the knee joint is vulnerable to deforming stresses from musculoskeletal pathology at either end of the lower extremity. This case report demonstrates how an excessive and fixed plantar flexed ankle can predispose a person to genu recurvatum. As depicted in Figure 13–42B, a relatively simple and inexpensive ankle orthotic device was used to treat the hyperextension deformity. Wearing a tennis shoe with a "built-up" heel provided excellent reduction in the severity of the genu recurvatum. The raised heel tilted the tibia and knee anteriorly, thereby significantly reducing the length of the deforming external moment arm at the knee. Body weight now produced a relatively small hyperextension torque at the knee, held in check by the anteriorly tilted tibia and by the rigidity provided by the fused ankle joint.

# REFERENCES

1. Andriacchi TP, Birac D: Functional testing in the anterior cruciate ligament-deficient knee. Clin Orthop 288:40–47, 1993.
2. Barber-Westin SD, Noyes FR, Heckmann TP, et al: The effect of exercise and rehabilitation on anterior-posterior knee displacements after anterior cruciate ligament autograft reconstruction. Am J Sports Med 27:884–893, 1999.
3. Basmajian JV, Lovejoy JF: Function of the popliteus muscles in man. J Bone Joint Surg 53A:557–562, 1971.
4. Beynnon BD, Johnson RJ, Fleming BC, et al: The strain behavior of the anterior cruciate ligament during squatting and active flexion-extension. Am J Sports Med 25:823–829, 1997.
5. Beynnon BD, Fleming BC: Anterior cruciate ligament strain in-vivo: A review of previous work. J Biomech 31:519–525, 1998.
6. Bohannon RW, Gajdosik RL, LeVeau BF: Isokinetic knee flexion and extension torque in the upright sitting and semireclined sitting positions. Phys Ther 66:1083–1086, 1986.
7. Boone DC, Azen SP: Normal range of motion of joints in male subjects. J Bone Joint Surg 61A:756–759, 1979.
8. Borges O: Isometric and isokinetic knee extension and flexion torque in men and women aged 20–70. Scand J Rehab 21:45–53, 1989.
9. Buchanan TS, Lloyd DG: Muscle activation at the human knee during isometric flexion-extension and varus-valgus loads. J Ortho Res 15:11–17, 1997.
10. Buff HU, Jones LC, Hungerford DS: Experimental determination of forces transmitted through the patello-femoral joint. J Biomech 21:17–23, 1988.
11. Butler DL, Noyes FR, Grood ES: Ligamentous restraints to anterior-posterior drawer in the human knee. J Bone Joint Surg 62A:259–270, 1980.
12. Bynum EB, Barrack RL, Alexander AH: Open versus closed chain kinetic exercises after anterior cruciate ligament reconstruction. Am J Sports Med 23:401–406, 1995.
13. Calmels PM, Nellen M, van der Borne I, et al: Concentric and eccentric isokinetic assessment of flexor-extensor torque ratios at the hip, knee, and ankle in a sample population of healthy subjects. Arch Phys Med Rehabil 78:1224–1230, 1997.
14. Clancy WG, Sutherland TB: Combined posterior cruciate ligament injuries. Clin Sports Med 13:629–647, 1994.
15. Covey DC, Sapega AA, Sherman GM: Testing for isometry during reconstruction of the posterior cruciate ligament. Am J Sports Med 24:740–746, 1996.
16. Crenshaw SJ, Pollo FE, Calton EF: Effects of lateral-wedged insoles on kinetics at the knee. Clinical Orthop 375:185–192, 2000.
17. Dahlkvist NJ, Mayo P, Seedhom BB: Forces during squatting and rising from a deep squat. Engineer Med 11:69–76, 1982.
18. Davies DV, Edwards DAW: The blood supply of the synovial membrane and intra-articular structures. Ann R Coll Surg 2:142–156, 1948.
19. deAndrade JR, Grant C, Dixon ASJ: Joint distension and reflex muscle inhibition in the knee. J Bone Joint Surg 47A:313–322, 1965.
20. DeHaven KE, Lintner DM: Athletic injuries: Comparison by age, sport, and gender. Am J Sports Med 14:218–224, 1986.
21. Desio SM, Burks RT, Bachus KN: Soft tissue restraints to lateral patellar translation in the human knee. Am J Sports Med 26:59–65, 1998.
22. DeVita P, Lassiter T, Hortobagyi T, et al: Functional knee effects during walking in patients with anterior cruciate ligament reconstruction. Am J Sports Med 26:778–784, 1998.
23. Dupont JY: Synovial plicae of the knee. Clin Sports Med 16:87–122, 1997.
24. Ernst GP, Saliba E, Diduch DR, et al: Lower-extremity compensations following anterior cruciate ligament reconstruction. Phys Ther 80:251–260, 2000.
25. Escamilla RF, Fleisig GS, Zheng N, et al: Biomechanics of the knee during closed kinetic chain and open kinetic chain exercises. Med Sci Sports Exerc 30:556–569, 1998.
26. Fisher NM, Pendergast DR, Calkins EC: Maximal isometric torque of knee extension as a function of muscle length in subjects of advancing age. Phys Med Rehabil 71:896–899, 1990.
27. Fitzgerald GK: Open versus closed kinetic chan exercises: After anterior cruciate ligament reconstructive surgery. Phys Ther 77:1747–1754, 1997.
28. Fitzgerald GK, Axe MJ, Snyder-Mackler L: The efficacy of perturbation training in nonoperative anterior cruciate ligament rehabilitation programs for physically active persons. Phys Ther 80:128–140, 2000.
29. Frank CB, Jackson DW: The science of reconstruction of the anterior cruciate ligament. J Bone Joint Surg 79A:1556–1576, 1997.
30. Frankel VH, Burstein AH, Brooks DB: Biomechanics of internal derangement of the knee. J Bone Joint Surg 53A:945–962, 1971.
31. Freeman BL: Recurrent dislocations. In Crenshaw AH (ed): Campbells' Operative Orthopaedics, 2nd vol, 8th ed. St. Louis, Mosby-Year Book, 1992.
32. Fulkerson JP, Hungerford DS: Disorders of the Patellofemoral Joint. Baltimore, Williams & Wilkins, 1990.
33. Fuss FK: Principles and mechanisms of automatic rotation during terminal extension in the human knee joint. J Anat 180:297–304, 1992.
34. Gilleard W, McConnell J, Parsons D: The effect of patellar taping on the onset of vastus medialis obliquus and vastus lateralis muscle activity in persons with patellofemoral pain. Phys Ther 78:25–32, 1998.
35. Gillquist J, Messner K: Anterior cruciate ligament reconstruction and long-term incidence of gonarthrosis. Sports Med 267:143–156, 1999.
36. Girgis FG, Marshall JL, Al Monajem ARS: The cruciate ligaments of the knee joint. Clin Orthop 106:216–231, 1975.
37. Goodfellow J, Hungerford DS, Zindel M: Patello-femoral joint mechanics and pathology. J Bone Joint Surg 58B:287–290, 1976.
38. Grabiner MD, Koh TJ, Draganich LF: Neuromechanics of the patello-femoral joint. Med Sci Sports Exerc 26:10–21, 1994.
39. Grace TG, Sweetser ER, Nelson MA, et al: Isokinetic muscle imbalance and knee-joint injuries. J Bone Joint Surg 66A:734–740, 1984.
40. Griffin JW, Tooms RE, Vander Zwaag R, et al: Eccentric muscle performance of elbow and knee muscle groups in untrained men and women. Med Sci Sports Exerc 25:936–944, 1993.
41. Harner CD, Xerogeanes JW, Livesay GA, et al: The human posterior cruciate ligament complex: An interdisciplinary study. Am J Sports Med 23:736–745, 1995.
42. Harner CD, Hoher J, Vogrin TM, et al: The effects of a popliteus muscle load on in-situ forces in the posterior cruciate ligament and on knee kinematics. Am J Sports Med 26:669–673, 1998.
43. Harris NL: Central quadriceps tendon for anterior cruciate ligament reconstruction. Am J Sports Med 25:23–28, 1997.
44. Heegaard J, Leyvraz PF, Van Kampen A, et al: Influence of soft structures on patellar three-dimensional tracking. Clin Orthop 299:235–243, 1994.
45. Heller L, Langman J: The menisco-femoral ligaments of the human knee. J Bone Joint Surg 46B:307–313, 1964.
46. Henning CE, Lynch MA, Glick KR: An in vivo strain gauge study of elongation of the anterior cruciate ligament. Am J Sports Med 13:22–26, 1985.
47. Hirokawa S, Solomonow M, Lu Y, et al: Anterior-posterior and rotational displacement of the tibia elicited by quadriceps contraction. Am J Sports Med 20:299–306, 1992.
48. Hoher J, Vogrin TM, Woo SLY, et al: In situ forces in the human posterior cruciate ligament in response to muscle loads: A cadaveric study. J Orthop Res 17:763–768, 1999.
49. Hollis JM, Takai S, Adams DJ, et al: The effects of knee motion and external loading on the length of the anterior cruciate ligament (ACL): A kinematic study. J Biomech Eng 113:208–214, 1991.
50. Hollister AM, Jatana S, Singh AK, et al: The axes of rotation of the knee. Clin Orthop 290:259–268, 1993.
51. Holm I, Ludvigsen P, Steen H: Isokinetic hamstrings/quadriceps ratios: Normal values and reproducibility in sport students. Isokin Exec Sci 4:141–145, 1994.
52. Horstmann T, Maschmann J, Mayer F, et al: The influence of age on isokinetic torque of the upper and lower leg musculature in sedentary men. Int J Sports Med 20:362–367, 1999.
53. Horton MG, Hall TL: Quadriceps femoris muscle angle: Normal values and relationships with gender and selected skeletal measures. Phys Ther 69:897–901, 1989.
54. Hoy MG, Zajac FE, Gordon ME: A musculoskeletal model of the human lower extremity: The effect of muscle, tendon, and moment arm on the moment angle relationship of musculotendon actuators at the hip, knee, and ankle. J Biomech 23:157–169, 1990.
55. Hubbard JK, Sampson HW, Elledge JR: Prevalence and morphology of the vastus medialis oblique muscle in human cadavers. Anat Rec 249:135–142, 1997.
56. Huberti HH, Hayes WC: Patellofemoral contact pressures. J Bone Joint Surg 66A:715–724, 1984.
57. Hungerford DS, Barry M: Biomechanics of the patellofemoral joint. Clin Orthop 144:9–15, 1979.

58. Inman VT, Saunders JB: Referred pain from skeletal structures. J Nerv Ment Dis 99:660–667, 1944.

59. Ishii Y, Terajima K, Terashima S, et al: Three-dimensional kinematics of the human knee with intracortical pin fixation. Clin Orthop 343:144–150, 1997.

60. Janousek AT, Jones DG, Clatworthy M, et al: Posterior cruciate ligament injuries of the knee joint. Sports Med 28:429–441, 1999.

61. Jenkins WL, Munns SW, Jayaraman G, et al: A measurement of anterior tibial displacement in the closed and open kinetic chain. J Orthop Sports Phys Ther 25:49–56, 1997.

62. Johnson F, Leitl S, Waugh W: The distribution of load across the knee. J Bone Joint Surg 62B:715–724, 1980.

63. Kaufer H: Mechanical function of the patella. J Bone Joint Surg 53A:1551–1560, 1971.

64. Keays SL, Bullock-Saxton J, Keays AC: Strength and function before and after anterior cruciate ligament reconstruction. Clin Orthop 373:174–183, 2000.

65. Kennedy JC, Alexander IJ, Hayes KC: Nerve supply of the human knee and its functional importance. Am J Sports Med 10:329–335, 1982.

66. Kellis E: Quantification of quadriceps and hamstring activity. Sports Med 25:37–62, 1998.

67. Kim YC, Yoo WK, Chung IH, et al: Tendinous insertion of semimembranosus muscle into the lateral meniscus. Surg Radiol Anat 19:365–369, 1997.

68. Krause WR, Pope MH, Johnson RJ, et al: Mechanical changes in the knee after meniscectomy. J Bone Joint Surg 58A:599–604, 1976.

69. Krauspe R, Schmidt M, Schaible HG, et al: Sensory innervation of the anterior cruciate ligament. J Bone Joint Surg 74A:390–397, 1992.

70. Laprade J, Culham E, Brouwer B: Comparison of five isometric exercises in the recruitment of the vastus medialis oblique in persons with and without patellofemoral pain syndrome. J Orthop Sports Phys Ther 27.197–204, 1998.

71. Last RJ: Some anatomical details of the knee joint. J Bone Joint Surg 30B:683–688, 1948.

72. Laubenthal KN, Smidt GL, Kettelkamp DB: A quantitative analysis of knee motion during activities of daily living. Phys Ther 52:34–42, 1972.

73. Li G, Rudy TW, Sakane M, et al: The importance of quadriceps and hamstring muscle loading on knee kinematics and in-situ forces in the ACL. J Biomechan 32:395–400, 1999.

74. Lieb FJ, Perry J: Quadriceps function. J Bone Joint Surg 50A:1535–1548, 1968.

75. Lieber RL: Skeletal Muscle Structure and Function. Baltimore, Williams & Wilkins, 1992.

76. Lindenfeld TN, Hewett TE, Andriacchi TP: Joint loading with valgus bracing in patients with varus gonarthrosis. Clin Orthop 344:290–297, 1997.

77. Liu W, Maitland ME: The effect of hamstring muscle compensation for anterior laxity in the ACL-deficient knee during gait. J Biomech 33:871–879, 2000.

78. Livingston LA: The quadriceps angle: A review of the literature. J Orthop Sports Phys Ther 28:105–109, 1998.

79. Lutz GE, Palmitier RA, An KN, et al: Comparison of tibiofemoral joint forces during open-kinetic-chain and closed-kinetic-chain exercises. J Bone Joint Surg 75A:732–739, 1993.

80. Maletius W, Messner K: Eighteen- to twenty-four-year follow-up after complete rupture of the anterior cruciate ligament. Am J Sports Med 27:711–717, 1999.

81. Markolf KL, Graff-Radford A, Amstutz HC: In vivo knee stability. J Bone Joint Surg 60A:664–674, 1978.

82. Matthews LS, Sonstegard DA, Henke JA: Load-bearing characteristics of the patellofemoral joint. Acta Orthop Scand 48:511–516, 1977.

83. McNair PJ, Marshall RN, Maguire K: Swelling of the knee joint: Effects of exercise on quadriceps muscle strength. Arch Phys Med Rehabil 77:896–899, 1996.

84. Morgan CD, Kalman VR, and Grawl DM: The anatomic origin of the posterior cruciate ligament: Where is it? Reference landmarks for PCL reconstruction. Arthroscopy 13:325–331, 1997.

85. Morrison JB: The mechanics of the knee joint in relation to normal walking. J Biomech 3:51–61, 1970.

86. Mossberg KA, Smith LK: Axial rotation of the knee in women. J Orthop Sports Phys Ther 4:236–240, 1983.

87. Muneta T, Takakuda K, Yamamoto H: Intercondylar notch width and its relation to the configuration and cross-sectional area of the anterior cruciate ligament. Am J Sports Med 125:69–72, 1997.

88. Nisell R, Ericson MO, Nemeth G, et al: Tibiofemoral joint forces during isokinetic knee extension. Am J Sports Med 17:49–54, 1989.

89. Osternig LR, Bates BT, James SL: Patterns of tibial rotary torque in knees of healthy subjects. Med Sci Sports Exerc 12:195–199, 1980.

90. Outerbridge RE: The etiology of chondromalacia patellae. J Bone Joint Surg 43B:752–757, 1961.

91. Paletta GA, Manning T, Snell E, et al: The effect of allograft meniscal replacement on intraarticular contact area and pressures in the human knee. Am J Sports Med 25:692–698, 1997.

92. Pandy MG, Shelburne KB: Dependence of cruciate ligament loading on muscle forces and external load. J Biomech 30:1015–1024, 1997.

93. Powers CM, Landel R, Perry J: Timing and intensity of vastus muscle activity during functional activities in subjects with and without patellofemoral pain. Phys Ther 76:946–955, 1996.

94. Powers CM: Rehabilitation of patellofemoral joint: A critical review. J Orthop Sports Phys Ther 28:345–354, 1998.

95. Powers CM: Patellar kinematics, part I: The influence of vastus muscle activity in subjects with and without patellofemoral pain. Phys Ther 80:956–964, 2000.

96. Powers CM: Patellar kinematics, part II: The influence of depth of the trochlear groove in subjects with and without patellofemoral pain. Phys Ther 80:965–973, 2000.

97. Raimondo RA, Ahmad CS, Blankevoort L, et al: Patella stabilization: A quantitative evaluation of the vastus medialis obliquus muscles. Orthopedics 21:791–795, 1998.

98. Rajala GM, Neumann DA, Foster C, et al: Quadriceps muscle performance in male speed skaters. J Strength Cond Res 8:48–52, 1994.

99. Rajendran K: Mechanism of locking at the knee joint. J Anat 143:189–194, 1985.

100. Reilly DT, Martens M: Experimental analysis of the quadriceps muscle force and patellofemoral joint reaction force for various activities. Acta Orthop Scand 43:126–137, 1972.

101. Roach KE, Miles TP: Normal hip and knee active range of motion: The relationship to age. Phys Ther 71:656–665, 1991.

102. Rispoli DM, Miller MD: Options in meniscal repair. Clin Sports Med 18:77–91, 1999.

103. Seedhom BB: Loadbearing function of the menisci. Physiotherapy 62:223–226, 1976.

104. Seering WP, Piziali RL, Nagel DA, et al: The function of the primary ligaments of the knee in varus-valgus and axial rotation. J Biomech 13:785–794, 1980.

105. Shelburne KB, Pandy MG: A musculoskeletal model of the knee for evaluating ligament forces during isometric contractions. J Biomech 30:163–176, 1997.

106. Shelbourne KD, Davis TJ, Klootwyk TE: The relationship between intercondylar notch width of the femur and the incidence of anterior cruciate ligament tears. Am J Sports Med 26:402–408, 1998.

107. Shoemaker SC, Markolf KL: In vivo rotatory knee stability: Ligamentous and muscular contributions. J Bone Joint Surg 64A:208–216, 1982.

108. Shrive NG, O'Connor JJ, Goodfellow JW: Load-bearing in the knee joint. Clin Orthop 131:279–287, 1978.

109. Sisk TD: Knee injuries. In Crenshaw AH (ed): Campbells' Operative Orthopaedics, 3rd vol, 8th ed. St. Louis, Mosby-Year Book, 1992.

110. Smidt GL: Biomechanical analysis of knee flexion and extension. J Biomech 6:79–92, 1973.

111. Smith KS, Weiss EL, Lehmkuhl LD: Brunnstrom's Clinical Kinesiology, 5th ed. Philadelphia, FA Davis, 1996.

112. Steinkamp LA, Dillingham MF, Markel MD, et al: Biomechanical considerations in patellofemoral joint rehabilitation. Am J Sports Med 21:438–444, 1993.

113. Stuart MJ, Meglan DA, Lutz GE, et al: Comparison of intersegmental tibiofemoral joint forces and muscle activity during various closed kinetic chain exercises. Am J Sports Med 24:792–799, 1996.

114. Snyder-Mackler L: Scientific rationale and physiological basis for the use of closed kinetic chain exercise in the lower extremity. J Sport Rehab 5:2–12, 1996.

115. Tipton CM, Vailas AC, Matthes RD: Experimental studies on the influences of physical activity on ligaments, tendons, and joints: A brief review. Acta Med Scand. Suppl 711:157–168, 1986.

116. Tyler TF, McHugh MP, Gleim GW, et al: The effect of immediate weightbearing after anterior cruciate ligament reconstruction. Clin Orthop 357:141–148, 1998.

117. Wada M, Imura S, Nagatani K, et al: Relationship between gait and clinical results after high tibial osteotomy. Clin Orthop 354:180–188, 1998.

118. Wang CJ, Walker PS, Wolf B: The effects of flexion and rotation on the length patterns of the ligaments of the knee. J Biomechan 6:587–596, 1973.

119. Wexler G, Hurwitz DE, Bush-Joseph CA, et al: Functional gait adaptations in patients with anterior cruciate ligament deficiency over time. Clin Orthop 348:166–175, 1998.

120. Williams PL, Bannister LH, Berry M, et al: Gray's Anatomy, 38th ed. New York, Churchill Livingstone, 1995.

121. Wojtys EM, Huston LJ: Longitudinal effects of anterior cruciate ligament injury and patellar tendon autograft reconstruction on neuromuscular performance. Am J Sports Med 28:336–44, 2000.

122. Woo SLY, Chan SC, Yamaji T: Biomechanics of knee ligament healing, repair and reconstruction. J Biomech 30:431–439, 1997.

123. Wood L, Ferrell WR, Baxendale RH: Pressures in normal and acutely distended human knee joints and effects on quadriceps maximal voluntary contractions. Physiol 73:305–314, 1988.

124. Wyatt MP, Edwards AM: Comparison of quadriceps and hamstring torque values during isokinetic exercise. J Orthop Sports Phys Ther 3:48–56, 1981.

125. Yack HJ, Riley LM, Whieldon TR: Anterior tibial translation during progressive loading of the ACL-deficient knee during weight-bearing and nonweight-bearing isometric exercise. J Orthop Sports Phys Ther 20:247–253, 1994.

126. Yasuda K, Sasaki T: Exercise after anterior cruciate ligament reconstruction. Clin Orthop 220:275–283, 1987.

127. Zakaria D, Harburn KL, Kramer JF: Preferential activation of the vastus medialis oblique, vastus lateralis, and hip adductor muscles during isometric exercises in females. J Orthop Sports Phys Ther 26:23–28, 1997.

## ADDITIONAL READING

Baker MM, Juhn MS: Patellofemoral pain syndrome in the female athlete. Clin Sports Med 19:315–329, 2000.

Baratta R, Solomonow M, Zhou H, et al: Muscle coactivation: The role of the antagonist musculature in maintaining knee stability. Am J Sports Med 16:113–122, 1988.

Beaupre A, Choukroun R, Guidouin R, et al: Knee menisci: Correlation between microstructure and biomechanics. Clin Orthop 208:72–75, 1986.

Grelsamer RP, Klein JR: The biomechanics of the patellofemoral joint. J Orthop Sports Phys Ther 28:286–298, 1998.

Grood ES, Suntay WJ, Noyes FR, et al: Biomechanics of the knee-extension exercise. J Bone Joint Surg 66A:725–734, 1984.

Hallen LG, Lindahl O: The "screw-home" movement in the knee joint. Acta Orthop Scand 37:97–106, 1966.

Harner CD, Hoher J: Evaluation and treatment of posterior cruciate ligament injuries. Am J Sports Med 23:736–745, 1995.

Hehne HJ: Biomechanics of the patellofemoral joint and its clinical relevance. Clin Orthop 258:73–85, 1990.

Hsieh YF, Draganich LF, Ho SH, et al: The effects of removal and reconstruction of the anterior cruciate ligament on patellofemoral kinematics. Am J Sports Med 26:201–209, 1998.

Kannus P, Jarvinen M, Johnson R, et al: Function of the quadriceps and hamstrings muscles in knees with chronic partial deficiency of the anterior cruciate ligament: Isometric and isokinetic evaluation. Am J Sports Med 20:162–168, 1992.

Lane JG, Irby SE, Kaufman K, et al: The anterior cruciate ligament in controlling axial rotation. Am J Sports Med 22:289–293, 1994.

Lunnen JD, Yack J, LeVeau BF: Relationship between muscle length, muscle activity, and torque of the hamstring muscles. Phys Ther 61:190–195, 1981.

McGinty G, Irrgang JJ, Pezzullo D: Biomechanical considerations for rehabilitation of the knee. Clin Biomech 15:160–166, 2000.

Noyes FR, Grood ES: The strength of the anterior cruciate ligament in humans and rhesus monkeys: Age-related and species-related changes. J Bone Joint Surg 58A:1074–1082, 1976.

Ogata K, Yasunaga M, Nomiyama H: The effect of wedged insoles on the thrust of osteoarthritic knees. Intern Orthopaed 21:308–312, 1997.

Scapinelli R: Vascular anatomy of the human cruciate ligaments and surrounding structures. Clin Anat 10:151–162, 1997.

Schutte MJ, Dabezies EJ, Zimny ML, et al: Neural anatomy of the human anterior cruciate ligament. J Bone Joint Surg 69A:243–247, 1987.

Snyder-Mackler L, Delitto A, Bailey SL, et al: Strength of the quadriceps femoris muscle and functional recovery after reconstruction of the anterior cruciate ligament. J Bone Joint Surg 77A:1166–1173, 1995.

Spoor CW, van Leeuwen JL: Knee muscle moment arms from MRI and from tendon travel. J Biomech 25:201–206, 1992.

Todo ST, Kadoya Y, Moilanen T, et al: Anteroposterior and rotational movement of the femur during knee flexion. Clin Orthop 362:162–170, 1999.

Van Eijden TMGJ, de Boer W, Weijs WA: The orientation of the distal part of the quadriceps muscles as a function of the knee flexion-extension angle. J Biomech 18:803–809, 1985.

# CHAPTER 14

# Ankle and Foot

## DONALD A. NEUMANN, PT, PhD

## TOPICS AT A GLANCE

## INTRODUCTION

The primary function of the ankle and foot is to absorb shock and impart thrust to the body during walking. While walking and running, the foot must be pliable enough to absorb the impact of millions of contacts throughout a lifetime. Pliability also allows the foot to conform to countless spatial configurations between it and the ground. Walking and running also require that the foot be relatively rigid to be able to withstand large propulsive thrusts. The healthy foot satisfies the seemingly paradoxical requirements of both shock absorption and thrust through an interaction of interrelated joints, connective tissues, and muscles. Although not emphasized in this chapter, the sensory functions of the healthy foot also offer important measures of protection and guidance to the lower extremity. This chapter sets forth a firm basis for an understanding of the evaluation and treatment of a multitude of disorders that affect the ankle and foot, many of which are kinesiologically related to the movement of the entire lower extremity.

Many of the kinesiologic issues addressed in this chapter are related specifically to the process of walking, or gait, a topic covered in greater detail in Chapter 15. Figure 15–12 should be consulted as a reference to the terminology used in this chapter to describe the different phases of the gait cycle.

## OSTEOLOGY

### Basic Terms and Concepts

#### NAMING THE JOINTS AND REGIONS

The term *ankle* refers primarily to the talocrural joint, but also includes two related articulations: the proximal and distal tibiofibular joints. The term *foot* refers to all the structures distal to the tibia and fibula. Note that this classification scheme includes the talus as part of both the ankle and the foot. The talus is an extremely important bone, having an essential role in both the local kinesiology of the ankle and foot and the kinesiology of the entire lower extremity.

Figure 14–1 depicts an overview of the terminology that describes the regions of the ankle and foot. The terms anterior and posterior have their conventional meanings when referring to the tibia and fibula (i.e., the leg). In reference to the ankle and foot, these terms are often used interchangeably with distal and proximal, respectively. The terms dorsal and plantar describe the superior (top) and inferior aspects of the foot, respectively.

Within the foot are three regions, each consisting of a set of bones and one or more joints. The *rearfoot* (hindfoot) consists of the talus, calcaneus, and subtalar joint; the *midfoot* consists of the remaining tarsal bones, including the transverse tarsal joint and the smaller distal intertarsal joints; and the *forefoot* consists of the metatarsals and phalanges, including all joints distal to and including the tarsometatarsal joints. Table 14–1 provides a summary of the organization of the bones and joints of the ankle and foot.

#### SIMILARITIES BETWEEN THE JOINTS OF THE DISTAL LEG AND DISTAL ARM

The ankle and foot have several features that are structurally similar to the wrist and hand. The radius in the forearm and the tibia in the leg each articulates with a set of small bones,

### TABLE 14–1. Structural Organization of the Bones and Joints of the Foot and Ankle

| Ankle | Foot |
|---|---|
| Bones | ***Rearfoot*** |
|   Tibia, fibula, and talus | Bones |
| Joints |   Calcaneus and talus* |
|   Talocrural | Joint |
|   Proximal and distal |   Subtalar (talocalcaneal) |
|     tibiofibular | |
| | ***Midfoot*** |
| | Bones |
| |   Navicular, cuboid, and cunei- |
| |     forms |
| | Joints |
| |   Transverse tarsal |
| |     Talonavicular |
| |     Calcaneocuboid |
| |   Distal intertarsal |
| |     Cuneonavicular |
| |     Cuboideonavicular |
| |     Intercuneiform and cuneo- |
| |       cuboid complex |
| | ***Forefoot*** |
| | Bones |
| |   Metatarsals and phalanges |
| | Joints |
| |   Tarsometatarsal |
| |   Intermetatarsal |
| |   Metatarsophalangeal |
| |   Interphalangeal |

\* The talus is included as a bone of the ankle and a bone of the foot.

the carpus and tarsus, respectively. When considering the pisiform of the wrist as a sesamoid, the carpus and tarsus each have seven bones. The general plan of the metatarsus and metacarpus, as well as the more distal phalanges, is nearly identical. A notable exception is that the first toe in the foot is not as functionally developed as the thumb in the hand.

As described in Chapter 12, the entire lower extremity internally or medially rotates during embryologic development. As a result, the first toe is positioned on the medial side of the foot, and the top of the foot is actually its dorsal surface. This orientation is similar to that of the hand when the forearm is fully pronated (Fig. 14–2). This plantigrade position of the foot is used for walking and standing.

### Individual Bones

#### FIBULA

The long and thin fibula is located lateral and parallel to the tibia (Figs. 13–2 and 13–3). The *fibular head* can be palpated just lateral to the lateral condyle of the tibia. The slender shaft of the fibula transfers a small fraction of the load through the leg, most of it being transferred through the thicker tibia. The shaft of the fibula continues distally to

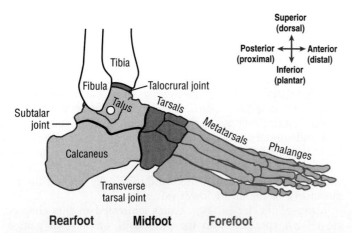

**FIGURE 14–1.** The essential terminology used to describe the regions of the foot and ankle.

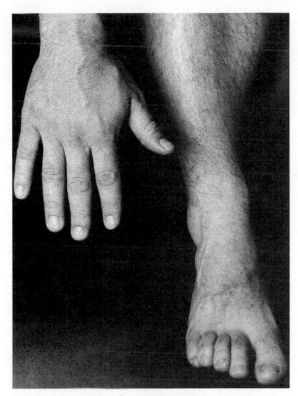

**FIGURE 14–2.** Topographic similarities between the pronated forearm and the foot. Note the thumb and great toe are both on the medial side of the respective extremity.

form the sharp and easily palpable *lateral malleolus* (from the Latin root *malleus*; a hammer). The lateral malleolus functions as a pulley for the tendons of the peroneus longus and brevis. The lateral malleolus also forms the lateral wall of the ankle or talocrural joint (Fig. 14–3).

| Osteologic Features of the Fibula and Distal Tibia |
|---|
| *Fibula* |
| • Fibular head |
| • Lateral malleolus |
| *Tibia* |
| • Medial malleolus |
| • Fibular notch |

## DISTAL TIBIA

The distal end of the tibia expands in size to accommodate loads transferred across the ankle. On the medial side of the distal shaft of the tibia is the prominent *medial malleolus*. On the lateral side is the *fibular notch*, a triangular concavity that accepts the distal end of the fibula at the distal tibiofibular joint (see Fig. 14–10).

### Torsion Angle of the Tibia

In adults, the distal end of the tibia is twisted about its long axis about 20 to 30 degrees relative to its proximal end.[57] Natural torsion is evident by the slight externally rotated position of the foot while standing. This twist of the leg is

referred to as lateral tibial torsion, based on the orientation of the bone's distal end relative to its proximal end.

## TARSAL BONES

The seven tarsal bones are shown in four different perspectives in Figures 14–4 through 14–7.

| Osteologic Features of the Tarsal Bones |
|---|
| *Talus* |
| • Trochlear surface |
| • Head |
| • Anterior, middle, and posterior facets |
| • Talar sulcus |
| • Lateral and medial tubercles |
| *Calcaneus* |
| • Tuberosity |
| • Lateral and medial processes |
| • Anterior, middle, and posterior facets |
| • Calcaneal sulcus |
| • Sustentaculum talus |
| *Navicular* |
| • Tuberosity |
| *Medial, intermediate, and lateral cuneiforms* |
| • Transverse arch |
| *Cuboid* |
| • Groove for the peroneus longus |

### Talus

The talus is the most proximal tarsal bone. Its dorsal or *trochlear surface* is a rounded dome, convex anterior-posteriorly and slightly concave medial-laterally (Fig. 14–6). Cartilage covers the trochlear surface and its adjacent sides, providing smooth articular surfaces for the talocrural joint. The prominent *head* of the talus projects forward and slightly medial toward the navicular. In the adult, the long axis of

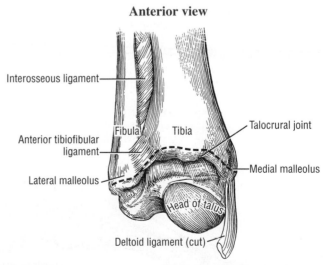

**Anterior view**

**FIGURE 14–3.** An anterior view of the distal end of the right tibia, fibula, and talus. The articulation of the three bones forms the talocrural (ankle) joint. The dashed line shows the attachment of the capsule of the ankle joint.

**Superior view**

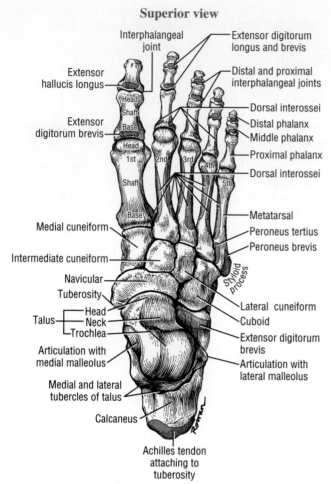

**FIGURE 14–4.** A superior (dorsal) view of the bones of the right ankle and foot. Proximal attachments of muscles are indicated in red, distal attachments in gray.

**Inferior view**

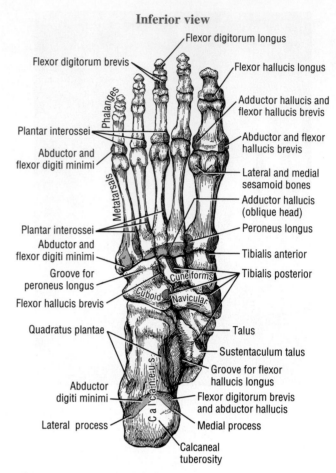

**FIGURE 14–5.** An inferior (plantar) view of the bones of the right ankle and foot. Proximal attachments of muscles are indicated in red, distal attachments in gray.

the *neck* of the talus positions the head about 30 degrees medial to the sagittal plane. In small children, the head is projected medially about 40 to 50 degrees, partially accounting for the often inverted appearance of their feet.

Figure 14–8 shows three articular facets on the plantar (inferior) surface of the talus. The *anterior* and *middle facets* are slightly curved and often continuous with each other. Note that the articular cartilage that covers these facets also

covers the adjacent head of the talus. The oval, concave *posterior facet* is the largest facet. As a functional set, the three facets articulate with the three facets on the dorsal (superior) surface of the calcaneus, forming the subtalar joint. The *talar sulcus* is an obliquely running groove located between the anterior-middle and posterior facets.

*Lateral* and *medial tubercles* are located on the posterior-medial surface of the talus (see Fig. 14–4). A groove formed

**Medial view**

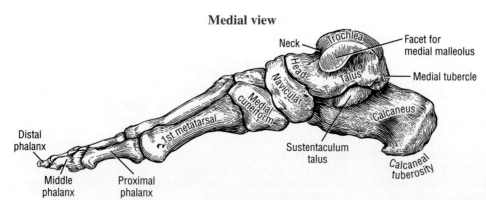

**FIGURE 14–6.** A medial view of the bones of the right ankle and foot.

**Lateral view**

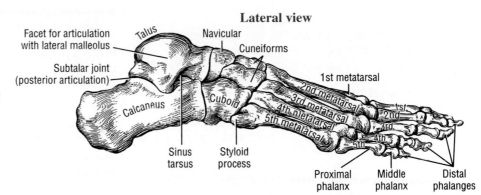

**FIGURE 14–7.** A lateral view of the bones of the right ankle and foot.

between these tubercles serves as a pulley for the tendon of the flexor hallucis longus (see Fig. 14–11).

### Calcaneus

The calcaneus, the largest of the tarsal bones, is well suited to accept the impact of heel contact during walking. The large and rough *calcaneal tuberosity* receives the attachment of the Achilles (calcaneal) tendon. The plantar surface of the tuberosity has *lateral* and *medial processes* that serve as attachments for many of the intrinsic muscles and the deep plantar fascia of the foot (see Fig. 14–5).

The calcaneus articulates with other tarsal bones on its dorsal and anterior surfaces. The dorsal surface contains three facets that join the "matching" facets on the talus (see Fig. 14–8). The *anterior* and *middle facets* are relatively small and nearly flat. The *posterior facet* is large and convex, conforming to the concave shape of the equally large posterior facet on the talus. Between the posterior and medial facet is a wide oblique groove called the *calcaneal sulcus*. This sulcus is filled with the attachments of several ligaments that bind the subtalar joint. With the subtalar joint articulated, the sulci of the calcaneus and talus form a tunnel within the subtalar joint, known as the *sinus tarsi* (see Fig. 14–7).

The relatively small anterior surface of the calcaneus joins the cuboid at the calcaneocuboid joint. The *sustentaculum talus* projects medially as a horizontal shelf from the dorsal surface of the calcaneus. (Sustentaculum talus literally means a "shelf for the talus.") The sustentaculum talus lies under and supports the middle facets of the subtalar joint (see Fig. 14–6).

### Navicular

The navicular bone is named for its resemblance to a ship (i.e., referring to "navy"). Its concave proximal surface (the "hull") accepts the head of the talus at the talonavicular joint (see Fig. 14–4). The distal surface of the navicular bone contains three relatively flat facets that articulate with the three cuneiform bones.

The medial surface of the navicular has a prominent *tuberosity*, easily palpable about 1 inch (2.5 cm) inferior and distal (anterior) to the tip of the medial malleolus. This tuberosity serves as one of several distal attachments of the tibialis posterior muscle.

### Medial, Intermediate, and Lateral Cuneiforms

As a set, the cuneiform bones act as a spacer between the navicular and three medial metatarsal bones (see Fig. 14–4).

The cuneiforms contribute to the *transverse arch* of the foot, accounting in part for the dorsal convexity to the middle region of the foot. The lateral cuneiform has a facet for articulation with a portion of the medial surface of the cuboid.

### Cuboid

As its name indicates, the cuboid has six surfaces, three of which articulate with adjacent tarsal bones (see Figs. 14–4, 14–5, and 14–7). The distal surface articulates with the bases of both the fourth and fifth metatarsals. The cuboid is therefore homologous to the hamate bone of the wrist.

The entire proximal surface of the cuboid articulates with the calcaneus. This surface is flat to slightly curved. The medial surface has an oval facet for articulation with the lateral cuneiform and, occasionally, a very small facet for articulation with the navicular. A distinct groove runs across the plantar surface of the cuboid, occupied by the tendon of the peroneus longus muscle.

**Superior view**

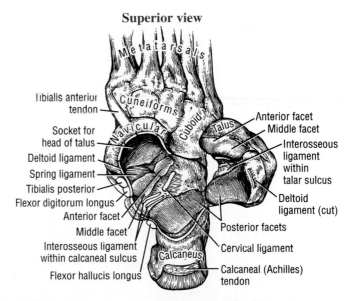

**FIGURE 14–8.** A superior view of the talus flipped laterally to reveal its plantar side as well as the dorsal side of the calcaneus. Observe the three articular facets located on the talus and on the calcaneus. (The interosseous and cervical ligaments and multiple tendons have been cut.)

## RAYS OF THE FOOT

A ray of the forefoot is defined as one metatarsal and its associated set of phalanges.

### Metatarsals

The five metatarsal bones link the distal row of tarsal bones with the proximal phalanges (see Fig. 14–4). Metatarsals are numbered 1 through 5, starting on the medial side. The first metatarsal is the shortest and thickest, and the second is usually the longest and the most rigidly attached to the distal row of tarsal bones. These morphologic characteristics reflect the larger forces that pass through the medial side of the forefoot during the push-off phase of gait. Each metatarsal has a *base* at its proximal end, a *shaft,* and a convex *head* at its distal end (see Fig. 14–4, first metatarsal). The bases of the metatarsals have small *articular facets* that mark the site of articulation with the bases of the adjacent metatarsals. The articular facet on the first metatarsal is occasionally lacking. Longitudinally, the shafts of the metatarsals are slightly concave on their plantar side. This arched shape enhances the load-supporting ability of the metatarsals (see Fig. 14–6). The plantar surface of the first metatarsal head has two small facets for articulation with two sesamoid bones that are imbedded within the tendon of the flexor hallucis brevis. The fifth metatarsal has a prominent *styloid process* just lateral to its base, marking the attachment of the peroneus brevis muscle (see Fig. 14–7).

---

**Osteologic Features of a Metatarsal**
- Base (with articular facets for articulation with the bases of adjacent metatarsals)
- Shaft
- Head
- Styloid process (on the fifth metatarsal only)

---

### Phalanges

As in the hand, the foot has 14 phalanges, named proximal, middle, and distal (see Fig. 14–4). The first toe—commonly called the great toe or hallux—has two phalanges, designated as proximal and distal. In general, each phalanx has a concave *base* at its proximal end, a *shaft,* and a convex *head* at its distal end.

---

**Osteologic Features of a Phalanx**
- Base
- Shaft
- Head

---

## ARTHROLOGY

The major joints of the ankle and foot are the *talocrural, subtalar,* and *transverse tarsal joints.* The talus is mechanically involved with all three of these joints. The multiple articulations made by the talus help to explain the bone's complex shape, with nearly 70% of its surface covered with articular cartilage. An understanding of the shape of the talus is crucial to an understanding of the arthrology of the ankle and foot.

### Terminology for Motions and Positions

The terminology used to describe the movements of the ankle and foot incorporates two sets of definitions: a fundamental set and an applied set. The *fundamental terminology* describes movement of the foot or ankle that occurs at right angles to the three standard axes of rotation (Fig. 14–9A). *Dorsiflexion* (extension) and *plantar flexion* describe the motion that is parallel to the sagittal plane, around a medial-lateral axis of rotation. *Eversion* and *inversion* describe the motion parallel to the frontal plane, around an anterior-posterior axis of rotation. *Abduction* and *adduction* describe motion in the horizontal (transverse) plane, around a vertical (superior-inferior) axis of rotation. At the major joints of the ankle and foot, however, the fundamental definitions are inadequate because most movements of the ankle and foot occur about an oblique axis rather than the three standard, orthogonal axes of rotation depicted in Figure 14–9A.

A second and more *applied terminology* or set of definitions is used to describe movements that occur perpendicular to an oblique axis of rotation (Fig. 14–9B). *Pronation* describes a motion that has elements of eversion, abduction, and dorsiflexion. *Supination,* in contrast, describes a motion that has elements of inversion, adduction, and plantar flexion. The orientation of the oblique axis of rotation depicted

**A. Fundamental movement definitions**    **B. Applied movement definitions**

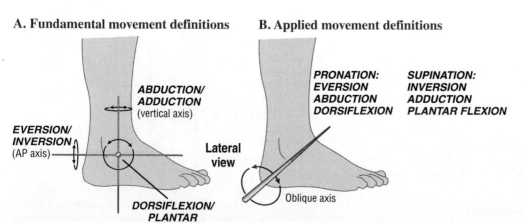

**ABDUCTION/ ADDUCTION** (vertical axis)

**EVERSION/ INVERSION** (AP axis)

**DORSIFLEXION/ PLANTAR FLEXION** (ML axis)

**Lateral view**

**PRONATION: EVERSION ABDUCTION DORSIFLEXION**

**SUPINATION: INVERSION ADDUCTION PLANTAR FLEXION**

Oblique axis

**FIGURE 14–9.** *A,* Fundamental movement definitions are based on the movement of any part of the ankle or foot in a plane perpendicular to the three standard axes of rotation: vertical, anterior-posterior (AP), and medial-lateral (ML). *B,* Applied movement definitions are based on the movements that occur at right angles to one of several oblique axes of rotation in the foot and ankle.

| TABLE 14–2. Terms that Describe Movements and Deformities of the Ankle and Foot | | | |
|---|---|---|---|
| **Motion** | **Axis of Rotation** | **Plane of Motion** | **Example of Fixed Deformity or Abnormal Posture** |
| Plantar flexion | Medial-lateral | Sagittal | Pes equinus |
| Dorsiflexion | | | Pes calcaneus |
| Inversion | Anterior-posterior | Frontal | Varus |
| Eversion | | | Valgus |
| Abduction | Vertical | Horizontal | Abductus |
| Adduction | | | Adductus |
| Supination | Oblique (varies by joint) | Varying elements of inversion, adduction, and plantar flexion | Inconsistent terminology—usually implies one or more of the components of supination |
| Pronation | | Varying elements of eversion, abduction, and dorsiflexion | Inconsistent terminology—usually implies one or more of the components of pronation |

in Figure 14–9B varies by major joint but, in general, has a pitch that is similar to that illustrated. The exact pitch of each major joint's axis of rotation is described in subsequent sections.

Pronation and supination are often called "triplanar" motions. Unfortunately, this description is confusing. The term triplane implies that the movement "cuts through" all three cardinal planes, not that the joint exhibiting this motion possesses three degrees of freedom. Pronation and supination occur in only one plane, about one (oblique) axis of rotation. Table 14–2 summarizes the terminology used to describe the movements of the ankle and foot, including the terminology that describes abnormal posture or deformity.

## Axes of Rotation

Movements at the ankle and foot are assumed to occur about axes of rotation that remain nearly stationary throughout the range of motion. Although this assumption does not hold for all joints, it does allow a rather complicated system to be explained in a relatively simple fashion. More complicated, and likely more accurate, axes of rotation and kinematic models of the ankle and foot are described elsewhere. (See references 1, 10, 45, and 48.)

## Structure and Function of Joints Associated with the Ankle

From an anatomic perspective, the ankle includes one articulation: the talocrural joint. Movement at the talocrural joint results in slight movement at the proximal and distal tibiofibular joints. Because of this functional association, all three joints are included under the topic of "ankle."

### TIBIOFIBULAR JOINTS

The fibula is bound to the lateral side of the tibia by two articulations: the proximal tibiofibular joint and the distal tibiofibular joint (see Fig. 13–2). The interosseous membrane—a sheet of connective tissue that runs between the tibia and fibula—also helps to bind the bones together. The interosseous membrane provides an attachment for many muscles that affect the foot and ankle.

### Proximal Tibiofibular Joint

The proximal tibiofibular joint is a synovial joint located just lateral to and below the knee. The joint is formed by the head of the fibula and the posterior-lateral aspect of the lateral condyle of the tibia (see Fig. 13–5). The joint surfaces are generally flat or slightly oval, covered by articular cartilage.

The proximal tibiofibular joint is enclosed by a capsule that is strengthened by anterior and posterior ligaments (see Figs. 13–7 and 13–10). The tendon of the popliteus muscle provides additional stabilization as it crosses just posterior to the joint. Firm stabilization is needed at the proximal tibiofibular joint so that forces within the biceps femoris and lateral collateral ligament of the knee can be transferred effectively from the fibula to the tibia.

> **Connective Tissues that Stabilize the Proximal Tibiofibular Joint**
> * Capsular ligaments
> * Popliteus tendon

### Distal Tibiofibular Joint

#### Articular Structure
The distal tibiofibular joint is formed by the articulation of the convex medial surface of the distal fibula, with the concave fibular notch of the tibia (Fig. 14–10). Anatomists typically classify this joint as a *synarthrosis* because it allows very slight movement and is filled with dense irregular connective tissue. The synovial membrane lining this joint is often continuous with the synovial membrane lining the talocrural joint.

#### Ligaments
The *interosseous ligament* provides the strongest bond between the distal ends of the tibia and fibula.[55] This ligament

**Anterior-lateral view**

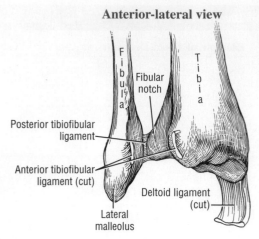

**FIGURE 14–10.** An anterior-lateral view of the right distal tibiofibular joint with the fibula reflected to show the articular surfaces.

is a distal extension of the interosseous membrane. The *anterior* and *posterior (distal) tibiofibular ligaments* also reinforce the distal tibiofibular joint (Figs. 14–10 and 14–11). A stable union between the distal tibia and distal fibula is essential to the stability and function of the talocrural joint.

---

**Ligaments of the Distal Tibiofibular Joint**
- Interosseous ligament
- Anterior tibiofibular ligament
- Posterior tibiofibular ligament

---

**Posterior view**

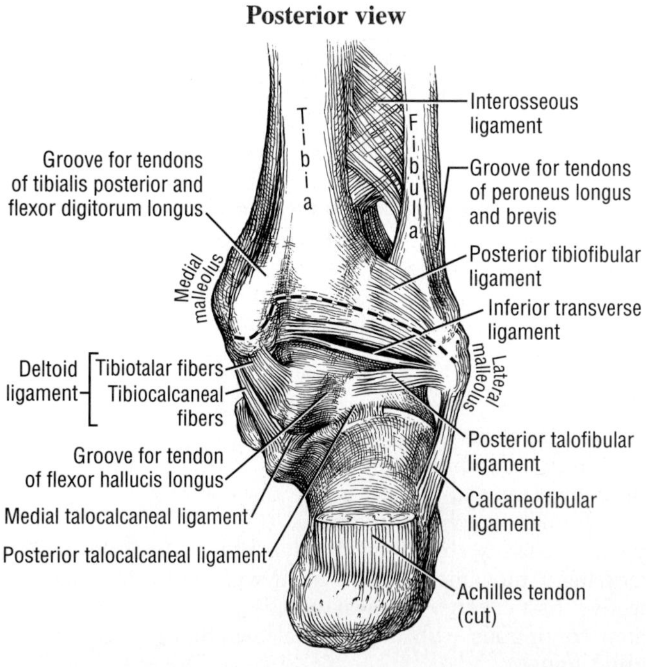

**FIGURE 14–11.** Posterior view of the right ankle region shows the major ligaments of the distal tibiofibular, talocrural, and subtalar joints. The dashed line indicates the attachments of the capsule of the talocrural (ankle) joint.

## TALOCRURAL JOINT

### Articular Structure

The talocrural joint is formed by the articulation of the trochlear surface and the sides of the talus, with the rectangular cavity formed by the distal end of the tibia and both malleoli (see Fig. 14–3). The talocrural joint is often referred to as the "mortise," owing its resemblance to the wood joint used by carpenters (Fig. 14–12). The concave shape of the proximal side of the ankle mortise is maintained by connective tissues that bind the tibia with the fibula. Interestingly, the total contact area within the talocrural joint is about 350 mm², which is relatively small compared with 1,120 mm² and 1,100 mm² for the knee and hip, respectively.[4]

### Ligaments

A thin *capsule* surrounds the talocrural joint. Externally, the capsule is reinforced by collateral ligaments that limit excessive inversion and eversion tilting of the talus within the rectangular concavity.

The medial collateral ligament of the talocrural joint is also referred to as the *deltoid ligament*. It is strong and expansive (Fig. 14–13). The apex of the triangular ligament is anchored to the medial malleolus, with its base fanning into three sets of superficial fibers. The distal attachments of these fibers are listed in the box. The deeper tibiotalar fibers blend with and strengthen the medial capsule of the talocrural joint.

---

**Distal Attachments of the Three Components of the Deltoid Ligament**
- Tibionavicular fibers attach to the navicular tuberosity.
- Tibiocalcaneal fibers attach to the sustentaculum talus.
- Tibiotalar fibers attach to the medial tubercle and adjacent side of the talus.

---

The primary function of the deltoid ligament is to limit eversion across the talocrural, subtalar, and talonavicular

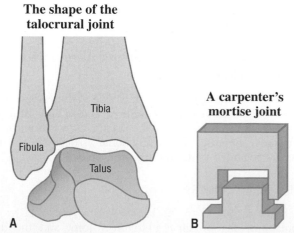

**FIGURE 14–12.** The similarity in shape of the talocrural joint (A) and a carpenter's mortise joint (B) is demonstrated.

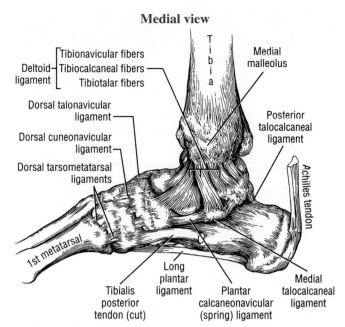

**Medial view**

Deltoid ligament
- Tibionavicular fibers
- Tibiocalcaneal fibers
- Tibiotalar fibers

Dorsal talonavicular ligament

Dorsal cuneonavicular ligament

Dorsal tarsometatarsal ligaments

1st metatarsal

Tibia

Medial malleolus

Posterior talocalcaneal ligament

Achilles tendon

Tibialis posterior tendon (cut)

Long plantar ligament

Plantar calcaneonavicular (spring) ligament

Medial talocalcaneal ligament

**FIGURE 14–13.** Medial view of the right ankle region highlights the medial collateral ligament.

joints. Sprains to the deltoid ligament are relatively uncommon due, in part, to the ligament's strength and to the fact that the lateral malleolus serves as a bony block against excessive eversion.

The *lateral collateral ligaments* of the ankle include the anterior and posterior talofibular and the calcaneofibular ligaments. Because of the relative inability of the medial malleolus to adequately block the medial side of the mortise, the majority of ankle sprains involve excessive inversion and subsequent injury to the lateral collateral ligaments.[12]

The *anterior talofibular ligament* attaches to the anterior aspect of the lateral malleolus and courses anteriorly and medially to the neck of the talus (Fig. 14–14). This ligament

is the most frequently injured of the lateral ligaments. Injury is often due to excessive inversion or adduction of the ankle, especially when combined with plantar flexion, for example, when inadvertently stepping into a hole.[7,46] The *calcaneofibular ligament* courses inferiorly and posteriorly from the apex of the lateral malleolus to the lateral surface of the calcaneus (see Fig. 14–14). This ligament resists inversion across the talocrural and subtalar joints. The calcaneofibular and anterior talofibular ligaments together limit inversion throughout most of the range of dorsiflexion and plantar flexion.[7]

> **Three Major Components of the Lateral Collateral Ligaments of the Ankle**
> - Anterior talofibular ligament
> - Calcaneofibular ligament
> - Posterior talofibular ligament

The *posterior talofibular ligament* originates on the posterior-medial side of the lateral malleolus and attaches to the lateral tubercle of the talus (Figs. 14–11 and 14–14). Its fibers run horizontally across the posterior side of the talocrural joint, in an oblique anterior-lateral to posterior-medial direction (Fig. 14–15). The primary function of the posterior talofibular ligament is to stabilize the talus within the mortise. In particular, it limits excessive abduction of the talus, especially when the ankle is fully dorsiflexed.[7]

The *inferior transverse ligament* is a small thick strand of fibers considered part of the posterior talofibular ligament (see Fig. 14–11). The fibers continue medially to the posterior aspect of the medial malleolus, forming part of the posterior wall of the talocrural joint.

In summary, the medial and lateral collateral ligaments of the ankle limit excessive inversion and eversion at every joint that the fibers cross. Because most ligaments course from anterior-to-posterior, they also limit anterior-to-posterior translation of the talus within the mortise. As described in the section on arthrokinematics, the movements of plantar

**FIGURE 14–14.** Lateral view of the right ankle region highlights the lateral collateral ligament.

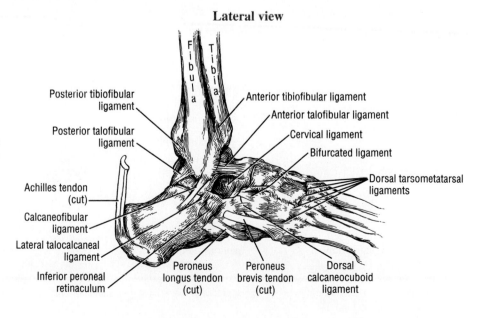

**Lateral view**

Posterior tibiofibular ligament

Posterior talofibular ligament

Achilles tendon (cut)

Calcaneofibular ligament

Lateral talocalcaneal ligament

Inferior peroneal retinaculum

Fibula

Tibia

Anterior tibiofibular ligament

Anterior talofibular ligament

Cervical ligament

Bifurcated ligament

Dorsal tarsometatarsal ligaments

Peroneus longus tendon (cut)

Peroneus brevis tendon (cut)

Dorsal calcaneocuboid ligament

**Superior view**

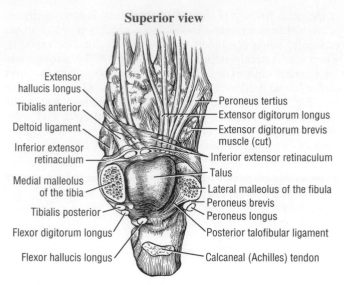

Extensor hallucis longus

Tibialis anterior

Deltoid ligament

Inferior extensor retinaculum

Medial malleolus of the tibia

Tibialis posterior

Flexor digitorum longus

Flexor hallucis longus

Peroneus tertius

Extensor digitorum longus

Extensor digitorum brevis muscle (cut)

Inferior extensor retinaculum

Talus

Lateral malleolus of the fibula

Peroneus brevis

Peroneus longus

Posterior talofibular ligament

Calcaneal (Achilles) tendon

**FIGURE 14–15.** A superior view displays a cross-section through the right talocrural joint. The talus remains, but the lateral and medial malleolus and all the tendons are cut.

flexion and dorsiflexion are kinematically linked to anterior and posterior translation of the talus, respectively. Table 14–3 summarizes movements that significantly stretch the major ligaments of the ankle. This information helps to explain the rationale behind several manual stress tests performed to evaluate the integrity of ligaments following ankle injury.

### Osteokinematics

The talocrural joint possesses one degree of freedom. Motion at this joint occurs about an axis of rotation that passes through the body of the talus and through the tips of the both malleoli. Because the lateral malleolus is inferior and posterior to the medial malleolus, which can be verified by palpation, the axis of rotation departs slightly from a pure

medial-lateral axis. As depicted in Figure 14–16A and B, the axis of rotation (red) is inclined slightly superior and anterior, as it crosses from the lateral to the medial side of the talus through both malleoli.[27] The axis deviates from a pure medial-lateral axis about 10 degrees in the frontal plane (see Fig. 14–16A), and 6 degrees in the horizontal plane (see Fig. 14–16B). Because of the pitch of the axis of rotation, dorsiflexion is associated with slight abduction and eversion, and plantar flexion with slight adduction and inversion. (These small secondary components are depicted in Fig. 14–16A and B.) The talocrural joint by definition, therefore, produces a movement of pronation and supination. As a result of relatively small differences in the orientation of the axis from the pure medial-lateral, the main components of pronation and supination at the talocrural joint are, by far, *dorsiflexion* and *plantar flexion* (Fig. 14–16D and E).[48]

An average of 26 degrees of dorsiflexion and 48 degrees of plantar flexion have been measured at the talocrural joint.[14] Associated movement at the subtalar joint may contribute to about 20% of this total motion. The 0-degree (neutral) position at the talocrural joint is defined by the foot held at 90 degrees to the leg. Dorsiflexion and plantar flexion at the talocrural joint need to be visualized when the foot is unloaded (i.e., off the ground and free to rotate) and when the foot is loaded during the stance phase of gait.

### Arthrokinematics

The following discussion assumes that the foot is unloaded and free to rotate, in a manner listed in Table 14–3. During *dorsiflexion,* the superior surface of the talus rolls forward relative to the leg as it simultaneously slides posteriorly (Fig. 14–17A). The simultaneous posterior slide allows the talus to rotate forward without much anterior translation. Figure 14–17A shows the calcaneofibular ligament becoming taut in response to the posterior sliding tendency of the talocalcaneal segment. As a general rule, any collateral ligament that becomes increasingly taut upon posterior translation of the talus also becomes increasingly taut at full dorsiflexion. Max-

### TABLE 14–3. Movements that Stretch and Elongate the Major Ligaments of the Ankle*

| Ligaments | Primary Joints | Movements that Stretch or Elongate Ligaments |
|---|---|---|
| Deltoid ligament (tibiotalar fibers) | Talocrural joint | Eversion, dorsiflexion with associated posterior slide of talus within the mortise |
| Deltoid ligament (tibionavicular fibers) | Talocrural joint | Eversion, plantar flexion with associated anterior slide of talus within the mortise |
| | Talonavicular joint | Eversion, abduction |
| Deltoid ligament (tibiocalcaneal fibers) | Talocrural joint *and* subtalar joint | Eversion |
| Anterior talofibular ligament | Talocrural joint | Plantar flexion with associated anterior slide of talus within the mortise, inversion, adduction |
| Calcaneofibular ligament | Talocrural joint | Dorsiflexion with associated posterior slide of talus within the mortise, inversion |
| | Subtalar joint | Inversion |
| Posterior talofibular ligament | Talocrural joint | Dorsiflexion with associated posterior slide of talus within the mortise, abduction, inversion |

* The information is based on movements of the unloaded foot relative to a stationary leg.

## Talocrural joint

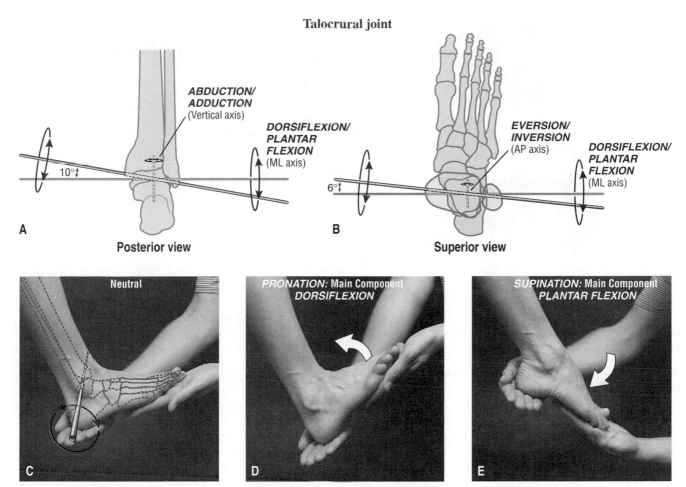

**A**  **Posterior view**

**B**  **Superior view**

**FIGURE 14–16.** The axis of rotation and osteokinematics at the talocrural joint. The slightly oblique axis of rotation at the talocrural joint (red) is shown from behind (*A*) and above (*B*). *C to E* show the primary active movement components of dorsiflexion and plantar flexion. Note that dorsiflexion (*D*) is combined with slight abduction and eversion, which are the other components of pronation; plantar flexion (*E*) is combined with slight adduction and inversion, which are the other components of supination.

imal dorsiflexion elongates the posterior capsule and all tissue capable of transmitting plantar flexion torque, such as the Achilles tendon.

During *plantar flexion,* the superior surface of the talus rolls backward as the bone simultaneously slides anteriorly,

stretching the anterior talofibular ligament (Fig. 14–17*B*). As a general rule, any collateral ligament that becomes increasingly taut upon anterior translation of the talus also becomes increasingly taut at full plantar flexion. Although not shown in Figure 14–17*B*, the tibionavicular fibers of the deltoid liga-

## Talocrural joint

**FIGURE 14–17.** A lateral view depicts the arthrokinematics at the talocrural joint during passive dorsiflexion (*A*) and plantar flexion (*B*). Stretched (taut) structures are shown as thin elongated arrows; slackened structures are shown as wavy arrows.

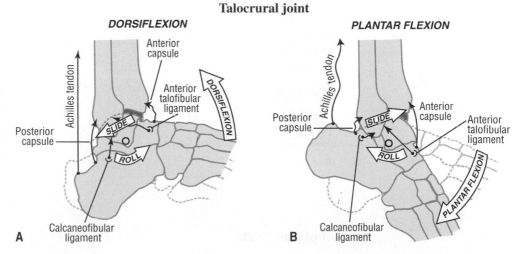

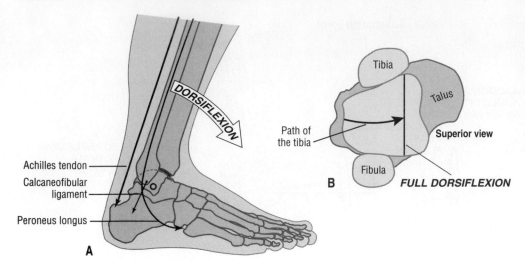

**FIGURE 14–18.** Factors that increase the mechanical stability of the fully dorsiflexed talocrural joint are shown. *A,* The increased passive tension in several connective tissues and muscles is demonstrated. *B,* The trochlear surface of the talus is wider anteriorly than posteriorly (red line). The path of dorsiflexion places the concave tibiofibular segment of the "mortise" in contact with the wider anterior dimension of the talus, thereby causing a wedging effect within the joint.

ment become taut at full plantar flexion (see Table 14–3). Plantar flexion also stretches the dorsiflexor muscles and the anterior capsule.

### Progressive Stabilization of the Talocrural Joint Throughout the Stance Phase of Gait

At initial heel contact, the ankle rapidly plantar flexes to lower the foot to the ground (see Fig. 15–15D). As soon as the foot flat phase of gait is reached, the leg starts to rotate forward (dorsiflex) over the foot. Dorsiflexion continues until

just after heel off phase. At this point in the gait cycle, the ankle becomes increasing stable owing to the greater tension in many stretched collateral ligaments and plantar flexor muscles (Fig. 14–18A). The dorsiflexed ankle becomes further stabilized as the wider anterior part of the talus wedges into the tibiofibular component of the mortise (Fig. 14–18B). The wedging effect causes the distal tibia and fibula to spread apart slightly. This action is resisted by tension in the distal tibiofibular ligaments and interosseous membrane. At the initiation of the push-off phase of walking, the talocrural

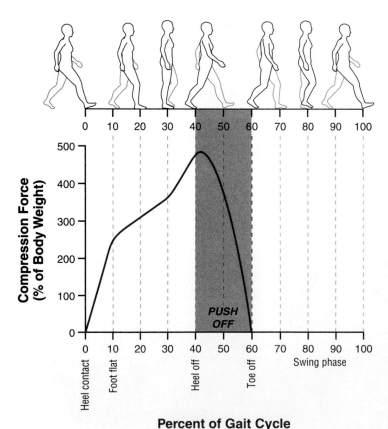

**FIGURE 14–19.** The compression force on the talocrural joint is plotted as a normal subject progresses through the stance phase of walking (0 to 60% of the gait cycle). The area shaded in red represents the push-off phase of walking. (Data from Stauffer RN, Chao EYS, Brewster RC: Force and motion analysis of the normal, diseased, and prosthetic ankle joint. Clin Orthop Rel Res 127:189–196, 1977.)

joint is well stabilized and prepared to accept compression forces that may reach over 4 times body weight (Fig. 14–19).[49]

The slight spreading of the concavity of the mortise at maximal dorsiflexion causes slight movement of the fibula. The line-of-force of the stretched anterior and posterior (distal) tibiofibular ligaments and interosseous membrane produces a slight superior translation of the fibula that is transferred superiorly to the proximal tibiofibular joint. For this reason, the proximal tibiofibular joint is more functionally related to the ankle (talocrural joint) than to the adjacent knee.

## SPECIAL FOCUS 14–1

### Ankle Injury Resulting from the Extremes of Dorsiflexion or Plantar Flexion

The proximal and distal tibiofibular joints and interosseous membrane are functionally and structurally related to the talocrural joint. This relationship becomes readily apparent following an injury related to extreme dorsiflexion; for example, landing from a fall. An extreme and violent dorsiflexion of the leg over the talus can cause the mortise to "explode" outward, rupturing many of the collateral ligaments. The explosive widening of the mortise can also injure the distal tibiofibular joint and interosseous membrane, the so-called high ankle sprain.

Full plantar flexion—the loose-packed position of the talocrural joint—slackens most collateral ligaments of the ankle and all plantar flexor muscles. Full plantar flexion also causes the distal tibia and fibula to "loosen its grip" on the talus. Plantar flexion places the narrower width of the talus between the malleoli, thereby releasing the tension within the mortise. Bearing all body weight over a fully plantar flexed ankle, therefore, places the talocrural joint at a relatively unstable position. Wearing high heels or landing from a jump in a plantar flexed, and usually inverted, position increases the likelihood of injuring the mortise.

## Structure and Function of the Joints Associated with the Foot

### SUBTALAR JOINT

The subtalar joint is the set of articulations formed by the posterior, middle, and anterior facets of the calcaneus and the talus (see Fig. 14–8). (Anatomy texts often limit the description of the subtalar joint to the prominent posterior facets only, referring to it as the talocalcaneal joint.[53])

To appreciate the extent of subtalar joint motion, one can firmly grasp the unloaded calcaneus and twist it in a side-to-side and rotary fashion. During this motion, the talus remains nearly fixed within the talocrural joint. Pronation and supination during non-weight-bearing activities occur as the calcaneus moves relative to the fixed talus. Most activities, however, occur as the calcaneus is relatively fixed under the load of body weight. This situation requires more complex kinematics involving the leg and talus rotating over a more stable calcaneus. Mobility at the subtalar joint allows the foot to assume positions that are independent of the orientation of the superimposed ankle and leg. This function is essential to activities such as walking across a steep hill, standing with feet held wide apart, and keeping one's balance on a rocking boat.

### *Articular Structure*

The prominent *posterior articulation* of the subtalar joint occupies about 70% of the total articular surface area (see Fig. 14–8). The concave posterior facet of the talus rests upon the convex posterior facet of the calcaneus. The articulation is normally held tightly opposed by its interlocking shape, body weight, interosseous ligaments, and activated muscle. The *anterior* and *middle articulations* consist of small, nearly flat joint surfaces.

### *Ligaments*

The posterior articulation within the subtalar joint is reinforced by a set of three slender ligaments, named by location as the *medial, posterior, and lateral talocalcaneal ligaments* (see Figs. 14–11, 14–13, and 14–14). These ligaments provide only secondary stability to the subtalar joint. Other larger ligaments provide the primary source of stability. The calcaneofibular ligament and the deltoid ligament are both discussed previously in reference to the talocrural joint. The most substantial ligaments to cross only the subtalar joint are the interosseous (talocalcaneal) and cervical ligaments. Broad and flat, these ligaments cross obliquely within the sinus tarsi and, therefore, are difficult to view unless the joint is opened, as in Figure 14–8. The *interosseous (talocalcaneal) ligament* has two distinct, flattened, anterior and posterior bands. These bands arise from the calcaneal sulcus and attach superiorly and medially on the talar sulcus and adjacent regions. The larger *cervical ligament* has an oblique fiber arrangement similar to the preceding ligament, but is located more laterally within the sinus tarsi. Distally, the cervical ligament courses superiorly and medially to attach primarily to the inferior-lateral surface of the neck of the talus (hence, the name "cervical") (see Fig. 14–14). As a group, the interosseous (talocalcaneal) and cervical ligaments provide the strongest connective tissue bond between the talus and calcaneus.[55]

The ligaments of the subtalar joint control the extremes of eversion and inversion (see the boxes).

---

**Ligaments that Limit the Extremes of *Eversion* at the Subtalar Joint**
- Medial fibers of the interosseous (talocalcaneal) ligament
- Tibiocalcaneal fibers within the deltoid ligament

---

**Ligaments that Limit the Extremes of *Inversion* at the Subtalar Joint**
- Cervical ligament
- Calcaneofibular ligaments

---

### Kinematics

#### Osteokinematics and Arthrokinematics

The arthrokinematics at the subtalar joint involve a sliding between the three sets of facets, yielding a curvilinear arc of movement between the calcaneus and the talus. The axis of rotation for this motion is described by several investigators. (See references 17, 19, 28, 44, and 56.) Although considerable variation exists from one subject to another, the axis of rotation is typically described as a line that pierces the lateral-posterior heel and courses through the subtalar joint in anterior, medial, and superior directions (Fig. 14–20 *A* to *C*, red). According to Manter,[28] the axis of rotation is typically positioned 42 degrees from the horizontal plane (see Fig. 14–20A) and 16 degrees from the sagittal plane (see Fig. 14–20B).

The calcaneus pronates and supinates about the talus (or vice versa when the foot is planted) in a path perpendicular to the axis of rotation (see the red circular arrows in Fig. 14–20 *A* to *C*). Given the general pitch to the axis, only two of the three main components of pronation and supination are readily evident at the subtalar joint: inversion and eversion, and abduction and adduction (see Fig. 14–20A and B). *Pronation*, therefore, has main components of *eversion* and *abduction* (Fig. 14–20D); *supination* has main components of *inversion* and *adduction* (Fig. 14–20E). The calcaneus can dorsiflex and plantar flex slightly relative to the talus; however, this motion is small.

For simplicity, the osteokinematics of the subtalar joint are demonstrated by rotating the calcaneus against a fixed and immobile talus. During walking, however, when the calcaneus is relatively immobile due to the load of body weight, pronation and supination at the subtalar joint occur primarily by rotation of the talus and leg.

#### Range of Motion

Grimston and colleagues[14] reported active range of motion across the ankle complex (combined talocrural joint and subtalar joint) in 120 subjects across multiple age groups. The range of motion for inversion and eversion and for abduction and adduction are listed in Table 14–4. Averaged across all age groups, total inversion exceeds eversion by nearly double: inversion, 22.6 degrees; eversion, 12.5 degrees. Although these data include slight motion from the talocrural joint, the ratio of inversion-to-eversion movement is consistent with data reported for the subtalar joint alone.[21] Eversion range of motion is naturally limited by the distal, projecting, lateral malleolus and the thick deltoid ligament. As shown in Table 14–4, the maximal range of abduction and adduction is nearly equivalent.

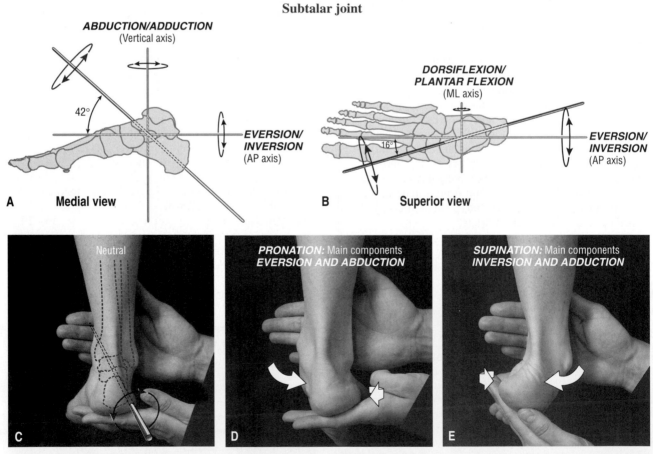

**FIGURE 14–20.** The axis of rotation and osteokinematics at the subtalar joint are shown. The axis of rotation (red) is shown from the side (*A*) and above (*B*); the axis of rotation is shown again in *C. D,* The movement of pronation, with the main components of eversion and abduction, is demonstrated. *E,* The movement of supination, with main components of inversion and adduction, is shown.

**Close-Packed and Loose-Packed Position of the Subtalar Joint**

In addition to controlling the position of the rearfoot, the subtalar joint also indirectly controls the stability of the more distal joints, especially the transverse tarsal joint. Although the relevance of this concept is discussed later in this chapter, *full supination at the subtalar joint restricts the overall flexibility of the midfoot.* A loosely articulated skeletal model helps to demonstrate this principle. With one hand stabilizing the forefoot, maximally "swing" the calcaneus into full inversion and note that the lateral aspect of the midfoot "drops" relative to the medial aspect. As a result, the talonavicular and calcaneocuboid joints become twisted longitudinally, thereby increasing the rigidity of the midfoot. For this reason, maximal supination at the subtalar joint is considered the close-packed position. The description does not imply maximal congruity at the joint, rather a position that increases the stability through the midfoot.

*Full pronation of the subtalar joint, in contrast, increases the overall flexibility of the midfoot.* Again, returning to a loosely articulated skeleton model, maximal eversion of the calcaneus untwists the medial and lateral aspects of the midfoot, placing them in a more or less parallel position. As a result, the talonavicular and calcaneocuboid joints untwist longitudinally, thereby increasing the flexibility of the midfoot. The loose-packed position of the subtalar joint is often described as maximal pronation, implying a reduced stability over the midfoot. Make the effort to "feel," on a partner, the increased flexibility of the midfoot as the calcaneus is gradually taken from maximal eversion to maximal inversion. As described in subsequent sections, the ability of the midfoot to change from greater to lesser flexibility has important mechanical implications during the stance phase of gait.

## TRANSVERSE TARSAL JOINT

As described earlier, the talocrural (ankle) joint permits motion primarily in the sagittal plane. The subtalar joint, however, permits a more oblique path of motion consisting of two primary components: inversion and eversion, and abduction and adduction. This section describes how the transverse tarsal joint allows even a more oblique path of motion, passing almost equally through all three cardinal planes. While weight bearing, the pronation and supination of the midfoot region allows the foot to adapt to a variety of surface contours (Fig. 14–21).

The transverse tarsal joint has a strong functional relationship to the subtalar joint. As subsequently described, these two major joints function cooperatively to control most of the pronation and supination posturing of the entire foot.

### Articular and Ligamentous Structure

The transverse tarsal joint, also known as the mid-tarsal or Chopart's joint, consists of two articulations: the *talonavicular joint* and the *calcaneocuboid joint*. Although functionally related, each joint is anatomically distinct. As a composite joint, the transverse tarsal joint is stabilized by the medial longitudinal arch, specialized ligaments, joint capsule, and, if needed, muscle.[55] The articular and ligamentous structure of the talonavicular and calcaneocuboid joints are described separately.

#### Talonavicular Joint
The talonavicular joint is the articulation between the convex head of the talus and the continuous concavity formed by the proximal side of the navicular bone and the dorsal sur-

**TABLE 14-4. The Mean and Standard Error\* for Active Range of Motion in Degrees for Inversion and Eversion and Abduction and Adduction at the Ankle Joint Complex†**

| Age (yr) | Inversion | Eversion | Abduction | Adduction |
|---|---|---|---|---|
| 9–13 | 26.7 (.7) | 10.5 (.4) | 41.6 (1.0) | 42.2 (1.7) |
| 14–16 | 28.8 (1.4) | 12.6 (.8) | 46.8 (1.5) | 42.4 (2.6) |
| 17–20 | 27.1 (1.3) | 11.9 (.7) | 45.0 (1.3) | 31.0 (13.6) |
| 21–39 | 20.5 (1.3) | 15.2 (.9) | 38.2 (1.9) | 34.5 (9.6) |
| 40–59 | 20.7 (1.5) | 13.8 (.9) | 33.2 (1.4) | 29.9 (1.7) |
| 60–69 | 17.1 (1.1) | 12.3 (.6) | 31.7 (1.0) | 27.9 (1.6) |
| 70–79 | 17.1 (1.0) | 11.4 (.6) | 31.3 (1.5) | 27.1 (1.3) |
| Average | 22.6 | 12.5 | 38.3 | 33.6 |

\* In parentheses.

† The subtalar and talocrural joint make up the ankle joint complex. The data were collected from healthy persons across different age groups, and the data were averaged across gender.[14]

**Standard Clinical Measurements of Subtalar Joint Range of Motion**

The range of motion at the subtalar joint is typically measured clinically by the use of a standard goniometer. To obtain a reliable and valid measurement through this means is difficult and, perhaps, impossible.[36] Causes of measurement error are due to the inability of a standard, rigid goniometer to follow the arc of pronation and supination, compounded by the movement in adjacent soft tissues and surrounding joints. As a method of improving the validly of this measurement, clinicians often report subtalar joint motion as a more simple motion of inversion and eversion of the rearfoot (calcaneus).

The rather strict terminology described for subtalar motion is not always adhered to in clinical and research settings. "Short-cuts" in terminology have evolved that, unfortunately, limit the ability to effectively communicate the precise details of foot and ankle kinesiology. For reasons such as those just described, pronation and supination at the subtalar joint are often referred to simply as "eversion and inversion" of the calcaneus, respectively. Eversion, for example, is only a component of, rather than a synonym for, pronation. Comparisons of range of motion data between studies are often made difficult, unless the motions are explicitly defined.

Clinically, the expression "subtalar joint neutral" is often used to establish a "baseline" or reference for evaluating a foot for an orthotic device.[9,30] The neutral, or 0 degree, position of the subtalar joint is attained by placing the subject's calcaneus in a position that allows both lateral and medial sides of the talus to be equally exposed for palpation within the mortise. In this position, the joint is typically one-third the distance from full eversion and two-thirds the distance from full inversion.

---

face of the plantar calcaneonavicular ("spring") ligament (Figs. 14–8 and 14–22). The *spring ligament* is thick and wide, spanning the gap between the sustentaculum talus of the calcaneus and the plantar surface of the navicular (Fig. 14–23). Functioning as the "floor" of the talonavicular joint, the spring ligament supports the head of the talus, thereby helping to explain the terminology "spring." Support is important during standing because body weight depresses the head of the talus toward the floor. The surface of the spring ligament that directly contacts the head of the talus is lined with smooth fibrocartilage.[55]

The talonavicular joint is enclosed by a thin, irregularly shaped capsule. Posteriorly, the capsule is thickened by the interosseous ligament of the subtalar joint (see Fig. 14–8). The capsule is strengthened dorsally by the *dorsal talonavicular ligament* and laterally by the calcaneonavicular fibers of the *bifurcated ligament* (see Figs. 14–13 and 14–14). Medi-

ally, the capsule of the talonavicular joint blends with the anterior edge of the *deltoid ligament.*

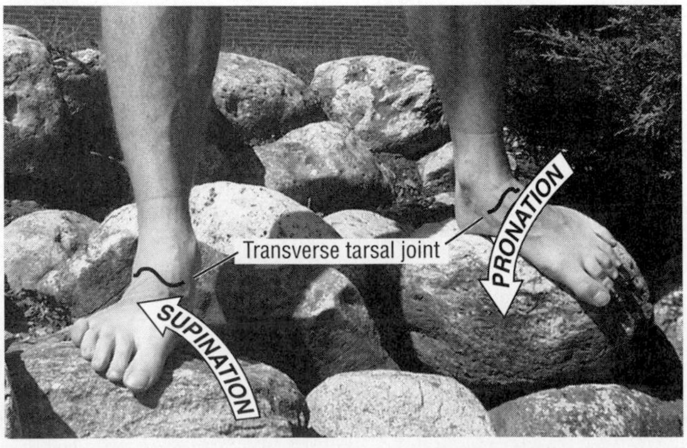

The ball-and-socket–like articulation of the talonavicular joint provides significant rotation to the medial side of the midfoot. The extent of this mobility becomes readily apparent by twisting the midfoot relative to the rearfoot.

*Calcaneocuboid Joint*

The calcaneocuboid joint is the lateral component of the transverse tarsal joint, formed by the junction of the anterior (distal) surface of the calcaneus and the proximal surface of the cuboid (see Fig. 14–22). Each articular surface has a slight concave and convex curvature that, when articulated, forms an interlocking wedge that resists sliding. The joint is therefore relatively inflexible, providing an element of rigidity to the lateral column of the foot. The limited mobility at the calcaneocuboid joint is in contrast to the ample movement permitted at the talonavicular joint.

The dorsal surface of the capsule of the calcaneocuboid joint is thickened by the *dorsal calcaneocuboid ligament* (see Fig. 14–14). The joint is further stabilized by three additional ligaments. The *bifurcated ligament* is a Y-shaped band of tissue with its stem attached to the calcaneus, just dorsal and lateral to the margin of calcaneocuboid joint. The stem of the ligament flares into lateral and medial fiber bundles. The medial (calcaneonavicular) fibers reinforce the dorsal-lateral side of the talonavicular joint. The lateral (calcaneocuboid) fibers cross dorsal to the calcaneocuboid joint, forming the primary bond between the two bones.[55] The long and short plantar ligaments reinforce the plantar side of the calcaneocuboid joint (see Fig. 14–23). The *long plantar ligament,* the longest ligament in the foot, arises from the plantar surface of the calcaneus, just anterior to the calcaneal tuberosity. The ligament inserts on the plantar surface of the bases of the lateral three or four metatarsal bones. The *short plantar ligament,* also called the plantar calcaneocuboid ligament, arises just anterior and deep to the long plantar liga-

**FIGURE 14–21.** The transverse tarsal joints allow for pronation and supination during standing on uneven surfaces.

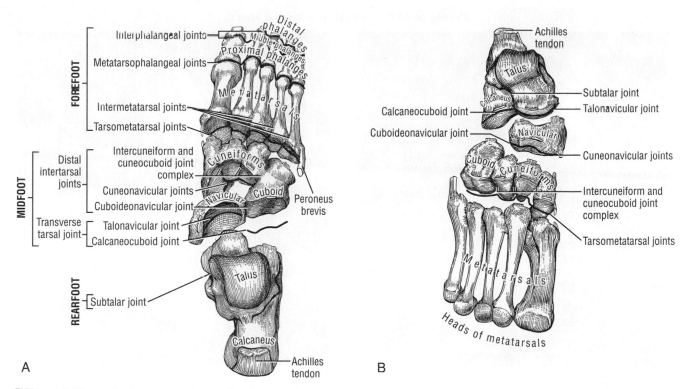

**FIGURE 14–22.** *A,* The bones and disarticulated joints of the right foot are shown from two perspectives: superior-posterior (*A*) and superior-anterior (*B*). *A* highlights the overall organization of the joints of the foot.

ment and inserts on the plantar surface of the cuboid bone. By passing perpendicularly to the calcaneocuboid joint, the plantar ligaments provide excellent structural stability to the lateral side of the foot.

### Kinematics

The transverse tarsal joint rarely functions without an associated movement at nearby joints, especially the subtalar joint. To appreciate the component of pronation and supination that occurs primarily at the transverse tarsal joint, hold the calcaneus firmly while maximally pronating and supinating the midfoot (Fig. 14–24*A* and *C*). During this motion, the navicular spins within the talonavicular joint. The combination of rotations at both subtalar and transverse tarsal joint accounts for most of the pronation and supination throughout the foot (Fig. 14–24*B* and *D*). As evident in the Figures, mobility of the forefoot also contributes to the pronation and supination postures of the foot.

### Osteokinematics

The description of the function of the transverse tarsal joint is complicated by three factors. First, two separate axes of rotation exist. Second, the amplitude and direction of movement at the transverse tarsal joint may be different during weight-bearing versus non-weight-bearing activities. Third, the stabilizing function of the transverse tarsal joint at the midfoot is influenced by the position of the subtalar joint. Each of these factors is considered in the upcoming sections.

**Axes of Rotation.** Manter[28] described two axes of rotation for movement at the transverse tarsal joint: *longitudinal* and *oblique*. Motion about the transverse tarsal joint occurs in a plane that is perpendicular to each of these axes. The

*longitudinal axis* is nearly coincident with the straight anterior-posterior axis (Fig. 14–25 *A* to *C*), with the primary component motions of *eversion* and *inversion* (Fig. 14–25*D* and *E*). The *oblique axis,* in contrast, has a strong vertical and medial-lateral pitch (Fig. 14–25 *F* to *H*). Motion about this axis, therefore, occurs freely as a combination of *abduction and dorsiflexion* (Fig. 14–25*I*) and *adduction and plantar flex-*

**Plantar view**

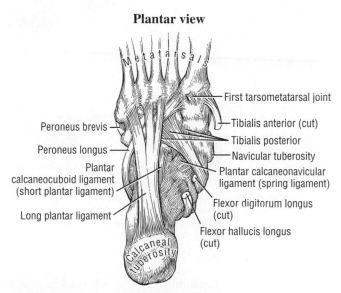

**FIGURE 14–23.** Ligaments and tendons deep within the plantar aspect of the right foot. Note the course of the tendons of the peroneus longus and tibialis posterior.

**Pronation of the foot (Dorsal-medial view)**

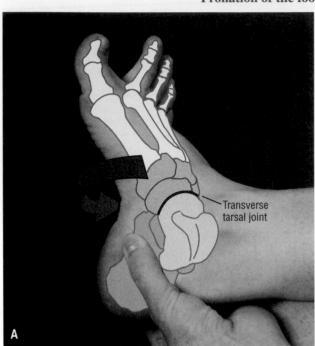

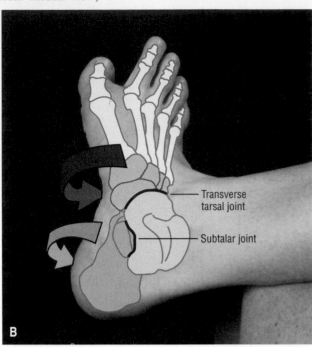

**Supination of the foot (Plantar-medial view)**

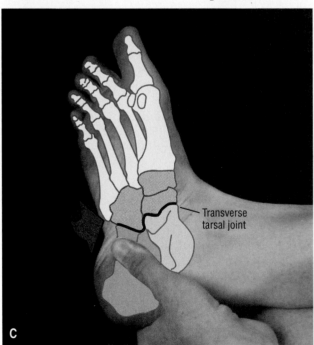

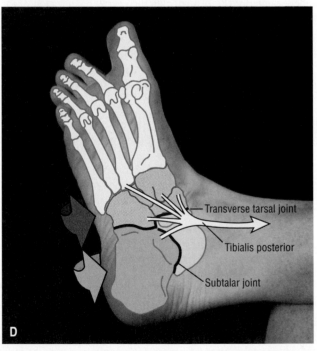

**FIGURE 14–24.** Pronation and supination of the unloaded right foot demonstrates the interplay of the subtalar and transverse tarsal joints. With the calcaneus held fixed, pronation and supination occur primarily at the midfoot (*A* and *C*). When the calcaneus is free, pronation and supination occur as a summation across both the rearfoot and midfoot (*B* and *D*). Rearfoot movement is indicated by gray arrows; midfoot movement is indicated by red arrows. The tibialis posterior is shown in *D* as it directs active supination over both the rearfoot and midfoot.

*ion* (Fig. 14–25*J*). Combining the movements produced about both axes produces the true form of pronation and supination (i.e., movement that maximally expresses components of all three cardinal planes). Movement at the

transverse tarsal joint makes the midfoot very adaptable in shape.

Range of motion at the transverse tarsal joint is difficult to measure and isolate from adjacent joints. By visual and

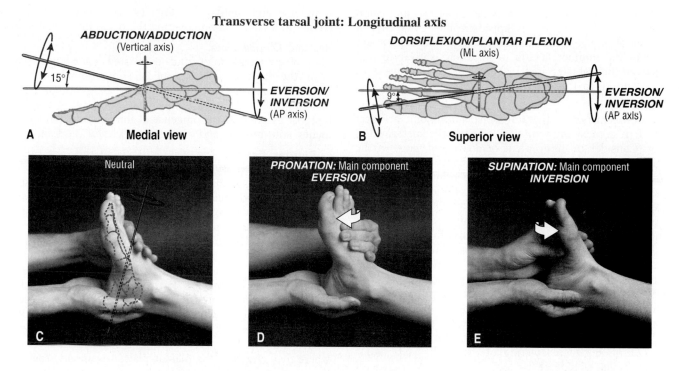

**Transverse tarsal joint: Longitudinal axis**

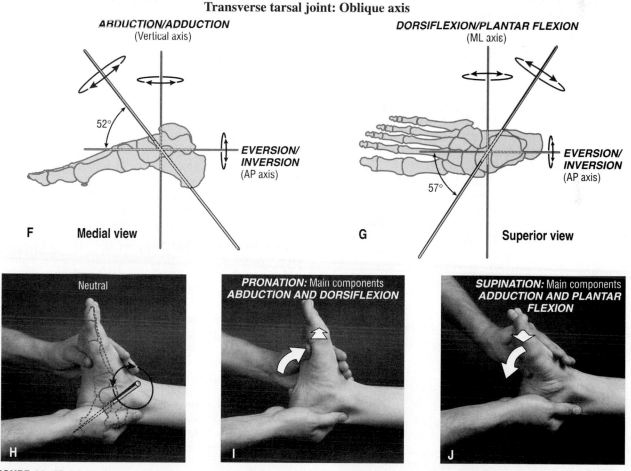

**Transverse tarsal joint: Oblique axis**

**FIGURE 14–25.** The axes of rotation and osteokinematics at the transverse tarsal joint. The *longitudinal axis* of rotation is shown in red from the side (*A* and *C*) and from above (*B*). Movements that occur about this axis (*D*) are *pronation* (with the main component of eversion) and (*E*) *supination* (with the main component of inversion). The *oblique axis* of rotation is shown in red from the side (*F* and *H*) and from above (*G*). Movements that occur about this axis are (*I*) *pronation* (with main components of abduction and dorsiflexion) and (*J*) *supination* (with main components of adduction and plantar flexion).

manual inspection, however, it is evident that the supination range of the midfoot region is approximately twice that of the pronation range. The amount of pure inversion and eversion of the midfoot occurs in a pattern similar to that observed at the subtalar joint: about 20 to 25 degrees of inversion and 10 to 15 degrees of eversion.

### Arthrokinematics

The arthrokinematics at the transverse tarsal joint are best described in context with motion of both the rearfoot and midfoot. Consider the movement of active *supination* of the unloaded foot (see Fig. 14–24D). The tibialis posterior muscle, with its multiple attachments, is the prime supinator of the foot. Because of the relatively rigid calcaneocuboid joint, an inverting and adducting calcaneus draws the lateral column of the foot "under" the medial column of the forefoot. An important pivot point for this motion is the talonavicular joint. The pull of the tibialis posterior contributes to the spin of the navicular, and to the raising of the medial arch (instep) of the foot. During this motion, the concave proximal surface of the navicular and spring ligament spin around the convex head of the talus.

*Pronation* of the unloaded foot occurs by similar but reverse kinematics as that described. The pull of the peroneus longus contributes to a lowering of the medial side and a raising of the lateral side of the foot.

### Medial Longitudinal Arch of the Foot

The characteristic concave in-step at the medial side of the foot is maintained primarily by the *medial longitudinal arch* (Fig. 14–26). The keystone of this arch is located near the talonavicular joint.

The medial longitudinal arch is the primary load-bearing and shock-absorbing structure in the foot. The bones that contribute to the medial arch are the calcaneus, talus, navicular, cuneiforms, and three medial metatarsals. Without the arched configuration, the large and rapidly acting forces produced during running, for example, may exceed the physiologic weight-bearing capacity of the bones. Additional structures that assist with reducing the forces acting on the foot are plantar fat pads, superficial plantar fascia, and sesamoid bones located at the plantar base of the first (great) toe.

In addition to the medial longitudinal arch, a secondary

transverse arch exists (see Fig. 14–26). This arch is discussed in a later section covering the distal intertarsal joints.

### Anatomic Considerations

The talonavicular joint and associated connective tissues form the keystone of the medial longitudinal arch. The height and general shape of the medial longitudinal arch are maintained by the thick plantar fascia, spring ligament, stability of the medial tarsometatarsal joints, short plantar ligaments, and intrinsic and extrinsic muscles of the foot.

**Plantar Fascia.** The plantar fascia of the foot provides the primary support of the medial longitudinal arch.[16] The fascia consists of an extensive series of thick, very strong longitudinal and transverse bands of collagen-rich tissue.[55] The plantar fascia covers the sole and sides of the foot and is organized into superficial and deep layers. The superficial fibers are attached primarily to the thick dermis, and they function to reduce shear forces and provide shock absorption. The more extensive deep plantar fascia attaches posteriorly to the medial process of the calcaneal tuberosity. From this origin, lateral, medial, and central sets of fibers course anteriorly, blending with and covering the first layer of the intrinsic muscles of the foot. The main, larger, central set of fibers extends anteriorly toward the metatarsal heads—where they attach to the plantar plates (ligaments) that cover the metatarsophalangeal joints and fibrous sheaths of the adjacent flexor tendons of the digits. Active toe extension, therefore, stretches the central band of deep fascia, adding tension to the medial longitudinal arch. The functional significance of this point is described later in this chapter.

### Functional Considerations

The medial longitudinal arch in the healthy foot is supported by two primary forces: (1) active muscle force and (2) passive force produced by the combined elasticity and tensile strength of connective tissues and the shape of the bones. When standing at ease, passive forces are generally sufficient to support the arch. Active forces are required, however, during more dynamic and stressful actions, such as standing on tiptoes, walking, and running. The following discussion is limited to passive forces that support the arch. The role of muscle forces are described later in this chapter.

**Passive Forces That Support the Medial Longitudinal Arch.** When standing, body weight crosses the mortise and is distributed across the medial longitudinal arch and, ultimately, to fat pads and the thick dermis located primarily at the heel and ball (metatarsal head region) of the foot. Body weight forces are distributed therefore, across a wide region of the foot (see the box).[6] The pressure under the forefoot is usually greatest in the region of the second and third metatarsal heads. Substantially greater pressure occurs during walking and even more so when running and jumping.

---

**Distribution of Compression Forces (by percent) Across the Foot while Standing**
- Rearfoot (heel), 60%
- Forefoot, 28%
- Midfoot, 8%

---

Body weight tends to depress the talus inferiorly and flatten the medial longitudinal arch. This action increases the distance between the calcaneus and metatarsal heads. Ten-

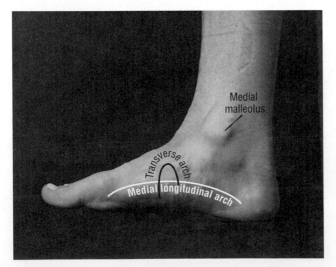

**FIGURE 14–26.** The medial side of a normal foot shows the medial longitudinal arch (white) and the transverse arch (black).

sion in stretched connective tissues, especially the deep plantar fascia, acts as a semielastic tie rod that yields slightly under load, allowing only a marginal drop in the arch (Fig. 14–27A, stretched spring). Acting like a truss, the tie rod supports and absorbs body weight. Experiments on cadaveric specimens indicate that the plantar fascia is the major structure that maintains the height of the medial longitudinal arch.[16] Sectioning of this fascia decreased arch stiffness by 25%.

While the arch is depressed, the rearfoot tends to pronate slightly. This is most evident from a posterior view as the calcaneus everts slightly relative to the tibia. As the foot is unloaded, such as when shifting body weight to the other leg, the naturally elastic and flexible arch returns to its preloaded raised height. The calcaneus inverts slightly back to its neutral position, allowing the mechanism to repeat its shock absorption function once again.

Standing at ease on healthy feet requires little or no activity of the intrinsic or extrinsic muscles of the foot.[2] The height and shape of the medial longitudinal arch is controlled primarily by passive restraints from the connective tissues depicted by the spring in Figure 14–27A. Active muscle support is required when one stands only as a "secondary line of support," for example, when holding heavy loads, or when the arch lacks inherent support because of overstretched connective tissues.[51] Basmajian and Stecko[2] showed significant EMG responses from the tibialis posterior and the intrinsic muscles, only after the healthy arch was loaded in excess of 400 pounds (1780 N).

*Abnormal Shape of the Medial Longitudinal Arch*

**Pes Planus—"Dropped" Medial Longitudinal Arch.** Pes planus or "flatfoot" describes a chronically dropped or abnormally low medial longitudinal arch.[24] The plantar fascia may be overstretched with the subtalar joint excessively pronated, causing a rearfoot valgus posture, where the calcaneus is everted away from the midline. The forefoot is usually abducted, and the talus and navicular bones are depressed, often causing a callus to develop on the adjacent skin. A foot with moderate-to-severe pes planus typically has a compromised ability to transfer loads throughout the foot. As depicted in Figure 14–27B, active forces from intrinsic and extrinsic muscles, such as the tibialis posterior, may be needed to compensate for the lack of tension produced in overstretched connective tissues. Increased muscular activity during standing may contribute to fatigue and various overuse symptoms, including pain, shin splints, bone spurs, and fascia and connective tissue inflammation.

Pes planus is often described as being either a rigid or flexible deformity.[41] The foot with *rigid pes planus* (see Fig. 14–27B) demonstrates a dropped arch even in non-weight-bearing. This deformity is often congenital, secondary to bony or joint malformation, such as tarsal coalition (i.e., partial fusion of the calcaneus with the talus fixed in eversion). Pes planus may also occur as a result of spastic paralysis. Because of the fixed nature and potential for producing painful symptoms, rigid pes planus may require surgical correction during childhood.

*Flexible pes planus* is the more common form of dropped arch. The medial longitudinal arch appears normal when unloaded, but drops excessively upon weight bearing. A flexible pes planus is often associated with other structural anomalies and/or compensatory mechanisms that cause excessive pronation of the foot. Surgical intervention is rarely

indicated for flexible pes planus. Treatment is usually in the form of orthoses, specialized footwear, and exercise.

**Pes Cavus—Abnormally "Raised" Medial Longitudinal Arch.** In its least complicated form, *pes cavus* describes an abnormally high medial longitudinal arch.[41] The condi-

**Normal arch**

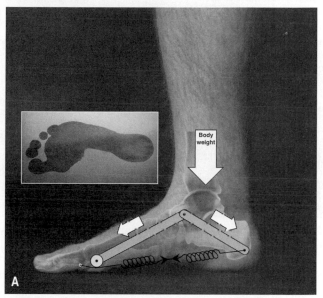

**Dropped arch**

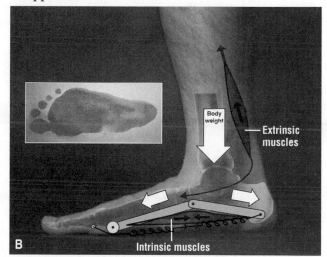

**FIGURE 14–27.** Models of the foot show a mechanism of accepting body weight while standing. *A,* With a normal medial longitudinal arch, body weight is accepted and dissipated through elongation of the plantar fascia, depicted as a red spring. The footprint illustrates the concavity of the normal arch. *B,* With an abnormally dropped medial longitudinal arch, the overstretched and weakened plantar fascia, depicted as an overstretched red spring, cannot adequately accept or dissipate body weight. As a consequence, various extrinsic and intrinsic muscles are active as a secondary source of support to the arch. The footprint illustrates the dropped arch and loss of a characteristic instep.

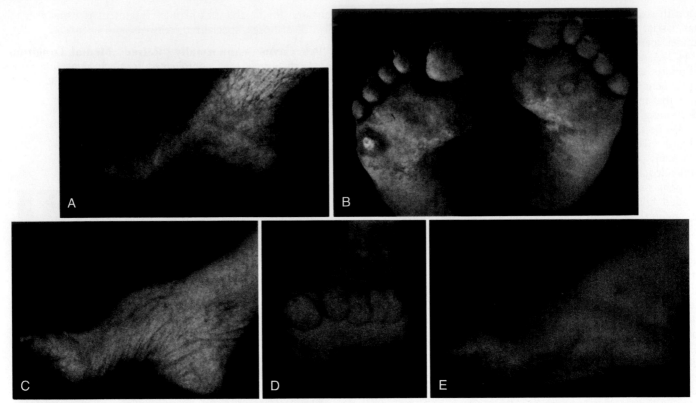

**FIGURE 14–28.** A case of a mild pes cavus deformity of unknown etiology is shown in *A. B* to *E* show signs or other deformities that may be associated with pes cavus: *(B)* callus formation under the metatarsal heads; *(C)* equinus (plantar flexion) deformity of the forefoot; *(D)* pronated forefoot relative to the rearfoot during weight bearing; *(E)* shortening of the medial column of the foot. (From Richardson EG: Neurogenic disorders. In Canale ST (ed): Campbell's Operative Orthopaedics, vol 4, 9th ed. St. Louis, Mosby-Year Book, 1998.)

tion is usually idiopathic and nonprogressive. As shown in Figure 14–28, a high arch tends to place the metatarsal heads more perpendicular to the ground. Callus formation under the metatarsal heads and metatarsalgia may result and is often treated with specialized footwear and orthoses. An abnormally high medial longitudinal arch is not as common as an abnormally low arch.

Severe cases of pes cavus may develop secondary to neuromuscular disorders, such as Charcot-Marie-Tooth disease, poliomyelitis, and cerebral palsy.[41] In these cases, pes cavus is often associated with other progressive problems, like "clawing" of the toes, tight plantar fascia, and compensatory overpronation of the forefoot. Treatment involves surgery and orthotic management.

---

### SPECIAL FOCUS 14–4

**A Possible Association Between a High Arch and Stress Fracture**

A study on 449 United States Navy Sea, Air, and Land (SEAL) candidates showed a higher incidence of stress fractures in feet with abnormally high arches.[21] The higher arch may involve a more supinated posture of the rearfoot and an associated increased rigidity throughout the foot. With a loss of pliability, the foot is subjected to a greater rate of stress, possibly contributing to the higher reported frequency of fracture. Interestingly, and probably for different reasons, the study also showed a higher incidence of stress fractures in the feet with abnormally low arches. Participants in the study were subjected to an extraordinarily high level of physical training, however.

---

## COMBINED ACTION OF THE SUBTALAR AND TRANSVERSE TARSAL JOINTS

### *Joint Interactions During the Stance Phase of Gait*

Generally, when the foot is unloaded (i.e., non-weight-bearing), pronation twists the sole of the foot outward, whereas supination twists the sole of the foot inward. During weight-bearing, however, pronation and supination of the foot permit the leg and talus to rotate in all three planes relative to a somewhat fixed calcaneus. This important kinesiologic function is orchestrated primarily through interaction among the subtalar joint, transverse tarsal joint, and medial longitudinal arch.

In the healthy foot, the medial longitudinal arch raises and lowers cyclically throughout the gait cycle. During most of the stance phase, the arch lowers slightly in response to the progressive loading of body weight (Fig. 14–29A).[5] Structures that resist the lowering of the arch help to absorb the stress of body weight and thus protect the foot, particularly its osseous structures. During the first 30 to 35% of the

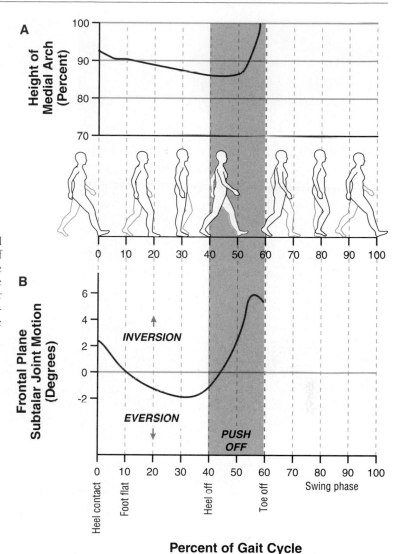

**FIGURE 14–29.** *A,* The percent change in height of the medial longitudinal arch throughout the stance phase (0 to 60%) of the gait cycle. On the vertical axis, the 100% value is the height of the arch when the foot is unloaded during the swing phase. *B,* Frontal plane range of motion at the subtalar joint (i.e., inversion and eversion of the calcaneus), throughout the stance phase. The area shaded in red represents the push-off phase of walking.

gait cycle, the subtalar joint pronates or everts, adding an element of flexibility to the midfoot (Fig. 14–29B).[8] By late stance, the arch rises as the supinated subtalar joint renders the midfoot relatively rigid. The foot is now well prepared to accept a large bending moment, created across the foot at the push-off phase of gait. The ability of the foot to repeatedly transform from a flexible and shock absorbent structure to a more rigid lever during each gait cycle is one of the most important and clinically relevant actions of the foot. As subsequently described, the subtalar joint is the principal joint that directs the pronation and supination kinematics of the foot.

### Early Stance Phase: Pronation at the Subtalar Joint

**Kinematic Mechanisms of Pronation.** Immediately following the heel contact phase of gait, the dorsiflexed talocrural joint and slightly supinated subtalar joint rapidly plantar flex and pronate, respectively. The pronation at the subtalar joint during stance is controlled by two mechanisms. First, the calcaneus tips into eversion as a result of the ground reaction force passing just lateral to the anterior-posterior axis of rotation through the calcaneus. The simultaneous impact of heel contact also pushes the head of the talus medially in the horizontal plane and inferiorly in the sagittal plane. Relative to the calcaneus, this motion of the talus abducts and dorsiflexes the subtalar joint. These motions are consistent with the definition of pronation. A loosely articulated skeletal model aids in the visualization of this motion. Second, during the early stance phase, the tibia and fibula, and to a lesser extent the femur, internally rotate after initial heel contact.[17,40] Because of the embracing configuration of the talocrural joint, the internally rotating lower leg steers the subtalar joint into further pronation. The argument is often raised that with the calcaneus in contact with the ground, pronation at the subtalar joint causes, rather than follows, internal rotation of the leg, and either perspective is valid.

The amplitude of pronation at the subtalar joint during early stance is relatively small—about 2 to 3 degrees on average—and lasts only about 1/4 of a second during average speed walking. The amount and the speed of the pronation influences the kinematics of the more proximal joints of

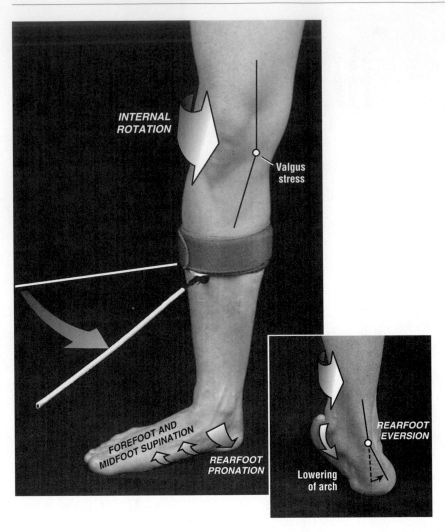

**FIGURE 14–30.** With the foot fixed, full internal rotation of the lower limb causes the following associated movements: rearfoot pronation (eversion), lowering of the medial longitudinal arch, and valgus stress at the knee. Note that as the rearfoot pronates, the floor "pushes" the forefoot and midfoot into a relatively supinated position.

the lower extremity. These effects can be appreciated by exaggerating and dramatically slowing the pronation action of the rearfoot during the initial loading phase of gait. Consider the demonstration depicted in Figure 14–30. While standing over a loaded and fixed foot, forcefully but slowly internally rotate the lower leg and note the associated pronation at the rearfoot (subtalar joint) and simultaneous lowering of the medial longitudinal arch. If forceful enough, this action also tends to internally rotate, slightly flex, and adduct the hip and to create a valgus strain on the knee (Table 14–5). These so-called mechanical events are exaggerated and do not all occur to this degree and precise pattern when the limb is loaded and at normal walking speed. Nevertheless, because of the linkages throughout the lower limb, excessive or uncontrolled pronation of the rearfoot could exaggerate one or more of these mechanically related joint actions. Clinically, a person who excessively pronates during early stance often complains of medial knee pain, apparently from a net genu valgus strain and subsequent overstretching on the medial collateral ligament. Whether the overpronation causes the knee valgus or vice versa is not always obvious.

Although widely accepted, a predictable kinematic relationship between the magnitude and timing of excessive pronation and excessive internal rotation of the lower limb has not been established conclusively.[40] Precise measurements of these kinematic relationships while a subject is walking are technically difficult. The kinematics themselves are highly variable and poorly defined. Some studies report the kinematics as a rotation of a single bone, and others report relative rotations between bones.[40] Additional studies are needed in this area before definite cause and effect relationships are known. These relationships are important for they

**TABLE 14–5. Associated Movements During an Exaggerated Pronation of the Subtalar Joint while Weight Bearing**

| Joint | Action |
| --- | --- |
| Hip | Internal rotation, flexion, and adduction |
| Knee | Valgus strain |
| Subtalar joint (rearfoot) | *Pronation* (and lowering of medial longitudinal arch) |
| Transverse tarsal joint (midfoot) | Inversion (supination) |

are the basis for many of the exercises and orthotics employed to reduce painful conditions related to excessive pronation.

## SPECIAL FOCUS 14–5

### Example of the Kinematic Versatility of the Foot

Earlier in this section, the point was made that pronation of the unloaded foot occurs primarily as a summation of the pronation at both the subtalar and transverse tarsal joints (see Fig. 14–24*B*). This summation of motion does not, however, necessarily occur when the foot is loaded while weight bearing. With the foot loaded or otherwise fixed to the ground, pronating the rearfoot may cause the midfoot and forefoot regions, which are receiving firm upward counterforce from the floor, to twist into relative supination (see Fig. 14–30). This reciprocal kinematic relationship between the rearfoot and more anterior regions of the foot demonstrates the versatility of the foot, amplifying the other's action when the foot is unloaded (see Fig. 14–24*B*), or counteracting each other's action when the foot is loaded (see Fig. 14–30).

**Kinesiologic Benefits of Controlling Normal Pronation.** From a kinesiologic perspective, controlled pronation of the subtalar joint at early stance has several useful mechanical effects. Pronation at the subtalar joint permits internal rotation of the talus, and the entire lower extremity, against a firmly planted calcaneus. The strong horizontal orientation of the facets at the subtalar joint certainly suggests this action. Without such a joint mechanism, the plantar surface of the calcaneus would otherwise "spin" like a child's top against the walking surface, along with the medially rotating leg. Eccentric activation of supinator muscles, such as the tibialis posterior, can help to decelerate the pronation and resist the lowering of the medial longitudinal arch. Controlled pronation of the subtalar joint favors relative flexibility throughout the midfoot, allowing the foot to accommodate to the varied shapes and contours of walking surfaces.

**Consequences of Excessive Pronation.** Innumerable examples exist on how malalignment of the foot affects the kinematics of walking. A common situation results from excessive or poorly controlled pronation at the subtalar joint during stance phase. This disorder has multiple causes, such as (1) laxity or weakness in the mechanisms that normally support and control the medial longitudinal arch, (2) abnormal shape or mobility of the tarsal bones, (3) excessive femoral anteversion, and (4) generalized muscle weakness and/or reduced flexibility. In each case, a structural fault causes the rearfoot to fall into excessive valgus (eversion) following heel contact.[29] Often, excessive subtalar joint pronation is a compensation for either excessive or restricted motion throughout the lower extremity, particularly in the frontal and horizontal planes. The most common structural deformity of the foot is *rearfoot varus.* (Varus describes a segment of the foot that is inverted toward the midline.) As a response to this deformity, the subtalar joint often overcompensates by excessively pronating, in speed and/or magnitude, to ensure that the medial aspect of the forefoot contacts the ground during stance phase.[30,38,52]

Similar compensations occur as a result of *forefoot varus.* The associated excessive internal rotation of the talus and leg may, in some cases, create a "chain reaction" of kinematic disturbances and compensations throughout the entire limb, such as those depicted in Figure 14–30. The abnormal kinematic sequence between the tibia and femur may cause an increased "Q angle" at the knee and an increased net lateral pull of the quadriceps or iliotibial band on the patella.[38] These situations may predispose the patient to patellofemoral joint dysfunction. For this reason, clinicians often note the position of the subtalar joint while the patient stands and walks in evaluation of the cause of patellofemoral joint pain.

## SPECIAL FOCUS 14–6

### Foot Orthoses

Clinicians generally agree that some form of foot orthosis or specialized footwear controls excessive pronation at the subtalar joint.[3,20,29,34] In general, a foot orthosis is a device inserted into the shoe in order to modify the foot's mechanics. Most often, a wedge is placed on the medial aspect of the orthosis, which in theory controls the rate, amount, and temporal sequencing of pronation at the subtalar joint. As an adjunct to orthoses, some clinicians also stress the need to improve the "eccentric control" of the muscles that decelerate pronation and other associated motions mechanically linked to pronation (see Table 14–5). These muscle groups include the supinators of the foot and the more proximal external rotators and abductors of the hip. This therapeutic approach strives to reduce the rate of pronation as well as the rate of loading on the foot.

The underlying pathomechanics of an excessively pronated foot are complex and not fully understood. The pathomechanics can involve many kinematic relationships, both within the joints of the foot or between the foot and the rest of the lower limb. Even if the pathomechanics are obviously located within the foot, abnormal motion in the forefoot can be compensated by abnormal motion in the rearfoot and vice versa. Furthermore, extrinsic factors, such as footwear, orthotics, terrain, and speed of walking or running, alter the kinematic relationships within the foot and lower extremity. An understanding of the complex kinesiology of the entire lower extremity is a definite prerequisite for the effective treatment of the painful or malaligned foot.

### Mid to Late Stance Phase: Supination at the Subtalar Joint

**Kinematic Mechanisms Related to Supination.** At about 15 to 20% into the gait cycle, the entire stance limb dramatically reverses its horizontal plane motion from inter-

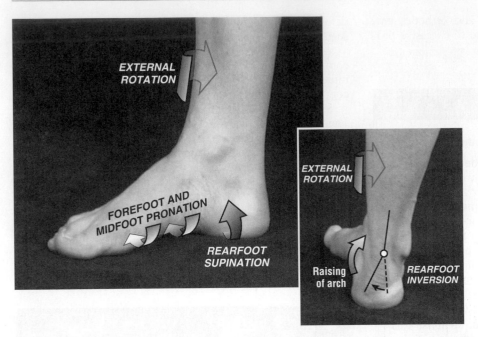

**FIGURE 14–31.** With the foot fixed, full external rotation of the lower limb causes the following associated movements: rearfoot supination (inversion) and raising of the medial longitudinal arch. Note that as the rearfoot supinates, the forefoot and midfoot pronate to maintain contact with the ground.

nal to external rotation.[17] External rotation of the leg, while the foot remains planted, coincides roughly with the beginning of the swing phase of the contralateral lower extremity. With the stance foot securely planted, external rotation of the femur, followed by the tibia, gradually reverses the direction of the talus from internal to external rotation. As a result, at about 35% into the gait cycle, the pronated (everted) subtalar joint starts to move toward supination (see Fig. 14–29B). As demonstrated in Figure 14–31, with the rearfoot supinating, the midfoot and forefoot must simultaneously twist into relative pronation in order for the foot to remain in full contact with the ground. By late stance, the fully supinated subtalar joint and elevated and tensed medial longitudinal arch convert the midfoot into a more rigid lever. Muscles such as the gastrocnemius and soleus use this stability to transfer forces from the Achilles tendon, through the midfoot, to the metatarsal heads during the push-off phase of walking or running.

A person who, for whatever reason, remains relatively pronated late into stance phase often has difficulty stabilizing the midfoot at a time when that is required. As a consequence, excessive activity may be needed from extrinsic and intrinsic muscles of the foot to reinforce the medial longitudinal arch. Over time, hyperactivity may lead to generalized muscle fatigue and painful syndromes, such as shin splints.

## DISTAL INTERTARSAL JOINTS

The distal intertarsal joints describe a collection of several joints or joint complexes (see Fig. 14–22 and the box). These joints are surrounded by a continuous capsule and synovial membrane. As a group, the distal intertarsal joints assist the transverse tarsal joint in the production of pronation and supination throughout the entire midfoot. Motions in these joints, however, are small. The primary function of these joints is to provide stability across the midfoot by formation of the transverse arch.

---

**Collection of Articulations within the Distal Intertarsal Joints Include**

- Cuneonavicular joints
- Cuboideonavicular joint
- Intercuneiform and cuneocuboid joint complex

---

### Basic Structure and Function

#### Cuneonavicular Joints

Three articulations are formed between the anterior side of the navicular and the posterior surfaces of the three cuneiform bones. Surrounding these articulations are plantar and dorsal ligaments. The slightly concave surface of each cuneiform fits into one of three slightly convex facets on the anterior side of the navicular. The large medial facet of the navicular accepts the large medial cuneiform. The major function of the cuneonavicular joints is to help transfer pronation and supination movements distally through the medial midfoot to the forefoot.

#### Cuboideonavicular Joint

A relatively small, fibrous cuboideonavicular joint is located between the lateral side of the navicular and proximal one-fifth of the medial side of the cuboid. This joint links the lateral and medial components of the transverse tarsal joint, thereby assisting in transferring pronation and supination movements across the more proximal regions of the midfoot. The cuboideonavicular joint is strengthened by dorsal, plantar, and interosseous ligaments.

#### Intercuneiform and Cuneocuboid Joint Complex

Three articulations are formed in this joint complex: two between the cuneiforms, and one between the lateral cuneiform and medial surface of the cuboid. Articular surfaces are essentially flat and aligned nearly parallel with the long axis of the metatarsals. The tarsal bones are held together by dorsal, plantar, and interosseous ligaments.

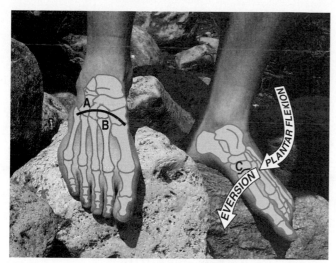

**FIGURE 14–32.** Structural and functional features of the midfoot and forefoot. *A,* The transverse arch is formed by the intercuneiform and cuneocuboid joint complex. *B,* The stable second ray is reinforced by the recessed second tarsometatarsal joint. *C,* Combined plantar flexion and eversion of the left tarsometatarsal joint of the first ray allow the forefoot to conform to the surface of the rock.

similar to the third ray in the hand (Fig. 14–32B). This stability is useful in late stance as the forefoot prepares for the dynamics of push off.

Mobility is greatest in the more peripheral tarsometatarsal joints, consisting primarily of dorsiflexion and plantar flexion, combined with inversion and eversion. At the first ray, dorsiflexion occurs naturally with inversion, and plantar flexion with eversion (Fig. 14–33A and B).[13] Note that these movement combinations are atypical in the ankle and foot because they do not fit the strict definition of pronation or supination. Nevertheless, movements at this joint provide useful functions, such as allowing the medial side of the foot to better conform around irregularities in the walking surface (Fig. 14–32C). The first tarsometatarsal joint provides an element of flexibility to the medial longitudinal arch. During the loading phase of walking, the first ray yields (dorsiflexes) slightly under the force of body-weight. Stiffness of the first ray limits the shock absorption ability of the medial longitudinal arch.[13]

The intercuneiform and cuneocuboid joint complex forms the *transverse arch* of the foot (Fig. 14–32A). This arch provides transverse stability to the midfoot. Under the load of body weight, the transverse arch depresses slightly, allowing body weight to be shared across all five metatarsal heads.[6] The arch receives dynamic support by intrinsic muscles; extrinsic muscles, such as the tibialis posterior and peroneus longus; connective tissues; and its keystone—the intermediate cuneiform.

## TARSOMETATARSAL JOINTS

### Anatomic Considerations

Five tarsometatarsal joints are formed by the articulation between the bases of the metatarsals and the distal surfaces of the three cuneiforms and cuboid (see Fig. 14–22). Specifically, the first metatarsal articulates with the medial cuneiform, the second with the intermediate cuneiform, and the third with the lateral cuneiform. The bases of the fourth and fifth metatarsal both articulate with the distal surface of the cuboid.

The articular surfaces of the tarsometatarsal joints are essentially flat. Dorsal, plantar, and interosseous ligaments add stability to these articulations. Of the five tarsometatarsal joints, only the first has a well-developed capsule.[55]

### Kinematic Considerations

The tarsometatarsal joints serve as base joints for each of the rays of the foot. Mobility is least at the second tarsometatarsal joint due, in part, to the wedged position of its base between the medial and lateral cuneiforms. Consequently, the second ray forms a stable central pillar through the foot,

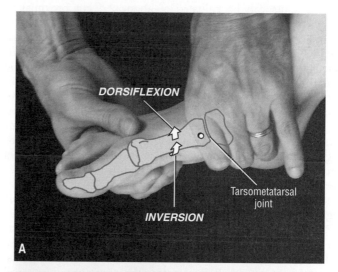

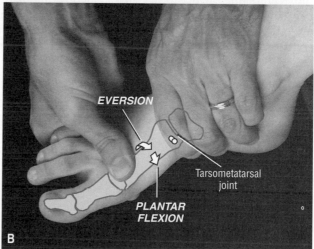

**FIGURE 14–33.** The osteokinematics of the first tarsometatarsal joint: Dorsiflexion and inversion (*A*) and plantar flexion and eversion (*B*).

## INTERMETATARSAL JOINTS

### *Structure and Function*

The bases of the four lateral metatarsals are interconnected by plantar, dorsal, and interosseous ligaments. Three small intermetatarsal synovial joints form at the points of contact between the bases of the second, third, and fourth metatarsals. Although interconnected by ligaments, a true joint does not typically form between the bases of the first and second metatarsals. This lack of articulation increases the relative movement of the first ray, in a manner similar to the hand.[55] Unlike the hand, however, the distal ends of all five metatarsals are interconnected by the deep transverse metatarsal ligaments. Slight motion at the intermetatarsal joints augments the flexibility at the tarsometatarsal joints.

## METATARSOPHALANGEAL JOINTS

### *Anatomic Considerations*

Five metatarsophalangeal joints are formed between the convex head of each metatarsal and the shallow concavity of the proximal end of each proximal phalanx (see Fig. 14–22). These joints can be palpated at about 2.5 cm proximal to the web of the toes.

*Articular cartilage* covers the distal end of each metatarsal head (Fig. 14–34). A pair of *collateral ligaments* spans each metatarsophalangeal joint, blending with and reinforcing the capsule. As in the hand, each collateral ligament courses obliquely from a dorsal-proximal to plantar-distal direction, forming a thick cord portion and a fanlike accessory portion.

The accessory portion attaches to the thick, dense *plantar plate*, located on the plantar side of the joint. The plate, or ligament, is grooved for the passage of flexor tendons. Fibers from the deep plantar fascia connect into the plantar plates and sheaths of the flexor tendons. Two *sesamoid bones* located within the tendon of the flexor hallucis brevis rest against the plantar plate of the first metatarsophalangeal joint (Fig. 14–35). Although not depicted in Figure 14–35, four deep *transverse metatarsal ligaments* blend with and join the adjacent plantar plates of all five metatarsophalangeal joints. By interconnecting all five plates, the transverse metatarsal ligaments help maintain the first ray in a similar plane as the lesser rays, thereby adapting the foot for propulsion and weight bearing rather than manipulation. In the hand, the

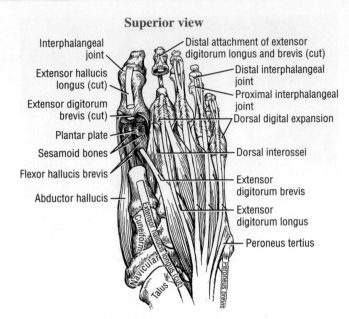

**Superior view**

FIGURE 14–35. Muscles and joints of the dorsal surface of the right forefoot. The distal half of the first metatarsal is removed to expose the concave surface of the first metatarsophalangeal joint. A pair of sesamoid bones is located deep within the first metatarsophalangeal joint. The proximal phalanx of the second toe is removed to expose the concave side of the proximal interphalangeal joint.

deep transverse metacarpal ligament connects only the fingers, freeing the thumb for opposition.

A *fibrous capsule* encloses each metatarsophalangeal joint and blends with the collateral ligaments and plantar plates. A poorly defined *extensor mechanism* covers the dorsal side of each metatarsophalangeal joint. This structure consists of a thin layer of connective tissue that is essentially inseparable from the dorsal capsule and extensor tendons.

### *Kinematic Considerations*

Movement at the metatarsophalangeal joints occurs in two degrees of freedom. *Extension* (dorsiflexion) and *flexion* (plantar flexion) occur approximately in the sagittal plane about a medial-lateral axis; *abduction* and *adduction* occur in the horizontal plane about a vertical axis. Both axes of rotation intersect at the center of each metatarsal head.

Most people demonstrate limited dexterity in movements at the metatarsophalangeal joints, especially in abduction and adduction. Passively, the toes can be hyperextended about 65 degrees and flexed about 30 to 40 degrees. The first toe typically allows greater hyperextension to near 85 degrees.

### *Deformities Involving the Metatarsophalangeal Joint of the First Toe*

**Hallux Rigidus and Hallux Valgus.** *Hallux rigidus,* or "limitus" in its less severe form, is a condition characterized by marked limitation of motion and by pain at the metatarsophalangeal joint of the first toe. Although the cause of the condition is not clear, degenerative changes frequently follow local trauma.[54] As the condition progresses, osteophytes formed on the dorsum of the metatarsal head may block hyperextension. The limitation of motion and the pain at

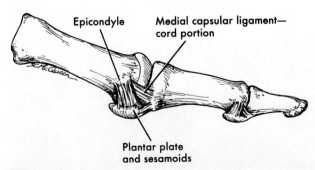

FIGURE 14–34. A medial view of the first metatarsophalangeal joint showing the cord and accessory portion of the medial (collateral) capsular ligaments. The accessory portion attaches to the plantar plate and sesamoid bones. (Redrawn from Haines R, McDougall A: Anatomy of hallux valgus. J Bone Joint Surg 36–B:272, 1954.)

this joint can have significant impact on walking. Normally, walking requires about 65 degrees of hyperextension at the metatarsophalangeal joints as the heel rises at late stance phase.[15] A person with hallux rigidus typically resorts to walking on the outer surface of the affected foot to avoid the necessity of hyperextending the first metatarsophalangeal joint at late stance. Those affected are advised to wear stiff soled shoes for walking and to avoid inclines or declines. Surgery is often recommended in more severe cases.[42]

The central feature of *hallux valgus* is a progressive lateral deviation of the first toe. Although the deformity appears to involve primarily the metatarsophalangeal joint, the pathomechanics of hallux valgus often involve the entire first ray (Fig. 14–36A and B). As depicted in the x-ray, hallux valgus is associated with *excessive adduction* of the first metatarsal about its tarsometatarsal joint. This is often referred to in the medical literature as "metatarsus primus varus."[11] The adducted position of the metatarsal bone eventually collapses the proximal phalanx into excessive abduction, thereby exposing the metatarsal head as a bunion. If the metatarsophalangeal joint assumes an abducted position in excess of 30 degrees, the proximal phalanx often begins to evert, or to rotate about its long axis.[42] The bunion deformity is also referred to as "hallux abducto-valgus" in order to account for the deviations in both horizontal and frontal planes.

The progressive axial rotation of the abducted proximal phalanx creates a muscular imbalance in the forces that normally align the metatarsophalangeal joint. The abductor hallucis muscle shifts toward the plantar aspect of the first metatarsophalangeal joint. The unopposed pull of the adductor hallucis and lateral head of the flexor hallucis brevis progressively increases the lateral deviation posture of the proximal phalanx. In time, the overstretched medial collateral ligament and capsule may weaken or rupture, removing an important source of reinforcement to the medial side of the joint.[26] Persons with marked hallux valgus often avoid

bearing weight over the first metatarsophalangeal joint, causing the lateral metatarsal bones to accept a greater proportion of the load. The pathomechanics of marked hallux valgus involve a zigzag-like collapse of the first ray, similar to the ulnar drift of the metacarpophalangeal joint in the rheumatoid hand (see Chapter 8).

Although the etiology of hallux valgus is not totally clear, genetics, incorrect footwear, pronated feet that cause valgus strain at the hallux, and asymmetry of the bones and joints all contribute to the condition. The full spectrum of severe hallux valgus is often associated with dislocation and osteoarthritis of the metatarsophalangeal joint, metatarsus varus (adductus), valgus of the first toe, bunion formation over the medial joint, hammer toe of the second digit, calluses, and metatarsalgia.[42] Surgical intervention is often indicated in cases of marked deformity and dysfunction.

## INTERPHALANGEAL JOINTS

As in the fingers, each toe has a *proximal interphalangeal* and a *distal interphalangeal joint*. The first toe, being analogous to the thumb, has only one *interphalangeal joint* (Fig. 14–22A).

All interphalangeal joints of the foot possess similar anatomic features. The joint consists of the convex head of the more proximal phalanx articulating with the concave base of the more distal phalanx. The proximal phalanx of the second toe is removed in Figure 14–35 to expose the concave side of the proximal interphalangeal joint. The structure and function of the connective tissues at the interphalangeal joints are generally similar to those described for the metatarsophalangeal joints. Collateral ligaments, plantar plates, and capsules are present, but smaller and less defined.

Mobility at the interphalangeal joints is limited primarily to flexion and extension. The amplitude of flexion generally exceeds extension, and motion tends to be greater at the proximal than the distal joints. Extension is limited primarily

**FIGURE 14–36.** Hallux valgus. *A,* Multiple features of hallux valgus and associated deformities. *B,* X-ray shows the pathomechanics often associated with hallux valgus: adduction of the first metatarsal evident by the increased angle between the first and second metatarsal bones; abduction of the proximal phalanx with subluxation of the metatarsophalangeal joint; displacement of the lateral sesamoid; rotation (eversion) of the phalanges; and exposed metatarsal head. (From Richardson EG: Disorders of the hallux. In Canale ST (ed): Campbell's Operative Orthopaedics, vol 4, 9th ed. St. Louis, Mosby-Year Book, 1998.)

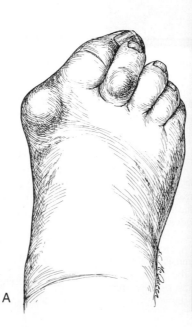

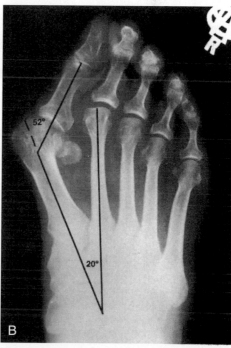

A

B

**Normal foot**

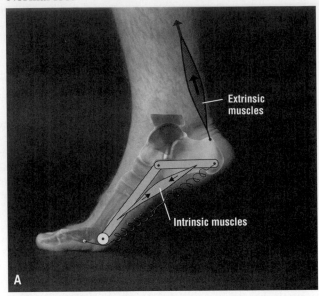

**Foot with pes planus**

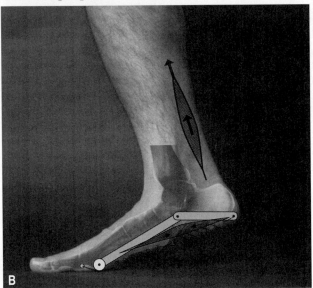

**FIGURE 14–37.** The "windlass effect" of the plantar fascia is demonstrated while standing on tiptoes. A windlass is a hauling or lifting device consisting of a rope wound around a cylinder that is turned by a crank. The rope is analogous to the plantar fascia, and the cylinder is analogous to the metatarsophalangeal joints. *A,* In the normal foot, contraction of the extrinsic plantar flexor muscles raises the calcaneus, thereby transferring body weight forward over the metatarsal heads. The resulting hyperextension of the metatarsophalangeal joints (shown collectively as the white disk) stretches (or winds up) the plantar fascia within the medial longitudinal arch (red spring). The increased tension from the stretch strengthens the midfoot and forefoot. Contraction of the intrinsic muscles provides additional reinforcement to the arch. *B,* The foot with pes planus (flat foot) typically has a poorly supported medial longitudinal arch. While attempting to stand up on tiptoes, the forefoot sags under the load of body weight. The reduced hyperextension of the metatarsophalangeal joints limits the usefulness of the windlass effect. Even with strong activation of the intrinsic muscles, the arch remains flattened and the midfoot and forefoot unstable.

by passive tension in the toe flexor muscles and plantar ligaments.

## ACTION OF THE JOINTS WITHIN THE FOREFOOT DURING THE LATE STANCE PHASE OF GAIT

The joints of the forefoot include all articulations associated with each ray, from the tarsometatarsal joint to the distal interphalangeal joints of the toe. Depending on the phase of gait, these joints provide an element of flexibility or stability to the forefoot.

During the later part of stance phase, the midfoot and forefoot must be relatively stable or rigid to accept the stresses that are associated with push off. In addition to activation of local intrinsic and extrinsic muscles, the foot is further stabilized by increased tension in the medial longitudinal arch. The increased tension occurs through a mechanism known as the "windlass effect," demonstrated by standing on tiptoes shown in Figure 14–37A. Because of the attachments of the plantar fascia on the proximal phalanges, hyperextension of the metatarsophalangeal joints increases the tension throughout the medial longitudinal arch. As the heel and most of the foot is raised, body weight shifts anteriorly toward the medial metatarsal heads, where fat pads and sesamoid bones and the rigidity of the second ray provide a suitable base of support for the action of the plantar flexor muscles.

In contrast to the healthy foot, consider the pathomechanics involved as a person with an unstable "flatfoot" (pes planus) attempts to rise up on tiptoes (Fig. 14–37B). Although the individual has no neuromuscular deficit, there is significant loss in the amount of lift of the heel, even upon maximal muscular effort. Without an effective medial longitudinal arch, the unstable, unlocked midfoot and forefoot sag under body weight. Consequently, the reduced hyperextension of the metatarsophalangeal joints limits the usefulness of the windlass effect for stretching the plantar fascia.

Table 14–6 summarizes the important functions of the ankle and foot during the stance phase of walking.

## MUSCLE AND JOINT INTERACTION

### Innervation of Muscles and Joints

#### INNERVATION OF MUSCLES

Extrinsic muscles of the ankle and foot have their proximal attachments in the leg, and a few extend as far proximal as the distal thigh. Intrinsic muscles, in contrast, have both proximal and distal attachments within the foot.

The extrinsic muscles are arranged in three compartments of the leg: anterior, lateral, and posterior. Each compartment is innervated by a different motor nerve. The anterior compartment is innervated by the deep branch of the peroneal nerve, the lateral compartment by the superficial branch of the peroneal nerve, and the posterior compartment by the tibial nerve. Each of these is a branch of the sciatic nerve, formed from the $L^4$-$S^3$ nerve roots of the sacral plexus.

Lateral to the head of the fibula, the common peroneal nerve ($L^4$-$S^2$) divides into a deep and superficial branch (Fig. 14–38). The *deep branch of the peroneal nerve* innervates the muscles within the anterior compartment: the tibialis ante-

**TABLE 14-6. Major Actions at Regions of the Ankle and Foot During the Stance Phase of Walking***

| Region | Representative Joint | Early Stance | | Mid to Late Stance | |
|---|---|---|---|---|---|
| | | *Action* | *Desired Function* | *Action* | *Desired Function* |
| Ankle | Talocrural | Plantar flexion | Allows rapid foot contact | Dorsiflexion followed by rapid plantar flexion | Produces a stable joint to accept body weight, followed by thrust needed for push off |
| Rearfoot | Subtalar | Pronation and lowering of the medial longitudinal arch | Permits internal rotation of lower limb<br>Allows the foot to function as a shock absorber<br>Produces a pliable midfoot | Continued pronation changing to supination, followed by a raising of the medial longitudinal arch | Permits external rotation of lower limb<br>Converts the midfoot to a rigid lever for push off |
| Midfoot | Transverse tarsal joint | Relative inversion as a response to counterforce from the ground | Allows full extent of subtalar joint pronation | Relative eversion | Allows the midfoot and forefoot to maintain firm contact with the ground |
| Forefoot | Metatarsophalangeal | Insignificant | — | Hyperextension | Increases tension in the plantar fascia<br>Through the windlass effect, raises the medial longitudinal arch and stabilizes the midfoot and forefoot for push off |

* Each region of the foot is represented by only one joint.

rior, extensor digitorum longus, extensor hallucis longus, and peroneus tertius. The deep branch continues distally to innervate the extensor digitorum brevis (i.e., an intrinsic muscle located on the dorsum of the foot). It also supplies sensory innervation to a triangular area of skin in the web space between the first and second toes. The *superficial branch of the peroneal nerve* innervates the peroneus longus and peroneus brevis within the lateral compartment. It then continues distally as a sensory nerve to much of the skin on the dorsal and lateral aspects of the leg and foot.

The *tibial nerve* ($L^4$-$S^3$) and its terminal branches innervate the remainder of the extrinsic and intrinsic muscle of the foot and ankle (Fig. 14-39). The muscles within the posterior compartment are divided into a superficial and deep set. The superficial set includes the calf muscles: the gastrocnemius and soleus, together known as the triceps surae, and the small plantaris. The deep set includes the tibialis posterior, flexor hallucis longus, and flexor digitorum longus. As the tibial nerve approaches the medial side of the ankle, it sends a sensory branch to the skin over the heel.

Just posterior to the medial malleolus, the tibial nerve bifurcates into the *medial plantar nerve* ($L^4$-$S^2$) and *lateral plantar nerve* ($L^4$-$S^3$). The plantar nerves supply sensation to the skin of most of the plantar side on the foot and motor innervation to all intrinsic muscles, except the extensor digitorum brevis. The organization of the innervation of the intrinsic muscles of the foot is similar to that in the hand. The medial plantar nerve is analogous to the median nerve, whereas the lateral plantar nerve is analogous to the ulnar

nerve. Tables 14-7 and 14-8 summarize the motor innervation of the extrinsic and intrinsic muscles of the ankle and foot.[23,55] As an additional reference, the motor nerve roots that supply all the muscles of the lower extremity are listed in Appendix IVA. Appendix IVB shows key muscles typically used to test the functional status of the $L^2$-$S^3$ ventral nerve roots.

## SENSORY INNERVATION TO THE JOINTS

The *talocrural joint* receives sensory innervation from the deep branch of the peroneal nerve. Detailed information on the sensory innervation to the more distal joints of the ankle however, is limited. In general, sensory innervation to the joints of the foot is supplied primarily through nerve branches that cross the region. Each major joint usually receives multiple sources of sensory innervation, traveling to the spinal cord primarily through $S^1$ and $S^2$ nerve roots.[18]

## Anatomy and Function of the Muscles

### EXTRINSIC MUSCLES

The primary functions of the muscles of the ankle and foot are to provide static control, dynamic thrust, and shock absorption to the distal lower extremity. These functions are performed by both intrinsic and extrinsic muscles. Additional discussion of the muscular interaction during the gait process follows in Chapter 15.

**Anterior view**

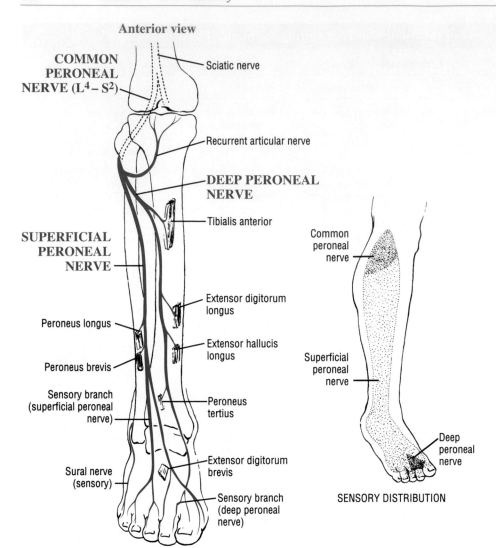

COMMON
PERONEAL
NERVE (L⁴ – S²)

Sciatic nerve

Recurrent articular nerve

**DEEP PERONEAL
NERVE**

Tibialis anterior

SUPERFICIAL
PERONEAL
NERVE

Peroneus longus

Extensor digitorum
longus

Extensor hallucis
longus

Peroneus brevis

Sensory branch
(superficial peroneal
nerve)

Peroneus
tertius

Sural nerve
(sensory)

Extensor digitorum
brevis

Sensory branch
(deep peroneal
nerve)

Common
peroneal
nerve

Superficial
peroneal
nerve

Deep
peroneal
nerve

SENSORY DISTRIBUTION

**FIGURE 14–38.** The path and general proximal-to-distal order of muscle innervation for the deep and superficial branches of the common peroneal nerve are illustrated. The primary nerve roots are in parentheses. (Modified with permission from de-Groot J: Correlative Neuroanatomy, 21st ed. Norwalk, Appleton & Lange, 1991.)

Because all the extrinsic muscles cross multiple joints, they possess multiple actions. Many actions can be appreciated by noting the point where the tendons cross the axes of rotation at the talocrural and subtalar joints (Fig. 14–40). Although Figure 14–40 is oversimplified (by lacking the transverse tarsal joint as well as other components of pronation and supination at the ankle and foot), it is useful for helping to understand the actions of the extrinsic muscles.

### Anterior Compartment Muscles

#### Muscular Anatomy

The four muscles of the anterior compartment are listed in the box. As a group, these pretibial muscles have their proximal attachments on the anterior and lateral aspects of the proximal half of the tibia, the adjacent fibula, and the interosseous membrane (Fig. 14–41). The tendons of these muscles cross the dorsal side of the ankle, restrained by a synovial-lined *superior* and *inferior extensor retinaculum*. Located most medially is the prominent tendon of the tibialis anterior that courses distally to the medial-plantar surface of the medial cuneiform. The tendon of the extensor hallucis longus passes just lateral to the tendon of the tibialis anterior, as it courses toward the dorsal surface of the first toe. Pro-

gressing laterally across the dorsum of the ankle are the tendons of the extensor digitorum longus and the peroneus tertius (or "third" peronei). The four tendons of the extensor digitorum longus attach to the dorsal surface of the middle and distal phalanges via the *dorsal digital expansion*. (This tissue is structurally analogous to the extensor mechanism in the fingers.) The peroneus tertius is part of the extensor digitorum longus muscle and may be considered as the toe-extensor's fifth tendon.[55] The peroneus tertius attaches to the base of the fifth metatarsal bone.

---

**Muscles of the Anterior Compartment of the Leg
(Pretibial "Dorsiflexors")**

*Muscles*
- Tibialis anterior
- Extensor digitorum longus
- Extensor hallucis longus
- Peroneus tertius

*Innervation*
- Deep portion of the peroneal nerve

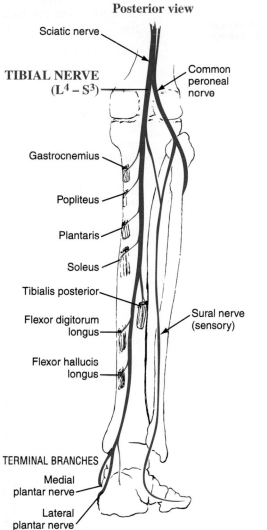

**Posterior view**

Sciatic nerve

**TIBIAL NERVE (L$^4$ – S$^3$)**

Common peroneal nerve

Gastrocnemius

Popliteus

Plantaris

Soleus

Tibialis posterior

Flexor digitorum longus

Flexor hallucis longus

Sural nerve (sensory)

TERMINAL BRANCHES

Medial plantar nerve

Lateral plantar nerve

Sural nerve

Tibial nerve

Lateral plantar nerve

Medial plantar nerve

**SENSORY DISTRIBUTION**

**FIGURE 14–39.** The path and general proximal-to-distal order of muscle innervation for the tibial nerve and its branches are shown. The primary nerve roots are in parentheses. (Modified with permission from deGroot J: *Correlative Neuroanatomy*, 21st ed. Norwalk, Appleton & Lange, 1991.)

**TABLE 14–7. Motor Innervation to the *Extrinsic* Muscles of the Ankle and Foot***

| Nerve | Muscles |
|---|---|
| Deep branch peroneal nerve | Tibialis anterior<br>Extensor digitorum longus<br>Peroneus tertius<br>Extensor hallucis longus |
| Superficial branch peroneal nerve | Peroneus longus and brevis |
| Tibial nerve | Plantaris<br>Tibialis posterior<br>Flexor digitorum longus<br>Flexor hallucis longus<br>Gastrocnemius and soleus |

* The muscles are listed in a general descending order of nerve root innervation.

**TABLE 14–8. Motor Innervation to the *Intrinsic* Muscles of the Foot***

| Nerve | Muscles |
|---|---|
| Deep branch of the peroneal nerve | Extensor digitorum brevis |
| Medial plantar nerve | Flexor digitorum brevis<br>Abductor hallucis<br>Flexor hallucis brevis<br>Lumbrical (second toe) |
| Lateral plantar nerve | Abductor digiti minimi<br>Quadratus plantae<br>Flexor digiti minimi<br>Adductor hallucis<br>Plantar interossei<br>Dorsal interossei<br>Lumbricals (third to fifth toes) |

* The muscles are listed in general descending order of nerve root innervation.

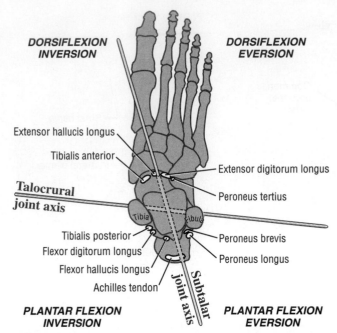

**FIGURE 14–40.** The multiple actions of muscles that cross the talocrural and subtalar joints, as viewed from above. The actions of each muscle are based on its position relative to the axes of rotation at the joints. Note that the muscles have multiple actions.

*Joint Action*

All four pretibial muscles are dorsiflexors because they cross anterior to the axis of rotation at the talocrural joint. The *tibialis anterior* also inverts the subtalar joint by passing just medial to the axis of rotation (see Fig. 14–40). The tibialis anterior inverts and adducts the talonavicular joint, as well as supports the medial longitudinal arch.

The primary actions of the *extensor hallucis longus* are dorsiflexion at the talocrural joint and extension of the first toe. Inversion at the subtalar joint is negligible due its small moment arm, at least when analyzed from the anatomic position. In addition to dorsiflexion of the ankle, the *extensor digitorum longus* and *peroneus tertius* evert the foot.

The pretibial muscles are most active during the early stance phase and again throughout the swing phase of gait (see Fig. 15–29, tibialis anterior). During early stance, the muscles are eccentrically active to control the rate of plantar flexion (i.e., the period between heel contact and foot-flat). Controlled plantar flexion is necessary for a soft landing of the foot. Through similar eccentric activation, the tibialis anterior decelerates the lowering of the medial longitudinal arch, including the pronation of the rearfoot. During the swing phase, the pretibial muscles actively dorsiflex the ankle and extend the toes to ensure that the entire foot clears the ground.

The ability to actively dorsiflex the entire foot in the near sagittal plane requires a rather exacting balance of forces from the pretibial muscles. The eversion and/or abduction influence of the extensor digitorum longus and peroneus tertius must counterbalance the inversion and adduction influence of the tibialis anterior. With isolated paralysis of the tibialis anterior muscle, although rare, the ankle can still be dorsiflexed, but the motion has a slight eversion-and-abduction bias.

### Lateral Compartment Muscles

*Muscular Anatomy*

The peroneus longus and the peroneus brevis muscles, often referred to as the evertors of the foot, occupy the lateral compartment of the leg muscles (Fig. 14–42). Both muscles attach proximally along the lateral fibula. The tendon of the peroneus longus, the more superficial of the two, courses distally a remarkable distance. After wrapping around the posterior side of the lateral malleolus, the tendon enters the plantar side of the foot through a groove in the cuboid bone. The tendon then travels between the long and short plantar ligaments to its final distal attachment on the plantar-lateral aspect of the first ray (Fig. 14–43).

**Anterior view**

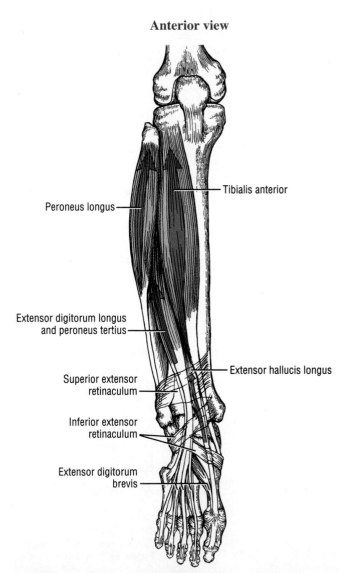

**FIGURE 14–41.** The pretibial muscles of the leg: tibialis anterior, extensor digitorum longus, extensor hallucis longus, and peroneus tertius. All four muscles dorsiflex the ankle.

**Lateral view**

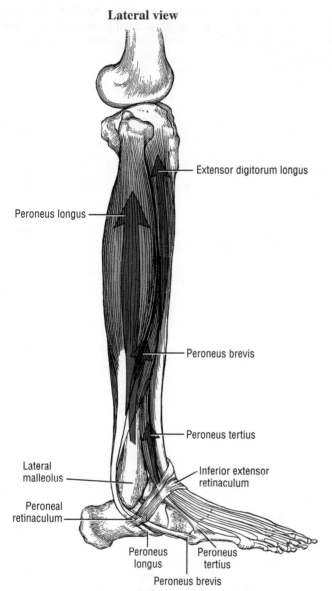

**FIGURE 14–42.** A lateral view of the muscles of the leg is shown. Note how both the peroneus longus and peroneus brevis (primary evertors) use the lateral malleolus as a pulley to change direction.

**Lateral Compartment of the Leg (the "Evertors")**

*Muscles*
- Peroneus longus
- Peroneus brevis

*Innervation*
- Superficial portion of the peroneal nerve

The tendon of the peroneus brevis muscle travels posterior to the lateral malleolus alongside the peroneus longus (see Fig. 14–15). Both peroneal tendons occupy the same synovial sheath as they pass under the *peroneal retinaculum*. It holds the tendons posterior to the lateral malleolus. The

**Plantar view**

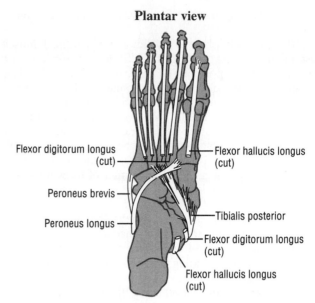

**FIGURE 14–43.** A plantar view of the right foot shows the distal course of the tendons of the peroneus longus, peroneus brevis, and tibialis posterior. The tendons of the flexor digitorum longus and flexor hallucis longus are cut.

tendon of the peroneus brevis separates from the peroneus longus tendon and courses toward its distal attachment on the styloid process of the fifth metatarsal.

*Joint Action*
The *peroneus longus* and *peroneus brevis* are the primary evertors of the joints of the foot (Fig. 14–40). Both muscles also plantar flex the talocrural joint. The lateral malleolus, serving as a fixed pulley, routes the peroneal tendons posterior to the axis of rotation at the talocrural joint. Although not evident in Figure 14–40, the peroneus longus and brevis also abduct the subtalar and transverse tarsal joints. The muscles provide stability to the lateral side of the talocrural joint. Strengthening exercises of the peroneal muscles are often advised for persons with histories of recurring inversion ankle sprains and injured lateral ligaments.

The distal attachment of the peroneus longus provides an ideal line-of-force for pronation of the forefoot. This is evident by the slight depression (plantar flexion) of the first ray during maximal-effort pronation of the unloaded foot. The peroneus longus also stabilizes the first tarsometatarsal joint against the medial pull of the tibialis anterior. Without this stability, the first ray would migrate medially, predisposing a person to a hallux valgus deformity.

The peroneus longus and brevis are most active throughout the mid to late stance phase,[50] when the subtalar joint is supinating and the dorsiflexed ankle joint is preparing to plantar flex. Activation of the peroneal muscles decelerates the rate and extent of supination at the subtalar joint. With the first ray fixed to the ground, the supinating rearfoot creates a relative pronated position at the midfoot and forefoot (see Fig. 14–31). With paralysis of the peroneus longus, the potent supination pull of the tibialis posterior is unopposed. As a result, the forefoot follows the rearfoot into supination, causing the person to walk on the lateral border of the foot.[22]

At the push-off phase of walking, the peroneal muscles assist other muscles with plantar flexion at the talocrural joint. The lateral position of the peroneal muscles helps neutralize the strong inversion (supination) bias of the remaining plantar flexors, including the tibialis posterior, the extrinsic toe flexors, and, to a limited degree, the gastrocnemius. Furthermore, as the heel is raised, contraction of the peroneal muscles, especially the peroneus longus, helps transfer body weight from the lateral to the medial side of the forefoot. This shifts the body's center-of-mass toward the opposite foot, which is entering the early stance phase of gait.

The eversion force of the peroneus longus stabilizes the foot by counteracting the potent medial pull of the many invertor-plantar flexor muscles. This is especially evident as the heel rises when standing on tiptoes (Figure 14–44). The strongly activated peroneus longus and tibialis posterior muscles neutralize one another as they form a functional "sling" that supports the transverse and medial longitudinal arches. The net effect of this muscle action slightly supinates the unloaded rearfoot, which provides further stability to the foot. This stability is necessary so that the plantar flexion torque required to stand on tiptoes can be effectively transferred forward over the metatarsal heads.

### Posterior Compartment Muscles

#### Anatomy

The muscles of the posterior compartment are divided into two groups. The superficial calf group includes the gastrocnemius, soleus (together known as triceps surae), and plantaris (Fig. 14–45A and B). The deep group includes the tibialis posterior, flexor digitorum longus, and flexor hallucis longus (Fig. 14–46).

---

**Muscles of the Posterior Compartment of the Leg**

*Superficial group* ("plantar flexors")
- Gastrocnemius
- Soleus
- Plantaris

*Deep group* ("invertors")
- Tibialis posterior
- Flexor digitorum longus
- Flexor hallucis longus

*Innervation*
- Tibial nerve

---

**Superficial Group.** The *gastrocnemius muscle* forms the prominent belly of the calf. This two-headed muscle attaches by separate heads from the posterior side of the medial and lateral femoral condyles. The larger medial head joins the lateral head midway down the leg to form a tendinous expansion that, after insertion of the tendon from the soleus muscle, forms the Achilles tendon. The broad flat *soleus muscle* lies deep to the gastrocnemius, arising primarily from the posterior side of the proximal fibula and middle tibia. The soleus blends with the Achilles tendon for its distal attachment to the calcaneal tuberosity. The gastrocnemius crosses the knee but the soleus does not. The functional significance of this anatomic arrangement is discussed later in the section. The *plantaris muscle* arises from the lateral supracondylar line of the femur. The fusiform muscle belly is only 7 to 10 cm long,[55] unusually small especially when compared with the surrounding muscles. The plantaris has a very long, slender tendon that courses between the gastrocnemius and soleus, eventually fusing with the medial margin of the Achilles tendon.

**Deep Group.** The tibialis posterior, flexor hallucis longus, and flexor digitorum longus muscles are located beneath the soleus muscle (see Fig. 14–46). As a group, these muscles arise from the posterior side of the tibia, fibula, and interosseous membrane. The more centrally located tibialis posterior muscle is framed and partially covered by the flexor hallucis longus laterally and the flexor digitorum longus medially. At their musculotendinous junctions, all three muscles with the juxtaposed tibial nerve and artery enter the plantar aspect of the foot from its medial side (see Fig. 14–43). The position of the tendons as they cross the ankle and foot explains the strong supination (inversion) component of

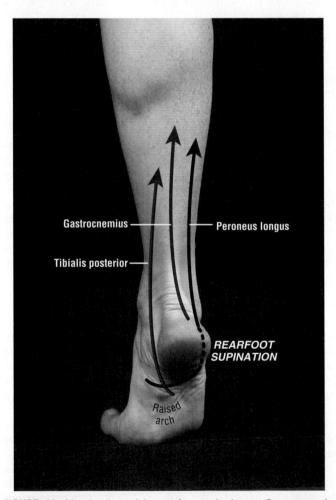

**FIGURE 14–44.** *The line-of-force of several plantar flexor muscles while rising on tiptoes. Note that the peroneus longus (black) and tibialis posterior (red) form a sling that supports the transverse and medial longitudinal arches. The pull of the gastrocnemius and tibialis posterior muscles causes a slight supination of the rearfoot, which adds further stability to the foot.*

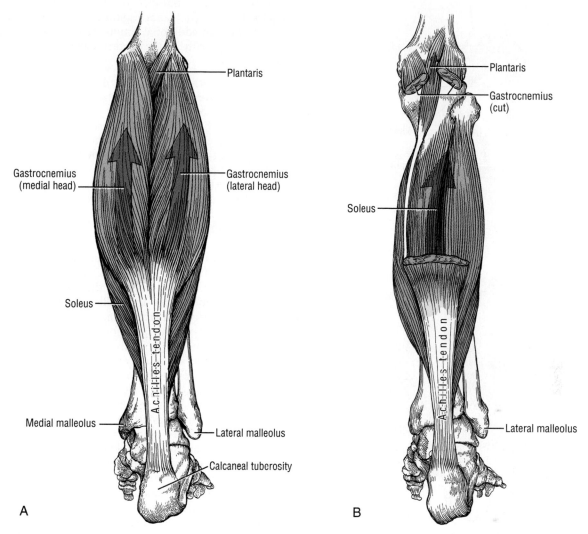

**FIGURE 14-45.** The superficial muscles of the posterior compartment of the right leg are shown: *A,* the gastrocnemius; *B,* the soleus and plantaris.

these muscles (see Fig. 14-40). The tibialis posterior, flexor digitorum longus, and aforementioned neurovascular bundle course through the tarsal tunnel, located just deep to the flexor retinaculum (Fig. 14-47). The tarsal tunnel is analogous to the carpal tunnel in the wrist. "Tarsal tunnel syndrome" (analogous to carpal tunnel syndrome) is characterized by entrapment of the tibial nerve beneath the flexor retinaculum and subsequent paresthesia over the plantar aspect of the foot.[43]

The tendon of the *flexor hallucis longus* courses distally through the ankle in a groove formed between the tubercles of the talus and the inferior edge of the sustentaculum talus (see Fig. 14-11). Fibrous bands convert this groove into a synovial-lined canal, anchoring the position of the tendon.[55] The somewhat deep (lateral) position of the tendon relative to the tibialis posterior and flexor digitorum longus explains why the flexor hallucis longus is not considered as a structure within the tarsal tunnel. Once in the plantar aspect of the foot, the tendon of the flexor hallucis longus courses between the two sesamoid bones of the first metatarsopha-

langeal joint, finally attaching to the plantar side of the base of the distal phalanx of the first toe (see Fig. 14-43).

The tendon of the *flexor digitorum longus* courses distally across the ankle posterior to the medial malleolus. At about the level of the base of the metatarsals, the main tendon of the flexor digitorum longus divides into four smaller tendons, each attaching to the base of the distal phalanx of the lesser toes (see Fig. 14-43).

The tendon of the *tibialis posterior muscle* lies just anterior to the tendon of the flexor digitorum longus in a shared groove on the posterior side of the medial malleolus (see Fig. 14-47). Once in the plantar aspect of the foot, the tendon of the tibialis posterior passes deep to the flexor retinaculum and superficial to the deltoid ligament. At this point, the tendon divides into superficial and deep parts, establishing attachments to every tarsal bone, except the talus, and to the bases of the several of the more central metatarsals (see Fig. 14-43). The extensive attachments support the medial longitudinal arch. A ruptured tendon may cause a collapse of the medial longitudinal arch and a drop

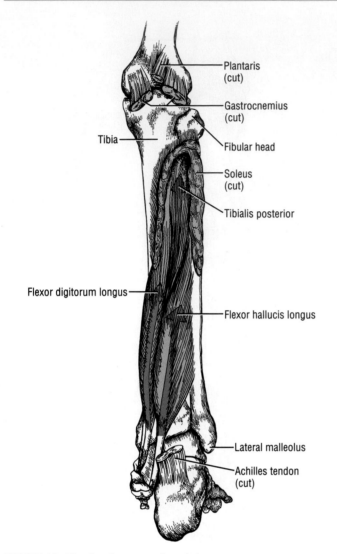

**FIGURE 14–46.** The deep muscles of the posterior compartment of the right leg: the tibialis posterior, flexor digitorum longus, and flexor hallucis longus.

in the height of the talus.[25,37] The most prominent, and readily palpable, distal attachment of the tibialis posterior is to the navicular tuberosity.

The tendons of both the tibialis posterior and the flexor digitorum longus use the medial malleolus as a fixed pulley to direct their force posterior to the axis of rotation at the talocrural joint. An analogous pulley is described for the peroneal tendons, as they pass posterior to the lateral malleolus (see Fig. 14–42). Tendons of the tibialis posterior and flexor digitorum longus are held posterior to the medial malleolus by the flexor retinaculum. Interestingly, the flexor hallucis longus uses a different plantar flexion pulley, formed by the medial and lateral tubercles of the talus and the sustentaculum talus.

*Joint Action: Plantar Flexion and Supination*
With the exception of the peroneus longus and brevis, all muscles that plantar flex the talocrural joint also supinate the subtalar or transverse tarsal joints. This strong inversion bias can be appreciated by noting the position of the poste-

rior compartment muscles relative to the subtalar joint in Figure 14–40. The flexor digitorum longus and flexor hallucis longus have additional actions at the more distal joints of the foot, especially at the metatarsophalangeal and interphalangeal joints.

**Active Plantar Flexion Used to Decelerate or Control Ankle Dorsiflexion.** The plantar flexor muscles are active throughout most of the stance phase of gait, particularly between foot-flat and toe-off phases (Fig. 15–29, gastrocnemius and soleus muscles). Normally, these muscles become active immediately after the dorsiflexor muscles relax. From foot-flat to just prior to about heel off, the plantar flexors act eccentrically to decelerate the forward rotation (dorsiflexion) of the leg over the fixed talus. Between the heel-off and toe-off phase, however, the muscle switches to a concentric activation to provide the thrust needed for push off.

**Active Plantar Flexion Used to Accelerate Ankle Plantar Flexion.** In healthy persons, maximal isometric plantar flexion torque exceeds the maximal torque of all other movements about the ankle and foot combined (Fig. 14–49).[47] A large plantar flexion torque reserve is needed to accelerate the body up and forward during brisk walking, running, jumping, and climbing. Plantar flexion torque is greatest with the ankle fully dorsiflexed (i.e., plantar flexor muscles elongated), and least with the ankle fully plantar flexed.[35] The fully dorsiflexed ankle is typically assumed as one prepares to sprint or jump. Interestingly, as the ankle vigorously plantar flexes at the "take off" of a sprint or jump, the contracting gastrocnemius is simultaneously elongated by the action of the extending knee. This biarticular arrangement prevents the gastrocnemius from overshortening, allowing greater torques throughout a larger range of ankle motion.[17] Because the soleus muscle does not cross the knee, its length-tension relationship is unaffected by the position of the knee. On the one hand, the slow-twitch soleus is more suited to control the relatively slow-changing postural movements of the leg over the talus during standing. The fast-twitch gastrocnemius, on the other hand, is apparently better suited for providing a propulsive plantar flexion torque for activities that also involve dynamic knee extension, such as jumping and sprinting.

Of all the plantar flexor muscles, the gastrocnemius and soleus are by far the most powerful, theoretically capable of producing about 80% of the total plantar flexion torque at the ankle.[32] The large torque potential of the triceps surae is due, in part, to the muscles' large cross-sectional area and relatively long moment arm (Table 14–9). The protruding calcaneal tuberosity provides the triceps surae with a moment arm of about 4.8 cm from the talocrural joint, roughly twice the average moment arm of the other plantar flexor muscles.

**Supination Potential of the Plantar Flexor Muscles.** The tibialis posterior, flexor hallucis longus, and flexor digitorum longus are the primary supinators of the foot. The tibialis posterior likely produces the greatest supination torque across the subtalar joint. The extensive distal attachments of the muscle, especially to the navicular bone, provide an effective supination twist of the midfoot (see Fig. 14–24D). As depicted in Figure 14–40, the triceps surae passes slightly medial to the subtalar joint's

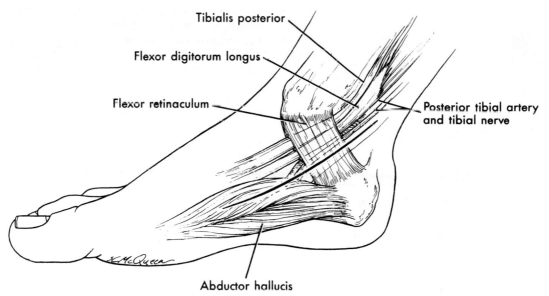

Tibialis posterior

Flexor digitorum longus

Flexor retinaculum

Posterior tibial artery and tibial nerve

Abductor hallucis

**FIGURE 14–47.** A medial view of the flexor retinaculum that covers the tendons of the tibialis posterior, flexor digitorum longus, and posterior tibial neurovascular bundle. (From Richardson EG: Neurogenic disorders. In Canale ST (ed): Campbell's Operative Orthopaedics, vol 4, 9th ed. St. Louis, Mosby-Year Book, 1998.)

---

**S P E C I A L   F O C U S   1 4 – 7**

### Plantar Flexor Muscles Acting as Extensors of the Knee

An important function of the plantar flexor muscles is to stabilize the knee in extension.[33] The importance of this function becomes evident when observing the gait of a person with weakened plantar flexor muscles. Without the muscle's necessary braking or decelerating action at the ankle, the lower leg advances via ankle dorsiflexion too rapidly and too far during the mid to late stance phase of gait. As shown with a weakened soleus while standing (Figure 14–48A), a forwardly rotated leg shifts the force of body weight posterior to the medial-lateral axis of rotation at the knee. This shift can create a sudden and often unexpected knee flexion torque. The dorsiflexed ankle, in this case, produces a flexion torque at the knee.

An important function of the soleus muscle is to resist excessive forward rotation of the leg, thereby maintaining body weight over or just anterior to the knee's medial-lateral axis of rotation. With the foot fixed to the ground, active plantar flexion at the ankle can extend the knee (Fig. 14–48B).[50] The soleus muscle is particularly well suited to stabilize the knee in extension. As a predominately slow-twitch muscle, the soleus can produce relatively low forces over a relatively long duration before fatiguing. Marked spasticity in the soleus muscle exerts a potent and chronic knee extension bias that, over time, contributes to genu recurvatum deformity.

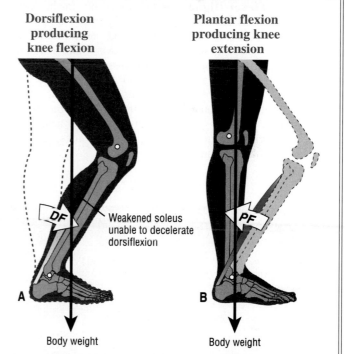

**Dorsiflexion producing knee flexion**

**Plantar flexion producing knee extension**

DF

Weakened soleus unable to decelerate dorsiflexion

PF

A

B

Body weight

Body weight

**FIGURE 14–48.** Two examples of how the ankle affects the position and stability of the knee while standing. *A*, Weakened soleus muscle is unable to decelerate ankle dorsiflexion (DF). With the foot fixed to the ground, ankle dorsiflexion occurs as a forward rotation of the leg over the talus. The forward position of the leg shifts the force of body weight posterior to the knee, causing it to "buckle" into flexion. *B*, A normal strength soleus muscle causes the ankle to plantar flex (PF). With the foot fixed to the ground, plantar flexion rotates the leg posteriorly, bringing the knee toward extension.

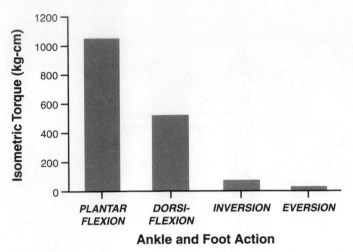

**Ankle and Foot Action**

**FIGURE 14–49.** The magnitude of maximal-effort isometric torque is shown for four actions of the ankle and foot. (N = 86 healthy men and women.) (Data from Sepic SB, Murray MP, Mollinger LA, et al: Strength and range of motion in the ankle in two age groups of men and women. Am J Phys Med 65: 75–84, 1986.)

axis of rotation, thereby providing this muscle with a potential to invert the rearfoot.

**Function of the Tibialis Posterior, Flexor Hallucis Longus, and Flexor Digitorum Longus.** The tibialis posterior, flexor hallucis longus, and flexor digitorum longus assist with the plantar flexion mechanics at the ankle during the late stance phase of walking. The flexor hallucis longus and flexor digitorum longus muscles are also flexors of the distal joints of the toes. During mid and especially late stance phase, active force in these muscles and in the lumbricals and interossei pulls the plantar surface of the hyperextending toes firmly against the ground. This action expands the weight-bearing surfaces of the toes, thereby minimizing contact pressures.[55]

The tibialis posterior, flexor hallucis longus, and flexor digitorum longus muscles also exert control of pronation and supination movements while walking. The tibialis posterior muscle is active during the stance phase longer than any other supinator muscle, from just before foot-flat to heel-off phase.[50] As the entire foot contacts the ground, the tibialis posterior decelerates the pronating rearfoot and, if needed, assists in a controlled lowering of the medial longitudinal arch. Through this eccentric action, the tibialis posterior absorbs some of the impact of loading. Persons who excessively and/or rapidly pronate during the stance phase may place excessive braking demands on the tibialis posterior, possibly explaining their complaints of muscle soreness in the lower medial leg.[53]

Throughout the mid to late stance, the tibialis posterior, flexor hallucis longus, and flexor digitorum longus help guide the rearfoot toward supination as the lower leg external rotates. During this time, the tibialis posterior, in particular, continues to support the medial longitudinal arch.

## MUSCULAR PARALYSIS FROM INJURY TO THE PERONEAL OR TIBIAL NERVES

### Injury to the Common Peroneal Nerve and Its Branches

The *common branch* of the peroneal nerve is located superficially as it winds around the lateral neck of the fibula, just deep to the peroneus longus. This nerve is injured frequently from lacerations or trauma that involves a fractured fibula. Injury to the *deep branch* of the peroneal nerve can result in paralysis of all the dorsiflexor (pretibial) muscles (see Fig. 14–38). With paralysis of the dorsiflexor muscles, the foot rapidly and uncontrollably plantar flexes following floor contact. During the swing phase, the hip and knee must excessively flex to ensure that the toes clear the ground.

Paralysis of the dorsiflexor muscles dramatically increases the likelihood of developing a fixed plantar flexion contracture at the talocrural joint. This deformity is called a *dropfoot* or *pes equinus*. In a surprisingly short period of time, a

**TABLE 14–9. A Comparison of the Maximal Plantar Flexion Torque Potential of Muscles at the Talocrural Joint**

| Muscle | Estimated Maximal Force Potential (kg) | Internal Moment Arm (cm) | Torque Potential* (kg-cm) |
| --- | --- | --- | --- |
| Gastrocnemius | 89.7 | 4.8 | 430.6 |
| Soleus | 78.0 | 4.8 | 374.4 |
| Tibialis posterior | 22.6 | 2.3 | 52.0 |
| Peroneus longus | 16.8 | 2.6 | 43.7 |
| Flexor hallucis longus | 17.6 | 2.3 | 40.5 |
| Peroneus brevis | 14.8 | 2.6 | 38.5 |
| Flexor digitorum longus | 10.9 | 2.3 | 25.1 |
| Total | 250.4 | — | 1004.8 |

Conversion: .098 N-m/kg-cm

* Torque potential is based on the muscles' estimated maximal force potential (physiologic cross-sectional area) and moment arm length.

## SPECIAL FOCUS 14–8

### Biomechanics of Raising up on Tiptoes

The functional strength of the plantar flexor muscles is often evaluated by requiring a subject to repeatedly stand on tiptoes. As shown in Figure 14–50, maximally raising the body requires an interaction of two concurrent torques, one at the talocrural joint and one at the metatarsophalangeal joints. The plantar flexor muscles, represented by the gastrocnemius, plantar flex the *talocrural joint* by rotating the calcaneus and talus within the mortise. The primary torque used to raise the body, however, is produced by extension across the *metatarsophalangeal joints.* Acting about these axes, the gastrocnemius has an internal moment arm that greatly exceeds the external moment arm owing to body weight (compare *B* and *C* in Fig. 14–50). Such a large mechanical advantage is rare in the musculoskeletal system. Acting as a second-class lever with the pivot point at the metatarsophalangeal joints, the gastrocnemius lifts the body using mechanics similar to those of a person lifting a large load with a wheelbarrow. If, for instance, the gastrocnemius functions with a mechanical advantage of 3:1 (i.e., ratio of the internal moment arm, or *B/C* in the Figure), the muscle needs to produce a lifting force of only one third, or 33%, of body weight to support the plantar flexed position. Rarely in the body does a muscle produce a force less than the load it is supporting. As a mechanical trade-off, however, the gastrocnemius, in theory, needs to shorten a distance three times greater than the vertical displacement of the body's center of mass (see Chapter 1). Maximal contraction of the gastrocnemius would produce a vertical displacement of the body only one-third the length of the muscle contraction. Nevertheless, the nature of this trade-off allows one to stand up on tiptoes with relative ease.

Figure 14–50 shows the importance of ample hyperextension range of motion at the metatarsophalangeal joints. Not only do the plantar flexion muscles use these joints to augment their internal moment arm, but, as described earlier, hyperextension of these joints pulls the plantar fascia taut via the windlass effect. This action helps the intrinsic muscles support the medial longitudinal arch and maintain a rigid forefoot, thereby allowing the foot to accept the load imposed by body weight.

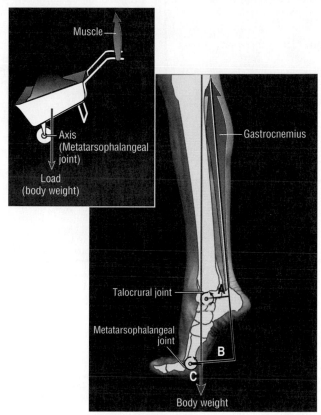

**FIGURE  14–50.** A mechanical model shows the biomechanics of standing on tiptoes. The force of a contracting gastrocnemius muscle acts with a relatively short internal moment arm from the talocrural joint (A), and a relatively long internal moment arm from the metatarsophalangeal joints (B). Once on tiptoes, the line-of-gravity due to body weight falls just posterior to the axis of rotation at the metatarsophalangeal joints. As a result, body weight acts with a relatively small external moment arm (C) from the metatarsophalangeal joints.

---

plantar flexed posture may lead to an adaptive shortening and tightening of the Achilles tendon. The relentless pull of gravity often contributes to a plantar-flexed posture, often requiring an orthosis to maintain adequate dorsiflexion while walking.

An injury to the *superficial branch* of the peroneal nerve may result in paralysis of the peroneus longus and peroneus brevis (see Fig. 14–38). Over time, paralysis may lead to a fixed supinated or inverted posture of the foot, a condition called *pes varus.* An injury to the common peroneal nerve may involve both deep and superficial nerve branches. The resulting paralysis of the dorsiflexor and peroneal muscles predisposes a person to a fixed deformity of combined plantar flexion of the talocrural joint and supination of the foot, a condition referred to as *pes equinovarus.*

### Injury to the Tibial Nerve

Injury to the tibial nerve may cause varying levels of weakness or paralysis in the muscles of the posterior compartment (see Fig. 14–39). Paralysis of the gastrocnemius and soleus results in profound diminution in plantar flexion torque. Over time, a fixed dorsiflexion posture may result at

**TABLE 14–10. Common Fixed Deformities or Abnormal Postures of the Ankle and Foot from Muscle Paralysis***

| Fixed Deformity or Abnormal Posture | Common Clinical Name | Muscle Paralysis and Associated Nerve Injury | Examples of Subsequent Musculotendinous Shortening |
|---|---|---|---|
| Plantar flexion of the talocrural joint | Drop-foot or pes equinus | Paralysis of pretibial muscles from injury to the *deep* branch of peroneal nerve | Gastrocnemius, soleus |
| Inversion (supination) of the foot | Pes varus | Paralysis of the peroneus longus and brevis from injury to the *superficial* branch of the peroneal nerve | Tibialis posterior |
| Plantar flexion of the talocrural joint and supination of the foot | Pes equinovarus | Paralysis of the dorsiflexor and peroneal muscles from injury to the *common* peroneal nerve | Gastrocnemius, soleus and tibialis posterior |
| Dorsiflexion of the talocrural joint | Pes calcaneus | Paralysis of the plantar flexor muscles from injury to the *tibial* nerve | Pretibial muscles |
| Eversion (pronation) of the foot | Pes valgus | Paralysis of the supinator muscles from injury to the *tibial* nerve | Peroneal muscles |
| Dorsiflexion of the talocrural joint and eversion of the foot | Pes calcaneovalgus | Paralysis of all the muscles in the posterior compartment of the leg from a severance of the tibial nerve just proximal to the popliteal fossa | Pretibial and peroneal muscles |

* The "foot" refers to the subtalar and transverse tarsal joints.

the talocrural joint, a condition known as *pes calcaneus*. The name calcaneus reflects the prominent heel pad that forms as a response to the heel of the dorsiflexed foot repeatedly striking the ground.

Paralysis involving primarily the supinator muscles may result in a fixed pronated deformity of the foot, primarily the result of the unopposed pull of the peroneus longus and brevis. The term *pes valgus* describes both eversion and abduction components of the pronation deformity. Paralysis involving all the muscles of the posterior compartment increases the potential for a fixed deformity called *pes calcaneovalgus*.

The common fixed deformities or abnormal postures of the ankle and foot are summarized in Table 14–10.

## INTRINSIC MUSCLES

### *Anatomic and Functional Considerations*

Intrinsic muscles are those that originate and insert within the foot. The following discussion highlights the primary attachments and actions of the intrinsic muscles. More detailed material is presented in Appendix IVC.

The dorsum of the foot has one intrinsic muscle, the extensor digitorum brevis, which is innervated by the deep branch of the peroneal nerve (see Figs. 14–35 and 14–41). The *extensor digitorum brevis* originates on the dorsal-lateral surface of the calcaneus, just proximal to the calcaneocuboid articulation. The muscle belly sends four tendons: one to the dorsal surface of the first toe, often designated as the exten-

sor hallucis brevis, and three that join the tendons of the extensor digitorum longus of the second through the fourth toes.[55] The extensor digitorum brevis assists the extensor hallucis longus and extensor digitorum longus muscles in extension of the toes.

The remaining intrinsic muscles of the foot originate and insert within the plantar aspect of the foot. Anatomically these muscles are organized in a fashion similar to the intrinsic muscles of the hand. One major difference, however, is that the foot does not contain muscles that oppose the first and fifth digits. The intrinsic muscles of the plantar aspect of the foot can be organized into four layers (Fig. 14–51A to C). The plantar fascia is located just superficial to the first layer of muscles.

### Layer 1

The intrinsic muscles in the first layer are the flexor digitorum brevis, abductor hallucis, and abductor digiti minimi (Fig. 14–51A). As a group, they originate on the lateral and medial processes of the calcaneal tuberosity and nearby connective tissues. The *flexor digitorum brevis* attaches distally to both sides of the middle phalanges of the four lesser toes. Proximal to this distal attachment, each tendon divides to allow passage of the tendons of the flexor digitorum longus. Note the similar relationship between the flexor digitorum superficialis and profundus of the hand. The flexor digitorum brevis assists the flexor digitorum longus in flexing the toes. The *abductor hallucis* forms the medial border of the foot, providing a covered passage for the plantar nerves that enter the plantar aspect of the foot. The abductor muscle

**Intrinsic muscles of the foot**

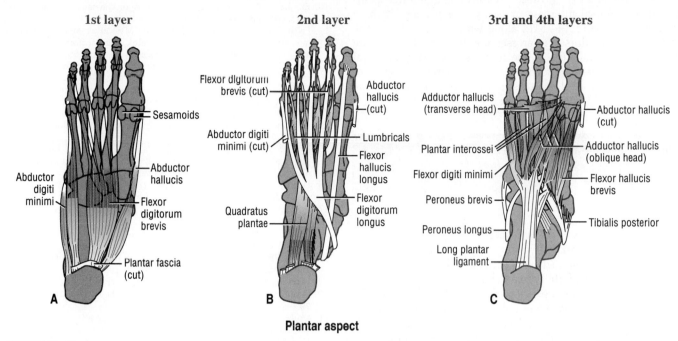

**Plantar aspect**

**FIGURE 14–51.** The intrinsic muscles of the plantar aspect of the foot are organized into four layers.

attaches distally to the medial border of the proximal phalanx of the first toe, together with the medial head of the flexor hallucis brevis (Fig. 14–51*C*). The *abductor digiti minimi* forms the lateral-plantar margin of the foot, attaching distally to the lateral border of the base of the proximal phalanx of the fifth toe. Each muscle abducts and flexes its respective digit.

> **Intrinsic Muscles of the Foot, Layer 1**
> • Flexor digitorum brevis
> • Abductor hallucis
> • Abductor digiti minimi

**Layer 2**

The intrinsic muscles in the second layer are the quadratus plantae and the lumbricals (Fig. 14–51*B*). Both muscles are functionally related to the tendons of the flexor digitorum longus. The *quadratus plantae* (flexor digitorum accessorius) attaches by two heads to the plantar aspect of the calcaneus. Both heads attach distally on the lateral edge of the common tendon of the flexor digitorum longus. The quadratus plantae helps to stabilize the tendons of the flexor digitorum longus, preventing them from migrating medially when under force. The four *lumbricals* have their proximal attachment from the tendons of the flexor digitorum longus. These small fleshy muscles pass on the medial side of the lesser toes to attach into the extensor digital expansion. They can flex the metatarsophalangeal joint and extend the interphalangeal joints.

> **Intrinsic Muscles of the Foot, Layer 2**
> • Quadratus plantae
> • Lumbricals

**Layer 3**

The intrinsic muscles in the third layer are the adductor hallucis, flexor hallucis brevis, and flexor digiti minimi (Fig. 14–51*C*). As a whole, these short muscles arise from the plantar aspect of the cuboid, cuneiforms, and bases of more central metatarsal bones, and from the local connective tissues. As in the hand, the *adductor hallucis* arises from two heads: oblique and transverse. Both heads attach to the lateral base of the proximal phalanx of the first toe and adjacent lateral sesamoid bone. The muscle flexes and adducts the metatarsophalangeal joint of the first toe. The *flexor hallucis brevis* has two heads that attach distally to the medial and lateral sides of the base of the proximal phalanx of the first toe. Medial and lateral sesamoid bones are located within the two tendons of this muscle, providing padding to the head of the first metatarsal. The *flexor digiti minimi* attaches to the lateral base of the proximal phalanx of the fifth toe, together with the abductor digiti minimi. Both muscles flex the metatarsophalangeal joint of their respective toes.

> **Intrinsic Muscles of the Foot, Layer 3**
> • Adductor hallucis
> • Flexor hallucis brevis
> • Flexor digiti minimi

## Layer 4

The fourth layer of intrinsic muscles contains three plantar and four dorsal interossei muscles. The *plantar interossei* are shown in Figure 14–51C, along with the muscles of the third layer. The dorsal interossei are illustrated in Figure 14–35. The overall plan of the interossei is nearly identical to that of the hand, except that the "reference digit" for abduction/adduction of the toes is the second, instead of the third.

---

**Intrinsic Muscles of the Foot, Layer 4**
- Plantar interossei (3)
- Dorsal interossei (4)

---

The *dorsal interossei* are two-headed, bipennate muscles. The second digit contains two dorsal interossei, whereas the third and fourth digit each contain one. All dorsal interossei insert on the base of the proximal phalanges; the first and second interossei insert on the medial and lateral side of the second digit, respectively, and the third and fourth dorsal interossei insert on the lateral side of the third and fourth digit (see Fig. 14–4). Each dorsal interosseus muscle abducts the metatarsophalangeal joint. The third, fourth, and fifth digit each contain a *plantar interosseus muscle*. Each muscle consists of one head and inserts on the medial side of the base of the corresponding proximal phalanx (see Fig. 14–5). These muscles adduct their respective metatarsophalangeal joint.

The actions assigned to each of the intrinsic muscles in the previous section are based on the assumption that the foot is unloaded and the toes are free to move. Although these unique actions allow the clinician to test the strength and dexterity of these muscles, the actions are not very relevant functionally. The intrinsic muscles of the foot are used less for manual dexterity, such as in the hand, and more for providing balance and, most notably, adding rigidity to the foot and stabilizing the medial longitudinal arch during push-off phase. This latter function explains why the intrinsic muscles are maximally active during late stance, just as the heel is rising off the floor (see Fig. 15–29).

## REFERENCES

1. Allinger TL, Ensberg JR: A method to determine the range of motion of the ankle complex: In vivo. J Biomechan 26:69–76, 1993.
2. Basmajian JV, Stecko G: The role of muscles in arch support of the foot. J Bone Joint Surg 45A:1184–1190, 1963.
3. Brown GP, Donatelli RD, Catlin PA, et al: The effect of two types of foot orthoses on rearfoot mechanics. J Orthop Sports Phys Ther 21:258–266, 1995.
4. Buckwalter JA, Saltzman CL: Ankle osteoarthritis: Distinctive characteristics. AAOS Instructional Course Lectures 48:233–241, 1999.
5. Cashmere T, Smith R, Hunt A: Medial longitudinal arch of the foot: Stationary versus walking measures. Foot Ankle Int 20:112–118, 1999.
6. Cavanagh PR, Rodgers MM, Iiboshi A: Pressure distribution under symptom-free feet during barefoot standing. Foot Ankle Int 7:262–276, 1987.
7. Colville MR, Marder RA, Boyle JJ, et al: Strain measurement in lateral ankle ligaments. Am J Sports Med 18:196–200, 1990.
8. Cornall MW, McPoil TG: Three-dimensional movement of the foot during the stance phase of walking. J Am Podiatr Med Assoc 89:56–66, 1999.
9. Elveru RA, Rothstein JM, Lamb RL, et al: Methods for taking subtalar joint measurements: A clinical report. Phys Ther 68:678–682, 1988.
10. Engsberg JR: A biomechanical analysis of the talocalcaneal joint—in vitro. J Biomechan 20:429–442, 1987.
11. Faber FWM, Kleinrensink GJ, Verhoog MW, et al: Mobility of the first tarsometatarsal joint in relation to hallux valgus deformity: Anatomical and biomechanical aspects. Foot Ankle Int 20:651–656, 1999.
12. Fallat L, Grimm DJ, Saracco JA: Sprained ankle syndrome: Prevalence and analysis of 639 acute injures. J Foot Ankle Surg 37:280–285, 1998.
13. Glasoe WM, Yack HJ, Saltzman CL: Anatomy and biomechanics of the first ray. Phys Ther 79:854–859, 1999.
14. Grimston SK, Nigg BM, Hanley DA, et al: Differences in ankle joint complex range of motion as a function of age. Foot Ankle Int 14:215–222, 1993.
15. Hopson MM, McPoil TG, Cornwall MW: Motion of the first metatarsophalangeal joint: Reliability and validity of four measurement techniques. J Am Podiatr Med Assoc 85:198–204, 1995.
16. Huang CK, Kitaoka HB, An KN, et al: Biomechanical evaluation of longitudinal arch stability. Foot Ankle Int 14:353–357, 1993.
17. Inman VT: The Joints of the Ankle. Baltimore, Williams & Wilkins, 1976.
18. Inman VT, Saunders JB: Referred pain from skeletal structures. J Nerv Ment Dis 99:660–667, 1944.
19. Isman RE, Inman VT: Anthropometric studies of the human foot and ankle. Bull Prosthet Res 10:97–129, 1969.
20. Johanson MA, Donatelli R, Wooden ML, et al: Effects of three different posting methods on controlling abnormal subtalar pronation. Phys Ther 79:149–158, 1994.
21. Kaufman KR, Brodine SK, Shaffer RA, et al: The effect of foot structure and range of motion on musculoskeletal overuse injuries. Am J Sports Med 27:585–593, 1999.
22. Kapandji IA: The Physiology of the Joints, vol 2, 5th ed., Edinburgh, Churchill Livingstone, 1982.
23. Kendall FP, McCreary AK, Provance PG: Muscles: Testing and Function, 4th ed. Baltimore, Williams & Wilkins, 1993.
24. Kitaoka HB, Luo ZP, An KN: Three-dimensional analysis of flatfoot deformity: Cadaver study. Foot Ankle Int 19:447–451, 1998.
25. Kitaoka HB, Patzer GL: Subtalar arthrodesis for posterior tibial tendon dysfunction and pes planus. Clin Orthop Rel Res 345:187–194, 1997.
26. Kura H, Luo ZP, Kitaoka HB, et al: Role of the medial capsule and transverse metatarsal ligament in hallux valgus deformity. Clin Orthop Rel Res 354:235–240, 1998.
27. Mann RA: Biomechanics of the foot. In American Academy of Orthopedic Surgeons (eds): Atlas of Orthotics: Biomechanical Principles and Application. St. Louis, Mosby, 1975, pp 257–266.
28. Manter JT: Movements of the subtalar joint and transverse tarsal joint. Anat Rec 80:397–410, 1941.
29. McCulloch MU, Brunt D, Vander Linden D: The effect of foot orthotics and gait velocity on lower limb kinematics and temporal events of stance. J Orthop Sports Phys Ther 17:2–10, 1993.
30. McPoil TG: The Foot and Ankle. In Malone TR, McPoil T, Nitz AJ (eds): Orthopedic and Sports Physical Therapy, 3rd ed. St. Louis, Mosby-Year Book, 1997.
31. McPoil TG, Knecht HG, Schuit D: A survey of foot types in normal females between ages of 18 and 30 years. J Orthop Sports Phys Ther 9:406–409, 1988.
32. Murray MP, Guten GN, Baldwin JM, et al: A comparison of plantarflexion torque with and without the triceps surae. Acta Orthop Scand 47:122–124, 1976.
33. Murray MP, Guten GN, Sepic SB, et al: Function of the triceps surae during gait. J Bone Joint Surg 60A:473–476, 1978.
34. Nigg BM, Khan A, Fisher V, et al: Effect of shoe insert construction on foot and leg movement. Med Sci Sports Exerc 30:550–555, 1998.
35. Nistor L, Markhede G, Grimby G: A technique for measurements of plantar flexion torque with the Cybex dynamometer. Scand J Rehab Med 14:163–166, 1982.
36. Pearce TJ, Buckley RE: Subtalar joint movement: Clinical and computed tomography scan correlation. Foot Ankle Int 20:428–432, 1999.
37. Pomeroy GC, Pike RH, Beals TC, et al: Acquired flatfoot in adults due to dysfunction of the posterior tibial tendon. J Bone Joint Surg 81A:1173–1182, 1999.
38. Powers CM, Maffucci R, Hampton S: Rearfoot posture in subjects with patellofemoral pain. J Orthop Sports Phys Ther 22:155–160, 1995.
39. Proctor P, Paul JP: Ankle joint biomechanics. J Biomechan 15:627–634, 1982.

40. Reischl SF, Powers CM, Rao S, et al: Relationship between foot pronation and rotation of the tibia and femur during walking. Foot Ankle Int 20:513–520, 1999.
41. Richardson EG: Pes planus. In Crenshaw AH (ed): Campbells' Operative Orthopaedics, vol 4, 8th ed. St. Louis, Mosby-Year Book, 1992.
42. Richardson EG: Disorders of the hallux. In Crenshaw AH (ed): Campbells' Operative Orthopaedics, vol 4, 8th ed. St. Louis, Mosby-Year Book, 1992.
43. Richardson EG: Neurogenic disorders. In Crenshaw AH (ed). Campbells' Operative Orthopaedics, vol 4, 8th ed. St. Louis, Mosby-Year Book, 1992.
44. Root ML, Weed JH, Sgarlato TE, et al: Axis of rotation of the subtalar joint. J Am Podiatr Med Assoc 56:149–155, 1966.
45. Scott SH, Winter DA: Biomechanical model of the human foot: Kinematics and kinetics during the stance phase of walking. J Biomechan 26:1091–1104, 1993.
46. Self BP, Harris S, Greenwald RM: Ankle biomechanics during impact landings on uneven surfaces. Foot Ankle Int 21:138–144, 2000.
47. Sepic SB, Murray MP, Mollinger LA, et al: Strength and range of motion in the ankle in two age groups of men and women. Am J Phys Med 65:75–84, 1986.
48. Siegler S, Chen J, Schneck CD: The three-dimensional kinematics and flexibility characteristics of the human ankle and subtalar joints. Part 1: Kinematics. Transactions of the ASME. J Biomech Eng 110:364–373, 1988.
49. Stauffer RN, Chao EYS, Brewster RC: Force and motion analysis of the normal, diseased, and prosthetic ankle joint. Clin Orthop Rel Res 127:189–196, 1977.
50. Sutherland DH: An electromyographic study of the plantarflexors of the ankle in normal walking on the level. J Bone Joint Surg 48A:66–71, 1966.
51. Thordarson DB, Schmotzer H, Chon J, et al: Dynamic support of the human longitudinal arch: A biomechanical evaluation. Clin Orthop Rel Res 316:165–172, 1995.
52. Tiberio D: Pathomechanics of structural foot deformities. Phys Ther 68:1840–1849, 1988.
53. Viitasalo JT, Kvist M: Some biomechanical aspects of the foot and ankle in athletes with and without shin splints. Am J Sports Med 11:4125–4130, 1983.
54. Weinfeld SB, Schon LC: Hallux metatarsophalangeal arthritis. Clin Orthop Rel Res 349:9–19, 1998.
55. Williams PL, Bannister LH, Berry M, et al: Gray's Anatomy, 4th ed. New York, Churchill Livingstone, 1995.
56. Wright DG, Desai SM, Henderson WH: Action of the subtalar and ankle joint complex during the stance phase of walking. J Bone Joint Surg 46A:361–382, 1964.
57. Yoshioka Y, Sui DW, Scudamore RA, et al: Tibial anatomy and functional axes. J Orthop Res 7:132–137, 1989.

## ADDITIONAL READINGS

Basmajian JV, Bentzon JW: An electromyographic study of certain muscles of the leg and foot in the standing position. Surg Gynecol Obstet 98:662–666, 1954.
Chan CW, Rudins A: Foot Biomechanics during walking and running. Mayo Clin Proc 69:448–461, 1994.
Cornwall MW, McPoil TG: Relative movement of the navicular bone during normal walking. Foot Ankle Int 20:507–512, 1999.
Eng JJ, Pierrynowski MR: The effect of soft foot orthotics on the three-dimensional lower limb kinematics during walking and running. Phys Ther 74:836–844, 1994.
Oatis CA: Biomechanics of the foot and ankle under static conditions. Phys Ther 68:1815–1821, 1988.

# Kinesiology of Walking

## GUY G. SIMONEAU, PT, PHD, ATC

### TOPICS AT A GLANCE

## INTRODUCTION

Walking (ambulation) serves an individual's basic need to move from place to place. As such, walking is one of the most common activities that people do on a daily basis. Ideally, walking is performed both efficiently, to minimize fatigue, and safely, to prevent falls and associated injuries. Years of practice provide a healthy person with the control needed to ambulate while carrying on a conversation, looking in various directions, and even handling obstacles and other destabilizing forces with minimal effort.

Although a healthy person gives walking the appearance of an effortless task, the challenge of ambulation can be recognized by looking at individuals at both ends of the lifespan (Fig. 15–1). Early in life, the young child needs several months to learn how to stand and walk. In fact, it is only by the age of 7 years that all the refinements of a mature gait pattern are completed.[76] Late in life, walking often becomes an increasingly greater challenge. Because of decreased strength, decreased balance, or disease, the elderly may require a cane or walker to ambulate safely. Patla[64] eloquently expressed the importance of ambulation in our lives: "Nothing epitomizes a level of independence and our perception of a good quality of life more than the ability to travel independently under our own power from one place to another. We celebrate the development of this ability in children and try to nurture and sustain it throughout the lifespan."

This chapter provides a description of the fundamental kinesiologic characteristics of gait (see the box). Unless indicated otherwise, the information provided refers to individuals with a normal and mature (age greater than 7 years) gait pattern, walking on level surfaces at a steady average speed. The chapter also provides enough details to be read independently of the rest of this book. The reading of chapters 12, 13, and 14, however, will facilitate a more thorough understanding of walking.

> **Major Topics**
> * Spatial and temporal descriptors
> * Control of the body's center of mass
> * Joint kinematics
> * Strategies to minimize energy expenditure
> * Energy expenditure
> * Muscle activity
> * Gait kinetics
> * Gait dysfunctions

The observation of gait, which is the focus of this chapter, provides information on the outcome of a complex set of "behind the scenes" interactions between sensory and motor functions. For a person to walk, the central nervous system must generate appropriate motor actions from the integration of visual, proprioceptive, and vestibular sensory

**Walking Child**          **Walking Adult**          **Walking Elder**

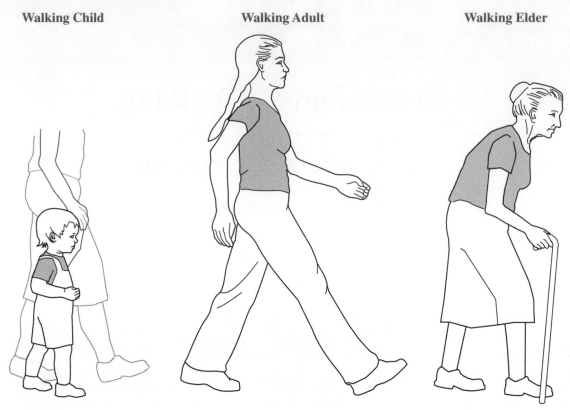

**FIGURE 15–1.** Walking at various stages in life.

inputs. Although this chapter covers the intricacy of limb and muscular actions performed during walking, it does not cover the concept of motor control. To gain a greater understanding of the complexity of the motor control of gait, the reader is advised to examine other sources on the topic, such as Shumway-Cook and Woollacott, 1995,[76] and Masdeu et al., 1997.[49]

## HISTORICAL PERSPECTIVE OF GAIT ANALYSIS

The Weber brothers (Wilhelm, a physicist/electrician, and Eduard, an anatomist/physiologist)[94] published the first scientific work on gait in 1836. Using instruments, such as a chronometer and a telescope with a scale, they described and measured elements of gait, such as step length, cadence, foot-to-ground clearance, and vertical excursion of the body. They also defined basic elements of the gait cycle, such as swing phase, stance phase, and double-limb support periods. Many of the terms they introduced remain in use today. The Webers hypothesized that the basic principle of walking is one of least muscular effort—a concept known to be true today, although the exact methods by which the body minimizes energy expenditure are still not fully understood. An extensive account of their work was published in 1894 and later translated in 1992.[95,96]

In the 19th century, other researchers, such as Marey and Vierordt, made use of ingenious technology to expand our knowledge of gait. Most often cited among Marey's many

novel methods of measurements are shoes that had air chambers attached to a recorder to indicate the swing and stance phase of gait (Fig. 15–2).[47,48] Another clever idea was the use of ink in small spray nozzles attached to the shoes and limbs.[87] The ink sprayed on the floor and wall as the

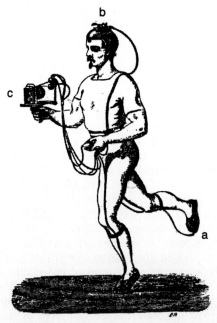

**FIGURE 15–2.** Marey's instrumented shoes used for the measurement of gait. (From Marey, 1873.)

individual walked and provided a permanent record of movement.

Concurrently, advances in the field of cinematography created a powerful medium to study and record the kinematic patterns of human's and animal's walking. Muybridge may be the most recognized individual of his time to use cinematography to document sequence of movements. Muybridge is most famous for settling an old controversy regarding a trotting horse. In 1872, using sequence photography, he showed that all four feet of a trotting horse are indeed simultaneously off the ground for very brief periods of time. Muybridge created an impressive collection of photographs on human and animal gait, which was initially published in 1887 and assembled and reproduced in 1979.[60,61]

Initially, the description of gait was limited to planar analyses; the motion was typically recorded in the sagittal plane and less frequently in the frontal plane. Braune and Fisher[6,7] are credited as being the first researchers, from 1895 to 1904, to perform a comprehensive three-dimensional analysis of a walking individual. By using four cameras (two pairs of cameras recording motion for each side of the body) and a number of light tubes attached to various body segments, they documented joint kinematics in three dimensions. They were also the first to use the principles of mechanics to measure dynamic quantities such as segmental acceleration, segmental inertial properties, and intersegmental loads (e.g., joint torques and forces). Their analysis of joint torques, limited to the swing phase of gait, dispelled the earlier concept, suggested by Weber and Weber in 1836, that lower extremity motion during the swing phase of gait was explained by a passive pendulum theory.

Throughout the 20th century, the understanding of walk-

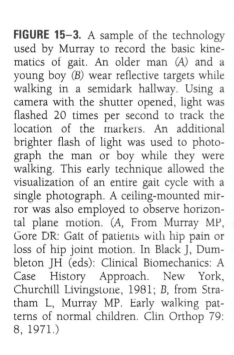

**FIGURE 15–3.** A sample of the technology used by Murray to record the basic kinematics of gait. An older man (A) and a young boy (B) wear reflective targets while walking in a semidark hallway. Using a camera with the shutter opened, light was flashed 20 times per second to track the location of the markers. An additional brighter flash of light was used to photograph the man or boy while they were walking. This early technique allowed the visualization of an entire gait cycle with a single photograph. A ceiling-mounted mirror was also employed to observe horizontal plane motion. (A, From Murray MP, Gore DR: Gait of patients with hip pain or loss of hip joint motion. In Black J, Dumbleton JH (eds): Clinical Biomechanics: A Case History Approach. New York, Churchill Livingstone, 1981; B, from Stratham L, Murray MP. Early walking patterns of normal children. Clin Orthop 79: 8, 1971.)

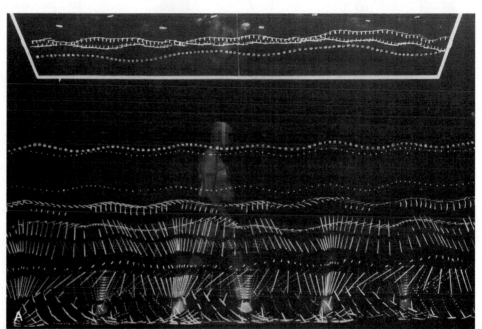

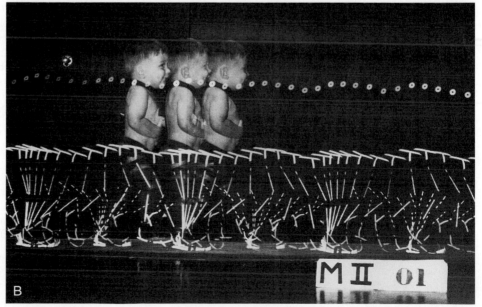

### The Gait Laboratory

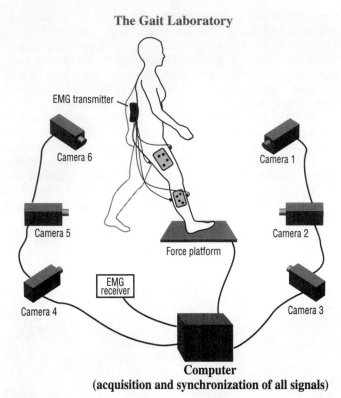

**FIGURE 15–4.** Instrumentation used in a typical laboratory to study gait.

ing was greatly enhanced by many scientific advances. Instrumentation to document kinematics evolved from simple video cameras, with film that required painstaking analysis with a ruler and protractor, to highly sophisticated infrared systems, with real-time coordinate data of limb segments. Notable researchers who contributed to the description of the kinematics of gait using a variety of imaging techniques include Eberhart (1947),[17] Murray (1967),[53,54] Inman (1981),[34] Winter (1991),[98] and Perry (1992).[67] Noteworthy is the work by Murray, a physical therapist and researcher, who published several papers in the 1960s, 1970s, and 1980s, describing the kinematics of many aspects of normal and abnormal gait (Fig. 15–3).[52,55,56,59] Among other accomplishments, data from her research—on the kinematics of walking in individuals with disabilities—influenced the design of artificial joints and lower extremity prosthetic limbs.

Similarly, a more extensive understanding of the kinetics of gait was made possible through the development of devices to measure the forces taking place at the foot-ground interface. Amar (1916),[3] Elftman (1938),[18] and Bresler and Frankel (1950)[8] all made significant contributions in this field. With the ability to measure the forces between the foot and the ground came computational methods to calculate the forces and torques taking place at the joints during ambulation.[65,77,100]

Surface and intramuscular electrodes can also be used to record the electrical activity pattern of muscles during gait. When this information is integrated with the kinematics of walking, the role that each muscle plays during gait is described. Many researchers, including Sutherland, Perry, Inman, and Winter, have made notable contributions to the study of electromyography (EMG) during walking. Knutson and Soderberg[41] provide a summary of the application of EMG in the study of gait.

Today, gait analysis is routinely performed in specialized biomechanics laboratories (Fig. 15–4). Three-dimensional kinematic data are obtained by using two or more synchronized high-speed cameras. Ground reaction forces are measured utilizing force platforms embedded in the floor. Muscle activity patterns are recorded by multichannel EMG systems. Ultimately, lower extremity joint forces, torques, and powers are calculated with a combination of kinematic data, ground reaction forces, and anthropometric characteristics of the individual (Fig. 15–5). These data are then used to describe normal and abnormal gait.

Patients with a variety of pathologies can benefit from instrumented gait analyses. The primary beneficiaries of this technology, however, are children with cerebral palsy. In this population, instrumented gait analysis is often used prior to surgery to help determine the proper intervention. It is employed again after surgery to objectively evaluate the outcome.[27] Comprehensive descriptions of the tools and methods used for gait analysis can be found in several other sources, such as Vaughan et al., 1992;[86] Whittle, 1996;[97] Harris and Smith, 1996;[33] and Allard et al., 1997.[2]

Sophisticated technology, such as that described here, provides detailed information that can enhance the ability to describe and understand gait. Such technology is rarely available in the typical clinical setting, however. Clinicians must routinely rely on direct visual observation to evaluate the gait characteristics of their patients. Such observational analysis requires a thorough knowledge and understanding of normal gait. Learning about gait, as presented here, is a

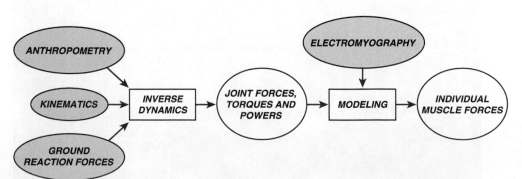

**FIGURE 15–5.** Typical approach used for the analysis of human motion. Variables in the shaded ovals can be precisely measured. Computational methods, in the rectangles, are used to calculate the variables in the non-shaded ovals.

**The Gait Cycle**

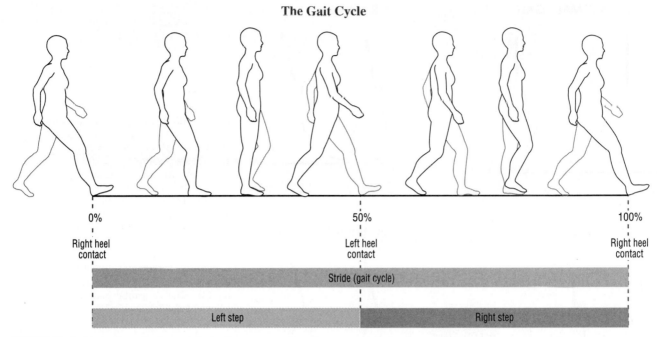

**FIGURE 15–6.** The gait cycle from right heel contact to the subsequent right heel contact.

more dynamic experience if the reading and studying of this chapter are combined with the observing of the gait patterns of relatives, friends, and neighbors.

## SPATIAL AND TEMPORAL DESCRIPTORS

This section describes measurements of distance and time as related to walking.

### Gait Cycle

Walking is the result of a cyclic series of movements. As such, it can be conveniently characterized by a detailed description of its most fundamental unit: a *gait cycle* (Fig. 15–6). The gait cycle is initiated as soon as the foot contacts the ground. Because foot contact is normally made with the heel, the 0% point or beginning of the gait cycle is referred to as *heel contact,* or *heel strike.* The 100% point or comple-

tion of the gait cycle occurs as soon as the same foot once again makes contact with the ground. A *stride* (synonymous with a gait cycle) is the sequence of events taking place between successive heel contacts of the same foot. In comparison, a *step* is the sequence of events that occurs within successive heel contacts of opposite feet, for example, between right and left heel contacts. A gait cycle, therefore, has two steps—a left step and a right step.

The most basic spatial descriptors of gait include the length of a stride and the length of a step (Fig. 15–7). *Stride length* is the distance between two successive heel contacts of the same foot. *Step length,* in contrast, is the distance between successive heel contacts of the two different feet. Comparing right with left step lengths can help to evaluate the symmetry of gait between the lower extremities (Fig. 15–8). *Step width* is the lateral distance between the heel centers of two consecutive foot contacts and normally ranges from 7 to 9 cm (Fig. 15–7). *Foot angle,* the degree of "toe-out," is the angle between the line of progression of the

**Spatial Descriptors of Gait**

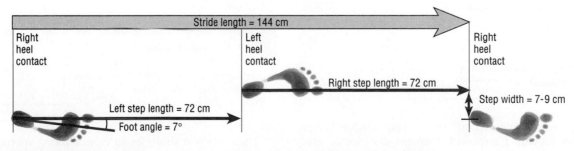

**FIGURE 15–7.** Spatial descriptors of gait and their normal values for a right gait cycle.

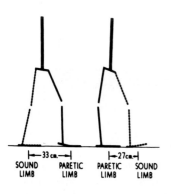

**A. NORMAL GAIT**

├─── 78 cm. ───┤   ├─── 78 cm. ───┤
RIGHT    LEFT      LEFT    RIGHT
LIMB     LIMB      LIMB    LIMB

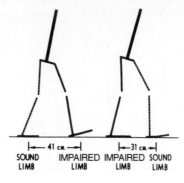

**B. PAINFUL HIP GAIT**

├── 41 cm. ──┤  ├── 31 cm. ──┤
SOUND   IMPAIRED  IMPAIRED  SOUND
LIMB     LIMB      LIMB     LIMB

**C. HEMIPARESIS GAIT**

├─33 cm.─┤  ├─27cm.─┤
SOUND   PARETIC  PARETIC   SOUND
LIMB     LIMB     LIMB      LIMB

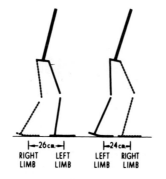

**D. PARKINSON'S DISEASE GAIT**

├─26cm.─┤  ├─24cm.─┤
RIGHT   LEFT   LEFT   RIGHT
LIMB    LIMB   LIMB   LIMB

**FIGURE 15–8.** Influence of impairment and pathology on step length. *A* illustrates the symmetrical step length expected in a healthy individual. *B* and *C* are examples of step length asymmetry often seen in those with an impairment or a pathology that affects a single lower extremity. Note that the unilateral pathology in *C* resulted in bilateral shortening of the normal step length, demonstrating the interdependence of the lower extremities during gait. *D* illustrates a relatively symmetrical bilateral reduction in step length secondary to Parkinson's disease, a pathology that often affects both lower extremities. (From Murray MP: Gait as a total pattern of movement. Am J Phys Med 46:290, 1967.)

body and the long axis of the foot. About 7 degrees is considered normal.[53]

---

**Spatial Descriptors of Gait**
- Stride length
- Step length
- Step width
- Foot angle

---

The most basic temporal descriptor of gait is *cadence,* the number of steps per minute, which is also called *step rate.* Other temporal descriptors of gait are *stride time* (the time for a full gait cycle) and *step time* (the time for the completion of a right or a left step). Note that in normal symmetrical gait, step time can be derived from cadence (i.e., step time is the reciprocal of cadence).

---

**Temporal Descriptors of Gait**
- Cadence
- Stride time
- Step time

**Spatial/Temporal Descriptor**
- Walking speed

---

*Walking speed* combines both spatial and temporal measurements by providing information on the distance covered in a given amount of time. The units of measurements are typically meters per second (m/s) or miles per hour (mph). Speed can be calculated by measuring the time it takes to cover a given distance, or the distance covered in a given amount of time, or by multiplying the step rate by the step length. Walking speed varies considerably between persons based on factors such as age and physical characteristics, such as height and weight.[15] Of all spatial and temporal measurements of gait, speed may be the best and most functional measure of an individual's walking ability.

Among normal adults, a gait cycle (i.e., two consecutive steps) takes slightly more than 1 second and covers approximately 1.44 meters (4.5 feet), representing a speed of 1.37 m/s. Data in Table 15–1 indicate that, at a freely chosen walking speed, women exhibit a slower walking speed, shorter step length, and faster cadence than men. These differences are likely in part reflective of anthropometric disparities between genders. Interestingly, even when anthropometrically matched with men, women demonstrate a higher cadence and shorter step length than men when walking at a standard speed.[21,56]

---

**Normal Values for Gait**
- Gait speed: 1.37 m/s (3 mph)
- Step rate: 1.87 steps/s (110 steps/min)
- Step length: 72 cm (28 inches)

---

There are two strategies to raise walking speed: increasing the stride, or step length, and increasing the cadence (Fig.

**TABLE 15-1. Normative Data for Walking Speed, Step Rate, and Step Length**

|  | Drillis (1961) (New York City) | Molen (1973) (Amsterdam) | Finley and Cody (1970) (Philadelphia) | Average Over Gender and City |
|---|---|---|---|---|
| Walking speed (m/s) | 1.46* | 1.39 (males) 1.27 (females) | 1.37 (males) 1.24 (females) | 1.37 |
| Step rate (steps/s) | 1.9* | 1.79 (males) 1.88 (females) | 1.84 (males) 1.94 (females) | 1.87 |
| Step length (m) | 0.76* | 0.77 (males) 0.67 (females) | 0.74 (males) 0.63 (females) | 0.72 |

\* Males and females are averaged together for these data.
Data obtained from 2300 pedestrians unaware of being observed as they walked.

15–9). Typically, an individual combines both strategies until the longest comfortable step length is reached. From that point on, a further increase in speed is solely related to increased cadence. *All measurements of gait (spatial, temporal, kinematic, and kinetic) depend on walking speed.* For proper reference and interpretation, therefore, reports of gait characteristics should include the walking speed at which the data were collected.

## Stance and Swing Phase

To help describe events taking place during the gait cycle, it is customary to subdivide the gait cycle from 0 to 100%. As stated earlier, heel or foot contact with the ground is considered the start of the gait cycle (0%) and the next ground contact made by the same foot is considered the end of the gait cycle (100%). Throughout this chapter, gait is described

using the right lower extremity as a reference. A full gait cycle for the right lower extremity can be divided into two major phases—stance and swing (Fig. 15–10). *Stance phase* (from right heel contact to right toe off) occurs as the right foot is on the ground, supporting the body's weight. *Swing phase* (from right toe off to the next right heel contact) occurs as the right foot is in the air, being advanced forward for the next contact with the ground. At normal walking speed, the stance phase occupies approximately 60% of the gait cycle, and the swing phase occupies the remaining 40%.

**Gait Cycle**
- Stance phase = 60% of gait cycle
- Swing phase = 40% of gait cycle

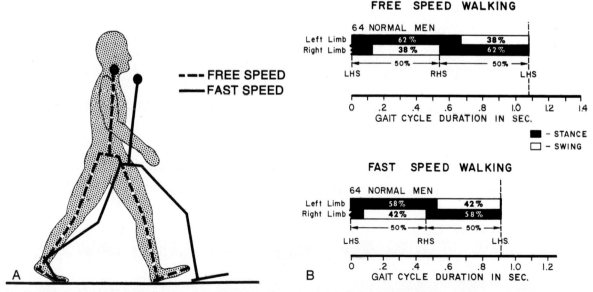

**FIGURE 15–9.** Methods to increase walking speed. *A* illustrates the longer step length used to increase walking speed; *B* illustrates the walking cadence used at a faster walking speed. The duration of the gait cycle is reduced from 1.08 seconds to 0.91 second. *B* also illustrates that at the faster walking speed, a smaller percentage of the gait cycle is spent in double-limb support (i.e., 16% at fast speed compared with 24% at free speed walking). (*A* from Murray MP, Kory RC, Clarkson BH, Sepic SB: Comparison of free and fast speed walking patterns of normal men. Am J Phys Med 45:8, 1966; *B* Modified from Murray MP, Gore DR, Clarkson BH: Walking patterns of patients with unilateral hip pain due to osteoarthritis and avascular necrosis. J Bone Joint Surg 53A:259, 1971.)

## SPECIAL FOCUS 15-1

### Simple Clinical Measurements of Gait

Sophisticated instrumentation, such as walkways and foot switches, exists to make spatial and temporal measurements of foot placement during gait.[88] For most clinical applications, this information can, however, be measured with readily available tools and a little imagination. Average walking speed can be measured using a stopwatch and a known distance. Step length and step width can be measured by the use of ink marks made by shoes or feet on a roll of paper covering the floor. This technique works especially well to document abnormal gait patterns, including asymmetry in step length.

Clinically, simple measurements of walking speed and distance can be helpful in monitoring functional progress or documenting functional limitations. Results obtained from a patient can be compared with normal values provided in Table 15–1, or with minimum standards required to perform a specific task, such as crossing a street within the time allowed by the stoplights.[22,23,45,71,90,91] The following are two proposed minimum standards, based on community-living activities: the ability to walk 300 m (1000 feet) in less than 11.5 minutes (walking speed of 0.45 m/s or 1 mph); the ability to walk at a speed of 1.3 m/s (3 mph) for 13 to 27 m (42 to 85 feet) in order to cross a street safely.

Within a gait cycle, the body experiences two periods of *double-limb support* (when both feet are in contact with the ground simultaneously) and two periods of *single-limb support* (when only one foot is on the ground) (see Fig. 15–10). We observe the first period of double-limb support between 0 and 10% of the gait cycle. During that time period, the body's weight is being transferred from the left to the right lower extremity. The right lower extremity is then in single-limb support until 50% of the gait cycle. During that time, the left lower extremity is in its swing phase, being advanced forward. The second period of double-limb support takes place between 50% and 60% of the gait cycle and serves the purpose of transferring the weight of the body from the right to the left lower extremity. Finally, from 60 to 100% of the gait cycle, the body is again in single-limb support, this time on the left lower extremity. This period of left single-limb support corresponds to the swing phase of the right lower extremity.

As gait speed increases, the percentage of the gait cycle spent in periods of double-limb support becomes shorter (see Fig. 15–9). Race walkers aim to walk as fast as possible while always keeping one foot in contact with the ground. For these athletes, greater speed is achieved by increasing cadence and stride length and by minimizing periods of double-limb support to the point where stance and swing phase times are about equal. Walking speed during race walking can be in excess of 3.3 m/s (7.5 mph).[58,80]

In running, the periods of double-limb support disappear altogether to be replaced by periods when both feet are off the ground simultaneously. The transition from walking to running normally takes place at a step rate of approximately

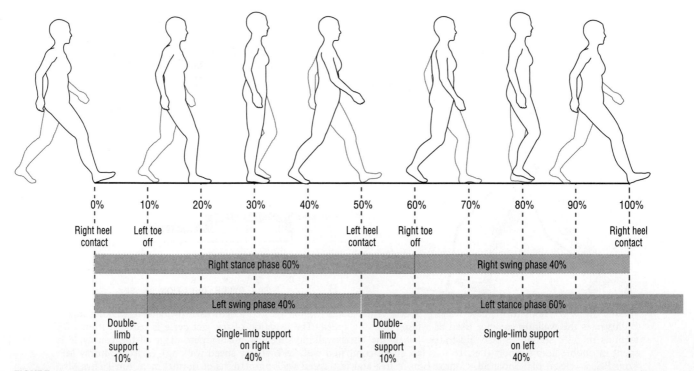

**FIGURE 15–10.** Subdivision of the gait cycle illustrates the phases of stance and swing and periods of single- and double-limb support.

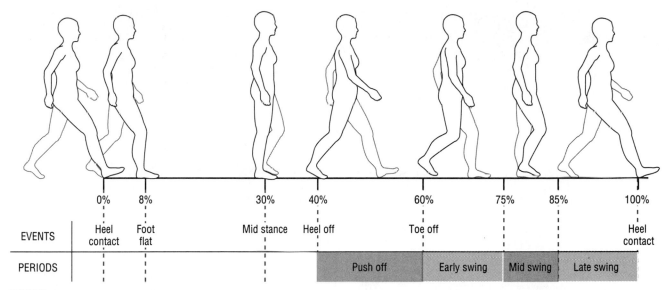

**FIGURE 15–11.** Traditional subdivisions of the gait cycle.

180 steps/minute or at a speed of approximately 2.0 m/s (4.5 mph). Above 2.0 m/s it is more energy efficient to run than walk.

Conversely, at a slow walking speed, the periods of double-limb support occupy an increasingly greater percentage of the gait cycle. A slower gait provides greater stability because both feet are on the ground simultaneously for a greater percentage of the cycle. In fact, the reduced speed, shorter step length, and slower cadence commonly seen in the elderly serve to improve gait stability and prevent falls.

*Subdivisions of stance and swing phases:* Traditionally, five events are defined to occur during stance phase: heel contact, foot flat, mid stance, heel off (or heel rise), and toe off (Fig. 15–11 and Table 15–2). *Heel contact* is defined as the instant the heel comes in contact with the ground, at 0% of the gait cycle. *Foot flat* corresponds to the instant the entire plantar surface of the foot comes in contact with the ground.

This event occurs at approximately 8% of the gait cycle. *Mid stance* is most often defined as the point where the body's weight passes directly over the supporting lower extremity. It is also defined as the time when the foot of the lower extremity in the swing phase passes the lower extremity in the stance phase (i.e., the feet are side by side). A third definition of mid stance is the time when the greater trochanter of the femur is vertically above the midpoint of the supporting foot in the sagittal plane. In reality, these three definitions all correspond to about 30% of the gait cycle or 50% of the stance phase. *Heel off,* which occurs at approximately 40% of the gait cycle, is the instant the heel comes off the ground. *Toe off* occurs at 60% of the gait cycle. It is defined as the instant the toes come off the ground.

A period referred to as *push off* is also often used. This period roughly corresponds to the movement of ankle plantar flexion from 40 to 60% of the gait cycle.

## TABLE 15-2. Common Terminology Defining the Subdivisions of the Gait Cycle

| Phases | Events | % of Cycle | Events of Opposite Limb |
|--------|--------|------------|-------------------------|
| Stance | Heel contact | 0 | |
| | Foot flat | 8 | |
| | | 10 | Toe off |
| | Mid stance | 30 | Mid swing (25–35%) |
| | Heel off | 40 | |
| | | 50 | Heel contact |
| | Toe off | 60 | |
| Swing | Early swing | 60–75 | |
| | Mid swing | 75–85 | Mid stance (80%) |
| | Late swing | 85–100 | |
| | | 90 | Heel off |
| | Heel contact | 100 | |

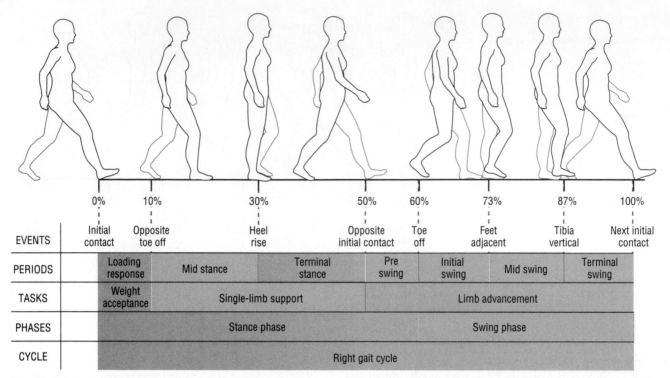

| | | | | | | | | | |
|---|---|---|---|---|---|---|---|---|---|
| | 0% | 10% | | 30% | | 50% | 60% | 73% | 87% | 100% |
| **EVENTS** | Initial contact | Opposite toe off | | Heel rise | | Opposite initial contact | Toe off | Feet adjacent | Tibia vertical | Next initial contact |
| **PERIODS** | Loading response | Mid stance | | | Terminal stance | Pre swing | Initial swing | Mid swing | | Terminal swing |
| **TASKS** | Weight acceptance | Single-limb support | | | | | Limb advancement | | | |
| **PHASES** | Stance phase | | | | | | Swing phase | | | |
| **CYCLE** | Right gait cycle | | | | | | | | | |

**FIGURE 15–12.** Terminology to describe the events of the gait cycle. *Initial contact* corresponds to the beginning of stance when the foot first contacts the ground at 0% of gait cycle. *Opposite toe off* occurs when the contralateral foot leaves the ground at 10% of gait cycle. *Heel rise* corresponds to the heel lifting from the ground and occurs at approximately 30% of gait cycle. *Opposite initial contact* corresponds to the foot contact of the opposite limb, typically at 50% of gait cycle. *Toe off* occurs when the foot leaves the ground at 60% of gait cycle. *Feet adjacent* takes place when the foot of the swing leg is next to the foot of the stance leg at 73% of gait cycle. *Tibia vertical* corresponds to the tibia of the swing leg being oriented in the vertical direction at 87% of gait cycle. The final event is, again, initial contact, which in fact is the start of the next gait cycle.

These eight events divide the gait cycle into seven periods. *Loading response,* between initial contact and opposite toe off, corresponds to the time when the weight is accepted by the lower extremity, initiating contact with the ground. *Mid stance* is from opposite toe off to heel rise (10 to 30% of gait cycle). *Terminal stance* begins when the heel rises and ends when the contralateral lower extremity touches the ground, from 30 to 50% of gait cycle. *Pre swing* takes place from foot contact of the contralateral limb to toe off of the ipsilateral foot, which is the time corresponding to the second double-limb support period of the gait cycle (50 to 60% of gait cycle). *Initial swing* is from toe off to feet adjacent, when the foot of the swing leg is next to the foot of the stance leg (60 to 73% of gait cycle). *Mid swing* is from feet adjacent to when the tibia of the swing leg is vertical (73 to 87% of gait cycle). *Terminal swing* is from a vertical position of the tibia to immediately prior to heel contact (87 to 100% of the gait cycle). The first 10% of the gait cycle corresponds to a task of weight acceptance—when body mass is transferred from one lower extremity to the other. Single-limb support, from 10 to 50% of the gait cycle, serves to support the weight of the body as the opposite limb swings forward. The last 10% of stance phase and the entire swing phase serve to advance the limb forward to a new location.

Although there is a significant amount of variation in the description of the swing phase of gait, this phase is traditionally subdivided into three sections: early, mid, and late swing (see Fig. 15–11). *Early swing* is the period from the time of toe off to mid swing (60 to 75% of the gait cycle). *Mid swing* corresponds to the mid stance event of the opposite lower extremity when the foot of the swing leg passes next to the foot of the stance leg (75 to 85% of the gait cycle). *Late swing* is the period from mid swing to foot contact with the ground (85 to 100% of the gait cycle).

An alternate and relatively more recent terminology, proposed by Perry,[67] consists of eight events to divide the gait cycle into seven periods (Fig. 15–12). The events are *initial contact, opposite toe off, heel rise, opposite initial contact, toe off, feet adjacent, tibia vertical,* and *initial contact* for the next stride. The four time periods during stance are *loading response, mid stance, terminal stance,* and *pre swing.* Swing phase has three time periods: *initial swing, mid swing,* and *terminal swing.* With a few exceptions, this terminology is in general agreement with the more traditional description of gait.

The existence of two different terminologies can be confusing, especially when many use them interchangeably. In this chapter, we predominantly use the terminology proposed by Perry in 1992.[67] And to eliminate any confusion, we describe the timing of the events during gait as a percentage of the gait cycle.

**SPECIAL FOCUS 15–2**

**Take Time to Develop Your Observation Skills**

The events of gait cycle described in this section can be observed by watching people walking in normal surroundings (streets, malls, airports). Like any clinical skill, observational gait analysis improves with practice. Repeated observation of individuals with normal gait patterns sharpens the ability to recognize normal gait variations and identify abnormal gait deviations.

Opportunities to practice this skill with a person already trained in observational gait analysis further sharpen these skills.

## DISPLACEMENT AND CONTROL OF THE BODY'S CENTER OF MASS

Walking can be defined as a series of losses and recoveries of balance. Ambulation is initiated by allowing the body to lean forward. To prevent a fall, momentary recovery of balance is achieved by moving either foot forward to a new location. Once gait is initiated, the body's forward momentum carries the center of mass (CoM) of the body beyond the foot's new location, necessitating a step forward with the other foot. Forward progression is then achieved by the successive and alternate relocations of the feet. The smooth, controlled transition between loss and recovery of balance continues as long as forward displacement of the body is desired. Ambulation stops when foot placement stops the forward momentum of the body and balance is regained over the static base of support. Although this description provides a useful and relatively accurate explanation of gait, it must be pointed out that walking also requires active participation of the musculature of the lower extremities.

### Displacement of the Center of Mass

The body's CoM is located just anterior to the second sacral vertebra, but the best visualization of the movement of the CoM is by tracking the displacement of the head or torso. Clearly, the most notable displacement of the body during gait is in the forward direction (Fig. 15–13). Superimposed on this forward displacement, however, are two sinusoidal patterns of movement that correspond to the movement of the CoM in the vertical and medial-lateral directions.

In the vertical direction, the CoM describes two full sine waves per gait cycle (Fig. 15–13A). This movement of the CoM is best understood by looking at the individual from the side. Minimum height of the CoM occurs at the midpoint of both periods of double-limb support (5% and 55% of the gait cycle). Maximum height of the CoM occurs at the midpoint of both periods of single-limb support (30% and 80% of the gait cycle). A total vertical displacement of approximately 5 cm is noted at the average walking speed in the adult male.

**Displacement of the Center of Mass**

- Total vertical displacement: 5 cm
- Total medial-lateral displacement: 4 cm

Side-to-side (medial-lateral) movement of the CoM also occurs during ambulation, creating a single sinusoidal pattern in the horizontal plane. This movement can be viewed from above the individual but is typically viewed from the rear or front (Fig. 15–13B). In this plane of movement, the CoM is alternately shifted from the right to the left lower extremity. Maximum position of the CoM to the right occurs at the midpoint of the stance phase on the right lower extremity (30% of the gait cycle), and maximum position of the CoM to the left occurs at the midpoint of the stance phase on the left lower extremity (80% of the gait cycle). A total medial-lateral displacement of approximately 4 cm occurs during normal ambulation.[34] The amount of displacement increases when the individual has a wider base of support during gait (i.e., walking with the feet wider apart) and decreases with a narrower base of support (i.e., walking with the feet closer together).

To summarize, consider the total pattern of motion of the CoM during a full gait cycle (see Fig. 15–13). Starting shortly after right heel contact, the CoM is moving forward, upward, and toward the right foot. This general direction of movement continues for the first 30% of the gait cycle—the body is essentially "climbing and shifting its mass" over the supporting lower extremity. At right mid stance, the CoM reaches its highest and most lateral position toward the right. Just after right mid stance, the CoM continues forward but starts moving in a downward direction and toward the left side of the body—the body is essentially "falling away" from the supporting lower extremity. This is a critical moment in the gait cycle. With the left limb in its swing phase, the body depends on the left lower extremity to make proper contact with the ground in order to accept the weight transfer and to prevent a fall. Shortly after left heel contact, during the double-limb support phase, the CoM is located midway between the feet and reaches its lowest position as it continues to move forward and toward the left lower extremity. From right toe off to mid stance on the left lower extremity (80% of the gait cycle), the CoM moves forward, upward, and toward the left lower extremity, which is now providing support. At 80% of the gait cycle, the CoM is again at its highest point, but in its most lateral position to the left. Shortly after left mid stance, the movement of the CoM shifts downward and toward the right side of the body. The gait cycle is completed when the right heel contacts the ground.

The body's CoM never directly falls over the body's base of support during single-limb support (Fig. 15–13B). This fact speaks to the relative imbalance of the body during gait. In the frontal plane, to avoid a loss of balance, the foot must be positioned just slightly lateral to the path of the body's CoM to control its medial-lateral movement. Proper location of the foot by hip frontal plane motion (i.e., hip abduction/adduction) is crucial considering the view of the limited ability of the subtalar joint musculature to generate a stabilizing torque in the frontal plane.[99]

## A. Vertical Displacement of CoM

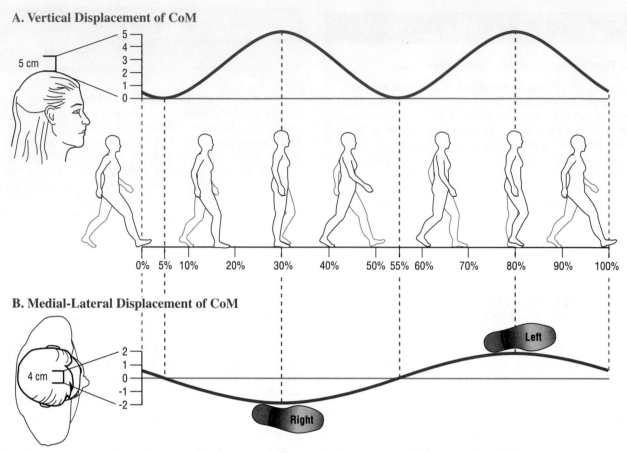

## B. Medial-Lateral Displacement of CoM

**FIGURE 15–13.** Center of mass (CoM) displacement during gait. The vertical and the medial-lateral displacements of the CoM are illustrated in A and B, respectively. The CoM is at its lowest and most central position, in the medial-lateral direction, in the middle of double-limb support (5% and 55% of the gait cycle)—a position of relative stability with both feet on the ground. Conversely, the CoM is at its highest and most lateral position at mid stance (30% and 80% of the gait cycle)—a position of relative instability. During single-limb support, the trajectory of the CoM is never directly over the base of support. This factor is illustrated in B, with the vertical projection of the CoM always medial to the footprints.

## Kinetic and Potential Energy Considerations

Although ambulation appears to take place at a steady forward speed, the body actually speeds up and slows down slightly with each step. When the supporting lower extremity is in front of the body's CoM, the body slows down. Conversely, when the supporting lower extremity is behind the body's CoM, the body speeds up. The body reaches its lowest velocity, therefore, at mid stance, once it has "climbed" on the supporting lower extremity, and its highest velocity during double-limb support, once it has "fallen away" from the supporting lower extremity and before "climbing" on the opposite limb. Because kinetic energy of the body during ambulation is a direct function of its velocity (equation 15–1), minimum kinetic energy is reached at mid stance (30% and 80% of the gait cycle) and maximum kinetic energy is reached at double-limb support (5% and 55% of the gait cycle) (Fig. 15–14).

$$\text{Kinetic energy} = 0.5 \, mv^2 \qquad 15{-}1$$

Where m is the mass of the body, and v the velocity of the CoM of the body.

Kinetic energy is complemented by potential energy (see

Fig. 15–14). Potential energy is a function of the mass of the body, the gravitational field acting on the body, and the height of the body's CoM (equation 15–2). During gait, maximum potential energy is achieved when the CoM reaches its highest points (30% and 80% of the gait cycle). Minimum potential energy of the body occurs at double-limb support (5% and 55% of the gait cycle), when the body's CoM is at its lowest points.

$$\text{Potential energy} = mgh \qquad 15{-}2$$

Where m is the mass of the body, g is the acceleration of the body due to the gravitational field, and h is the height of the body's CoM.

In a graphic representation of the changes in kinetic and potential energy during gait, a relationship between the curves is readily observed (see Fig. 15–14). The times of maximum potential energy correspond to the times of minimum kinetic energy and vice versa. As potential energy is lost from mid stance to double-limb support (the CoM of the body going from its highest to its lowest location), kinetic energy is gained (the CoM of the body going from its minimum to maximum speed). Conversely, as kinetic energy

**Transfer of Energy During Gait**

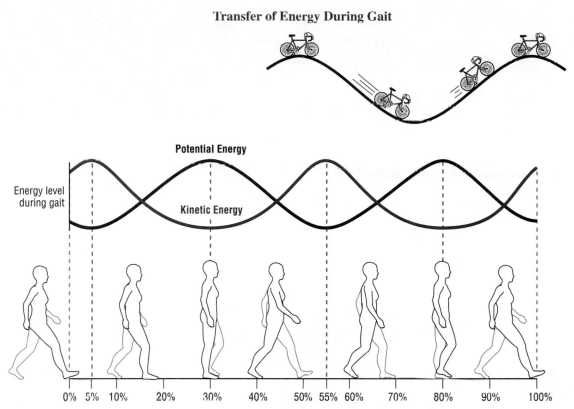

**FIGURE 15–14.** Transfer between potential and kinetic energy during gait. The minimum potential energy exists when the center of mass (CoM) is at its lowest points (5% and 55% of the gait cycle). The maximum potential energy occurs when the CoM is at its highest points (30% and 80% of the gait cycle). The reverse occurs for kinetic energy. For example, a bicycle that gains speed while going down a hill and loses speed while it climbs up the next hill illustrates the transfer between potential and kinetic energy.

is lost from double-limb support to mid stance, potential energy is gained. This cyclic transfer between kinetic and potential energy minimizes the metabolic cost of walking.

Despite the ability of the body to efficiently transfer and thereby conserve energy while walking, a net energy cost still occurs. This cost is proportional to the amount of medial-lateral and vertical displacement of the CoM.

## JOINT KINEMATICS

During gait, the body's CoM is displaced linearly as a result of the summation of the angular rotation of the joints of the lower extremities, which is not unlike a car moving forward owing to the rotation of its tires. Movements at the joints of the lower extremities, therefore, are described as a function of angular rotation. Although joint angular rotation occurs primarily in the sagittal plane, important motion, although of smaller magnitude, occurs in the frontal and horizontal planes.

> **Gait Kinematics are Described for the**
> * Sagittal plane
> * Frontal plane
> * Horizontal plane

Most often, the angular rotation that takes place at the joint itself is described (i.e., the relative motion of one bone compared with another). In some instances (e.g., for the sagittal plane motion of the pelvis), the movement of the bones in space is described without regard to the other bones that make up the adjacent joints. The reader must therefore be careful to recognize when a discussion pertains to joint kinematics and when it pertains to bone kinematics.

## Sagittal Plane Kinematics

Sagittal plane movement of the pelvis is small and is described here as movement of the bony structure itself. Conversely, the sagittal plane kinematics of the hip, knee, ankle, and first metatarsophalangeal joints are of larger magnitude and are described as joint motion. In this section, as in the entire chapter, the gait cycle is described from right heel contact to the subsequent right heel contact.

**Pelvis.** Movement of the pelvis in the sagittal plane is described in terms of anterior and posterior pelvic tilt about a medial-lateral axis (see Chapter 12). Neutral pelvis position is used as a reference. This neutral position (0 degrees) is defined as the orientation of the pelvis in relaxed stance. Because the pelvis is a relatively rigid structure, both iliac crests are considered as moving together. During gait at normal speed, the amount of anterior and posterior pelvic tilt is small (i.e., a total of approximately 2 to 4 degrees). Although the movement of the pelvis is described as an independent "detached" structure, this small movement takes place both at the hips (pelvic-on-femoral flexion/extension) and at the lumbosacral joint (pelvic-on-lumbar flexion/extension).

The pattern of motion of the pelvis over the full gait cycle resembles a sine wave with two full cycles (Fig. 15–15A). At

right heel contact, the pelvis is near neutral. From 0 to 10% of the gait cycle, a period of double-limb support, a small amount of posterior pelvic rotation (tilt) occurs. Then the pelvis starts tilting anteriorly during the period of single-limb support, reaching a slight anterior pelvic tilted position just after mid stance (30% of the gait cycle). In the second half of the stance phase, the pelvis tilts posteriorly until just after toe off. During initial and mid swing (60 to 87% of gait),

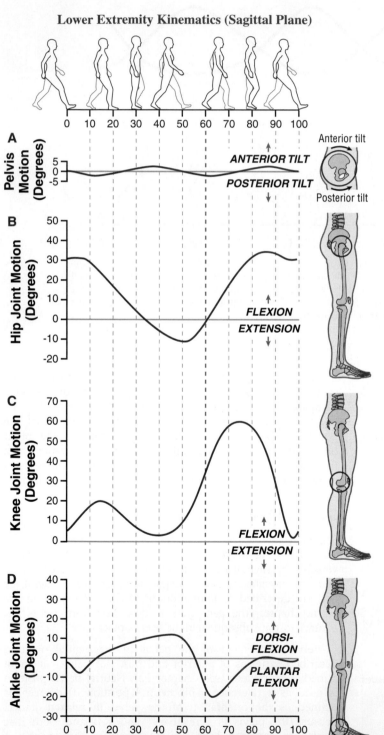

**Lower Extremity Kinematics (Sagittal Plane)**

**FIGURE 15–15.** Sagittal plane angular rotation of the pelvis (*A*), hip (*B*), knee (*C*), and ankle (*D*) during a gait cycle.

the pelvis again tilts anteriorly before starting to tilt in the posterior direction in terminal swing.

In general, pelvic motion increases when speed of ambulation increases.[34] Variability in the amount, timing, and direction of tilt, however, has been noted across walking speed. The greater magnitude of pelvic tilt with faster walking speed serves to increase functional leg length, which in turn serves to increase step length.

The sagittal plane tilt of the pelvis while walking is caused by the sum of the passive and active forces produced by the hip joint capsule and the hip flexor and extensor muscles. In pathologic situations, persons with marked hip flexion contractures show an exaggerated anterior tilt of the pelvis in the second half of the stance phase (i.e., between 30 and 60% of the gait cycle). The large passive tension in the shortened anterior hip structures creates a potent anterior tilting tendency often associated with an increased lumbar lordosis.

**Hip.** At a typical walking speed, the hip is flexed approximately 30 degrees at heel contact (Fig. 15–15B). As the body moves forward over the fixed foot, the hip extends. Maximum hip extension of approximately 10 degrees is achieved prior to toe off. Flexion of the hip is initiated during pre swing, and the hip is at about 0 degrees of flexion/extension by toe off (60% of gait). During the swing phase, the hip further flexes to bring the lower extremity forward for the next foot placement. Maximum flexion (slightly more than 30 degrees) is achieved just prior to heel contact. Note that at heel contact, the hip has already started to extend in preparation for weight acceptance. Overall, approximately 30 degrees of flexion and 10 degrees of extension, from anatomic neutral position, are needed at the hip for normal walking. As for all of the joints of the lower extremities, the magnitude of hip movement is proportional to walking speed.

Individuals with limited hip mobility may appear to walk without gait deviations. The movement of the pelvis and lumbar spine, compensating for reduced hip motion, may remain unnoticed. Apparent hip extension can be achieved through an anterior pelvic tilt and associated increase in lumbar lordosis. Conversely, a posterior pelvic tilt accompanied by a flattening of the lumbar spine provides apparent hip flexion. To ambulate, individuals with a fused (i.e., ankylosed) hip use an exaggerated posterior and anterior pelvic tilt to compensate for the absence of hip mobility (Fig. 15–16). Because the pelvis and lumbar spine motions are mechanically linked at the sacroiliac joint, exaggerated pelvic

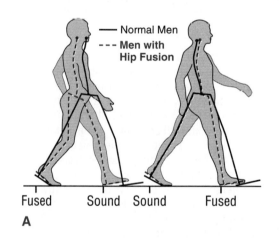

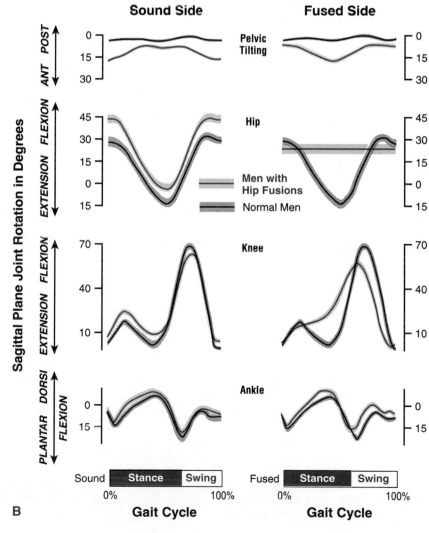

**FIGURE 15–16.** Body diagram (A) and average sagittal plane kinematic patterns (B) of men with unilateral hip fusion (red lines) compared with men with normal hip motion. The lack of mobility of one hip drastically affects motion of the pelvis, the ipsilateral knee, and the contralateral hip. Less significant effects are noted at the contralateral knee and at both ankles. This figure illustrates how impairment (i.e., reduced mobility of the hip) that affects a single joint will affect motion of the other joints. (Modified from Gore DR, Murray MP, Sepic SB, Gardner GM: Walking patterns of men with unilateral surgical hip fusion. J Bone Joint Surg 57A:759, 1975.)

### Abnormal Pelvic Motion as an Indicator of Hip Pathology

Although a completely fused hip is a relatively rare occurrence, limited hip range of movement due to orthopedic and neurologic disorders is not uncommon. Tight hip flexors, which limit hip extension, may be present in the elderly with a hip flexion contracture as well as in individuals with cerebral palsy and hip flexor spasticity. Limited hip motion may also be present in those with advanced hip osteoarthritis. Clinically, pelvic motion is evaluated during observational gait analysis because excessive pelvic tilt is a clue to a possible pathology that limits hip motion.

tilting may increase the stress at the lumbar spine. These stresses could eventually irritate the structures within this region, resulting in low back pain.

**Knee.** The kinematic pattern of the knee is a little more complex than that of the hip (Fig. 15–15C). At heel contact, the knee is flexed approximately 5 degrees and it continues to flex an additional 10 to 15 degrees, during the initial 15% of the gait cycle. This slight knee flexion, controlled by eccentric action of the quadriceps, serves the purpose of shock absorption and weight acceptance as body weight is progressively transferred to this lower extremity. Following initial flexion, the knee extends to nearly full extension until about heel off (40% of the gait cycle). At this point the knee starts flexing, reaching approximately 35 degrees of flexion by the time of toe off (60% of gait). Maximum knee flexion of approximately 60 degrees is assumed by the beginning of mid swing (73% of gait). Knee flexion during initial swing serves to shorten the length of the lower limb, facilitating toe clearance. In mid and terminal swing, the knee extends to just short of full extension in preparation for heel contact.

Normal function of the knee during gait on a level surface requires range of motion from nearly full extension to approximately 60 degrees of flexion. A limitation of knee extension (i.e., knee flexion contracture) results in a functionally shorter leg, affecting the kinematics of both the stance leg and the swing leg. The stance leg, lacking full knee extension, must assume a "crouched" position, involving the hip, knee, and ankle, and the normal swing leg needs greater knee and, possibly, hip flexion to clear the toes. The uneven functional leg length also leads to excessive trunk and CoM movement, increasing the metabolic demands of walking. A flexed knee posture during gait also increases the muscular demand on the knee extensors, resulting in further metabolic costs.

A lack of sufficient knee flexion during the swing phase of gait interferes with toe clearance as the foot moves forward. To compensate, the hip must flex excessively. If the knee is immobilized in full extension with an orthosis or a cast, more noticeable compensations, such as hip "hiking" and hip circumduction, are required.

**Ankle (Talocrural Joint).** At the ankle, heel contact occurs with the talocrural joint in a slightly plantar flexed position (between 0 and 5 degrees) (Fig. 15–15D). Shortly after heel contact (the first 8% of the gait cycle), the foot is positioned flat on the ground by the movement of plantar flexion controlled eccentrically by the ankle dorsiflexors. Then, up to 10 degrees of ankle dorsiflexion occurs as the tibia moves forward over the planted foot (from 8 to 45% of the gait cycle). Shortly after heel off (40% of the gait cycle), the ankle starts to plantar flex, reaching a maximum of 15 to 20 degrees of plantar flexion just after toe off. During the swing phase, the ankle is again dorsiflexed to a neutral position to allow the toes to clear the ground.

Average speed of ambulation requires approximately 10 degrees of dorsiflexion and 20 degrees of plantar flexion. Interestingly, greater dorsiflexion is needed during the stance phase than during the swing phase of gait. Similar to the knee and the hip, limitation of motion at the ankle leads to an abnormal gait pattern. For example, limited ankle plantar flexion may result in a decreased push off, possibly leading to a shorter step length.

### Summary of Sagittal Plane Kinematics

Several underlying principles govern sagittal plane motion of the joints of the lower extremities. At heel contact, the joints of the lower extremity are aligned to "reach forward," or to elongate the lower extremity, in order to position the foot on the ground. Shortly after heel contact, controlled knee flexion and ankle plantar flexion cushion loading for a smooth weight acceptance. All the joints of the supporting lower extremity then extend in order to support the weight of the body at the necessary height so that the foot of the contralateral swing leg can clear the ground. During swing, all the joints of the swing leg participate in shortening the lower extremity to bring the foot forward without tripping on the ground. In terminal swing, the lower extremity again "reaches forward" for the next heel contact.

The level of control of the lower limbs during ambulation is remarkable.[98] During swing, typical toe clearance (the minimum distance between the toes and the floor) is only 0.8 to 0.9 cm. This minimum clearance occurs at mid swing, when the foot actually has its greatest linear horizontal speed (4.5 m/s). The transition from the swing to the stance phase is also amazingly well controlled. To provide smooth contact with the ground, vertical heel speed slows just prior to heel contact to only 0.05 m/s. This level of control is the basis of the argument against using the term heel "strike" to describe the typically well-controlled heel contact with the ground. Further evidence of the fine control taking place during walking is expressed by the small clearance observed between the edge of the steps and the foot during stair descent.[78]

Conversely, a lack of adequate dorsiflexion mobility during stance, due to a tight heel cord, for example, may cause a premature heel off, resulting in a "bouncing"-type gait. Interestingly, limited dorsiflexion may also lead to a shorter step length because the body is "bouncing" excessively up and down instead of moving forward. A "toeing-out" gait pattern can somewhat compensate for limited ankle dorsiflexion. With excessive toeing-out of the foot, the individual rolls off the medial aspect of the foot in the second half of stance phase. Although toeing-out reduces the need for ankle dorsiflexion, it increases the stress applied to the medial structures of the foot and the knee.

In extreme cases where there is a pes equinus deformity (i.e., fixed plantar flexion of the ankle), the individual may walk on hyperextended toes and the heel never comes in contact with the ground. This condition is most often observed in individuals with cerebral palsy.

Limited ankle dorsiflexion also intereferes with clearing the toes during swing phase. To compensate, increased knee and/or hip flexion may be needed. Limited dorsiflexion in swing may be due to plantar flexor tightness, calf spasticity, or ankle dorsiflexor weakness.

**First Tarsometatarsal Joint.** The first tarsometatarsal joint, the function of which is described in Chapter 14, has a slight amount of plantar and dorsiflexion that contributes to the overall flexibility of the foot's medial longitudinal arch during gait.[28]

**First Metatarsophalangeal Joint.** The metatarsophalangeal (MTP) joint of the hallux (great toe) is crucial to normal gait. At heel contact, the MTP joint is slightly hyperextended. From shortly after heel contact to heel off, the MTP joint is in a relatively neutral position. Between heel off to just prior to toe off, the MTP joint hyperextends approximately 45 to 55 degrees. (This is the angle measured between the long axis of the first metatarsal and the proximal phalanx of the hallux.[34]) During the late part of stance phase and initial swing, the joint flexes and returns to the neutral position.

Limited MTP joint hyperextension due to a soft tissue injury, such as a joint sprain (turf-toe) or degeneration of the joint (hallux rigidus), typically results in an exaggerated toeing-out gait. One consequence of this abnormal gait pattern is a less efficient push off. Toeing-out also creates increased stress to the medial structures of the knee and foot, including the hallux, as mentioned earlier.

## Frontal Plane Kinematics

Joint rotations within the frontal plane are of smaller amplitude compared with those in the sagittal plane. Yet, these rotations are important, especially at the hip and subtalar joints.

**Pelvis.** Frontal plane motion of the pelvis during walking is best observed from in front of or behind the individual, watching the iliac crests rise and fall. The pelvis rotates through a total excursion of about 10 to 15 degrees as a result of pelvic-on-femoral (hip) adduction and abduction on the stance limb. During weight acceptance on the right lower extremity (i.e., the first 15 to 20% of the gait cycle), the pelvis drops on the swing (left) side owing to pelvic-on-femoral adduction of the right stance hip (Fig. 15–17A).

**FIGURE 15–17.** Frontal plane pelvis and hip motion for a full gait cycle starting with right heel contact. *A* illustrates that during right stance phase, the left iliac crest initially drops before progressively moving upward in late stance. The relatively higher left iliac crest during right swing phase reflects the drop of the right iliac crest when the right foot is off the ground. *B* illustrates frontal plane hip motion, accounting for the frontal plane motion of the pelvis and the femur. (Data from Ounpuu S: Clinical gait analysis. In Spivack BS (ed): Evaluation and Management of Gait Disorders. New York, Marcel Dekker, 1995.)

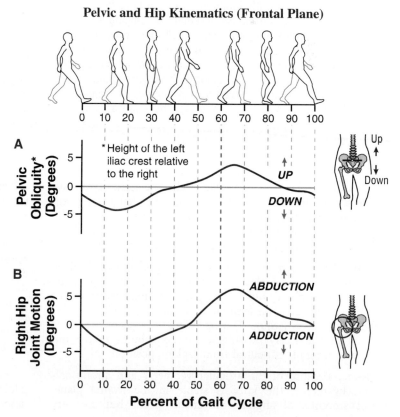

Pelvic and Hip Kinematics (Frontal Plane)

Percent of Gait Cycle

## SPECIAL FOCUS 15-5

**Possible Causes For Excessive Hip Frontal Plane Motion**

Excessive frontal plane movement of the stance hip is quite common, causing exaggerated medial-lateral shifts in the CoM. There are at least three reasons why excessive movement of the pelvis and hip in the frontal plane may be observed: weakness of the hip abductors, reduced "shortening" of the swing leg, and a discrepancy in leg length.

The drop of the contralateral iliac crest (i.e., hip adduction) during early to mid stance is normally controlled by an eccentric activation of the hip abductor muscles of the stance leg. Inadequate abduction torque from these muscles often leads to excessive frontal plane motion during stance.[62] While standing on one limb, a person with moderate hip abductor weakness demonstrates an excessive drop of the pelvis to the side of the lifted leg (Fig. 15–18). This action is referred to as a positive Trendelenburg sign. Typically, however, a person with weakened hip abductors, especially if severe, compensates by leaning the trunk to the side of the weakened muscle during any single-limb support activities, whether standing or walking. While walking, this is called a "compensated" Trendelenburg gait or gluteus medius limp. Leaning of the trunk to the side of weakness minimizes the external torque demands, due to body weight, on the abductor muscles of the stance leg.

Another deviation that is observed by looking at the movement of the pelvis in the frontal plane is called hip hiking. Hip hiking on the side of the swing leg compensates for the inability of the knee and/or ankle of the lower extremity to sufficiently shorten the limb for clearance of the foot. The classic example is walking with a knee orthosis, keeping the knee in full extension. Hip hiking is more accurately described as the excessive elevation of the iliac crest on the side of the swing leg. Elevation results from pelvic-on-femoral abduction of the stance leg. Muscles involved in this movement include the primary abductors of the stance leg, the quadratus lumborum of the swing leg, and possibly the abdominals and back extensors on the side of the swing leg.

A significant leg length difference also affects movement of the pelvis in the frontal plane. Leg length discrepancy can be severe, secondary to a fracture of the femur or a unilateral coxa valga, or it can be slight (<0.5 cm) owing to natural variability. During periods of double-limb support, the iliac crest of the longer leg is positioned higher than the iliac crest of the shorter leg. This pelvic obliquity, which is occurring for every gait cycle, results in increased side bending of the lumbar spine.

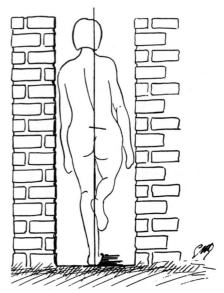

**FIGURE 15–18.** Excessive drop of the right iliac crest and lean of the trunk toward the left stance leg are characteristic of weakness of the left gluteus medius. (From Calve J, Galland M, De Cagny R: Pathogenesis of the limp due to coxalgia: The antalgic gait. J Bone Joint Surg 21A:12, 1939.)

---

Between 20 and 60% of the gait cycle, the right stance hip progressively abducts, thereby elevating the left (swing leg) iliac crest. Throughout most of the right swing phase, the right iliac crest progressively drops as a consequence of the pelvic-on-femoral hip adduction of the left stance hip.

**Hip.** The pattern of elevation and depression of the iliac crests reflects frontal plane hip motion (Fig. 15–17B). During the stance phase, hip frontal plane motion results almost entirely from pelvic-on-femoral movement (see Chapter 12, pelvis moving on femur). During swing, motion of the pelvis as well as the freely moving femur contributes to the hip joint returning to its neutral frontal plane position.

**Knee.** Because of the articular geometry and strong collateral ligaments, the knee is stable in the frontal plane. Small amounts of angular movement occur but are very difficult to quantify. Pins inserted in the cortices of the femur and the tibia demonstrate that at a walking speed of 1.2 m/sec, an average of 1.2 degrees of knee abduction (valgus) is present at the time of heel contact (Fig. 15–19).[44] This alignment remains unchanged throughout the stance phase. The knee usually abducts an additional 5 degrees during initial swing. This maximum abduction occurs when the knee is near its maximum flexion angle in the sagittal plane. The knee returns to its slightly abducted position prior to the next heel contact. Advanced osteoarthritic changes and abnormal lower extremity alignments (e.g., genu valgum) may affect frontal plane motion of the knee.

**Ankle (Talocrural Joint).** The primary motion of the talocrural joint is dorsiflexion/plantar flexion. Although as described in Chapter 14, the ankle everts and abducts

**Knee Kinematics (Frontal Plane)**

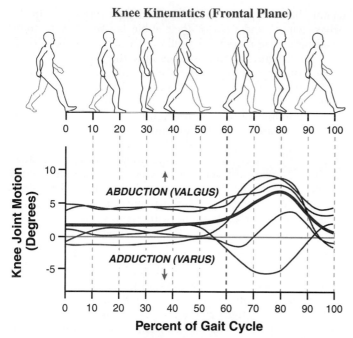

**FIGURE 15–19.** Frontal plane angular motion of the knee is illustrated. The red line is the average of four of the five subjects. The gray lines are each subject's individual data. (Data from Lafortune MA, Cavanagh PR, Sommer III HJ, Kalenak A: Three-dimensional kinematics of the human knee during walking. J Biomech 25:347, 1992.)

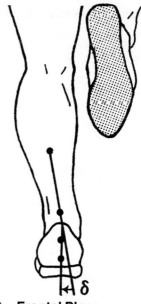

**δ = Frontal Plane
Subtalar Joint Angle**

**FIGURE 15–20.** Method to measure rear foot (subtalar joint) motion. The inversion/eversion angle, made by the lines bisecting the lower leg and the calcaneus, is measured as a simplified indicator of the amount of foot pronation/supination. This measurement can be made using a video system. (Modified from McClay IS: The use of gait analysis to enhance the understanding of running injuries. In Craik RL, Oatis CA (eds): Gait Analysis: Theory and Application. St. Louis, Mosby, 1995.)

slightly with dorsiflexion and inverts and adducts slightly with plantar flexion, these secondary frontal and horizontal plane motions are very small and are ignored here.

**Foot/Subtalar Joint.** The triplanar motions of pronation and supination occur through interaction of the subtalar and transverse tarsal joints. Pronation combines components of eversion, abduction, and dorsiflexion; supination combines inversion, adduction, and plantar flexion. This chapter considers the frontal plane motions of subtalar joint eversion and inversion to represent the more global motions of foot pronation and supination, respectively. Subtalar motions are typically measured as the angle made between the posterior aspect of the calcaneus and the posterior aspect of the lower leg (Fig. 15–20).

The subtalar joint is inverted approximately 2 to 3 degrees at the time of heel contact (Fig. 15–21). Immediately after heel contact, rapid eversion of the calcaneus begins and continues until mid stance (30 to 35% of the gait cycle), where a maximally everted position of approximately 2 degrees is reached. At that time, the subtalar joint reverses its direction of movement and starts toward inversion. Normally, a relatively neutral position of the calcaneus is reached at about 40 to 45% of the gait cycle, at approximately heel off. Between heel off and toe off, calcaneal inversion continues until it reaches a value of approximately 6 degrees of inversion.[14] During swing, the calcaneus returns to a slightly inverted position in preparation for the next heel contact. This pattern of motion is generally agreed upon in the literature; however, the reported amount of foot pronation during gait varies based on the techniques and preferences for measurement. Reischl and coworkers,[70] using a

three-dimensional model of the foot, report a mean peak pronation of 10.5 ± 3.4 degrees, occurring at 26.8 ± 8.7% of the gait cycle, on their sample of 30 subjects.

The movement of foot pronation/supination during walking is accompanied by changes in height of the foot's medial longitudinal arch. A detailed review of foot kinesiology and function, including the fall and rise of the medial longitudinal arch during gait, is provided in Chapter 14.

**SPECIAL FOCUS 15–6**

**Summary of Frontal Plane Kinematics**

The best location to observe frontal plane kinematics of the joints of the lower extremities is from behind the individual. Hip motion plays an important role in minimizing the vertical displacement of the body's CoM. The rapid pronation (eversion) of the foot after heel contact participates in the process of weight acceptance and provides a flexible and adaptable structure for making contact with the ground. Later in the stance phase, between heel off and toe off, the inversion of the calcaneus associated with supination of the foot provides a more rigid foot structure, which helps propel the body forward.

## Subtalar Joint Kinematics (Frontal Plane)

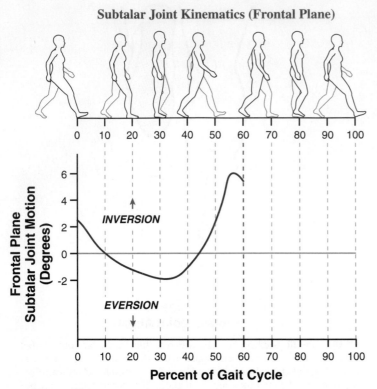

**FIGURE 15–21.** Frontal plane inversion/eversion of the calcaneus as an indicator of subtalar joint motion while walking. (Data from Cornwall MW, McPoil TG: Three-dimensional movement of the foot during the stance phase of walking. J Am Podiatr Med Assoc 89:56, 1999.)

## Horizontal Plane Kinematics

Information currently available about lower extremity kinematics in the horizontal plane is provided by a limited number of studies. To improve the accuracy of measurements, inves-

tigators have on some occasions fixed rigid metal pins in the pelvis, femur, and tibia of their subjects. Attached to these metal pins were markers that allowed video cameras to track bone movement. In some studies only the movement of the bony structures in space was observed; other researchers described the relative motion that took place at the joint itself.[35,44]

In the following section, rotation of the pelvis, femur, and tibia describes horizontal plane movement of the bone itself. Conversely, movement of the hip and knee refers to the rotation taking place at these articulations. Most of the studies that describe horizontal plane kinematics include a small number of typically healthy young individuals. Generalization to a larger population and a population with gait deviations, therefore, must be done with some degree of reservation.

**Pelvis.** During walking, the pelvis rotates in the horizontal plane about a vertical axis of rotation through the hip joint of the stance leg. The following description of pelvic rotation is based on a top view for a right gait cycle. At right heel contact, the right anterior-superior iliac spine (ASIS) is forward compared with the left ASIS. For the initial 15 to 20% of gait, counterclockwise rotation of the pelvis takes place (Fig. 15–22). Throughout the rest of stance on the right lower extremity, a clockwise rotation of the pelvis occurs as the left ASIS progressively moves forward along with the advancing left swing leg. At right toe off, the right ASIS is now behind the left. During swing of the right lower extremity, the right ASIS progressively moves forward. Throughout the gait cycle, the pelvis rotates 3 to 4 degrees in each direction. A greater amount of rotation of the pelvis occurs with increasing walking speed to increase step length.

**Femur.** After heel contact, the femur rotates internally for the first 15 to 20% of the gait cycle (see Fig. 15–22). At about 20% of the gait cycle, it reverses its direction and rotates externally until shortly after toe off. Internal rotation of the femur takes place throughout most of the swing phase. Overall, the femur rotates approximately 6 to 7 degrees in each direction during gait.[11]

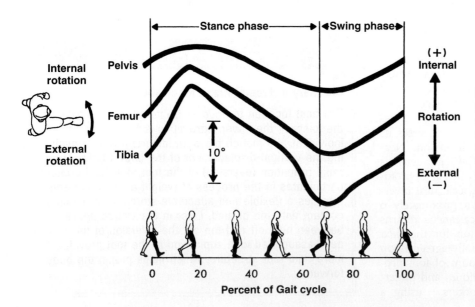

**FIGURE 15–22.** Pattern of horizontal plane motion of the pelvis, femur, and tibia. The pattern of motion is similar for the three bony structures, with progressively larger amplitude of movement for the more distal structures. For the right lower extremity, the clockwise motion corresponds to external rotation. (From Mann RA: Biomechanics of the foot. In American Academy of Orthopedic Surgeons (ed): Atlas of Orthotics: Biomechanical Principles and Application. St. Louis, Mosby, 1975.)

**Tibia.** The pattern of movement of the tibia is very similar to the movement described for the femur (see Fig. 15–22). The magnitude of the rotation is about 8 to 9 degrees in each direction.

**Hip.** Both the femur and the pelvis rotate simultaneously. At right heel contact, the right hip is in slight external rotation based on the relative posterior position of the contralateral (left) ASIS (Fig. 15–23). A net internal rotation movement of the right hip occurs during most of stance on the right lower extremity as the contralateral (left) ASIS is brought forward. A maximum internally rotated position is achieved by 50% of gait. External rotation of the right hip occurs from 50% of gait until mid swing, as the right leg is picked up and brought forward. From mid swing to right heel contact, a slight amount of right hip internal rotation takes place.[84]

**Knee.** At the time of heel contact, the knee is in a position of 2 to 3 degrees of relative external rotation (i.e., the tibia is externally rotated relative to the femur). Throughout stance, the knee progressively internally rotates by virtue of the greater internal rotation of the tibia as compared with the femur. By toe off, the knee approaches about 5 degrees of relative internal rotation. Again, the tibia being relative to the femur. During swing, the joint externally rotates in preparation for the next heel contact (Fig. 15–24).[44]

Disruption of synchrony of movement between the tibia and femur (e.g., as a result of excessive pronation of the foot) may cause knee pain with walking and running. Validation of this concept is impeded by the difficulty of accurately measuring the knee's horizontal plane rotation during gait.

### Knee Kinematics (Horizontal Plane)

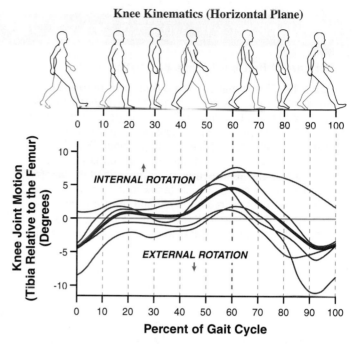

**FIGURE 15–24.** Horizontal plane angular motion of the knee. The red line is the average of the five subjects. The gray lines are each subject's individual data. (Data from Lafortune MA, Cavanagh PR, Sommer III HJ, Kalenak A: Three-dimensional kinematics of the human knee during walking. J Biomech 25:347, 1992.)

**Ankle and Foot.** Horizontal plane rotation of the talocrural joint is slight and is not considered here. The primary movement of the subtalar joint (inversion and eversion) is in the frontal plane and is described earlier.

## Trunk and Upper Extremity Kinematics

The role of the trunk and upper extremities in maintaining balance and minimizing energy expenditure during gait must be recognized.

**Trunk.** During ambulation, translation of the CoM follows the general pattern of translation of the trunk (see Fig. 15–13). In addition to its translational movement, the trunk rotates in the horizontal plane, about a vertical axis. The shoulder girdle rotates in the opposite direction of the pelvis. The average total rotational excursion of the shoulder girdle is approximately 7 degrees.[54] This pattern of movement of the trunk is believed to be important to the overall efficiency of gait. Restriction of trunk motion increases energy expenditure during walking by as much as 10%.[68]

**Shoulder.** In the sagittal plane, the shoulder exhibits a sinusoidal pattern of movement that is out of phase with hip flexion/extension. As the hip (femur) moves toward extension, the ipsilateral shoulder (humerus) moves toward flexion and vice versa. At heel contact, the shoulder is in its maximally extended position of approximately 25 degrees from the anatomically neutral position. The shoulder then progressively rotates forward to reach a maximum of 10 degrees of flexion by 50% of the gait cycle. In the second half of the gait cycle, as the ipsilateral hip moves forward

### Hip Kinematics (Horizontal Plane)

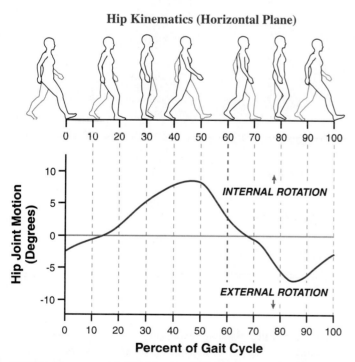

**FIGURE 15–23.** Horizontal plane angular motion of the hip. (Data from Sutherland DH, Kaufman KR, Moitoza JR: Kinematics of normal human walking. In Rose J, Gamble JG (eds): Human Walking, 2nd ed. Philadelphia, Williams & Wilkins, 1994.)

### SPECIAL FOCUS 15–7

**Summary of Horizontal Plane Kinematics**

Figure 15–25 summarizes the direction of horizontal plane rotation of the major bones of the lower extremity and subtalar joint during walking, using different sets of data.[14,30,46] The pelvis, femur, and tibia rotate internally, well after heel contact (i.e., through about 15 to 20% of the gait cycle). This mass internal rotation is accompanied by subtalar joint eversion. As described in Chapter 14, an everting subtalar joint tends to increase the pliability of the midfoot region, including the transverse tarsal joint. A pliable midfoot serves to cushion the impact of limb loading. After about 15 to 20% of the gait

cycle, the pelvis, femur, and tibia all begin to externally rotate until toe off. Simultaneously, after a slight delay, the subtalar joint starts moving toward inversion, which tends to increase the stability of the midfoot region. This stability enables the midfoot to serve as a rigid lever in terminal stance and pre swing, allowing the plantar flexors to lift the calcaneus without the midfoot collapsing under the body's weight. Further investigation, such as that performed by Reischl and colleagues,[70] is needed to clearly elucidate the exact relationship that exists between the timing and magnitude of pronation of the foot and rotation of the femur and tibia.

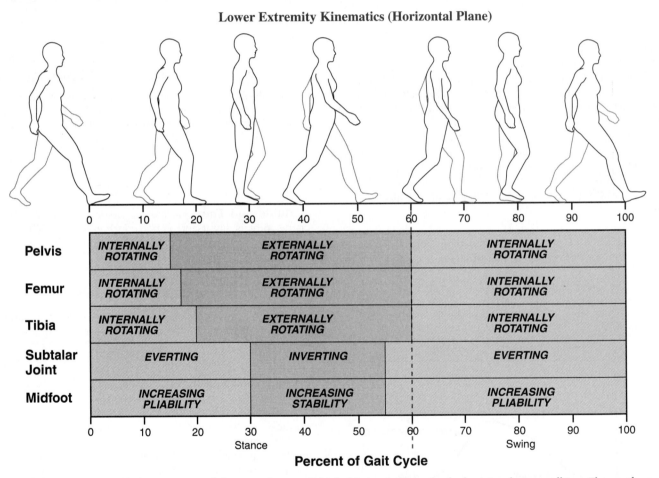

**FIGURE 15–25.** Horizontal plane rotation of the major bones of the lower extremity and subtalar joint during walking. The graph shows the direction of rotation, which is not necessarily the same as the absolute joint position.

toward flexion, the shoulder extends to return to 25 degrees of extension by the next heel contact.

The pattern of movement of the shoulder is consistent across individuals, although the magnitude of movement varies greatly. In general, the amplitude of shoulder movement increases with greater speed. Arm swing is partly active,

rather than fully passive, especially for the movement of extension that requires activation of the posterior deltoid muscle.[93] The major function of arm swing is to balance the rotational forces in the trunk.[19] Restriction of arm motion has not been shown to have a significant effect on the energy cost of ambulation.[68]

**Elbow.** The elbow is in approximately 20 degrees of flexion at heel contact. As the shoulder moves into flexion in the first 50% of the gait cycle, the elbow flexes to a maximum of approximately 45 degrees. In the second half of the gait cycle, as the shoulder extends, the elbow extends to return to 20 degrees of flexion.[54]

## Kinematic Strategies to Minimize Energy Expenditure

During gait, five kinematic strategies are used to minimize the displacement of the CoM. In turn, they optimize energy efficiency. Vertical displacement of the CoM is reduced by the combined actions of the first four strategies. The fifth strategy serves to minimize the medial-lateral displacement of the CoM (Table 15–3). The strategies detailed in this chapter are based on the six determinants of gait originally described by Saunders and colleagues in 1953.[73] A detailed account of the determinants is found in Inman and colleagues.[34,35]

To appreciate the usefulness of these five strategies, envision gait without such mechanisms. This can be duplicated by using two pencils connected at the eraser ends (Fig. 15–26A). When walking, a large vertical oscillation of the eraser end of the pencils (the body's CoM) is readily observed. The eraser end is highest when the pencils are side by side in a vertically oriented position (i.e., mid stance). Conversely, the eraser end is lowest when the pencils are maximally angled (i.e., double-limb support). This gait pattern results in a large displacement of the CoM.

### MINIMIZING VERTICAL DISPLACEMENT OF THE CENTER OF MASS

Limiting the downward displacement of the CoMs is achieved by horizontal plane pelvic rotation and sagittal plane ankle rotation. Horizontal plane rotation of the pelvis advances the entire swing leg forward, thereby minimizing the amount of hip flexion and extension needed for a given step length (compare Fig. 15–26A with Fig. 15–26B). As a consequence of the lower extremities remaining closer to a vertical orientation throughout the gait cycle, the lowest points of the CoM trajectory are raised, which reduces the downward displacement of the CoM. Sagittal plane ankle rotation makes use of the inverted T-shaped configuration of the ankle/foot complex (Fig. 15–26C). At heel contact, the

alignment of the ankle places the large protruding calcaneus in contact with the ground, functionally elongating the lower extremity. Near the end of stance, as the hip extends and the knee starts to flex, the lower extremity is elongated by plantar flexion of the ankle (i.e., heel rise). This functional elongation of the lower extremity at both ends of stance phase further reduces the downward displacement of the CoM (compare Fig. 15–26B with Fig. 15–26C).[39]

Limiting the upward displacement of the CoM is partially achieved by stance phase knee flexion, when the lower extremity is in its most vertical orientation (Fig. 15–26D). Frontal plane pelvic rotation further assists in minimizing upward displacement of the CoM (Fig. 15–26E). During stance phase, the contralateral iliac crest falls as the ipsilateral iliac crest rises. Throughout a complete gait cycle, therefore, the iliac crests alternately rise and fall like the ends of a see saw, but the point just anterior to S2 (i.e., the point representing the body's CoM) remains relatively stationary, as would the pivot point of a seesaw. This frontal plane seesaw action of the iliac crests minimizes the vertical oscillation of the body's CoM.

As shown in Figure 15–27, the combination of the four strategies minimizes the total net vertical displacement of the CoM. The downward displacement of the CoM is reduced by horizontal plane pelvic rotation and sagittal plane ankle rotation. The upward displacement of the CoM is reduced by stance phase knee flexion and frontal plane pelvic rotation.

### MINIMIZING MEDIAL-LATERAL DISPLACEMENT OF THE CENTER OF MASS

While a person walks, his or her CoM shifts side to side and remains within the dynamic base of support provided by the feet (see Fig. 15–13). A person strives to minimize the amplitude of this medial-lateral displacement by reducing step width, which is a function of frontal plane hip motion (i.e., hip abduction/adduction).

Although reduced step width minimizes side-to-side displacement and therefore energy expenditure, it also decreases the size of the dynamic base of support. The average step width of 7 to 9 cm represents a mechanical compromise of being narrow enough to reduce side-to-side shifts of the CoM, but wide enough to provide an adequate base of support. A greater or lesser step width is associated with a trade-off in either energy expenditure or stability. Persons with balance disorders, for example, may choose a wider

**TABLE 15–3. Kinematic Strategies to Minimize Energy Expenditure During Gait**

| Direction of Action | Name of Strategy | Action |
|---|---|---|
| Vertical | Horizontal plane pelvic rotation | Minimizes the downward displacement of the center of mass (CoM) |
| Vertical | Sagittal plane ankle rotation | Minimizes the downward displacement of the CoM |
| Vertical | Stance phase knee flexion | Minimizes the upward displacement of the CoM |
| Vertical | Frontal plane pelvic rotation | Minimizes the upward displacement of the CoM |
| Medial-lateral | Frontal plane hip rotation (step width) | Minimizes the side-to-side excursion of the CoM |

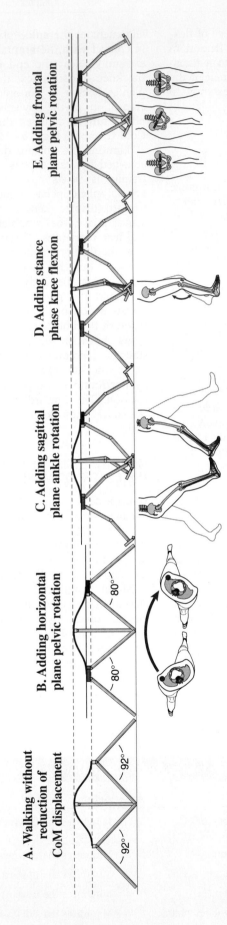

**FIGURE 15–26.** This series illustrates the individual and additive effects of four kinematic strategies to reduce vertical CoM excursion. *A* illustrates the large vertical oscillation of the CoM while walking without the strategies. *B* illustrates that rotation of the pelvis in the horizontal plane functionally lengthens the lower extremities and reduces the magnitude of the hip flexion-extension angle required for a given step length, thereby reducing the downward displacement of the CoM. *C* illustrates that further reduction of the downward displacement of the CoM is achieved by rotation of the ankle in the sagittal plane. *D* illustrates that the small amount of knee flexion present during stance reduces the functional length of the lower extremity and, therefore, the upward displacement of the CoM. *E* shows that the contralateral pelvic drop during stance also minimizes the net overall elevation of the CoM. The angle values in *A* and *B* are for illustrative purposes only and do not represent the actual hip angles during walking.

**A. Walking without reduction**
**of CoM displacement**

**B. Walking with reduction of**
**CoM displacement**

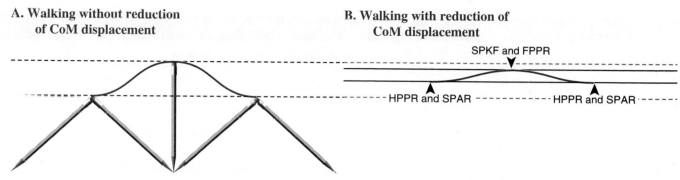

**FIGURE 15–27.** Combined action of the four kinematic strategies to reduce vertical CoM excursion. Without these strategies, a large vertical displacement of the body's CoM (red) would occur when walking (*A*). *B* illustrates the combined action of horizontal plane pelvic rotation (HPPR) and sagittal plane ankle rotation (SPAR) to minimize the downward displacement of the CoM during double-limb support. It also shows the action of stance phase knee flexion (SPKF) and frontal plane pelvic rotation (FPPR) to minimize the upward displacement of the CoM at mid stance.

base of support. They must pay for this benefit, however, by the associated increased energy cost of walking.

## ENERGY EXPENDITURE

Energy expenditure during gait is measured by the amount of energy used in kilocalories per meter walked per kilogram of body weight (kcal/m/kg). Typically, energy expenditure is measured indirectly by quantifying oxygen consumption.[72] When walking, the body strives to minimize energy cost. Conservation of energy is achieved by minimizing the excursion of the CoM, controlling the body momentum, and taking advantage of the intersegmental transfers of energy.

The gait speed at which optimal energy conservation occurs is approximately 1.33 m/s, or 80 m/min or 3 mph.[72]

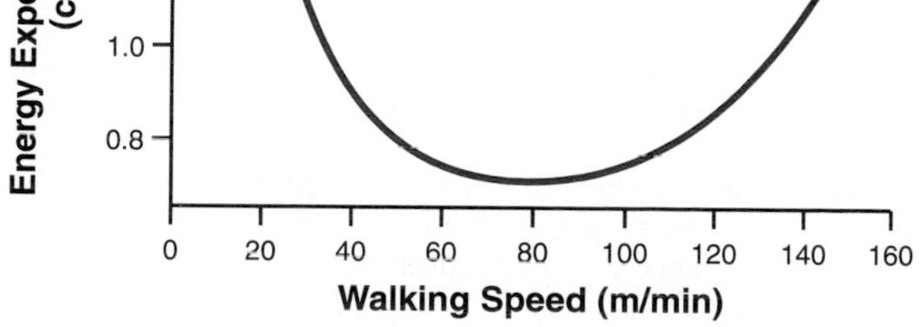

**Energy Expenditure During Walking**

FIGURE with graph: Y-axis "Energy Expenditure Per Meter (cal/kg/m)" with values 0.8, 1.0, 1.2, 1.4, 1.6; X-axis "Walking Speed (m/min)" with values 0, 20, 40, 60, 80, 100, 120, 140, 160.

**FIGURE 15–28.** Energy expenditure as a function of walking speed. The lowest energy expenditure per meter walked is at a speed of approximately 1.33 m/s (80 m/min). (Data from Ralston HJ: Effects of immobilization of various body segments on energy cost of human locomotion. Ergonomics Suppl:53, 1965.)

Not surprisingly, the speed at which the body is most energy efficient roughly corresponds to the walking speed freely adopted by individuals ambulating on the street (see Table 15–1). Walking faster or slower than that optimal speed increases the energy cost of ambulation (Fig. 15–28).

Walking speed is equal to the product of step length and cadence (step rate). Maximum energy efficiency at the optimal walking speed is achieved by the body's innate ability to adopt the ultimate combination of step length and step rate. Amazingly, this ability is demonstrated across all walking speeds. While the energy cost of ambulation changes across walking speeds, a standard and optimal ratio of step length to step rate of 0.0072 m/steps/min for men and 0.0064 m/steps/min for women is maintained.[102] At any given walking speed, imposition of a different step length or step rate increases energy expenditure.

With abnormal gait the energy cost of ambulation increases (Table 15–4). As a consequence of increased energy cost per distance walked, individuals with disability tend to walk slower so as to keep the rate of energy consumption per minute at a comfortable aerobic level. They naturally adopt a walking speed that is most efficient and comfortable for them. Further discussion of the energetics of walking in individuals with pathologic gaits can be found in Perry's textbook[67] and reviews of the literature by Gonzalez and Corcoran[29] and Waters and Mulroy.[92]

## MUSCLE ACTIVITY

During a gait cycle, most muscles of the lower extremities have one or two short bursts of electrical activity lasting from 100 to 400 msec (10 to 40% of the gait cycle). Like all other elements of gait, phasic muscular activation is repeated at each stride. Knowledge of when muscles are active during the gait cycle provides insight into their specific roles. Gait deviations can be more easily understood and treated when the clinician has a thorough knowledge of specific muscle function during ambulation.

Activity of the lower extremity musculature has been studied extensively using electromyography (EMG). Most often, muscular activity is expressed on a temporal basis; the

**TABLE 15-4. Increased Energy Cost of Walking Associated with Specific Conditions**

| Conditions | Increased Energy Cost (%) | Authors |
|---|---|---|
| Immobilization of one ankle | 3–6 | Ralston, 1965; Waters et al., 1988 |
| Immobilization of one knee in full extension | 23–33 | Kerrigan et al., 1995; Waters et al., 1982 |
| Immobilization of one knee at 45 degrees of flexion | 37 | Ralston, 1965 |
| Immobilization of one hip, arthrodesis | 32 | Waters et al., 1988 |
| Unilateral transtibial amputation, walking with prosthesis | 20–38 | Fisher and Gullickson, 1978 |
| Unilateral transfemoral amputation, walking with prosthesis | 20–60 | Fisher and Gullickson, 1978 |
| Postcerebrovascular accident, moderate-to-severe residual deficits | 55 | Corcoran et al., 1970 |

Percentage increase based on energy cost of normal gait.

muscle is simply considered "ON" or "OFF." The muscle is said to be ON when its EMG activity level reaches a predetermined value above the resting level. Otherwise, the muscle is considered to be OFF. The red horizontal bars used in Figure 15–29 illustrate when selected muscles are ON during the gait cycle. Another method to report muscular activity (the lighter shaded areas in Fig. 15–29) is to express the intensity of the EMG signal during gait as a percentage of the amount of EMG recorded during maximum voluntary contraction of the same muscle.[98] This type of analysis provides insight into the relative level of activation of the muscle (i.e., an index of muscular effort) throughout the gait cycle.

## Hip

Three muscle groups at the hip play a critical role during normal ambulation: the hip extensors, such as the gluteus maximus and the hamstrings; the hip flexors, such as the iliacus and the psoas; and the hip abductors, such as the gluteus medius and minimus. Less well documented is the role of the hip adductors and rotators.

**Hip Extensors.** Activation of the gluteus maximus starts in an eccentric manner at terminal swing. This mild muscular activation serves two purposes—decelerating hip flexion and preparing the musculature for weight acceptance at the beginning of stance. At heel contact, the gluteus maximus is strongly activated in order to extend the hip and prevent forward "jackknifing," or uncontrolled trunk flexion over the femur. This abnormal "jackknifing" occurs if pelvic motion were slowed following heel contact while the trunk continues its forward displacement. The gluteus maximus remains active from heel contact to mid stance (i.e., first 30% of the gait cycle) to support the weight of the body and produce hip extension. Strong activation of the gluteus maximus when the foot is firmly planted on the ground also assists indirectly with knee extension.

The hamstrings assist the gluteus maximus during the first 10% of the gait cycle. Similar to the gluteus maximus, the hamstrings serve to generate hip extension and to support the weight of the body to prevent the collapse of the lower extremity during early stance.

**Hip Flexors.** The iliacus and psoas become active prior to toe off to decelerate hip extension. Eccentric muscle activation is followed by concentric muscle activation to bring the hip into flexion just prior to toe off and into initial swing. Despite the movement of hip flexion continuing into terminal swing, the hip flexors are considered active only in the first 50% of swing. Hip flexion in the second half of the swing phase is a result of the forward momentum that the thigh gains in initial swing. The rectus femoris also acts as a hip flexor and therefore assists with the aforementioned actions. The key roles of the hip flexors are to advance the leg forward during swing in preparation for the next step and to lift the leg to allow for toe clearance during swing. The action of the sartorius is similar to that of the iliacus and psoas.

**Hip Abductors.** While hip flexors and extensors have their primary role in the sagittal plane, the hip abductors—gluteus medius, gluteus minimus, and tensor fascia lata—stabilize the pelvis in the frontal plane. The gluteus medius is active toward the very end of the swing phase in preparation for heel contact. The gluteus medius and minimus, the two primary hip abductors, are most active during the first 40% of the gait cycle, especially during single-limb support. The primary function of the abductors is to control the slight dropping of the pelvis to the side of the swing leg (see Fig. 15–17). Following this eccentric activation, these muscles act concentrically to initiate the relative abduction of the hip that occurs in later stance. As described earlier in this chapter, adequate frontal plane torque from the hip abductor muscles is crucial for frontal plane stability during gait (see Fig. 15–18). A cane used in the hand contralateral to the weak hip abductors is an effective way to reduce the demands placed on the weakened abductors, thereby reducing frontal plane instability of the pelvis due to body weight (see Chapter 12).

The hip abductors also control the alignment of the femur in the frontal plane. Inadequate muscular activation may result in excessive adduction of the femur, producing an excessive valgus torque at the knee during the stance phase. Other accessory roles of the gluteus medius include assisting with hip flexion and internal rotation, using anterior fibers, and assisting with hip extension and external rotation, using posterior fibers.

## Timing and Relative Intensity of EMG During Gait

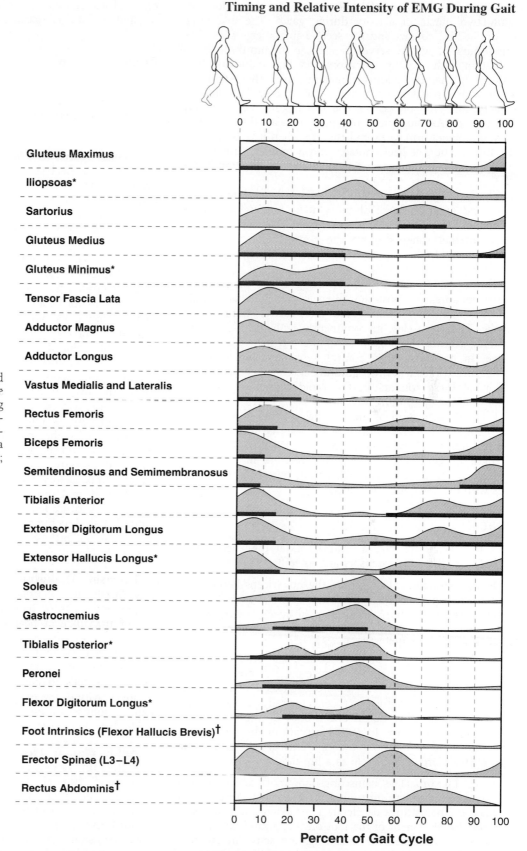

**FIGURE 15–29.** Timing (dark red bars) and relative intensity of muscle activation (light red shading) during gait. (Muscle timing data from Knutson and Soderberg, 1995; relative intensity of muscle activation data from Winter, 1991; Bechtol,* 1975; Carlsoo,† 1972.)

**Hip Adductors and Hip Rotators.** The hip adductors show two bursts of activity during gait.[98] The first burst occurs at heel contact and the second just after toe off. The initial burst of activity serves to stabilize the hip through co-activation with the hip extensors and hip abductors. It is also likely that the adductor magnus and other adductors assist with hip extension at that time. The second burst of activity, after toe off, assists the hip flexors with initiating hip flexion. As illustrated in Figure 12–36, the adductors have a moment arm to extend the hip when it is flexed (i.e., the hip position at heel contact) and a moment arm to flex the hip when it is in extension (i.e., the hip position at toe off).

The hip internal rotators (tensor fascia lata, gluteus minimus, and anterior fibers of the gluteus medius) are active throughout much of the stance phase. During this time, these internal rotators move the contralateral side of the pelvis forward, thereby assisting with advancement of the swing leg (see Fig. 12–39).

The hip external rotators, consisting of the six short external rotators, the posterior fibers of the gluteus medius, and the gluteus maximus, are most active during early stance. These muscles, in conjunction with the hip internal rotators, control the alignment of the hip in the horizontal plane. In particular, they control pelvic rotation while the lower limb is fixed to the ground. Consider the important action of these rotators in the rapid change of direction while walking or running.

Eccentric activation of the external rotators may be especially important to the control of the internal rotation of the lower limb in early stance (see Fig. 15–25). Inadequate strength or control of the external rotators may result in excessive internal rotation of the femur, especially in individuals with excessive foot pronation.

## Knee

Two muscle groups play a critical role at the knee during ambulation: the knee extensors and knee flexors.

**Knee Extensors.** As a group, the quadriceps become active in the very late stage of swing in preparation for heel contact. The major burst of activity, however, occurs shortly after heel contact. The function of the quadriceps at this time is to control the knee flexion that takes place in the first 10% of the gait cycle. Eccentric activation serves to cushion the rate of weight acceptance on the lower extremity (i.e., shock absorption) and to prevent excessive knee flexion. The quadriceps then act concentrically to extend the knee and support the weight of the body during mid stance. Some individuals show increased activity of the rectus femoris immediately following toe off. This action reflects the role of this biarticular muscle as a hip flexor.

**Knee Flexors.** The hamstrings are most active from a period just before to just after heel contact. Before heel contact, the hamstrings decelerate knee extension in preparation for the placement of the foot on the ground. During the initial 10% of stance, the hamstrings are active in order to assist with hip extension and to provide stability to the knee through co-activation. The short head of the biceps femoris may also assist with knee flexion during the swing phase. Most of the knee flexion during pre swing and the swing

phase of gait results from passive intersegmental dynamics of the limb and a small gastrocnemius activation.[75,98]

## Ankle and Foot

At the ankle, several muscles play a crucial role in normal gait: the tibialis anterior, extensor digitorum, extensor hallucis longus, gastrocnemius, soleus, tibialis posterior, and peroneals.

**Tibialis Anterior.** The tibialis anterior has two periods of activity. At heel contact, a strong eccentric activation is present to decelerate the passive plantar flexion of the ankle caused by the weight of the body being applied on the most posterior section of the calcaneus. Unopposed by the eccentric activation of the tibialis anterior and other ankle dorsiflexors, this large, passive plantar flexion torque results in the gait deviation referred to as "foot slap." This term is derived from the characteristic sound made by the foot slapping the ground just after heel contact. From heel contact to foot flat, the tibialis anterior may also assist with decelerating foot pronation, also an eccentric muscle activation. The poor mechanical advantage of the muscle to invert the foot, however, raises some doubt with regard to the effectiveness of the tibialis anterior in strongly controlling foot pronation.

The second action of the tibialis anterior is the dorsiflexion of the ankle during swing. The purpose of this muscle action is to clear the toes from the ground. Extreme weakness of the tibialis anterior and the other ankle dorsiflexors is expressed by the inability to dorsiflex the ankle during swing. This problem, known as "drop foot," causes an individual to excessively flex the knee and hip during swing. Other compensatory maneuvers, such as vaulting, hip circumduction, and hip hiking, may also be adopted to clear the toes. A drop foot causes the forefoot to contact the ground first. A common remedy for a drop foot is a posterior ankle-foot orthosis that passively maintains ankle dorsiflexion during swing.

**Extensor Digitorum and Extensor Hallucis Longus.** Similar to the tibialis anterior, the extensor digitorum longus and extensor hallucis longus decelerate plantar flexion of the ankle at heel contact. These muscles, however, lack the line-of-force to decelerate foot pronation during loading response and mid stance. During the swing phase, the toe extensors assist with dorsiflexion of the ankle and extend the toes to ensure that the toes clear the ground. Minor activity of the extensor digitorum longus and extensor hallucis longus during push off may provide stability to the ankle through co-activation with the ankle plantar flexors.[98]

**Ankle Plantar Flexors.** The soleus and gastrocnemius are active throughout most of the stance phase. From about 10 through 40% of the gait cycle (i.e., opposite toe off to heel off), the ankle plantar flexors eccentrically control the forward movement of the tibia on the foot (i.e., ankle dorsiflexion). Excessive or uncontrolled forward movement of the tibia results in exaggerated ankle dorsiflexion and possibly uncontrolled knee flexion. The major burst of activity of the ankle plantar flexors occurs near heel off and decreases rapidly to near zero at toe off. During that brief period, shortening of the muscles creates an ankle plantar flexion torque that participates in the forward propulsion of the body. This action is referred to as push off.

The gastrocnemius also generates low-level muscular activity in initial swing, presumably to help with knee flexion. Note that since the rectus femoris is also active during initial swing, a small amount of co-activation of the knee flexors and extensors is taking place.[90]

The other plantar flexors of the ankle (tibialis posterior, flexor hallucis longus, flexor digitorum longus, and peroneals) assist the gastrocnemius-soleus group in the previously described actions. Some additional actions of these muscles are noteworthy.

**Tibialis Posterior.** The tibialis posterior, a potent supinator muscle of the foot, is active between 5 and 55% of the gait cycle. Tibialis posterior decelerates pronation of the foot between 5 and about 35% of the cycle and supinates the foot between 35% and 55% (mid stance to toe off) of the cycle.[37]

The tibialis posterior receives special attention in the treatment of people with cerebral palsy. The often hyperactive tibialis posterior along with the soleus muscle may cause an equinovarus deformity of the foot and ankle, resulting in the individual's walking on a foot that is plantar flexed and supinated.

Active individuals with flat, overly pronated feet may develop a syndrome known as shin splints. This syndrome is due to overuse and subsequent strain of the tibialis posterior and/or anterior ankle muscles. The overuse is secondary to the increased work demands placed on the supinator muscles as they attempt to control the excessive pronation bias of the foot during early stance.

**Peronei.** The peroneus brevis and longus are active from about 20 to 30% of the gait cycle to just after heel off. In addition to their function as plantar flexors, these pronator (evertor) muscles help counteract the inversion of the foot caused by activation of the tibialis anterior and posterior leg muscles. The peronei help with the alignment and stabilization of the subtalar joint. The peroneus longus assists in the overall kinematics of the foot by placing the first ray rigidly on the ground, which provides a firm base of support for the action of the foot as a rigid lever during the terminal stance and pre swing phases of gait.

**Intrinsic Muscles of the Foot.** The intrinsic muscles of the foot are typically active from mid stance to toe off (30 to 60% of the gait cycle), particularly if the foot is not supported by well-fitting shoes. These muscles stabilize the forefoot and raise the medial longitudinal arch, thereby providing a rigid lever for ankle plantar flexion in terminal stance and pre swing.

## Trunk

Only the actions of the erector spinae and the rectus abdominis are discussed here.

**Erector Spinae.** The erector spinae at the level of the mid-lumbar region (L³-L⁴) show two periods of activity. The first period is from slightly before heel contact to about 20% of the gait cycle. The second period is from 45 to 70% of the gait cycle, which corresponds to opposite heel contact.

These two bursts of activity control the forward momentum of the trunk shortly after heel contact for each step.

**Rectus Abdominis.** This muscle has very low activity throughout the gait cycle. Nevertheless, increased activity occurs at 20% and again at 70% of the gait cycle. This activity may reflect a period of co-activation with the erector spinae for the purpose of trunk stability in the sagittal plane. The activity of the trunk flexors also coincides with the time when the hip flexors actively flex the hip. Increased activity of the rectus abdominis, therefore, may be used to stabilize the pelvis and lumbar spine and to provide a stable fixation for the hip flexor muscles, principally the iliopsoas and rectus femoris.

The role of the trunk musculature during gait may in fact be underestimated. Based on the evolution of the vertebrate spine, Gracovetsky[31,32] proposed his theory of the "spinal engine," in which walking was first achieved by motion of the spine. The hypothesis that the lumbar spine actually plays an important role to move the pelvis during walking may deserve consideration in future research.

## GAIT KINETICS

Understanding the forces that are responsible for movement during gait plays a critical role in understanding normal and pathologic movement. Although the kinetics (study of forces) of walking are not visually observable, they are responsible for the observed kinematics.

### Ground Reaction Forces

During ambulation, forces are applied under the surface of the foot every time a person takes a step (Fig. 15–30A and B). The forces applied to the ground by the foot are called *foot forces*. The forces applied to the foot by the ground are called *ground (or floor) reaction forces*. These forces are of equal magnitude but opposite direction. (Newton's Third Law—the law of action and reaction—states that forces are always present in pairs that are equal in magnitude and opposite in direction.) In this chapter, ground reaction forces are consistently referred to because in most instances the interest is in the forces applied to the body, as opposed to those applied to the ground.

The description of the ground reaction forces follows a Cartesian coordinate system, with the forces being expressed along three orthogonal axes: vertical, anterior-posterior, and medial-lateral. The vector summation of the three forces gives a single resultant force vector between the foot and the ground. Such vector summation performed for the vertical and anterior-posterior components of the ground reaction forces leads to the classic butterfly representation of the ground reaction forces for a single step (Fig. 15–31).

---

**Ground Reaction Forces**
- Vertical: peak value = 120% body weight (BW)
- Anterior-posterior: peak value = 20% BW
- Medial-lateral: peak value = 5% BW

**Ground Reaction Forces During Gait**

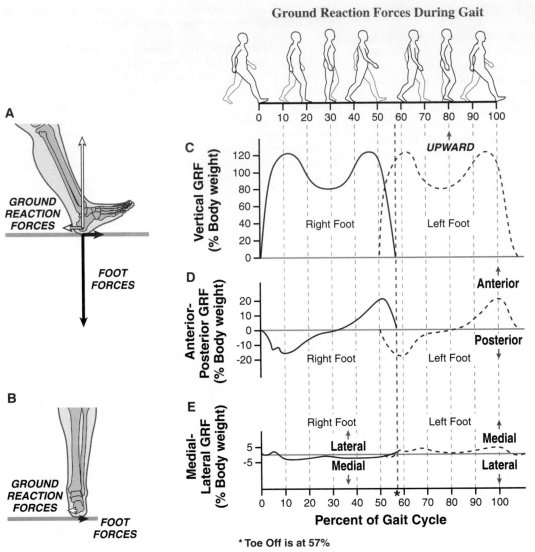

**A**

**GROUND REACTION FORCES**

**FOOT FORCES**

**B**

**GROUND REACTION FORCES**

**FOOT FORCES**

**C** Vertical GRF (% Body weight)

120 100 80 60 40 20 0

Right Foot    Left Foot

UPWARD

**D** Anterior-Posterior GRF (% Body weight)

20 10 0 -10 -20

Right Foot    Left Foot

Anterior

Posterior

**E** Medial-Lateral GRF (% Body weight)

Right Foot    Left Foot

5 -5

Lateral    Medial

Medial    Lateral

0 10 20 30 40 50 60 70 80 90 100

**Percent of Gait Cycle**

\* Toe Off is at 57%

**FIGURE 15–30.** Ground reaction forces (GRFs) during gait. *A* illustrates the vertical and anterior-posterior GRF (black and white arrows, respectively) and foot forces (filled arrows) at 10% of gait cycle. *B* illustrates the medial-lateral forces at 10% of gait cycle. *C, D,* and *E* show the GRF for a gait cycle. Dashed lines are data for left foot contact. (Data from Whittle M: Gait Analysis: An Introduction, 2nd ed. Oxford, Butterworth-Heinemann Ltd., 1996.)

**Vertical Forces.** The vertical forces are those directed perpendicular to the supporting surface. In the vertical direction, the ground reaction forces peak twice in a given gait cycle. Forces are slightly greater than body weight at the time of the loading response and again at the time of terminal stance (Fig. 15–30C). During mid stance, the ground reaction forces are slightly lower than body weight. This slight fluctuation in force is due to the vertical acceleration of the body's CoM. (Force is a function of mass as well as acceleration: F = ma.) At the time of loading response, the body's CoM is moving downward (see Fig. 15–13). A vertical ground reaction force greater than one's body weight, therefore, is needed to initially decelerate the downward movement of the body and then accelerate it upward. This is similar to jumping on a bathroom scale and briefly reading a weight that is higher than static body weight. At mid stance, the vertical ground reaction forces are less than body weight as a result of a relative "unweighting," caused by the upward momentum of the body gained during the early part of stance. The higher ground reaction force at terminal stance reflects the combined push provided by the plantar flexors

and the need to reverse the downward movement of the body that occurs in terminal stance through pre swing.

**Anterior-Posterior Forces.** In the anterior-posterior direction, shear forces are applied parallel to the supporting surface. At heel contact, the ground reaction force is in the posterior direction (i.e., the foot applies an anteriorly directed force to the ground) (Fig. 15–30D). At that time, sufficient friction is required between the foot and the ground to prevent the foot from slipping forward (picture the classic cartoon of a person falling to the ground after slipping on a banana peel). The magnitude of the ground reaction forces increases with longer steps. This is the reason people often take shorter steps when walking on an icy surface—they are decreasing the demand for friction.

During terminal stance and pre swing, the ground reaction force is directed anteriorly, with the foot applying a posteriorly directed force to the ground in order to propel the body forward. The magnitude of the propulsive force depends on walking speed and, especially, attempts to accelerate. Inadequate friction between the foot and the ground at

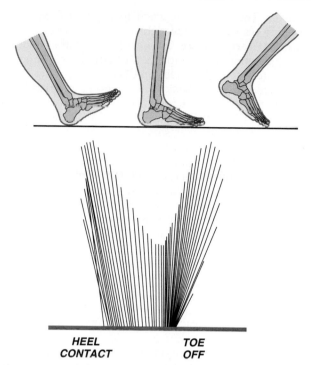

**FIGURE 15–31.** Classic "butterfly" representation of the ground reaction forces for a step. Each line represents the resultant force from the vector addition of the vertical and anterior-posterior forces at regular time intervals (i.e., every 10 ms in this case). Progression from heel contact to toe off takes place from left to right. (Data from Whittle M: Gait Analysis: An Introduction, 2nd ed. Oxford, Butterworth-Heinemann Ltd., 1996.)

**HEEL CONTACT**  **TOE OFF**

from one lower extremity to the other at the time of double-limb support. Slowing down requires a greater braking force than propulsive force, and speeding up requires the opposite.

**Medial-Lateral Forces.** The magnitude of the ground reaction force in the medial-lateral direction is relatively small (i.e., less than 5% of body weight) and more variable across individuals (Fig. 15–30E). As with anterior-posterior shear force, the magnitude and direction of this shear force depends mostly on the relationship between the position of the body's CoM and the location of the foot. During the initial 5 to 10% of the gait cycle, a small, laterally directed ground reaction shear force is produced to stop the small lateral-to-medial velocity of the foot that is typically present at the time of heel contact. During the rest of stance phase, however, the CoM of the body is medial to the foot (see Fig. 15–13), causing a laterally directed force to be applied to the ground by the foot and, therefore, a medially directed ground reaction force. These medially directed ground reaction forces throughout stance initially decelerate the lateral movement of the CoM. Then, these ground reaction forces accelerate CoM medially toward the contralateral lower extremity, which is swinging forward and preparing to make the next foot contact with the ground.

Although the action of the medial-lateral ground reaction forces may not be easily felt during normal gait, they can be readily felt when walking while using very large steps or when jumping from side to side. In fact, greater peak values in medial-lateral ground reaction forces are often seen in individuals with wider step widths. The need for friction can again be appreciated by observing someone walking on ice. Individuals walking on icy surfaces reduce their step widths almost as if they were walking on a tightrope. This learned adaptation is intended to keep the body's CoM directly over the feet to minimize the medial-lateral ground reaction forces and, therefore, the need for friction. Ice skaters make use of these medial-lateral ground reaction forces to propel their bodies forward. This is achieved by using a blade that digs into the ice, providing an adequate resistance for propulsion.

## Path of the Center of Pressure

The path of the center of pressure (CoP) under the foot throughout stance follows a relatively reproducible pattern (Fig. 15–32). At heel contact, the CoP is located just lateral to the midpoint of the heel. It then moves progressively to the lateral midfoot region at mid stance, and to the medial forefoot region (under the first/second metatarsal head) during heel off to toe off. The location of the CoP, acting as the point of application of the ground reaction forces at heel contact, helps to explain the tendency for the ankle and foot to plantar flex and evert, respectively (Fig. 15–33). Both tendencies are partially controlled by eccentric activation of ankle muscles, namely the ankle dorsiflexors and the tibialis posterior.

## Joint Torques and Powers

During gait, the ground reaction forces applied under the foot generate an external torque on the joints of the lower

this time often causes the foot to slide backward without propelling the body forward. This explains the difficulty experienced when accelerating quickly while walking on a slippery surface.

The peak anterior-posterior ground reaction force is typically equal to about 20% of body weight. These shear forces are in large part the result of the CoM of the body being either posterior (at heel contact) or anterior (at terminal stance and pre swing) to the foot. The larger the step length, the greater the shear forces because of the greater angle between the lower extremity and the floor. Inertial properties of the body, such as momentum, also contribute to anterior-posterior ground reaction forces.

The posteriorly directed ground reaction force at heel contact momentarily slows the forward progression of the body. Conversely, the body is momentarily accelerated forward at toe off as a result of an anteriorly directed ground reaction force. Note that the propulsive force of one limb is applied simultaneously to the braking force of the opposite limb during the times of double-limb support (see Fig. 15–30D). When walking at a constant velocity, the propulsive force occurring late in stance balances the braking force occurring early in stance. Because these forces are of relatively equal magnitude but of opposite direction, they provide balance to the body when the weight is transferred

### Path of the Center of Pressure on the Plantar Surface of the Foot

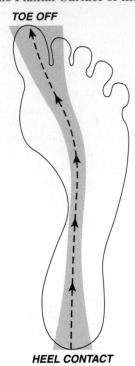

**TOE OFF**

**HEEL CONTACT**

**FIGURE 15–32.** Path of the center of pressure (CoP) under the foot from heel contact to toe off. The shaded area is representative of individual variability of the CoP path. (Data from Katoh Y, Chao EYS, Laughman RK, et al: Biomechanical analysis of foot function during gait and clinical applications. Clin Orthop 177:23, 1983.)

### Torques Generated by Ground Reaction Forces at Heel Contact

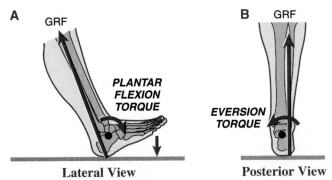

**A**    GRF

**PLANTAR FLEXION TORQUE**

**Lateral View**

**B**    GRF

**EVERSION TORQUE**

**Posterior View**

**FIGURE 15–33.** At heel contact, the point and direction of application of the ground reaction forces on the calcaneus behind the center of rotation of the ankle (black circle) create a plantar flexion torque at the ankle (*A*). This external torque requires the generation of an opposing dorsiflexion internal torque by the ankle dorsiflexors. In *B*, the lateral location of the ground reaction force on the calcaneus produces subtalar joint eversion and, therefore, foot pronation. This tendency is controlled by action of the tibialis posterior. (From Adams JM, Perry J: Gait analysis: Clinical application. In Rose J, Gamble JG: Human Walking, 2nd ed. Philadelphia, Williams & Wilkins, 1994.)

extremities. This fact is illustrated in Figure 15–34. During the loading response on the right limb, the line of action of the ground reaction force is located behind the ankle and knee but anterior to the hip. As a consequence, the ground reaction forces at heel contact produce ankle plantar flexion, knee flexion, and hip flexion. To prevent collapse of the lower extremity, these external torques are resisted by internal joint torques created by the ankle dorsiflexors, the knee extensors, and the hip extensors.

Knowledge of ground reaction force and length of the external moment arms (see Fig. 15–34) allows for an estimate of the torques imposed on the joints of the lower extremity during stance phase. This simplified analysis assumes a condition of static equilibrium. Accurate calculation of joint torques during gait requires the use of the inverse dynamic approach, which takes into account the dynamic nature of the action.[4] This approach requires the knowledge of the anthropometric characteristics of the individual's segment masses, location of the segments' center of mass, and segments' mass center inertia matrix, and precise measurements of body motion (each segment's linear and angular velocity) and ground reaction forces throughout the gait cycle (see Fig. 15–5).

In the following description, internal joint torques refer to those created by the body. Most often these torques can be related to the activity of the surrounding musculature. Muscles do generate most of the internal torques necessary to keep the body upright and move the body forward. Description of joint torque, therefore, should match the description of muscular activation provided earlier in this chapter. In some cases, especially with pathologic conditions, joint torques can be the result of passive forces generated by the deformation of soft tissues, such as the capsule and ligaments. Joint torques can be generated, therefore, even in the absence of EMG activity of the surrounding musculature. In fact, many patients without normal muscular function learn to use passive forces to generate the joint torques necessary to ambulate.

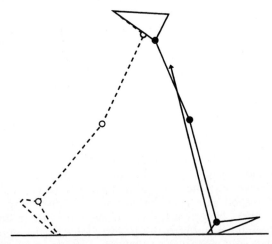

**FIGURE 15–34.** During the loading response, the line of action of the ground reaction forces (posterior to the ankle, posterior to the knee, and anterior to the hip) promotes ankle plantar flexion, knee flexion, and hip flexion. (From Whittle M: Gait Analysis: An Introduction, 2nd ed. Oxford, Butterworth-Heinemann Ltd., 1996.)

**Joint Torques**
- Internal joint torques: produced by the body
- External joint torques: applied to the body

The term net joint torques reflects the fact that the inverse dynamic approach used to calculate internal joint torques does not take into account co-activation of agonist-antagonist muscle groups. Note, too, that the net torque produced by muscles does not necessarily reflect the direction of movement of that joint. As illustrated in Figure 15–34, during the loading response, a net internal dorsiflexion torque exists while the ankle is moving in plantar flexion. This combination of dorsiflexion torque and plantar flexion movement indicates an eccentric activation of the ankle dorsiflexors.

The concept of net internal torque provides valuable insight into the role of particular muscles in controlling a joint during walking. Internal net torque does not, however, provide the answer to the rate of muscle activation. Understanding the rate of work performed by the controlling muscles requires knowledge of power. Joint power is the product of the net joint torque and the joint angular velocity. Joint power reflects the net rate of generating or absorbing energy by all muscles and other connective tissues crossing a joint. A positive value indicates power generation, which reflects a concentric muscle activation, whereas a negative value indicates power absorption, which reflects an eccentric muscle activation. The concept of power generation and absorption may be understood with the example of performing a jump. During the initial squatting movement preceding a jump, most muscles of the lower extremities work eccentrically, absorbing energy. This energy is then released by a concentric muscle activation during the upward movement of the body. Application of this concept in the field of athletic strength building is known as plyometric training.

**Joint Power is the Product of the Net Joint Torque and the Joint Angular Velocity**
- Power is generated by concentric muscle activation
- Power is absorbed by eccentric muscle activation

Analysis of joint torques and powers gives a more complete picture of the biomechanics of gait. These variables help establish the relative contribution of various joints and muscle groups to tasks such as generation of forward velocity, support of body weight, and control of balance during gait. In the healthy adult, for example, the ankle plantar flexors are suggested as the primary source of forward velocity of the body.[38] The understanding and treatment of pathologic gait benefit from this type of information.

The following sections highlight the primary torques and powers generated during walking. These sections also provide the figures that summarize the kinematics and kinetics of the hip, knee, and ankle in the sagittal plane and the hip in the frontal plane. Careful study of these figures should provide an increased understanding of the relationships

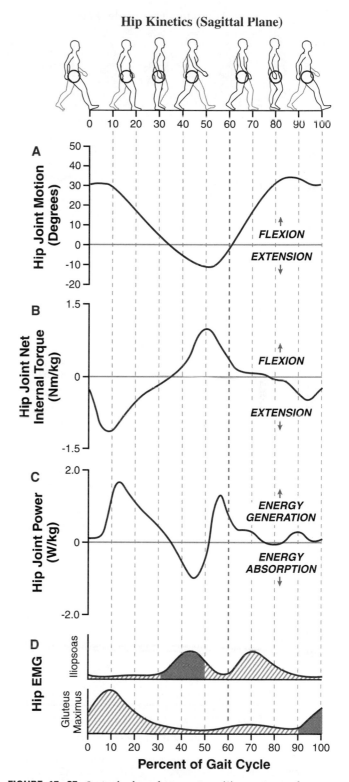

**Hip Kinetics (Sagittal Plane)**

**FIGURE 15–35.** Sagittal plane hip motion (*A*), net internal torques (*B*), powers (*C*), and electromyographic (EMG) activity (*D*) for a gait cycle. The EMG curves represent the relative intensity of the muscle activation during the gait cycle, with the shaded and hatched areas indicating eccentric and concentric muscle activation, respectively. (Torque and power data normalized to body mass from Winter et al, 1996, and EMG data from Winter, 1991, and Bechtol, 1975.)

## Hip Kinetics (Frontal Plane)

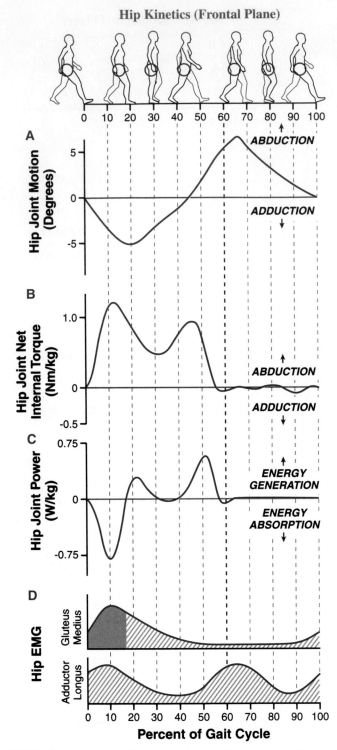

**FIGURE 15-36.** Frontal plane hip motion (A), net internal torques (B), powers (C), and electromyographic (EMG) activity (D) for a gait cycle. The EMG curves represent the relative intensity of the muscle activation during the gait cycle, with the shaded and hatched areas indicating eccentric and concentric muscle activation, respectively. (Torque and power data normalized to body mass from Winter et al, 1996, and EMG data from Winter, 1991.)

among joint motion, torque, power, and muscle activation during gait.

**Hip.** In the early stance, in the *sagittal plane,* the hip musculature generates a hip extension torque that serves to accept the weight of the body, control the trunk, and extend the hip (Fig. 15–35A and B). In the second half of stance, a flexion torque is generated to decelerate hip extension. This hip flexion torque is the result of passive forces from the anterior capsule and activity of the hip flexors. In initial swing, a small hip flexion torque, corresponding to the concentric activation of the flexors, initiates hip flexion. In terminal swing, an extensor torque is needed to decelerate the movement of hip flexion.

Figure 15–35C shows the power curve for the hip in the *sagittal plane.* Power is generated to support the body, raise the CoM, control the trunk, and propel the body forward in the first 35% of the gait cycle. Power is then absorbed until 50 to 55% of the gait cycle is reached, reflecting the deceleration of hip extension secondary to resistance provided by the anterior capsule of the hip and the eccentric activation of the hip flexors. In pre swing and initial swing, power is generated to flex the hip.

## Hip Kinetics (Horizontal Plane)

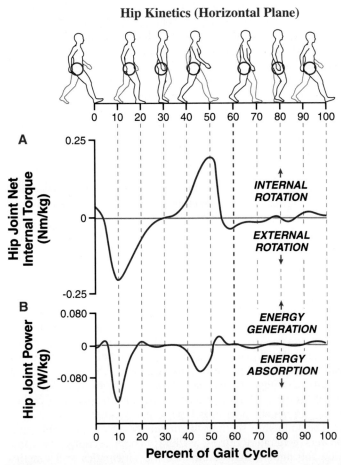

**FIGURE 15-37.** Horizontal plane net internal torques (A) and powers (B). (Data normalized to body mass from Winter et al, 1996.)

To complete the description of sagittal plane hip movement during gait, Figure 15–35D illustrates the relative intensity of activity of two primary antagonistic muscles of the hip. The areas of the EMG curve that are shaded indicate an eccentric muscle activation. The hatched areas indicate a concentric muscle activation. In general, the muscular activations correlate with power absorption and power generation.

In the *frontal plane,* a large abduction torque occurs during stance to support the mass of the body that is located medial to the hip joint (Fig. 15–36A and B). Power absorption during the initial lowering of the opposite side of the pelvis (Fig. 15–36C) reflects the eccentric activation of the hip abductors (Fig. 15–36D). Power generation is seen at 20 and 60% of the gait cycle, as the contralateral pelvis is raised (Fig. 15–36C).

In the *horizontal plane,* an external rotation torque is used to decelerate the internal rotation of the femur in the first 20% of the gait cycle (Fig. 15–37A). This torque is followed by an internal rotation torque that advances the contralateral side of the pelvis forward during the remainder of stance. Notice the small magnitude of these torques, approximately 15% of those in the sagittal and frontal planes. The eccentric activation of the hip external rotators in the initial 20% of the gait cycle accounts for the power absorption noted at that time (Fig. 15–37B).

**Knee.** In the *sagittal plane,* at heel contact, a very brief (first 4% of the gait cycle) initial flexion torque presumably ensures that the knee is flexed to provide an adequate knee alignment for shock absorption (Fig. 15–38A and B). A large extensor torque needed for the loading response quickly follows this flexion torque. This extensor torque continues until 20% of gait, initially to eccentrically control knee flexion, then to extend the knee. Between 20 and 50% of the gait cycle, a net flexor torque is present as the knee flexes before toe off. Because little activity of the hamstrings is present at that time, the net flexor torque likely results from passive tension in the posterior capsule of the knee. Just before toe off, however, a small extensor torque occurs to control knee flexion. In terminal swing, a flexion torque is generated to decelerate knee extension.

The power curve for the sagittal plane reflects the action of the musculature surrounding the knee (Fig. 15–38C and D). The short duration power generation at early stance shows that the net knee flexion torque creates flexion of the knee. Then, power absorption momentarily takes place, reflecting the eccentric action of the quadriceps. This is followed by another brief moment of power generation, indicating the start of knee extension. Just prior to toe off, power is absorbed by the knee extensors that control the flexion of the knee. In terminal swing, the hamstrings are absorbing energy as the swing leg is decelerated.

In the *frontal plane* (Fig. 15–39A), an internal abductor torque at the knee counters the external adductor (varus) torque created by the resultant ground reaction force passing medial to the stance knee (Fig. 15–40). The internal abductor torque is created by a combination of active and passive structures, including the iliotibial tract, the tensor fascia latae, and the lateral ligaments of the knee. Power values in this plane are very low because of the low knee angular velocities in the frontal plane (Fig. 15–39B).

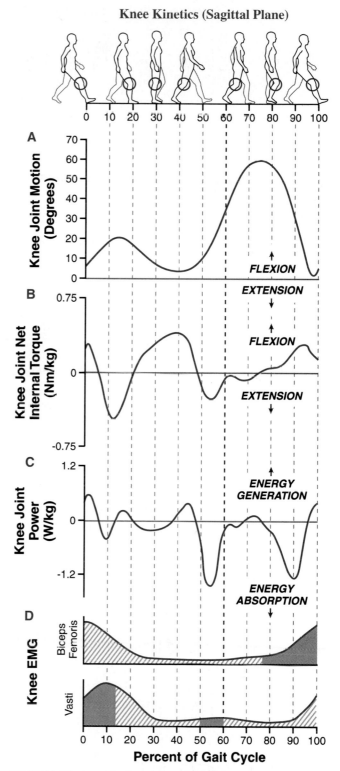

**Knee Kinetics (Sagittal Plane)**

**FIGURE 15–38.** Sagittal plane knee motion (A), net internal torques (B), powers (C), and electromyographic (EMG) activity (D) for a gait cycle. The EMG curves represent the relative intensity of the muscle activation during the gait cycle, with the shaded and hatched areas indicating eccentric and concentric muscle activation, respectively. (Torque and power data normalized to body mass from Winter et al, 1996, and EMG data from Winter, 1991.)

## Knee Kinetics (Frontal Plane)

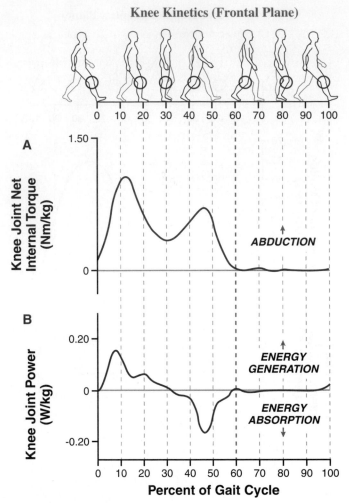

**FIGURE 15-39.** Frontal plane net internal torques (A) and powers (B) for the knee. (Data normalized to body mass from Winter et al, 1996.)

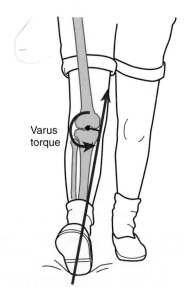

**FIGURE 15-40.** Weight application on the foot during gait creates a varus torque at the knee. Greater loading of the medial femoral condyle and tibial plateau explains the greater incidence of joint deterioration of the medial aspect of the knee. This varus torque also tends to "open" the lateral aspect of the knee. This tendency is resisted by the lateral structures of the knee.

In the *horizontal plane* that describes tibial on femoral motion, the joint torques are similar to those at the hip, with an external rotation torque in the first half of stance and an internal rotation torque in the second half (Fig. 15–41A). These torques are generated by knee ligaments in response to the active hip torques in the horizontal plane.[20] During loading response, a small amount of power is absorbed as the knee's capsular and ligamentous structures resist the internal rotation motion of the tibia (Fig. 15–41B).

**Ankle and Foot.** In the *sagittal plane,* a small dorsiflexion torque is generated at the ankle immediately after heel contact (Fig. 15–42A and B). This torque serves to eccentrically control the movement of plantar flexion generated by the application of body weight on the calcaneus (see Fig. 15–33). A plantar flexion torque prevails throughout the rest of stance, initially to eccentrically control the tibia advancing over the foot, then to plantar flex the ankle at push off. A very small dorsiflexion torque is present during swing to keep the ankle dorsiflexed in order to clear the toes.

## Knee Kinetics (Horizontal Plane)

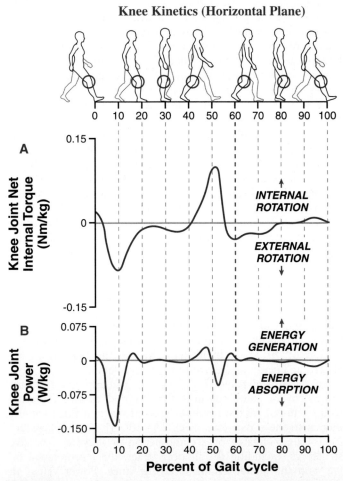

**FIGURE 15-41.** Horizontal plane net internal torques (A) and powers (B) for the knee. (Data normalized to body mass from Winter et al, 1996.)

## Ankle Kinetics (Sagittal Plane)

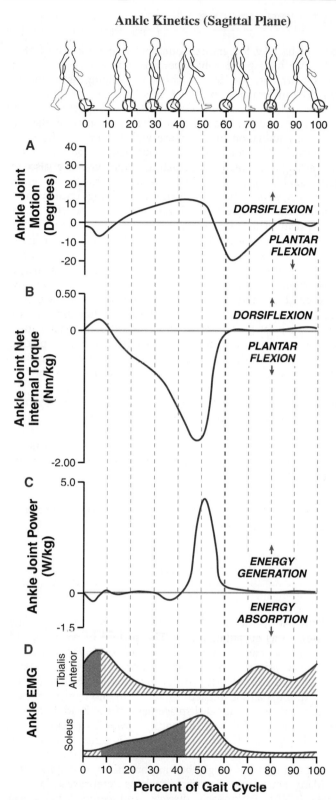

**FIGURE 15–42.** Sagittal plane ankle motion (*A*), net internal torques (*B*), powers (*C*), and electromyographic (EMG) activity (*D*) for a gait cycle. The EMG curves represent the relative intensity of the muscle activation during the gait cycle, with the shaded and hatched areas indicating eccentric and concentric muscle activation, respectively. (Torque and power data normalized to body mass from Winter et al, 1996, and EMG data from Winter, 1991.)

In the sagittal plane, power is absorbed prior to push off (Fig. 15–42*C*), reflecting the eccentric nature of the action of the plantar flexors (Fig. 15–42*D*). This is followed by a large generation of energy from the plantar flexors at push off. This power generation is responsible for a large portion of the propulsive forces pushing the body forward during gait.[38]

The torques and especially the power values in the *frontal and horizontal planes* are very small and exhibit large variation among people (Figs. 15–43 and 15–44). In the frontal plane, stance phase is characterized by a small initial eversion torque (from 0 to 20% of gait) followed by an inversion torque (from 20 to 45% of gait) and a smaller eversion torque just prior to toe off.[101] In the horizontal plane, an external rotation torque is present during the stance phase. This external rotation torque should in fact be called an abduction torque based on the description of ankle movement provided in Chapter 14.

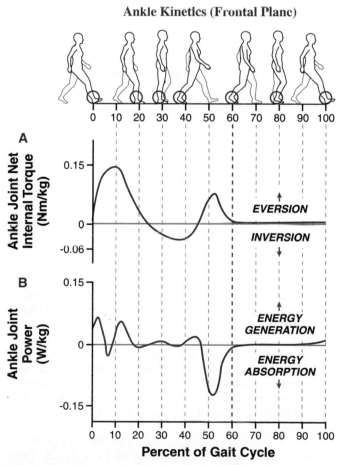

**FIGURE 15–43.** Frontal plane net internal torques (*A*) and powers (*B*) for the ankle. (Data normalized to body mass from Winter et al, 1996.)

**Ankle Kinetics (Horizontal Plane)**

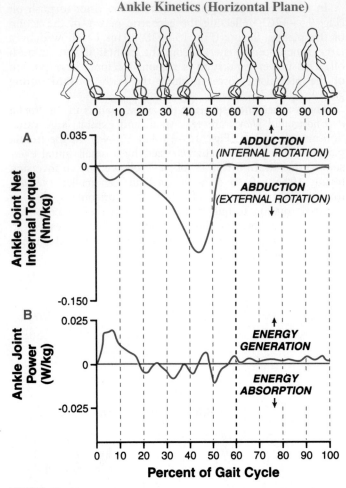

**FIGURE 15–44.** Horizontal plane net internal torques (A) and powers (B) for the ankle. (Data normalized to body mass from Winter et al, 1996.)

## Joint and Tendon Forces

Joint surfaces, ligaments, and tendons are all subjected to large tensile, compressive, or shear forces during walking. Knowledge of the magnitude of these forces is of interest, especially to the clinician, orthopedic surgeon, and bioengineer. The design of surgical joint implants, in particular, requires these types of data. Direct measurements in men and women are obviously not readily obtainable; therefore, these forces are typically calculated indirectly through biomechanical analysis including modeling and optimization techniques.

Forces applied to various structures of the lower extremities during ambulation are presented in Table 15–5. These forces can be surprisingly large. Consider, for example, that the compressive bone-on-bone force at the hip during ambulation at 1.4 m/s is equal to 6.4 times body weight.[79]

## GAIT DYSFUNCTIONS

Most of us take for granted our ability to walk. The fact is, unless we have personally experienced an injury or a physical impairment, we do not think of walking as a difficult task. The information provided thus far in this chapter, however, reminds us of the complexity of ambulation. Many actions must occur simultaneously at each part of the gait cycle for ambulation to take place with maximum efficiency.

Normal ambulation requires sufficient range of motion and strength at each participating joint. Walking also requires sophisticated control of movement through the central nervous system. The complexity of walking creates many opportunities for the normal gait pattern to be affected by impairment. The adaptability of the system, however, does create many opportunities to modify the gait pattern in order to walk—despite even severe impairments. In these cases, a normal gait pattern is sacrificed for the ability to move from one location to another independently. We have all used this ability to adapt gait, even if for only a painful blister under the foot or for walking on hot sand at the beach. In essence, an abnormal or a pathologic gait pattern reflects an effort to preserve ambulation through adaptation. The cost of gait deviation is, typically, increased energy expenditure and application of abnormal stresses to the body.

Three common causes of pathologic gait patterns are listed in the box. Each includes many specific and general pathologies. The observed deviations may be the direct response to a specific impairment or may in fact be a compensation. The features of pathologic gait, therefore, depend on the nature of the impairment as well as the ability of the individual to compensate for that impairment.

| **Causes of Pathologic Gait Patterns** |
| --- |
| • Pain |
| • Central nervous system disorders |
| • Musculoskeletal system impairments |

Pain can cause an abnormal gait pattern that is often referred to as an antalgic gait. The pattern of weight avoidance on the painful limb often leads to characteristic features. The primary findings are a shorter step length, stance time on the painful side, and swing time on the uninvolved side. If the pain is related to hip joint compression from muscle activation, lateral displacement of the head and trunk toward the painful weight-bearing lower extremity occurs (see Chapter 12). If the source of pain is other than the hip, the trunk may lean slightly toward the swing leg in an attempt to alleviate weight bearing on the injured stance leg.

Many neurologic disorders, such as cerebrovascular accidents (CVA), Parkinson's disease, and cerebral palsy, can cause abnormal gait patterns.[83] Spasticity of muscles, defined as increased tone and resistance to stretch, often affects the extensor musculature of individuals with cerebral palsy and CVA. As a result, the gait pattern appears stiff-legged and is often accompanied by a tendency to circumduct and scuff the feet. A scissoring gait pattern due to hyperactive hip adductors may also be noted. Parkinson's disease often causes a hurried small-step gait pattern, also called festinat-

**TABLE 15–5. Forces Applied to the Lower Extremity Structures During Ambulation**

| Structures (Types of Force) | Speed | Authors | Magnitude (BW) |
|---|---|---|---|
| *Ankle* | | | |
| Talocrural joint (peak compression) | 1.4 m/s | Simonsen et al. (1995) | 4.2 |
| Talocrural joint (peak compression) | 114 s/min | Collins (1995) | 4.0 |
| Talocrural joint (peak compression) | 4.2 m/s (r) | Scott and Winter (1990) | 12.0 |
| Talocrural joint (peak anterior shear*) | 116 s/min | Stauffer et al. (1977) | 0.6 |
| Talocrural joint (peak posterior shear*) | 116 s/min | Stauffer et al. (1977) | 0.3 |
| Achilles tendon (peak tension) | 1.5 m/s | Finni et al. (1998) | 2.0 |
| Achilles tendon (peak tension) | 1.7 m/s | Finni et al. (1999) | 4.0 |
| Achilles tendon (peak tension) | 4.2 m/s (r) | Scott and Winter (1990) | 7.0 |
| Ankle dorsiflexors (peak tension) | 114 s/min | Collins (1995) | 1.0 |
| Plantar fascia (peak tension) | 4.2 m/s (r) | Scott and Winter (1990) | 2.1 |
| *Knee* | | | |
| Tibiofemoral joint (peak compression) | 1.4 m/s | Simonsen et al. (1995) | 4.6 |
| Tibiofemoral joint (peak compression) | 114 s/min | Collins (1995) | 5.0 |
| Patellofemoral joint (peak compression) | 1.0 m/s | Komistek et al. (1998) | 0.3 |
| Patellofemoral joint (peak compression) | 1.5 m/s | Kuster et al. (1993) | 1.5 |
| Patellofemoral joint (peak compression) | 1.0 m/s | Taylor et al. (1998) | 0.8 |
| Patellofemoral joint (peak compression) | 4.2 m/s (r) | Scott and Winter (1990) | 9.0 |
| Anterior cruciate ligament (peak tension) | 114 s/min | Collins (1995) | 1.5 |
| Posterior cruciate ligament (peak tension) | 114 s/min | Collins (1995) | 0.4 |
| Patellar tendon (peak tension) | 1.7 m/s | Finni et al. (1999) | 3.0 |
| Patellar tendon (peak tension) | 4.2 m/s (r) | Scott and Winter (1990) | 5.8 |
| Hamstrings (peak tension) | 114 s/min | Collins (1995) | 1.1 |
| *Hip* | | | |
| Hip (peak compression) | 1.4 m/s | Simonsen et al. (1995) | 6.4 |
| Hip (peak compression) | 0.9 m/s | Pedersen et al. (1997) | 3.1 |
| Hip (peak compression) | 114 s/min | Collins (1995) | 3.8 |
| Adductor magnus (peak tension) | 0.9 m/s | Pedersen et al. (1997) | 0.3 |
| Gluteus medius (peak tension) | 0.9 m/s | Pedersen et al. (1997) | 0.5 |

BW, units in number of body weights; s/min, steps per minute; m/s, meters per second; * direction of shear of tibia on talus; (r), running speed.

ing gait. Apraxia, defined as a disorder of voluntary movement, occurs in some disease processes affecting the elderly. Gait apraxia may result in an ambulation pattern characterized by a wide base of support, short stride, and shuffling. Individuals with impaired sensory function and balance may show an unstable gait pattern.[76] With neurologic disorders, the primary cause of gait dysfunction is an inability to generate and control an appropriate level of muscle force. Eventually, muscle weakness and joint contracture may compound the primary neuromotor deficit.

Deficits in the musculoskeletal system also result in a wide variety of gait deviations. Abnormal (excessive or limited) joint range of motion and/or limited muscle strength can cause gait deviations. Abnormal joint range of motion may occur secondary to injuries, tightness or contracture of connective tissues and muscles, abnormal joint structure, joint instability, or congenital connective tissue laxity. In most cases, abnormal range of motion in one joint leads to some form of compensation in one or more surrounding joints. Muscular weakness may be due to disuse atrophy following an injury or a limited neural drive secondary to a peripheral neural injury. Whatever the cause, weakness ultimately leads to modification of the gait pattern. Tables 15–6 through 15–11 and Figures 15–45 through 15–51 present some of the most common gait deviations observed in the general population.

**TABLE 15–6. Gait Deviations at the Ankle/Foot Secondary to Specific Ankle/Foot Impairments***

| Observed Gait Deviation at the Ankle/Foot | Likely Impairment | Selected Pathologic Precursors | Mechanical Rationale and/or Associated Compensations |
|---|---|---|---|
| "Foot slap": rapid ankle plantar flexion occurs following **heel contact**.† The name foot slap is derived from the characteristic noise made by the forefoot hitting the ground. | Mild weakness of ankle dorsiflexors | Common peroneal nerve palsy and distal peripheral neuropathy | Ankle dorsiflexors have sufficient strength to dorsiflex the ankle during swing but not enough to control ankle plantar flexion after heel contact. |
| Entire plantar aspect of the foot touches the ground at **initial contact**,‡ followed by normal, passive ankle dorsiflexion during the rest of stance. | Marked weakness of ankle dorsiflexors | Common peroneal nerve palsy and distal peripheral neuropathy | Sufficient strength of the dorsiflexors to partially, but not completely, dorsiflex the ankle during swing. Normal dorsiflexion occurs during stance as long as the ankle has normal range of motion. |
| **Initial contact** with the ground is made by the forefoot followed by the heel region. Normal passive ankle dorsiflexion occurs during stance. | Severe weakness of ankle dorsiflexors | Common peroneal nerve palsy and distal peripheral neuropathy | No active ankle dorsiflexion is possible during swing. Normal dorsiflexion occurs during stance as long as the ankle has normal range of motion. |
| **Initial contact** is made with the forefoot, but the heel never makes contact with the ground during stance. | Heel pain | Calcaneal fracture, plantar fasciitis | Purposeful strategy to avoid weight bearing on the heel |
| | Plantar flexion contracture (pes equinus deformity) or spasticity of ankle plantar flexors | Upper motor neuron lesion/cerebral palsy, cerebrovascular accident (CVA) | To maintain the weight over the foot, the knee and hip are kept in flexion throughout stance, leading to a "crouched gait." |
| **Initial contact** is made with the forefoot, and the heel is brought to the ground by a posterior displacement of the tibia (Fig. 15–45) | Plantar flexion contracture (pes equinus deformity) or spasticity of ankle plantar flexors | Upper motor neuron lesion (cerebral palsy, CVA) Ankle fusion in a plantar flexed position | Knee hyperextension occurs during stance owing to the inability of the tibia to move forward over the foot. Hip flexion and excessive forward trunk lean during terminal stance occur to shift the weight of the body over the foot. |
| Premature elevation of the heel in **mid stance** | Lack of ankle dorsiflexion | Congenital or acquired muscular tightness of ankle plantar flexors | Characteristic bouncing gait pattern |
| Heel remains in contact with the ground late in **terminal stance** | Weakness or flaccid paralysis of plantar flexors with or without a fixed dorsiflexed position of the ankle (pes calcaneus deformity) | Peripheral or central nervous system disorders Excessive surgical lengthening of the Achilles tendon | Excessive ankle dorsiflexion results in prolonged heel contact, reduced push off, and a shorter step length. |
| Supinated foot position and weight bearing on the lateral aspect of the foot during **stance** | Pes cavus deformity | Congenital structural deformity | A high medial longitudinal arch is noted with reduced midfoot mobility throughout swing and stance. |
| Excessive foot pronation occurs during **stance** with failure of the foot to supinate in mid stance. Normal medial longitudinal arch noted during swing. | Rearfoot varus and/or forefoot varus | Congenital or acquired structural deformity | Excessive foot pronation and associated flattening of the medial longitudinal arch may be accompanied by a general internal rotation of the lower extremity during stance. |
| Excessive foot pronation with weight bearing on the medial portion of the foot during **stance**. The medial longitudinal arch remains absent during **swing**. | Weakness (paralysis) of ankle invertors | Upper motor neuron lesion | An overall excessive internal rotation of the lower extremity during stance is possible. |
| | Pes planus deformity | Congenital structural deformity | |

| Observed Gait Deviation at the Ankle/Foot | Likely Impairment | Selected Pathologic Precursors | Mechanical Rationale and/or Associated Compensations |
| --- | --- | --- | --- |
| Excessive inversion and plantar flexion of the foot and ankle occur during **swing** and at **initial contact**. | Pes equinovarus deformity due to spasticity of the plantar flexors and invertors | Upper motor neuron lesion (cerebral palsy, CVA) | Contact with the ground is made with the lateral border of the forefoot. Weight bearing on the lateral border of the foot during stance. |
| Ankle remains plantar flexed during **swing** and can be associated with dragging of the toes, typically called drop foot (Fig. 15–46). | Weakness of dorsiflexors and/or pes equinus deformity | Common peroneal nerve palsy | Hip hiking, hip circumduction, or excessive hip and knee flexion of the swing leg or vaulting of the stance leg may be noted to lift the toes off the ground and prevent the toes from dragging during swing. |

\* An impairment is a loss or an abnormality in physiologic, psychologic, or anatomic structure or function.

† The terms in bold indicate the time in the gait cycle when the gait deviation is expressed.

‡ Initial contact is often used instead of heel contact to reflect the fact that with many gait deviations the heel is not the section of the foot that makes initial contact with the ground.

TABLE **15-7.** Gait Deviations Seen at the Ankle/Foot as a Compensation for an Impairment of the Ipsilateral Knee, Ipsilateral Hip, or Contralateral Lower Extremity

| Observed Gait Deviation at the Ankle/Foot | Likely Impairment | Mechanical Rationale |
| --- | --- | --- |
| Vaulting: compensatory mechanism demonstrated by exaggerated ankle plantar flexion during **mid stance**; leads to excessive vertical movement of the body (Fig. 15–47). | Any impairment of the contralateral lower extremity that reduces hip flexion, knee flexion, or ankle dorsiflexion during swing. | Strategy used to allow the foot of a functionally long, contralateral lower extremity to clear the ground during swing. |
| Excessive foot angle during **stance** that is called toeing-out. | Retroversion of the neck of the femur or tight hip external rotators | Foot is in excessive toeing-out due to excessive external rotation of the lower extremity. |
| Reduction of the normal foot angle during **stance** that is called toeing-in. | Excessive femoral anteversion or spasticity of the hip adductors and/or hip internal rotators | General internal rotation of the lower extremity |

The terms in bold indicate the time in the gait cycle when the gait deviation is expressed.

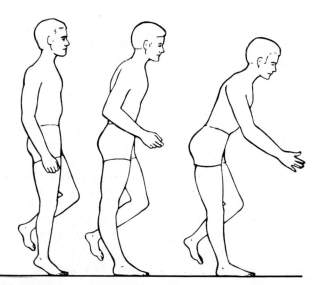

**FIGURE 15–45.** Knee hyperextension and forward trunk lean with an ankle plantar flexion contracture. (From Perry J: Contractures: A historical perspective. Clin Orthop 219:8, 1987.)

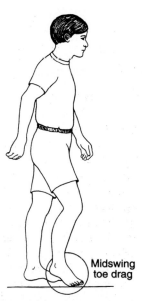

Midswing toe drag

**FIGURE 15–46.** Drop foot during swing phase, reflective of weak dorsiflexors. (From Shumway-Cook A: Motor Control: Theory and Practical Applications. Baltimore, Williams & Wilkins, 1995.)

**TABLE 15-8. Gait Deviations at the Knee Secondary to Specific Knee Impairments**

| Observed Gait Deviation at the Knee | Likely Impairment | Selected Pathologic Precursors | Mechanical Rationale and/or Associated Compensations |
|---|---|---|---|
| Rapid extension of the knee (knee extensor thrust) immediately after **initial contact** | Spasticity of the quadriceps | Upper motor neuron lesion | Depending on the status of the posterior structures of the knee, may occur with or without knee hyperextension. |
| Knee remains extended during the **loading response**, but there is no extensor thrust. | Weak quadriceps | Femoral nerve palsy, L³–L⁴ compression neuropathy | Knee remains fully extended throughout stance. An associated anterior trunk lean in the early part of stance moves the line of gravity of the trunk, slightly anterior to the axis of rotation of the knee (Fig. 15–48). This keeps the knee extended without action of the knee extensors. This gait deviation may lead to an excessive stretching of the posterior capsule of the knee and eventual knee hyperextension (genu recurvatum) during stance. |
| | Knee pain | Arthritis | Knee is kept in extension to reduce the need for quadriceps activity and associated compressive forces. It may be accompanied by an antalgic gait pattern characterized by a reduced stance time and shorter step length. |
| Genu recurvatum (hyperextension) during **stance** | Knee extensor weakness (see the two previously described gait deviations in this table) | Poliomyelitis | Secondary to progressive stretching of the posterior capsule of the knee |
| Varus thrust during **stance** | Laxity of the posterior and lateral ligamentous joint structures of the knee | Traumatic injury or progressive laxity | Rapid varus deviation of the knee during mid stance, typically accompanied by knee hyperextension |
| Flexed position of the knee during **stance** and lack of knee extension in **terminal swing** (Fig. 15–49) | Knee flexion contracture >10° (genu flexum) Hamstring overactivity (spasticity) | Upper motor neuron lesion | Associated increase in hip flexion and ankle dorsiflexion during stance |
| | Knee pain and joint effusion | Trauma or arthritis | Knee is kept in flexion since this is the position of lowest intraarticular pressure. |
| Reduced or absent knee flexion during **swing** | Spasticity of knee extensors | Upper motor neuron lesion | Compensatory hip hiking and/or hip circumduction could be noted. |
| | Knee extension contracture | Immobilization (cast, brace) or surgical fusion | |

The terms in bold indicate the time in the gait cycle when the gait deviation is expressed.

**TABLE 15-9. Gait Deviations Seen at the Knee as a Compensation for an Impairment of the Ipsilateral Ankle, Ipsilateral Hip, or Contralateral Lower Extremity**

| Observed Gait Deviation at the Knee | Likely Impairment | Mechanical Rationale |
|---|---|---|
| Knee is kept in flexion during **stance** despite the knee having normal range of motion on examination. | Impairments at the ankle or the hip including a pes calcaneus deformity, plantar flexor weakness, and hip flexion contracture. | Exaggerated ankle dorsiflexion or hip flexion during stance forces the knee in a flexed position. The contralateral (healthy) swing leg shows exaggerated hip and knee flexion to clear the toes owing to the functionally shorter stance leg. |
| Hyperextension of the knee (genu recurvatum) from **initial contact to pre swing** | Ankle plantar flexion contracture (pes equinus deformity) or spasticity of ankle plantar flexors | Knee must hyperextend to compensate for the lack of forward displacement of the tibia during stance (see Fig. 15–45). |
| Antalgic gait | Painful stance leg | This is characterized by a shorter step length and stance time on the side of the painful lower extremity; it may be accompanied by ipsilateral trunk lean, if hip pain, contralateral trunk lean occurs with knee and foot pain. |
| Excessive knee flexion in **swing** | Lack of ankle dorsiflexion of the swing leg or a short stance leg | Strategy to increase toe clearance of the swing leg and is typically accompanied by increased hip flexion. |

The terms in bold indicate the time in the gait cycle when the gait deviation is expressed.

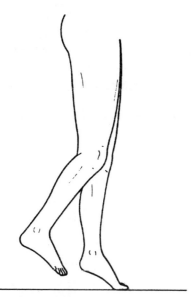

**FIGURE 15–47.** Vaulting on unaffected side to compensate for limited functional shortening of the swing leg. (From Whittle M: Gait Analysis: An Introduction, 2nd ed. Oxford, Butterworth-Heinemann Ltd., 1996.)

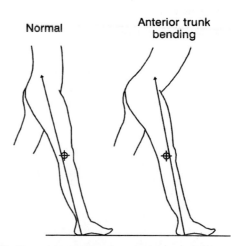

Normal        Anterior trunk bending

**FIGURE 15–48.** Weak quadriceps leading to anterior trunk lean. (From Whittle M: Gait Analysis: An Introduction, 2nd ed. Oxford, Butterworth-Heinemann Ltd., 1996.)

**TABLE 15-10. Gait Deviations at the Hip/Pelvis/Trunk Secondary to Specific Hip/Pelvis/Trunk Impairments**

| Observed Gait Deviation at the Hip/Pelvis/Trunk | Likely Impairment | Selected Pathologic Precursors | Mechanical Rationale and/or Associated Compensations |
|---|---|---|---|
| Backward trunk lean during **loading response** | Weak hip extensors | Paralysis or poliomyelitis | This action moves the line of gravity of the trunk behind the hip and reduces the need for hip extension torque. |
| Lateral trunk lean toward the **stance** leg; since this movement compensates for a weakness, it is often called "compensated" Trendelenburg gait and is referred to as a waddling gait if bilateral. | Marked weakness of the hip abductors | Guillain-Barré or poliomyelitis | Shifting the trunk over the supporting limb reduces the demand on the hip abductors. |
| | Hip pain | Arthritis | Shifting the trunk over the supporting lower extremity reduces compressive joint forces associated with the action of hip abductors (see Fig. 15–18). |
| Excessive downward drop of the contralateral pelvis during **stance.** (Referred to as positive Trendelenburg sign if present during single-limb standing.) | Mild weakness of the gluteus medius of the stance leg | Guillain-Barré or poliomyelitis | While the Trendelenburg sign may be seen in single-limb standing, a compensated Trendelenburg gait is often seen in severe weakness of the hip abductors. |
| Forward bending of the trunk during **mid** and **terminal stance,** as the hip is moved over the foot. | Hip flexion contracture | Hip osteoarthritis | Forward trunk lean is used to compensate for lack of hip extension. An alternative adaptation could be excessive lumbar lordosis. |
| | Hip pain | Hip osteoarthritis | Keeping the hip at 30 degrees of flexion minimizes intraarticular pressure. |
| Excessive lumbar lordosis in **terminal stance** | Hip flexion contracture | Arthritis | Lack of hip extension in terminal stance is compensated for by increased lordosis. |
| Trunk lurches backward and toward the unaffected stance leg from **heel off** to **mid swing.** | Hip flexor weakness | $L^2$-$L^3$ nerve compression | Hip flexion is passively generated by a backward movement of the trunk. |
| Posterior tilt of the pelvis during **initial swing** | Hip flexor weakness | $L^2$-$L^3$ nerve compression | Abdominals are used during initial swing to advance the swing leg. |
| Hip circumduction: semicircle movement of the hip during **swing**—combining hip flexion, hip abduction, and forward rotation of the pelvis (Fig. 15–50). | Hip flexor weakness | $L^2$-$L^3$ nerve compression | Hip abductors are used as flexors. |

* The terms in bold indicate the time in the gait cycle when the gait deviation is expressed.

**TABLE 15–11. Gait Deviations Seen at the Hip/Pelvis/Trunk as a Compensation for an Impairment of the Ipsilateral Ankle, Ipsilateral Knee, or Contralateral Lower Extremity**

| Observed Gait Deviation at the Hip/Pelvis/Trunk | Likely Impairment | Mechanical Rationale |
| --- | --- | --- |
| Forward bending of the trunk during the **loading response** | Weak quadriceps | Trunk is brought forward to move the line of gravity anterior to the axis of rotation of the knee, thereby reducing the need for knee extensors (see Fig. 15–48). |
| Forward bending of the trunk during **mid** and **terminal stance** | Pes equinus deformity | Lack of ankle dorsiflexion during stance results in knee hyperextension and forward trunk lean to move the weight of the body over the stance foot (see Fig. 15–45). |
| Excessive hip and knee flexion during **swing** (Fig. 15–51) | Often due to lack of ankle dorsiflexion of the swing leg; may also be due to a functionally or anatomically short contralateral stance leg. | Used to clear the toes of the swing leg |
| Hip circumduction during **swing** (Fig. 15–50) | Lack of shortening of the swing leg secondary to reduced hip flexion, reduced knee flexion, and/or lack of ankle dorsiflexion | Used to lift the foot of the swing leg off the ground and provide toe clearance |
| Hip hiking (elevation of the ipsilateral pelvis during **swing**) | Lack of shortening of the swing leg secondary to reduced hip flexion, reduced knee flexion, and/or lack of ankle dorsiflexion<br>Functionally or anatomically short stance leg | Used to lift the foot of the swing leg off the ground and provide toe clearance |
| Excessive backward horizontal rotation of the pelvis on the side of the stance leg in terminal stance | Ankle plantar flexor weakness | Ankle plantar flexor weakness leads to prolonged heel contact and lack of push off. An increased pelvic horizontal rotation is used to lengthen the limb and maintain adequate step length. |

\* The terms in bold indicate the time in the gait cycle when the gait deviation is expressed.

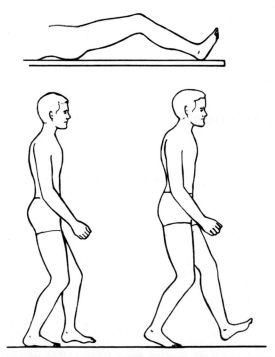

**FIGURE 15–49.** Knee flexion contracture causing a crouched gait of the stance leg. (From Perry J: Contractures: A historical perspective. Clin Orthop 219:8, 1987.)

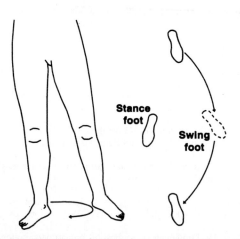

**FIGURE 15–50.** Hip circumduction during swing. (From Whittle M: Gait Analysis: An Introduction, 2nd ed. Oxford, Butterworth-Heinemann Ltd., 1996.)

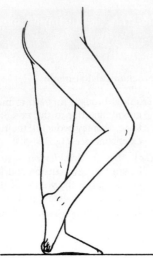

**FIGURE 15–51.** Excessive hip and knee flexion to compensate for foot drop. (From Whittle M: Gait Analysis: An Introduction, 2nd ed. Oxford, Butterworth-Heinemann Ltd., 1996.)

## REFERENCES

1. Adams JM, Perry J: Gait analysis: clinical application. In Rose J, Gamble JG (eds): Human Walking, 2nd ed. Philadelphia, Williams & Wilkins, 1994.
2. Allard P, Cappozzo A, Lundberg A, Vaughan CL: Three-Dimensional Analysis of Human Locomotion. New York, John Wiley & Sons, 1997.
3. Amar J: Trottoir dynamographique. Comptes rendus hebdomadaires des séances de l'Académie des Sciences 163:130, 1916.
4. Andrews JG: Euler's and Lagrange's equations for linked rigid-body models of three-dimensional human motion. In Allard P, Stokes IAF, Blanchi JP (eds): Three-Dimensional Analysis of Human Movement. Champaign, IL, Human Kinetics, 1995.
5. Bechtol CO: Normal human gait. In Bowker JH, Hall CB (eds): Atlas of Orthotics: American Academy of Orthopaedic Surgeons. St. Louis, Mosby, 1975.
6. Braune W, Fisher O: Der Gang des Menschen [The human gait]. Leipzig, Germany, B.G. Teubner, 1895–1904.
7. Braune W, Fisher O: The Human Gait (translation by Maquet P, Furlong R). Berlin, Springer-Verlag, 1987. (Original work published 1895–1904.)
8. Bresler B, Frankel JP: Forces and moments in the leg during walking. Am Soc Mech Engrs Trans 72:27, 1950.
9. Calve J, Galland M, De Cagny R: Pathogenesis of the limp due to coxalgia: The antalgic gait. J Bone Joint Surg 21:12, 1939.
10. Carlsoo S: How man moves: Kinesiological methods and studies. New York, Crane, Russak & Company, 1972.
11. Chan CW, Rudins A: Foot biomechanics during walking and running. Mayo Clin Proc 69:448, 1994.
12. Collins JJ: The redundant nature of locomotor optimization laws. J Biomech 28:251, 1995.
13. Corcoran PJ, Jebsen RH, Brengelmann GL, Simons BC: Effects of plastic and metal leg braces on speed and energy cost of hemiparetic ambulation. Arch Phys Med Rehabil 51:69, 1970.
14. Cornwall MW, McPoil TG: Three-dimensional movement of the foot during the stance phase of walking. J Am Podiatr Med Assoc 89:56, 1999.
15. Craik RL, Dutterer L: Spatial and temporal characteristics of foot fall patterns. In Craik RL, Oatis CA (eds): Gait Analysis: Theory and Application. St. Louis, Mosby-Year Book, Inc, 1995.
16. Drillis R: The influence of aging on the kinematics of gait. In Geriatric Amputee (NAS-NRC pub. No. 919). Washington, DC, NAS-NRC, 1961.
17. Eberhart H: Fundamental studies of human locomotion and other information relating to design of artificial limbs. Report to US Veterans' Association. Berkeley, CA, University of California, 1947.
18. Elftman H: The measurement of the external force in walking. Science 88:152, 1938.
19. Elftman H: The function of the arms in walking. Hum Biol 11:529, 1939.
20. Eng JJ, Winter DA: Kinetic analysis of the lower limbs during walking: What information can be gained from a three-dimensional model? J Biomech 28:753, 1995.
21. Finley F, Cody K, Finizie R: Locomotion patterns in elderly women. Arch Phys Med Rehabil 50:140, 1969.
22. Finley F, Cody K: Locomotive characteristics of urban pedestrians. Arch Phys Med Rehabil 51:423, 1970.
23. Finley FR, Cody KA, Sepic SB: Walking patterns of normal women. Arch Phys Med Rehabil 51:637, 1970.
24. Finni T, Komi PV, Lukkariniemi J: Achilles tendon loading during walking: Application of a novel optic fiber technique. Eur J Appl Physiol 77:289, 1998.
25. Finni T, Lepola V, Komi PV: Tendomuscular loading in normal locomotion conditions. In Kyrolainen H, Avela J, Takala T (eds): Limiting Factors of Human Neuromuscular Performance. Jyvaskyla, Finland, University of Jyvaskyla, 1999.
26. Fisher SV, Gullickson G: Energy cost of ambulation in health and disability: A literature review. Arch Phys Med Rehabil 59:124, 1978.
27. Gage JR: Gait analysis in cerebral palsy. In Clinic in Developmental Medicine, 121. London, Mac Keith Press, 1991.
28. Glasoe WM, Yack HJ, Saltzman CL: Anatomy and biomechanics of the first ray. Phys Ther 79:854, 1999.
29. Gonzalez EG, Corcoran PJ: Energy expenditure during ambulation. In Downey JA, Myers SJ, Gonzalez EG, Lieberman JS: The Physiological Basis of Rehabilitation Medicine, 2nd ed. Boston, Butterworth-Heinemann, 1994.
30. Gore DR, Murray MP, Sepic SB, Gardner GM: Walking patterns of men with unilateral surgical hip fusion. J Bone Joint Surg 57A:759, 1975.
31. Gracovetsky S: An hypothesis for the role of the spine in human locomotion: A challenge to current thinking. J Biomed Eng 7:205, 1985.
32. Gracovetsky S: The Spinal Engine. New York, Springer-Verlag, 1988.
33. Harris G, Smith P: Human Motion Analysis: Current Applications and Future Directions. New York, IEEE Press, 1996.
34. Inman VT, Ralston HJ, Todd F: Human Walking. Baltimore, Williams & Wilkins, 1981.
35. Inman VT, Ralston HJ, Todd F: Human locomotion. In Rose J, Gamble JG (eds): Human Walking. Philadelphia, Williams & Wilkins, 1994.
36. Katoh Y, Chao EYS, Laughman RK, et al: Biomechanical analysis of foot function during gait and clinical applications. Clin Orthop 177: 23, 1983.
37. Kaye RA, Jahss MH: Tibialis posterior: A review of anatomy and biomechanics in relation to support of the medial longitudinal arch. Foot Ankle 11:244, 1991.
38. Kepple TM, Siegel KL, Stanhope SJ: Relative contributions of the lower extremity joint moments to forward progression and support during gait. Gait Posture 6:1, 1997.
39. Kerrigan DC, Croce UD, Marciello M, Riley PO: A refined view of the determinants of gait: Significance of heel rise. Arch Phys Med Rehabil 81:1077, 2000.
40. Kerrigan DC, Viramontes BE, Corcoran PJ, LaRaia PJ: Measured versus predicted vertical displacement of the sacrum during gait as a tool to measure biomechanical gait performance. Am J Phys Med Rehabil 74: 3, 1995.
41. Knutson LM, Soderberg GL: EMG: Use and interpretation in gait. In Craik RL, Oatis CA (eds): Gait Analysis: Theory and Application. St. Louis, Mosby-Year Book, Inc, 1995.
42. Komistek RD, Stiehl JB, Dennis DA, et al: Mathematical model of the lower extremity joint reaction forces using Kane's method of dynamics. J Biomech 31:185, 1998.
43. Kuster M, Wood GA, Sakurai S, Blatter G: Stress on the femoropatellar joint in downhill walking—a biomechanical study, Z Unfallchirurgie Versicherungsmedizin 86:178, 1993.
44. Lafortune MA, Cavanagh PR, Sommer III HJ, Kalenak A: Three-dimensional kinematics of the human knee during walking. J Biomech 25: 347, 1992.
45. Lerner-Frankiel MB, Vargas S, Brown MB, et al: Functional community ambulation: What are your criteria? Clin Management 6:12, 1990.
46. Mann RA: Biomechanics of the foot. In American Academy of Ortho-

paedic Surgeons (ed): Atlas of Orthotics. Biomechanical Principles and Application. St. Louis, Mosby, 1975.

47. Marey EJ: La machine animal. Paris, Librairie Germer Bailliere, 1873.
48. Marey EJ: Movement. London, W. Heinemann, 1895.
49. Masdeu JC, Sudarsky L, Wolfson L: Gait disorders of aging: Falls and therapeutic strategies. Philadelphia, Lippincott-Raven, 1997.
50. McClay IS: The use of gait analysis to enhance the understanding of running injuries. In Craik RL, Oatis CA (eds): Gait analysis: Theory and application. St Louis, Mosby-Year Book, Inc, 1995.
51. Molen HH: Problems on the evaluation of gait. Amsterdam, Free University, 1973.
52. Murray MP, Kory RC, Clarkson BH, Sepic SB: Comparison of free and fast speed walking patterns of normal men. Am J Phys Med 45:8, 1966.
53. Murray MP: Gait as a total pattern of movement. Am J Phys Med 46:290, 1967.
54. Murray MP, Sepic SB, Barnard EJ: Patterns of sagittal rotation of the upper limbs in walking: Study of normal men during free and fast speed walking. Phys Ther 47:272, 1967.
55. Murray MP, Gore DR, Clarkson BH: Walking patterns of patients with unilateral hip pain due to osteoarthritis and avascular necrosis. J Bone Joint Surg 53A:259, 1971.
56. Murray M, Kory R, Sepic S: Walking patterns of normal women. Arch Phys Med Rehabil 51:637, 1979.
57. Murray MP, Gore DR: Gait of patients with hip pain or loss of hip joint motion. In Black J, Dumbleton JH (eds): Clinical Biomechanics: A Case History Approach. New York, Churchill Livingstone, 1981.
58. Murray MP, Guten GN, Mollinger LA, Gardner GM: Kinematic and electromyographic patterns of Olympic race walkers. Am J Sports Med 11:68, 1983.
59. Murray MP, Gore DR, Sepic SB, Mollinger LA: Antalgic maneuvers during walking in men with unilateral knee disability. Clin Orthop 199:192, 1985.
60. Muybridge E: Animal Locomotion, vols. 1–11. Philadelphia, University of Pennsylvania, 1887.
61. Muybridge E: Human and animal locomotion, vols. 1–3. New York, Dover, 1979.
62. Neumann DA: Biomechanical analysis of selected principles of hip joint protection. Arthritis Care Res 2:146, 1989.
63. Ounpuu S: Clinical gait analysis. In Spivack BS (ed): Evaluation and Management of Gait Disorders. New York, Marcel Dekker, 1995.
64. Patla A: A framework for understanding mobility problems in the elderly. In Craik RL, Oatis CA (eds): Gait Analysis: Theory and Application. St. Louis, Mosby-Year Book, Inc, 1995.
65. Paul JP: Forces transmitted by joints in the human body. Proc Inst Mech Eng 181:8, 1966.
66. Pederson DR, Brand RA, Davy DT: Pelvic muscle and acetabular contact forces during gait. J Biomech 30:959, 1997.
67. Perry J: Gait analysis: Normal and pathological function. Thorofare, NJ, Slack, Inc, 1992.
68. Ralston HJ: Effects of immobilization of various body segments on energy cost of human locomotion. Ergonomics Suppl:53, 1965.
69. Ralston HJ: Energetics of human walking. In Herman RM, Grillner S, Stein PSG, Stuart DG (eds): Neural Control of Locomotion. New York, Plenum, 1976.
70. Reischl SF, Powers CM, Rao S, Perry J: Relationship between foot pronation and rotation of the tibia and femur during walking. Foot Ankle Int 20:513, 1999.
71. Robinett CS, Vondran MA: Functional ambulation velocity and distance requirements in rural and urban communities. Phys Ther 68:1371, 1988.
72. Rose J, Ralston HJ, Gamble JG: Energetics of walking. In Rose J, Gamble JG (eds): Human Walking, 2nd ed. Philadelphia, Williams & Wilkins, 1994.
73. Saunders JB de CM, Inman VT, Eberhart HD: The major determinants in normal and pathological gait. J Bone Joint Surg 35A:543, 1953.
74. Scott SH, Winter DA: Internal forces of chronic running injury sites. Med Sci Sports Exer 22:357, 1990.
75. Shiavi R: Electromyographic patterns in adult locomotion: A comprehensive review. J Rehabil 22:85, 1985.
76. Shumway-Cook A, Woollacott M: Motor control: Theory and practical applications. Philadelphia, Williams & Wilkins, 1995.
77. Siegler S, Liu W: Inverse dynamics in human locomotion. In Allard P, Cappozzo A, Lundberg A, Vaughan CL (eds): Three-dimensional analysis of human locomotion. New York, John Wiley & Sons, 1997.
78. Simoneau GG, Cavanagh PR, Ulbrecht JS, et al: The influence of visual factors on fall-related kinematic variables during stair descent by older women. J Gerontol Med Sci 46:M188, 1991.
79. Simonsen EB, Dyhre Poulsen P, Voigt M, et al: Bone-on-bone forces during loaded and unloaded walking. Acta Anat 152:133, 1995.
80. Smidt GL: Rudiments of gait. In Smidt GL (ed): Gait in Rehabilitation. New York, Churchill Livingstone, 1990.
81. Statham L, Murray MP: Early walking patterns of normal children. Clin Orthop 79:8, 1971.
82. Stauffer RN, Chao EYS, Brewster RC: Force and motion analysis of the normal, diseased and prosthetic ankle joint. Clin Orthop 127:189, 1977.
83. Sudarsky L: An overview of neurological diseases causing gait disorder. In Spivack BS (ed): Evaluation and Management of Gait Disorders. New York, Marcel Dekker, 1995.
84. Sutherland DH, Kaufman KR, Moitoza JR: Kinematics of normal human walking. In Rose J, Gamble JG (eds): Human Walking, 2nd ed. Philadelphia, Williams & Wilkins, 1994.
85. Taylor SJ, Walker PS, Perry JS, et al: The forces in the distal femur and the knee during walking and other activities measured by telemetry. J Arthroplasty 13:428, 1998.
86. Vaughan CL, Davis BL, O'Connor JC: Dynamics of human gait. Champaign, IL, Human Kinetics Publishers, Inc, 1992.
87. Vierordt KH: Das Gehen des Menschen in Gesunden und Kranken Zuständen nach Selbstregistrirenden Methoden Dargestellt. Tubingen, Germany, Laupp, 1881.
88. Walsh JP: Foot fall measurement technology. In Craik RL, Oatis CA (eds): Gait Analysis: Theory and Application. St. Louis, Mosby-Year Book, Inc, 1995.
89. Waters R, Campbell J, Thomas L, et al: Energy cost of walking in lower-extremity plaster casts. J Bone Joint Surg 64A:896, 1982.
90. Waters RL, Barnes G, Husserel T, et al: Energy expenditure following hip and ankle arthrodesis. J Bone Joint Surg 70A:1032, 1988.
91. Waters RL, Lunsford BR, Perry J, Byrd R: Energy-speed relationship of walking: Standard tables. J Orthop Res 6:215, 1988.
92. Waters RL, Mulroy S: The energy expenditure of normal and pathologic gait. Gait Posture 9:207, 1999.
93. Webb D, Tuttle RH, Baksh M: Pendular activity of human upper limbs during slow and normal walking. Am J Phys Anthropol 93:477, 1993.
94. Weber W, Weber E: The mechanics of human motion. Gottingen, Germany, Dieterischen Buchhandlung, 1836.
95. Weber W, Weber E: Mechanik der Menschlichen Gewerkzeuge. [Mechanics of the human walking apparatus]. Berlin, Germany, Springer-Verlag, 1894.
96. Weber W, Weber E: Mechanics of the human walking apparatus. (Translation by Maquet P, Furlong R.) Berlin, Germany, Springer-Verlag, 1992. (Original work published in 1894.)
97. Whittle M: Gait Analysis: An Introduction, 2nd ed. Oxford, Butterworth-Heinemann Ltd, 1996.
98. Winter DA: The Biomechanics and Motor Control of Human Gait: Normal, Elderly and Pathological, 2nd ed. Waterloo, Canada, University of Waterloo Press, 1991.
99. Winter DA: Anatomy, biomechanics and control of balance during standing and walking. Waterloo, Ontario, Canada, Waterloo Biomechanics, 1995.
100. Winter DA, Eng JJ, Ishac MG: A review of kinetic parameters in human walking. In Craik RL, Oatis CA (eds): Gait Analysis: Theory and Application. St. Louis, Mosby-Year Book, Inc, 1995.
101. Winter DA, Eng JJ, Ishac M: Three-dimensional moments, powers and work in normal gait: Implications for clinical assessments. In Harris GF, Smith PA (eds): Human Motion Analysis: Current Applications and Future Directions. New York, IEEE Press, 1996.
102. Zarrugh MY, Todd FN, Ralston HJ: Optimization of energy expenditure during level walking. Eur J Appl Physiol 33:293, 1974.

## Part A: Nerve Root Innervation of the Lower Extremity Muscles

| | Nerve Root | | | | | | | |
| | Lumbar | | | | | Sacral | | |
| Muscle | L$^1$ | L$^2$ | L$^3$ | L$^4$ | L$^5$ | S$^1$ | S$^2$ | S$^3$ |
|---|---|---|---|---|---|---|---|---|
| Psoas minor | X | X | | | | | | |
| Psoas major | *X* | X | X | *X* | | | | |
| Iliacus | (x) | X | X | *X* | | | | |
| Pectineus | | X | X | *X* | | | | |
| Sartorius | | X | X | (x) | | | | |
| Quadriceps | | X | X | X | | | | |
| Adductor brevis | | X | X | X | | | | |
| Adductor longus | | X | X | *X* | | | | |
| Gracilis | | X | X | X | | | | |
| Obturator externus | | | X | X | | | | |
| Adductor magnus | | *X* | X | X | *X* | *X* | | |
| Gluteus medius | | | | X | X | X | | |
| Gluteus minimus | | | | X | X | X | | |
| Tensor fascia lata | | | | X | X | X | | |
| Gluteus maximus | | | | | X | X | X | |
| Piriformis | | | | | (x) | X | X | |
| Gemellus superior | | | | | X | X | X | |
| Obturator internus | | | | | X | X | X | |
| Gemellus inferior | | | | X | X | X | (x) | |
| Quadratus femoris | | | | X | X | X | (x) | |
| Biceps (long head) | | | | | *X* | X | X | *X* |
| Semitendinosus | | | | *X* | X | X | X | |
| Semimembranosus | | | | *X* | X | X | *X* | |
| Biceps (short head) | | | | | X | X | X | |
| Tibialis anterior | | | | X | X | *X* | | |
| Extensor hallucis longus | | | | *X* | X | X | | |
| Extensor digitorum longus | | | | X | X | X | | |
| Peroneus tertius | | | | X | X | X | | |
| Extensor digitorum brevis | | | | *X* | X | X | | |
| Peroneus longus | | | | *X* | X | X | | |
| Peroneus brevis | | | | *X* | X | X | | |
| Plantaris | | | | *X* | X | X | (x) | |
| Gastrocnemius | | | | | | X | X | |
| Popliteus | | | | X | X | X | | |

| Muscle | Nerve Root | | | | | | | |
|---|---|---|---|---|---|---|---|---|
| | Lumbar | | | | | Sacral | | |
| | L¹ | L² | L³ | L⁴ | L⁵ | S¹ | S² | S³ |
| Soleus | | | | | *X* | **X** | **X** | |
| Tibialis posterior | | | | (x) | **X** | **X** | | |
| Flexor digitorum longus | | | | | **X** | **X** | (x) | |
| Flexor hallucis longus | | | | | **X** | **X** | **X** | |
| Flexor digitorum brevis | | | | *X* | **X** | **X** | | |
| Abductor hallucis | | | | *X* | **X** | **X** | | |
| Flexor hallucis brevis | | | | *X* | **X** | **X** | | |
| Lumbrical I | | | | *X* | **X** | **X** | | |
| Abductor digiti minimi | | | | | | **X** | *X* | |
| Quadratus plantae | | | | | | **X** | **X** | |
| Flexor digiti minimi | | | | | | **X** | **X** | |
| Abductor digiti minimi | | | | | | **X** | **X** | |
| Adductor hallucis | | | | | | **X** | **X** | |
| Plantar interossei | | | | | | **X** | **X** | |
| Dorsal interossei | | | | | | **X** | **X** | |
| Lumbricals II, III, IV | | | | (x) | (x) | **X** | **X** | |

(x), minimal literature support; *X*, moderate literature support; **X**, strong literature support.

Modified from Kendall FP, McCreary AK, and Provance PG: Muscles: Testing and Function, ed. 4. Baltimore, Williams & Wilkins, 1993. Data based on a compilation from several anatomical sources.

## Part B: Key Muscles for Testing the Function of Ventral Nerve Roots (L²-S³)

The table shows the key muscles typically used to test the function of individual ventral nerve roots of the lumbosacral plexus (L²-S³) in the clinic. Reduced strength in a key muscle may indicate an injury to the associated nerve root.

| Key Muscles | Ventral Nerve Root | Sample Test Movements |
|---|---|---|
| Iliopsoas | L² | Hip flexion |
| Adductor longus | L² | Hip adduction |
| Quadriceps femoris | L³ | Knee extension |
| Tibialis anterior | L⁴ | Ankle dorsiflexion |
| Extensor digitorum longus | L⁵ | Toe extension |
| Gluteus medius | L⁵ | Hip abduction |
| Gluteus maximus | S¹ | Hip extension with knee flexed |
| Semitendinosus | S¹ | Knee flexion and internal rotation |
| Gastrocnemius/soleus | S² | Ankle plantar flexion |
| Flexor hallucis longus | S² | Flexion of the hallux |
| Dorsal and plantar interossei | S³ | Abduction and adduction of the toes |

## Part C: Attachments and Innervations of the Lower Extremity Muscles

### HIP AND KNEE MUSCULATURE

**Adductor Brevis**
*Proximal attachment:* anterior surface of the inferior pubic ramus
*Distal attachment:* proximal one third of the linea aspera of the femur
*Innervation:* obturator nerve

**Adductor Longus**
*Proximal attachment:* anterior surface of the body of the pubis
*Distal attachment:* middle one third of the linea aspera of the femur
*Innervation:* obturator nerve

**Adductor Magnus**
***Anterior (Adductor Head)***
*Proximal attachment:* ischial ramus
*Distal attachment:* entire linea aspera of the femur
*Innervation:* obturator nerve

***Posterior (Extensor Head)***
*Proximal attachment:* ischial tuberosity
*Distal attachment:* adductor tubercle on femur
*Innervation:* tibial portion of sciatic nerve

**Articularis Genu**
*Proximal attachment:* anterior surface of the distal femoral shaft
*Distal attachment:* proximal synovial membrane of the knee
*Innervation:* femoral nerve

**Biceps Femoris**
*Long Head*
*Proximal attachments:* from a common tendon with the semitendinosus; originating from a medial impression on the posterior surface of the ischial tuberosity and part of the sacrotuberous ligament.
*Distal attachment:* head of the fibula
*Innervation:* tibial portion of the sciatic nerve

*Short Head*
*Proximal attachment:* lateral lip of the linea aspera below the gluteal tuberosity
*Distal attachment:* head of the fibula
*Innervation:* common peroneal portion of the sciatic nerve

**Gemellus Inferior**
*Proximal attachment:* tuberosity of the ischium
*Distal attachment:* blends with the tendon of the obturator internus
*Innervation:* nerve to the quadratus femoris

**Gemellus Superior**
*Proximal attachment:* dorsal surface of the ischial spine
*Distal attachment:* blends with the tendon of the obturator internus
*Innervation:* nerve to the obturator internus

**Gluteus Maximus**
*Proximal attachments:* outer ilium, posterior gluteal line, aponeurosis of the erector spinae and gluteus medius muscles, posterior side of sacrum and coccyx, and part of sacrotuberous and posterior sacro-ilac ligaments
*Distal attachments:* gluteal tuberosity and iliotibial band
*Innervation:* inferior gluteal nerve

**Gluteus Medius**
*Proximal attachment:* outer surface of the ilium, above the anterior gluteal line
*Distal attachment:* lateral surface of the greater trochanter
*Innervation:* superior gluteal nerve

**Gluteus Minimus**
*Proximal attachment:* outer surface of the ilium between the anterior and inferior gluteal lines, as far posterior as the greater sciatic notch
*Distal attachment:* anterior aspect of the greater trochanter
*Innervation:* superior gluteal nerve

**Gracilis**
*Proximal attachments:* anterior aspect of lower body of pubis and inferior ramus of pubis
*Distal attachment:* proximal medial surface of the tibia just posterior to the upper end of the attachment of the sartorius
*Innervation:* obturator nerve

**Iliopsoas**
*Psoas Major*
*Proximal attachments:* transverse processes and lateral bod-

ies of the last thoracic and all lumbar vertebrae including the intervertebral discs
*Distal attachment:* lesser trochanter of the femur

**Iliacus**
*Proximal attachments:* superior two thirds of the iliac fossa, inner lip of the iliac crest, and small region of the sacrum across the sacroiliac joint
*Distal attachment:* lesser trochanter of the femur via the lateral side of psoas major tendon
*Innervation:* femoral nerve

**Obturator Externus**
*Proximal attachments:* external surface of the obturator membrane and surrounding external surfaces of the inferior pubic ramus and ischial ramus
*Distal attachment:* medial surface of the greater trochanter at the trochanteric fossa
*Innervation:* obturator nerve

**Obturator Internus**
*Proximal attachments:* internal side of the obturator membrane and immediately surrounding surfaces of the inferior pubic ramus and ischial ramus; bony attachments extend superiorly within the pelvis to the greater sciatic notch.
*Distal attachment:* medial surface of the greater trochanter just anterior and superior to the trochanteric fossa
*Innervation:* nerve to the obturator internus

**Pectineus**
*Proximal attachment:* pectineal line on superior pubic ramus
*Distal attachment:* pectineal (spiral) line on the posterior surface of the femur
*Innervation:* femoral nerve and occasionally a branch from the obturator nerve

**Piriformis**
*Proximal attachment:* anterior side of the sacrum between the sacral foramina; blends partially with the capsule of the sacroiliac joint
*Distal attachment:* apex of the greater trochanter
*Innervation:* nerve to the piriformis

**Popliteus**
*Proximal attachment:* by an intracapsular tendon that attaches to the lateral aspect of the lateral femoral condyle
*Distal attachment:* posterior surface of the posterior side of the proximal tibia above the soleal line
*Innervation:* tibial nerve

**Psoas Minor**
*Proximal attachments:* transverse processes and lateral bodies of the last thoracic and the first lumbar vertebrae including the intervertebral disc
*Distal attachment:* pubis near the pectineal line
*Innervation:* femoral nerve

**Quadratus Femoris**
*Proximal attachment:* lateral surface of the ischial tuberosity just anterior to the attachments of the semimembranosus

*Distal attachment:* quadrate tubercle (middle of intertrochanteric crest)

*Innervation:* nerve to the quadratus femoris

**Rectus Femoris**

*Proximal attachment:* straight tendon: anterior-inferior iliac spine, and reflected tendon: groove around the superior rim of the acetabulum and into the capsule of the hip

*Distal attachment:* base of the patella and, via ligamentum patella, to the tibial tuberosity

*Innervation:* femoral nerve

**Sartorius**

*Proximal attachment:* anterior-superior iliac spine

*Distal attachment:* along a line on the proximal medial surface of the tibia

*Innervation:* femoral nerve

**Semimembranosus**

*Proximal attachment:* lateral impression on the posterior surface of the ischial tuberosity

*Distal attachments:* posterior aspect of the medial condyle of the tibia. Additional attachments include the medial collateral ligament, oblique popliteal ligament, and popliteus muscle.

*Innervation:* tibial portion of the sciatic nerve

**Semitendinosus**

*Proximal attachments:* from a common tendon with the long head of the biceps femoris originating from a medial impression on the posterior surface of the ischial tuberosity and part of the sacrotuberous ligament

*Distal attachment:* proximal medial surface of the tibia just posterior to the lower end of the attachment of the sartorius

*Innervation:* tibial portion of the sciatic nerve

**Tensor Fasciae Lata**

*Proximal attachment:* outer surface of the iliac crest just posterior to the anterior-superior iliac spine

*Distal attachment:* proximal one third of the iliotibial band of the fascia lata

*Innervation:* superior gluteal nerve

**Vastus Intermedius**

*Proximal attachment:* anterior-lateral regions of the upper two thirds of the femoral shaft

*Distal attachments:* medial capsule, base of the patella, and via ligamentum patella, to the tibial tuberosity

*Innervation:* femoral nerve

**Vastus Lateralis**

*Proximal attachments:* upper region of intertrochanteric line, anterior and inferior border of the greater trochanter, lateral region of the gluteal tuberosity, lateral lip of the linea aspera

*Distal attachment:* lateral capsule, base of the patella, and via ligamentum patella, to the tibial tuberosity

*Innervation:* femoral nerve

**Vastus Medialis**

*Proximal attachments:* lower region of intertrochanteric line, medial lip of linea aspera, proximal medial supracondylar line, fibers from adductor magnus

*Distal attachment:* medial capsule, base of the patella and via ligamentum patella, to the tibial tuberosity

*Innervation:* femoral nerve

## ANKLE AND FOOT MUSCULATURE

**Extensor Digitorum Longus**

*Proximal attachments:* lateral condyle of tibia, proximal two thirds of the medial surface of the fibula, and adjacent interosseous membrane

*Distal attachments:* by four tendons that attach to the proximal base of the dorsal surface of the middle and distal phalanges via the dorsal digital expansion

*Innervation:* deep branch of the peroneal nerve

**Extensor Hallucis Longus**

*Proximal attachments:* middle section of the medial surface of the fibula and adjacent interosseous membrane

*Distal attachments:* dorsal base of the distal phalanx of the great toe

*Innervation:* deep branch of the peroneal nerve

**Flexor Digitorum Longus**

*Proximal attachments:* posterior surface of the middle one third of the tibia just medial to the proximal attachment of the tibialis posterior

*Distal attachments:* by four separate tendons to the base of the distal phalanx of the four lesser toes

*Innervation:* tibial nerve

**Flexor Hallucis Longus**

*Proximal attachment:* distal two thirds of most of the posterior surface of the fibula

*Distal attachment:* plantar surface of the base of the distal phalanx of the great toe

*Innervation:* tibial nerve

**Gastrocnemius**

*Proximal attachments:* by two separate heads from the posterior aspect of the lateral and medial femoral condyle

*Distal attachment:* calcaneal tuberosity via the Achilles tendon

*Innervation:* tibial nerve

**Peroneus Brevis**

*Proximal attachment:* distal two thirds of the lateral surface of the fibula

*Distal attachment:* styloid process of the fifth metatarsal

*Innervation:* superficial branch of the peroneal nerve

**Peroneus Longus**

*Proximal attachments:* lateral condyle of tibia, head, and proximal two thirds of the lateral surface of the fibula

*Distal attachment:* lateral surface of the medial cuneiform and lateral side of the base of first metatarsal bone

*Innervation:* superficial branch of the peroneal nerve

**Peroneus Tertius**

*Proximal attachments:* distal one third of the medial surface of the fibula and adjacent interosseous membrane

*Distal attachment:* dorsal surface of the base of the fifth metatarsal

*Innervation:* deep branch of the peroneal nerve

**Plantaris**

*Proximal attachments:* most inferior part of lateral supracondylar line of the femur and oblique popliteal ligament of the knee

*Distal attachment:* joins the medial aspect of Achilles tendon to insert on the calcaneal tuberosity

*Innervation:* tibial nerve

### Soleus

*Proximal attachments:* posterior surface of the fibula head and proximal one third of its shaft and from the posterior side of the tibia near the soleal line

*Distal attachment:* calcaneal tuberosity via the Achilles tendon

*Innervation:* tibial nerve

### Tibialis Anterior

*Proximal attachments:* lateral condyle and proximal two thirds of the lateral surface of the tibia and the interosseous membrane

*Distal attachment:* medial and plantar aspects of the medial cuneiform and the base of the first metatarsal

*Innervation:* deep branch of the peroneal nerve

### Tibialis Posterior

*Proximal attachments:* proximal two thirds of posterior surface of the tibia and fibula and adjacent interosseous membrane

*Distal attachments:* tendon attaches to every tarsal bone but the talus plus the bases of the second through the fourth metatarsal bones. The main insertion is on the navicular tuberosity and the medial cuneiform bone.

*Innervation:* tibial nerve

## INTRINSIC MUSCLES OF THE FOOT

### Extensor Digitorum Brevis

*Proximal attachment:* lateral-distal aspect of the calcaneus just proximal to the calcaneocuboid joint

*Distal attachments:* by three tendons that blend with the tendons of the extensor digitorum longus of the second through fifth toes. A fourth tendon inserts on the dorsal base of the proximal phalanx of the great toe.

*Innervation:* deep branch of the peroneal nerve

## LAYER 1

### Abductor Digiti Minimi

*Proximal attachments:* medial and lateral processes of the calcaneal tuberosity, plantar aponeurosis, and plantar surface of the base of the fifth metatarsal bone with flexor digiti minimi

*Distal attachment:* lateral side of the proximal phalanx of the fifth toe sharing an attachment with the flexor digiti minimi

*Innervation:* lateral plantar nerve

### Abductor Hallucis

*Proximal attachments:* flexor retinaculum, medial process of the calcaneus and plantar fascia

*Distal attachments:* medial side of the base of proximal phalanx of the hallux sharing an attachment with the medial tendon of the flexor hallucis brevis

*Innervation:* medial plantar nerve

### Flexor Digitorum Brevis

*Proximal attachments:* medial process of calcaneal tuberosity and central part of the plantar fascia

*Distal attachments:* each of four tendons inserts on the sides of the plantar aspect of the base of the middle phalanx of the lesser toes.

*Innervation:* medial plantar nerve

## LAYER 2

### Lumbricals

*Proximal attachments:* from the tendons of the flexor digitorum longus muscle

*Distal attachments:* each muscle crosses the medial side of each metatarsophalangeal joint to insert into the dorsal digital expansion of the four lesser toes

*Innervation:* to second toe—medial plantar nerve; to third through fifth toes—lateral plantar nerve

### Quadratus Plantae

*Proximal attachments:* by two heads from the medial and lateral aspect of the plantar surface of the calcaneus, distal to the calcaneal tuberosity

*Distal attachment:* lateral border of the flexor digitorum longus common tendon

*Innervation:* lateral plantar nerve

## LAYER 3

### Adductor Hallucis

*Proximal Attachment*

**Oblique head:** plantar aspect of the base of the second through fourth metatarsal and the fibrous sheath of the peroneus longus tendon

**Transverse head:** plantar aspect of the ligaments that support the metatarsophalangeal joints of the third through fifth toes

*Distal attachments:* both heads converge to insert on the lateral base of the proximal phalanx of the great toe along with the lateral tendon of the flexor hallucis brevis

*Innervation:* lateral plantar nerve

### Flexor Digiti Minimi

*Proximal attachments:* plantar surface of the base of the fifth metatarsal bone and fibrous sheath covering the tendon of the peroneus longus

*Distal attachment:* lateral surface of the base of the proximal phalanx of the fifth toe blending with the tendon of the abductor digiti minimi

*Innervation:* lateral plantar nerve

### Flexor Hallucis Brevis

*Proximal attachment:* plantar surface of the cuboid and lateral cuneiform bones and from parts of the tendon of the tibialis posterior muscle

*Distal attachment:* by two tendons in which the lateral tendon attaches to the lateral base of the proximal phalanx of the great toe with the adductor hallucis; the medial tendon attaches to the medial base of the proximal phalanx of the great toe with the abductor hallucis. A pair of sesamoid bones is located within the tendons of this muscle.

*Innervation:* medial plantar nerve

# LAYER 4

## Dorsal Interossei

*Proximal Attachments*

First: adjacent sides of the first and second metatarsal
Second: adjacent sides of the second and third metatarsal
Third: adjacent sides of the third and fourth metatarsal
Fourth: adjacent sides of the fourth and fifth metatarsal

*Distal Attachments\**

First: medial side of the base of the proximal phalanx of the second toe
Second: lateral side of the base of the proximal phalanx of the second toe
Third: lateral side of the base of the proximal phalanx of the third toe
Fourth: lateral side of the base of the proximal phalanx of the fourth toe
*Innervation:* lateral plantar nerve

## Plantar Interossei

*Proximal Attachments*

First: medial side of the third metatarsal
Second: medial side of the fourth metatarsal
Third: medial side of the fifth metatarsal

*Distal Attachments\**

First: medial side of the proximal phalanx of the third toe
Second: medial side of the proximal phalanx of the fourth toe
Third: medial side of the proximal phalanx of the fifth toe
*Innervation:* lateral plantar nerve

---

\*Attaches into the dorsal digital expansion of the toes.

# INDEX

Note: Page numbers followed by the letter f refer to figures; those followed by the letter t refer to tables, and those followed by the letter b refer to boxed material.